D1611458

Textbook of Assisted Reproductive Techniques

Fifth Edition

Volume 1: Laboratory Perspectives

The editors would like to dedicate this edition to the late Professor Robert G. Edwards and the late Queenie V. Neri.

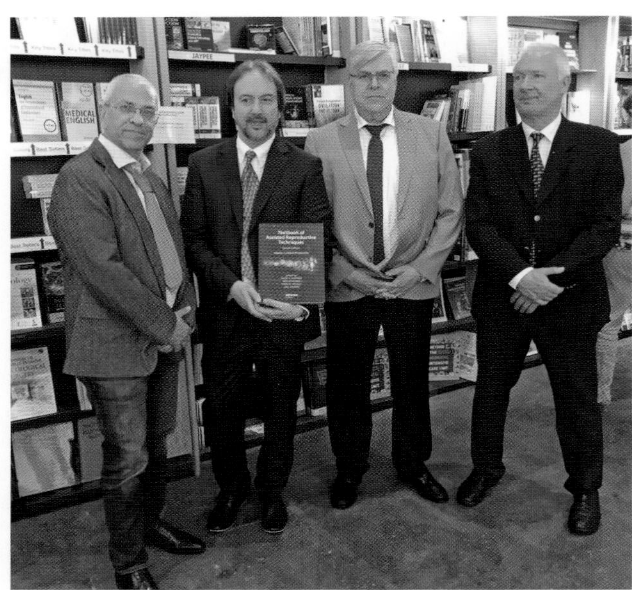

The editors (from left to right: Ariel Weissman, David K Gardner, Zeev Shoham, Colin M Howles) at the annual meeting of ESHRE, Geneva, July 2017.

Textbook of Assisted Reproductive Techniques

Fifth Edition

Volume 1: Laboratory Perspectives

Edited by

David K. Gardner DPhil, FAA
Professor, School of Biosciences, University of Melbourne
Scientific Director, Melbourne IVF, Melbourne, Australia

Ariel Weissman MD
Senior Physician, IVF Unit, Department of Obstetrics and Gynecology,
Edith Wolfson Medical Center
Holon and Sackler Faculty of Medicine, Tel Aviv University, Tel Aviv, Israel

Colin M. Howles PhD, FRSM
Aries Consulting SARL, Geneva, Switzerland
Honorary Fellow, University of Edinburgh, UK

Zeev Shoham MD
Director, Reproductive Medicine and Infertility Unit,
Department of Obstetrics and Gynecology,
Kaplan Medical Center, Rehovot, Israel

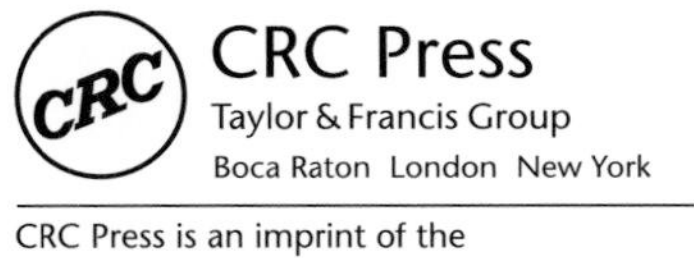

CRC Press is an imprint of the
Taylor & Francis Group, an **informa** business

CRC Press
Taylor & Francis Group
6000 Broken Sound Parkway NW, Suite 300
Boca Raton, FL 33487-2742

Printed and bound in India by Replika Press Pvt. Ltd.

Printed on acid-free paper

International Standard Book Number-13: 978-1-4987-4014-2 (Pack- Hardback and eBook)

Visit the Taylor & Francis Web site at
http://www.taylorandfrancis.com

and the CRC Press Web site at
http://www.crcpress.com

Contents

Contributors

Ashok Agarwal
American Center for Reproductive Medicine
Cleveland Clinic
Cleveland, Ohio

Gulfam Ahmad
American Center for Reproductive Medicine
Cleveland Clinic
Cleveland, Ohio
and
Department of Physiology
University of Health Sciences
Lahore, Pakistan
and
College of Medicine
Prince Sattam bin Abdulaziz University
AlKharj, Kingdom of Saudi Arabia

Pilar Alamá
IVI
Valencia, Spain

Mina Alikani
Tyho-Galileo Research Laboratories
Livingston, New Jersey

Janell Archer
Reproductive Services/Melbourne IVF
Royal Women's Hospital
Melbourne, Australia

Natalia Basile
IVI
Madrid, Spain

Itziar Belil
Reproductive Medicine Service
Hospital Universitari Dexeus
Barcelona, Spain

Andrea Borini
9.baby—Family and Fertility Center
Bologna, Italy

Harold Bourne
Reproductive Services/Melbourne IVF
Royal Women's Hospital
Melbourne, Australia

Andrea Rodrigo Carbajosa
Clínica Tambre
Madrid, Spain

Ching-Chien Chang
Reproductive Biology Associates
Atlanta, Georgia

Ana Cobo
IVI
Valencia, Spain

Jacques Cohen
ART Institute of Washington
and
Tyho-Galileo Research Laboratories
Livingston, New Jersey

Tyler Cozzubbo
The Ronald O. Perelman and Claudia Cohen Center for Reproductive Medicine
Weill Cornell Medical College
New York City, New York

Nava Dekel
Department of Biological Regulation
The Weizmann Institute of Science
Rehovot, Israel

Alfonso P. Del Valle
The Toronto Institute for Reproductive Medicine—ReproMed
Toronto, Canada

Francisco Domínguez
Valencia University
INCLIVA
Valencia, Spain

Thomas Ebner
Kepler University
Kinderwunsch Zentrum
Linz, Austria

Robert G. Edwards (Deceased)
Duck End Farm
Cambridge, United Kingdom

Aisaku Fukuda
IVF Osaka Clinic
Higashi-Osaka, Osaka, Japan

David K. Gardner
School of BioSciences
University of Melbourne
and
Melbourne IVF
Victoria, Australia

Antonia Gilligan
Alpha Environmental
Livingston, New Jersey

Veronica Gold
Sara Racine In Vitro Fertilization Unit
Tel Aviv Sourasky Medical Center
Tel Aviv, Israel

Irit Granot
IVF Unit
Herzliya Medical Center
Herzliya, Israel

Kelsey M. Grieve
Institute of Cell Biology and Centre for Integrative Physiology
and
MRC Centre for Reproductive Health
Queen's Medical Research Institute
University of Edinburgh
Edinburgh, United Kingdom

James Grifo
Department of Obstetrics and Gynecology
NYU Langone Medical Center
New York City, New York

Johan Guns
Centre for Reproductive Medicine
UZ Brussel
Brussels, Belgium

Liran Hiersch
Department of Obstetrics and Gynecology
Lis Maternity Hospital
Tel Aviv Sourasky Medical Center
and
Sackler Faculty of Medicine
Tel Aviv University
Tel Aviv, Israel

Ronny Janssens
Centre for Reproductive Medicine
UZ Brussel
Brussels, Belgium

Martin H. Johnson
Department of Physiology, Development & Neuroscience
School of Anatomy
University of Cambridge
and
Christ's College
Cambridge, United Kingdom

María José de los Santos
IVI, Valencia, Spain

Junaid Kashir
College of Biomedical and Life Sciences
Cardiff University
Cardiff, United Kingdom
and
College of Medicine
Alfaisal University
and
Department of Comparative Medicine
King Faisal Specialist Hospital and Research Centre
Riyadh, Saudi Arabia

Mandy Katz-Jaffe
Colorado Center for Reproductive Medicine
Lone Tree, Colorado

Jason Kofinas
Kofinas Fertility Group
New York City, New York

Masashige Kuwayama
Repro-Support Medical Research Centre
ReproLife, Inc.
Tokyo, Japan

Michelle Lane
Department of Obstetrics and Gynecology
University of Adelaide
Adelaide, Australia
and
Repromed
Dulwich, Australia

Jonathan Lewin
Nuffield Department of Obstetrics
and Gynaecology
University of Oxford
Oxford, United Kingdom

Willy Lissens
Center for Medical Genetics/Research Center
Reproduction and Genetics
Vrije Universiteit Brussel (VUB)
Universitair Ziekenhuis Brussel (UZ Brussel)
Brussels, Belgium

Reda Z. Mahfouz
THOR Department
Cleveland Clinic Lerner College of Medicine
Case Western Reserve University
Cleveland, Ohio

Mira Malcov
Sara Racine In Vitro Fertilization Unit
Tel Aviv Sourasky Medical Center
Tel Aviv, Israel

José María de los Santos
IVI
Valencia, Spain

Caroline McCaffrey
Department of Obstetrics and Gynecology
NYU Langone Medical Center
New York City, New York

Marius Meintjes
Frisco Institute for Reproductive Medicine
Frisco, Texas

Marcos Meseguer
IVI Valencia
Valencia, Spain

Markus Montag
ilabcomm GmbH
Sankt Augustin, Germany

Yoshiharu Morimoto
HORAC Grand Front Osaka Clinic
Osaka City, Japan

Zsolt Peter Nagy
Reproductive Biology Associates
Atlanta, Georgia

Queenie V. Neri (Deceased)
The Ronald O. Perelman and Claudia Cohen Center for Reproductive Medicine
Weill Cornell Medical College
New York, New York

Gianpiero D. Palermo
The Ronald O. Perelman and Claudia Cohen Center for Reproductive Medicine
Weill Cornell Medical College
New York, New York

Sagit Peleg-Schalka
Sara Racine In Vitro Fertilization Unit,
Tel Aviv Sourasky Medical Center
Tel Aviv, Israel

Nigel Pereira
The Ronald O. Perelman and Claudia Cohen Center for Reproductive Medicine
Weill Cornell Medical College
New York, New York

José Remohí
IVI
Valencia, Spain

Laura F. Rienzi
GENERA Centres for Reproductive Medicine
Roma, Marostica, Umbertide, Napoli, Italy

Zev Rosenwaks
The Ronald O. Perelman and Claudia Cohen Center for Reproductive Medicine
Weill Cornell Medical College
New York City, New York

Maria Ruiz-Alonso
Igenomix
Valencia, Spain

Tamer M. Said
The Toronto Institute for Reproductive Medicine—ReproMed
Toronto, Canada

Denny Sakkas
Boston IVF
Waltham, Massachusetts

Manabu Satou
IVF Namba Clinic
Nishi-ku, Osaka, Japan

Heide Schatten
Department of Veterinary Pathobiology
University of Missouri
Columbia, Missouri

Tim Schimmel
ART Institute of Washington
and
Tyho-Galileo Research Laboratories
Livingston, New Jersey

Sara Seneca
Center for Medical Genetics/Research Center Reproduction and Genetics
Vrije Universiteit Brussel (VUB)
Universitair Ziekenhuis Brussel (UZ Brussel)
Brussels, Belgium

Rakesh Sharma
American Center for Reproductive Medicine
Cleveland Clinic
Cleveland, Ohio

Kaylen M. Silverberg
Texas Fertility Center
Ovation Fertility
Austin, Texas

Carlos Simón
Igenomix
Valencia, Spain

Cecilia Sjöblom
Westmead Fertility Centre
Institute of Reproductive Medicine
University of Sydney
Westmead, Australia

Katrien Stouffs
Center for Medical Genetics/Research Center
Reproduction and Genetics
Vrije Universiteit Brussel (VUB)
Universitair Ziekenhuis Brussel (UZ Brussel)
Brussels, Belgium

Qing-Yuan Sun
State Key Laboratory of Reproductive Biology
Institute of Zoology
Chinese Academy of Sciences
Beijing, China

Jason E. Swain
CCRM IVF Network
Lone Tree, Colorado

Karl Swann
College of Biomedical and Life Sciences
Cardiff University
Cardiff, United Kingdom

Evelyn E. Telfer
Institute of Cell Biology and Centre for Integrative Physiology
University of Edinburgh
Edinburgh, United Kingdom

Tom Turner
Texas Fertility Center
Ovation Fertility
Austin, Texas

Filippo M. Ubaldi
GENERA Centres for Reproductive Medicine
Rome, Italy

Gábor Vajta
RVT Australia
Queensland, Australia

Anna Veiga
Reproductive Medicine Service
Hospital Universitari Dexeus
and
Barcelona Stem Cell Bank
Centre of Regenerative Medicine in Barcelona
Barcelona, Spain

Felipe Vilella
Igenomix
Valencia, Spain

Dagan Wells
Nuffield Department of Obstetrics & Gynaecology
University of Oxford
Oxford, United Kingdom

Yuval Yaron
Prenatal Genetic Diagnosis Division, Genetic Institute
and
Department of Obstetrics and Gynecology
Lis Maternity Hospital
Tel Aviv Sourasky Medical Center
and
Sackler Faculty of Medicine
Tel Aviv University
Tel Aviv, Israel

Carlotta Zacà
9.baby—Family and Fertility Center
Bologna, Italy

The beginnings of human *in vitro* fertilization

ROBERT G. EDWARDS

In vitro fertilization (IVF) and its derivatives in preimplantation diagnosis, stem cells, and the ethics of assisted reproduction continue to attract immense attention scientifically and socially. All these topics were introduced by 1970. Hardly a day passes without some public recognition of events related to this study, and clinics spread ever further worldwide. Now that we must be approaching 1.5 million IVF births, it is time to celebrate what has been achieved by so many investigators, clinical, scientific, and ethical.

While much of this "Introduction" chapter covers the massive accumulation of events between 1960 and 2000, it also briefly discusses new perspectives emerging in the twenty-first century. Fresh advances also increase curiosity about how these fields of study began and how their ethical implications were addressed in earlier days. As for me, I am still stirred by recollections of those early days. Foundations were laid in Edinburgh, London, and Glasgow in the 1950s and early 1960s. Discoveries made then led to later days in Cambridge, working there with many PhD students. It also resulted in my working with Patrick Steptoe in Oldham. Our joint opening of Bourn Hall in 1980, which became the largest IVF clinic of its kind at the time, signified the end of the beginning of assisted human conception and the onset of dedicated applied studies.

INTRODUCTION

First of all, I must express in limited space my tributes to my teachers, even if inadequately. These include investigators from far-off days when the fundamental facts of reproductive cycles, surgical techniques, endocrinology, and genetics were elicited by many investigators. These fields began to move in the twentieth century, and if one pioneer of these times should be saluted, it must be Gregory Pincus. Famous for the contraceptive pill, he was a distinguished embryologist, and part of his work dealt with the maturation of mammalian oocytes *in vitro*. He was the first to show how oocytes aspirated from their follicles would begin their maturation *in vitro*, and how a number matured and expelled a first polar body. I believe his major work was done in rabbits, where he found that the 10–11-hour timings of maturation *in vitro* accorded exactly with those occurring *in vivo* after an ovulatory stimulus to the female rabbit.

Pincus et al. also studied human oocytes (1). Extracting oocytes from excised ovaries, they identified chromosomes in a large number of oocytes and interpreted this as evidence of the completion of maturation *in vitro*. Many oocytes possessed chromosomes after 12 hours, with the proportion remaining constant over the next 30 hours and longer. Twelve hours was taken as the period of maturation. Unfortunately, chromosomes were not classified for their meiotic stage. Maturing oocytes would be expected to display diakinesis or metaphase I chromosome pairs. Fully mature oocytes would display metaphase II chromosomes, signifying they were fully ripe and ready for fertilization. Nevertheless, it is well known that oocytes can undergo atresia in the ovary, involving the formation of metaphase II chromosomes in many of them. These oocytes complicated Pincus' estimates, even in controls, and were the source of his error, which led later workers to inseminate human oocytes 12 hours after collection and culture *in vitro* (2,3). Work on human fertilization *in vitro*, and indeed comparable studies in animals, remained in abeyance from then and for many years. Progress in animal IVF had also been slow. After many relatively unsuccessful attempts in several species in the 1950s and 1960s, a virtual dogma arose that spermatozoa had to spend several hours in the female reproductive tract before acquiring the potential to bind to the zona pellucida and achieve fertilization. In the late 1960s, Austin and Chang independently determined the need for sperm capacitation, identified by a delay in fertilization after spermatozoa had entered the female reproductive tract (4,5). This discovery was taken by many investigators as the reason for the failure to achieve fertilization *in vitro*, and why spermatozoa had to be exposed to secretions of the female reproductive tract. At the same time, Chang reported that rabbit eggs that had fully matured *in vitro* failed to produce normal blastocysts, with none of them implanting normally (6).

MODERN BEGINNINGS OF HUMAN IVF, PREIMPLANTATION GENETIC DIAGNOSIS, AND EMBRYO STEM CELLS

My PhD began at the Institute of Animal Genetics, Edinburgh University, in 1952, encouraged by Professor Conrad Waddington, the inventor of epigenesis, and supervised by Dr. Alan Beatty. At the time, capacitation was gaining in significance. My chosen topic was the genetic control of early mammalian embryology, specifically the growth of preimplantation mouse embryos with altered chromosome complements.

Achieving these aims included a need to expose mouse spermatozoa to x-rays, ultraviolet light, and various chemicals *in vitro*. This would destroy their chromatin and prevent them from making any genetic contribution to the embryo, hopefully without impairing their capacity to fertilize eggs *in vivo*. Resulting embryos would become gynogenetic haploids. Later, my work changed to exposing ovulated mouse oocytes to colchicine *in vivo* in order to destroy their second meiotic spindle *in vivo*. This treatment freed all chromosomes from their attachment to the meiotic spindle, and they then became extruded from the egg into tiny artificial polar bodies. The fertilizing spermatozoon thus entered an empty egg, which resulted in the formation of androgenetic haploid embryos with no genetic contribution from the maternal side. For three years, my work was concentrated in the mouse house, working at midnight to identify mouse females in estrus by vaginal smears, collecting epididymal spermatozoa from males, and practicing artificial insemination with samples of treated spermatozoa. This research was successful, as mouse embryos were identified with haploid, triploid, tetraploid, and aneuploid chromosomes. Moreover, the wide range of scientific talent in the Institute made it a perfect place for fresh collaborative studies. For example, Julio Sirlin and I applied the use of radioactive DNA and RNA precursors to the study of spermatogenesis, spermiogenesis, fertilization, and embryogenesis, and gained knowledge unavailable elsewhere.

An even greater fortune beckoned. Allen Gates, who was newly arrived from the United States, brought commercial samples of Organon's pregnant mares' serum (PMS) rich in follicle-stimulating hormone (FSH), and human chorionic gonadotropin (hCG) with its strong luteinizing hormone (LH) activity to induce estrus and ovulation in immature female mice. Working with Mervyn Runner (7), he had used low doses of each hormone at an interval of 48 hours to induce oocyte maturation, mating, and ovulation in immature mouse females. He now wished to measure the viability of three-day embryos from immature mice by transferring them to an adult host to grow to term (8). I was more interested in stimulating adult mice with these gonadotropins to induce estrus and ovulation at predictable times of the day. This would help my research, and I was by now weary of taking mouse vaginal smears at midnight. My future wife, Ruth Fowler, and I teamed up to test this new approach to superovulating adult mice. We chose PMS to induce multifolliculation and hCG to trigger ovulation, varying the doses and times from those utilized by Allen Gates. PMS became obsolete for human studies some time later, but its impact has stayed with me from that moment, even until today.

Opinion in those days was that exogenous hormones such as PMS and hCG would stimulate follicle growth and ovulation in immature female mammals, but not in adults because they would interact badly with an adult's reproductive cycles. In fact, they worked wonderfully well. Doses of 1–3 IU of PMS induced the growth of numerous follicles, and similar doses of hCG 42 hours later invoked estrus and ovulation a further 6 hours later in almost all of them. Often, 70 or more ovulated oocytes crowded the ampulla, most of them being fertilized and developing to blastocysts (9). Oocyte maturation, ovulation, mating, and fertilization were each closely timed in all adults, another highly unusual aspect of stimulation (10). Diakinesis was identified as the germinal vesicle regressed, with metaphase I a little later and metaphase II—expulsion of the first polar body—and ovulation at 11.5–12 hours after hCG. Multiple fertilization led to multiple implantation and fetal growth to full term, just as similar treatments in anovulatory women resulted in quintuplets and other high-order multiple pregnancies a few years later. Years afterward, germinal vesicle breakdown and diakinesis were to prove equally decisive in identifying meiosis and ovulation in human oocytes *in vivo* and *in vitro*. Even as these results were gained, Ruth and I departed in 1957 from Edinburgh to the California Institute of Technology, where I switched over to immunology and reproduction, a topic that was to dominate my life for five or six years on my return to the United Kingdom.

The Institute at Edinburgh had given me an excellent basis not only in genetics, but equally in reproduction. I had gained considerable knowledge about the endocrine control of estrus cycles, ovulation, and spermatozoa; the male reproductive tract; artificial insemination; the stages of embryo growth in the oviduct and uterus; superovulation and its consequences; and the use of radiolabeled compounds. Waddington had also been deeply interested in ethics and the relationships between science and religion, and instilled these topics in his students. I had been essentially trained in reproduction, genetics, and scientific ethics, and all of this knowledge was to prove to be of immense value in my later career. A visit to the California Institute of Technology widened my horizons into the molecular biology of DNA and the gene, a field then in its infancy.

After a year in California, London beckoned me to the National Institute for Medical Research to work with Drs. Alan Parkes and Colin (Bunny) Austin. I was fortunate indeed to have two such excellent colleagues. After two intense years in immunology, my curiosity returned to maturing oocytes and fertilization *in vitro*. Since they matured so regularly and easily *in vivo*, it should be easy to stimulate maturation in mouse oocytes *in vitro* by using gonadotropins. In fact, to my immense surprise, when liberated from their follicles into culture medium, oocytes matured immediately in vast numbers in all groups, with exactly the same timing as those maturing *in vivo* following an injection of hCG. Adding hormones made no difference. Rabbit, hamster, and rat oocytes also matured within 12 hours, each at their own species' specific rates. But to my surprise, oocytes from cows, sheep, and rhesus monkeys, and the occasional baboon, did not mature *in vitro* within 12 hours. Their germinal vesicles persisted unmoved, arrested in the stage known as diffuse diplotene. Why had they not responded like those of rats, mice, and rabbits? How would human oocytes respond? A unique opportunity emerged to collect pieces of human ovary and to aspirate human oocytes from their occasional follicles. I grasped it with alacrity.

MOVING TO HUMAN STUDIES

Molly Rose was a local gynecologist in the Edgware and District Hospital who delivered two of our daughters. She agreed to send me slivers or wedges of ovaries such as those removed from patients with polycystic disease, as recommended by Stein and Leventhal, or with myomata or other disorders demanding surgery. Stein–Leventhal wedges were the best sources of oocytes, with their numerous small Graafian follicles lined up in a continuous rim just below the ovarian surface. Though samples were rare, they provided enough oocytes to start with. These oocytes responded just like the oocytes from cows, sheep, and pigs, their germinal vesicles persisting and diakinesis being absent after 12 hours *in vitro*.

This was disappointing, and especially so for me, since Tjio, Levan, and Ford had identified 46 diploid chromosomes in humans, while studies by teams in Edinburgh and France had made it clear that many human beings were heteroploid. This was my subject, because chromosomal variations mostly arose during meiosis, and this would be easily assessed in maturing oocytes at diakinesis. Various groups also discovered monosomy or disomy in many men and women. Some women were XO or XXX; some men were XYY and XYYY. Trisomy 21 proved to be the most common cause of Down's syndrome, and other trisomies were detected. All this new information reminded me of my chromosome studies in the Edinburgh mice.

For human studies, I would have to obtain diakinesis and metaphase I in human oocytes, and then continue this analysis to metaphase II when the oocytes would be fully mature, ready for fertilization. Despite being disappointed at the current failure with human oocytes, it was time to write my findings for *Nature* in 1962 (11). There was so much to write regarding the animal work and in describing the new ideas then taking shape in my mind. I had heard Institute lectures on infertility, and realized that fertilizing human oocytes *in vitro* and replacing embryos into the mother could help to alleviate this condition. It could also be possible to type embryos for genetic diseases when a familial disposition was identified. Pieces of tissue, or one or two blastomeres, would have to be excised from blastocysts or cleaving embryos, but this did not seem to be too difficult. There were few genetic markers available for this purpose in the early 1960s, but it might be possible to sex embryos by their XX or XY chromosome complement by assessing mitoses in cells excised from morulae or blastocysts. Choosing female embryos for transfer would avert the birth of boys with various sex-linked disorders such as hemophilia. Clearly, I was becoming totally committed to human IVF and embryo transfer.

While looking in the library for any newly published papers relevant to my proposed *Nature* manuscript, I discovered those earlier papers of Pincus and his colleagues. They had apparently succeeded 30 years earlier in maturing human oocytes cultured for 12 hours where I had failed. My *Nature* paper (11) became very different from that originally intended, even though it retained enough for publication. Those results of Pincus et al. had to be repeated. After trying hard, I failed completely to repeat them, despite infusing intact ovaries *in vitro* with gonadotropin solutions, using different culture media to induce maturation, and using joint cultures of maturing mouse oocytes and newly released human oocytes. Adding hormones to culture media also failed. It began to seem that menstrual cycles had affected oocyte physiology in a different manner than in non-menstruating mammalian species. Finally, another line of inquiry emerged after two years of fruitless research on the precious few human oocytes available. Perhaps the timing of maturation in mice and rabbits differed from that of those oocytes obtained from cows, baboons, and humans. Even as my days in London were ending, Molly Rose sent a sliver of human ovary. The few oocytes were placed in culture just as before. Their germinal vesicles remained static for 12 hours as I already knew, and then, after 20 hours *in vitro*, three oocytes remained, and I waited to examine them until they had been *in vitro* for 24 hours. The first contained a germinal vesicle, and so did the second. There was one left and one only. Its image under the microscope was electrifying. I gazed down at chromosomes in diakinesis and at a regressing germinal vesicle. The chromosomes were superb examples of human diakinesis with their classical chiasmata. At last, I was on the way to human IVF, to completion of the maturation program and the onset of studies on fertilization *in vitro*.

This was the step I had waited for, a marker that Pincus had missed. He never checked for diakinesis, and apparently confused atretic oocytes, which contained chromosomes, with maturing oocytes. Endless human studies were opening. It was easy now, even on the basis of one oocyte in diakinesis, to calculate the timing of the final stages of maturation because the post-diakinesis stages of maturation were not too different from normal mitotic cycles in somatic cells. This calculation provided me with an estimate of about 36 hours for full maturation, which would be the moment for insemination. All these gaps in knowledge had to be filled. But now, my research program was stretching far into the future.

At this wonderful moment, John Paul, an outstanding cell biologist, invited me to join him and Robin Cole at Glasgow University to study differentiation in early mammalian embryos. This was exciting, to work in biochemistry with a leading cell biologist. He had heard that I was experimenting with very early embryos, trying to grow cell lines from them. He also wanted to grow stem cells from mammalian embryos and study them *in vitro*. This began one of my most memorable 12 months of research. John's laboratory had facilities unknown anywhere else, with CO_2 incubators, numerous cell lines in constant cultivation, cryopreservation facilities, and the use of media droplets held under liquid paraffin. We decided to start with rabbits. Cell lines did not grow easily from cleaving rabbit embryos. In contrast, stem cells migrated out in massive numbers from cultures of rabbit blastocysts, forming muscle, nerves, phagocytes, blood islands, and other tissues *in vitro* (12). Stem cells were differentiating *in vitro* into virtually all the tissues of the body. In contrast, dissecting the inner cell mass from blastocysts and culturing it intact or as disaggregated cells produced lines of cells that divided and divided, without ever differentiating. One line of these embryonic stem cells expressed specific enzymes, diploid chromosomes, and a fibroblastic structure as it grew over 200 and more generations. Another was epithelioid and had different enzymes but was similar in other respects. The ability to make whole-embryo cultures producing differentiating cells was now combined with everlasting lines of undifferentiated stem cells that replicated over many years without changing. Ideas of using stem cells for grafting to overcome organ damage in recipients began to emerge. My thoughts returned constantly to growing stem cells from human embryos to repair defects in tissues of children and adults.

Almost at my last moment in Glasgow, with this new set of ideas in my mind, a piece of excised ovary yielded several oocytes. Being placed *in vitro*, two of them had reached metaphase II and expelled a polar body at 37 hours. This showed that another target on the road to human IVF had been achieved as the whole pattern of oocyte maturation continued to emerge but with increasing clarity.

Cambridge University, my next and final habitation, is an astonishing place. Looking back on those days, it seems that the Physiological Laboratory was not the ideal place to settle in that august university. Nevertheless, a mixture of immunology and reproduction remained my dominant theme as I rejoined Alan Parkes and Bunny Austin there. I had to do immunology to obtain a grant to support my family, but thoughts of human oocytes and embryos were never far away. One possible model of the human situation was the cow and other agricultural species, and large numbers of cow, pig, and sheep oocytes were available from ovaries given to me by the local slaughterhouse. Each species had its own timing, all of them longer than 12 hours (13). Pig oocytes were closest to humans, requiring 37 hours. In each species, maturation timings *in vitro* were exactly the same as those arising *in vivo* in response to an hCG injection. This made me suspect that a woman ovulated 36–37 hours after an injection of hCG. Human oocytes also trickled in, improving my provisional timings of maturation, and one or two of them were inseminated, but without signs of fertilization.

More oocytes were urgently needed to conclude the timings of oocyte meiosis. Surgeons in Johns Hopkins Hospital, Baltimore, performed the Stein–Leventhal operation, which would allow me to collect ovarian tissue, aspirate oocytes from their follicles, and retain the remaining ovarian tissues for pathology if necessary.

I had already met Victor McKusick, who worked in Johns Hopkins, at many conferences. I asked for his support for my request to work with the hospital gynecologists for six weeks. He found a source of funds, made laboratory space available, and gave me a wonderful invitation that introduced me to Howard and Georgeanna Jones. This significant moment was equal to my meeting with Molly Rose. The Joneses proved to be superb and unstinting in their support. Sufficient wedges and other ovarian fragments were available to complete my maturation program in human oocytes. Within three weeks, every stage of meiosis was classified and timed (14). We also undertook preliminary studies on inseminating human oocytes that had matured *in vitro*, trying to achieve sperm capacitation by using different media or adding fragments of ampulla to the cultures, and even attempting fertilization in rhesus monkey oviducts. Two nuclei were found in some inseminated eggs, resembling pronuclei, but sperm tails were not identified, so no claims could be made (15). During those six weeks, however, oocyte maturation was fully timed at 37 hours, permitting me now to predict with certainty that women would ovulate at 37 hours after an hCG injection.

A simple means of access to the human ovary was now essential in order to identify human ovarian follicles *in vivo* and to aspirate them 36 hours after hCG, just before the follicular rupture. Who could provide this? And how about sperm capacitation? Only in hamsters had fertilization *in vitro* been achieved, using *in vivo*-matured oocytes and epididymal spermatozoa (16). I met Victor Lewis, my third clinical colleague, and we noticed what seemed to be anaphase II in some inseminated eggs. Again, no sperm tails were seen within the eggs.

An attempt to achieve human capacitation in Chapel Hill, North Carolina, working with Robert McGaughey and his colleagues, also failed (17). A small intrauterine chamber lined with porous membrane was filled with washed human spermatozoa, sealed, and inserted overnight into the uterus of human volunteers at mid-cycle. Molecules entering it could react with the spermatozoa. No matured human eggs were fertilized. Later evidence indicated that the chamber contained inflammatory proteins, perhaps explaining the failure.

DECISIVE STEPS TO CLINICAL HUMAN IVF

Back in the United Kingdom, my intention to conceive human children *in vitro* had grown even stronger. So many medical advantages could flow from it. A small number of human embryos had been flushed from human oviducts or uteri after sexual intercourse, providing slender information on these earliest stages of human embryology. It was time to attain human fertilization *in vitro*, in order to move close to working with infertile patients. Ethical issues and moral decisions would emerge, one after the other, in full public view. Matters such as cloning and sexing embryos, the risk of abnormalities in the children, the clinical use of embryo stem cells, the ethics of oocyte donation and surrogate pregnancy, and the right to initiate human embryonic life *in vitro* would never be very far away. These issues were all acceptable, since I was confident that studies of human conception were essential for future medicine, and correct ethically, medically, and scientifically. The increasing knowledge of genetics and embryology could assist many patients if I could achieve human fertilization and grow embryos for replacement into their mothers.

Few human oocytes were available in the United Kingdom. Despite this scarcity, one or two of those matured and fertilized *in vitro* possessed two nuclei after insemination. But there were no obvious sperm tails. I devised a cow model for human fertilization, using *in vitro*-matured oocytes and insemination *in vitro* with selected samples of highly active, washed bull spermatozoa extracted from neat semen. It was a pleasure to see some fertilized bovine eggs, with sperm tails and characteristic pronuclei, especially using spermatozoa from one particular bull. Here was a model for human IVF and a prelude to a series of events that implied that matters in my research were suddenly changing. A colleague had stressed that formalin fixatives were needed to detect sperm tails in eggs. Barry Bavister joined our team to study for his PhD and designed a medium of high pH, which gave excellent fertilization rates in hamsters. We decided to collaborate by using it for trials on human fertilization *in vitro*.

Finally, while browsing in the library of the Physiological Laboratory, I read a paper in *The Lancet* that instantly caught my attention. Written by Dr. P.C. Steptoe of the Oldham and District General Hospital (18), it described laparoscopy, with its narrow telescope and instruments and its minute abdominal incisions. He could visualize the ampulla and place small amounts of medium there, in an operation lasting 30 minutes or less and maybe even without using anesthesia. This is exactly what I wanted, because access to the ampulla was equivalent to gaining access to ovarian follicles. Despite advice to the contrary from several medical colleagues, I telephoned him about collaboration and stressed the uncertainty in achieving fertilization *in vitro*. He responded most positively, just as Molly, Howard and Georgeanna, and Victor had done. We decided to get together.

Last but by no means least, Molly Rose sent a small piece of ovary to Cambridge. Its dozen or more oocytes were matured *in vitro* for 37 hours, then Barry and I added washed spermatozoa suspended in his medium. We examined them a few hours later. To our delight, spermatozoa were pushing through the zona pellucida, into several of the eggs. Maternal and paternal pronuclei were forming beautifully. We saw polar bodies and sperm tails within the eggs. That evening in 1969, we watched in delight virtually all the stages of human fertilization *in vitro* (Figure I.1). One fertilized egg had fragments, as Chang had forecast from his work on oocyte maturation and fertilization *in vitro* of rabbit eggs. This evidence strengthened the need to abandon oocyte maturation *in vitro* and replace it with stimulating maturation by means of exogenous hormones. Our 1969 paper in *Nature* surprised a world unaccustomed to the idea of human fertilization *in vitro* (19).

Incredibly fruitful days followed in our Cambridge laboratory. Richard Gardner, another PhD candidate, and I excised small pieces of trophectoderm from rabbit blastocysts and sexed them by staining the sex chromatin body. Those classified as female were transferred into adult females and were all correctly sexed at term. This work transferred my theoretical ideas of a few years earlier into the practice of preimplantation diagnosis of inherited disease, in this case for sex-linked diseases (20). Alan Henderson, a cytogeneticist, and I analyzed chiasmata during diakinesis in mouse and human eggs, and explained the high frequencies of Down's syndrome in offspring of older mothers as a consequence of meiotic errors arising in oocytes formed last in the fetal ovary, which were then ovulated last at later maternal ages (21). Dave Sharpe, a lawyer from Washington, joined forces with me to write an article in *Nature* (22) on the ethics of IVF, the first ever paper in the field. I followed this up with a detailed analysis of ethics and law in IVF covering scientific possibilities, oocyte donation, surrogacy by embryo transfer, and other matters (22). So the first ethical papers were written by scientists and lawyers and not by philosophers, ethicists, or politicians.

THE OLDHAM YEARS

Patrick and I began our collaboration six months later in the Oldham and District General Hospital, almost 200 miles north of Cambridge. He had worked closely with two pioneers, Palmer in Paris (23) and Fragenheim in Germany (24). He improved the pneumoperitoneum to gain working space in the abdominal cavity and used carbon fibers to pass cold light into the abdomen from an external source (25). By now, Patrick was waiting in the wings, ready to begin clinical IVF in distant Oldham. We had a long talk about ethics and found our stances to be very similar.

Work started in the Oldham and District General Hospital and moved later to Kershaw's Hospital, set up by my assistants, especially Jean Purdy. We knew the routine. It was based on my Edinburgh experiences with mice. Piero Donini from Serono Laboratories in Rome had purified urinary human menopausal gonadotropin (hMG) as a source of FSH and the product was used clinically to stimulate follicle growth in anovulatory women by Bruno Lunenfeld (26). It removed the need for PMS, thus avoiding the use of nonhuman hormones. We used low dosage levels in patients; that is, two to three vials (a total of 150–225 IU) given on days 3 and 5, and 5000–7000 IU of hCG on day 10. Initially, the timing of oocyte maturation *in vitro* was confirmed by performing laparoscopic collections of oocytes from ovarian follicles at 28 hours after hCG to check that they were in metaphase I (27). We then moved to 36 hours to aspirate mature metaphase II oocytes for fertilization. Those beautiful oocytes were surrounded by masses of viscous cumulus cells and were maturing exactly as predicted. We witnessed follicular rupture at 37 hours through the laparoscope. Follicles could be classified from their appearance as ovulatory or nonovulatory, this diagnosis being confirmed later by assaying several steroids in the aspirated follicular fluids (Figure I.2).

It was a pleasure and a new duty to meet the patients searching for help to alleviate their infertility. We did our best, driving from Cambridge to Oldham and arriving at

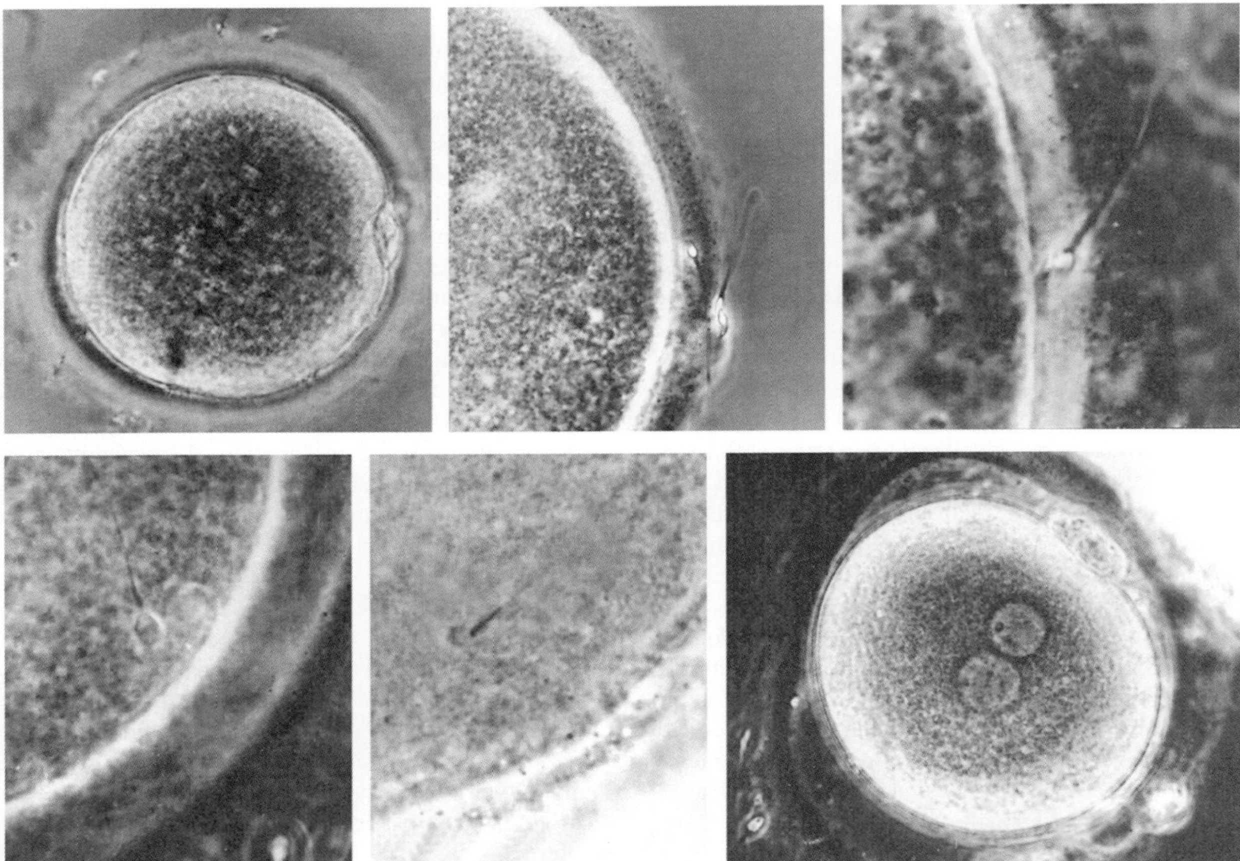

Figure I.1 A composite picture of the stages of fertilization of the human egg. (*Upper left*) An egg with a first polar body and spermatozoa attached to the outer zona pellucida. (*Upper central*) Spermatozoa are migrating through the zona pellucida. (*Upper right*) A spermatozoon with a tail beating outside the zona pellucida is attaching to the oocyte vitelline membrane. (*Lower left*) A spermatozoon in the ooplasm, with enlarging head and distinct mid-piece and tail. (*Lower central*) Further development of the sperm head in the ooplasm. (*Lower right*) A pronucleate egg with two pronuclei and polar bodies. Notice that the pronuclei are apparently aligned with the polar bodies, although more dimensions must be scored to ensure that polarity has been established in all axes.

noon to prepare the small laboratory there. Patrick had stimulated the patients with hMG and hCG, and he and his team led by Muriel Harris arrived to prepare for surgery.

Patrick's laparoscopy was superb. Ovarian stimulation, even though mild, produced five or six mature follicles per patient, and ripe oocytes came in a steady stream into my culture medium for insemination and overnight incubation. The next morning, the formation of two pronuclei and sperm tails indicated fertilization had occurred, even in simple media, now with a near-neutral pH. Complex culture media, Ham's F10 and others, each with added serum or serum albumin, sustained early and later cleavages (28), and even more fascinating was the gradual appearance of morulae and then light, translucent blastocysts (Figure I.3) (29). Here was my reward—growing embryos was now a routine, and examinations of many of them convinced me that the time had come to replace them into the mother's uterus. I had become highly familiar with the teratologic principles of embryonic development, and knew many teratologists. The only worry I had was the chance of chromosomal monosomy or trisomy, on the basis of our mouse studies, but these conditions could be detected later in gestation by amniocentesis. Our human studies had surpassed work on all animals, a point that was highlighted even more when we grew blastocysts to day 9 after they had hatched from their zona pellucida (Figure I.4) (30). This beautifully expanded blastocyst had a large embryonic disc that was shouting that it was a potential source of embryonic stem cells.

When human blastocysts became available, we tried to sex them using the sex chromatin body as in rabbits. Unfortunately, they failed to express either sex chromatin or the male Y body so we were unable to sex them as female or male embryos. Human preimplantation genetic diagnosis would have to wait a little longer.

During these years there were very few plaudits for us, as many people spoke against IVF. Criticism was mostly aimed at me, as usual when scientists bring new challenges to society. Criticism came not only from the Pope and archbishops, but also from scientists who should have known better, including James Watson (who testified to a U.S. Senate Committee that many abnormal babies would

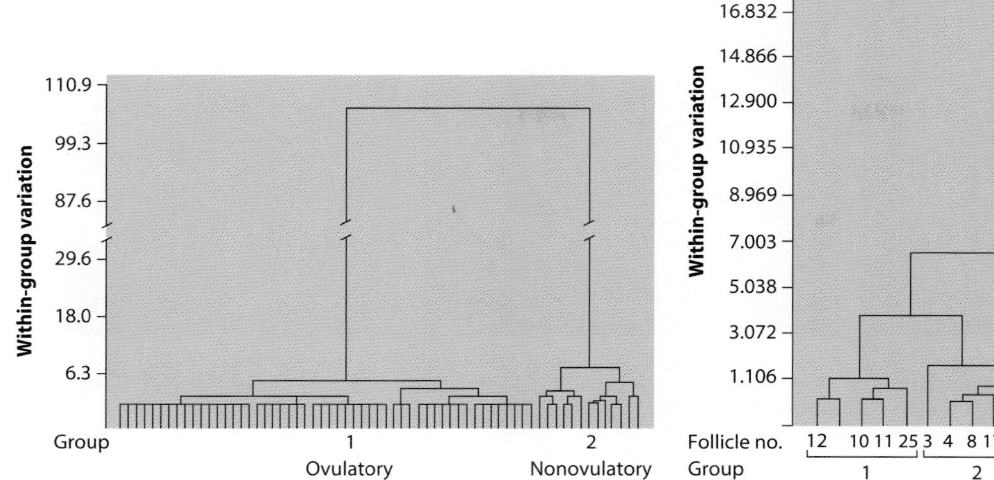

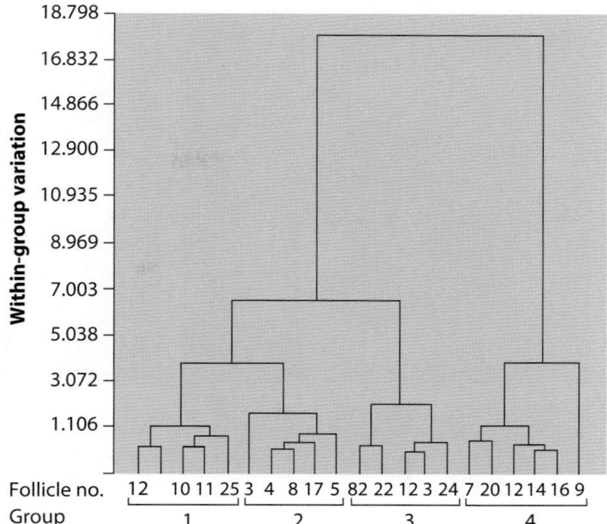

Figure I.2 Eight steroids were assayed in fluids extracted from human follicles aspirated 36–37 hours after the human chorionic gonadotropin (hCG) shot. The follicles had been classified as ovulating or non-ovulating by laparoscopic examination *in vivo*. Data were analyzed by cluster analysis, which groups follicles with similar features. The upper illustration shows data collected during the natural menstrual cycle. Note that two sharply separated groups of follicles were identified, each with very low levels of within-group variance. Attempting to combine the two groups resulted in a massive increase of within-group variation, indicating that two sharply different groups had been identified. These different groups accorded exactly with the two groups identified by means of steroid assays. The lower figure shows the same analysis during stimulated cycles on fluids collected 36–37 hours after injecting hCG. With this form of stimulation, follicle growth displays considerable variation within groups. Attempts to combine all the groups result in a moderately large increase in variation. This evidence suggests that follicles vary considerably in their state of development in simulated cycles using human menopausal gonadotropin (hMG) and hCG.

be born), and Max Perutz, who supported him. These scientist critics knew virtually nothing about my field, so who advised them to make such ridiculous charges? Cloning football teams or intelligentsia was always raised by ethicists, which clearly dominated their thoughts rather than the intense hopes of our infertile patients. Yet one theologian, Gordon Dunstan, who became a close friend, knew all about IVF from us, and wrote an excellent book on its ethics. He was far ahead of almost every scientist in my field of study. Our patients also gave us their staunch support, and so did the Oldham Ethical Committee, Bunny Austin back home in Cambridge, and Elliott Philip, a colleague of Patrick's.

Growing embryos became a routine, so we decided to transfer one each to several patients. Here again we were in untested waters. Transferring embryos via the cervical canal, the obvious route to the uterus, was virtually a new and untested method. We would have to do our best. From now on, we worked with patients who had seriously distorted tubes or none whatsoever. This step was essential, since no one would have believed we had established a test-tube baby in a woman with near-normal tubes. This had to be a condition of our initial work. Curiously, it led many people to make the big mistake of believing that we started IVF to bypass occluded oviducts. Yet we already knew that embryos could be obtained for men with oligozoospermia or antibodies to their gametes, and for women in various stages of endometriosis.

One endocrinological problem did worry me. Stimulation with hMG and hCG shortened the succeeding luteal phase, leaving only a very short time for embryos to implant before the onset of menstruation. Levels of urinary pregnanediol also declined soon after oocyte collection. This condition was not a result of the aspiration of granulosa and cumulus cells, and luteal support would be needed, preferably progesterone. Csapo et al. stressed how this hormone was produced by the ovaries for the first 8–10 weeks before the placenta took over this function (31). Injections of progesterone in oil given over that long period of time seemed unacceptable since it would be extremely uncomfortable for patients. While mulling over this problem, my attention turned to those earlier endocrinologists who believed that exogenous hormones would distort the reproductive cycle, although I doubt they even knew anything about a deficient luteal phase.

This is how we unknowingly made our biggest mistake in the early IVF days. Our choice of Primolut® (Sigma Chemical Co., St. Louis, Missouri) depot, a progestogen, meant it should be given every five days to sustain pregnancies, since it was supposed to save threatened abortions. So, we began embryo transfers to patients in stimulated cycles, giving this luteal phase support. Even though our work was slowed down by having to wait to see whether pregnancies arose in one group of patients before stimulating the next, enough patients had accumulated after two to three years. None of our patients was pregnant, and

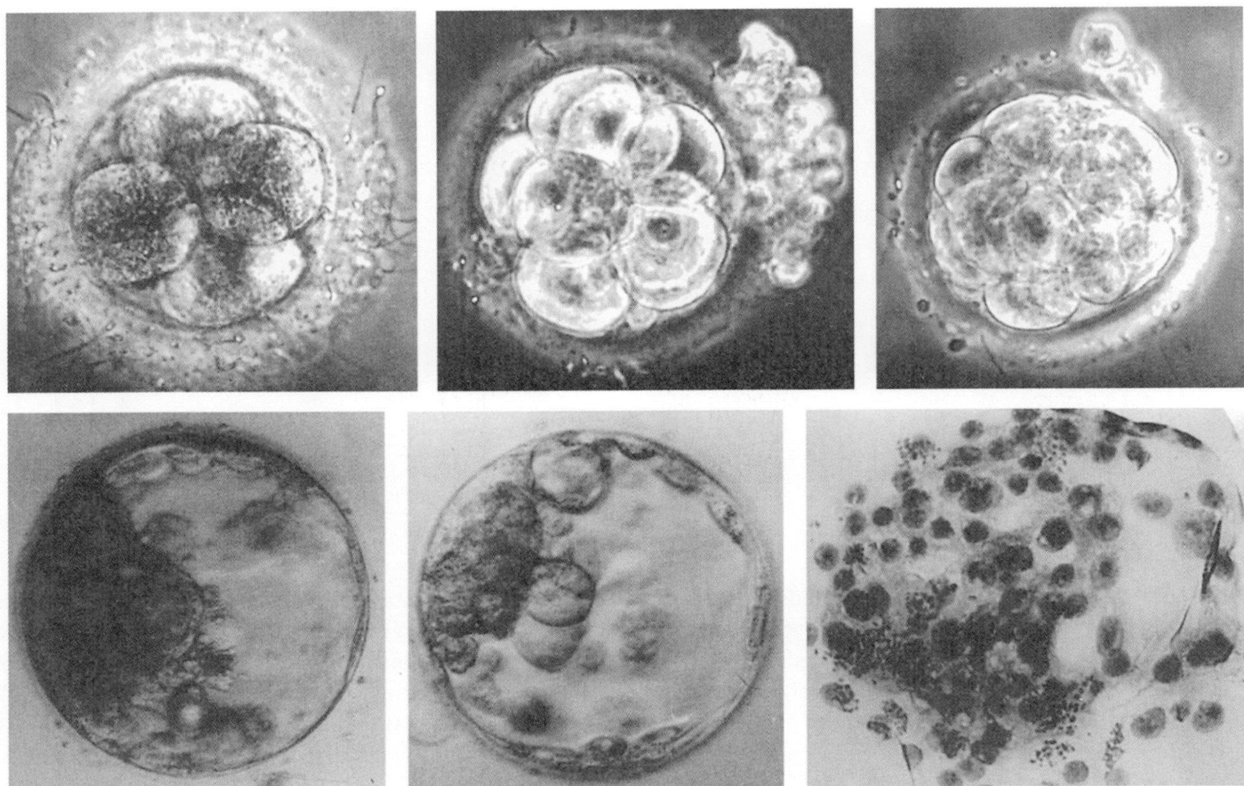

Figure I.3 Successive stages of human preimplantation development *in vitro* in a composite illustration made in Oldham in 1971. (*Upper left*) Four-cell stage showing the crossed blastomeres typical of most mammals. (*Upper middle*) Eight-cell stage showing the even outline of blastomeres and a small piece of cumulus adherent to the zona pellucida. (*Upper right*) A 16–32-cell stage showing the onset of compaction of the outer blastomeres. Often, blastocelic fluid can be seen accumulating between individual cells to give a "stripy" appearance to the embryo. (*Lower left and middle*) Two living blastocysts showing a distinct inner cell mass, single-celled trophectoderm, blastocelic cavity, and thinning zona pellucida. (*Lower right*) A fixed preparation of a human blastocyst at five days, showing more than 100 even-sized nuclei and many mitoses.

disaster loomed. Our critics were even more vociferous as the years passed, and the mutual support between Patrick and I had to pull us through.

Twenty or more different factors could have caused our failure; for example, cervical embryo transfers, abnormal embryos, toxic culture dishes or catheters, inadequate luteal support, incompatibility between patients' cycles and that imposed by hMG and hCG, inherent weakness in human implantation, and many others. We had to glean every scrap of information from our failures. I knew Ken Bagshawe in London, who was working with improved assay methods for gonadotropic hormones. He offered to measure blood samples taken from our patients over the implantation period using his new hCG assay. He telephoned: three or more of our patients previously undiagnosed had actually produced short-lived rises of hCG over this period. Everything changed with this information. We had established pregnancies after all, but they had aborted very early. We called them biochemical pregnancies, a term that still remains today. It had taken us almost three years to identify the cause of our failure, and the finger of suspicion pointed straight at Primulot. I knew it was luteolytic, but it was apparently also an abortifacient, and our ethical decision to use it had caused much heartache, immense loss of work and time, and despair for some of our patients. The social pressures had been immense, with critics claiming our embryos were dud and our whole program was a waste of time; but we had come through it and now knew exactly what to do next.

We accordingly reduced the levels of Primulot depot, and utilized hCG and progesterone as luteal aids. Suspicions were also emerging that human embryos were very poor at implanting. We had replaced single embryos into most of our patients, rarely two. Increasingly we began to wonder whether more should be replaced, as when we replaced two in a program involving transfer of oocytes and spermatozoa into the ampulla so that fertilization could occur *in vivo*.

This procedure was later called gamete intrafallopian transfer (GIFT) by Ricardo Asch. We now suspected that single embryo transfers could produce a 15%–20% chance of establishing pregnancy, just as our first clinical pregnancy arose after the transfer of a single blastocyst in a patient stimulated with hMG and hCG (32). Then came the fantastic news—a human embryo fertilized and grown *in vitro* had produced a pregnancy. Everything seemed fine, even with ultrasound images. My culture protocols

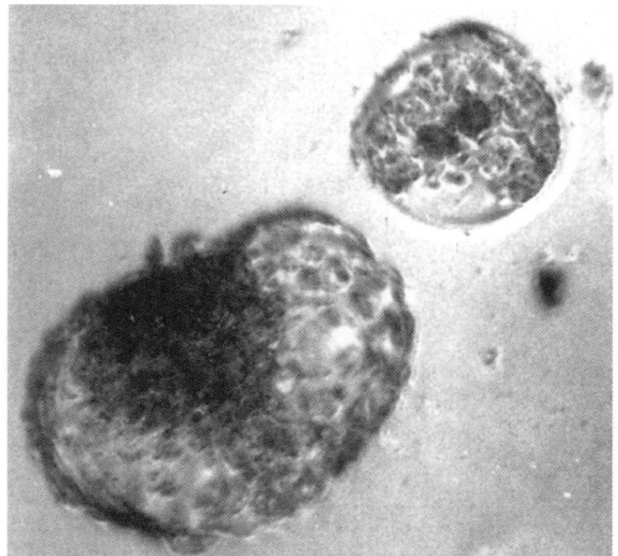

Figure I.4 A hatched human blastocyst after nine days in culture. Notice the distinct embryonic disc and the possible bilaminar structure of the membrane. The blastocyst has expanded considerably, as shown by comparing its diameter with that of the shed zona pellucida. The zona contains dying and necrotic cells and its diameter provides an estimate of the original oocyte end embryo diameters.

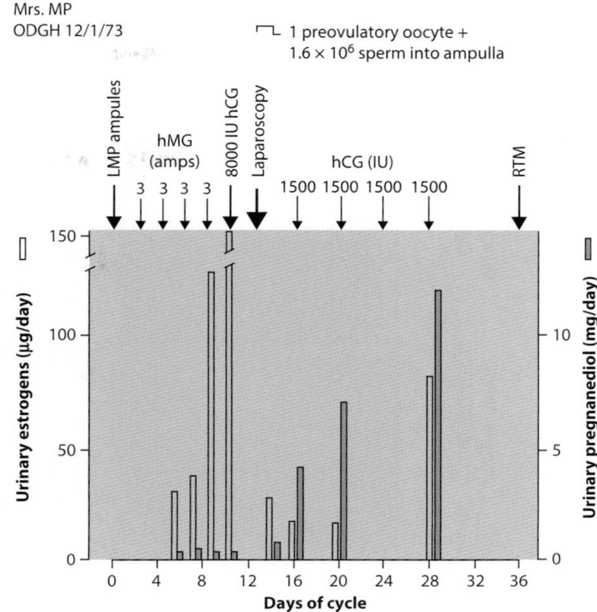

Figure I.5 The first attempts at gamete intrafallopian transfer (GIFT) were called oocyte recovery with tubal insemination (ORTI). In this treatment cycle, using human menopausal gonadotropin (hMG) and human chorionic gonadotropin (hCG), including additional injections of hCG for luteal support, a single preovulatory oocyte and 1.6 million sperm were transferred into the ampulla. Return to menstruation (RTM) indicates stages of the menstrual cycle. *Abbreviations*: LMP, last menstrual period; ODGH, Oldham and District General Hospital.

were satisfactory after all. Patrick rang: he feared the pregnancy was ectopic and he had to remove it sometime after 10 gestational weeks. Every new approach we tested seemed to be ending in disaster, yet we would not stop, since the work itself seemed highly ethical, and conceiving a child for our patients was perhaps the most wonderful thing anyone could do for them. In any case, ectopic pregnancies are now known to be a regular feature with assisted conception.

I sensed that we were entering the final phase of our Oldham work, seven years after it began. We had to speed up, partly because Patrick was close to retiring from the National Health Service. Four stimulation protocols were tested in an attempt to avoid problems with the luteal phase: hMG and hCG; clomiphene, hMG, and hCG to gain a better luteal phase; bromocriptine, hMG, and hCG because some patients had high prolactin concentrations; and hCG alone at mid-cycle. We also tested what came to be known as GIFT, calling it oocyte recovery with tubal insemination [ORTI] by transferring one or two eggs and spermatozoa to the ampulla) (Figure I.5). Natural-cycle IVF was introduced, based on collections of urine samples at regular intervals eight times daily, to measure exactly the onset of the LH surge, using a modified HiGonavis assay (Figure I.6). Cryopreservation was also introduced by freezing oocytes and embryos that looked to be in good condition when thawed. A recipient was given a donor egg fertilized by her husband's spermatozoa, but pregnancy did not occur.

Lesley and John Brown came as the second entrants for natural-cycle IVF. Lesley had no oviducts. Her egg was aspirated in a few moments and inseminated simply and efficiently. The embryo grew beautifully and was transferred an hour or so after it became eight cells. Their positive pregnancy test a few days after transfer was another milestone—surely nothing could now prevent their embryo developing to full term in a normal reproductive cycle, but those nine months lasted a very long time. Three more pregnancies were established using natural-cycle IVF as we abandoned the other approaches. A triploid embryo died *in utero*—more bad luck. A third pregnancy was lost through premature labor on a mountain walking holiday, two weeks after the mother's amniocentesis (32,33). It was a lovely, well-developed boy. Louise Brown's birth, and then Alistair's, proved to a waiting world that science and medicine had entered human conception. Our critics declared that the births were a fake, and advised against attending our presentation on the whole of the Oldham work at the Royal College of Obstetricians and Gynaecologists.

IVF WORLDWIDE

The Oldham period was over. Good facilities were now needed, with space for a large IVF clinic. Bourn Hall was an old Jacobean house in lovely grounds near Cambridge (Figure I.7). The facilities on offer for IVF in Cambridge were far too small, so we purchased it mostly with venture capital. It was essential to conceive 100 or 1000 IVF babies

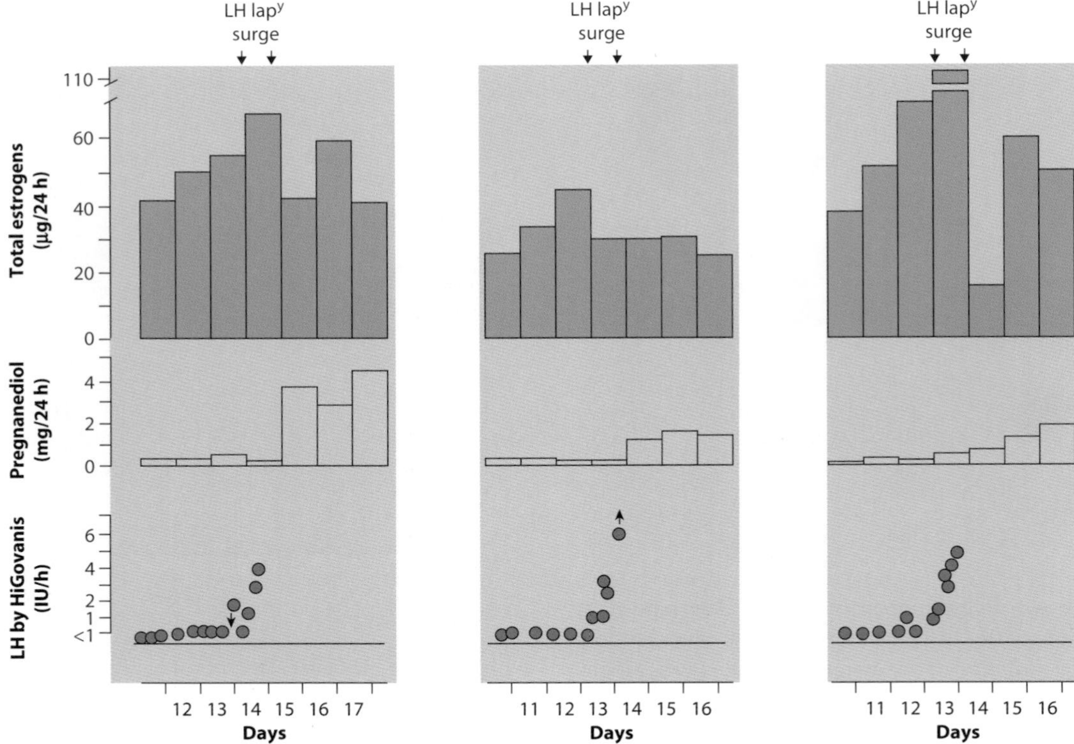

Figure I.6 Recording the progress of the human natural menstrual cycle for *in vitro* fertilization (IVF). Three patients are illustrated. All three displayed rising 24-hour urinary estrogen concentrations during the follicular phase and rising urinary pregnanediol concentrations in the luteal phase. Luteinizing hormone (LH) levels were measured several times daily and the data clearly reveal the exact time of onset of the LH surge.

to ensure that the method was safe and effective clinically. The immense delays in establishing Bourn Hall delayed our work by two years after Louise's birth. Finally, on minimal finance, Bourn Hall was opened in September 1980 on a shoestring, supported by our own cash and loans. The delay gave the rest of the world a chance to join in IVF. Alex Lopata delivered an IVF baby in Australia, and one or two others were born elsewhere. Natural-cycle IVF was chosen initially at Bourn Hall since it had proved successful in Oldham, and we became experts in it. Pregnancies flowed, at 15% per cycle. An Australian team of Alan Trounson and Carl Wood announced the establishment of several IVF pregnancies after stimulation by clomiphene and hCG and replacing two or three embryos (34), so they had moved ahead of us

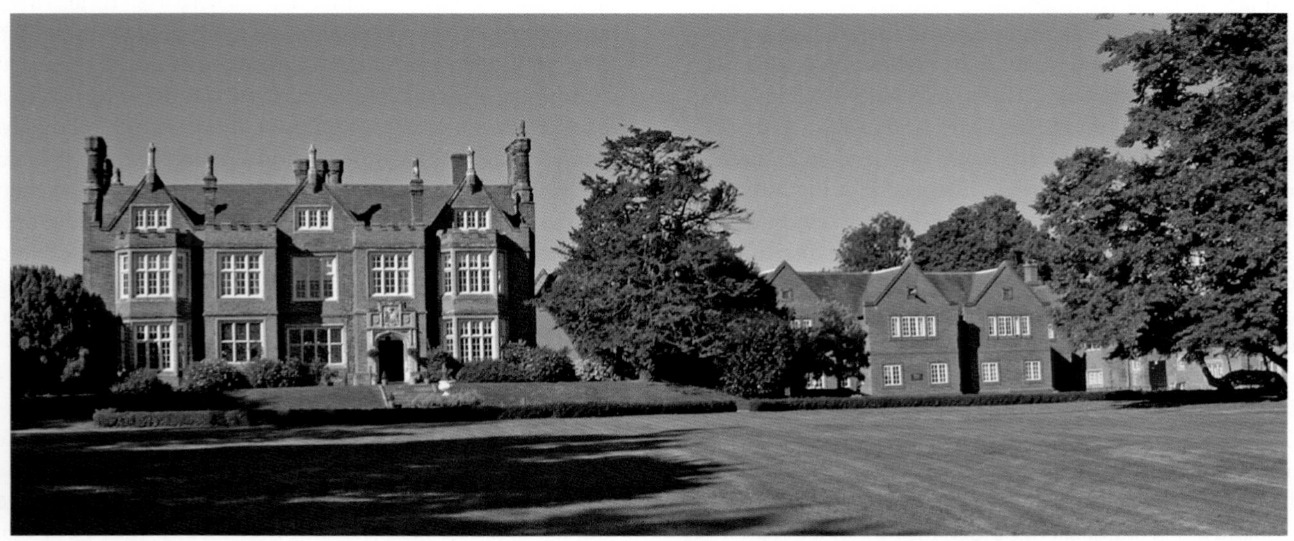

Figure I.7 Bourn Hall (courtesy of Dr. P Brinsden).

during the delayed opening of Bourn Hall. Our own effort now expanded prodigiously. Thousands of patients queued for IVF. Simon Fishel, Jacques Cohen, and Carol Fehilly joined the embryology team among younger trainees, and new clinicians joined Patrick and John Webster. Patients and pregnancies increased rapidly, and the world was left standing far behind. Howard and Georgeanna Jones began in Norfolk using gonadotropins for ovarian stimulation. Jean Cohen began in Paris, Wilfred Feichtinger and Peter Kemeter in Vienna, Klaus Diedrich and Hans van der Venn in Bonn, Lars Hamberger and Matts Wikland in Sweden, and Andre van Steirteghem and Paul Devroey in Brussels. IVF was now truly international.

The opening of Bourn Hall had not deterred our critics. They put up a fierce rearguard action against IVF, alongside LIFE, Society for the Unborn Child, individual gynecologists, and others.

Objections raised against IVF included low rates of pregnancy (no one mentioned the similar low rates of pregnancy with natural conception), the possibilities of oocyte and embryo donation, surrogate mothers, unmarried parents, one-sex parents, embryo cryopreservation, cloning, and endless other objections.

LIFE issued a legal action against me for the abortion of an embryo grown for 14 days and longer *in vitro*. Their action was rejected by the U.K. Attorney General since the laws of pregnancy began after implantation. We fully respected the intense ethical nature of our proceedings. We also recognized the need for research, and the necessity to protect or cryopreserve the best embryos for later replacement into their mothers. Those not replaced had to be used for research under strict controls, combined with open publication and discussion of our work.

Each year, 1000—rising to almost 2000—patients passed through Bourn Hall. Different stimulation regimens or new procedures could be tested in very little time.

Clomiphene/hMG was reintroduced. Bourn babies increased: 20, 50, 100–1000 after five to six years. This was far more than half of the world's entire IVF babies, including the first born in the U.S.A., Germany, Italy, and many other countries. Detailed studies were performed on embryo culture, implantation, and abortion. We even tried aspirating epididymal spermatozoa for IVF, without achieving successful fertilization.

Among the immense numbers of patients, people with astonishingly varied conditions of infertility emerged. Some were poor responders in whom immense amounts of endocrine priming were essential, some were women with a natural menstrual cycle that was not as it should have been, some had previous misdiagnoses that had laid the cause of infertility on the wife when the husband had never even been investigated, and some were men bringing semen samples that we discovered had been obtained from a friend. The collaboration between nurses, clinicians, and scientists was remarkable. Yet trouble—ethical trouble—was never far away. I purchased a freezing machine to resume our Oldham work, but, unknown to me, Patrick talked to officers of the British Medical Association (BMA) and for some reason agreed to delay embryo cryopreservation. Apparently, the BMA felt it would be an unwelcome social development. I did not approve of these reservations: David Whittingham had shown how low-temperature cryostorage was successful with mouse embryos, without causing genetic damage. "Freezing and cloning" became a term of intense approbation at this time. I unwillingly curtailed our cryopreservation program.

One weekend, major trouble erupted as a result of this difference between Patrick and me. My duties in Bourn Hall prevented me from attending a conference in London. Trying to be helpful, I telephoned my lecture to London. Reception at the other end was apparently so poor as to lead to misinterpretations of what I had said. Next morning, the press furor about my supposed practice of cryopreserving embryos after IVF was awful; so bad, indeed, that legal action had to be taken. Luckily, my lecture had been recorded, and listening to the tapes with a barrister revealed nothing contentious. I had said nothing improper in my lecture or during the question-and-answer session. That day, I issued seven libel actions against the cream of British society: the BMA and its secretary, the BBC, *The Times*, and other leading newspapers. There were seven in one day and another one later! If only one was lost, I could be ruined and disgraced. However, they were all won, even though it took several years with the BMA and its secretary. These legal actions had inhibited our research, with the cryopreservation program being shut down for more than a year. Every single embryological note of mine from those days in Oldham and from Bourn Hall was examined in detail for my opponents by someone who was clearly an embryologist. Nothing was found to incriminate me.

That wretched period passed. The number of babies kept on growing, embryo cryopreservation was resumed, and Gerhard Zeilmaker in The Netherlands beat us and the world to the first "ice" baby (35). Colin Howles and Mike McNamee joined us in endocrinology and Mike Ashwood-Smith and Peter Holland's joined us in embryology as the old team faded away. Fascinating days had returned. Working with barristers, we designed consent forms that were far in advance of those used elsewhere. Oocyte donation and surrogacy by embryo transfer were introduced. The world's first paper on embryo stem cells appeared in *Science* in 1984, sent from Bourn Hall, and the world's first paper on human preimplantation diagnosis in 1987 appeared in *Human Reproduction*. However, embryo research faltered as all normal embryos were cryopreserved for their parents, so almost none were available for study. Alan Handyside, one of our Cambridge PhDs, joined Hammersmith Hospital in London to make major steps in introducing preimplantation genetic diagnosis (36). As we reached 1000 pregnancies, our data showed the babies to be as normal as those conceived *in vivo*.

Test-tube babies (an awful term) were no longer unique and were accepted worldwide, exactly as Patrick and I had hoped. Our work was being recognized (Figure I.8). Clinics sprang up everywhere. Ultrasound was introduced to detect follicles for aspiration by the Scandinavians (37),

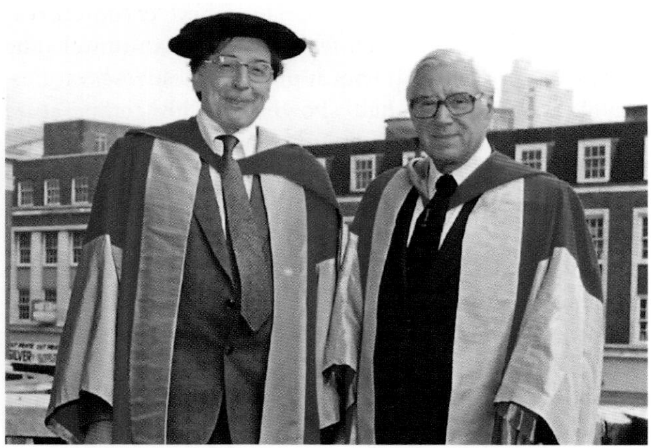

Figure I.8 A happy picture of Patrick and I, standing in our robes after being granted our Hon. DSc by Hull University.

making laparoscopy for oocyte recovery largely redundant. Artificial cycles were introduced in Australia and intracytoplasmic sperm injection (ICSI) was introduced in Belgium (38), and gonadotropin-releasing hormone agonists were used to inhibit the LH surge. Ian Craft in London showed how postmenopausal women aged 52 or more could establish pregnancies using oocyte donation and endocrine support. Women over 60 years of age conceived and delivered children. This breakthrough was especially welcome to me, since older women surely have the right to have children at ages almost the same as those possible for men.

Ethics continued side by side with advancing science and medicine. The U.K. governmental Warnock report recommended permitting embryo research and proposed a Licensing Authority for IVF. A year or so later, the U.K. House of Lords, in all its finery, responded with a 3:1 vote in favor, decisive support for all we had done in Mill Hill, Cambridge, and Oldham. What a wonderful day! The British House of Commons passed a liberal IVF law after intense debate, and so did the Spanish government, although elsewhere things were not so liberal. Ten years after the birth of Louise Brown, the British Parliament had therefore accepted IVF, research on human embryos until day 14, and establishing research embryos. Cloning and embryo stem cells still bothered the politicians of 1988, only to re-emerge in 1998, gray shadows of my earlier times in Glasgow. IVF had also become fundamental to establishing embryonic stem cells for organ repair, or cloning. During all this activity, tragedy struck all of us in Bourn Hall. Jean Purdy died in 1986 and Patrick Steptoe in 1988. They at least saw IVF come of age.

By the 1990s, burgeoning medical science was digging deeper into endless aspects of human conception *in vitro*. The intracytoplasmic injection of a single spermatozoon into an oocyte to achieve fertilization, ICSI, was one of the greatest advances since IVF was introduced. It transformed the treatment of male infertility, enabling severely oligozoospermic men to father their own children. It did not stop there, since epididymal spermatozoa and even those aspirated from the testis could be used for ICSI. Spermatids have also been used. ICSI became so simple that many clinics reduced IVF to fewer and fewer cases. New gonadotropin-releasing hormone antagonists introduced novel ways to control the cycle, enabling many oocytes to be stimulated by hMG and, subsequently, by using recombinant human FSH. Treatment in the natural cycle could be improved, since these antagonists control LH levels and prevent premature LH surges. My own interests were returning to embryology, as the molecular biology revolution influenced our thinking. I am convinced that the oocyte and egg must be highly programmed, timewise, in embryonic polarities and integrating genetic systems such that the tight systems place every new gene product in its right place in the one-cell egg and cleaving embryo. This must be right; there can surely be no other explanations for the fabulous modification in embryonic growth in the first week or two of embryonic life. I have been delighted to work with Chris Hansis on identifying a gene (for hCG-*) in one blastomere of four- and eight-cell human embryos, providing evidence of blastomere differentiation at this early stage of embryogenesis (39).

This topic returns me to my scientific origins studying mouse embryos in the Institute of Animal Genetics in Edinburgh, where Waddington reported the amazing story of the gene *Aristapedia* in *Drosophila*, which he had induced to grow legs in place of eyes. These unusual flies then bred true, showing he had uncovered a gene that had been silenced for millions of years and how this could be an essential component of normal differentiation. He called it epigenesis, and we fear today that some aspects of IVF may lead to deleterious epigenetic changes in children such as Angelman or Beckwith–Wiedemann syndrome. Risks of epigenetic changes in cattle embryos and those of other species may be heightened by adding serum to media used to culture embryos to cause, for example, large-calf syndrome. It would be wise to be well aware of these findings when practicing human IVF; for example, by assessing the role of sera in human culture media.

IVF OUTLOOK

In one sense, opening up human conception *in vitro* was perhaps among the first examples of applied science in modern "hi tech." Human IVF has since spread throughout the world, with apparently more than 3.5 million such babies born worldwide by 2008—yet Louise Brown is only just 30 years of age. The need for IVF and its derivatives is greater than ever, since up to 10% of couples may suffer from some form of infertility. Major advances in genetic technologies now identify hundreds of genes in a single cell, and diagnosing genetic disease in embryos promises to help avoid desperate genetic diseases in newborn children. Indeed, the ethics of this field have now become even more serious, since the typing of embryo genotypes provides detailed predictions of future life and health.

IVF has now combined closely with genetics to eliminate disease or disability genes, or lengthen the life span.

But most of all, practicing IVF teaches a wider understanding of the desire and love for a child and a partner, the wonderful and ancient joys of parenthood, the pain of failure, and the deep motivation needed in donating and receiving an urgently needed oocyte or a surrogate uterus. Parenthood is more responsible than ever before. Its complex choices are gathered before couples everywhere by the information revolution, placing family responsibilities on patients themselves, where it really matters. And IVF now reveals more and more about miracles preserved in embryogenesis from flies and frogs to humankind, over 600 million years of evolution.

The Human Genome Project is now complete and will inevitably assist IVF since we will soon understand the genetic aspects of early embryo growth and how to detect abnormal genes in embryos. This textbook contains chapters that describe in detail the several advances and developments that have expanded the possibilities of treating diverse causes of human infertility as well as numerous genetic disorders.

Already it is clear that a staggering array of genes operate in preimplantation stages in mammalian including human embryos, and new methods are being introduced to deal with such highly multigenic embryonic systems. We are indeed enmeshed in a field embracing some of the most fundamental evolutionary stages of our existence as we pass from oocyte to blastocyst and to implantation.

REFERENCES

1. Pincus G, Saunders B. The comparative behavior of mammalian eggs *in vivo* and *in vitro*. VI. The maturation of human ovarian ova. *Anat Rec* 1939; 75: 537–45.
2. Menkin MF, Rock J. *Am J Obstet Gynecol* 1949; 55: 440.
3. Hayashi M. Seventh International Conference of the International Planned Parenthood Federation. *Excerpta Medica* 1963: 505.
4. Austin CR. *Adv Biosci* 1969; 4: 5.
5. Chang M. *Adv Biosci* 1969; 4: 13.
6. Chang MC. The maturation of rabbit oocytes in culture and their maturation, activation, fertilization and subsequent development in the fallopian tubes. *J Exp Zool* 1955; 128: 379–405.
7. Runner M, Gates AH. Sterile, obese mothers. *J Hered* 1954; 45: 51–5.
8. Gates AH. Viability and developmental capacity of eggs from immature mice treated with gonadotrophins. *Nature* 1954; 177: 754–5.
9. Fowler RE, Edwards RG. Induction of superovulation and pregnancy in mature mice by gonadotrophins. *J Endocrinol* 1957; 15: 374–84.
10. Edwards RG, Gates AH. Timing of the stages of the maturation divisions, ovulation, fertilization and the first cleavage of eggs of adult mice treated with gonadotrophins. *J Endocrinol* 1959; 19: 292–304.
11. Edwards RG. Meiosis in ovarian oocytes of adult mammals. *Nature (London)* 1962; 196: 446–50.
12. Cole R, Edwards RG, Paul J. Cytodifferentiation and embryogenesis in cell colonies and tissue cultures derived from ova and blastocysts of the rabbit. *Dev Biol* 1966; 13: 385–407.
13. Edwards RG. Maturation *in vitro* of mouse, sheep, cow, pig, rhesus monkey and human ovarian oocytes. *Nature* 1965; 208: 349–51.
14. Edwards RG. Maturation *in vitro* of human ovarian oocytes. *Lancet* 1965; 2: 926–9.
15. Edwards RG, Donahue R, Baramki T, Jones H, Jr. Preliminary attempts to fertilize human oocytesmatured *in vivo*. *Am J Obstet Gynecol* 1966; 96: 192–200.
16. Yanagimachi R, Chang MC. *J Exp Zool* 1964; 156: 361–76.
17. Edwards RG, Talbert L, Israestam D et al. Diffusion chamber for exposing spermatozoa to human uterine secretions. *Am J Obstet Gynecol* 1968; 102: 388–96.
18. Steptoe PC. Laparoscopy and ovulation. *Lancet* 1968; 2: 913.
19. Edwards RG, Bavister BD, Steptoe PC. Early stages of fertilisation *in vitro* of human oocytes matured *in vitro*. *Nature (London)* 1969; 221: 632–5.
20. Gardner RL, Edwards RG. Control of the sex ratio at full term in the rabbit by transferred sexed blastocysts. *Nature (London)* 1968; 218: 346–8.
21. Henderson SA, Edwards RG. Chiasma frequency and maternal age in mammals. *Nature (London)* 1968; 218: 22–8.
22. Edwards RG, Sharpe DJ. Social values and research in human embryology. *Nature (London)* 1971; 231: 81–91.
23. Palmer R. *Acad Chir* 1946; 72: 363.
24. Fragenheim H. *Geburts Frauenheilkd* 1964; 24: 740.
25. Steptoe PC. *Laparoscopy in Gynaecology*. Edinburgh: Livingstone, 1967.
26. Lunenfeld B. In: Inguilla W, Greenblatt RG, Thomas RB, eds. *The Ovary*. Springfield, IL: CC Thomas, 1969.
27. Steptoe PC, Edwards RG. Laparoscopic recovery of preovulatory human oocytes after priming of ovaries with gonadotrophins. *Lancet* 1970; 1: 683–9.
28. Edwards RG, Steptoe PC, Purdy JM. Fertilization and cleavage *in vitro* of preovulatory human oocytes. *Nature (London)* 1970; 227: 1307–9.
29. Steptoe PC, Edwards RG, Purdy JM. Human blastocysts grown in culture. *Nature (London)* 1971; 229: 132–3.
30. Edwards RG, Surani MAH. The primate blastocyst and its environment. *Uppsala J Med Sci* 1978; 22: 39–50.
31. Csapo AI, Pulkkinen MO, Kaihola HL. The relationship between the timing of luteectomy and the incidence of complete abortions. *Am J Obstet Gycecol* 1974; 118: 985–9.
32. Steptoe PC, Edwards RG. Reimplantation of a human embryo with subsequent tubal pregnancy. *Lancet* 1976; 1: 880–2.
33. Edwards RG, Steptoe PC, Purdy JM. Clinical aspects of pregnancies established with cleaving embryos grown *in vivo*. *Br J Obstet Gynaecol* 1980; 87: 757–68.

34. Trounson AO, Leeton JF, Wood C et al. Pregnancies in humans by fertilization *in vitro* and embryo transfer in the controlled ovulatory cycle. *Science* 1981; 212: 681–2.
35. Zeilmaker GH, Alberda T, Gent I et al. Two pregnancies following transfer of intact frozen–thawed embryos. *Fertil Steril* 1984; 42: 293–6.
36. Handyside A, Kontogianni EH, Hardy K, Winston RML. Pregnancies from biopsied human preimplantation embryos sexed by Y-specifi c DNA application. *Nature (London)* 1990; 344: 768–70.
37. Wikland M, Enk L, Hamberger L. Transvesical and transvaginal approaches for the aspiration of follicles by use of ultrasound. *Ann NY Acad Sci* 1985; 442: 182–94.
38. Palermo G, Joris H, Devroey P et al. Pregnancies after intracytoplasmic injection of single spermatozoon into an oocyte. *Lancet* 1992; 340: 17–18.
39. Hansis C, Edwards RG. Cell differentiation in the preimplantation human embryo. *Reprod BioMed Online* 2003; 6: 215–20.

Robert G. Edwards and the thorny path to the birth of Louise Brown: A history of *in vitro* fertilization and embryo transfer

MARTIN H. JOHNSON MA, PHD, FRCOG, FRSB, FMEDSCI, FRS

INTRODUCTION

Robert G. Edwards was awarded the 2010 Nobel Prize for Physiology or Medicine "for the development of *in vitro* fertilization" (1). There is a variety of accounts of the events leading up to this discovery and its acceptance, most of them by participants (2), but historical scholarship is rarer (3). This article is based on research undertaken partly in preparation for the introductory lecture to the Nobel Symposium celebrating the award of the 2010 Nobel Prize in Physiology or Medicine to Robert G. Edwards, and partly conducted since then. It is based on a paper published originally in 2011 (1), but adds considerably to that paper by use of verifiable sources to produce a historical narrative of the path to *in vitro* fertilization (IVF) and the birth of Louise Brown that differs in a number of places from the conventionally accepted version and adds further detail. It tries to make clear what a difficult birth IVF had, something often overlooked by current practitioners.

Primary sources used were the publications by Edwards and Steptoe between the 1950s and 1980s; the National Archives, the archives of the Royal Society of Medicine, Cambridge University, the British Medical Association, Churchill College, Cambridge, the Physiology Library at Cambridge, the National Institute for Medical Research (NIMR) at Mill Hill and the personal papers of Robert G. Edwards (courtesy of the Edwards family); transcripts of interviews with Robert G. Edwards (unpublished), with K. Elder and R.L. Gardner (available from the British Library Oral History Section), and with Grace MacDonald (4), Noni Fallows, Sandra Corbertt, and John Webster (5); personal recollections from the late 1970s by Edwards and Steptoe as recalled in interviews with Danny Abse for the autobiographical account *A Matter of Life* and on film with Peter Williams; and members of Robert G. Edwards' family and his colleagues and former students and staff members for clarificatory evidence about personal recollections by Edwards, for additional verifiable information and with whom to test some new interpretations.

CHILDHOOD BACKGROUND

Robert G. Edwards was born on September 27, 1925 into a working-class family in the small Yorkshire mill town of Batley. Edwards, who was known by his middle name of Geoff until he was 18, was the second of three brothers, between an older brother, Sammy, and the younger, Harry (2). Sammy was named after his father, Samuel, who was frequently away from home working on the railways, maintaining the track in the Blea Moor tunnel on the Carlisle–Settle line. It was an unhealthy place to work, filled with coal-fired smoke that exacerbated Samuel's bronchitis, a consequence of being gassed in World War I. Edwards' mother, Margaret, was a machinist in a local mill. She came originally from Manchester, to where the family relocated when Edwards was about five, having been offered the relative security of a council house in the suburb of Gorton. It was in Manchester that Edwards received his education: bright working-class children could take a scholarship exam at age 10 or 11 to compete for the few coveted places at a grammar school, the potential pathway out of poverty and even to university. All three brothers passed the exam, but Sammy decided against grammar school, preferring to leave education as soon as he could to earn. His mother was reportedly furious at this wasted opportunity, and so when her two younger sons passed the exam, there was no doubting that they would continue in education, and so it was that that Geoff/Bob progressed in 1937 to Manchester Central Boy's High School, which also claims James Chadwick FRS (1891–1974) as an alumnus. Chadwick, like Edwards, became a Cambridge professor and was awarded the 1935 Nobel Prize in Physics for discovering the neutron (6). The Edwards family's summers were spent in the Yorkshire Dales, to where their mother took her sons to be closer to their father's place of work. There, Edwards labored on the farms and developed an enduring affection for the Dales. These early experiences were formative for Edwards in three ways. Thus, Edwards became a life-long egalitarian, for five years a Labour Party councilor and almost selected as the Labour parliamentary candidate for Cambridge (7), willing to listen to and talk with all and sundry, regardless of class, education, status, and background. Second he also developed an enduring curiosity about agricultural and natural history and especially the reproductive patterns among the Dales' sheep, pigs, and cattle. Finally, he claimed great pride in being a "Yorkshire man," traditionally having attributes of affability and generosity of spirit combined with no-nonsense blunt speaking. Indeed, following his only meeting with Gregory Pincus (1903–1967 [8]) at a conference in Venice in May 1966, at which Edwards, the young pretender, clashed with the "father of the pill" over the timing of egg maturation in humans, he paid

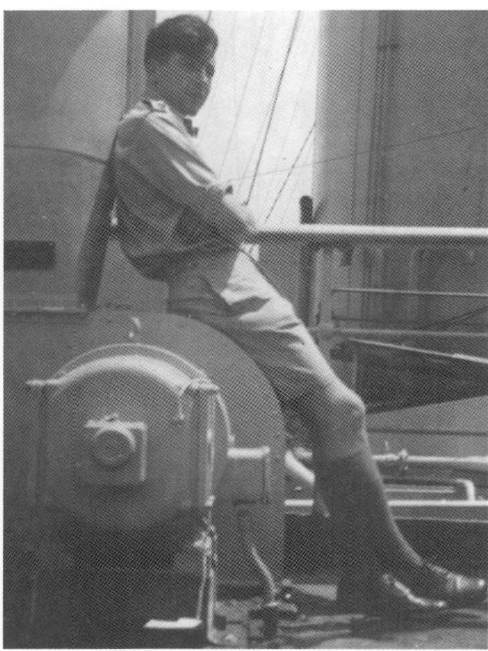

Figure II.1 Edwards on National War Service in the 1940s (courtesy of the Edwards family).

Pincus the biggest compliment he could then imagine, saying, "He would have made a fine Yorkshireman!" (2).

The intervention of World War II provided an unwelcome interruption to Edwards' education, for, after leaving school in 1943, he was conscripted for war service into the British Army for almost four years (Figure II.1). To his surprise, as someone from a working-class family, he was identified as potential officer material and sent on an officer-training course, before being commissioned in 1946. However, his army experiences were broadly negative, the alien lifestyle of the officers' mess reinforcing his socialist ideals. The one positive feature of his war service was the chance to travel overseas; he particularly appreciated his time in the Middle East. The years in the army were broken by nine months' compassionate leave back in the Yorkshire Dales, for which he was released to help run a farm when his farmer friend there fell ill. So engaged did he become in farming life that, after discharge from the army in 1948, he returned home to Gorton, from where he applied to read agricultural sciences at the University College of North Wales at Bangor and gained both a place and a government grant to fund it. However, he was disappointed in the course offered at Bangor, describing it as not "scientific," and he was bored through two tedious years of agricultural descriptions. For his third year, he transferred to zoology, a course much more to his style and led by the more intellectually challenging Rogers Brambell FRS (1901–1970 [9]). However, that year was insufficient to salvage his honors degree, and in 1951, aged 26, he gained a simple pass. Unbeknown to him at the time, he was not alone in this undistinguished academic embarrassment, as neither "Tibby" Marshall FRS (1878–1949 [10]), the founder of the reproductive sciences, nor Sir Alan Parkes FRS (1900–1990 [11]), the first Professor of Reproductive Sciences at Cambridge, who was later to recruit Edwards there, distinguished themselves as undergraduates. In 1951, however, Edwards "was disconsolate. It was a disaster. My grants were spent and I was in debt. Unlike some of the students I had no rich parents … I could not write home, 'Dear Dad, please send me £100 as I did badly in the exams'" (2).

However, his low spirits did not last long. He learnt that John Slee (12), a life-long friend he had made at Bangor, had been accepted on a postgraduate diploma course in animal genetics at Edinburgh University under Conrad Waddington FRS (1905–1975 [13]), who had moved there in 1947 from Christ's College in Cambridge, home also to both Marshall and Parkes. Edwards applied and, despite his pass degree and to his amazement, he was accepted. That summer, he worked harvesting hay, portering bananas, heaving sacks of flour, and in a menial job with a newspaper, all to earn enough to pay his way in Edinburgh (2).

FAMILY LIFE

In Edinburgh, Edwards not only started to map out his scientific career, but importantly also met Ruth Fowler (Figure II.2), who was to become his life-long scientific collaborator and whom he was to marry in 1954, with their five daughters arriving between 1959 and 1964. When they met, Edwards claims that he was initially somewhat overwhelmed, even "intimidated" by Ruth's august family background. Her father, Sir Ralph Fowler FRS (1889–1944 [14]), and her maternal grandfather, Lord Ernest Rutherford FRS (1871–1937 [15]), were not only both "titled," but both also had the most impressive academic credentials imaginable: a world away from a working-class Northern family. Ralph Fowler was an exceptionally talented Plummer Professor of Mathematical Physics in Cambridge from 1932 to 1944 (14). Back in Cambridge in 1919 after World War I, he was stimulated to work with Rutherford, who had recently arrived there to take the chair of Experimental Physics. Rutherford was the first Nobel laureate in Ruth's family, having been awarded the 1908 Nobel Prize for Chemistry "for his investigations

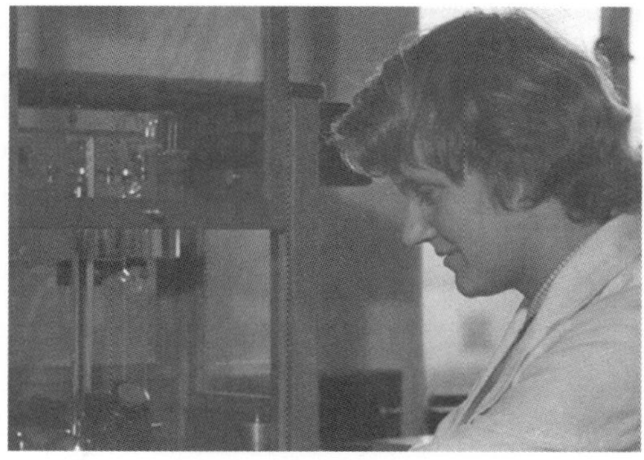

Figure II.2 Ruth Fowler in the laboratory, Edinburgh, in the 1950s (courtesy of the Edwards family).

into the disintegration of the elements, and the chemistry of radioactive substances" (15). Ralph Fowler not only worked under Rutherford, but, in the course of doing so, met his only daughter, Eileen, whom he married in 1921. They had four children, of whom Ruth was the last, born in December 1930. Tragically her mother died shortly afterwards and her father, although himself unwell, undertook such grueling high-security war work, much of it away in North America, that his health deteriorated and he died at the relatively young age of 55 when Ruth was 13. Thus, Ruth was to know only Mrs. Phyllida Cook as her parent (14).

EDWARDS, THE RESEARCH SCIENTIST

The intellectual spirit of scientific enquiry that Edwards experienced in Edinburgh fitted his aptitudes well, for Waddington rewarded his Diploma year with a three-year PhD place (1952–1955), followed by two years of postdoctoral research, and funded it with a salary of the princely sum of £240 per year (2). His chosen field of research was the developmental biology of the mouse. Edwards realized that to understand development involved engaging in an interdisciplinary mix, not just of embryology and reproduction—the conventional view at the time—but also of genetics. Given the increasing scientific and social emphasis on genetics over the last 50 years, it is important to understand how advanced this view was in the 1950s, when genetic knowledge was still rudimentary and largely alien to the established developmental and reproductive biologists of the day, as Edwards himself was later to recall (16). For example, it was in the 1950s that DNA was established as the molecular carrier of genetic information (17–20), that it was first demonstrated that each cell of the body carried a full set of DNA/genes (21–23), and that genes were selectively expressed as mRNA to generate different cell phenotypes (24). Moreover, it was only by the late 1950s that cytogenetic studies led to the accepted human karyotype as 46 chromosomes (25,26), that agreement was reached on the Denver system of classification of human chromosomes (27), and that the chromosomal aneuploidies underlying developmental anomalies such as Down, Turner, and Klinefelter syndromes were described (28–31). The dates of these discoveries make Edwards' research between 1952 and 1957 all the more remarkable. Working under his supervisor Alan Beatty, he generated haploid, triploid, and aneuploid mouse embryos and studied their potential for development. In order to undertake what were, in effect, early attempts at "genetic engineering" in mammals, he needed to be able to manipulate the chromosomal composition of eggs, spermatozoa, and embryos.

In mice, spermatozoa were abundant, and were studied in experiments mostly undertaken with a visiting Argentinean postdoc, Julio Sirlin (Figure II.3) (2). Together they labeled spermatozoa radioactively *in vivo* in order to study the kinetics of spermatogenesis and then to follow the radioactive products post-fertilization, thereby to demonstrate the fate of the male contributions during

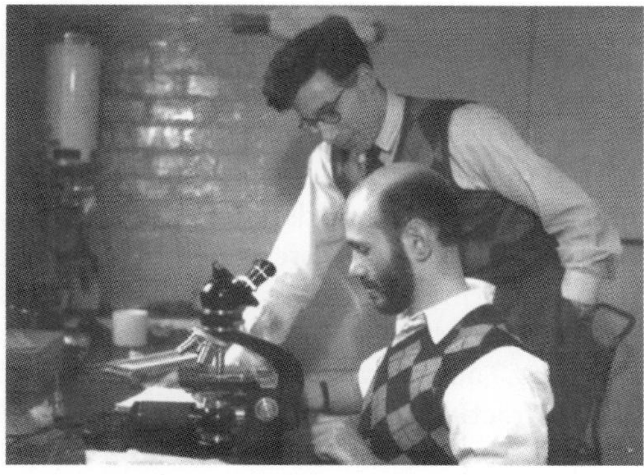

Figure II.3 Julio Sirlin with Edwards in the 1950s (courtesy of Julio Sirlin).

early development. They also exposed males and/or their spermatozoa to various chemical mutagens and UV or x-ray irradiation, and examined the effects on sperm-fertilizing capacity and, where it was shown to be present, how the treatments impacted on development. In some cases, sperm activation of the egg was evident, but in the absence of any functional sperm chromatin, and so gynogenetic embryos were formed. These experiments resulted in 14 papers, including four in *Nature*, between 1954 and 1959 (see Gardner and Johnson [32] for a full bibliographic record of Edwards).

Eggs and embryos were not as abundant as spermatozoa, and overcoming this problem led Edwards to two discoveries that proved to be of particular significance for his later IVF work. First, working with his wife Ruth, he devised ways of increasing the numbers of synchronized eggs recoverable from adult female mice through a series of papers, the first published in 1957 (33), on the control of ovulation induced by use of exogenous hormones. In doing so, they overturned the conventional wisdom that superovulation of adults was not possible. Second, working with an American postdoc, Alan Gates (34), Edwards described the remarkable timed sequence of egg chromosomal maturation events that led up to ovulation after injection of the ovulatory hormone, human chorionic gonadotropin.

His six years in Edinburgh, between 1951 and 1957, give an early taste of his prodigious energy, resulting in 38 papers (32). Indeed, so productive was this period that the last of the Edinburgh-based papers did not appear in print until 1963. These papers firmly placed the young Edwards at the forefront of studies on the genetic manipulation of development and started to attract attention. It was also in Edinburgh that Edwards' interest in ethics was first sparked by the interdisciplinary debates among scientists and theologians that Waddington organized, and, as a result, he went on what he describes as a "church crawl," trying the 10 or so variants of Christianity on offer in 1950s Edinburgh. He did not emerge from his consumer testing "God-intoxicated" (2), but convinced that man held his own future in his own hands. Edwards' humanist ethical sympathies and antipathy to the "revealed truths" of religion were to be developed further in all his later encounters (32).

AN AMERICAN DIVERSION

These 1950s studies in science and ethics were to form the platform on which Edwards' later IVF work was to be based, but before that his interests and life took a diversion to the California Institute of Technology for the year 1957–1958. He describes his year at Caltech as being "a bit of a holiday," but it was a holiday that with hindsight had both distracting and significant consequences. He went there to work with Albert Tyler (1906–1968 [35]), an influential elder statesman of American reproductive science, working on spermatozoon–egg interactions. Caltech was then a hotbed of developmental biology, and Tyler had clustered around him an exciting group of young scientists, which included that year a visit by the then English doyen of fertilization, Lord Victor Rothschild FRS (1910–1990 [36]). Rothschild was later to clash scientifically with Edwards over his IVF work (37), a clash in which the younger man triumphed again (38), just as he had with Pincus. Tyler was exploring the molecular specificity of egg–spermatozoon interactions and had turned for a model to immunology. Immunology was then at an exciting phase in its development, with the engaging Sir Peter Medawar FRS (1915–1987, Nobel laureate in Physiology or Medicine, 1960 [39]), influentially for Bob, extending his ideas on immunological tolerance to the paradox of the "fetus as an allograft": a semi-paternal graft nonetheless somehow protected from maternal immune attack inside the mother's uterus (40). This confluence of reproduction and immunology excited Edwards' restless curiosity and hence the choice of Tyler. Significantly, the subject also offered funding possibilities via the Ford and Rockefeller Foundations and the Population Council, which were increasingly concerned about world population growth and the need for better methods to control fertility (41–43). Immuno-contraception then seemed to offer tantalizingly specific possibilities, alas not much closer to being realized today (44).

So when Edwards returned to the United Kingdom from Caltech in 1958 at Alan Parkes' invitation to join him at the Medical Research Council (MRC) National Institute for Medical Research (NIMR) in north London, it was to work on the science of immuno-contraception (7). This period in the U.S.A. initiated a series of 23 papers on the immunology of reproduction between 1960 and 1976 (32). It also prompted Edwards' first involvement in founding an international society in 1967 in Varna, Bulgaria, when the International Coordinating Committee for the Immunology of Reproduction was created (45). Immuno-reproduction was, in retrospect, to prove a distracting diversion from what was to become Edwards' main work, albeit one that continued to enthuse and stimulate his imagination for many years. Indeed, it was his research into immuno-reproduction that led serendipitously to his first meeting with Patrick Steptoe (see later). The period at Mill Hill, between 1958 and 1962, seems to have been a period of increasing intellectual conflict for him. While being enthusiastic about the science underlying immuno-contraception, his old interests in eggs, fertilization, and, in particular, the genetics of development were gradually reasserting themselves. His day job was therefore increasingly supplemented by evening and weekend flirtations with egg maturation.

THE CRUCIAL EGG MATURATION STUDIES

The stimulus that reawakened Edwards' interest in eggs was provided by the then recent consensus about the number of human chromosomes and, more particularly, the descriptions in 1959 of the pathologies in man that resulted from chromosomal anomalies (28–31). Thus, his 1962 *Nature* paper begins: "Many of the chromosomal anomalies in man and animals arise through non-disjunction or lagging chromosomes during meiosis in the oocyte. Investigation of the origin and primary incidence of such anomalies would be greatly facilitated if meiotic stages etc., were easily available" (46). The idea that these aneuploidies in humans might result from errors in the complex chromosomal dance that he and Gates had observed in maturing mouse eggs drove his thinking. The possible clinical relevance of his work on egg maturation and aneuploidy in the mouse was becoming significant. So Edwards resumed his experimenting with mice, trying to mimic *in vitro* the *in vivo* maturation of eggs, one rationale being that this route would open the possibility of similar studies in humans, in which not even induced ovulation had then been described (47). He tried releasing the immature mouse eggs from their ovarian follicles into culture medium containing the ovulatory hormone human chorionic gonadotropin, to explore whether he could simulate their *in vivo* development. Amazingly, he found it worked first time; the eggs seemed to mature at the same rate as they had *in vivo*. However, they did so whether or not the hormone had been added. The eggs evidently were maturing spontaneously when released from their follicles. The same happened in rats and hamsters. If this were to happen in humans too, then the study of the chromosomal dance during human egg maturation was a realistic practical possibility, as was IVF and thereby studies on the genetics of early human development. Edwards' excitement at seeing eggs mature spontaneously was temporarily blunted by his library discovery that Pincus in the 1930s (48,49) and M.C. Chang (1908–1991 [50,51]) earlier in the 1950s had been there before him, using both rabbit and, Pincus claimed, human eggs.

In order to pursue his cytogenetic studies on the maturation of human eggs, he needed a reliable supply of human ovarian tissue from which to retrieve and mature eggs. This requirement posed difficulties for a scientist with no medical qualification, given the elitist attitudes and lack of scientific awareness then prevalent amongst most of the U.K. gynecological profession (3,52,53). His first breakthrough came with Molly Rose, who was a gynecologist at the Edgware General Hospital, northwest London, near Mill Hill. Edwards was introduced to her through John

Humphrey FRS (1915–1997 [54]), who was the medically qualified Head of Immunology at Mill Hill. Humphrey, notwithstanding his more privileged social background, was a kindred spirit for Edwards, sharing his passion for science, its social application and utility, as well as his left-wing politics; indeed, he had been a Marxist until 1940 and was for many years denied entry to the U.S.A. in consequence. Edwards asked Humphrey if he knew anyone who might be helpful, and he not only suggested Rose, but also offered to arrange an introduction. Rose was to provide biopsied ovarian samples intermittently for the next 10 years.

Between 1960 and 1962, Edwards used human ovarian biopsies provided by Rose to try to repeat and extend Pincus' observations from the 1930s. Given the sporadic supply of human material, he also tried dog, monkey, and baboon ovarian eggs, but in all cases with limited success compared with smaller rodents. In the 1962 *Nature* paper (46), he cautiously interprets the few maturing human (3/67), monkey (10/56), and baboon (13/90) eggs that he had observed as most likely arising from *in vivo* stimulation, rendering them partially matured at the time of their recovery from the biopsy. He suggests that Pincus' observations on human eggs are also likely to be similarly artefactual, the source of his Venice spat with Pincus some four years later (*vide supra*). This 1962 paper ends with the report of an ingenious experimental approach to try and persuade the reluctant human eggs to mature. Thus, the ovarian arteries of patients undergoing ovarian removal were cannulated and perfused with hormones post-removal, perhaps unsurprisingly in retrospect, without success.

However, by this time, his quest for human eggs, and his dreams of IVF and studying the genetics and development of early human embryos, had reached the ears of the then Director of the Institute, Sir Charles Harington FRS (1897–1972 [55]), who, Edwards alleged (2), banned any work on human IVF at NIMR. Alan Parkes was no longer able to defend Edwards, having left in 1961 to take up his chair in Cambridge and, although he had asked Edwards to join him there, funding was not available until 1963. So by the time Edwards left Mill Hill in 1962 for a year in Glasgow, he had encountered a taste of the opposition to human IVF that was to come.

GLASGOW AND STEM CELLS

Edwards had accepted an invitation from John Paul to spend a year in the biochemistry department at Glasgow University. Paul was then the acknowledged master of tissue culture in the U.K. and had got wind of some experiments that Edwards had been doing at NIMR attempting to generate stem cells from rabbit embryo cultures (56,57). The objective of this strategy was to use these stem cells to study early developmental mechanisms, either *in vitro* or *in vivo* after their incorporation into embryos. Paul had proposed that they work together, with fellow Glasgow biochemist Robin Cole, to see what progress might be made. This must have been an attractive invitation, not simply because the challenge was scientifically interesting, but also because Edwards could learn more about culture media for his eggs and hopefully later embryos, then an uncertain prospect, with successful mouse embryo culture only recently having been described (58). However, by this time, the Edwards family was growing, so Ruth remained in north London with their young daughters, while her husband commuted to Glasgow for the working week.

The collaboration was to result in two papers (56,57), remarkable for their prescience. They described the production of embryonic stem cells from both rabbit blastocysts and the inner cell masses dissected from them. The cells were capable of proliferating through over 100 generations and of differentiating into various cell types. These experiments were initiated some 20 years before Evans and Kaufman (59) described the derivation of embryonic stem cells from mice. That this work has largely been ignored by those in the stem cell field is probably mainly attributable to its being too far ahead of its time (60). Thus, reliable molecular markers for different types of cells were not available then, nor were appropriate techniques with which to critically test the developmental potential of the cultured cells.

THE MOVE TO CAMBRIDGE

Edwards arrived in Cambridge from Glasgow in 1963 as a Ford Foundation Research Fellow, and settled with Ruth and his five daughters in a house in Gough Way, off the Barton Road. He had previously visited Cambridge at least once, as "a recently graduated PhD" in the late 1950s for a conference on reproduction held in Trinity College (Figure II.4), where he recalls meeting some of the big names in the subject, including John Hammond, Alan Parkes, M.C. Chang, Thaddeus Mann, Rene Moricard, Bunny Austin, and Charles Thibault (16). Although Edwards was to remain in Cambridge for the rest of his career, in 1963 his initial reactions to the place were mixed. He describes how he immediately reacted against the then extant "misogynist public-school traditions; the exclusivity," "the privileges given to the already privileged." But he set against that the "sheer beauty of the place," "the concern with the truth and high seriousness," "the ambience of scientific excellence … I was surrounded by so many talented young men and women" (2).

Edwards worked in a cluster of seven smallish rooms at the top of the Physiological Laboratory backing onto Downing Place, which were collectively known as the "Marshall laboratory" and were to be shared eventually with two other groups. One group was led initially by Sir Alan Parkes, the first Mary Marshall, and Arthur Walton, Professor of Reproductive Physiology at the University (11), who had arrived in 1961. His group included scientists with mainly zoological or comparative interests, such as his wife Ruth Deansley, Bunny Austin, and Dick Laws FRS, who was often away "in the field" with Parkes collecting material, especially in Uganda at the Nuffield Unit of Tropical Animal Ecology (11). Parkes was also much involved at this time in writing and committee work,

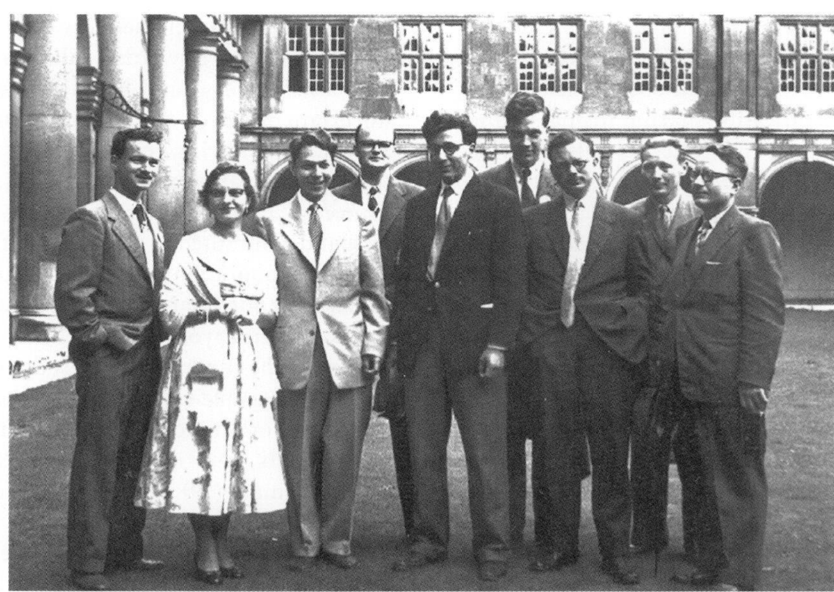

Figure II.4 Edwards as "a very recent PhD student" (center) and Alan Gates (extreme left) at a meeting in Trinity College Cambridge in the late 1950s (courtesy of the Edwards family).

especially with the World Health Organization, which was then becoming concerned about world population growth and ways to curb it (11). Parkes was also acting as an unpaid company secretary to the then fledgling *Journal of Reproduction and Fertility* (called *Reproduction* since 2001 [61–63]). In 1967, Parkes retired. Edwards applied for his chair on January 6, 1966 (64), but was unsuccessful, the chair passing instead to Thaddeus Mann FRS (1908–1993 [65]), who worked on the biochemistry of semen. Mann decided not to relocate to the Physiology Laboratory from his Cambridge base at the Agricultural Research Council Unit of Reproductive Physiology and Biochemistry at Huntingdon Road, where he was Director. Neither was the leadership of the Marshall laboratory to pass to Edwards, as the University appointed as its head his more senior colleague and friend Colin "Bunny" Austin (1914–2004 [66]), who had been in Cambridge intermittently since 1962 (Figure II.5). Austin was elected the first Charles Darwin Professor of Animal Embryology (1967–1981) and began attracting several upcoming reproductive biologists to the Marshall laboratory, including John Marston, David Whittingham, and Matthew Kaufmann. In addition, a new group was formed in 1967 with the arrival from the Strangeways laboratory of Denis New (1929–2010) as university lecturer in histology (67). New built a group comprising initially PhD students Chris Steele and David Cockroft, later joined by postdoc Frank Webb (1976–1977), and visiting scientists such as Joe Daniels Jr, on leave from the University of Colorado.

It was against this varied scientific background that Edwards, who was already 38 when he arrived in Cambridge, began for the first time to assemble his own group. He recruited as his technician Jean Purdy (Figure II.6) in 1968, one of her attractions being her nursing qualification, a sign of the increasing importance that his forays into the use of clinical material was assuming. Purdy was to stay with him until her early death at age 39 in 1985 (68). He also recruited his first two graduate students: Richard Gardner and this author in 1966 (69,70). Gardner studied early mouse embryology from 1966 to 1971 and until 1973 as a postdoctoral worker, before moving to zoology in Oxford. This author worked on immunoreproduction from 1966 to 1969, returning as a postdoc between 1971 and 1974 after two years in the U.S.A., before moving to the Anatomy Department in Cambridge.

From 1969 onwards, Edwards' group increased in size substantially as more accommodation was made available

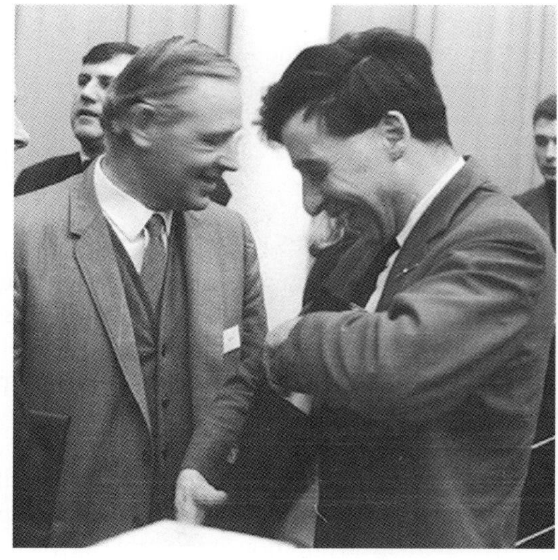

Figure II.5 Edwards with "Bunny" Austin (1960s) (courtesy of the Edwards family).

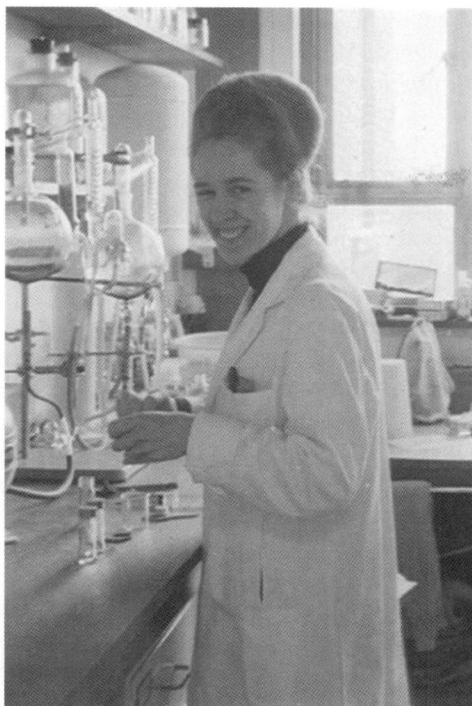

Figure II.6 Jean Purdy (1946–1985) (courtesy of Barbara Rankin).

to the Marshall laboratory. David Griffin (now retired from the World Health Organization) was to join as Head Technician between 1970 and 1975, with junior technicians including Sheila Barton (1936–2013) in addition to Jean Purdy. Early graduate students recruited included Roger Gosden (1970–1974), Carol Readhead (1972–1976), and Rob Gore-Langton (1973–1978), all working on follicle growth; Craig Howe (1971–1974) working on immuno-reproduction; and Azim Surani (1975–1979) working on implantation. A "third generation" of graduate students also arrived; for example, Janet Rossant (from 1972) studied with Gardner, and Alan Handyside (from 1974), Peter Braude (from 1975), and Ginny Bolton (from 1976) studied with Johnson. Postdoctoral workers also arrived, including Ginny Papaioannou (1971–1974), and Ruth Fowler-Edwards resumed working in the laboratory, developing hormonal assays and studying the endocrine aspects of follicle development and early pregnancy. Thus, slowly until 1969, and more rapidly thereafter, Edwards built a lively group, its members working in diverse areas of reproductive science that reflected his own broad interests and knowledge. Moreover, Edwards encouraged a spirit of open communication and egalitarianism, which extended across all three groups, with sharing of resources, space, equipment, knowledge, and ideas, as well as social activities.

Through the 1960s and 1970s, Edwards' work was funded by the Ford Foundation via grants first to Parkes and then to Austin (71) to continue work on basic reproductive mechanisms, with an eye to developing new methods of fertility control, and he continued to pursue the immunology of reproduction. However, he also worked on egg maturation, collecting pig, cow, sheep, the odd monkey, and some human eggs. He showed that eggs of all these species would indeed mature *in vitro*, but that the eggs of larger animals simply needed a longer time than those of smaller ones, with human eggs taking up to 36 hours rather than the 12 hours or less erroneously reported by Pincus. These cytogenetic studies were reported in two seminal papers in 1965 (72,73), both of which are primarily concerned with understanding the kinetics of the meiotic chromosomal events during egg maturation. In its discussion, the *Lancet* paper displays a breathtaking clarity of vision as Edwards sets out a program of research that predicted the events of the next 20 years and beyond (Table II.1). Significantly, if not surprisingly given his research interests, the early study and detection of genetic disease is afforded a heavy focus compared with the slight emphasis on infertility

Table II.1 Key points in the program of research laid out in the discussion to Edwards' 1965 *Lancet* paper

1. Studies on non-disjunction of meiotic chromosomes as a cause of aneuploidy in humans[a]
2. Studies on the effect of maternal age on non-disjunction in relation to the origins of trisomy 21[a]
3. Use of human eggs in *in vitro* fertilization (IVF) to study fertilization
4. Study of culture methods for human eggs fertilized *in vitro*
5. Use of priming hormones to increase the number of eggs per woman available for study/use
6. Study of early IVF embryos for evidence of (ab)normality—especially aneuploidies arising prior to or at fertilization[a]
7. Control of some of the genetic diseases in man[a]
8. Control of sex-linked disorders by sex detection at the blastocyst stage and transfer of only female embryos[a]
9. Intracervical transfer of IVF embryos into the uterus
10. Use of IVF embryos to circumvent blocked tubes[b]
11. Avoidance of a multiple pregnancy (as observed after hormonal priming and *in vivo* insemination) by transfer of a single IVF embryo

Source: Edwards RG. *Lancet* 1965; 286: 926–9.

[a] Five aims relating specifically to genetic disease.

[b] One aim relating specifically to infertility relief.

alleviation. This genetic focus continues in his research papers over the next four years. Thus, within three years, working with his graduate student Richard Gardner, he provided proof of principle for preimplantation genetic diagnosis (PGD) in a paper on rabbit embryo sexing published in 1968 (74), a paper that was to anticipate the development of PGD clinically by some 22 years (75). Likewise, working with the Cambridge geneticist Alan Henderson, Edwards was to develop his "production line theory" of egg production to explain the origins of maternal aneuploidy in older women. Thus, the earliest eggs to enter meiosis in the fetal ovary were shown to have more chiasmata and to be ovulated earlier in adult life than those entering meiosis later in fetal life (76,77).

THE PROBLEM OF FERTILIZATION OF THE HUMAN EGG

Notwithstanding his broad range of scientific interests, Edwards' ambitions to achieve IVF in humans remained undiminished. In 1966, this was no trivial task, having been accomplished convincingly only in rabbits and hamsters (78,79). In trying to achieve this aim, he was engaging in two struggles: the first being simply but critically the continuing practical difficulty in obtaining a regular supply of human ovarian tissue. Local Cambridge sources proved unreliable and Molly Rose was now two to three hours' drive away in London; so, during the summer of 1965, Edwards turned to the U.S.A. for help and approached Victor McKusick, a leading American cytogeneticist at the Johns Hopkins University. There he initiated his longstanding contact with Howard and Georgeanna Jones in obstetrics and gynecology (80). The supply of American eggs they generated during his six-week stay allowed him to confirm the maturation timings that were published the same year.

However, it was the second scientific struggle that was then occupying most of his attention, namely that in order to fertilize these *in vitro*-matured eggs, he had to "capacitate" the spermatozoa, a final maturation process that spermatozoa undergo physiologically in the uterus and that is essential for the acquisition of fertilizing competence. The requirement for sperm capacitation had been discovered in the early 1950s by Austin, and independently by M.C. Chang (81,82). Failing to achieve this convincingly at Johns Hopkins, he made a second transatlantic summer journey in 1966 to visit Luther Talbot and his colleagues at Chapel Hill. He tried a variety of ways (83) to overcome the problem of "sperm capacitation," one of the most ingenious of which was to construct a 2.5 cm-long chamber from a nylon tube, plugged at each end, and with holes drilled in the walls that were encased in panels made of Millipore membrane (84). The chamber, which had a short thread attached to it, fitted snugly inside the inserter tube of an intrauterine device and so could be placed into the volunteer woman's uterus intracervically at mid-cycle, where it sat for up to 11 hours before being recovered by gently pulling on the thread, exactly as was being done routinely for the insertion and removal of intrauterine devices. By placing spermatozoa within the chamber, the membrane of which permitted equilibration of its contents with uterine fluid, he hoped to expose them to a capacitating environment. However, this ingenious approach, like the many others, failed—in this case most probably because the chamber itself induced an inflammatory response or a local bleed. For all the ingenuity of his various experimental approaches to achieving capacitation, and despite the occasional evidence of early stages of fertilization using such spermatozoa, no reliable evidence for the completion of the process was forthcoming. Then, in 1968, both struggles began to resolve.

THE MEETING WITH PATRICK STEPTOE

Patrick Steptoe (1913–1988; Figure II.7) had been a consultant obstetrician at Oldham General Hospital since 1951 (85), where for several years he had been pioneering the development and use of the laparoscope in gynecological surgery (85,86). Much to his frustration, his progress had fallen on the largely deaf ears of the conservative gynecological hierarchy, and indeed incited considerable opposition and some outright hostility (87). Edwards' claimed that he was scanning the medical and scientific journals in the library, and in a "eureka" moment occurring in "one autumn day in 1967" (2), came across a paper by Steptoe describing his experiences with laparoscopy (2,85,88). Edwards goes on to describe how he rang Steptoe to discuss a possible collaboration, but was "warned off" Steptoe by London gynecological colleagues (2,89). This warning and the daunting prospect of collaboration in far-away Oldham deterred him from following through. Finally, Edwards reported actually meeting Steptoe the following spring of 1968 at a meeting at the Royal Society of Medicine, at which, ironically, Edwards was talking about his work on immuno-reproduction, not his attempts at IVF.

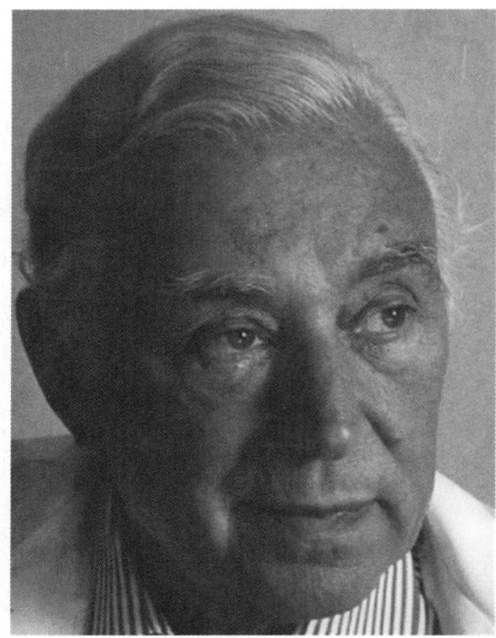

Figure II.7 Patrick Steptoe (1913–1988) (courtesy of Andrew Steptoe).

The Steptoe paper that Edwards found that day in the library was cited in his later tributes to the then deceased Steptoe (85,88) as being a *Lancet* paper entitled "Laparoscopy and ovulation" (90). However, these later recollections do not withstand scrutiny. Thus, the *Lancet* paper cited was published in October 1968, but their first meeting was in fact earlier that year, on Wednesday February 28, 1968, at a joint meeting of the Section of Endocrinology of the Royal Society of Medicine with the Society for the Study of Fertility held at 1 Wimpole Street (1,91). Moreover, according to Steptoe (92), they had already commenced collaborating prior to October 1968; indeed, their first paper together was submitted for publication later that year in December 1968 (see next section). Clearly, the paper read by Edwards must have been another, earlier than October 1968, one that preceded February 1968 by several months. The "paper" by Steptoe that Edwards most likely saw was his book on gynecological laparoscopy (1,86,93,94), and the feature that probably caught his attention, according to two earlier accounts (1,2,89), was his realization that laparoscopy could provide a way of recovering capacitated spermatozoa from the oviduct by flushing with a small volume of medium: "a practical way … of letting spermatozoa be in contact with the secretions of the female tract" (2). Indeed, Edwards says he actually rang Steptoe to ask whether this really was possible and was reassured by him that this was the case. Steptoe explicitly lays out this possibility in his book (86). Thus, on page 27 he reports: "By means of laparoscopy, Sjovall (1964) has carried out extended post-coital tests and has recovered spermatozoa from the fimbriated end of the tubes … "; and on page 70 he writes: "An extended post-coital test can be done by aspirating fluid from the tubal ostium … " Steptoe's book arrived in the Cambridge University library in March 1967 (1) and it is possible that Edwards' attention was drawn to the book by a review of it in the *British Medical Journal* on November 11, 1967 (1,95). This conclusion conflicts with the later memories of Edwards (85,88) that he contacted Steptoe initially because of his ability to recover eggs laparoscopically. However, it is possible that by time they met, some six months later, this had become more of a concern to Edwards, given the emerging reports of the failure of *in vitro*-matured rabbit eggs to produce viable embryos. Indeed, a letter, written admittedly on July 30, 2003, by Eliot Philipp, recalls that at the actual meeting Edwards had said it was eggs that he wanted Steptoe to recover (Figure II.8), albeit for making human stem cells (96), an enduring interest of Edwards.

FERTILIZATION OF THE HUMAN EGG ACHIEVED AT LAST

Despite the initiation of the collaboration with Steptoe, the actual solution to the capacitation problem existed nearer to home than Oldham, in the laboratories shared with Austin. In the early 1950s, Austin had co-discovered the requirement for sperm capacitation (81,82), and after his appointment to the Cambridge chair, Austin's first graduate student (1967–1972) was Barry Bavister, who set

You asked me to write to you about my recollections of your first meeting with Patrick Steptoe. This is what I remember:-

You went up to him and said "You're Patrick Steptoe" and he answered "Yes". You went on "I am Bob Edwards, we spoke on the 'phone six months ago"
Patrick Said "You never called back". Characteristically he asked, "What is it you want?"
You answered "Human eggs, and I believe you can get them for me". Patrick said "Yes I could by laparoscopy, but why do you want them?" You answered "Because I want to be able to develop stem cells". Patrick said "What is the use of them, what would you do with them?"
You answered "If you, Patrick Steptoe, had a heart attack, some of you heart muscle cells will be damaged and it would be wonderful to be able to replace them with new specially designed cells and that is the reason why I want stem cells."

Patrick answered "Well I have another reason; for wanting to fertilise eggs outside the uterus". He went on "I think that if we make an embryo outside the body and re-introduce it in to the uterus we could bypass blocked Fallopian tubes."

There was a short silence when one of you said, "Yes, that might be easier than making stem cells and you said "Yes, that might be easier than making stem cells, but I really would like stem cells."

You both agreed however, that making an embryo or several embryos outside the human body and replacing them within the uterus would be a good way of bypassing blocked Fallopian tubes and that is what you decided on, rather than your initial request of making stem cells.

Figure II.8 Extract from a letter, written on July 30, 2003, by Eliot Philipp to Edwards, recalling his memories of the words used at the first meeting between Edwards and Steptoe (courtesy of the Edwards family).

Table II.2 Summary of data

Egg type	Experimental	Control
Initially assigned	56	17
Survived	54/56	17/17
Matured to metaphase II	34/54	7/17
Evidence of sperm penetration	18/34	
Sperm within the zona pellucida	6/18	
Sperm inside the zona pellucida (~7 hours post-insemination)	5/18	
Evidence of pronuclei (~11 hours post-insemination)	7/18	0/7
With two pronuclei	2/18	

Source: Edwards RG, Bavister BD, Steptoe PC. *Nature* 1969; 221: 632–5.

to work to try and define the factors influencing the capacitation of hamster spermatozoa *in vitro*. By 1968, Bavister had discovered a key role for pH, showing how higher rates of fertilization could be obtained by simply increasing the alkalinity of the medium (97). Edwards seized on this observation and co-opted Bavister to his project. That proved to do the trick, and in December 1968 Edwards, together with Bavister and Steptoe, submitted the paper to *Nature* in which IVF in humans was described convincingly for the first time (38).

This 1969 *Nature* paper makes modest claims. Only 18 of 56 eggs assigned to the experimental group showed evidence of "fertilization in progress," of which only two were described as having the two pronuclei to be expected if fertilization were occurring normally (Table II.2). However, like Edwards' other papers, this one is a model of clarity, describing well-controlled experiments, cautiously interpreted. Despite the relatively small numbers, this paper convinced eventually, although some doubts were expressed at the time (37,98). That this paper convinced where previous claims had failed (99–104) was precisely because the skilled hands and creative intellect that were behind it are so evident from its text.

The provenance of the eggs described in the 1969 paper is not immediately clear from the paper itself. All were obtained by *in vitro* maturation after ovarian biopsy, but in addition to Steptoe's co-authorship, four other gynecologists are thanked in the acknowledgements section of the paper: Molly Rose, Norman Morris (1920–2008; Professor of Obstetrics and Gynecology at Charing Cross Hospital, London from 1958 to 1985 [105]), Janet Bottomley (1915–1995; Consultant Obstetrician and Gynecologist at Addenbrooke's Hospital, Cambridge from 1958 to 1976), and Sanford Markham (b. 1934; Chief of the Section of Obstetrics and Gynaecology at the U.S. Air Force Hospital, South Ruislip, to the northwest of London from 1967 to 1972). An analysis described by Johnson (1) reasonably concludes that those eggs described in the paper as "undergoing fertilization" were provided in roughly equal numbers by Rose and Steptoe.

However, with Steptoe now on board, Rose no longer featured as a supplier of eggs (2). While the initial attraction of laparoscopy for Edwards had been the recovery of capacitated spermatozoa from the oviduct, once working with Steptoe, he rapidly exploited the wider possibilities for the recovery of *in vivo*-matured eggs from the ovary (90). Indeed, the 1969 paper includes the following statement: "Problems of embryonic development are likely to accompany the use of human oocytes matured and fertilized *in vitro*. When oocytes of the rabbit and other species were matured *in vitro* and fertilized *in vivo*, the pronuclear stages appeared normal but many of the resulting embryos had subnuclei in their blastomeres, and almost all of them died during the early cleavage stages … When maturation of rabbit oocytes was started *in vivo* by injecting gonadotropins into the mother, and completed in the oviduct or *in vitro*, full term rabbit fetuses were obtained" (98). The paper goes on to discuss how the use of hormonal priming to stimulate intrafollicular egg maturation might be achieved and reports: "Preliminary work using laparoscopy has shown that oocytes can be recovered from ovaries by puncturing ripening follicles *in vivo* … "

Through these preliminary collaborative studies, Edwards and Steptoe were already building a research partnership. Although both had very different personalities and brought very different skills to the project, they shared energy, commitment, and vision. Both were also marginalized by their professional peers, a marginalization that also perhaps helped to cement their partnership (3). With the paper's publication, announced to the media on St. Valentine's Day (106), all hell was let loose. The impossible tangle of TV cables and pushy reporters trying to force their way up the stairs to the fourth floor laboratories proved a major disruption to the physiological laboratory in general and to the members of the Marshall laboratory in particular. It was something that was to recur episodically over the next 10 years.

THE BATTLES BEGIN

However, 1969 seemed to be a good year for Edwards. Not only did IVF succeed at long last and his partnership with Steptoe seemed set to flourish, but also so impressed were the Ford Foundation with his work that in late 1968 they had established, at Austin's prompting (107), an endowment fund with the University of Cambridge to cover the salary cost of a Ford Foundation Readership (a halfway step to a professorship [108]). Elated by Edwards' promotion and their achievement, Edwards and Steptoe pressed on, with the latter's laparoscopic skills coming to the fore, first in 1970 with the collection of *in vivo*-matured eggs from follicles after mild hormonal stimulation (4,109), and then achieving regular fertilization of these eggs and their early development through cleavage to the blastocyst stage (110–112). So well was the work going that in late 1970 and early 1971 they confidently applied to the U.K. Medical Research Council (MRC) for long-term funding (2).

However, any illusions that Edwards may have had that their achievements would prove a turning point in his fortunes were soon shattered. The hostility to his work of much of the media coverage in 1969 heralded the dominant pattern of scientific and medical responses for the next 10 years and resulted just two months later in the MRC rejecting the grant application (3). The practical consequences of this rejection were profound—both psychologically and physically—not least that for the next seven years, Edwards and Purdy shuttled on the 12-hour round trip between Cambridge and Oldham, Greater Manchester, paradoxically just north of his schoolboy haunts of Gorton, where the two of them had set up a small laboratory and clinic in Dr. Kershaw's cottage hospital (113), all the while leaving Ruth and his five daughters in Cambridge. The one bright feature in undertaking this heroic task was the unswerving financial support provided by an American heiress—Lillian Lincoln Howell (71)—that at least ameliorated the MRC decision.

The professional attacks on Edwards and his work took a number of forms (3), and one must try to make a mental time trip back to the 1960s and 1970s to understand their basis. Despite the nature of the political and religious battles to come in the 1980s, his scientific and medical colleagues did not then focus on the special status of the human embryo as an ethical issue. Ethical issues were raised professionally, but took quite a different form. It is perhaps difficult now to comprehend the complete absence of infertility from the consciousness of most gynecologists in the U.K. at the time, of whom Steptoe was a remarkable exception (85). Indeed, even Edwards' strong commitment to treating infertility came to the fore only after he had teamed up with Steptoe, with his previous priority being the study and prevention of genetic and chromosomal disorders.

In the several reports from the Royal College of Obstetricians and Gynaecologists (RCOG) and the MRC during the 1960s examining the areas of gynecological ignorance that needed academic attention, infertility simply did not feature (52,53). Overpopulation and family planning were seen as dominant concerns and the infertile were ignored as, at best, a tiny and irrelevant minority and, at worst, as a positive contribution to population control. This was a values system that Edwards did not accept (114), and the many encouraging letters he received from infertile couples spurred him on and provided a major stimulus to his continued work later, despite so much professional and press antagonism. For his professional colleagues, however, the fact that infertility was not seen as a significant clinical issue meant that any research designed to alleviate it was viewed not as experimental treatment, but as using humans in experiments. Given the sensitivity to the relatively recent Nazi "medical experiments," the formal acceptance of the Helsinki Declaration (115,116), and the public reaction and disquiet surrounding the recent publication of "human guinea-pigs" (117), this distinction was critical. The MRC, in rejecting the grant application, took the position that what was being proposed was human experimentation, and so were very cautious, emphasizing risks rather than benefits, of which they saw few if any (3,5).

Edwards and Steptoe were also attacked for their willingness to talk with the media. It is difficult nowadays, when the public communication of science is embedded institutionally, to understand how damaging to them this was. The massive press interest of the late 1960s was unabated in the ensuing years, and so Edwards was faced with a choice: either he could keep his head down and allow press fantasies and speculations to go unanswered and unchallenged, or he could engage, educate, and debate. For him this was no choice, regardless of the consequences professionally (32). His egalitarian spirit demanded that he trust common people's common sense. His radical political views demanded that he fought the corner of the infertile: the underdog with no voice. The Yorkshireman in him relished engagement in the debate and argument. In Edwards and Sharpe (114), he sets out his reasons for public engagement and acknowledges the risk to his own interests:

> Scientists may have to make disclosures of their work and its consequences that run against their immediate interests; they may have to stir up public opinion, even lobby for laws before legislatures (114).

And risky it was. One of the scientific referees on their MRC grant application started his referee's report by declaring the media exposure distasteful:

> Dr. Edwards feels the need to publicise his work on radio and television, and in the press, so that he can change public attitudes. I do not feel that an ill-informed general public is capable of evaluating the work and seeing it in its proper perspective. This publicity has antagonised a large number of Dr. Edwards' scientific colleagues, of whom I am one (3).

Edwards' pioneering role in the public communication of science proved to be disadvantageous to his work.

The Edwards and Sharpe (114) paper is a tour de force in its survey of the scientific benefits and risks of the science of IVF, in the legal and ethical issues raised by IVF, and in the pros and cons of the various regulatory responses to them. It sets out the issues succinctly and anticipates social

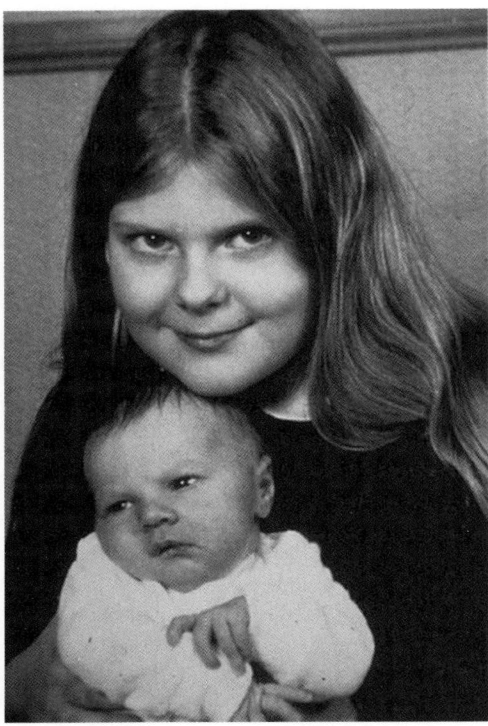

Figure II.9 Louise Brown holding the thousandth Bourn Hall baby, 1987 (courtesy of Bourn Hall Clinic).

Table II.3 Some of challenges that had to be overcome before the first successful live births after *in vitro* fertilization and embryo transfer were achieved

1. Technical aspects of follicle aspiration laparoscopically ("new suction gadget")
2. Ovulation induction
3. Timing of laparoscopy in relation to induction of ovulation
4. Ovarian stimulation
5. Cycle monitoring
6. Oocyte culture
7. Sperm preparation
8. Insemination procedure: medium and timing
9. Culture for embryo cleavage: medium and assessment
10. Technical aspects of embryo transfer, including route of transfer, medium, and timing
11. Luteal support
12. Monitoring of early pregnancy

Source: Elder K, Johnson MH. *Reprod Biomed Soc Online* 2015; 1: 19–33.

responses that were some 13–19 years into the future. Edwards built on his strong commitment to social justice based on a social ethic in subsequent years, as he engaged at every opportunity with ethicists, lawyers, and theologians, arguing, playing "devil's advocate" (literally, in the eyes of some), and engaging in what would now be called practical ethics as he hammered out his position and felt able to fully justify his instincts intellectually (118). However, the establishment was, with few exceptions, unwilling to engage seriously in ethical debates (118,119) in advance of the final validation of IVF that was to come in 1978 with the birth of Louise Brown (Figure II.9) (120).

THE BIRTH OF LOUISE BROWN

It is difficult now to comprehend the sheer magnitude of the task facing Edwards, Steptoe, and Purdy in 1969. Not only did they suffer almost complete isolation from their peers, they also faced a massive scientific and clinical mountain to climb to get from a fertilized egg to a baby, given the paucity of knowledge at the time (see Table II.3). In fact, their progress on reaching the point where transfer of embryos was possible (stage 9 in Table II.3) was impressively rapid, with the first embryo transfer being attempted in December 1971, just two years from the start of their collaboration. This rapid progress was achieved probably because the end point of each task from stage 1 to stage 9 was easily measurable in relation to controlled changes made to the protocols (112). However, for the 97 women who underwent laparoscopy between 1969 and December 1971, when egg recovery, fertilization, and *in vitro* culture were being perfected, there was no chance of a pregnancy, and so they were "experimental subjects," as the MRC had claimed. Moreover, 76 of them (27% of the total number of women who volunteered as patients between 1969 and 1978) did not subsequently undergo embryo transfer attempts in Oldham up to 1978 (5). However, all the evidence suggests that these patients were well informed about the risks and benefits (5), but nonetheless they, as much as Edwards, Purdy, and Steptoe, deserve recognition for their pioneering role in the development of IVF.

After the first transfer in December 1971, most viable embryos were transferred, with a total of 112 transfers occurring between that first one and the last in June 1978 (4,112). Once transfer was being attempted, the task became much more difficult, however, and this difficulty was behind the delay in achieving a successful pregnancy. There were essentially two types of problem to be grappled with. The first was that multiple features of the system could have been responsible for the failure to establish a pregnancy: the transfer technique and timing (both of which had proved difficult to get right in cattle) (120), the quality of the embryos, and the receptivity of the endometrium. Moreover, varying the latter two of these systematically was difficult, and, given the absence of a reliable and sensitive test for human chorionic gonadotropin until late in 1977, there was no immediate way of assessing the impact of any changes that were made. The second problem was the suspicion that the endocrine conditions established as being ideal for the production of eggs and embryos may have been deleterious for the receptivity of the endometrium. Indeed, it was this latter suspicion that drove most of their experimental variations to the treatment schedules, and that ultimately resulted in the two successful

Oldham pregnancies, both of which came, heroically, from single egg collections in natural cycles (4,112).

Only with the live births did the U.K. social, scientific, and medical hierarchies, such as the MRC, the RCOG, the British Medical Association, the Royal Society, and Government moved, albeit gradually, from their almost visceral reactions against IVF and its possibilities to serious engagement with the issues (121). Thus, both the MRC and the RCOG started to move to consider funding of work on IVF, perhaps somewhat surprisingly, given that only two live births resulted from a total of 112 transfers (4), although again the MRC declined to fund a second grant proposal from Edwards. Moreover, the National Health Service declined to provide facilities in Cambridge for Edwards and Steptoe to relocate to on Steptoe's retirement from Oldham, hence the setting up of the Bourn Hall clinic in 1982. The Thatcher Government of the time started to seriously consider the issues and set up the Warnock committee of enquiry in 1982 that reported in 1984, to a storm of parliamentary criticism, which Edwards and others had to battle to turn around over the next five years with a fierce campaign of both public and parliamentary education to counter the increasingly shrill voice of the anti-embryo research lobby (121,122). In addition, Edwards' personal battles continued, with legal suites issued during the 1980s against both the British Medical Association and various members of the national press for defamation. Thus, it was not until 1989, 24 years after Edwards' 1965 visionary paper in *The Lancet*, 20 years after IVF had first been described, and 11 years after the birth of Louise Brown that the U.K. Parliament finally gave its stamp of approval to his vision.

However, Edwards' role was realized and recognized professionally at last by the awards of fellowships of the RCOG in 1984 and of the Royal Society in 1983 (and an FRS for Steptoe followed in 1987). But despite being awarded the Albert Lasker prize in 2001, the Nobel Prize and a knighthood did not come his way until 2010—some 40 years after the *Nature* paper that started the whole IVF story in earnest.

DISCUSSION

This chapter describes some of the early years of Edwards' life and work in order to provide a context for the events leading up to the 1969 *Nature* paper describing IVF and the final validation of the claims made in that paper with the birth of Louise Brown in 1978. It is evident even from the earliest stages of his late entry into research that Edwards is a man of extraordinary energy and drive, qualities sustained throughout his long career, as witnessed in his prodigious output of papers between 1954 and 2008 (32). Indeed, several of the referees on the unsuccessful 1971 MRC grant application specifically criticized his "overenthusiasm," doubting that he could achieve the program he sets out therein as "too ambitious" (3). Tenacity of purpose comes through clearly in Edwards' work, a trait he was inclined to attribute to his Yorkshire origins, but that may also have been fueled by his working-class determination to show himself to be as good as the next (wo)man. The influences of Waddington's Edinburgh Institute, of Waddington himself, and of his supervisor, Alan Beatty, on Edwards' interests and values are also clear from the dominant role that developmental genetics played in his thinking, especially until the time he met Steptoe. Indeed, from examination of Edwards' papers and interests, his passionate conversion to the cause of the infertile seems directly attributable to Steptoe's influence. Admittedly, Edwards' forays into immuno-reproduction did involve consideration of immunological causes of infertility, but these were more usually of interest to him as models for developing new contraceptive agents. Indeed, Edwards was as captured as most reproductive biologists of the time by the 1960s' consensus on the need for better methods of world population control. This position was understandable given the reality of those concerns, as is demonstrated now in the problem of global warming that is attributable at least in part to a failure to control population growth. It is a measure of his imagination and empathy that he could grasp so rapidly Steptoe's understanding of the plight of the infertile and so flexibly incorporate this understanding into his plans. That empathy clearly reflects his underprivileged origins, with his espousal of the cause of the junior, the disadvantaged, the ill-informed, and the underdog being a thread running through his career. Edwards can be very critical, but I have found no one who can remember him ever being nasty or vindictive. Even when he disagrees with someone passionately, he never loses his respect for them as people. That Steptoe tapped into this sentiment is clear.

The way in which Edwards met Steptoe has been absorbed into folklore, but an examination of the evidence seems to warrant some revision to commonly held later reminiscences. It remains uncertain exactly which publication(s) by Steptoe it was that Edwards read in 1967, but seems likely that he did read Steptoe's book. Thus, it was spermatozoa, not eggs, that were exercising Edwards in 1967, and it was the problem of sperm capacitation, not egg retrieval, to which Steptoe and his laparoscope seemed to offer a solution in 1967. The book is the only place that this issue is specifically addressed. Their actual meeting at the Royal Society of Medicine in 1968 is also re-evaluated: Edwards was an invited speaker lecturing about his work on immuno-reproduction; so paradoxically, what has been seen as a sidetrack to his main work was, albeit serendipitously, the reason for their actual meeting.

The early collaboration between them involved the recovery of ovarian biopsies, just like those Rose and others had been providing. However, the attractions of pre-ovulatory follicular egg recovery were already clear to them both by 1968, and became, with embryo replacement, the central planks of their partnership. Steptoe and Edwards were in many ways an unlikely partnership. Their personal styles were very different, and there are clear hints in his writings that Edwards found their early days together difficult. But like most successful partnerships, their differences were sunk in a mutual respect for the other's pioneering skills and willingness to take on

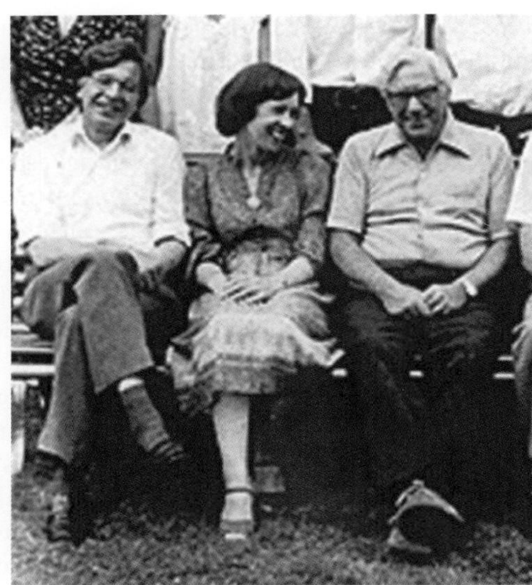

Figure II.10 Edwards, Purdy, and Steptoe at Bourn Hall, 1981 (courtesy of Bourn Hall Clinic).

the established conventions. In Jean Purdy, they also had a partner who worked quietly away in the background, smoothing the bumps on the path of their work together (Figure II.10) (113).

However, it remains Edwards' extraordinary foresight that marks him out so distinctively. His combination of vision and intellectual rigor is evident not just in his work on stem cells, PGD, and, with Steptoe, infertility, but also in his pioneering work in the public communication of science, in how ethical discourse about reproduction is conducted, in consideration of regulatory issues, and in the dissemination of IVF internationally, the latter largely a consequence of his key role in both the establishment of the European Society for Human Reproduction and Embryology in 1984 and in the founding of five journals: *Human Reproduction* (in 1986), *Human Reproduction Update* and *Molecular Human Reproduction* (both in 1996), *Reproductive BioMedicine Online* (in 2000) and *Reproductive BioMedicine and Society* (in 2015). The epithet "the father of assisted reproduction" is surely deservedly appropriate.

ACKNOWLEDGMENTS

I thank the Edwards family for their help in writing this account, plus Kay Elder, Sarah Franklin, Nick Hopwood, and Allen Packwood for their unfailing wisdom and help, and Barry Bavister, Richard Gardner, Roger Gosden, David Griffin, Ginny Papaioannou, Barbara Rankin, Carol Readhead, Sarah Howlett, Pat Tate, and Frank Webb for contributing their own memories from their own papers and for correcting mine. However, I take full responsibility for the contents of this article. I thank the Edwards family for permission to reproduce Figures II.1, II,2, II.4, II.5, and II.8, Julio Sirlin for permission to reproduce Figure II.3, Barbara Rankin for permission to reproduce Figure II.6, Andrew Steptoe for permission to reproduce Figure II.7, and Bourn Hall Clinic for permission to reproduce Figures II.9 and II.10. The research was supported by grants from the Wellcome Trust (088708 to Nick Hopwood, Martin Johnson et al., 100606 to Sarah Franklin, and 094985 to Allen Packwood and Martin Johnson), which otherwise had no involvement in the research or its publication.

REFERENCES

1. Johnson MH. Robert Edwards: The path to IVF. *Reprod Biomed Online* 2011; 23: 245–62.
2. Edwards RG, Steptoe PC. *A Matter of Life: The Story of a Medical Breakthrough*. London: Hutchinson, 1980.
3. Johnson MH, Franklin SB, Cottingham M, Hopwood N. Why the medical research council refused Robert Edwards and Patrick Steptoe support for research on human conception in 1971. *Hum Reprod* 2010; 25: 2157–74.
4. Elder K, Johnson MH. The Oldham Notebooks: An analysis of the development of IVF 1969–1978. II. The treatment cycles and their outcomes. *Reprod Biomed Soc Online* 2015; 1: 9–18.
5. Johnson MH, Elder K. The Oldham Notebooks: An analysis of the development of IVF 1969–1978. IV. Ethical aspects. *Reprod Biomed Soc Online* 2015; 1: 34–45.
6. Massey H, Feather N. James Chadwick: 20 October 1891–24 July 1974. *Biogr Mems Fell R Soc* 1976; 22: 10–70.
7. Ashwood-Smith M. Robert Edwards at 55. *Reprod Biomed Online* 2002; 4(Suppl 1): 2–3.
8. Ingle DJ. Gregory Goodwin Pincus. April 9, 1903–August 22, 1967. *Biogr Mems Natl Acad Sci USA* 1971; 229–70.
9. Oakley CL. Francis William Rogers Brambell. 1901–1970. *Biogr Mems Fell R Soc* 1973; 19: 129–71.
10. Parkes AS. Francis Hugh Adam Marshall. 1878–1949. *Biogr Mems Fell R Soc* 1950; 7: 238–51.
11. Polge C. Sir Alan Sterling Parkes. 10 September 1900–17 July 1990. *Biogr Mems Fell R Soc* 2006; 52, 263–83.
12. Slee J. *RGE* at 25—Personal reminiscences. *Reprod Biomed Online* 2002; 4(Suppl 1): 1.
13. Robertson A. Conrad Hal Waddington. 8 November 1905–26 September 1975. *Biogr Mems Fell R Soc* 1977; 23: 575–622.
14. Milne EA. Ralph Howard Fowler. 1889–1944. *Biogr Mems Fell R Soc* 1945; 5: 60–78.
15. Eve AS, Chadwick J. Lord Rutherford. 1871–1937. *Biogr Mems Fell R Soc* 1938; 2: 394–423.
16. Edwards RG. An astonishing journey into reproductive genetics since the 1950's. *Reprod Nutr Dev* 2005; 45: 299–306.
17. Watson JD, Crick FH. Genetical implications of the structure of deoxyribonucleic acid. *Nature* 1953; 171: 964–7.
18. Watson JD, Crick FH. Molecular structure of nucleic acids: a structure for deoxyribose nucleic acid. *Nature* 1953; 171: 737–8.
19. Franklin R, Gosling R. Molecular configuration in sodium thymonucleate. *Nature* 1953; 171: 740–1.

20. Wilkins MHF, Stokes AR, Wilson HR. Molecular structure of deoxypentose nucleic acids. *Nature* 1953; 171: 738–40.
21. Gurdon JB. The developmental capacity of nuclei taken from intestinal epithelium cells of feeding tadpoles. *Development* 1962a; 10: 622–40.
22. Gurdon JB. Adult frogs derived from the nuclei of single somatic cells. *Dev Biol* 1962b; 4: 256–73.
23. Gurdon JB, Elsdale TR, Fischberg M. Sexually mature individuals of *Xenopus laevis* from the transplantation of single somatic nuclei. *Nature* 1958; 182; 64–5.
24. Weinberg AM. Messenger RNA: Origins of a discovery. *Nature* 2001; 414: 485.
25. Ford CE, Hamerton JL. The chromosomes of man. *Nature* 1956; 178: 1020–23.
26. Tjio JH, Levan A. The chromosome number of man. *Hereditas* 1956; 42: 1–6.
27. Lejeune J, Levan A, Böök M et al. A proposed standard system of nomenclature of human mitotic chromosomes. *Lancet* 1960; 275: 1063–65.
28. Ford CE, Jones KW, Polani PE, De Almeida JC, Briggs JH. A sex chromosome anomaly in a case of gonadal dysgenesis (Turner's syndrome). *Lancet* 1959; 273: 711–13.
29. Ford CE, Polani PE, Briggs JH, Bishop PM. A presumptive human XXY/XX mosaic. *Nature* 1959; 183: 1030–32.
30. Jacobs PA, Strong JA. A case of human intersexuality having a possible XXY sex-determining mechanism. *Nature* 1959; 183: 302–3.
31. Lejeune J, Gautier M, Turpin R. Etude des chromosomes somatiques de neuf enfants mongoliens. *Comptes Rendus Hebd Seances Acad Sci* 1959; 248: 1721–22.
32. Gardner RL, Johnson MH. Bob Edwards and the first decade of *Reproductive BioMedicine Online*. *Reprod Biomed Online* 2011; 22: 106–24.
33. Fowler RE, Edwards RG. Induction of superovulation and pregnancy in mature mice by gonadotrophins. *J Endocr* 1957; 15: 374–84.
34. Edwards RG, Gates AH. Timing of the stages of the maturation divisions, ovulation, fertilization and the first cleavage of eggs of adult mice treated with gonadotrophins. *J Endocr* 1959; 18: 292–304.
35. Horowitz NH, Metz CB, Piatigorsky J, Piko L, Spikes JD, Ycas M. Albert Tyler. *Science* 1969; 163: 424.
36. Reeve S. Nathaniel Mayer Victor Rothschild, G.B.E., G.M. Third Baron Rothschild. 31 October 1910–20 March 1990. *Biogr Mems Fell R Soc* 1994; 39: 364–80.
37. Rothschild D. Did fertilization occur? *Nature* 1969; 221: 981.
38. Edwards RG, Bavister BD, Steptoe PC. Early stages of fertilization *in vitro* of human oocytes matured in vitro. *Nature* 1969; 221: 632–5.
39. Mitchison NA. Peter Brian Medawar. February 1915–2 October 1987. *Biogr Mems Fell R Soc* 1990; 35: 282–301.
40. Medawar PB. Some immunological and endocrinological problems raised by the evolution of viviparity in vertebrates. *Symp Soc Exp Biol* 1953; 7: 320–38.
41. Clarke AE. *Disciplining Reproduction: Modernity, American Life Sciences, and the Problems of Sex*. Berkeley, CA: University of California Press, 1998.
42. Connelly M. *Fatal Misconception: The Struggle to Control World Population*. Cambridge, MA: Harvard University Press, 2008.
43. Marks LV. *Sexual Chemistry: A History of the Contraceptive Pill*. New Haven, CT: Yale University Press, 2001.
44. Naz RK, Gupta SK, Gupta JC, Vyas HK, Talwar GP. Recent advances in contraceptive vaccine development: A mini-review. *Hum Reprod* 2005; 20: 3271–83.
45. Rukavina D. The history of reproductive immunology: My personal view. *Am J Reprod Immunol* 2008; 59: 446–50.
46. Edwards RG. Meiosis in ovarian oocytes of adult mammals. *Nature* 1962; 196: 446–50.
47. Gemzell CA. The induction of ovulation with human pituitary gonadotrophins. *Fertil Steril* 1962; 13: 153–68.
48. Pincus G, Enzmann EV. The comparative behavior of mammalian eggs *in vivo* and *in vitro*: I. The activation of ovarian eggs. *J Exp Med* 1935; 62: 665–75.
49. Pincus G, Saunders B. The comparative behavior of mammalian eggs *in vivo* and *in vitro*: VI. The maturation of human ovarian ova. *Anat Rec* 1939; 75: 537–45.
50. Greep RO. Min Chueh Chang. October 10, 1908–June 5, 1991. *Biogr Mems Natl Acad Sci USA* 2010.
51. Chang MC. The maturation of rabbit oocytes in culture and their maturation, activation, fertilization and subsequent development in the Fallopian tubes. *J Exp Zool* 1955; 128: 379–405.
52. MRC. *Research in Obstetrics and Gynaecology: Report to the Secretary of the Council by Section A1, General Clinical Medicine*. National Archives, FD 7/912, 1969.
53. RCOG. *Macafee Report*. The Training of Obstetricians and Gynaecologists in Britain, and Matters Related Thereto: The Report of a Select Committee to the Council of the Royal College of Obstetricians and Gynaecologists. London: RCOG, 1967.
54. Askonas BA. John Herbert Humphrey. 16 December 1915–25 December 1987. *Biogr Mems Fell R Soc* 1990; 36: 274–300.
55. Himsworth H, Pitt-Rivers R. Charles Robert Harington. 1897–1972. *Biogr Mems Fell R Soc* 1972; 18, 266–308.
56. Cole RJ, Edwards RG, Paul J. Cytodifferentiation in cell colonies and cell strains derived from cleaving ova and blastocysts of the rabbit. *Exp Cell Res* 1965; 37: 501–4.

57. Cole RJ, Edwards RG, Paul J. Cytodifferentiation and embryogenesis in cell colonies and tissue cultures derived from ova and blastocysts of the rabbit. *Dev Biol* 1966; 13: 385–407.
58. McLaren A, Biggers JD. Successful development and birth of mice cultivated *in vitro* as early embryos. *Nature* 1958; 182: 877–8.
59. Evans MJ, Kaufman MH. Establishment in culture of pluripotential cells from mouse embryos. *Nature* 1981; 292: 154–6.
60. Edwards RG. IVF and the history of stem cells. *Nature* 2001; 413: 349–51.
61. Parkes AS. *Off-beat Biologist*. Cambridge: The Galton Foundation, 1985.
62. Cook B. *JRF*—The first 100 volumes. *Reproduction* 1994; 100: 2–4.
63. Clarke J. The history of three scientific societies: the Society for the Study of Fertility (now the Society for Reproduction and Fertility) (Britain), the Societe 'Francaise pour l'Etude de la Fertilite', and the Society for the Study of Reproduction (USA). *Stud Hist Phil Biol Biomed Sci* 2007; 38: 340–57.
64. Edwards RG. Letter to Cambridge University Registrary, plus supporting documents, applying for the Mary Marshall and Arthur Walton Professorship of the Physiology of Reproduction. Edwards' papers, 6 Jan 1966. Uncatalogued, Churchill College Archive.
65. Polge C. Obituary: Professor Thaddeus Mann. The Independent, 9 December 1993.
66. Short R. Colin Austin. *Aust Acad Sci Newslett* 2004; 60: 11.
67. Arechaga J. Technique as the basis of experiment in developmental biology: An interview with Denis A.T. New. *New Int J Dev Biol* 1997; 41: 139–52.
68. Edwards RG, Steptoe PC. Preface. In: Edwards RG, Purdy JM, Steptoe PC (eds). *Implantation of the Human Embryo*. London: Academic Press, 1985: vii–viii.
69. Gardner RL. Bob Edwards—2010 Nobel laureate in physiology or medicine. *Physiology News* 2011; 82: 18–22.
70. Gardner RL, Johnson MH. Robert Edwards. *Hum Reprod* 1991; 6: iii–iv.
71. Johnson MH, Elder K. The Oldham Notebooks: An analysis of the development of IVF 1969–1978. VI. Sources of support and patterns of expenditure. *Reprod Biomed Soc Online* 2015: 1, 58–70.
72. Edwards RG. Maturation *in vitro* of human ovarian oocytes. *Lancet* 1965; 286: 926–9.
73. Edwards RG. Maturation *in vitro* of mouse, sheep, cow, pig, rhesus monkey and human ovarian oocytes. *Nature* 1965; 208: 349–51.
74. Gardner RL, Edwards RG. Control of the sex ratio at full term in the rabbit by transferring sexed blastocysts. *Nature* 1968; 218: 346–9.
75. Theodosiou AA, Johnson MH. The politics of human embryo research and the motivation to achieve PGD. *Reprod Biomed Online* 2011; 22: 457–71.
76. Edwards RG. Are oocytes formed and used sequentially in the mammalian ovary? *Phil Trans R Soc B* 1970; 259: 103–5.
77. Henderson SA, Edwards RG. Chiasma frequency and maternal age in mammals. *Nature* 1968; 218: 22–8.
78. Chang MC. Fertilization of rabbit ova *in vitro*. *Nature* 1959; 184: 466–7.
79. Yanagimachi R, Chang MC. Fertilization of hamster eggs *in vitro*. *Nature* 1963; 200: 281–2.
80. Jones Jr HW. From reproductive immunology to Louise Brown. *Reprod Biomed Online* 2002; 4(Suppl 1): 6–7.
81. Austin CR. Observations of the penetration of sperm into the mammalian egg. *Aust J Sci Res B* 1951; 4: 581–96.
82. Chang MC. Fertilizing capacity of spermatozoa deposited into the fallopian tubes. *Nature* 1951; 168: 697–8.
83. Edwards RG, Donahue RP, Baramki TA, Jones Jr HW. Preliminary attempts to fertilize human oocytes matured *in vitro*. *Am J Obstet Gynecol* 1966; 96: 192–200.
84. Edwards RG, Talbert L, Israelstam D, Nino HN, Johnson MH. Diffusion chamber for exposing spermatozoa to human uterine secretions. *Am J Obstet Gynecol* 1968; 102: 388–96.
85. Edwards RG. Patrick Christopher Steptoe, C. B. E. 9 June 1913–22 March 1988. *Biogr Mems Fell R Soc* 1996; 42: 435–52.
86. Steptoe PC. *Laparoscopy in Gynaecology*. Edinburgh: E and S. Livingstone, 1967.
87. Philipp E. Obituary: P C Steptoe CBE, FRCSED, FRCOG, FRS. *Br Med J* 1988; 296: 1135.
88. Edwards RG. Tribute to Patrick Steptoe: Beginnings of laparoscopy. *Hum Reprod* 1989; 4(Suppl): 1–9.
89. Edwards RG. Interviewed in: To Mrs. Brown a daughter. Peter Williams TV: The Studio, Boughton. Faversham, UK, 1978.
90. Steptoe PC. Laparoscopy and ovulation. *Lancet* 1968; 292: 913.
91. Hunting P. *The History of the Royal Society of Medicine*. London: The Royal Society of Medicine Press Ltd, 2002.
92. Steptoe PC. Laparoscopy: Diagnostic and therapeutic uses. *Proc Roy Soc Med* 1969; 62: 439–41.
93. Steptoe PC. A new method of tubal sterilisation. In: Westin B, Wiqvist N, eds. *Amsterdam: Fertility and Sterility: Proc 5th World Congress June 16–22, 1966*. Stockholm: International Congress Series no. 133, Excerpta Medica Foundation, 1967; 1183–4.
94. Steptoe PC. Laparoscopic studies of ovulation, its suppression and induction, and of ovarian dysfunction. In: Wood C, Walters WAW (eds). *Fifth World Congress of Gynaecology and Obstetrics, held in Sydney, Australia, 1967*. Sydney: Butterworths, 1967; 364.
95. Morrison DL. Laparoscopy. *BMJ* 1967; 4: 34.

96. Letter from Eliot Philipp to Edwards dated July 2003, setting out his memory of the exchange of remarks when Steptoe and Edwards first met in the spring of 1967. Uncatalogued Edwards' papers, Churchill College Archive. *General Letters, file 146.*
97. Bavister BD. Environmental factors important for *in vitro* fertilization in the hamster. *J Reprod Fertil* 1969; 18: 544–5.
98. Edwards RG, Bavister BD, Steptoe PC. Did fertilization occur? *Nature* 1969; 221: 981–2.
99. Hayashi M. Fertilization *in vitro* using human ova. In: *Proceedings of the 7th International Planned Parenthood Federation, Singapore. Excerpta Medica International Congress Series No. 72*. Amsterdam, The Netherlands, 1963.
100. Petrov GN. Fertilization and first stages of cleavage of human egg *in vitro. Arkhiv Anatomii Gistologii i Embriologii* 1958; 35: 88–91.
101. Petrucci D. Producing transplantable human tissue in the laboratory. *Discovery* 1961; 22: 278–83.
102. Rock J, Menkin M. *In vitro* fertilization and cleavage of human ovarian eggs. *Science* 1944; 100: 105–7.
103. Shettles LB. A morula stage of human ovum developed *in vitro. Fertil Steril* 1955; 9: 287–9.
104. Yang WH. The nature of human follicular ova and fertilization *in vitro. J Jpn Obstet Gynecol Soc* 1963; 15: 121–30.
105. Anon, 2008. Morris, Prof. Norman Frederick. In: *Who Was Who 1920–1980.* A & C Black and Oxford University Press. [Available from: http://www.ukwhoswho.com/view/article/oupww/whowaswho/U28190].
106. Anon. New step towards test-tube babies. Nature—Times News Service; *The Times* 14 February, 1969.
107. Holmes RF. Letter to D Kellaway (Sec Fac Board Biol. B), dated 21 May. University of Cambridge Archives, 1968; 731.020.
108. Hankinson GS. Letter (G.B.6812.534) from the General Board of the Faculties, the Old Schools, Cambridge to RG Edwards detailing some aspects of the Ford Foundation endowment fund, 20 December 1968. Edwards' papers uncatalogued, Churchill College Archive.
109. Steptoe PC, Edwards RG. Laparoscopic recovery of preovulatory human oocytes after priming of ovaries with gonadotrophins. *Lancet* 1970; 295: 683–9.
110. Edwards RG, Steptoe PC, Purdy JM. Fertilization and cleavage *in vitro* of preovulatory human oocytes. *Nature* 1970; 227: 1307–9.
111. Steptoe PC, Edwards RG, Purdy JM. Human blastocysts grown in culture. *Nature* 1971; 229: 132–3.
112. Elder K, Johnson MH. The Oldham Notebooks: An analysis of the development of IVF 1969–1978. III. Variations in procedures. *Reprod Biomed Soc Online* 2015; 1: 19–33.
113. Johnson MH, Elder K. The Oldham Notebooks: An analysis of the development of IVF 1969–1978. V. The role of Jean Purdy reassessed. *Reprod Biomed Soc Online* 2015; 1: 46–57.
114. Edwards RG, Sharpe DJ. Social values and research in human embryology. *Nature* 1971; 231: 87–91.
115. Rickham PP. Human Experimentation: Code of Ethics of World Medical Association. Declaration of Helsinki. *Br Med J* 1964; 2: 177.
116. Hazelgrove J. The old faith and the new science. The Nuremberg Code and human experimentation ethics in Britain 1946–73. *Soc Hist Med* 2002; 15:109–35.
117. Pappworth MH. *Human Guinea-pigs.* London: Routledge and Keegan Paul, 1967.
118. Edwards RG. Fertilization of human eggs *in vitro*: morals, ethics and the law. *Q Rev Biol* 1974; 49: 3–26.
119. Jones A, Bodmer WF. *Our Future Inheritance: Choice or Chance?* London: Oxford University Press, 1974.
120. Edwards RG, Steptoe PC. Birth after the reimplantation of a human embryo. *Lancet* 1978; 312: 366.
121. Johnson MH, Theodosiou AA. PGD and the making of the genetic embryo as a political tool. In: McLean S (ed.). *Regulating PGD: A Comparative and Theoretical Analysis.* London: Routledge, 2011.
122. Mulkay M. *The Embryo Research Debate: Science and the Politics of Reproduction.* Cambridge: Cambridge University Press, 1997.

New guidelines for setting up an assisted reproduction technology laboratory

1

JACQUES COHEN, MINA ALIKANI, ANTONIA GILLIGAN, and TIM SCHIMMEL

There are a number of ways to set up and operate a successful assisted reproduction technology (ART) laboratory; one set-up may have little in common with another but prove to be equally successful. This is important to remember as one ventures into establishing a new clinic. Facilities for ART range from a makeshift *in vitro* fertilization (IVF) laboratory with a minimum of equipment to a fully equipped laboratory specifically designed for ART and with additional space dedicated to clinical care and research. This chapter does not cover makeshift laboratories, which may incorporate retrieval and transport of gametes and embryos from other locations. While such models can be successful under some circumstances, compelling evidence showing that they produce optimal results is still lacking (1,2). Both IVF and intracytoplasmic sperm injection (ICSI) can be applied to transported oocytes, and in certain situations "transport IVF" is a welcome alternative for those patients whose reproductive options have been limited by restrictive governmental regulations (3,4). This chapter discusses the more typical purpose-built, all-inclusive laboratories that are adjacent or in close proximity to oocyte retrieval and embryo transfer facilities, with an emphasis on the special problems of construction. For choices of culture system, culture medium, supplementation, viability assays, and handling and processing of gametes and embryos, including freezing and vitrification, the reader is referred to other relevant chapters in this textbook.

PERSONNEL AND EXPERIENCE

While the environment, physical plant, and equipment require special consideration in the design of an integrated gamete and embryo culture facility, it is the staff that will carry out the procedures and is essential to the success of the entire operation. Successful clinical practice in general, and ART in particular, is almost entirely dependent on the skill and experience level of medical and laboratory personnel. For the laboratory staff, enthusiasm is another key factor to success, especially because there are still few formal teaching and skills examination programs in place for a specialty in ART. Most clinical embryologists are trained using an apprenticeship program, but such institutions are rare and there are no internationally accepted guidelines. Good clinical outcome requires a cautious and rational assessment of individual abilities, so laboratory staff, directors, and embryologists must consider their experience in the context of what will be required of them (5).

This chapter aims to provide information necessary for experienced practitioners to set up a new laboratory. Setting up a new laboratory or thoroughly renovating an existing facility is very much an art, as is the practice of ART itself. We do not recommend that new laboratories and ART clinics are built by administrators, engineers, or architects without considerable input from experienced embryologists.

Programs should develop a strong (though friendly) system of tracking individual performances for crucial clinical and laboratory procedures such as embryo transfer efficiency, ICSI, and biopsy proficiency, among others. Certain regulatory bodies such as the College of American Pathologists (CAP) in the U.S.A. and the Human Fertilisation and Embryology Authority (HFEA) in the U.K. provide guidelines and licensing for embryologists, sometimes even for subspecialties such as the performance of ICSI, the practice of embryo biopsy, and directing IVF and andrology laboratories. So far, such licensing has done little more than provoke debate, because licensing does not necessarily guarantee skill (or success) and the licenses are not valid across borders from one country to another.

Tradition also plays its role. For example, in some Asian countries embryology directors are usually medical professionals. Thus academic titles are often seen as being more important than actual qualifications. What then qualifies someone to be a laboratory director or an embryologist? The answer is not a simple one. In general, current licensing authorities including the American Board of Bioanalysis (ABB) consider individuals trained in general pathology or reproductive medicine and holding an MD degree as well as individuals holding a PhD degree qualified to be laboratory directors if they meet some other requirements. However, pathologists do not necessarily have experience in gamete and embryo cell culture, and some reproductive medicine specialists, such as urologists and immunologists, may have never worked with gametes and embryos. It is possible for a medical practitioner to direct a laboratory in certain countries without ever having practiced gamete and embryo handling! "*Eppur si muove*" ("And yet it moves"), as Galileo said when condemned by the Roman inquisition for the heresy of accepting Copernican astronomy. Once there are rules, even silly ones, it may be hard to change them.

EMPIRICAL AND STATISTICAL REQUIREMENTS FOR STAFF

There is considerable disagreement about what should be required experience for embryologists. Hands-on experience in all facets of clinical embryology is an absolute requirement when starting a new program. Even highly experienced experimental embryologists and animal scientists should be directly supervised by experienced clinical personnel. The period during which close supervision must continue depends on the types of skills required, the daily caseload, and time spent performing procedures. Clearly, performing 100 cases over a one-year period is a very different circumstance than performing the same number over six weeks; the period of supervision then should be adjusted accordingly.

The optimal ratio of laboratory staff to the expected number of procedures is debatable, and unfortunately, economics play an all too important role here. However, with the incorporation of new technologies and treatment modalities in routine care, the complexity of IVF laboratory operations has increased substantially over the past decade, in turn requiring more careful consideration of staffing levels (6). According to some calculations, while a "traditional" IVF cycle required roughly nine personnel hours, a contemporary cycle can require up to 20 hours for completion. Thus the number of embryologists required for safe and efficient operation of the laboratory has also increased. Recently, based on a comprehensive analysis of laboratory tasks and their complexity, an Interactive Personnel Calculator was introduced to help laboratory directors and administrators determine staffing needs (6). Overall, it is safe to say that the ratio of laboratory staff to caseload should be high so that embryologists can not only safely perform procedures but dedicate time to quality control and continued education and training in order to maintain the high standards required for success. The challenge of keeping these standards within national health systems or in the face of insurance mandates that must provide a wide range of services on a minimal budget is real, but should not be insurmountable. Needless to say, patients usually do not benefit from such constraints, as a comparison of results in different health service systems in Western countries would suggest. There are limitations to such comparisons, but live births per embryo and cumulative data from fresh and cryopreservation cycles are considered objective assessments (7).

The job description for the embryologist ideally includes all embryology and andrology tasks, except for medical and surgical procedures. Embryologists are often involved in other important tasks as well, including patient management, follicular monitoring, genetic counseling, marketing, and administration. However, it should be realized that these tasks seriously detract from their main responsibilities. First and foremost, the embryologist's duty is to perform gamete and embryo handling and culture procedures. Secondly, but equally important, the embryologist should maintain quality control standards, both by performing routine checks and tests and by maintaining detailed logs of incidents, changes, unexpected events, and corrective measures. Across all these duties, the following seven positions can be clearly defined: director, supervisor, senior embryologist, embryologist, trainee, assistant, and technician. There may also be positions for others to do preimplantation genetic diagnosis, research, quality control supervision, or administrative work. Obviously, not all of these separate positions are necessary for smaller centers and important tasks can be combined.

Although a seemingly unimportant detail, one of the most important jobs in the IVF laboratory at Bourn Hall Clinic in Cambridge, U.K., during the first few years of operation was that of a professional witness and embryology assistant. This position was the brainchild of Jean Purdy, the third partner who was involved in the work that led to the birth of Louise Brown. The embryology assistant effectively enforced and oversaw the integrity of the chain of custody of gametes and embryos during handling, particularly when large numbers of patients were being treated simultaneously. The "witness" also ensured that embryologists performed only those procedures for which they were qualified. Interestingly, recent literature suggests that this crucial concept has not been universally and fully understood or adopted by all IVF laboratories. In one group of laboratories (8), "limited and consequently virtually ineffective" witnessing processes were only abandoned in favor of a more robust witnessing program after implementation of a failure mode and effects analysis (FMEA) showed a high risk of error in gamete and embryo identification. The authors stated that, "Only after FMEA optimization has the witness embryologist been formally recognized as a committed role, specifically trained for witnessing shift work." Hopefully, the publication of this and other similar studies (9) that show the effectiveness of a witnessing system will encourage more laboratories to re-examine their practices and allocate adequate resources to ensuring the safety and efficiency of all procedures performed by the laboratory.

FACILITY, DESIGN, AND BUDGET

In the early days of IVF some clinics were built in remote areas, based on the premise that environmental factors such as stress could affect the patient and thereby the outcome of treatment. Today's laboratories are commonly placed in city centers and large metropolitan areas in order to service large populations locally. It is important that patients understand that there have been millions of others like them before and that in general IVF is a routine, though complex, medical procedure. It is clear that the choice of a laboratory site is of great importance for a new program. The recent development of better assays for determining the baseline quality of the environment facilitates site selection. There is now awareness that some buildings or building sites could be intrinsically harmful to cell tissue culture (10–12). The direct effect of poor air quality and the presence of volatile organic compounds (VOCS) on IVF outcomes has been demonstrated by recent studies of novel filtration systems and other countermeasures (13,14). A laboratory design should be based on the anticipated caseload and any subspecialty. Local building and practice permits must be assessed prior to engaging and completing a design. There are five basic types of design:

1. Laboratories using only transport IVF
2. Laboratories adjacent to clinical outpatient facilities that are only used part of the time

3. Full-time clinics with intra-facility egg transport using portable warming chambers
4. Fully integrated laboratories with clinical areas
5. Moveable temporary laboratories

Before developing the basic design for a new laboratory, environmental factors must be considered. While air quality in modern laboratories can be controlled to a degree, it can never be fully protected from the exterior environment and adjoining building spaces. Designers should first determine if the building or the surrounding site is scheduled to undergo renovations, demolition, or major changes of any kind in the foreseeable future. City planning should also be reviewed. Historical environmental data and trends, future construction, and the ability of maintenance staff to maintain and service the IVF laboratory need to be determined. Activity related to any type of construction can have a significant negative impact on any proposed laboratory. Prevalent wind direction, industrial hazards, and general pollution reports such as ozone measurements should also be determined. Even when these factors are all deemed acceptable, basic air sampling and determination of VOC concentrations is necessary inside and outside the proposed building area. The outcome of these tests will determine which design requirements are needed to remove VOCs from the laboratory area. In most cases, an over-pressured laboratory (at least 0.10–0.20 inches of water) that uses a high number (7–15) of fresh air changes per hour is the best solution, because it also provides for proper medical hygiene. The laboratory walls and ceiling should have the absolute minimum number of penetrations. This generally requires a solid ceiling, sealed lighting, and airtight utility connections. Contrary to many vendors' representations, commercial suspended ceilings using double-sided tape and clips are not ideal. Doors will require seals and sweeps, and should be lockable. Ducts and equipment must be laid out in such a way that routine and emergency maintenance and repair work can be performed outside the laboratory with minimal disruption to the laboratory. Air handling must not use an open plenum design. In the ideal case, 100% outside air with chemical and physical filtration will be used with sealed supply and return ducts.

While providing cleaner air, 100% outside air sourcing will maximize the life of a chemical filter and will provide a lower concentration of VOCs in the IVF laboratory's air. In climates where temperatures routinely exceed 32°C with 85%-plus relative humidity, 100% outside air could result in an unacceptable level of humidity (>60%), which could allow mold growth. In these cases the use of limited return air from the lab is acceptable. A 50% outside air system with 15–30 total air changes per hour does work well and the relative humidity becomes very controllable. To place this in perspective, traditional medical operating room design calls for 10%–15% outside air.

The air supply equipment may supplement outside air with recirculated air, with processing to control the known levels of VOCs. On rare occasions, laboratories will require full-time air recirculation, while most may actually find the outside air to be perfectly clean at least most of the time. Outside air is often erroneously judged to be polluted without proper chemical analysis, while inside air is usually considered "cleaner" because it may "smell" better (10). In most laboratory locations, conditions are actually the reverse, and designers should not "follow their instincts" in these matters. Humidity must also be completely controlled according to climate and seasonal variation. The system must be capable of supplying the space with air with a temperature as high as 30°C–35°C at less than 40% relative humidity. Air inlets and outlets should be carefully spaced to avoid drafts that can change local "spot" temperatures, or expose certain equipment to relatively poor air or changes in air quality. Laminar flow hoods and micromanipulation workstations should not be located too close to air supply fixtures to avoid disruption of the sterile field and to minimize cooling on the microscope stage. Semi-enclosed workstations based on Class 2 cabinets or neonatal isolette incubators can be considered to optimize the work environment and bridge the gap between the incubator and the workstation. A detailed layout and assessment of all laboratory furniture and equipment is therefore essential prior to construction and has many other benefits.

Selection of an experienced and sub-specialized (and flexible) architect and a mechanical engineer for the project is essential. Confirm what their past experience has been in building biologically clean rooms. The use of "environmentally friendly" or "green" products has been suggested by some designers. The reliance on "natural" products does not ensure a clean laboratory. In one case, wood casework with a green label was found to be a major source of formaldehyde. Floor coverings using recycled vinyl and rubber were selected for their low environmental impact, without considering the significant release of trapped gases by the material.

Supervision of the construction is also critical. Skilled tradesmen using past training and experience may not follow all of the architect's instructions. The general contractor and the builders must be briefed on why these novel construction techniques are being used. They must understand that the use of untested methods and products can compromise the project (and the payment of their fees!). Contractual agreement is recommended.

Just as the organization and flow of traffic in a world-class restaurant results in a special ambience where more than just the food is the attraction, appropriate modular placement of equipment ensures safety and comfort in the over-pressured IVF laboratory. Placement of stacks of incubators, gamete handling areas (laminar flow units or isolettes), and micromanipulation stations should minimize distances that dishes and tubes need be moved. Ideally, an embryologist should be able to finish one complete procedure without moving more than three meters in any direction; not only is this efficient, but also it minimizes accidents in a busy laboratory. Design and implementation of a work area incorporating product, gas and liquid nitrogen supplies, and a workstation, refrigerator, and incubators is feasible even without the embryologists having to walk between storage cabinets and equipment. Such a modular design can be duplicated multiple times within a larger air handling area allowing the handling of large numbers of gametes and embryos. For logistical reasons, sperm preparation and cryopreservation may be placed in adjacent areas. The number of modules can easily be determined by the expected number of cases and procedure types, the average number of eggs collected, and the number of embryologists expected to work simultaneously. Each person should be provided with sufficient workspace to perform all procedures without delay. Additional areas can contain simple gamete handling stations or areas for concentrating incubators. Cryopreservation and storage facilities are often located in a separate space, although this is not strictly necessary; if separated, these areas should always be adjacent to the main laboratory. Storage spaces could be separated further using closets or rooms with negative pressure. Another separate laboratory or module may contain an area for culture medium preparation, sterilization, and water treatment; however, the need for such an area is diminishing now that commercial manufacturers provide all the basic needs of an IVF laboratory. Administration should be performed in separate offices on a different air handling system from the main laboratories.

Last but not least, it is preferable to prepare semen in a separate laboratory altogether, adjacent to one or more collection rooms. The semen laboratory should have ample space for microscopes, freezing, and sterile zoning. Proper separation of patient samples during processing is essential and some elemental design features may be considered before the first procedures are carried out. Some thought should go into planning the semen collection area. This small room should be at the end of a hallway preferably with its own exit; it should be soundproofed, not too large, and with a sink. Clear instructions on how to collect semen for ART should be provided in the room. The room should also be adjacent to the semen preparation laboratory, preferably with a double-door pass-through for samples. This pass-through should have a signaling device so the patient can inform the embryologist that the sample is ready; it also permits male patients to leave the area without having to carry a specimen container.

EQUIPMENT AND STORAGE

A detailed list of equipment should be prepared and checked against the planned location of each item; it can later be used as the basis of maintenance logs. It is important to consider the inclusion of crucial equipment and spare tools in the laboratory design, to allow for unexpected malfunction. Similarly, two or more spare incubators should not be seen as excessive; at least one spare follicle aspiration pump and micromanipulation station (equipped with a laser) should also be included. There are many other instruments and equipment pieces the malfunction of which would jeopardize patient care, although some spares need not be kept on hand as manufacturers may have them available; however, such details need to be repeatedly checked as suppliers' stocks continue to change. It may also be useful to team up with other programs or an embryology research laboratory locally so that a crucial piece of equipment can be exchanged in case of unexpected failure.

Some serious thought is needed when contemplating the number and type of incubators (for a comprehensive review, see [15]). The ratio of incubators to patient procedures depends on incubator size and capacity and it varies considerably from program to program. It is clear that the number and type of incubator, as well as the length and number of incubator door openings, affect results. In principle, the number of cases per incubator should be kept to a minimum; we prefer a limit of four cases per large standard box incubator. The smaller box incubators should not handle more than two to three cases. In benchtop incubators, the use of one dish slot per patient is not recommended. Several other incubators can be used for general purposes during micromanipulation and for other generic uses to limit further the number of incubator openings. Strict guidelines must be implemented and adhered to when maintaining distinct spaces for separating culture dishes or tubes of different patients. Tracking of incubators and even shelves within each incubator is recommended so their performance can be evaluated on an ongoing basis. Separate compartments within an incubator may be helpful and can be supplied by certain manufacturers. Servicing and cleaning of equipment such as incubators may have to be done when the laboratory is not performing procedures. Placement of incubators and other pieces of equipment on large castors may be helpful in programs where downtime is rare. Pieces of equipment can then be serviced outside the laboratory. New incubators and equipment pieces that come in contact with gametes and embryos must be "burned-in" or "off-gassed." Protocols vary per equipment type and manufacturer.

When there are several options available to the laboratory designer, supply and evacuation routes should be planned in advance. One of the most susceptible aspects of ART is cryopreservation. In case of an emergency such as a fire or power failure, it may be necessary to relocate the liquid nitrogen-filled dewars without using an elevator, or to relocate the frozen samples using a temporary container. This may seem an extreme consideration, especially in the larger laboratories that stockpile thousands of samples, but plans should be made. It may be possible to keep a separate storage closet or space near the building exit, where long-term samples, which usually provide the bulk of the storage, can be kept; this would require repeated checking of a facility that is not part of the laboratory. Liquid nitrogen tank alarms with remote notification capability should be installed on all dewars holding gametes and embryos. The route of delivery of liquid nitrogen and other gas cylinders must be relatively easy, without stairways between the laboratory and the delivery truck, and should be sensibly planned in advance. Note that the flooring of this route is usually destroyed within months because of liquid nitrogen spills and wear caused by delivery containers, so the possibility of an alternative delivery corridor should be considered for these units.

Liquid nitrogen containers and medical gas cylinders are preferentially placed immediately adjacent to the laboratory in a closet or small, ventilated room with outside access. Pipes and tubes enter the laboratory from this room, and cylinders can be delivered to this room without compromising the laboratory area in any way. Providing liquid nitrogen and even liquid oxygen vapor to triple gas incubators is nowadays a preferred option since vapor is cleaner than compressed gas. This allows liquid nitrogen vapor to be pumped into the cryopreservation laboratory using a manifold system and minimal piping. Lines should be properly installed and insulated to ensure that they do not leak or allow condensation and conserve energy at the same time. Medical gases can be directed into the laboratory using pre-washed vinyl/Teflon-lined tubing such as fluorinated ethylene propylene, which has high humidity, temperature, and UV radiation stability. Lines should be properly marked every meter indicating the incubators supplied in order to facilitate later maintenance. Alternatively, solid manifolds made from stainless steel with suitable compression fittings can be used. Avoid the soldered or brazed copper lines used in domestic plumbing applications wherever possible; copper lining can be used but should be cleaned and purged for a prolonged period prior to use in the laboratory. Copper line connections should not be soldered as this could cause continuous contamination. This recommendation may conflict with existing building codes, but non-contaminating alternatives can be found. A number of spare lines hidden behind walls and ceilings should be installed as well, in case of later renovation or facility expansion.

Large programs should consider the use of exterior bulk tanks for carbon dioxide and liquid nitrogen. This removes the issues of tanks for incubators or cryopreservation. These tanks are located where delivery trucks can hook onto and deliver directly to the tank. Pressurized gas lines or cryogenic lines then run the carbon dioxide or liquid nitrogen to the IVF laboratory for use.

Placement of bulky and difficult pieces of equipment should be considered when designing doorways and electrical panels. Architects should be fully informed of all equipment specifications to avoid the truly classic door-width mistake. Emergency generators should always be installed, even where power supplies are usually reliable. The requirements can be determined by an electrical engineer. Thankfully, these units can be removed from the laboratory, but must be placed in well-ventilated areas that are not prone to flooding. Additional battery "uninterruptible power systems" may be considered as well, but are of very limited capability. Buildings should also be checked for placement of the main power inlets and distribution centers, especially because sharing power lines with other departments or companies may not be advisable. Circuit breakers should be easily accessible to embryologists or building maintenance staff. General knowledge of the mechanical and electrical engineering of the building and the laboratory specifically will always be advantageous. Leaving all the building mechanics and facilities to other individuals is often counterproductive. Embryologists need to be involved with facilities management and be updated with construction decisions inside and outside the building in a timely manner.

Ample storage spaces should always be planned for IVF laboratories. In the absence of dedicated storage space, laboratory space ends up being used instead, filling all cabinets and negating any advantages of the original design. The dedicated storage area should be used to stock all materials in sufficient quantity to maintain a steady supply. A further reason to include storage areas in laboratory design—sufficient on its own to justify the space—is that new supplies, including sterile disposable items, release multiple compounds for prolonged periods. This "out-gassing" has been determined to be a major cause of air pollution in a number of laboratories in which supplies were stored inside the lab. Separate storage space therefore provides the best chance of good air quality, especially when it is supplied by separate air handling system. It should be large enough to handle bulky items as well as mobile shelving for boxes. One should be careful to avoid the natural inclination to save extra trips by bringing too many items into the laboratory, or the gains made by careful design may be lost. As a possible makeshift solution, storage cabinetry in the laboratory can be designed with separate negative pressure air handling in order to minimize release of VOCs from off-gassing package materials.

MICROSCOPES AND VISUALIZATION OF CELLS

Though dissecting microscopes are crucial for the general handling of gametes and embryos, many people still consider inverted microscopes to be a luxury even though they are in regular use with micromanipulation systems. Proper visualization of embryos is key to successful embryo selection for transfer or freezing; if the equipment is first class, visualization can be done quickly and accurately (16). Even so, appropriately detailed assessment is still dependent on the use of an oil overlay system to prevent damage by prolonged exposure. Each workstation and microscope should be equipped with a still camera and/or video camera and monitor. Still photos can be placed in the patient file and video footage permits speedy review of embryonic features with colleagues after the gametes are safely returned to the incubator; this is also helpful for training of new embryologists. Interference optics such as Hoffman and Nomarski are preferable because they permit the best measure of detail and depth. Novel visualization of internal elements such as spindles using polarized microscopy requires additional equipment, but can be incorporated into routine operation (17). Ideally, the captured photos should be digitally stored for recall in the clinic's medical database.

Development of new time-lapse microscopy technologies has made continuous and uninterrupted monitoring of embryo development a reality. This is an invaluable teaching and learning tool. However, equipment costs are high and, for many laboratories, prohibitive. Equipment for time-lapse technology can be sizable and may require separate consideration in terms of lab design and bench space.

CONSTRUCTION, RENOVATION, AND BUILDING MATERIALS

Construction and renovation can introduce a variety of compounds into the environment of the ART laboratory, either temporarily or permanently. Either can have major adverse effects on the outcome of operations (10–12,18,19). The impact of the exterior environment on IVF success has been demonstrated. Pollutants can have a significant negative effect on success in an IVF laboratory (10,20). These effects can range from delayed or abnormal embryonic development, reduced or failed fertilization, and reduced implantation rates to pregnancy loss and failure of a treatment cycle. Many of the damaging materials are organic chemicals that are released or out-gassed by paint, adhesives from flooring, cabinets, and general building materials, as well as from laboratory equipment and procedures. It is important to realize that the actual construction phase of the laboratory can cause permanent problems. Furthermore, any subsequent renovation activity in adjacent areas can also cause similar, or even greater problems. Neighboring tenants can be informed of the sensitivity of gametes and embryos in culture. At the very least, changes undertaken in adjacent areas should be supervised by IVF laboratory personnel to minimize potential damage. However, new construction immediately outside the building is considerably more problematic. City works such as street construction are very hard to predict and nearly impossible to control. A good relationship with the neighbors should be maintained and a working relationship with building owners and city planners should be established so that the IVF laboratory is kept informed of upcoming changes.

For the construction of a new laboratory or if changes are to be made to areas adjacent to the IVF facility, the following guidelines should be followed. First, the area to be demolished and reconstructed needs to be physically isolated from the IVF laboratory (if this is not the new IVF laboratory itself). The degree of isolation should be equivalent to an asbestos or lead abatement project. The isolation should be done through: (1) physical barriers, consisting of poly-sheeting supported by studding where needed; (2) limited access to the construction area and the use of an access passageway with two doors in series; (3) removal of all construction waste via an exterior opening or proper containment of waste before using an interior exit; (4) negative air pressure in the construction area, exhausting to the exterior, far removed from the laboratory's air intake, and properly located with regard to the prevailing winds and exterior airflow; (5) extra interior fans during any painting or the use of adhesives to maximize removal of noxious fumes; and (6) compiling and logging of Material Safety Data Sheets (MSDS) for all paints, solvents, and adhesives in use.

Follow-up investigations with manufacturers and their representatives may be helpful because specifications of equipment may be changed without notice. The negative pressurization of the laboratory space requires continuous visual confirmation via a ball and tube pressure indicator or simply paper strips. Periodic sampling for particulates, aldehydes, and organics could be done outside the demolition and construction site, provided this is economically feasible. Alternatively, tracer gas studies can be done to verify containment. The general contractor of the demolition and construction should be briefed in detail on the need to protect the IVF facility and techniques to accomplish this. When possible, the actual members of the construction crew themselves should be selected and briefed in detail. Large filter units using filter pellets of carbon and permanganate can be placed strategically. Uptake of organics can be assayed, but the frequency of routine filter changes should be increased during periods of construction activity.

SELECTION OF BUILDING MATERIALS

Many materials release significant amounts of VOCs and a typical list includes paints, adhesives, glues, sealants, and caulking, which release alkanes, aromatics, alcohols, aldehydes, ketones, and other classes of organic materials. This section outlines steps to be taken in order to reduce these out-gassing chemicals. Any and all interior painting throughout the facility should only be done on prepared surfaces with water-based paint formulated for low VOC potential. During any painting, auxiliary ventilation should be provided using large industrial construction fans, with exhaust vented to the exterior. Paints that can significantly influence air quality should be emission tested (some suppliers already have these test results available). Safety Data Sheets (SDS; previously MSDS) are generally available for construction materials. Suppliers should be encouraged to conduct product testing for emission potential. The variety of materials and applications complicates the testing process, but several procedures have been developed to identify and quantify the compounds released by building materials and furnishings. Interior paints must be water-based, low-volatile paints with acrylic, vinyl acrylic, alkyd, or acrylic latex polymers. Paints meeting this specification can also contain certain inorganic materials. Low-volatile paints may still contain low concentrations of certain organics. No interior paint should contain formaldehyde, acetaldehyde, isocyanates, reactive amines, phenols, and other water-soluble volatile organics. Adhesive glues, sealants, and caulking materials present some of the same problems as paints. None of these materials used in the interior should contain formaldehyde, benzaldehyde, phenol, and similar substances. Although water-based versions of these are generally not available, their composition varies widely. Silicone materials are preferred whenever possible, particularly for sealants and caulking work. A complete list of guidelines for material use during the construction of a tissue culture laboratory is available elsewhere (21).

"BURNING IN" OF THE FINISHED FACILITY

New IVF laboratories and new facilities around existing laboratories have often been plagued by complaints of occupants who experience discomfort from the chemicals released by new construction and furnishings. The ambient levels of many of these materials can be reduced by "burning in" the facility. A typical burn-in consists of increasing the temperature of the new area by 10°C–20°C and increasing the ventilation rate; even higher temperatures are acceptable. The combination of elevated temperature and higher air exchange aids in the removal of the volatile organics. Upon completion of the construction, the air handling system should be properly configured for the burn-in of the newly constructed area. As previously stated, the system must be capable of supplying the space with air with a temperature of 30°C–35°C, at less than 40% relative humidity. The burn-in period can range from 10 to 28 days, and the IVF laboratory should be kept closed during this time. If these temperatures cannot be reached by the base system, use auxiliary electrical heating to reach the minimum temperature. During burn-in, all lighting and some auxiliary equipment should be turned on and left running continuously. Naturally, ventilation is critical if redistribution of irritants is to be avoided; the whole purpose is to purge the air repeatedly. Auxiliary equipment should of course be monitored during the burn-in.

The same burn-in principle applies to newly purchased incubators or other laboratory equipment. Removal of volatile organics is especially important in the critical microenvironment of the incubator. Whenever possible, it is advantageous to purchase incubators months in advance of their intended initial use and to operate them at an elevated temperature in a clean, protected location. An existing embryology laboratory is not a good space for the burn-in of a new incubator.

Most of the equipment available for use in an ART laboratory has not been designed or manufactured to be VOC-free. Special attention must be invested in new laboratory equipment to eliminate or reduce VOC levels by as much as possible before first use.

Most manufacturers do not address the issues of VOC out-gassing in product manuals, even if the equipment has been expressly designed for the IVF field. Unpacking, cleaning, and operating equipment prior to final installation in a lab for out-gassing the "new car smell" is always recommended.

Incubators should be unpacked, inspected, cleaned, outgassed, operated, re-cleaned, calibrated, and tested well in advance. The process can take several months to accomplish, but is generally a very essential task that is rewarded with the most suitable culture system that the selected incubator model can provide. When possible, operating incubators at elevated temperatures above the typical culture temperature will hasten the release or burn-off of VOCs. Extended operation at between 40°C–45°C works well to burn off VOCs if this is within the manufacturer's recommended temperature range. Incubator model VOC loads can vary greatly. Accurate VOC testing may be expensive and time consuming, but it is recommended to test a specific incubator model to determine the new unit's typical VOC characteristics and how much time outgassing may require.

Handheld VOC testing devices are available and can be used to help monitor the decline of total VOCs, but cannot match the level of accuracy of an environmental organic chemist's testing. Handheld VOC meter technology generally is not sensitive enough to monitor low-molecular-weight classes of VOCs. They are reasonably affordable, easily used, and can provide a means of monitoring VOC reduction to help determine if the out-gassing time may be sufficient to observe a reduction of VOCs.

New incubators are generally tested with a mouse embryo assay (MEA), replicating a culture system as part of a new incubator commissioning process. Most laboratories today use some variation of an oil culture system. The oil can serve as an excellent filter against potential VOCs, but may not protect a culture system from the full range of VOC exposure, particularly low-molecular-weight compounds such as aldehydes. Incubator MEA commissioning should include both an oil and an open exposed media test to help evaluate the success of preparing the incubator. The dual MEA approach works well for humidified incubator systems, but may not be applicable if a dry, non-humidified culture system is used. Most dry, non-humidified culture systems are designed to recirculate chamber air and incorporate a VOC filtration strategy. Open culture generally cannot be used with non-humidified incubators. The manufacturer's recommendations should be followed. Non-humidified incubators may require extended off-gassing and should be tested prior to use in order to confirm that they do not have a VOC issue. Chemical VOC filters should be replaced after burn-off prior to any MEA testing.

Laminar flow hoods and isolettes are also important potential VOC sources that should not be overlooked. They should be given ample time to operate and out-gas as they can contribute to a lab's VOC contamination load. High-efficiency particulate air (HEPA) and chemical filters should be selected for low-VOC manufacturing traits and also may require off-gassing. Care must be taken when out-gassing laminar flow hoods and isolettes as they require a HEPA-filtered environment or replacement of their filters when transferred to an IVF lab.

After the burn-in is complete, commissioning of the IVF suite should be conducted to verify that the laboratory meets the design specifications. The ventilation and isolation of the laboratory should be verified by a series of tests using basic airflow measurements and tracer gas studies. The particulate levels should be determined to verify that the HEPA system is functional. Particulate sampling can be performed using U.S. Federal Standard 209E. Microbial sampling for aerobic bacteria and fungi is often done in new facilities using an Andersen sampler followed by microbiological culturing and identification. The levels of VOC contamination should be determined. Possible methods are included in the U.S. Environmental

Protection Agency protocols using gas chromatography/mass spectroscopy and high-performance liquid chromatography that is sensitive at the microgram per cubic meter level (22–25).

MAINTENANCE PLANNING AND STERILIZATION

Even the best systems and designs will eventually fail unless they are carefully maintained. The heating, ventilation, and air conditioning (HVAC) will require filter changes, coil cleaning, replacement of drive belts, and chemical purification media. The most prevalent failure concerns the initial particulate filter. These are inexpensive filters designed to keep out large dust particles, plant debris, and insects, among others. If such filters are not replaced promptly and regularly, they will fail, allowing the HVAC unit to become contaminated. The HEPA filters and chemical media also require inspection and periodic replacement. Maintenance staff should report their findings to the IVF laboratory.

The IVF laboratory must have a cleaning facility for surgical instruments. Ongoing use of an autoclave is not a problem as long as the released steam is rapidly exhausted to the outside. This keeps the relative humidity in the facility to controllable limits. Autoclaves should not be placed on the IVF laboratory's HVAC system, but rather in a room that is built using tight construction and is exhausted directly outside of the building. The use of cold sterilizing agents is not advised. Aldehydes such as glutaraldehyde and *ortho*-pathaldehyde from the autoclave can be transported inside the IVF laboratory.

INSURANCE ISSUES

ARTs have become common practice worldwide and are regulated by a combination of legislation, regulations, or committee-generated practice standards. The rapid evolution and progress of ART reveal new legal issues that require consideration. Even the patients themselves are changing, as it becomes more acceptable for single women and homosexual couples to seek and receive treatment. Donation of gametes, embryos, and gamete components, enforcement of age limits for treatment, selective fetal reduction, preimplantation genetic diagnosis, surrogacy, and many other practices in ART present practitioners and society at large with challenges, which are often defined by social norms, religion, and law and are specific to each country.

Furthermore, financial and emotional stresses often burden patients seeking treatment in countries where medicine is not socialized and infertility treatment is not covered by insurance. This translates into an increasing number of ART lawsuits related to failed treatments in spite of generally improved success rates. Laboratory personnel and the laboratory owner should therefore obtain an insurance policy of a sufficiently high level and quality commencing prior to the first day of operations. Litigation-prone issues need special consideration, and include:

- Cancellation of a treatment cycle prior to egg retrieval
- Failure to become pregnant
- Patient identification errors
- Cryostorage mishaps

These issues occur even if experienced practitioners consider themselves at low risk of exposure. Prior to engaging in the practice of ART, protocols must be established to identify potential problem areas and establish countermeasures.

CONCLUSIONS

It may be surprising how many professionals continue to pursue the establishment of new ART clinics at a time when competition is fierce, financial benefits are small, and existing ART services may appear to be approaching saturation in many areas and countries. Appearances can be misleading, however, and ART centers of excellence that deserve the trust and confidence of patients and serve as models for other practices are always needed.

This chapter provides some guidance for those who aspire to establish such outstanding, well thought out and planned ART practices. Although it cannot safeguard practitioners against adverse events, it introduces concepts in the proper design, construction, and operation of ART facilities that are of fundamental importance to treatment success; these guidelines have been painstakingly compiled through decades of practical experience and research. The approach is best adopted as a whole rather than dissected into its components and adopted in part or selectively. Keep in mind that resisting the urge to cut corners in the wrong places avoids future headaches and positions you and your patients on the path to success.

REFERENCES

1. Jansen CA, van Beek JJ, Verhoeff A, Alberda AT, Zeilmaker GH. *In vitro* fertilisation and embryo transfer with transport of oocytes. *Lancet* 1986; 22: 676.
2. Verhoeff A, Huisman GJ, Leerentveld RA, Zeilmaker GH. Transport in vitro fertilization. *Fertil Steril* 1993; 60: 187–8.
3. Coetsier T, Verhoeff A, De Sutter P, Roest J, Dhont M. Transport *in vitro* fertilization/intracellular sperm injection: A prospective randomized study. *Hum Reprod* 1997; 12: 1654–6.
4. De Sutter P, Dozortsev D, Verhoeff A et al. Transport intracytoplasmic sperm injection (ICSI): A cost-effective alternative. *J Assist Reprod Genet* 1996; 13: 234–7.
5. Kovačič B, Plas C, Woodward BJ, Verheyen G, Prados FJ, Hreinsson J, De los Santos MJ, Magli MC, Lundin K, Plancha CE. The educational and professional status of clinical embryology and clinical embryologists in Europe. *Hum Reprod* 2015; 30: 1755–62.
6. Alikani M, Go KJ, McCaffrey C, McCulloh DH. Comprehensive evaluation of contemporary assisted reproduction technology laboratory operations to determine staffing levels that promote patient safety and quality care. *Fertil Steril* 2014; 102: 1350–6.

7. Abdalla HI, Bhattacharya S, Khalaf Y. Is meaningful reporting of national IVF outcome data possible? *Hum Reprod* 2010; 25: 9–13.
8. Intra G, Alteri A, Corti L, Rabellotti E, Papaleo E, Restelli L, Biondo S, Garancini MP, Candiani M, Viganò P. Application of failure mode and effect analysis in an assisted reproduction technology laboratory. *Reprod Biomed Online* 2016; 33: 132–9.
9. Cimadomo D, Ubaldi FM, Capalbo A, Maggiulli R, Scarica C, Romano S, Poggiana C, Zuccarello D, Giancani A, Vaiarelli A, Rienzi L. Failure mode and effects analysis of witnessing protocols for ensuring traceability during PGD/PGS cycles. *Reprod Biomed Online* 2016; 33: 360–9.
10. Cohen J, Gilligan A, Esposito W, Schimmel T, Dale B. Ambient air and its potential effects on conception *in vitro*. *Hum Reprod* 1997; 12: 1742–9.
11. Cohen J, Gilligan A, Willadsen S. Culture and quality control of embryos. *Hum Reprod* 1998; 13(Suppl 3): 137–44.
12. Merton JS, Vermeulen ZL, Otter T et al. Carbon-activated gas filtration during in vitro culture increased pregnancy rate following transfer of *in vitro*-produced bovine embryos. *Theriogenology* 2007; 67: 1233–38.
13. Heitmann RJ, Hill MJ, James AN, Schimmel T, Segars JH, Csokmay JM, Cohen J, Payson MD. Live births achieved via IVF are increased by improvements in air quality and laboratory environment. *Reprod Biomed Online* 2015; 31: 364–71.
14. Esteves SC, Bento FC. Implementation of cleanroom technology in reproductive laboratories: The question is not why but how. *Reprod Biomed Online* 2016; 32: 9–11.
15. Swain JE. Decisions for the IVF laboratory: Comparative analysis of embryo culture incubators. *Reprod Biomed Online* 2016; 28: 535–47.
16. Alikani M, Cohen J, Tomkin G et al. Human embryo fragmentation in vitro and its implications for pregnancy and implantation. *Fertil Steril* 1999; 7: 836–42.
17. Navarro PA, Liu L, Trimarchi JR et al. Noninvasive imaging of spindle dynamics during mammalian oocyte activation. *Fertil Steril* 2005; 83(Suppl 1): 1197–205.
18. Hall J, Gilligan A, Schimmel T, Cecchi M, Cohen J. The origin, effects and control of air pollution in laboratories used for human embryo culture. *Hum Reprod* 1998; 13(Suppl 4): 146–55.
19. Boone WR, Johnson JE, Locke AJ, Crane MM4th, Price TM. Control of air quality in an assisted reproductive technology laboratory. *Fertil Steril* 1999; 71: 150–4.
20. Morbeck DE. Air quality in the assisted reproduction laboratory: A mini-review. *J Assist Reprod Genet* 2015; 32: 1019–24.
21. Gilligan A. *Guidelines for material use in the USA during construction of a tissue culture laboratory.* Emerson, NJ: Alpha Environmental, 2015.
22. Seifert B. Regulating indoor air. Presented at the 5th International Conference on Indoor Air Quality and Climate, Toronto, Canada, 1990; 5: 35–49.
23. Sarigiannis DA, Karakitsios SP, Gotti A et al. Exposure to major volatile organic compounds and carbonyls in European indoor environments and associated health risk. *Environ Int* 2011; 37: 743–65.
24. Federal Standard 209E. Washington, DC: General Services Administration, US Federal Government, 1992.
25. Compendium of Methods for the Determination of Toxic Organic Compounds in Ambient Air, US EPA 600/4-84-041, April 1984/1988. [Available from the U.S. EPA through the Superintendent of Government Documents, Washington, DC.]

Quality control

Maintaining stability in the laboratory

2

RONNY JANSSENS and JOHAN GUNS

INTRODUCTION

It has now been almost 40 years since *in vitro* fertilization (IVF) was developed by Edwards and Steptoe. Over these decades, practice in assisted reproductive technology (ART) has evolved from a new experimental procedure into a well-established routine treatment of infertility driven by the development of new procedures such as intracytoplasmic sperm injection (ICSI), extended culture, preimplantation genetic diagnosis (PGD) and preimplantation genetic screening (PGS), vitrification, ongoing research, the development of better and safer products and culture media, more stringent quality control programs by commercial companies, and a better understanding of possible factors that might have an impact on the outcome of the procedure. Although success rates have improved over time, it is hard to define which laboratory practices contribute to this success (1). In a survey of U.S. high-performing centers, factors that were identified were experience of physicians, embryologists, and staff members, as well as consistency of approach, attention to detail, and good communication as being vital to excellent outcomes.

Together with the evolution from research towards worldwide routine application, we have seen increasing regulatory requirements and the development of professional standards for embryology laboratories. In the beginning of this century, both U.S. and European authorities issued regulations to ensure the quality and safety of human tissues and cells, and now the European Union Tissues & Cells Directive 2004/23/EC (EUTCD) (2) has been implemented in all EU member states.

Although the legislation differs between the U.S.A. and Europe and the interpretation and translation into national legislation of the EUTCD in the EU member states is different from country to country, there is a common requirement to implement a quality management system (QMS) in an ART laboratory.

All is well, until disaster strikes you. Remember Captain Smith, a very experienced captain on the helm of the Titanic when it sunk in 1912. Sometimes things do not go as expected and disasters or errors occur. All embryologists are or will be confronted with Murphy's Law: if anything can go wrong, it will go wrong. It is our challenge and professional duty to beat Murphy's Law and be better than Captain Smith and here, quality management can help.

Although sometimes seen as a burden, quality management supports a successful clinic. It is a tool to avoid unwanted and uncontrolled fluctuations in a process and ensures the consistency of approach and attention to detail so that stable results can be achieved over time. Essential elements of quality management (and relevant standards for quality management) leading to standardization are risk management, validation, standard operating procedures, communication, and training.

Risk management

Treatment is influenced by internal and external factors that create uncertainty in achieving the desired outcome. The effect of this uncertainty is "risk." Risk management (3) is an instrument dealing with the possibility that some future event might cause harm (4). It includes strategies and techniques for recognizing and confronting any such threat and provides a disciplined environment for proactive decision-making (or beating Murphy's Law). Risk management is now an essential element of accreditation or certification standards and is even mandatory for some regulatory authorities such as the Human Fertilisation and Embryology Authority (HFEA) (5) in the U.K. In a risk assessment procedure, you identify what the risks are, what would be the cause, what would be the consequence, and what controls could be in place to minimize risk. There are many risk assessment techniques (6), but the two most commonly used are failure mode and effects analysis (proactive) and fault tree analysis (retrospective). It is good practice to perform a proactive risk assessment before introducing or changing a procedure. Once risks are identified, they can be controlled or treated so that the likelihood or the consequence (impact) of an event is reduced. A good example of proper risk treatment in the IVF laboratory is the installation of a real-time equipment monitoring system (EMS). The EMS increases the detection of equipment malfunctioning and reduces the consequence by warning in time so that loss of valuable biological material can be prevented. Although there is an important investment cost to installing a real-time EMS, it has been demonstrated that, even for a small laboratory, an automated system can represent not just increased functionality, but it also saves money within three years (7). Monitoring and alarming is an essential tool for quality control and maintaining stability in the laboratory and is also required by EU directive 2006/86/EC (8), ISO 15189:2012 (9), and the HFEA code of practice (5).

Validation

In ISO 15189:2012 (9), the standard for accreditation of medical laboratories, validation is defined as "confirmation, through the provision of objective evidence, that the requirements for a specific intended use or application have been fulfilled." IVF is a process (a set of interrelated or interacting activities that transform inputs into outputs). A basic objective of validation is to ensure that each step and each variable of the process is identified and controlled and process variability is reduced so that the finished product meets customer requirements (consistent high pregnancy rates).

The U.S. Food and Drug Administration (FDA) published guidelines (10) that outline the general principles for process validation. Quality, risks, safety, and efficacy should be considered from the design phase of a process. Certainly in IVF, the quality of the "end product" cannot be measured, so each contributing factor (infrastructure, equipment, and utilities) and all the steps of the process need to be known and controlled.

Ideally, prospective validation is preferred, but certainly in existing IVF clinics this is not always possible, and then validation is done by analysis of historical data and prospective and concurrent product testing.

Validation should be performed for new premises, laboratory equipment, utilities, and processes and procedures and should result in written reports. During the validation, in-process controls should be defined in order to monitor the process.

Process validation is needed before the introduction (process design) of a new method into routine use, whenever the conditions change for which a specific method has been validated (other instruments, changes in environment, etc.) and whenever the method is changed (10,11).

During routine use, continuous process verification is necessary to ensure that the process remains in a state of control. Examples of laboratory processes that need to be validated are cleaning and decontamination procedures, sperm processing, IVF/ICSI, egg collection, embryo culture, cryopreservation, and embryo replacement.

In addition, equipment needs to be validated in order to provide a high degree of assurance that it will consistently meet its predetermined specifications with minimal variation. Equipment validation is broken down into three phases: installation qualification (IQ), operational qualification (OQ), and performance qualification (PQ). IQ is the first step and ensures that the equipment is correctly installed according to the manufacturer's specifications. As an example, a new incubator needs to be installed on a solid, vibration-free surface, the room temperature should be within a defined range, and the instrument should be connected to CO_2 and main power. During the next step, OQ, the equipment is calibrated and tests are performed in order to document a baseline of the critical parameters of the equipment. For an incubator, this is defining set points for CO_2, temperature, and oxygen and a verification of these parameters with independent, calibrated measuring equipment. The PQ phase then tests the ability of the incubator to perform over long periods within an acceptable tolerance range. The equipment, utility, and system should then be maintained, monitored, and calibrated according to a regular schedule by responsible personnel with appropriate qualifications and training. Parameters of calibration and equipment verification should be traceable to international standards. Calibrated equipment should be labeled, coded, or identified so that the calibration status and recalibration due date are clear. If equipment is not used for a certain period of time, then the calibration status needs to be verified before use.

Documentation

Good documentation is an essential part of any QMS. The process and equipment validation and laboratory standard operating procedures need to be correctly and completely documented. These documents should be approved by the laboratory director, regularly reviewed, and updated. Before any new or changed procedure may be introduced into routine, staff should be trained; the training should be specific and focused on the role of the employee.

Change control

The core principle of quality management is about change; change for continual improvement or the plan, do, check, act cycle. Whenever processes or procedures are changed, the impact of the change should be justified and documented in order to prove that the change does not adversely affect the process.

Change control is a systematic approach that is used to ensure that any intended modification to the process, equipment, instruments, facility, and so on, are introduced in a coordinated manner and to reduce the possibility that unwanted or unnecessary changes will be introduced into the culture system (12).

Unplanned deviation from these approved process or documents with potential impacts on quality, safety, or efficacy should be registered as non-conformity in the QMS.

The key principle of change control is to understand and document what was done, why, when, where, by whom, how, and what were the results.

Changes requiring revalidation are changes of facilities and installations, which may influence the process (cleanrooms or heating, ventilation, and air conditioning [HVAC]), changes in materials (puncture needles or transfer catheters) or reagents (culture media), changes in the process itself (implementation of new technology or findings based on current knowledge), changes in equipment, or support system changes (cleaning, supply, or information technology). All changes that have the potential to impact quality, safety, and efficacy should be justified, documented, approved (or rejected), communicated, and made known to laboratory staff and implemented in practice.

A change request procedure should be incorporated into the QMS.

QUALITY CONTROL AND QUALITY ASSURANCE

Having established in detail what aspects of the process are important to delivering the required quality (by proper validation), it is necessary that in-process controls are properly monitored. Regular monitoring of key performance indicators for fertilization, embryo development, and implantation provides good evidence of a clinic's performance, but unfortunately, a real decline in pregnancy rates may only be detected very late. It is therefore crucial to establish strict quality control procedures, routines, and controls to ensure that procedures and pieces of equipment operate appropriately and the process remains "in control."

This section will focus on the instruments and techniques used to document environmental and process parameters such as temperature and gas concentrations, and will discuss the quality control and quality assurance of laboratory personnel, infrastructure, equipment, culture media, and contact materials.

Infrastructure and environment

Cleanrooms and air quality

The relation between environmental toxicants and fertilization and embryo development has been reported by several authors (13,14). More recently, positive pressure in the lab, high-efficiency particulate air (HEPA) filtration of laboratory air, filtration for volatile organic compounds (VOCs), and use of chemical active compounds are identified as factors that are common in high-performing IVF programs (1). Most modern IVF centers are now located in cleanrooms.

HVAC functioning of a cleanroom should be monitored by a building monitoring system (BMS). The air quality requirement can vary from country to country, but most modern IVF laboratories are housed in cleanrooms classified ISO 8 to ISO 7 or EU GMP D to C. Once the clinic has specified its air quality requirements, compliance with the designated classification has to be demonstrated in the formal process of qualification (or validation). Qualification is mostly done on a yearly basis by a testing organization that performs normative tests compliant with the ISO 14644-1 and ISO 14644-2 standards (15,16). Qualification is followed by monitoring in order to control performance, both in rest state and in operation.

Air quality monitoring (17) consists of the enumeration of particles and microorganisms, both in rest and in activity. Before starting, a monitoring program needs to establish the sampling frequency and locations, the number of samples per location, the sample volume, and the test methods. This way of working, which is not yet familiar to ART and other tissue/cell establishments, derives from pharmaceutical guidelines. The EU directive refers to annex 1 of the EU GMP (18) that specifies the techniques for particle and microbial testing, similar to those described in the U.S. cGMP (17) and the U.S. Pharmacopeia for the production of medicines for human use (19). These pharmaceutical guidelines can guide the ART establishments in the setting up of a monitoring program.

Furthermore, the EU GMP makes a distinction between environmental monitoring at rest state and monitoring of the aseptic process in operation. Environmental monitoring verifies at rest state whether the environment is ready for the forthcoming activity, while aseptic process monitoring aims to ensure that the people, processes, and environment remain under control during operation.

Particle counters can be part of a BMS or an EMS. It is possible to monitor VOCs in laboratory air. Photo ion VOC detectors, measuring in the ppm range and with a 4–20-mV output, are commercially available and can easily be connected to any real-time EMS. Monitoring VOCs may lead to the detection of non-compliance of cleaning and disinfection procedures by cleaning staff out of working hours and can avoid the introduction of dangerous and toxic products released by non-approved cleaning agents.

The maintenance schedule for serving and filter replacement should be defined (by particle count for HEPA filters and analysis of filter saturation for active carbon and chemical VOC filters) and records should be kept of filter replacement dates and batch numbers. The preventive maintenance schedule should be defined in a service-level agreement between the laboratory and the company performing the maintenance.

Temperature—relative humidity

The absolute value of ambient temperature in the cleanroom is not really important (occupational health and safety rules should be respected) but should not exceed 25°C. If the environment of a cleanroom is cold and dry, microbiological contaminants will not grow. If the ambient relative humidity and temperature of the cleanroom environment exceeds 50% and 25°C, the risk of bacteria growth increases. On the other hand, humidity that is below 35% promotes static electricity, personal discomfort, and irritation of mucous membranes and eyes. An ambient relative humidity between 40% and 50% minimizes the impact of bacteria and respiratory infections and provides a comfortable working environment. Also, incubators do not function well if ambient temperature is above 30°C. However, for optimal lab performance, it is important to keep ambient temperature constant to avoid fluctuations in the surface temperature of equipment (heated stages and incubators), and therefore the ambient temperature should be monitored and alarmed.

During the design phase of a new cleanroom, attention should be given to the positioning of workstations and incubators so that they are not located directly in front of or below HEPA filtered air conditioning outlets.

Ambient temperature and relative humidity (RH) are usually monitored by a BMS.

Light

The effect of direct sunlight and hard white fluorescent light on mammalian zygotes and embryos is well documented (20,21) and most laboratories limit the amount of light exposure to gametes and embryos. In total, 95% of this light energy originates from microscope halogen lamps during manipulation and handling (22), and in particular, the blue region (400–500 nm) of light is harmful (23). Therefore, the use of green filters on microscopes is recommended.

Gas supplies

There is now convincing evidence that low oxygen concentrations for embryo culture are associated with increase live birth rates (24). IVF incubators depend on a supply of gas in order to regulate their internal atmospheres. Depending on the incubator's design, this is either 100% CO_2 and 100 N_2 for incubators with integrated gas mixing units, or custom-made mixtures of 5%–6% CO_2, 5% O_2 and 89%–90% N_2 for incubators without integrated gas mixing capacity (MINCTM benchtop incubator, Cook Medical; BT37 benchtop incubator, Origio/Planer). All gases should be of the highest quality and VOC filters should be installed on gas lines. Incubators with gas mixing units do have sensors and can give an alarm when the gas supply is failing, but this is not the case with incubators that run on premixed gasses. The latter can be monitored by placing a small Petri dish-sized infrared CO_2 sensor (25) inside an incubator chamber.

Laboratory equipment and real-time monitoring

Real-time monitoring (RTM) has long been seen as simply impractical because of the lack of accurate CO_2 sensors, the difficulty in connecting too many points, and the cost of cabling and adding sensors and data transmitters. Today, with the universal availability of low-cost wireless technology, the internet, smartphones, and tablets, this is no longer the case, and there are now affordable solutions that provide vital information in real time to monitoring systems and the people who need it, such as the laboratory manager. RTM systems can reduce "loss" by equipment failure and thus provide the manager with increased safety and reliability. Also, regulators see the benefits of monitoring; this requirement is now integrated into professional guidelines (26), regulatory requirements (8), and accreditation standards (9).

It is possible to connect analog sensors for temperature and gas levels (CO_2, O_2, and VOCs). If feasible, sensors that are independent from the equipment to monitor should be used. This makes it possible to detect equipment sensor drift, allows verification of manufacturers' performance claims, and may detect environmental factors such as electrical failure.

Air pressure, RH, airflow sensors, and particle counters can be connected to a RMS, but these parameters are usually integrated into a BMS. Laboratory ambient air monitoring should be part of the EMS since deviations in ambient temperate have consequences on the temperature regulation of microscope heated stages.

Digital signals that can be monitored in real time include door status and equipment alarm signals. It is even possible to read digital Recommended Standard (RS) 232 or RS 485 interphases.

Modern web-based systems provide accurate and effective control of equipment. The data are accessible remotely over a secure internet connection and intelligent alarms warn the laboratory manager in case of an unexpected event or equipment malfunctioning or failure. To increase reliability, technical alarms (sensor break, monitoring equipment failure, or network failure) should be possible, and this aspect should be taken into account when a monitoring system is chosen. Of course, with modern technology, it is possible to send alarms by telephone, email, or SMS, but the alarm messaging program should be bi-directional so that alarm acknowledgement is possible (and logged). In case of no reaction within a predefined timeframe, an automatic cascading system should be activated.

Culture system

Temperature issues

Although the optimal temperature for oocyte handling and embryo culture is not really known, limited decreases in temperature can alter the cytoskeleton (27) and spindle (28) of oocytes, and there is limited recovery after cooling and rewarming (29), indicating that human meiotic spindles are exquisitely sensitive to alterations in temperature and that the maintenance of temperature at 37°C during *in vitro* manipulations is important for normal fertilization and subsequent embryo development. These temperature effects are irreversible so it is important to avoid suboptimal temperatures. Temperature issues can occur during follicle puncture, during manipulations on heated stages on stereo microscopes and injection microscopes, in incubators, and during embryo transfer. Temperature should be measured in culture dishes under oil and in tubes with calibrated probes. The choice of measuring probe is important. Thin, fast-responding, non-shielded type T thermocouples can be used to detect small temperature gradients and are excellent at detecting hotspots on heating stages, while more precise, small probes fixed in culture dishes are more suitable for precise temperature measurements in incubators. While the most stable and accurate sensors are resistance temperature detectors (Pt100 and Pt1000), they are not easily available in small sizes for fixing inside a culture dish. For this purpose, thermistor probes are probably a better choice. Thermistors with 0.1°C accuracy are now widely available and at a very reasonable price. They have a fast response time and because of their high sensitivity are ideal for detecting temperature changes in culture dishes. Of course, accurate temperature measurement is only possible through the use of suitably calibrated sensors and instruments, and the accuracy of these measurements will be meaningless unless the equipment and sensors are correctly used. Good knowledge of measurement science is a basic requirement, one that is lacking in many laboratories.

Culture media and pH

The choice of culture medium is beyond the scope of this chapter. There is no ideal pH for culture media, as this varies from medium to medium and manufacturer to manufacturer, but it usually fluctuates within a range of 7.2 to 7.4. The pH of bicarbonate-buffered medium is regulated by the concentration of CO_2 dissolved in the culture

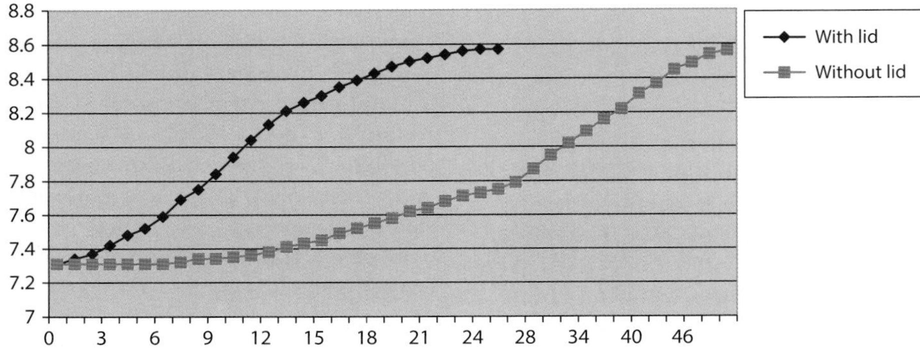

Figure 2.1 pH of culture medium under oil in ambient air over time (minutes).

medium, and this is regulated by the partial pressure of CO_2 in the incubator air. It is therefore important to carefully monitor incubator performance by RTM. In large-volume standard incubators, it is easy to integrate infrared CO_2 sensors. In small-volume desktop incubators, this is more challenging, but in some brands it is possible. While with modern and well-controlled incubators it is possible to maintain stable pH values, pH will increase while culture media are outside the incubator. To slow down this pH increase, oil is often layered over culture media. Besides this protective effect on pH, an oil overlay also reduces evaporation and heat loss and provides protection from particulate air contaminants.

The protective effect on pH is, however, quite limited in time, as shown in Figure 2.1. When culture medium is directly exposed to ambient air, the pH rise starts immediately. When a culture dish is removed from the incubator and the lid is left on the dish, then the pH starts to rise after 10 minutes. It is therefore good practice to leave lids on culture dishes during zygote and embryo scoring. These pH problems can be avoided by working in isolators with CO_2 (and temperature) regulation.

For quality control purposes, the pH of each batch of culture medium after proper equilibration should be measured and should be within the range specified on the certificate of analysis. A conventional pH meter with a glass electrode is technically challenging (samples for measurement have to be removed from the incubator, measurements should be done at 37°C, and measurements have to be done in ambient air) and time consuming. Better solutions are the continuous pH recorders in incubators or the use of a point-of-care blood gas analyzer.

Osmolality

The osmolality of commercial media ranges from 255 to 298 mOsm/kg (30). Most IVF labs culture embryos in droplets of media under oil overlay. Microdrop preparation can influence culture media osmolality, which can impair embryo development (31), so this technique should be standardized and staff should be trained in culture dish preparation. With recent developments such as non-humidified benchtop incubators and single-step media with prolonged culture without medium change, monitoring osmolality has become an important part of quality control (after opening and during storage) and process control (measurement of spend culture medium and after five to six days of culture). For this purpose, each laboratory should have a freezing point depression osmometer.

Contact materials

Disposables such as oocyte retrieval needles, culture dishes, ICSI needles, and transfer catheters are used extensively throughout the whole IVF procedure and the choice of disposable should be defined and its performance documented in a validation procedure. Disposables for embryo culture are available from many different manufacturers. Unfortunately, some have been shown to have toxic effects on gametes and embryos by sperm motility assay (32) or mouse embryo assay (MEA) (33).

The American Society for Reproductive Medicine (ASRM) practice guidelines (34) require that material that comes into contact with sperm, eggs, or embryos should be non-toxic and should be tested by the vendor with an appropriate bioassay or animal model. This includes, but is not limited to, aspiration needles, transfer catheters, plastic ware, glassware, culture media, and protein sources. The European Society of Human Reproduction and Embryology (ESHRE) guidelines (26) require that culture media should be mouse embryo tested, and the European Directives require that these disposables should be tested with an adequate bioassay by the supplier, but there is no consensus or standard on how this MEA test should be performed. Variables that have an effect on MEA sensitivity (35) are the starting point (oocytes, zygotes, or two-cell embryos), number of embryos per volume of culture medium, culture medium and use of albumin, exposure protocol of the disposable (medium volume and duration of exposure), and the use of an oil overlay, so manufacturers can easily modify their assay conditions and either aim to maximize sensitivity (with a high rejection rate) or reduce sensitivity (with a low rejection rate). Product inserts or certificates of analysis are not informative and the end-user cannot judge the real value of the company's statement "MEA tested." Laboratories should therefore request this information and select suppliers based on their transparency in providing information on test conditions, exposure protocols, and acceptance criteria.

Laboratory personnel

The number and qualifications of laboratory personnel are critical factors for maintaining stability in the laboratory. The recommended staffing levels are one full-time equivalent "bench" or "hand-on" embryologist per 120 stimulation cycles per year (36). As in any discipline in which technical proficiency can directly influence a measurable outcome, monitoring performance is essential to confirming that a procedure is carried out correctly and optimally and to discovering departures from protocol and opportunities for correction and improvement. Examples of performance parameters are number of two pronuclei and number of degenerated oocytes per total number of mature eggs injected (ICSI), number of embryos recovered intact and viable per number cryopreserved and per number thawed (cryopreservation or vitrification), number of clinical pregnancies per number of embryo transfers (embryo transfer), number of embryos continuing development per number of embryos biopsied, number of embryos with molecular signals per number of embryos biopsied (embryo biopsy), number of oocytes survived and intact per number of oocytes vitrified (oocyte vitrification), and number of gestation sacs per total number of hatched embryos (37).

Witnessing

One of the definitions of quality is to satisfy stated or implied needs or, in other words, to meet patients' expectations. Traceability of cells during IVF is a fundamental aspect of treatment, and involves witnessing protocols. Failure mode effect analysis of a human double-witness system has clearly demonstrated the loopholes and risks of manual witnessing (38). Automated electronic systems based on barcodes or radiofrequency identification tags can replace manual witnessing (39) and reduce the risk of gamete exchange. It is our experience that such an electronic witnessing system reduces staff distraction and stress, increasing staff efficiency.

REFERENCES

1. Van Voorhis B, Thomas M, Surrey E, Sparks A. What do consistently high-performing *in vitro* fertilization programs in the U.S. do? *Fertil Steril* 2010; 94: 1346–9.
2. Directive 2004/23/EC of the European Parliament and of the Council of 31 March 2004 on setting standards of quality and safety for the donation, procurement, testing, processing, preservation, storage and distribution of human tissues and cells. Official Journal of the European Union 7.4.2004.
3. ISO 31000:2009. Risk management—Principles and guidelines, 2009.
4. Mortimer D, Mortimer ST. *Quality and Risk Management in the IVF Laboratory*. Cambridge: Cambridge University Press, 2005.
5. Human Fertilisation and Embryology Authority. *Code of Practice*, 8th edition. http://www.hfea.gov.uk/code.html
6. ISO 31010:2009. Risk management—Risk assessment techniques. 2009.
7. Mortimer D, Di Berardino T. To alarm or monitor? A cost–benefit analysis comparing laboratory dial-out alarms and a real-time monitoring system. *Alpha Newsletter* 2008; August: 1–7.
8. Directive 2006/86/EC implementing Directive 2004/23/EC of the European Parliament and of the Council as regards traceability requirements, notification of serious adverse reactions and events and certain technical requirements for the coding, processing, preservation, storage and distribution of human tissues and cells. Official Journal of the European Union 25.10.2006.
9. ISO 15189:2012. Medical laboratories—Requirements for quality and competence, 2012.
10. FDA (CDER, CBER, CVM). Process Validation: General Principles and Practices, 2011.
11. Huber Ludwig. Validation of Analytical Methods and Procedures. http://www.labcompliance.com/tutorial/methods/
12. OECD Principles of Good Laboratory Practices. http://www.oecd.org/chemicalsafety/testing/oecdserieson-principlesofgoodlaboratorypracticeglpandcomplianc-emonitoring.htm
13. Cohen J, Gilligan A, Esposito W, Schimmel T, Dale B. Ambient air and its potential effects on conception. *Hum Reprod* 1997; 12: 742–9.
14. Johnson JE, Boone WR, Bernard RS. The effects of volatile compounds (VC) on the outcome of *in vitro* mouse embryo culture. *Fertil Steril* 1993; (Suppl 1): S98–9.
15. International Standard Organisation. Cleanrooms and associated controlled environments—Part 1: Classification of air cleanliness, ISO 14644-1, 1999.
16. International Standard Organisation. Cleanrooms and associated environments—Part 2: Specifications for testing and monitoring to prove continued compliance with ISO 14644-1, ISO 14644-2:2000, 2000.
17. Guns J, Janssens R, Vercammen M. Air quality management. In: *Practical Manual of In Vitro Fertilization: Advanced Methods and Novel Devices*. Nagy ZP, Varghese AC, Ashok A (eds.). pp. 17–25, 2012.
18. European Union. EU Good Manufactering Practice. Medicinal Products for Human and Veterinary Use. Annex 1: Manufacture of Sterile Medicinal Products (corrected version), 91/356/EEC, 2008.
19. USP29-NF24. *Microbiological Evaluation of Clean Rooms and Other Controlled Environments*. Baltimore, MA: United States Pharmacopeia, 2010.
20. Schumacher A, Fischer B. Influence of visible light and room temperature on cell proliferation in preimplantation rabbit embryos. *J Reprod Fertil* 1988; 84: 197–204.

21. Takahashi M, Saka N, Takahashi H, Kanai Y, Schultz RM, Okano A. Assessment of DNA damage in individual hamster embryos by comet assay. *Mol Reprod Dev* 1999; 54: 1–7.
22. Ottosen LDM, Hindkjar J, Ingerslev J. Light exposure of the ovum and preimplantation embryo during ART procedures. *J Assist Reprod Genet* 2007; 24: 99–103.
23. Korhonen K, Sjövall S, Viitanen J, Ketoja E, Makarevich A, Pëippo J. Viability of bovine embryos following exposure to the green filtered or wider bandwidth light during in vitro embryo production. *Hum Reprod* 2009; 24: 308–14.
24. Bontekoe S, Mantikou E, vanWely M, Seshadri S, Repping S, Mastenbroek S. Low oxygen concentrations for embryo culture in assisted reproductive technologies. *Cochrane Database Syst Rev* 2012; 7: CD008950.
25. https://planer.com/products/petrisense-ph-co2-sensor.html
26. Magli MC, Van den Abbeel E, Lundin K, Royere D, Van der Elst J, Gianaroli L. Revised guidelines for good practice in IVF laboratories. *Hum Reprod* 2008: 23: 1253–62.
27. Almeida PA, Bolton VY. The effect of temperature fluctuations on the cytoskeletal organization and chromosome constitution of the human oocyte. *Zygote* 1995; 3: 357–65.
28. Pickering SJ, Braude PR, Johnson MH, Cant A, Currie J. Transient cooling to room temperature can cause irreversible disruption of the meiotic spindle in the human oocyte. *Fertil Steril* 1990; 54: 102–8.
29. Wang WH, Meng L, Hackett RJ, Odenbourg R, Keefe DL. Limited recovery of meiotic spindles in living human oocytes after cooling-rewarming observed using polarized light microscopy. *Hum Reprod* 2001; 16: 2374–8.
30. Swain JE, Pool TB. Culture media in IVF: Decisions for the laboratory. In: *Practical Manual of In Vitro Fertilization: Advanced Methods and Novel Devices.* Zsolt PN, Alex CV, Ashok A (eds.). New York, NY: Springer, 2012.
31. Swain J.E, Cabrera L, Xu X, Smith GD. Microdrop preparation factors influence culture-media osmolality, which can impair mouse embryo preimplantation development. *Reprod Biomed Online* 2012; 24: 142–7.
32. Nijs M, Franssen K, Cox A, Wissmann D, Ruis H, Ombelet W. Reprotoxicity of intrauterine insemination and *in vitro* fertilization-embryo transfer disposables and products: A 4-year survey. *Fertil Steril* 2009: 92: 527–35.
33. Van den Abbeel E, Vitrier S, Lebrun F, Van Steirteghem A. Optilized bioassay for the detection of embryology contaminants. *Hum Reprod* 1999; 114.
34. The Practice Committee of the American Society for Reproductive Medicine and the Practice Committee of the Society for Assisted Reproductive Technology. Revised guidelines for human embryology and andrology laboratories. *Fertil Steril* 2008; 90(Suppl 3): S45–S59.
35. Boone WR, Higdon HL, Johnson JE. Quality management issues in the assisted reproduction laboratory. *J Reprod Stem Cell Biotechnol* 2010; 1: 30–107.
36. Alpha Scientists in Reproductive Medicine. The Alpha Consensus Meeting on the professional status of the clinical embryologist: Proceedings of an expert meeting. *Reprod Biomed Online* 2015; 30: 451–61.
37. Go KJ. 'By the work, one knows the workman': The practice and profession of the embryologist and its translation to quality in the embryology laboratory. *Reprod Biomed Online* 2015; 31: 449–58.
38. Rienzi L, Bariani F, Dalla Zorza M, Romano S, Scarica C, Maggiulli R, Nanni Costa A, Ubaldi FM. Failure mode and effects analysis of witnessing protocols for ensuring traceability during IVF. *Reprod Biomed Online* 2015; 31: 516–22.
39. Thornhill AR, Brunetti XO, Bird S, Bennett K, Rios LM, Taylor J. Reducing human error in IVF with electronic witnessing. *Fertil Steril* 2011; 96(3): S179.

The assisted reproduction technology laboratory 3

Current standards

CECILIA SJÖBLOM

INTRODUCTION

Quality assurance (QA), quality control (QC), and accreditation are concepts that seem to touch on a wide range of functions in our society. QC systems and standardization are especially needed in units for assisted reproduction technology (ART) to ensure the reproducibility of all methods and that all members of staff are competent to perform their duties. The necessity of a QC system becomes even clearer when considering the possible risks of ART.

Over the years that ARTs have been practiced, extensive knowledge has been gained on how to run an ART laboratory and what methods to use in order to achieve ultimate success. Facing the future, we encounter other variables such as the safety and efficiency of the laboratory, and quality and standardization become key features. Professional, national, and international guidelines on how ART should be performed have been established over the years, and many countries have legislation concerning how ART should be practiced (1–3). Among others, England, Australia, and the U.S.A. have instituted a system whereby the ART clinics have to be licensed to practice these techniques and the clinic as well as the laboratory are audited by a third-party authority in order to ensure correct practice (4–7). However, with the increased knowledge of the importance of implementing quality systems, most clinics choose to conform to any of a range of available standards.

This chapter first provides an overview of the most common laboratory standards together with some regional/national guidelines and regulation. Then it provides a simple "how-to" guide for laboratories seeking to conform to internationally recognized standardization. Then, most importantly, it goes beyond the standards to establish some key determinants of success, which are interdependent for maintaining high quality standards, safety, and improved results in the *in vitro* fertilization (IVF) laboratory.

STANDARDS

International standards and regulatory frameworks

International Organization for Standardization (ISO) 9001 (8) is the most widely used standard in ART clinics and involves the quality system of the whole organization. This standard covers the need for quality management and the provision of resources (both personnel and equipment), and a substantial section involves customer satisfaction and how to improve services. A more detailed overview of ISO 9001:2015 is presented in Chapter 32 (9).

ISO 17025:2005, specifying general requirements for the competence of testing and calibration laboratories (10), is the main international standard for laboratory accreditation. It is based on the European norm (EN) 45001 (11), and was originally modeled on the corresponding ISO/International Electrotechnical Commission (IEC) guide (12). The scope of this standard is specialized and is aimed toward assurance of methods and includes both the quality system and the technical part of the activities such as validations of methods, QA, QC, and calibration of equipment. In 1997, Fertility Centre Scandinavia became the first IVF laboratory to be accredited according to this international standard (13).

With an increase in laboratory accreditation it was evident that ISO 17025, aiming to standardize testing and calibration laboratories, could not fully accommodate and cover the complexities of a medical testing laboratory. ISO 15189, on medical laboratories, particular requirements for quality, and competence, was issued to aid the accreditation of methods used in medical testing. It was first issued in 2003, with the current second edition issued in 2012 (14). It is used for the accreditation of medical laboratories and brings together the quality system requirements of ISO 9001 and the competency requirements of ISO 17025, and addresses the specific needs of medical laboratories.

Most medical laboratories in Europe and Australia are accredited according to ISO 15189:2012. There are differences between the two laboratory standards, with ISO 15189 focusing on patient outcome without downgrading the need for accuracy, and it emphasizes not only the quality of the measurement, but also the total service provided by a medical lab. The language and terms are familiar to the medical profession, and it highlights important features of pre- and post-investigational issues while addressing ethics and the information needs of the medical laboratory. ISO 15189:2012 addresses the need for equivalency of quality management systems and competency requirements between laboratories. The need for this becomes more obvious at a time when potential and actual patients are increasingly mobile—the systems to collect medical data on these patients must be standardized independently from their location.

IVF laboratories located in the EU are required to adhere to the Directive on setting standards of quality and safety for the donation, procurement, testing, processing, preservation, storage, and distribution of human tissues and cells, usually called the European Union Tissue and Cells Directive (EUTCD) and its guide/supporting documents (15–19). The European Society of Human Reproduction and Embryology (ESHRE) have issued a position paper on the EUTCD (20), and it is important to underline that regardless of ESHRE's recommendations, each EU country interprets the Directive differently. However, one part of the EUTCD is very clear: the demand for a quality system. The Directive states that "Tissue establishments shall take all necessary measures to ensure that the quality system includes at least the following documentation; standard operating procedures (SOPs), guidelines training and reference manuals." Certainly, by achieving accreditation to ISO 15189, this demand will be fulfilled, along with several other demands of the Directive.

Joint Commission (JC; U.S.A.) and Joint Commission International (JCI) accredit and certify hospitals and healthcare organizations worldwide. It is a non-profit organization with the main focus on improving patient safety. JCI have a range of standards including Accreditation Standards for Clinical Laboratories (21). The World Health Organization (WHO) in collaboration with JC and JCI has developed a core program for patient safety solutions. It brings attention to patient safety and practices, which can help reduce the risks involved with medical procedures. The most recent advice builds on "nine patient safety solutions" including patient identification, and recommends actions in four basic categories: (i) risk management and quality management systems; (ii) policies, protocols, and systems; (iii) staff training and competence; and (iv) patient involvement (22).

The Clinical and Laboratory Standards Institute (CLSI) is another global not-for-profit standards development organization, and while mostly applicable to the U.S.A., the CLSI standards are of great help for improving laboratory quality and safety (for further information, see Chapter 2 [23,24]).

Other standards that might be less suitable for the IVF laboratory are the Good Manufacturing Practice/Good Laboratory Practice (GMP/GLP) guides. These standards apply to research laboratories and the pharmaceutical production industry. They include demands on the laboratory facilities that will be difficult to meet with the limited resources that many IVF clinics have (25,26).

In addition to these quality system-driven standards, there are many IVF-specific standards and guidelines including WHO laboratory manuals for the examination and processing of human sperm (27) and the Alpha/ESHRE consensus on embryo assessment (28). The Alpha consensus group has published a consensus for cryopreservation establishing key performance indicators (KPIs) and benchmarks for both slow freezing and vitrification (29).

National/regional standards

While the ISO standards cover the fundamental needs for quality systems in the IVF laboratory, many regions and countries have specific guidelines, laws, and regulations. It is important to note that while some of these regulatory frameworks are standards and others are license requirements or law, when it comes to inspections and audits, the laboratory is expected to conform.

Europe

With the EUTCD in place, all IVF laboratories handling gametes and embryos are required to have a quality system and to fulfill the demands of the Directive and the national interpretation of it. This has led to most of the IVF laboratories in the EU holding or working toward formal accreditation to ISO 15189 or ISO 17025. ESHRE have recently published revised guidelines for good practice in IVF laboratories, providing an easy-to-navigate guide to support laboratory specialists and also to fulfill some of the demands of the Directive (30). In the U.K., where all IVF clinics are required to be licensed by the Human Fertilisation and Embryology Authority (HFEA) (31), there are further guidelines regulating the IVF laboratory as detailed in the HFEA code of practice (HFEA CoP) (32). Specifically, the CoP contains demands for risk management, sample identification, and embryology staffing as described later in this chapter.

Australia and New Zealand

In Australia, the Reproductive Technology Accreditation Committee (RTAC) undertakes the licensing of IVF clinics. While the RTAC CoP (7) is far less comprehensive than its U.K. counterpart, it contains critical criteria with a focus on risk management, staffing, and sample identification, as well as further guidelines covering the requirement of a quality management system. In addition to the code, Fertility Society Australia issues technical bulletins, which act as educational communication to all units and certifying bodies, offering advice and guidance. It is not enforceable (33). In New Zealand, RTAC licensing is optional, but most clinics hold an RTAC license. While the majority of IVF clinics hold an ISO 9001 certification, most are also accredited by National Association of Testing Authorities (NATA) to ISO 15189 for some of the crucial methods such as semen analysis. However, very few laboratories hold ISO 15189 accreditation for the overall IVF laboratory processes.

Asia

At the time of publication, there were few, if any, IVF laboratories in Asia accredited according to ISO 15189 or similar standards and the laboratory accreditation was not widespread. However, there is an increased interest and need for standardization. Many private IVF centers throughout the region have ISO 9001 certification.

Memorial Hospital in Istanbul, Turkey, was the first IVF laboratory in the region to achieve ISO 15189 accreditation (acknowledging that Turkey is a transcontinental country at the junction of Europe and Asia).

With the introduction of strict regulations of ART in China, it has become increasingly challenging to obtain approval to operate an ART center. The Ministry of Health issued the first series of regulations on ART in 2001 and these have been regularly revised, with the latest updates issued in 2015 (34). These regulations have detailed requirements with respect to facilities, staff, equipment, clinic management, QA/QC, indication and contraindication of IVF, intracytoplasmic sperm injection (ICSI), egg donation, and preimplantation genetic diagnosis, among others, as well as the ethical aspects of various issues. In addition, since 2006 the department requires control inspections of ART providers to be done every two years and that there is provision for accredited training of ART specialists. The Chinese Society of Reproductive Medicine of the Chinese Medical Association is actively engaged in detailed ART treatment guideline establishment and implementation.

The Indian health authorities are working on an ART Bill, with the 2014 draft still to be legislated. The Indian Council of Medical Research (ICMR) have issued National Guidelines for Accreditation, Supervision, and Regulation of ART Clinics (not legislated) (35). The guidelines cover issues such as staff qualifications and laboratory procedures, but neither the draft Bill nor the ICMR Guidelines have a formal demand for quality systems. The PNDT Act (Prenatal Diagnostic Techniques) prohibits sex selection pre- and post-conception. ISO certification is not widespread for individual IVF clinics, but larger hospitals that have IVF departments are commonly ISO certified.

In Japan, the Japan Society of Obstetrics and Gynecology have created guidelines for IVF treatments and clinics. They do not, however, comprehensively cover laboratory practices and the need for quality systems. As a result, some clinics have created their own umbrella organizations for implementing common quality practices within IVF called the Japanese Institution for Standardising Assisted Reproductive Technology (JIS-ART).

In Singapore, the Ministry of Health has introduced stringent licensing requirements for assisted reproduction services in private hospitals and clinics. It covers demands for QC, facilities, embryology training, and sample identification (36). All IVF providers in Singapore are accredited according to the international version of the RTAC CoP (37).

Middle East

ART in many Muslim countries is covered by a number of fatwas (religious opinion concerning an Islamic law issued by an Islamic scholar) (38). The first fatwa relating to ART was issued in 1980 by His Excellency Gad El Hak Ali Gad El Hak, the Grand Sheikh of Egypt's Al-Azhar University. The core requirement is that the couple is married, and the use of donor sperm or oocytes is prohibited (39).

Apart from the fatwas, there are very few regulations and standards for IVF laboratories in the Middle East and few laboratories are formally accredited to international standards, but many larger hospitals hold JCI and ISO accreditations.

Saudi Arabia has a comprehensive fatwa containing demands for documented SOPs, safeguarding of sample ID, and prevention of mix-ups, among others. The Ministry of Health has started setting standards and some centers have had their first audit by the authorities (38).

The United Arab Emirates (UAE) has stringent laws regulating IVF and all laboratories have audits by the UAE health authority. There are also requirements that all laboratories should obtain an international accreditation within 3 years of starting up. The law includes demands on the embryology staff degrees and training, laboratory facilities, documented protocols and procedures, and QC. The regulations have on and off prohibited cryopreservation of embryos (currently illegal); however, there are indications that this legislation will be changed in the near future (40).

Latin America

The Latin American Network of Assisted Reproduction (RED) covers most of the Latin American clinics. While membership in the organization is voluntary, over 90% of clinics participate in the data collection, accreditation, and continuous professional development training programs. The accreditation includes external audits and follows the Standard Rules for the Accreditation of the ART center and its laboratories of embryology and andrology (41) involving, among others, QC, KPIs, staff requirements, equipment, and materials.

Russia

There are no IVF laboratories in Russia accredited to ISO 15189. However, with the growing interest in IVF tourism and with the prospect of attracting patients from Europe, many clinics in Russia are working toward implementing European standards. So far, four centers hold ISO 9001:2015 certification and at least one of those is in the process of achieving ISO 15189. One large center holds full College of American Pathology (CAP) accreditation. Russia has limited standards and regulations for IVF and separates between state-owned and private clinics. The state clinics are required to report data to the Ministry of Health, but there are no formal audits and so implementation of the rules is not widespread.

North America

In 2004, the Canadian Federal Government passed the Assisted Human Reproduction (AHR) Act and created the Federal agency Assisted Reproduction Canada (42,43). The Act is divided into prohibited activities, including cloning, non-medically indicated sex selection, and the payment of donors, and controlled activities, covering the performance of all procedures involved in IVF. The Act was challenged by the province of Quebec, leading to a lengthy, complicated legal battle ending with the Supreme Court of Canada ruling that much of the AHR Act was unconstitutional and that the regulation of clinics is the responsibility of provinces (44). Quebec has passed an Act of its own, with breaches resulting in hefty fines; however, Ontario, which has a high number of IVF clinics, does not have any regulation. A handful of clinics are accredited through Accreditation Canada and the audits include a laboratory expert assessing laboratory space and environment, procedures, and safety aspects. The Canadian Fertility and Andrology Society

(CFAS) have published a number of clinical practice guidelines and are working toward comprehensive professional standards concerning the laboratory activities involved in IVF prepared by its ART Lab Special Interest Group, as well as training and competency requirements that include the continuing professional development of all ART laboratory scientists (45).

In the U.S.A., the practice committee of the American Society for Reproductive Medicine and the practice committee of the Society for Assisted Reproductive Technology have issued guidelines for human embryology and andrology laboratories (46,47). A comprehensive overview of the U.S. standards and regulations for IVF laboratories can be found in Chapter 2 (24).

HOW TO ACHIEVE LABORATORY ACCREDITATION

It is important to underline that in no way are all the quality standards independent of each other. ISO 17025:2005 is basically the same standard as ISO 15189:2012, with the major difference being the medical laboratory terminology used in ISO 15189. The quality system requirements of both standards are based on ISO 9001:2000. As a result of this, laboratories within ISO 9001-certified clinics seeking accreditation will have major parts of the system requirements of the two laboratory standards already in place. It could be recommended that the first step toward accreditation is to get the clinic certified to ISO 9001; further details on this subject are found in Chapter 30 (9). The requirements discussed throughout the continuation of this part of the chapter will be for laboratory accreditation to ISO 15189 or ISO 17025 on top of (over and above) what is already required for certification to ISO 9001. For example, scope, organization and document control are found in all the standards and many of the demands are the same, but the requirements discussed in these sections below will be what ISO 15189 has (hereinafter referred to as the standard) in addition to what has already been implemented through ISO 9001 certification. Correlation tables for ISO 9001, 17025, and 15189 can be found in the standards themselves.

GETTING STARTED

The first step toward an accreditation is to make sure that everyone in the organization wants to achieve the same goal. The full understanding of how everyone benefits from an accreditation will make the process easier. A good way to ensure this is to have staff meetings throughout the process and involve all staff from the very beginning. The most frequent mistake organizations make when trying to implement a QC system is not to involve everyone. Divide the project into smaller sections and give out personal responsibilities enabling all staff to be included in the preparation work. This will also make the implementation easier.

A good way to make sure that all demands in the standard are covered is to make up a table of contents—using the ISO 15189:2012 standard table of contents as a template (Table 3.1). An assessment can then be made of what needs to be added to the quality manual and other documentation. It is important to note that while the standards have demands for management structure, internal audit, or document control, the laboratory standards have some more specified demands not found in ISO 9001, and these need to be added to the specific procedures.

Table 3.1 Table of contents for ISO 15189:2012

1 Scope
2 Normative references
3 Terms and definitions
4 Management requirement
4.1 Organization and management
4.2 Quality management system
4.3 Document control
4.4 Service agreements
4.5 Examination by referral laboratories
4.6 External services and supplies
4.7 Advisory services
4.8 Resolution of complaints
4.9 Identification and control of nonconformities
4.10 Corrective action
4.11 Preventive action
4.12 Continual improvement
4.13 Control of records
4.14 Evaluations and audits
4.15 Management review
5 Technical requirements
5.1 Personnel
5.2 Accommodation and environmental conditions
5.3 Laboratory equipment, reagents, and consumables
5.4 Pre-examination process
5.5 Examination process
5.6 Ensuring quality of examination results
5.7 Post-examination process
5.8 Reporting of results
5.9 Release of results
5.10 Laboratory information management

METHODS AND SOPS

Examination process (ISO 15189:2012; 5.5)

The methods and processes we use in the embryology laboratory and their efficacy has a direct impact on the pregnancy results of the clinic. It is therefore hugely important that we standardize these methods and make sure that they are reproducible. In simple words, an ICSI should be done in the same way using the same disposals and equipment by all embryologists in the lab, ensuring that an ICSI done by embryologist A on a Monday is performed in exactly the same way and with the same level of skill as an ICSI done by embryologist B on a Friday. Ensuring the performance of correct methods is achieved through several steps. First, we need to make sure that the processes and methods we use are correct and up to date with the latest developments in ART. Hence, a clear starting point should be a literature search, together with the knowledge gained from workshops, external training, and visits to other clinics. Once the details of the methods have been agreed between the embryology team members, they need to be documented. A document describing a method or process used in a laboratory is commonly called an SOP. A good SOP should follow a set format and ISO 15189:2012; 5.5.3 contains a very good guide for SOP layouts. The SOP title should be followed by a short clinical description of the method. The analytic principles need to include a theoretical description of the method and review of the current literature. The SOP should outline the competence demands on embryologists performing the process. Collection and handling of gametes and embryos should include the sampling procedures and the physical environmental issues such as temperature. Remember that all variables in the SOP, such as those referring to the measurement of temperature, have to give a precise range, followed by a description of how the temperature is measured, the accuracy of the thermometer, and how often and how it is calibrated. There should be clear descriptions of how the sample is labeled and, considering the risks associated with the work in an IVF laboratory (48), the marking should be logical and clear in order to eliminate completely the risk of mixing of samples (for further details, refer to the "Sample identification, witnessing, and prevention of misidentification" section). The description of the procedural steps should be written in an uncomplicated way so that they can be easily followed by any new member of staff under supervision.

All equipment used for the method should be listed with references to handling instructions and calibration protocols. Any safety routines and occupational hazards involved should be discussed and clearly known by the embryologists. References to any textbooks or publications concerning the method should be included last.

The standard demands that the procedures used should meet the requirements of the users of the laboratory service, preferably using methods that have been published in established/authoritative textbooks, peer-reviewed texts, or journals. If in-house methods are used, these need to be appropriately validated for the intended use and fully documented by the laboratory.

When the SOP is written, it needs to be communicated to all members of the embryology team, and it is important to allow them to comment, give feedback, and suggest changes before the document is formally issued and implemented. The way to check that all embryologists follow the new SOP is to undertake audits and it is suggested to audit all processes three months after the issue of the SOP. If the audit findings include discrepancies between the written SOP and the embryologists' hands-on working procedure, then either the SOP needs to be changed to reflect the actual hands-on procedure or the member of staff needs to be retrained and reminded of the importance of following the agreed SOP. No embryologists can insist on doing things "their own way" in a standardized high-quality IVF laboratory.

Once the SOPs are fully implemented and the audits show that we have achieved the required reproducibility, then we need to ask: is it working? Is the method we agreed upon successful? The standard calls this "validation" and it is the process that confirms that the techniques and methods used in the IVF laboratory are suitable for the production of good embryos, viable pregnancies, and live births. All methods have to be validated regularly, and the SOP should include information on how often and how validations are done. The EUCTD includes demands for validation, and in the U.K., the HFEA CoP (32) requires that all processes in the IVF laboratory should be validated. Some methods and techniques used in the laboratory can be difficult to validate, and it is acceptable to use retrospective analysis of fertilization, damage, and pregnancy rates to validate ICSI and IVF. Appropriate validation of new techniques can become very difficult when considering the sample size needed to prove a null hypothesis or small increase in pregnancy rates. An accurate validation of a new culture medium will need hundreds of patients in each study group. Adding to the complexity of validation practice is the fine line between validation and research, and questions are raised regarding the need for ethical approval to undertake validations (49). However, it is highly recommended to regularly validate other practices in the lab, such as changes of osmolarity during preparation of dishes, temperature fluctuation during denudation, and temperature distribution in incubators. Validation of temperature in a culture medium in different types of dishes on all heated stages in the laboratory should confirm the appropriate range of surface temperature of the heated stage.

HANDLING OF GAMETES AND EMBRYOS

Pre- and post-examination process (ISO 15189:2012; 5.4, 5.7)

The standard has specific demands on how the sample—that is, gametes and embryos—should be collected and stored. The samples have to be correctly and safely identified and any laws regulating the identification of patient samples have to be taken into account (for further details, refer to the "Identification, witnessing, and prevention of misidentification" section). The sample should be accompanied by a written, standardized request of what procedure the sample should be used for. It is a common occurrence that the requests for treatment are unclear and that couples who could have had normal IVF end up having ICSI due to poor communication. Senior embryologists with considerable experience in assessing sperm samples are more suitable to making the final decision on IVF or ICSI in conjunction with the couple on the day of treatment when the sample has been washed than the referring doctor who takes the decision on IVF or ICSI based solely on a semen analysis report. Other procedures where clear requests are crucial are frozen embryo transfer cycles to ensure that the embryo is thawed on the correct day. For collection of sperm, the date and time of collection should be noted by the patient and the date and time of receipt should be recorded by the laboratory.

Usually, the procedures for collecting samples at pre- and post-examination are documented in the applicable laboratory SOPs for sperm processing and oocyte collection. However, it is important to include the specific demands of the standards for these procedures and the documentation of them.

LABORATORY SHEETS AND REPORTS

Reporting and releasing results (ISO 15189:2012; 5.8, 5.9)

The details from assessments of gametes and embryos we document in the laboratory on lab sheets are referred to in the standard as reports. The reporting of results should always be accurate, clear, unambiguous, and objective. This requires that the lab sheets be standardized and follow a set format. They should be filled out in a neat manner—no scribbling allowed. All entries and comments on a lab sheet should be accompanied by a date and signature. For sperm assessment, sources of errors and uncertainty of measurements should be stated and properly calculated for each method. Formal reports, such as seminal fluid analysis reports, should also be checked and signed off by the senior andrologist/embryologist before being issued.

Many laboratories have computerized databases and enter the information from the lab sheets into the database. It is important to understand that the handwritten lab sheet is considered source data and therefore needs to be archived correctly, not destroyed after computer entry. If the laboratory wants to go paper free it has to indeed be paper free and allow for direct data entry onto the computer without an in-between paper sheet. When considering the need for signatures and witnessing, a complete paperless IVF laboratory could be difficult to create.

THE EMBRYOLOGY LABORATORY

Facilities (ISO 15189:2012; 5.2)

A laboratory needs to ensure that the environmental conditions of the laboratory are suitable for the safe handling of gametes and embryos and do not invalidate the results or adversely affect the quality of any procedure. In simple words, this means that the IVF laboratory has to be designed in such a way that the outcome of any procedure is optimal and not affected by environmental parameters.

Live birth results following IVF treatment vary from country to country and from clinic to clinic, and often within a clinic from month to month. It is a general consensus that patient demographics, such as age and cause of infertility, are the main factors affecting the outcome. Considering a varying population of patients, it is of great importance that parameters in the laboratory are stable. Defining the environment and setting limits for acceptable working conditions will help with reducing variables and result in the patient being the only factor that varies. Exactly what this encompasses will always be down to interpretation and international, national, or regional regulations; however, the standard has some clear demands, and some environmental factors cannot be ignored.

General laboratory layout

The theater for oocyte retrieval and embryo transfer should be in close vicinity to the laboratory. The laboratory layout should further ensure safe handling of gametes and embryos; small, crowded laboratories impose a significant risk for accidents, resulting in loss of gametes and embryos.

The laboratory should never double as an embryologist office. There needs to be a minimal allowance of paper in the laboratory as this can increase the amount of particles in the air. Therefore, only patient records necessary for ongoing treatment should be kept in the laboratory. Also, the laboratory is not the place for cardboard boxes as these involve a high risk of fungus infections. Furthermore, the laboratory is not a storage room for disposables; only a weekly stock of disposables should be kept inside the lab, and further storage can be managed elsewhere. The equipment held in the laboratory should be limited to only that which is absolutely necessary; again, the laboratory is not a storage room for old lab equipment.

Access rules

The laboratory should have limited access ensured by use of locks, swipe cards, or other access controls. It should also hold documentation verifying who has access to the laboratory. There should be documented and implemented rules for what is required for access to the laboratory including demands for change of clothes and shoes, the use of hair cover and masks, and the washing of hands. While some embryologists insist that changing clothes and covering hair are of no importance, it is important to understand that embryology and handling of gametes and embryos are sterile processes with a need to protect the samples from microbes and contaminants. The correct degree of cleanliness is impossible to reach if the embryologists are using their own clothes or only minimal cover such as laboratory coats. Best practice is to change clothes and preferably use scrubs, which are made of low-lint, no shedding material; cotton is high lint and not advisable. Many embryologists complain that these types of scrubs are uncomfortable and that they will not use them as cotton is comfortable, but it is important to understand that we did not become embryologists to be comfortable—we need to do what is best for gametes and embryos. Further, all hair should be covered, and again some might see the cap as a fashion item that looks much better if hair is allowed outside it, but they need to be reminded to tuck in all hair before entering the laboratory. Changing into cleanroom shoes goes without saying. Best practice is to have all-white shoes with white soles in the laboratory. This makes it easy to spot any spillage on them. Also, the rack for these shoes should be designed so that the shoes are hung up with soles facing out, allowing for daily inspection of the cleanliness of the shoes. If colored shoes are used outside the laboratory it will be easy to spot anyone who has forgotten to change shoes. Hands should be washed using a proper disinfectant soap before entering the laboratory. Furthermore, jewelry, nail polish, long fingernails, and perfumes should not be worn in the laboratory.

Health and safety

The laboratory is required to ensure the safety of its entire staff. This includes providing an environment that minimizes the risk of transfer of any contagious contaminants through the use of class II biosafety cabinets when handling unscreened patient materials.

Temperature

The optimal IVF laboratory temperature is a matter of great debate; however, it has to be defined to a limited range. Some embryologists argue that an elevated laboratory temperature benefits the embryos through reduced risk of cooling during transport from the incubator to the heated stage. However, high laboratory temperatures will provide a perfect environment for microbes and contaminants. All laboratory equipment is designed to operate at room temperature, usually defined as 22 ± 2°C, and unless the laboratory can show process verification at a different temperature, this range will be the one demanded by the standard. A laboratory without temperature control cannot be accredited.

Light

The embryo is extremely sensitive to light exposure; however, there is a wide range of opinions on whether light in the laboratory or from microscopes will harm embryos or not. It has been very elegantly demonstrated in a large study on hamster and mouse embryos that cool fluorescent light increases the reactive oxygen species production and apoptosis in blastocysts and reduces the development of live-term fetuses (50). The embryos were handled under minimal light conditions and the test groups were exposed to 5–30 minutes of cool white, warm white, or midday sunlight. A total of 44% of blastocysts exposed to cool white light and transferred to recipients developed to term of pregnancy (day 19), compared with 73% in the control; 58% of blastocysts exposed to warm white light developed to term (day 19). When embryos were exposed to only one minute of sunlight, only 25% of embryos developed to term, with 35% being resorbed. In light of these findings, best practice should be to have a dim light in the laboratory and to close out any daylight.

Air quality

Another area of great debate is the demands of clean air in the laboratory, and this has also been affected by regional interpretation of the EUCTD. The standard requires that attention is paid to sterility and presence of dust and it is highly recommended that laboratories periodically monitor the particle count and presence of volatile organic compounds (VOCs) in the air, together with microbial monitoring using contact plates for surfaces, such as replicate organism detection and counting containing Sabouraud dextrose agar (SDA; for detection of fungus) and trypticase soy agar (TSA; for detection of bacteria) and similar (TSA and SDA) settlement plates for air sampling. The plates should be exposed in key positions in the laboratory, theater, and treatment rooms for four hours. Acceptable limits are zero colonies inside the flow hoods or handling chambers and <10 colonies outside the hoods in the laboratory.

General cleanliness

An IVF laboratory should always be clean and the laboratory standards demand that documented frequent cleaning procedures are implemented and that cleaning is confirmed by active signatures. The use of harsh detergents is not recommended and cleaning should be undertaken using 70% alcohol and sterile water or other products tested for embryology use such as Oosafe® (SparMED, Stenløse, Denmark) (51). Steam cleaners are suitable for the cleaning of floors.

CULTURE MEDIUM, DEVICES, AND DISPOSABLES (ISO 15189:2012 4.6, 5.3)

All devices used in ART, such as culture media and consumables, will affect the outcome of the treatment. First, the laboratory needs to decide on their own requirements for culture medium, oocyte collection needles, culture dishes, and so on. This includes limits in toxicity and results from mouse embryo assays for culture media, oocyte pickup needles, or plastic ware. There is solid evidence that many of the devices and disposables we use in the embryology laboratory are indeed reprotoxic and it is our duty to make sure that we do not use items that will expose the embryos to stress (52). It is important to take into account any national, regional, or local regulation that applies. EUTCD stipulates that all devices that come into contact with cells, gametes, or embryos need to be tested according to the EU devices directives (53,54) and be Conformité Européenne (CE) marked. The laboratory also has to define requirements for the safe transport of devices from supplier to the laboratory, and how they will be inspected when they arrive to ensure they meet the limits specified. For example, there has to be a system to ensure that the box containing the culture medium is still cold when it arrives. This can easily be done by inserting a temperature probe into the box upon arrival, or requesting that the medium provider pack a temperature data logger with the medium, which you can attach to your computer when the medium arrives and ascertain that the temperature inside has been constant and correct throughout the transport. Moreover, consumables then have to be verified before taken into use. Some laboratories choose to culture excess embryos or undertake sperm survival assays in new batches of culture medium; however, this type of verification is not demanded by the standard, and it could be argued if it is really necessary (for testing methods, see Chapter 2) (24). If all the devices conform to the EU devices regulation, they should already have been stringently tested. ISO 15189 only demands that the laboratory actively checks the test reports issued by the manufacturer and confirms that the reports comply with their own limits for use.

When the devices have been accepted for use, it is crucial that they are stored correctly to ensure their continued suitability for use. The laboratory has to safeguard correct storage by defining the exact storage environment. Limits for temperature in refrigerators and freezers are crucial and culture medium should be stored in a pharmaceutical refrigerator that guarantees a constant temperature throughout, whereas a normal kitchen refrigerator is not acceptable (Chapter 2). The environment in general storage rooms is also important as plastic ware stored at high temperatures will not be suitable for use.

All purchased supplies, reagents, and consumables should be included in the laboratory inventory. Information in the inventory shall include lot number (batch number), date of reception, and date taken into use. The inventory for equipment should include unique identification, date of arrival, date placed in service, last calibration or service, and periodicity of service and calibration. The laboratory is required to keep a list of approved suppliers and to critically evaluate all suppliers on an annual basis.

The batch or LOT number of any device that comes into contact with a given patient's gametes or embryos needs to be recorded on that individual patient's records.

It is not appropriate to have a list of batches currently used in the lab and to draw conclusions from this using the date and guesswork of what device was used for what patient.

It is of great advantage to have a computerized case file system whereby each cycle has a batch record page attached. This page includes a full list of culture media and laboratory ware and the batches in use, and with a simple mouse click, it marks what materials were used in every step of the cycle, from culture media down to pipette tips.

EQUIPMENT (ISO 15189:2012; 5.3)

A laboratory should have all the equipment needed to ensure provision of the best service. The standards require a documented program for preventive maintenance and it is the responsibility of the laboratory manager to regularly monitor and ensure appropriate service, calibration, and function of all equipment. All equipment used in an accredited laboratory has to be clearly labeled with a unique identifier, date of last calibration or service, and date or expiration criteria as to when recalibration/service is due. Together with this, all equipment used should be included in an equipment record containing information listed in ISO 15189:2012; 5.3.1.7. There should be clearly documented processes for validation of equipment function before it is taken into use. The standard of equipment used in IVF laboratories is generally very high, but even the best equipment can fail and not function optimally if it is not appropriately maintained. All embryologists should have solid knowledge of how to operate all equipment and there should be written implemented procedures in place for action taken if there happens to be an equipment failure. Crucial equipment such as incubators should always be connected to auto-dialers enabling staff to promptly respond to any faults out of hours.

Equipment should be verified by test runs; for example, before a new centrifuge is taken into use in the laboratory, a series of mock sperm preparations have to be undertaken and documented.

MONITORING AND TRACEABILITY (ISO 15189:2012; 5.2, 5.3, 5.5)

Chapter 2 presents a detailed report of the monitoring of equipment and laboratory parameters and the traceability of reference equipment (24).

Monitoring of KPIs

Most clinics that have a quality system in place monitor KPIs. Similar to the monitoring of laboratory environmental parameters, each clinic has to agree on documented limits of performance. Usually, when monitoring parameters such as live birth, clinical pregnancy, and fertilization, there is no upper limit; however, a lower limit is necessary, as well as documented plans for immediate action whenever a KPI falls under the agreed limit.

The KPIs that are essential for monitoring in connection with the laboratory include, but are not limited to, fertilization rates for IVF and ICSI, damage rates for ICSI, survival of embryos after thawing, and pregnancy results from embryo transfer. Benchmarking and KPI monitoring are hotly debated topics and it must be underlined that trying to benchmark against a different laboratory's KPIs is a futile exercise, as laboratory performance is affected by factors such as patient selection, among others. The best benchmarking for KPIs is done against an in-house-determined "gold standard." This is a subsection of good-prognosis patients and the indicators for this group should be very much constant. For example, a drop in the overall KPI for fertilization with no drop in the corresponding "gold standard" indicate that the issue is related to the material coming into the laboratory. However, a drop in the KPI for the "gold standard" definitely suggests that there might be a problem with performance.

KPIs should be monitored for the whole laboratory and for each embryologist and doctor. It is important to underline the importance of confidentiality when monitoring individual performance, taking into account the need for the training of any embryologist falling under the given limit, but not ignoring the stress and decrease in self-confidence this can lead to. All members of staff need to understand that the monitoring is not a way of punishing people, but rather to ensure that all embryologists perform to the same high standard, minimizing variables. Another important outcome of individual performance monitoring is to identify persons with exceptionally high results so that others can learn more and thereby increase the overall success.

QUALITY ASSURANCE

Ensuring quality (ISO 15189:2012; 5.6)

QA makes sure that you are doing the right thing in the right way and QC makes sure that what you have done is what you expected. In short, QA is process oriented and QC is product oriented. When discussing QA/QC it is easy to get confused; however, the terminology is not important—what is important is that the laboratory has control mechanisms in place to ensure that they perform according to the SOPs and to the highest standard. ISO 15189:2012 demands that the laboratory has QC and QA systems in place for monitoring of the validity of the methods used. This includes the demand of internal and external controls and inter/intra-laboratory comparisons and validations. The laboratory is required to determine the uncertainty of results. This can be difficult with a subjective parameter such as embryo scoring; however, it can easily be done for the assessment of sperm. Through assessment of a series of sperm samples by all laboratory staff involved in the preparation of sperm, a coefficient of variance can be calculated, usually resulting in a 10%–15% variance.

The standard also demands that all embryologists/andrologists assess sperm samples and photos or movies of embryos on a regular basis, usually at least every three months. It is the responsibility of the laboratory manager to document the results from these comparisons, calculate variations, and address any deviance. To collect samples and photos and arrange these types of intra-laboratory comparisons takes time and, over and above this, the standards also demand that the laboratory participates in inter-laboratory comparisons. A laboratory can share photos of embryos and samples of sperm with other centers and set up an inter-laboratory comparison scheme, although the standard clearly states that self-developed programs like this should not be used when organized external schemes are available. In the U.K., most laboratories participate in the U.K. National External Quality Assessment Service (UKNEQAS) andrology and embryology morphology scheme, which uses online resources, DVDs, and/or formalin-fixed samples for assessment (55).

A web-based inter-laboratory comparison scheme is run by Dr. James Stanger and includes schemes for the assessment of all stages of human preimplantation embryos, sperm morphology and concentration, and ultrasound measurement of follicles (www.fertaid.com). The scheme provides monthly assessments of embryos and sperm and allows the laboratory manager to use the information for intra-laboratory comparison. As each of the different schemes has some 200–300 participants around the world, the intra-laboratory comparison scheme provides a solid reference for the laboratory management to implement corrective actions when deviations are found (56). This comparison program is in substantial agreement with the ISO/IEC guide 43-1, which is a requirement by the standard (57).

PATIENT CONTACT

Advisory services (15189:2012 4.7)

In most IVF clinics, the embryologists have no or very little contact with the patient and also very little input into the exact treatment options. In an accredited laboratory, the standard demands that the laboratory actively provides advice on choice of treatment and clarification of any laboratory outcomes. As discussed previously, some decisions such as fertilizing oocytes using IVF or ICSI should be taken by a senior embryologist rather than a doctor. The ultimate approach is to have the couple/patient sit down with the embryologist after oocyte and sperm collection for a "post-oocyte pick up (OPU) chat." This gives the opportunity for the embryologist to discuss with the couple/patient issues such as the quality and numbers of sperm and oocytes, and advise them on the best procedure ahead. This short chat should also include reminding the couple/patient of risk and success; that is, there is always a risk for failed fertilization, failed cleavage, or failed blastocyst development. If the couple/patient has been reminded of these risks, it makes it somewhat less stressful to make a call to them in the unlikely event of a failed fertilization. ISO 15189 even demands that the embryologist should take part in the clinical rounds (i.e., meeting with the patients), enabling the provision of advice and guidance on embryology in general and in individual cases.

AUDITS

(ISO 15189:2012 4.14)

Audits can be internal or external, vertical or horizontal, or process oriented or system oriented. Therefore, it is easy to get confused and caught up in terminology, and to miss out on the great opportunity that audits provide for improving the system and our service to patients. To find nonconformities at an audit is not bad—it is proof that the system is working and we are capable of recognizing our weaknesses and faults and ready to learn and improve on them. For general internal audit principles, see Chapter 32 (9).

Internal audits

The laboratory standards are more precise in what exactly should come out of an audit and what is needed for a correct audit process. When preparing, writing, and implementing internal audit procedures, ISO 15189 is very precise and elaborate on what exactly is needed. In relation to ISO 9001 internal audit demands, the laboratory standards are more stringent with how often internal audits need to be undertaken, and it requires all accredited methods and procedures to be audited on an annual basis.

External audits

If the laboratory aims to seek formal accreditation to ISO 15189, the National Authority for Conformity Assessment performs the external audits. A formal accreditation is always advantageous, but in many countries this option is not available, and as it is a rather pricey process, some laboratories choose to state that they adhere to the standard without formal accreditation.

When a laboratory is ready to be formally accredited they need to apply for accreditation and the national authority will assess whether they have the appropriate expertise to perform the audit. If not, they can seek help from other members of the International Laboratory Accreditation Cooperation (ILAC) or European Cooperation for Accreditation who have the appropriate experienced auditors. Together with the application, the laboratory has to supply evidence of a fully compliant quality system and it is essential that all methods for which accreditation is sought have gone through a series of internal audits. Result documentation from these audits is supplemental to the application. The accreditation body then arranges a pre-audit to assess the readiness of the laboratory and, pending the outcome of this pre-audit, an accreditation audit will be arranged. When the accreditation audit has been done, the lead auditor or any technical experts can only recommend that the laboratory be awarded accreditation. This recommendation is then passed on to the board of the accreditation body, which will decide if the laboratory is to be awarded accreditation.

BEYOND THE STANDARDS

While the embryology laboratory could be seen as any other clinical medical laboratory, there are some major differences to do with the delicacy of the samples it handles. While a mistake in the day-to-day pathology laboratory can mostly be rectified by resampling, a mistake in the embryology laboratory can lead to major irreparable trauma for the patients (48). Therefore, it is of great importance that we acknowledge these differences and implement processes that help safeguard us from incidents. While some national and regional guidelines acknowledge these differences, IVF laboratories worldwide need to understand and address this. There are three major areas concerning the safeguarding of patients' gametes and embryos, but also aiming to protect the embryologists working in the laboratory: (i) training of embryologists to make sure that the staff handling these delicate samples and undertaking the complex IVF processes are properly trained; (ii) appropriate sample identification processes; and (iii) implementation of risk management processes.

Training and accreditation of embryologists

Personnel (ISO 15189:2012; 5.1)

Clinical embryology is a highly skilled profession and the main contributors to IVF success are the skills and knowledge of the embryologists. When considering the impact that the training of embryologists has on results, it is evident that there is a need for formalized training programs in every clinical IVF laboratory.

When looking at the international ISO standards, the requirement for personnel is not clearly defined. They state that the laboratories need to define all personnel groups within the laboratory in respect of education and experience and the areas of responsibility should be clearly outlined together with duties in the documented job descriptions. The quality manual should include documentation on how proof of competence is issued and how introduction of new personnel is performed, and the management of the laboratory should formulate goals for each member of staff with respect to further education and training. These goals should be assessed and discussed at annual appraisals, which should be documented but kept confidential. There should be clearly documented procedures in place for the introduction and training of new staff and the reintroduction of staff after long periods of absence or leave.

In recent years, there has been an increased focus on the training and accreditation/certification of clinical embryologists. In the U.K., there has been a formal training program in place for embryologists since 1995 through Association of Clinical Embryologists (ACE) (58). The original program (ACE Certificate) included a minimum of two years and had both practical and theoretical components (58). The current training program is managed under the National Health Service (NHS) Scientist Training Program (59). This is a three-year graduate entry program that is covered by a fixed-term employment and, upon finalization, awards the holder a Master's degree in reproductive science from an accredited university. Post-training, clinical embryologists follow a career pathway including gaining certification from the Association of Clinical Sciences (ACS; state registration and membership of the Royal Collage of Pathologists). ACE also provide an online continual professional development scheme.

In 2008, ESHRE introduced a certification for embryologists with the aim of certifying the competence of clinical embryologists working in IVF and of developing a formal recognition for embryologists (60). It provides two different pathways to certification: a senior track and a clinical track. All ESHRE members who meet the requirements can apply. The assessment includes a logbook outlining the procedures included in the training and the minimum cases done, and passing a multiple-choice examination. ESHRE also offer a continuous embryology education credit system, with the credits being needed for three-yearly renewal of the certificate.

The Canadian Fertility and Andrology Society have issued guidelines for an applied training program and evaluation and development of competencies for ART laboratory professionals and will in the near future implement formal certification/accreditation (45).

For a comprehensive overview of embryologist requirements in the U.S.A., see Chapter 2 (24).

In Australia, Scientists in Reproductive Technologies (SIRT) are in the process of formalizing embryology training, aiming for a future certification and continuous professional development system.

With the U.K. career development pathway being available for U.K. embryologists only and with the ESHRE certification, while available for all ESHRE members, requiring the embryologist to travel to the annual ESHRE conference to sit the exam, there is still a need for clinics to find ways of formalizing training for their embryologists. Every clinic should have documented training procedures clearly stating the minimum of supervised procedures a trainee has to undertake before being signed off for independent work. For the ESHRE certification this includes 50 procedures of each of OPU, semen analysis and preparation, insemination, ICSI, zygote and embryo evaluation, embryo transfer (ET), cryopreservation of oocytes/embryos, and thawing of oocytes/embryos. Obviously the outcome of those procedures needs to be evaluated too, and the trainees have to meet the set KPIs of the clinic to be approved. To ensure the theoretical component—that the trainee knows why, and not only how—it is suggested that essays set on subjects such as preimplantation genetic diagnosis and embryo development are included along with a small examination. It is also crucial to fulfill the need for continued professional development, allowing embryologists to attend conferences and workshops and to participate in research.

Sample identification, witnessing, and prevention of misidentification

One of the most crucial tasks in the IVF lab is to ensure the correct identity of gametes and embryos. Over the years, there have been numerous reports of misidentification resulting at best in a cancelled cycle if the mistake is identified before embryo transfer, and at worst in tragedy if realized after the embryo transfer or indeed birth. These errors are generally the result of trained personnel not following the known procedure for reasons such as distraction, tiredness, or being rushed (61,62). Alternatively, it is caused by poorly written or nonexistent policies and protocols (active failure vs. latent condition). The solution to misidentification is the development of robust identification procedures that are risk assessed (for further details, see the "Risk identification, management, and prevention" section).

The EU tissue directive includes demands for appropriate sample identification with the core being a unique identifier for each sample. However, the most stringent guidelines involving safe sample identification procedures are provided by the HFEA CoP (32). In the U.K., it is a licensing requirement to have robust ID systems (Mandatory Requirement T71, HFEA CoP) and all IVF laboratories have to put in place processes to ensure that no mismatches of gametes or embryos or identification errors occur. With this comes a demand for double witnessing of the identification at all critical prints of the IVF laboratory process. The witnessing has to be signed at the time of the checked step and records must be kept in each patient's case file. Together with this license requirement, the guidelines stipulate that all samples of gametes and embryos be labeled with at least the patient's name and a unique identifier such as a clinic or cycle-specific couple identifying number. Most clinics interpret this as using the surname and a clinic or cycle-specific couple identifying a number such as couple number. It is important to note that a patient's name or date of birth is not a unique identifier. The witnessing is mandatory and required every time gametes or embryos change vessel (dish or tube) and the person checking should have full understanding of the process they are witnessing, allowing only clinic staff named on the HFEA license to undertake the check. At semen sample handover, oocyte retrieval, and embryo transfer, the patient is required as an active participant in the identification.

In Australia, RTAC have issued a technical bulletin on Patient and Sample Identification (Technical Bulletin 4), and while this document is very detailed and provides robust guidelines for identification, it is not enforceable (33). Similarly, the recently updated ESHRE laboratory guidelines include a section on identification of patients and traceability of their reproductive cells (30).

While most laboratories use manual double witnessing, identification checks can also be electronic, with several witnessing systems being available for embryology purposes. The most commonly used are based on barcodes (Matcher, fertqms.com; Trusty, optimalivf.com.au; OCTAXFerti Proof™, www.mtg-de.com) or using radiofrequency technology (RI Witness™, www.research-instruments.com). The advantages of automated systems are that their accuracy is not affected by lack of concentration or poor protocols (62), and they have a significantly lower error rate than human error (0.001% compared with 1%–3%) (63). So by introducing electronic witnessing we can possibly reduce errors in misidentification and potentially add an extra level of patient safety (63,64). But at the same time it is important to underline that all the current electronic witnessing systems are based on some type of sticker being attached to the tubes and dishes and mistakes can certainly occur in printing and labeling. Moreover, while the systems are not foolproof, they are expensive and some are bulky, taking up a substantial space. The development of electronic witnessing systems for IVF is only at its infancy and the technology will more than likely be refined in the future.

In addition to the HFEA CoP, RTAC bulletin, and ESHRE guidelines, which are IVF specific, there are several standards and recommendations on the subject of patient and sample identification. The CLSI guideline on Accuracy in Patient and Sample Identification (64) describes the essential components of processes and systems that need to be implemented for accurate patient and sample identification. It covers the whole process from the pre-examination phase to the reporting of results, underlining the importance of staff training, risk assessment, and the use of unique identifiers, and it relates to both manual and electronic systems. The previously mentioned "nine-patient safety solutions" from WHO/JCI have patient identification at its core (22). The ISO standards also have demands of correct sample labeling; however, they offer little information on safe solutions.

There are certainly huge advantages to the use of manual double witnessing, but there is always a slight risk that a procedure like this can cause mistakes, as we cannot double the embryologist workforce. One major source of incidents in the IVF laboratory is insufficient staffing, and to be interrupted while working with embryos can have disastrous consequences. In a busy IVF lab setting, scientists need to switch repeatedly between the patients' material they are working on to the patients' material they are being asked to check (65,66). In practice, the principle operator interrupts their workflow to locate a "witness" and the "witness" is interrupted from their own task to carry out the double check. Daniel Brison (67) estimated that, in a well-staffed IVF lab, each embryologist was witnessing 15–20 other procedures in a morning on top of their own workload. Many laboratories today have very few embryologists, and with a witnessing routine in place this will not only increase the workload, but will also add a heightened risk of distraction when an embryologist has to interrupt others' work to get them to witness a certain step in the procedure. Moreover, human beings and systems under stress will underperform in rushed situations and stress is known to affect human performance in many sectors, including the IVF laboratory. Most clinics have periods when patient throughput is increased without compensation in relation to staffing levels. Systematic overtime, overloaded work schedules, high cognitive loads, and chronic staff shortages contribute to error-inducing environments (68–70). In addition, other forms of stress such as inadequate training and lack of guidance have been identified as sources of identification errors (71).

When introducing a robust, safe ID system in the laboratory, the best way of starting is to avoid reinventing the wheel. Even if your laboratory is located outside the U.K., the HFEA CoP Section 18 provides a great guide on how to ensure that the correct gametes are mixed and the right embryos transferred (32). To make it simple, the IVF laboratory has to have written protocols for witnessing and each step involved has to be risk assessed (documented). As a part of the standardization introduced into a laboratory, there will be written SOPs and flowcharts, and it is easy to identify each step where a gamete or embryo changes tube or dish. Simply add a witnessing signature to the laboratory sheet to each of those steps (the procedure itself should already have a signature on the sheet). An exception to the witnessing requirements is the so-called "forced functions," such as when a clinic receives only one sperm sample on a given day, and so there will be a forced function when the sample is transferred from one tube to another. If the clinic makes use of this it has to be risk assessed.

With the first step in the process being reception of gametes, semen samples, or oocytes and the last step being embryo transfer, the HFEA CoP underlines the need for the patient to be involved in this crucial identification step. Here it is important to implement a process that involves positive patient identification, which is the foundation for error prevention (72). In simple words, the embryologist will ask the patient to audibly read out his/her name and any other identifier you have chosen such as date of birth, and at the same time have a witness—the doctor or nurse—to confirm this positive identification step being done.

The witnessing action itself also needs to be done correctly. It should include three major components: (i) the ID-labeled vessel that holds the gametes or embryos; (ii) the new vessel that the sample is being moved in to, labeled with the same ID; and (iii) the patient documentation (i.e., the laboratory sheet containing the full identification of the patient). In addition to these three components, the embryologist performing the "move" (principle operator) reads the name and unique identifier aloud from the sample vessel, the new vessel, and the laboratory sheet, followed by the witness reading aloud the same.

Other hugely important factors are the strength and quality of the identifier itself. The need for a strong unique identifier together with the name is paramount. With the date of birth being too weak and not considered unique, the clinic or laboratory needs to create a couple-specific identifying number such as a unit number or couple number. A patient-specific number such as a medical records number is not advisable as the embryo mostly belongs to the couple, not one patient only. This identification, name, and couple number then need to be affixed to the vessel in a clear, safe manner. The most widely used labeling is handwriting with a nontoxic pen. Usually, the ID is written on the side of tubes and bottom of dishes (mirrored from the outside) to allow easy noticing. Printed stickers are also being used; however, it should be made clear that stickers contain glue and, when placed in a humidified incubator, this results in an increase of VOCs, which in turn can be toxic to the embryo. Another way of labeling is etching the ID into the plastic using a small syringe, but scratching of plastic will also increase VOCs and can be toxic to the embryo. Moreover, the etched details appear very faint and cannot be considered safe from a clear witnessing point of view. Finally, the ID should always be affixed to the part of the vessel actually carrying the sample. Labeling the lid of a dish or a tube is not acceptable.

If a process involves gametes or embryos changing vessel several times during a short time period, such as sperm preparation or embryo freezing/thawing, then it can be acceptable to witness the whole area. For example, a laboratory preparing sperm can have multiple biosafety cabinets with one designated centrifuge and other equipment assigned to a specific defined work area. Note that each work area has to have a designated centrifuge and two samples cannot be centrifuged together if this approach is adapted. When a sample is being brought into this area, all tubes involved can be witnessed at the same time with the prospect that only one sample will be handled through the whole process from start to finish (Figure 3.1). Obviously this process needs to be risk assessed if adapted.

Correct labeling together with witnessing procedures will help minimize the risk of misidentification, but it is also absolutely imperative that only one couple's samples are handled at any one time. Preparation of a number of sperm samples, or cryopreservation or thawing of multiple patients' embryos at the same time, poses a huge risk for mix-ups and should never be done.

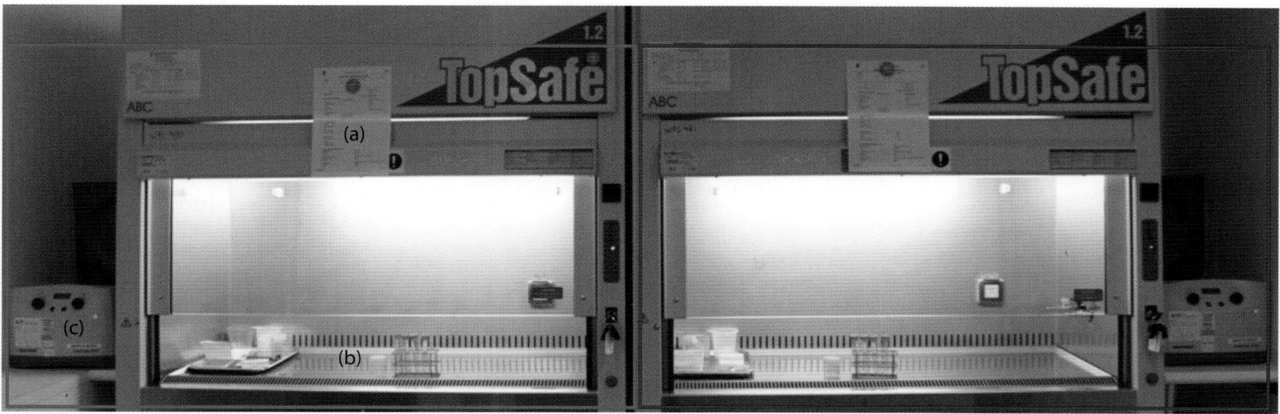

Figure 3.1 Sperm preparation areas RED and BLUE each containing all equipment needed for complete sperm preparation. (a) Documentation for the patient, assigning work area RED to this patient. (b) Labeled sample pot and preparation tubes are double witnessed when brought into the area. (c) Only the sample currently being prepared in area RED is centrifuged in the area's designated centrifuge. When the preparation is complete, the area is sterilized before being assigned to the next patient.

Risk identification, management, and prevention

According to the WHO, one in six couples experience difficulties in conceiving and would need some form of assisted reproduction method (73). Worldwide, over 3.75 million children have been born as a result of an ART treatment and it is estimated that over 800,000 treatment cycles are undertaken annually (74–76). With the increase in IVF cycle number worldwide, it has become evident that just like in other areas of medicine and healthcare, errors are inherent. But it is important to remember that these errors most often result from a complex interplay of multiple factors; only rarely are they due to the carelessness or misconduct of single individuals. Historically, rather than addressing the source of errors, prevention strategies have relied almost exclusively on enhancing the carefulness of the caregiver (77). A culture of blame and finding a scapegoat has commonly been the response to adverse events, and this is an approach that can never improve the system and prevent the incident form reoccurring. The portioning of blame to an individual usually comes with a promise that "it will never happen again" (78). The crucial changes in the approach to risk management in IVF clinics are presented in Table 3.2.

In order to prevent errors and identify risks, IVF laboratories must introduce robust risk management including an analysis of systems and structures in advance of those risks actually materializing, thus embedding risk management into the daily routine for embryologists. The international standard ISO 31000:2009 Risk Management—Principles and Guidelines (79) is the most widely acknowledged tool for addressing, managing, and preventing risk. Implementing this standard will vastly decrease the risk of adverse events and near misses, but also provides tools for how to learn from incidents when they happen and prevent them from happening again. ISO 31000 will provide a clear guide on how to set up a risk management policy and clearly outlines what needs to be included.

Errors and incidents result from failures and these can be categorized as active failures or latent conditions (80,81). Active failures result from violation of the agreed protocols, lapses, or mistakes. Latent conditions or errors include error-provoking conditions such as workload, fatigue, knowledge, supervision, and equipment and weaknesses in defense including unworkable procedures or switching off a malfunctioning alarm. Latent conditions are embedded in all systems as it is not possible to foresee all error-producing situations. However, as they pre-exist, active failures may be able to be identified prior to adverse events occurring. Therefore, these conditions tend to be the targets of risk management systems.

The first step toward risk management in the laboratory is to have a clear overview of the protocols and procedures undertaken by the embryologists. This should be provided already as part of the quality system and demand for SOPs. With the use of process maps and flow charts for the procedures, it will be easy to identify areas and procedures that could be high risk, but total risk management has to include all processes and procedures. Mortimer and Mortimer (82) provide a simple summary of risk management by asking and answering three basic questions: what can go wrong? What will we do? If something happens, how will we resolve it? There are three core tools for helping us address risk and to answer those questions: failure mode and effects analysis (FMEA), root cause analysis, and audit.

A comprehensive way of proactively addressing risk is to make use of FMEA. Like many approaches that improve quality and safety, FMEA has its origins in the army, space, and aviation industry, but is now used as a tool for error prevention in a wide range of industries, including healthcare. The aim of FMEA is to try to think of every possible way a process can go wrong, how serious it would be, and how the process can be improved to avoid failure. It is important that all embryologists in the team are involved in assessing each process using FMEA. A simple format for FMEA is illustrated in Table 3.3.

Table 3.2 Shift in approaches to risk management in *in vitro* fertilization clinics

Outdated approach	Modern approach
Main goal	
To protect the IVF clinic's reputation	To improve patient safety and minimize risk of harm to and misidentification of embryos and gametes through better understanding of systemic factors that affect the risk for incidents
Reporting	
Acknowledge only reports submitted in writing	Variety of methods to report: paper form, electronic form, telephone call, anonymous reporting, person-to-person reporting
Investigation	
Investigate only the serious occurrences	Encourage reporting of "near misses" and investigate and discuss the potential causes
Interview staff one on one when there is an adverse incident	Have root cause analysis meetings with the entire team
Corrective/preventive action	
Blame and train (or dismissal)	Perform a criticality analysis chart and determine the root cause of the "near miss" or the adverse occurrence
Work with department involved to develop corrective action	Work with the team to develop a safety improvement plan
Information from investigation kept confidential	Develop corrective action and share with the whole IVF team
Communication	
Talk to the patients only if necessary and be vague about incident/findings	Advise clinic director to speak directly with the patients and talk with them about any unexpected outcome and error; keep them appraised of steps taken to make the environment safe for the next patient
Long-term follow-up	
Assume that action is taken to correct the problem that occurred, notice only when it happens again that no action is taken	Monitor and audit to determine that changes have been initiated and that the changes have made a difference

Source: Adapted form Kuhn AM, Youngberg BJ. *Qual Saf Health Care* 2002; 11: 158–62.
Abbreviations: IVF, *in vitro* fertilization.

The first step is to identify the process to be assessed, using the examples of insemination, mixing of oocytes, and sperm for IVF. Then identify what could go wrong (potential failure mode); for example, an embryologist forgets to inseminate, mixing the wrong oocytes and sperm, losing oocytes, bumping a dish, and so on. Then ask "what could be the result of this failure?" It could be failed fertilization, creation of an embryo or indeed child with the "wrong parents," and decreasing the chances of pregnancy. Then assess the seriousness of the suggested failures using a 1–10 scale with 1 being no effect and 10 being critical. For failed fertilization one could argue a seriousness of 8, but the creation of a mixed-up embryo has a severity of 10. Once severity has been established, address the different causes of the failure; in this case, being rushed, low staffing levels, poor processes, lack of checklists, and no witnessing system. Then rate how often this would happen from 1 being no known occurrences (has never happened in any IVF clinic) and 10 being very high risk (with this happening regularly). Forgetting to inseminate happens in all clinics, but one could argue that it is very rare, so an occurrence of 2 or 3 would be appropriate. Then discuss and list the current controls (e.g., use of daily worksheets or reminders) followed by assessing what chance there is that we would detect the failure. With forgetting to inseminate, this will be evident the morning after when the oocytes are found without sperm and are unfertilized, and we can assign this a 1 representing detection every time it happens. However, with the case of a mix-up, this could go completely undetected and should be assigned a 9–10; the fault will be passed to the customer undetected or, in IVF terms, the resulting embryo will be transferred leaving the patient or child to detect the failure. Then calculate the risk priority number (RPN) by multiplying the severity, occurrence, and detection; for forgetting to inseminate, this

Table 3.3 Failure mode and effects analysis worksheet

Item/ function	Potential failure mode	Potential effects of failure	S Severity rating 1–10	Potential cause (s)	O Occurrence rating 1–10	Current controls	D Detection rating 1–10	RPN Risk priority number	Recommendations and action	Action taken	**New S** 1–10	**New O** 1–10	**New D** 1–10	**New RPN**

is 8 × 3 × 1 = 24. Now the initial analysis is done and the embryology team has the task of lowering the RPN. There needs to be an active discussion on how we can change the procedure, allowing everyone in the team to come up with suggestions. Remember that we can sometimes grow accustomed to our own best practices but should consider the suggestions from trainees, who after all provide us with a fresh pair of eyes. Preventing failure in insemination could include the introduction of daily worksheets and checklists together with witnessing and improved ID checks. For example, Westmead Fertility Centre in Sydney, Australia, has a system where each insemination is noted on the database and if one patient's oocytes have not been inseminated by 4 p.m., an automated text message will be sent to the senior embryologists and scientific director. When these suggested changes have been discussed, documented, and implemented, a new value for severity, occurrence, and detection is assigned and the new RPN should hopefully be significantly lower than the original.

The FMEA exercise is not only a mathematical exercise resulting in reduced risk through the actions taken, but is also a great way of making all embryologists aware of what risks are involved in each step of the IVF process, and this awareness itself can help reduce risks.

Even the best risk management systems have incidents and near misses. So what can be done when an incident occurs? The answer is root cause analysis, which is the reactive component in a risk management system. A root cause analysis is simply an analysis of the very reason for the incident occurring. A simple example is when recently trialing a new incubator, the lid accidentally fell over the hand of the embryologist while placing dishes inside, resulting in spillage of the medium and loss of one out of 23 oocytes. The root cause analysis included discussing the incident at the lab meeting. Had it happened before? Were there any near misses previously where the lid had been falling without incident? But also we discussed how we place dishes in the incubators. Are we sometimes carrying more than one dish? We further contacted the supplier to see whether it was a fault of the incubator itself. It was concluded that the lid of our trial incubator did not recline and was a risk if left open without holding on to it. We implemented a procedure where only one dish could be carried and placed in the incubator at any one time, always allowing one hand to be free to hold up the lid. At no time is it appropriate to revert to the old, outdated way of thinking where we apportion blame; this can never result in improvement. More complex root cause analyses could focus on the failure to inseminate as used for the FMEA, but instead of looking at it proactively, doing a root cause analysis after the fact. Mortimer and Mortimer (82) provide an interesting example of root cause analysis of poor fertilization results, with the outcome being a complete reformulation of the fertilization medium.

Many root cause analyses I have been involved in concluded that the level of staffing was inappropriate. It is important to underline that staffing issues such as overworking and poor training are the main contributors to incidents. There is also the issue with staff who are not accepting professional responsibility and do not take enough care to undertake their duties or follow protocols; they should not continue to work in the laboratory (82).

Finally, a very effective tool in addressing and analyzing risk is audits. All incidents followed by a root cause analysis will include suggestions for change and continuous improvement. To ensure these have been implemented and are indeed effective, one needs to undertake internal audits (see the "Audits" section).

Another side to safe practice is to have robust contingency plans. There should always be a documented, agreed plan B. This will include having a backup for all equipment, such as a minimum of two microscopes, heated stages, centrifuges, and so on. For more expensive equipment such as ICSI rigs, oocyte aspiration pumps, and controlled freezers, where sometimes the clinic cannot afford to have two sets, there needs to be a written agreement with another IVF clinic regarding utilization of their equipment.

CONCLUDING REMARKS AND FUTURE ASPECTS

Throughout completing the long and work-intensive process of applying standardized systems in an embryology laboratory, one might ask what it has meant for the embryologists and the results of the clinic. There is no doubt that introducing and fully implementing a quality system standardizes methods and the ways in which embryologists perform their work. The troubleshooting, maintenance of equipment, and milieu are improved and standardized. This guarantees optimal handling of a couple's gametes and embryos and inevitably will lead to improved outcome.

The number of ART treatment cycles undertaken worldwide is increasing every year and with the improvement of the techniques we use, more babies are born as a result of IVF. With the outcome improving, we are aiming toward a future where more focus will be on the safety of treatment and indeed the long-term health of children resulting from ART. With this comes a demand for standardization and improvement of quality. The introduction of quality management systems will ensure reproducibility and traceability, which will be crucial for the future follow-up of these children.

To face the future we need to improve our understanding of the long-term effects of our laboratory procedures on embryo health, acknowledging that some of our methods might deliver in numbers but might be detrimental when considering the adult health of children conceived through IVF. A review of the follow-up of children born from IVF over 25 years in Sweden has revealed that in contrast to cleavage-stage transfer, children born after blastocyst transfer exhibited a higher risk of preterm birth and congenital malformations (83). This report clearly underlines that suboptimal culturing and handling of embryos have long-reaching effects far beyond blastocyst development, successful pregnancy, and live birth. It indicates that what we do in the clinical embryology laboratory is closely connected to the adult health of children born from IVF. This further highlights the importance of standardization, as well as implementing processes that go beyond the standards; working toward improved risk management, robust and thorough training of clinical embryologists, and processes to ensure correct identification and prevention of mix-ups.

Finally, it is important to acknowledge that quality management together with a never-ending commitment to improve our service, beyond standards, is the only way forward toward a future where we can guarantee safe, efficient IVF treatment for all patients and the birth of children who go on to live a healthy life.

ACKNOWLEDGEMENTS

Thanks to Dr. Diego Ezcurra for commenting on the layout of this chapter. Deep gratitude goes to the friends who have helped with the information on national and regional regulations; in no specific order, David Mortimer, Ann-Sofie Forsberg, Helen Priddle, Devika Gunasheela, Lyndsay Devlin, Meishan Jin, Marcus Hedenskog, CT Yeong, Ahmad Suleiman, Rosemary Cullinan, Nader Abdelmonheim, Semra Kahraman, Irina Burkina, and Amal Atared.

REFERENCES

1. ISO/IEC Guide 2: *Standardization and Related Activities—General Vocabulary.* Geneva: International Organization for Standardization. 2004. [Available from: www.iso.org]
2. Hazekamp JT. Current differences and consequences of legislation on practice of assisted reproductive technology in the Nordic countries. The Nordic Committee on Assisted Reproduction of the Scandinavian Federation of Societies of Obstetrics and Gynecology. *Acta Obstet Gynecol Scand* 1996; 75: 198–200.
3. Clinical and laboratory guidelines for assisted reproductive technologies in the Nordic Countries: NFOG bulletin supplement. *NFOG* 1997; 3.
4. Dawson KJ. Quality control and quality assurance in IVF laboratories in the UK. *Hum Reprod* 1997; 12: 2590–1.
5. Pool TB. Practices contributing to quality performance in the embryo laboratory and the status of laboratory regulation in the US. *Hum Reprod* 1997; 12: 2591–3.
6. Lieberman BA, Matson PL, Hamer F. The UK Human Fertilisation and Embryology Act 1990. How well is it functioning? *Hum Reprod* 1994; 9: 1779–82.
7. Code of Practice for Assisted Reproductive Technology Units. Fertility Society of Australia Reproductive Technology Accreditation Committee (RTAC) revised March 2014. [Available from: http://www.fertilitysociety.com.au/wp-content/uploads/RTAC-COP-Final-20141.pdf]
8. ISO 9001. *Quality Management Systems—Requirements.* 5th edition. Geneva: International Organization for Standardization, 2015.
9. Keck C, Sjoblom C, Fischer R, Baukloh V, Alper M. Quality management in reproductive medicine. In: *Textbook of Assisted Reproductive Techniques.* 4th edition, Gardner D (ed.). London: Informa, 2012.
10. ISO 17025. *General Requirements for the Competence of Testing and Calibration Laboratories.* Geneva: International Organization for Standardization. 2005.
11. EN 45001. *General Criteria for the Operation of Testing Laboratories.* Geneva: International Organization for Standardization. 1989.
12. ISO/IEC Guide 25. *General Requirements for the Competence of Calibration and Testing Laboratories.* 3rd edition. Geneva: International Organization for Standardization, 1990.
13. Wikland M, Sjoblom C. The application of quality systems in ART programs. *Mol Cell Endocrinol* 2000; 166: 3–7.
14. ISO 15189. *Medical laboratories—Requirements for Quality and Competence.* 3rd edition. Geneva: International Organization for Standardization, 2012.
15. Directive 2004/23/EC of the European Parliament and of the Council of 31 March 2004 on setting standards of quality and safety for the donation, procurement, testing, processing, preservation, storage and distribution of human tissues and cells. *Off J Eur Union* 2004; 102: 48–58. [Available from: http://eur-lex.europa.eu/Lex-UriServ/LexUriServ.do?uri=OJ:L:2004:102:0048:0058:en:PDF]
16. Guide to the Quality and Safety of Tissues and Cells for Human Application. 1st edition. *Council of Europe European Directorate for the Quality of Medicines & HealthCare (EDQM).* https://www.edqm.eu/sites/default/files/foreword_list_of_contents_tissues_cell_guide_2nd_edition_2015.pdf
17. Commission Directive 2006/17/EC of 8 February 2006 implementing Directive 2004/23/EC of the European Parliament and of the Council as regards certain technical requirements for the donation, procurement and testing of human tissues and cells (Text with EEA relevance). *Off J Eur Union* 2006; 38: 40–52. [Available from: http://eur-lex.europa.eu/legal-content/EN/TXT/?uri=celex%3A32006L0017]
18. Commission Directive 2006/86/EC of 24 October 2006 implementing Directive 2004/23/EC of the European Parliament and of the Council as regards

traceability requirements, notification of serious adverse reactions and events and certain technical requirements for the coding, processing, preservation, storage and distribution of human tissues and cells (Text with EEA relevance). *Official J Eur Union* 2006; 294: 32–50. [Available from: http://eur-lex.europa.eu/legal-content/EN/TXT/PDF/?uri=CELEX:32012L0039]

19. Commission Directive 2012/39/EU of 26 November 2012 amending Directive 2006/17/EC as regards certain technical requirements for the testing of human tissues and cells (Text with EEA relevance). *Official J Eur Union* 2012; 327: 24–25. [Available from: http://eur-lex.europa.eu/legal-content/EN/TXT/?qid=1463631863044&uri=CELEX:32012L0039]
20. ESHRE position paper on the EU Tissues and Cells Directive EC/2004/23, November, 2007. [Available from: https://www.eshre.eu/~/media/sitecore-files/Guidelines/Guidelines/Position-Papers/Tissues-and-cells-directive.pdf?la=en]
21. Joint Commission International Accreditation Standards for Clinical Laboratories, 2nd edition. Joint Commission International, 2010. [Available from: www.jointcommissioninternational.org]
22. WHO Collaborating Centre for Patient Safety Solutions. Patient Safety Solutions. [Available from: http://www.ccforpatientsafety.org/Patient-Safety-Solutions/]
23. Clinical and Laboratory Standards Institute. [Available from: http://www.clsi.org/]
24. McCulloh D. Quality control: Maintaining stability in the laboratory. In: Gardner D. ed. *Textbook of Assisted Reproductive Techniques*. 4th edition. London: Informa. 2012.
25. The Commission of the European Communities. Commission Directive 2003/94/EC, Laying down the principles and guidelines of good manufacturing practice in respect of medicinal products for human use and investigational medicinal products for human use. *Off J Eur Union* 2003; 14: L262/22–6.
26. European Commission. EC Guide to Good Manufacturing Practice, Revision to Annex 1. *Manufacture of Sterile Medicinal Products*. Brussels: Enterprise and Industry Directorate-General, 2008.
27. *WHO Laboratory Manual for the Examination and Processing of Human Sperm*. 5th edition, 2010. [Available from: http://www.who.int/reproductive-health/publications/infertility/9789241547789/en/]
28. Balaban B, Brison D, Calderon G et al. The Istanbul consensus workshop on embryo assessment; proceedings of an expert meeting. *Hum Reprod* 2011; 26: 1270–83.
29. Alpha Scientists in Reproductive Medicine. The Alpha consensus meeting on cryopreservation key performance indicators and benchmarks: Proceedings of an expert meeting. *Reprod Biomed Online* 2012; 25(2): 146–67.
30. ESHRE Guideline Group on good laboratory practice in IVF labs. Revised guidelines for good practice in IVF laboratories 2015. [Available from: www.eshre.eu/Guidelines-and-Legal/Guidelines/Revised-guidelines-for-good-practice-in-IVF-laboratories-%282015%29.aspx]
31. Human Fertilisation and Embryology Authority (HFEA). [Available from: www.HFEA.gov.uk]
32. *Human Fertilisation and Embryology Authority (HFEA) Code of Practice*, 8th edition, published 2009, revised 2015. [Available from: http://www.hfea.gov.uk/code.html]
33. Reproductive Technology Accreditation Committee RTAC Technical Bulletins. [Available from: http://www.fertilitysociety.com.au/rtac/technical-bulletins/]
34. Chinese ART laws and regulations can be obtained by contacting the National Health and Family Planning Commission of the PRC. [Available from: http://en.nhfpc.gov.cn/]
35. National Guidelines for Accreditation, Supervision & Regulation of ART Clinics in India. Indian Council of Medical Research National Academy of Medical Sciences (India), 2005. [Available from: http://icmr.nic.in/art/art_clinics.htm]
36. Licensing terms and conditions on assisted reproduction services. Section 6(5) of the private hospitals and medical clinics act (CAP248). [Available from: https://www.moh-ela.gov.sg/ela/]
37. Code of Practice for Assisted Reproductive Technology Units, International Edition. Fertility Society of Australia Reproductive Technology Accreditation Committee (RTAC) revised March 2014. [Available from: http://www.fertilitysociety.com.au]
38. Inhorn MC. Making Muslim babies: IVF and gamete donation in Sunni v. Shi'a Islam. *Cult Med Psychiatry* 2006; 30: 427–50.
39. Ali A. The Conditional Permissibility of *In Vitro* Fertilisation under Islamic Jurisprudence. Al-Ghazzali awareness paper, Al-Ghazzali centre for Islamic sciences and human development, 2004. [Available from: http://alghazzali.org/]
40. Cabinet decision (36) of 2009 issuing the implementing regulation of federal law No. (11) of concerning licensing of fertilisation centres in the State. *Health Authority Abu-Dhabi (HAAD)* 2008. [Available from: http://www.haad.ae/haad/tabid/852/Default.aspx]
41. Normas para la acreditacion de centros de reproduccion asistida y sus laboratorios de embriologia y andrologia. Version 12, 2007. [Available from: http://redlara.com/aa_ingles/default.asp]
42. Department of Justice Canada. Assisted Human Reproduction Act. S.C. c.2 2004. [Available from: http://laws-lois.justice.gc.ca/eng/acts/A-13.4/]
43. Federal agency Assisted Reproduction Canada (AHRC). [Available from: http://www.ahrc-pac.gc.ca]
44. Supreme Court of Canada Citation: Reference re Assisted Human Reproduction Act. BETWEEN: Attorney General of Canada Appellant and Attorney General of Quebec. [Available from: scc.lexum.org/en/2010/2010scc61/2010scc61.html]

45. Canadian Fertility and Andrology Society (CFAS), ART Lab Special Interest Group. [Available from: http://www.cfas.ca/index.php?option=com_content&view=article&id=742&Itemid=522]
46. American Society for Reproductive Medicine. Revised minimum standards for in vitro fertilization, gamete intrafallopian transfer, and related procedures. *Fertil Steril* 1998; 70(4 Suppl 2): 1S–5S.
47. American Society for Reproductive Medicine. Revised guidelines for human embryology and andrology laboratories. *Fertil Steril* 2008; 90: S45–59.
48. Van Kooij JR, Peeters MF, Te Velde ER. Twins of mixed races: Consequences for Dutch IVF laboratories. *Hum Reprod* 1997; 12: 2585–7.
49. Hartshorne GM, Baker H. Fads and foibles in ART; Where is the evidence? *Hum Fertil (Camb)* 2006; 9: 27–35.
50. Takenaka M, Horiuchi T, Yanagimachi R. Effects of light on development of mammalian zygotes. *Proc Natl Acad Sci USA* 2007; 104: 14289–93.
51. Oosafe MEA tested IVF laboratory disinfectants. Denmark, Sparmed, Stenlose. [Available from: http://www.sparmed.dk/en/products/disinfectants/]
52. Nijs M, Franssen K, Cox A et al. Reprotoxicity of intrauterine insemination and *in vitro* fertilization-embryo transfer disposables and products: A 4-year study. *Fertil Steril* 2009; 92: 527–35.
53. Council Directive 93/42/EEC of 14 June 1993 concerning medical devices, OJ L 169, 12.7.1993. Directive last amended by Regulation (EC) No 1882/2003 of the European Parliament and of the Council (OJ L 284, 31.10.2003).
54. Directive 98/79/EC of the European Parliament and of the Council of 27 October 1998 on *in vitro* diagnostic medical devices. OJ L 331, 7.12.1998, Directive as amended by Regulation (EC) No 1882/2003.
55. United Kingdom National External Quality Assessment Service (NEQUAS). [Available from: www.ukneqas.org.uk]
56. QAP online FertAid. [Available from: www.fertaid.com]
57. ISO/IEC guide 43-1. Geneva: International Organization for Standardization, 1997.
58. The Association of Clinical Embryologists (ACE). [Available from: https://www.embryologists.org.uk/]
59. NHS Scientist Training Programme (STP). [Available from: https://www.healthcareers.nhs.uk/explore-roles/life-sciences/reproductive-science/training-development-and-registration]
60. European Society of Human Reproduction and Embryology (ESHRE) Certification for Embryologists. [Available from: https://www.eshre.eu/Accreditation-and-Certification/Certification-for-embryologists.aspx]
61. *Australian Commission on Safety and Quality in Health Care (ACSQHC).* Technology Solutions to Patient Misidentification—Report of Review ACSQHC, 2008.
62. Lusky K. Patient ID systems offer smart start. *Collage of American Pathologists Periodical, CAP Today,* 2005. [Available from: http://www.captodayonline.com/Archives/feature_stories/1005_Patient_ID_systems.html]
63. Aller R. Positive patient identification. More than a double check (positive patient identification systems and products). *Collage of American Pathologists Periodical, CAP Today,* 2005: 26–34. [Available from: http://www.captodayonline.com/Archives/surveys/1005_System_Survey.pdf]
64. Clinical and Laboratory Standards Institute (CLSI). *Accuracy in Patient and Sample Identification.* Approved Guideline (GP33-A). Wayne, PA: CLSI, 2010.
65. Adams S, Carthey J. IVF Witnessing and electronic systems. HFEA commissioned report comparing the relative risks of witnessing systems. [Available from: www.hfea.gov.uk/docs/Witnessing_samples_id_report.pdf]
66. Kerr A. A problem shared…? Teamwork, autonomy and error in assisted conception. *Soc Sci Med* 2009; 69: 1741–9.
67. Brison D. Reducing risk in the IVF laboratory: Implementation of a double witnessing system. *Clin Risk* 2004; 10: 176–80.
68. Amalberti R, Auroy Y, Berwick D et al. Five system barriers to achieving ultrasafe health care. *Ann Intern Med* 2005; 142: 756–64.
69. Leape LL, Berwick DM. Safe health care: Are we up to it? *BMJ* 2000; 320: 7256.
70. Toft B, Mascie-Taylor H. Involuntary automaticity: A work-system induced risk to safe health care. *Health Serv Manage Res* 2005; 18: 211–16.
71. Kennedy CR, Mortimer D. Risk management in IVF. *Best Pract Res Clin Obstet Gynaecol* 2007; 21: 691–712.
72. Lippi G, Blanckaert N, Bonini P et al. Causes, consequences, detection, and prevention of identification errors in laboratory diagnostics. *Clin Chem Lab Med* 2009; 47: 143–53.
73. Edi-Osagie E, Hooper L, Seif MW. The impact of assisted hatching on live birth rates and outcomes of assisted conception: A systematic review. *Hum Reprod* 2003; 18: 1828–35.
74. Zegers-Hochschild F, Adamson GD, de Mouzon J. International Committee for Monitoring Assisted Reproductive Technology (ICMART) and the World Health Organization (WHO) revised glossary of ART terminology. *Fertil Steril* 2009; 92: 1520–4.
75. Capri Workshop Group for the European Society of Human Reproduction and Embryology (ESHRE). Intrauterine insemination. *Hum Reprod Update* 2009; 1: 1–13.
76. Connolly M, Hoorens S, Chambers GM. The costs and consequences of assisted reproductive technology: An economic perspective. *Hum Reprod Update* 2010; 16: 603–13.

77. Kuhn AM, Youngberg BJ. The need for risk management to evolve to assure a culture of safety. *Qual Saf Health Care* 2002; 11: 158–62.
78. Wu AW. Medical error: The second victim. The doctor who makes the mistake needs help too. *BMJ* 2000; 320: 726–7.
79. ISO 31000:2009. *Risk Management—Principles and Guidelines*. Geneva: International Organization for Standardization, 2009.
80. Reason J. The contribution of latent human failures to the breakdown of complex systems. *Philos Trans R Soc Lond B Biol Sci* 1990; 327: 475–84.
81. Reason J. Human error: Models and management. *BMJ* 2000; 320: 768.
82. Mortimer D, Mortimer ST. *Quality and Risk Management in the IVF Laboratory*. Cambridge: Cambridge University Press, 2005.
83. Finnström O, Källén B, Lindam A et al. Maternal and child outcome after in vitro fertilization–a review of 25 years of population-based data from Sweden. *Acta Obstet Gynecol Scand* 2011; 90: 494–500.

n of sperm

4

KAYLEN M. SILVERBERG and TOM TURNER

INTRODUCTION

Abnormalities in sperm production or function, alone or in combination with other factors, account for 35%–50% of all cases of infertility. Although a battery of tests and treatments have been described and continue to be used in the evaluation of female infertility, the male has been essentially neglected. It would appear that the majority of programs offering advanced assisted reproduction technologies (ARTs) employ only a cursory evaluation of the male—rarely extending beyond semen analysis and antisperm antibody detection. Several factors certainly account for this disparity. First, most practitioners of ARTs are gynecologists or gynecologic subspecialists who have little formal training in the evaluation of the infertile or subfertile men. Second, the urologists, who perhaps theoretically should have taken the lead in this area, have devoted little of their literature or research budgets to the evaluation of the infertile male. Third, and perhaps most important, is the inescapable fact that sperm function testing remains a very controversial area of research. Many tests have been described, yet few have been extensively evaluated in a proper scientific manner. Those that have continue to be criticized for poor sensitivity or specificity, a lack of standardization of methodology, suboptimal study design, problems with outcome assessment, and the lack of long-term follow-up. Although many of these same criticisms could also be leveled against most diagnostic algorithms for female infertility, in that arena, the tests continue to prevail over their critics. Fourth, like female infertility, male infertility is certainly multifactorial. It is improbable that one sperm function test will prove to be a panacea, owing to the multiple steps involved in fertilization. In addition to arriving at the site of fertilization, sperm must undergo capacitation and the acrosome must allow for the penetration of the cumulus cells and the zona pellucida so the sperm head can fuse with the oolemma. In addition, the sperm must activate the oocyte, undergo nuclear decondensation, form the male pronucleus, and then fuse with the female pronucleus. Finally, with the advent and the rapid continued development of micro-assisted fertilization, sperm function testing has assumed a role of even less importance. As fertilization and pregnancy rates improve with procedures such as intracytoplasmic sperm injection (ICSI), more and more logical questions are being asked about the proper role for sperm function testing. This chapter reviews the most commonly employed techniques for sperm evaluation and examines the issues surrounding their utilization in the modern ART program.

PATIENT HISTORY

A thorough history of the infertile couple at the time of the initial consultation will frequently reveal conditions that could affect semen quality. Some of the important factors to consider are as follows:

1. Reproductive history, including previous pregnancies with this and other partners.
2. Sexual interaction of the couple, including frequency and timing of intercourse as well as the duration of their infertility.
3. Past medical and surgical history: specific attention should be paid to sexually transmitted diseases, prostatitis, or epididymitis, as well as scrotal trauma or surgery—including varicocele repair, vasectomy, inguinal herniorrhaphy, and vasovasostomy.
4. Exposure to medication, drugs, toxins, and adverse environmental conditions such as temperature extremes in occupational and leisure activities, either in the past or in the present.

SEMEN ANALYSIS

The hallmark of the evaluation of the male remains the semen analysis. It is well known that the intrapatient variability of semen specimens from fertile men can be significant over time (1). This variability decreases the diagnostic information that can be obtained from a single analysis, often necessitating additional analyses. What is also apparent from literature that analyzes samples from "infertile" patients is that the deficiencies revealed may not be sufficient to prevent pregnancy from occurring. Rather, they may simply lower the probability of pregnancy, resulting in so-called "subfertility." Clearly, the overall prognosis for a successful pregnancy is dependent on the complex combination of variables in semen quality coupled with the multiple factors inherent in the female reproductive system that must each function flawlessly. The commonly accepted standard for defining the normal semen analysis is the criteria defined by the World Health Organization (WHO). These parameters for both the fourth and the fifth edition are listed in Table 4.1.

The normal or reference values for semen analyses have been altered with each new edition of the WHO. The values from the current (fifth) edition have been derived from a retrospective look at the semen parameters of men with two to seven days of abstinence whose partner conceived within 12 months after the cessation of the use of contraception (2,3). There are significant changes in the parameters listed in the current edition compared with past editions. Some of these changes are due to observations

Table 4.1 World Health Organization reference values for semen analysis

	Reference values	
Parameter	**Fourth edition**	**Fifth edition**
Volume	>2.0 mL	1.5 (1.4–1.7)
Sperm concentration	20×10^6	$15\ (12–16) \times 10^6$
Total sperm count	40×10^6	$39\ (33–46) \times 10^6$
Total motility	50%	40% (38–42)
Progressive motility	25%	32% (31–34)
Vitality	50%	58% (55–63)
pH	7.2	7.2
Morphology	15%	4% (3.0–4.0)

Source: Data from World Health Organization. *WHO Laboratory Manual for the Examination of Human Semen and Sperm–Cervical Mucus Interaction*, 4th edition. New York, NY: Cambridge University Press, 1999; 60–1; World Health Organization. *WHO Laboratory Manual for the Examination of Human Semen*, 5th edition. Geneva: WHO Press, 2010: 223–5.

Note: Liquefaction: Complete within 60 minutes at room temperature. Appearance: Homogeneous, gray, and opalescent. Consistency: Leaves pipette as discrete droplets. Leukocytes: Fewer than 1 million/mL.

made of the semen samples from the patients mentioned above. These real differences in declining sperm concentrations, motility, and normal morphology are thought to be due to environmental influences. However, the drastic changes in the morphology reference values are primarily due to the suggested use of the Kruger strict morphology method in the fifth edition. Many labs prefer to continue using the fourth edition because of the suggested use of the Kruger strict morphology. The value of this method will be discussed in the sperm morphology section of this chapter.

COLLECTION OF THE SPECIMEN

When the semen analysis is scheduled, instructions should be given to the couple to ensure collection of an optimum semen sample. Written instructions are useful, especially if the patient is collecting the specimen outside of the clinical setting. During the initial infertility evaluation, a semen specimen should be obtained following a two- to seven-day abstinence from sexual activity (1). A shorter period of time may adversely affect the semen volume and sperm concentration, although it may enhance sperm motility. A longer period of abstinence may reduce the sperm motility. In light of the natural variability in semen quality that all men exhibit, the initial semen collection may not accurately reflect a typical ejaculate for that patient. A second collection, with a two- to seven-day abstinence period, can eliminate the tension associated with the initial semen collection, as well as provide a second specimen from which a typical set of semen parameters can be determined. An additional cause of variable semen quality can be the site of collection. Understandably, many men are inhibited by collecting their semen sample at the clinic. Although collecting at home is less intimidating, it is not always practical due to distance or schedules. In the case where the semen sample is collected at the clinic, the second and subsequent collections are usually better than the first due to an increase in the patient's comfort level. The second collection may also be used to determine the optimal abstinence period for this particular patient. Masturbation is the preferred method of collection. The use of lubricants is discouraged since most are spermicidal. However, some mineral oils and a few water-based lubricants are acceptable. Since masturbation may present significant difficulty for some men, either in the clinic or at home, an alternative method of collection must be available. The use of certain silastic condoms (seminal collection devices) during intercourse may be an acceptable second choice. Interrupted intercourse should not be considered, as this method tends to lose the sperm-rich initial few drops of semen while transferring many bacteria to the specimen container (1,4).

CARE OF THE SPECIMEN

Appropriate care of the ejaculate between collection and examination is important. Specimens should be collected only in approved, sterile, plastic, disposable cups. Many other plastic containers are toxic to sperm, especially if the sperm is allowed to remain in the containers for the duration of time that it takes to deliver the specimen from off-site. Washed containers may contain soap or residue from previous contents, which can kill or contaminate the sperm. Delivery of the semen to the laboratory should occur within 60 minutes of collection, and the specimen should be kept at room temperature during transport. These recommendations are designed to maintain optimal sperm viability until the time of analysis.

CONTAINER LABELING

The information recorded on the specimen container label should include the male's name as well as a unique identifying number. Typically, a social security number, birth date, or a clinic-assigned patient number is used. Other helpful information recorded on the label should include the date and time of collection and the number of days since the last ejaculation. When the specimen is received from the patient, it is important to confirm that the information provided on the label is complete and accurate.

EXAMINATION OF THE SPECIMEN

Liquefaction and viscosity

When the semen sample arrives in the laboratory, it is checked for liquefaction and viscosity. Although similar, these factors are distinct from each other (5,6). Liquefaction is a natural change in the consistency of semen from a semi-liquid to a liquid. Before this process is completed, sperm are contained in a gel-like matrix that prevents their homogeneous distribution. Aliquots taken from this uneven distribution of sperm for the purpose of determining concentration, motility, or morphology may not be truly representative of the specimen as a whole. As liquefaction occurs over 15–30 minutes, sperm are released and distributed throughout the semen. Incomplete liquefaction may adversely affect the accuracy of the semen analysis by preventing this even distribution of sperm within the sample. The coagulum that characterizes freshly ejaculated semen results from secretions from the seminal vesicles. The liquefaction of this coagulum is the result of enzymatic secretions from the prostate. Watery semen, in the absence of a coagulum, may indicate the absence of the ejaculatory duct or nonfunctional seminal vesicles. Inadequate liquefaction, in the presence of a coagulum, may indicate a deficiency of prostatic enzymes (7,8).

Viscosity refers to the liquefied specimen's tendency to form drops from the tip of a pipette. If drops form and fall freely, the specimen has a normal viscosity. If drops will not form or the semen cannot be easily drawn up into a pipette, viscosity is high. This high viscosity remains, even after liquefaction has taken place. Highly viscous semen may also prevent the homogeneous distribution of sperm. Treatment with an enzyme, such as chymotrypsin (9), or aspiration of semen through an 18-gauge needle may reduce the viscosity and improve the distribution of sperm before an aliquot is removed for counting. Any addition of medium containing enzymes should be recorded, as this affects the actual sperm concentration. The new volume must be factored in when calculating the total sperm count.

Semen volume

Semen volume is best measured with a serological pipette that is graduated to 0.1 mL. This volume is recorded and later multiplied by the sperm concentration in order to obtain the total count of sperm in the sample. A normal seminal volume before dilution is considered to be >1.4 mL (2).

Sperm concentration

A variety of counting chambers are available for determining sperm concentration. Those more commonly used include the hemocytometer, the Makler counting chamber, and the MicroCell. Regardless of the type of chamber used, an aliquot from a homogeneous, mixed semen sample is placed onto a room temperature chamber. The chamber is covered with a glass coverslip, which allows the sperm to distribute evenly in a very thin layer. Sperm within a grid are counted, and a calculation is made according to the formula for the type of chamber used. Accuracy is improved by including a greater number of rows, squares, or fields in the count. Sperm counts should be performed immediately after loading semen onto the chamber. Waiting until the heat from the microscope light increases the speed of the sperm may inaccurately enhance the count. As indicated earlier, a particular patient's sperm count may vary significantly from one ejaculate to another. This observation holds true for both fertile and infertile males, further complicating the definition of a normal range for sperm concentration. Demographic studies employing historic controls were used to define a sperm concentration of <15 million/mL as abnormal (fifth edition) (2). Several investigators had observed that significantly fewer pregnancies occurred when men had sperm counts <15 million/mL; however, the prognosis for pregnancy did not increase proportionately with sperm concentrations above this threshold.

Sperm motility

Sperm motility may be affected by many factors:

- Patient's age and general health
- Length of time since the last ejaculation
- Patient's exposure to outside influences such as excessive heat or toxins
- Method of collection
- Length of time and adequacy of handling from collection to analysis

When the aliquot of semen is placed on the room temperature counting chamber, the count and motility should be determined immediately. As previously stated, this will prevent the effect of the heat from the microscope light source from influencing the results. If a chamber with a grid is used to count the sperm, the motility can be determined at the same time as the concentration by using a multiple-click cell counter to tally motile and non-motile sperm and then totaling these numbers to arrive at the true sperm concentration. The accuracy of the concentration and of the motility improves as more sperm are counted. If a wet-mount slide is used to determine motility, more than one area of the slide should be used, and each count should include at least 200 sperm. Prior to examining the specimen for motility, the slide or counting chamber should be examined for signs of sperm clumping. Sperm clumping to other sperm head to head, head to tail, or tail to tail may indicate the presence of sperm antibodies in the semen. This should not be confused with clumping of sperm to other cellular debris in the semen, which is not associated with the presence of antibodies. In either case, sperm clumping may affect the accuracy of both the sperm count and the motility (1,4).

Motility is one of the most important prerequisites for achieving fertilization and pregnancy. The head of the sperm must be delivered a great distance *in vivo* through the barriers of the reproductive tract to the site of the egg. Sperm must have sufficient motility in order to penetrate both the layers of coronal cells and the zona pellucida before fusing with the egg's cell membrane (oolemma). An exact threshold level of motility that is required to accomplish fertilization and pregnancy, however, has never been described (10). This may be due to variables in the equipment and techniques used in assessing motility.

Progression

While sperm motility represents the quantitative parameter of sperm movement expressed as a percentage, sperm progression represents the quality of sperm movement expressed on a subjective scale. A typical scale, such as the one below, attempts to depict the type of movement exhibited by most of the sperm visualized on a chamber grid. Progression of sperm may also be calculated with sperm motility as a percentage of sperm exhibiting "progressive motility." With the advent of successful micro-assisted fertilization, progression has assumed more limited utility. Nevertheless, for those laboratories that quantify progression of motility separately, a score of 0 means no motility; 1 means motility with vibratory motion without forward progression; 2 means motility with slow, erratic forward progression; 3 means motility with relatively straightforward motion; and 4 is motility with rapid forward progression (4).

Sperm vitality

When a motility evaluation yields a low proportion of moving sperm (less than 50%), a vitality stain may be beneficial. This is a method used to distinguish non-motile sperm that are living from those that are dead. This technique will be discussed later in the sperm function section.

Additional cell types

While observing sperm in a counting chamber or on a slide, additional cell types may also be seen. These include endothelial cells from the urethra, epithelial cells from the skin, immature sperm cells, and white blood cells. The most common and significant of these cell types is referred to collectively as "round cells." These include immature sperm cells and white blood cells. In order to distinguish between them, an aliquot of semen can be placed in a thin layer on a slide and air-dried. The cells are fixed to the slide and stained using a Wright–Giemsa or Bryan–Leishman stain. When viewed under 400× or 1000× power, cell types may be differentiated primarily by their nuclear morphology. Immature sperm have one to three round nuclei within a common cytoplasm. Polymorphonuclear leukocytes may also be multinucleate, but the staining method will typically reveal characteristic nuclear bridges between their irregularly shaped nuclei (1). A peroxidase stain may be used to identify granulocytes and to differentiate them from the immature sperm. The presence of greater than 1 million white blood cells per one milliliter of semen may indicate an infection in the urethra or accessory glands, which provide the majority of the seminal plasma. Such infections could contribute to infertility (1,11). As such, these samples must be cultured so that the offending organism can be identified and appropriate treatment can be instituted. Besides bacteria, white blood cells on their own can contribute to infertility. They can especially be a detrimental factor in the *in vitro* fertilization (IVF) process. Even though the white blood cells can be removed by centrifugation of the semen sample through a layer of silica beads, the toxins produced by the cells, called leukokines, may pass through the layer and concentrate in the medium below containing the sperm. If this sperm is to be used in the insemination of oocytes, the concentrated toxins will be in contact with the oocytes for several hours. These toxins may cause detrimental effects to the oocytes and to the embryos that develop from fertilization.

Sperm morphology

Sperm morphology can be assessed in several ways. The most common classification systems are the fourth edition and the fifth edition of the WHO standard, the latter of which incorporates Kruger strict criteria (Figure 4.1) (12). Two easy methods of preparing slides for assessing normal morphology include the following: first, a 5–10-μL drop of semen is placed on a slide and a second slide is used to smear the sample in a very thin, smoothly distributed layer. The slide is then air-dried. A 5–10-μL drop of stain (typically hematoxylin or methylene blue) is placed on the dried sample and a coverslip is placed over the specimen. Alternatively, the drop of semen may be mixed with an equal volume of fixative plus stain prior to placing it on the slide. With either method, at least 200 sperm must be counted using phase contrast microscopy. If the fourth edition of WHO is used, 400× is sufficient magnification. However, when using the fifth edition of WHO, 100× is recommended in order to obtain an accurate measurement of the sperm. WHO fourth edition criteria for assessing normal forms include the following:

- Head: Oval and smooth heads are normal; round, pyriform, pin, double, and amorphous heads are all abnormal.
- Mid-piece: A normal mid-piece is straight and slightly thicker than the tail.
- Tail: Single, unbroken, straight tails without kinks or coils are normal.

A normal semen analysis should contain at least 15% normal sperm using WHO fourth edition criteria.

- Head: Smooth; oval configuration; length, 5–6 μm, diameter 2.5–3.5 μm; acrosome, must constitute 40%–70% of the sperm head.
- Mid-piece: Slender, axially attached; <1 μm in width and approximately 1.5 μm in head length; no cytoplasmic droplets, >50% of the size of the sperm head.
- Tail: Single, unbroken, straight, without kinks or coils, approximately 45 μm in length (Figure 4.2) (12,13,14).

As described by Kruger et al., sperm forms that are not clearly normal should be considered abnormal. The presence of 4% or greater normal sperm morphology should be interpreted as a normal result. Normal morphology of <4% is abnormal (13,14). Normal sperm morphology has been reported to be directly related to fertilization potential. This may be due to the abnormal sperm's inability to deliver normal genetic material to the cytoplasm of the egg. From video recordings, it appears that abnormal sperm are more likely to have diminished, aberrant, or absent motility. This reduced or unusual motility may result from hydrodynamic inefficiency due to the head shape, abnormalities in the tail structure that prevent normal motion, and/or deficiencies in energy production necessary for

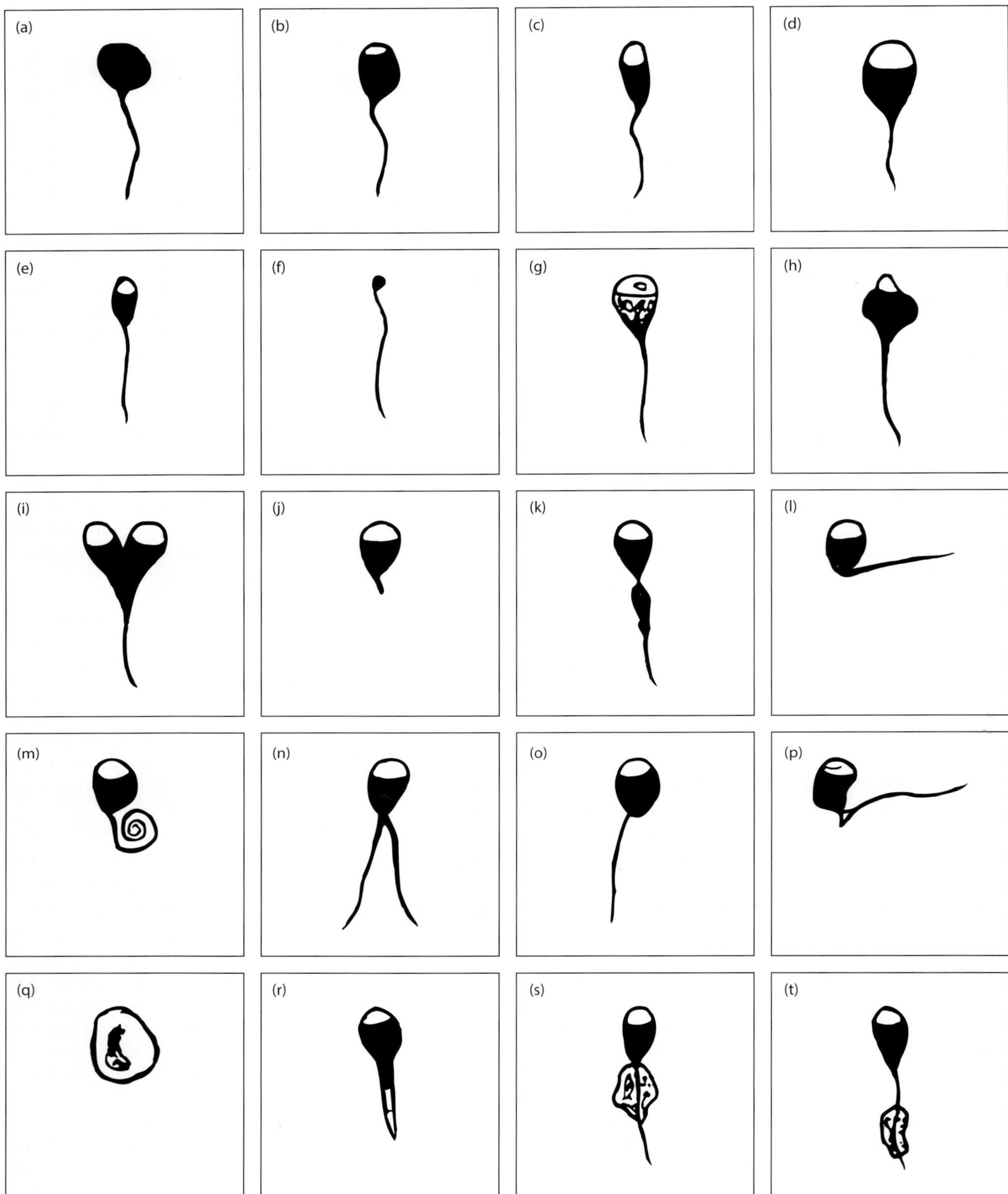

Figure 4.1 Different types of sperm malformations. (a) Round head/no acrosome; (b) small acrosome; (c) elongated head; (d) megalo head; (e) small head; (f) pinhead; (g) vacuolated head; (h) amorphous head; (i) bicephalic; (j) loose head; (k) amorphous head; (l) broken neck; (m) coiled tail; (n) double tail; (o) abaxial tail attachment; (p) multiple defects; (q) immature germ cell; (r) elongated spermatid; (s) proximal cytoplasmic droplet; and (t) distal cytoplasmic droplet. (From Sathananthan AH, ed. *Visual Atlas of Human Sperm Structure and Function for Assisted Reproductive Technique*. Melbourne: La Trobe and Monash Universities, Singapore: National University, 1996, with permission.)

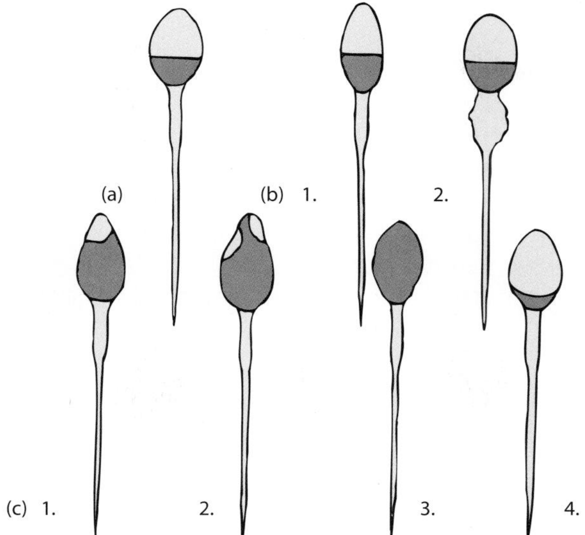

Figure 4.2 A diagrammatic representation of quick-stained spermatozoa. (a) Normal form; (b.1) slightly amorphous head; (b.2) neck defect; (c.1 and 2) abnormally small acrosome; (c.3) no acrosome; and (c.4) acrosome 70% of sperm head. (From Sathananthan AH, ed. *Visual Atlas of Human Sperm Structure and Function for Assisted Reproductive Technique*. Melbourne: La Trobe and Monash Universities, Singapore: National University, 1996, with permission.)

motility (15,16). In addition to compromised motility, abnormal sperm do not appear to bind to the zona of the egg as well as normal sperm. This has been demonstrated in studies employing the hemizona binding assay (17). IVF has helped further to elucidate the role that normal sperm morphology plays in the fertilization process and in pregnancy. Both the fourth edition WHO method and the Kruger strict method of determining normal sperm morphology have been used to predict a patient's fertility.

Several studies have concluded that the Kruger method of strict morphology determination shows the most consistent prediction of fertilization *in vitro* following conventional insemination (11,18,19). This method of assessing normal sperm morphology, because of its precise, non-subjective nature, establishes a threshold below which abnormal morphology becomes a contributing factor in infertility. While Kruger strict morphology provides a repeatable, objective method of analyzing sperm morphology based on precise measurements, some IVF labs prefer to use the WHO fourth edition of sperm morphology (15%) as a cutoff point below which ICSI is used and above which insemination may be used. The opinion in those labs is that the 15% level of morphology, while not as precise as the Kruger method, is more realistic for determining patients who will do well with insemination. In addition, the Kruger strict scale ensures that some patients will be diagnosed as having 0% normal morphology. This can give the false impression that the patient has no normal sperm with which to accomplish fertilization by insemination or by ICSI.

COMPUTER-ASSISTED SEMEN ANALYSIS

Computer-assisted semen analysis (CASA) was initially developed to improve the accuracy of manual semen analysis. Its goal is to establish a standardized, objective, reproducible test for sperm concentration, motility, and morphology. The technique also attempts, for the first time, to actually characterize sperm movement. The automated sperm movement measurements—known as kinematics—include straight-line velocity, curvilinear velocity, and mean angular displacement (Table 4.2). The use of CASA requires specialized equipment, including a phase contrast microscope, video camera, video recorder, video monitor, computer, and printer.

To perform CASA, sperm are placed on either a Makler or a MicroCell chamber and they are then viewed under a microscope. The video camera records the moving images of the sperm cells and the computer digitizes them. The digitized images consist of pixels whose changing locations are recorded frame by frame. A total of 30–200 frames per minute are produced. The changing locations of each sperm are recorded and their trajectories are computed (Figure 4.3) (20). In this manner, hyperactive motion can also be detected and recorded. Hyperactive sperm exhibit a whip-like, thrashing movement, which is thought to be associated with sperm that are removed from seminal plasma and ready to fertilize the oocytes (20,21). Persistent questions about the validity and reproducibility of results have kept CASA from becoming a standard procedure in the andrology laboratory. The accuracy of sperm concentration appears to be diminished in the presence of either severe oligospermia or excessive numbers of sperm. In cases of oligospermia, counts may be overestimated due to the machine counting debris as sperm. High concentrations of sperm may be underestimated in the presence of clumping. High sperm concentrations can also cause overestimations in counting due to the manner in which the software handles collisions between motile sperm and non-motile sperm. In these cases, diluting the sample may improve the accuracy of the count (21,22). Sperm concentration also appears to be closely related to the type of counting chamber employed. Similar to the challenges reported with manual counting, sperm counts may vary with regard to whether one is using a Makler or a MicroCell.

Sperm motion parameters identified by CASA have been assessed by several investigators for their ability to predict fertilization potential. Certain types of motion have been determined to be important in achieving specific actions related to fertilization, such as cervical mucus penetration and zona binding. However, the overall potential of CASA for predicting pregnancy is still a subject of much debate. In summary, persistent questions about results and their interpretation continue to limit the routine use of CASA. As reproducibility improves overall ranges of sperm concentration, CASA may become the standard for semen analysis.

The use of fluorescent DNA staining with CASA may also improve its reliability. In addition, as the kinematics of sperm motion becomes better understood, CASA may

Table 4.2 Kinematic measurements in computer-assisted semen analysis

Symbol	Name	Definition
VSL	Straight-line velocity	Time average velocity of the sperm head along a straight line from its first position to its last position
VCL	Curvilinear velocity	Time average velocity of the sperm head along its actual trajectory
VAP	Average path velocity	Time average velocity of the sperm head along its average trajectory
LIN	Linearity	Linearity of the curvilinear trajectory (VSL/VCL)
WOB	Wobble	Degree of oscillation of the actual sperm head trajectory around its average path (VAP/VCL)
STR	Straightness	Straightness of the average path (VSL/VAP)
ALH	Amplitude of lateral head	Amplitude of variations of the actual sperm head trajectory about its average trajectory displacement (the average trajectory is computed using a rectangular running average)
RIS	Riser displacement	Point-to-point distance of the actual sperm head trajectory to its average path (the average path is computed using an adaptive smoothing algorithm)
BCF	Beat-cross frequency	Time average rate at which the actual sperm trajectory crosses the average path trajectory
HAR	Frequency of the fundamental	Fundamental frequency of the oscillation of the curvilinear trajectory around its average harmonic path (HAR is computed using the Fourier transformation)
MAG	Magnitude of the amplitude	Squared height of the HAR spectral peak (MAG is a measure of the peak to fundamental harmonic peak dispersion of the raw trajectory about its average path at the fundamental frequency)
VOL	Area of fundamental harmonic	Area under the fundamental harmonic peak in the magnitude spectrum (VOL is a harmonic measure of the power-bandwidth of the signal)
CON	Specimen concentration	Concentration of sperm cells in a sample in millions of sperm per mL of plasma or medium
MOT	Percentage motility	Percentage of sperm cells in a suspension that are motile (in manual analysis, motility is defined by a moving flagellum; in computer-assisted semen analysis, motility is defined by a minimum VSL for each sperm)

Source: Data from Enginsu MF et al. *Hum Reprod* 1992; 7: 1136–40.

play an integral role in determining the optimal method of assisted reproductive technique that should be utilized for specific types of male factor patients.

SPERM ANTIBODIES

Because mature spermatozoa are formed after puberty, they can be recognized as foreign protein by the male immune system. In the testicle, the sperm are protected from circulating immunoglobulins by the tight junctions of the Sertoli cells. As long as the sperm are contained within the lumen of the male reproductive tract, they are sequestered from the immune system, and no antibodies form to their surface antigens. If there is a breach in this so-called "blood–testis barrier," an immune response may be initiated. The most common causes of a breach in the reproductive tract, which could initiate antibody formation, include vasectomy, varicocele repair, testicular biopsy, torsion, trauma, and infection (23,24). Once formed, antibodies are secreted into the fluids of the accessory glands, specifically the prostate and seminal vesicles. At the time of ejaculation, the fluids from these glands contribute most of the volume to the seminal plasma. These antibodies can then come into contact with the sperm and may cause them to clump. In women, the atraumatic introduction of sperm into the reproductive tract as a result of intercourse or artificial insemination does not appear to be a factor in the production of sperm antibodies. However, events that induce trauma or introduce sperm to the mucous membranes outside of the reproductive tract can induce antibody formation. Proposed examples of such events include trauma to the vaginal mucosa during intercourse or the deposition of sperm into the gastrointestinal tract by way of oral or anal intercourse (24). There are several tests currently employed for detecting the presence of sperm antibodies. The two most common are the mixed agglutination reaction (MAR) and the immunobead binding test.

The MAR

This test is performed by mixing semen, IgG- or IgA-coated latex beads or red blood cells, and IgG or IgA antiserum on a microscope slide. The slides are incubated and observed at 400× magnification. At least 200 sperm are counted. If antibodies are present, the sperm will form

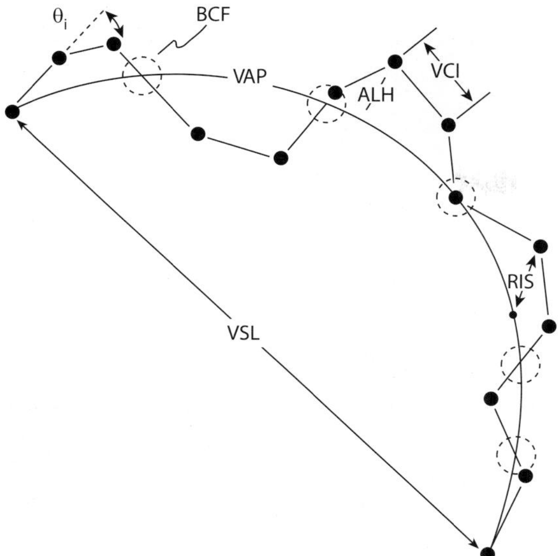

Figure 4.3 Examples of kinematic measurements involved in a single-sperm tracing. *Abbreviations*: ALH, amplitude of lateral head; BCF, beat-cross frequency; RIS, riser displacement; VAP, average path velocity; VCL, curvilinear velocity; VSL, straight-line velocity. (Reproduced from data from Enginsu MF et al. *Hum Reprod* 1992; 7: 1136–40.)

clumps with the coated latex beads or coated red blood cells. If antibodies are absent, the sperm will swim freely. The level of antibody concentration considered to be clinically relevant must be established by each center conducting the test. The WHO considers a level of binding of ≥50% to be clinically significant. This test is used only for detection of direct antibodies in men, and is not specific for the location of bead attachment to the sperm.

The immunobead binding test

This test is performed by combining IgG- or IgA-coated latex beads and washed sperm on a slide. The sperm must be removed from the seminal plasma by washing the sample with media plus bovine serum albumin (BSA). The presence of human protein on the surface of the sperm interferes with the binding of the immunobeads to the sperm, and thus may mask a positive result. After washing, the sperm is placed on a slide with IgG- or IgA-coated latex beads and is read at 200× or 400× magnification. If antibodies are present, the small beads will attach directly to the sperm. This test provides potentially greater information than the MAR, as results consider the number of sperm bound by beads, the type of antigen involved in binding, and the specific location where the bead is bound to the sperm.

If antibodies are absent, the beads will not attach. Like the MAR test, this test can be used for the detection of direct antibodies in men. However, it may also be used to detect antibodies produced in a woman's serum, follicular fluid, or cervical mucus by incubating these bodily fluids with washed sperm that have previously tested negative for antibodies. To perform an indirect test, known direct antibody-negative sperm are washed free of seminal plasma and resuspended in a small volume of media plus BSA. They are incubated for one hour at 37°C with the bodily fluid to be tested. The sperm are then washed free of the bodily fluid, resuspended in media plus BSA, and mixed on a slide with IgG- or IgA-coated latex beads. The test is interpreted by noting the percentage and location of the bead attachment. The third edition WHO standard considers the level of binding of ≥20% as representing a positive test, whereas the fourth edition WHO standard considers a level of ≥50% to be a positive test. The level of binding of ≥50% is commonly considered to be clinically significant (10,25). The clinical value of antisperm antibody testing is predicated on the observation that the presence of a significant concentration of antibodies may impair fertilization. It has been reported that antibody-positive sperm may have difficulty penetrating cervical mucus. Although in these cases intrauterine insemination or IVF may improve the prognosis for fertilization, antibody levels >80%, coupled with subpar concentration, motility, or morphology, may necessitate the addition of ICSI in order to achieve the highest percentage of fertilization (26). As suggested by the literature, andrology laboratories may do a significantly better job of preparing sperm if they are aware of the presence of antibodies. Specifically, it has been demonstrated that the use of increased concentrations of protein in the media used for sperm preparation will reduce the adverse effect of antisperm antibodies on sperm motility. In summary, antisperm antibodies have been demonstrated to be a contributing factor in infertility. While their presence alone may not be sufficient to prevent pregnancy, their detection should encourage the andrologist to pursue additional appropriate action.

SPERM VITALITY

An intact plasma membrane is an integral component of, and possibly a biologic/diagnostic indicator for, sperm viability. The underlying principle is that viable sperm contain intact plasma membranes that prevent the passage of certain stains, whereas nonviable sperm have defects within their membranes that allow for staining of the sperm. Several so-called "vital stains" have been employed for this purpose. They include eosin Y, trypan blue, and/or nigrosin (27). When viewed with either bright field or phase contrast microscopy, these stains allow for the differentiation of viable, non-motile sperm from dead sperm. This procedure may, therefore, play a significant role in determining the percentage of immotile sperm that are viable and available for ICSI. Unfortunately, dyes such as eosin Y are specific DNA probes that may have toxic effects if they enter a viable sperm or oocyte, which precludes the use of these sperm that have been exposed to the dyes for ICSI or insemination. Flow cytometry has also been utilized for the determination of sperm viability. Like vital staining, flow cytometry is based on the principle that an intact plasma membrane will prevent the passage of nucleic acid-specific stains. Some techniques, such as the one described by Noiles et al., employ dual staining, which can differentiate between an intact membrane and a damaged membrane (28). There are no studies that prospectively evaluate sperm viability staining as a predictor of ART outcome.

HYPO-OSMOTIC SWELLING TEST

Another means of assessing the sperm plasma membrane is the hypo-osmotic swelling test (HOST). This assay is predicated upon the observation that all living cells are permeable to water, although to different degrees. The human sperm membrane has one of the highest hydraulic conductivity coefficients (2.4 μL/min/atm at 22°C) of any mammalian cell (29).

As originally described, the HOST involves placing a sperm specimen into hypotonic conditions of approximately 150 mOsmol (30). This environment, while not sufficiently hypotonic to cause cell lysis, will cause swelling of the sperm cells. As the tail swells, the fibers curl, and this change can be detected by phase contrast microscopy, differential interference contrast, or Hoffman optics. The normal range for a positive test is typically considered to be a score ≥60%; that is, at least 60% of the cells demonstrate curling of the tails. A negative test is defined as <50% curling (31). This test generated a significant amount of initial interest, and several investigators compared it to the sperm penetration assay (SPA) as an *in vitro* surrogate for fertilization, reporting good correlation (32,33). In the 1990s, several investigators reported using the test as a predictor of ART outcome, with conflicting results. Although one group reported a favorable correlation, another found no predictive value for the test (34,35). It has also been suggested that, owing to sperm morphology changes in response to the test, the HOST may facilitate an embryologist's ability to select sperm that is appropriate for injection. Regardless, as evidenced by the fact that there have been essentially no new human studies on the HOST in the past 15 years, it is likely that the use of the HOST is not increasing significantly. In our program at the Texas Fertility Center, we use the HOST to identify sperm that is suitable for use in ICSI cases where all sperm is non-motile. In summary, the HOST currently lacks sufficient critical evaluation to determine its true role in the assessment and/or treatment of the infertile male.

ASSAYS OF THE SPERM ACROSOME

The acrosome is an intracellular organelle, similar to a lysosome, which forms a cap-like structure over the apical portion of the sperm nucleus (36). The acrosome contains multiple hydrolytic enzymes, including hyaluronidase, neuraminidase, proacrosin, phospholipase, and acid phosphatase, which, when released, are thought to facilitate sperm passage through the cumulus mass, and possibly the zona pellucida as well (Figure 4.4). In fact, only acrosome-reacted sperm is capable of penetrating the zona pellucida, binding to the oolemma, and fusing with the oocyte (37). Once sperm undergoes capacitation, it is capable of an acrosome reaction. This reaction is apparently triggered by fusion of the sperm plasma membrane with the outer acrosomal membrane at multiple sites, leading to diffusion of the acrosomal enzymes into the extracellular space. This leads to the dissolution of the plasma membrane and acrosome, leaving the inner acrosomal membrane exposed over the head of the sperm (Figure 4.5). Although electron microscopy has produced many elegant pictures of acrosome-intact and acrosome-reacted sperm, it is not always possible to know whether sperm that fail to exhibit an acrosome have truly acrosome reacted, or could possibly be dead. In addition, electron microscopy is not a technique that is available to all andrologists.

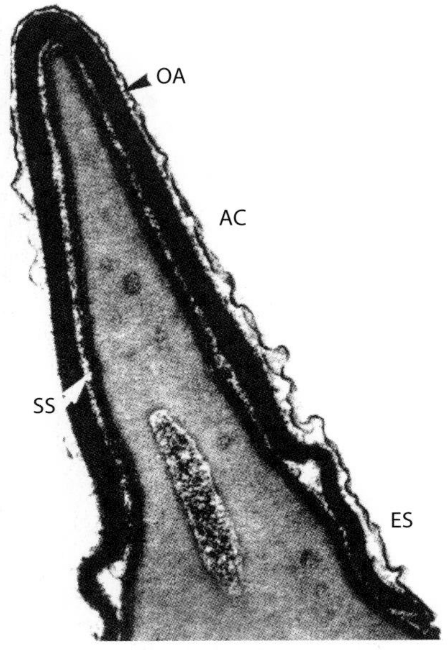

Figure 4.4 Sperm head with intact acrosome. *Abbreviations*: AC, acrosomal cap; ES equatorial segment; OA, outer acrosomal membrane; SS, subacrosomal space. (From Sathananthan AH, ed. *Visual Atlas of Human Sperm Structure and Function for Assisted Reproductive Technique*. Melbourne: La Trobe and Monash Universities, Singapore: National University, 1996, with permission.)

This has led to the necessity for the development of biochemical markers for the acrosome reaction. Throughout the 1970s, 1980s, and 1990s, multiple biochemical tests were described using a variety of lectins, antibodies, and stains. Although they apparently correlated well with electron microscopy, the tests were still time consuming and difficult to perform (38,39). Contemporary assays for the determination of acrosomal status employ fluorescent plant lectins or monoclonal antibodies, which can be detected much more easily with fluorescence microscopy (40,41). These assays may prove to be of value if they can truly identify males who manifest deficiencies in their ability to undergo the acrosome reaction. Evidence in support of the value of this test includes the finding that defective zona-induced acrosome reactions are present in a high percentage of subfertile men who have a normal semen analysis (42). Hypothetically, such patients may need to have their sperm specially preincubated—such

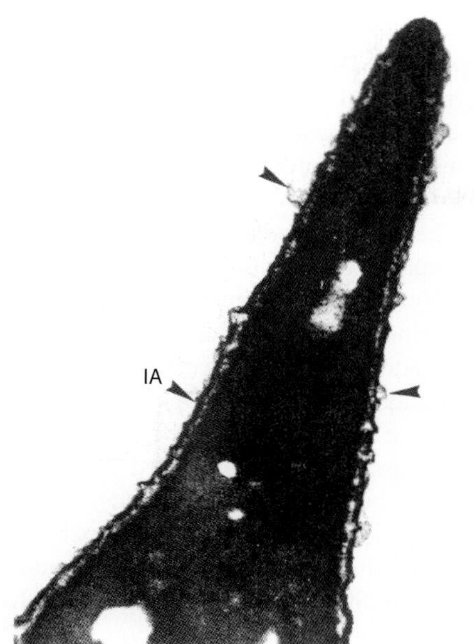

Figure 4.5 Acrosome-reacted sperm. *Abbreviation*: IA, inner acrosomal membrane. (From Sathananthan AH, ed. *Visual Atlas of Human Sperm Structure and Function for Assisted Reproductive Technique*. Melbourne: La Trobe and Monash Universities, Singapore: National University, 1996, with permission.)

as with follicular fluid or calcium ionophore—prior to insemination if they fail to acrosome react on their own. Conversely, this test may help to identify a small subpopulation of males who prematurely acrosome react. Several studies have reported an association between ejaculated sperm with low percentages of acrosome-intact sperm and poor subsequent fertilization (43). Therefore, ICSI should be considered for men with abnormal acrosome reaction testing. A published meta-analysis has demonstrated a high predictive value of tests of acrosomal reactivity for the prediction of fertilization *in vitro* (44). These areas certainly await additional study.

OTHER BIOCHEMICAL TESTS

As noted above, one of the predominant enzymes that is present in the acrosome is proacrosin. The enzymatic action of acrosin is not necessarily correlated to the presence of an intact acrosome; therefore, assays for the presence of acrosin have been described (45). Acrosin activity has been reported to be greater in fertile men than in infertile men (46); however, there are no prospective evaluations correlating acrosin activity to fertilization rates in ART patients. Like all other tissues that require energy synthesis and transport, spermatozoa contain measurable levels of creatinine phosphokinase. Two isomers, CK-M and CK-B, have been described, and differences have been noted in the levels of these isomers in semen specimens from fertile and infertile men. Specifically, CK-M levels exceed CK-B levels in normospermic males, while CK-B levels are greater in spermatozoa from oligospermic males (47). In this same study, researchers found that semen samples in which CK-M/CK-B ratios exceeded 10% exhibited higher fertilization rates in IVF than specimens with lower ratios. Few other studies have addressed this topic.

SPERM PENETRATION ASSAY

The SPA or hamster egg penetration assay was initially described by Yanagimachi et al. in 1976 (48). It measures the ability of sperm to undergo capacitation and the acrosome reaction, penetrate the oolemma, and then decondense. In this test, oocytes from the golden hamster are first treated in order to remove the zona pellucida. As one of the functions of the zona is to confer species specificity, its presence would preclude performance of this test. However, zona removal obviously prohibits the SPA from being able to assess sperm for the presence of zona receptors.

Following zona removal, human sperm are incubated for 48 hours with the hamster oocytes, and the number of penetrations with nuclear decondensation is calculated. As originally described, it was hoped that the test would correlate with the ability of human sperm to fertilize human oocytes *in vitro*. Although the test was designed to assess the ability of sperm to fuse to the oolemma, it also indirectly assesses sperm capacitation, the acrosome reaction, and the ability of the sperm to be incorporated into the ooplasm. Unfortunately, however, intrinsic in the design of the test is its inability to assess the sperm's ability to bind to—and penetrate through—the zona pellucida. This factor continues to be one of the major criticisms that plague this test. Throughout the 1980s, multiple modifications of the SPA were published. These included modifications of the techniques for sperm preparation prior to the performance of the assay, such as inducing the acrosome reaction or incubation with TEST yolk buffer (Irvine Scientific, Irvine, CA), changes in the protocol methodology itself, and modifications of the scoring system (49,50). Published reports demonstrated widely varying conclusions, such as the finding that the SPA could identify anywhere from 0% to 78% of men whose sperm would fail to fertilize oocytes in ART procedures (51). Most criticisms of the SPA literature center on the poor standardization of the assay, the poor reproducibility of the test, and the lack of a standard normal range.

Although some reports suggest a correlation between the SPA and fertility, neither a large literature review (51) nor a prospective long-term (five-year) follow-up study demonstrated such a correlation (52). In fact, a meta-analysis of 2906 subjects from 34 prospective, controlled studies suggested that the SPA is a poor predictor of fertilization (53). In light of these considerations, support for this test has gradually waned.

HEMIZONA ASSAY

Over the past several years, a growing body of research has demonstrated a significant correlation between tests of sperm–zona pellucida binding and subsequent fertilization in ART. This led the European Society for Human Reproduction and Embryology (ESHRE) Andrology Special Interest Group to recommend inclusion of such tests in the advanced evaluation of the male (54). Like the SPA, the hemizona assay (HZA) employs sperm and nonviable oocytes in an *in vitro* assessment of fertilization (55). In this test, however, both gametes are human in origin. As described, the HZA assesses the ability of sperm to undergo capacitation, acrosome react, and bind tightly to the zona. Classically, oocytes that failed to fertilize during an ART procedure are bisected, and then sperm from a proven fertile donor (500,000/mL) is added to one hemizona, while sperm from the subject male is added to the other hemizona. Following a four-hour incubation, each hemizona is removed and pipetted in order to dislodge loosely attached sperm. A comparison or hemizona index (HZI) is then calculated by dividing the number of test sperm tightly bound to the hemizona by the number of control (fertile) sperm bound to the other hemizona:

$$\text{HZI} = \frac{\text{Number of test sperm bound}}{\text{Number of control sperm bound} \times 100}$$

This test assesses the ability of sperm to bind to the zona itself. Although the HZA is relatively expensive, labor intensive, and difficult to perform, there are some data that suggest that the HZA may help to identify individuals with a poor prognosis for success with ART (Figure 4.6) (56,57). A more recent prospective study employing receiver operating characteristic curve analysis has also suggested that HZA results may be used to predict subsequent fertilization in ART procedures with both high sensitivity and specificity (58). Unlike several other tests of sperm function, a cutoff value (35%) has been identified as a predictor of IVF success. In addition, pregnancy rates in patients with values over 30 have been shown to be significantly higher than those in patients with values under 30 (40.6% vs. 11.1%, $p < 0.05$) (59).

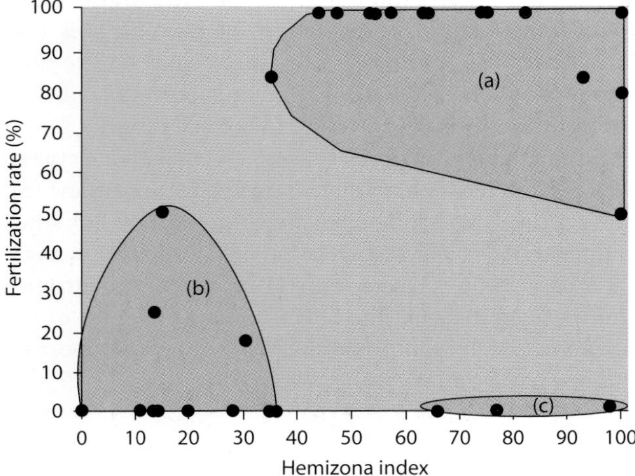

Figure 4.6 Cluster analysis of hemizona assay index and fertilization rate. (a) Good fertilization; (b) poor fertilization; and (c) false-positive hemizona assay index. (From Burkman LJ et al. *Fertil Steril* 1988; 49: 688–97, with permission.)

MANNOSE BINDING ASSAY

Another test has been developed in order to assess the ability of sperm to bind to the zona. This *in vitro* procedure is based on a series of observations that suggest that sperm–oocyte interaction involves the recognition by a sperm surface receptor of a specific complementary receptor on the surface of the zona pellucida. This zona receptor appears to be a glycoprotein, the predominant sugar moiety of which is mannose (60). In an elegant series of experiments, Mori et al. determined that sperm–zona binding could be curtailed by the addition of a series of sugars to the incubating media. Although many sugars impaired binding, the addition of mannose totally inhibited sperm–oocyte interaction (61). *In vitro* assays in which labeled probes of mannose conjugated to albumin are co-incubated with semen specimens allow for the differential staining of sperm (Figure 4.7). Those that bind the probe are thought to possess the sperm surface receptor for the mannose-rich zona glycoprotein. Several investigators, including our group, have subsequently demonstrated that sperm from fertile populations exhibit greater mannose binding than do sperm from infertile males (62–64). This new area shows promise in the area of sperm function testing, but also invites further study.

ASSAYS OF SPERM DNA INTEGRITY

The most current area of investigation into sperm function involves the assessment of sperm DNA integrity. Sperm chromatin has been demonstrated to be packaged very differently from chromatin in somatic cells. Specifically, the DNA is organized in such a manner that it remains very compact and stable (65). As there are many ways in which this DNA organization or the sperm chromatin itself can be damaged, several assays of sperm chromatin assessment have been developed. There are two basic types of assay: direct assays, such as the "Comet" and "Terminal deoxynucleotidyl transferase dUTP nick end labeling (TUNEL)" assays; and indirect assays, such as the sperm chromatin structure assay or acridine orange assay (66). The direct assays detect actual breakages in the DNA, while the indirect assays measure

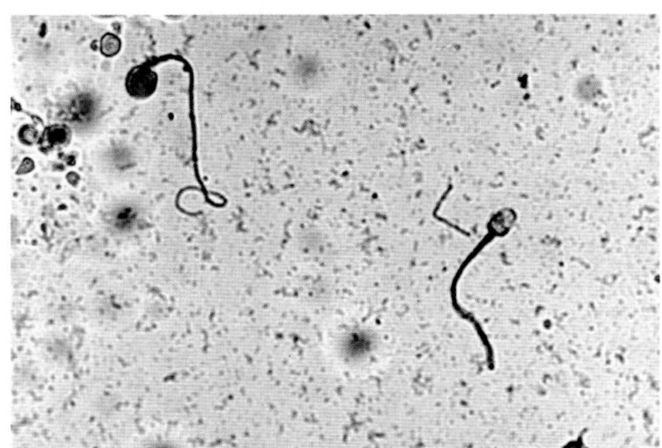

Figure 4.7 Mannose-positive (brown) and mannose-negative (clear) sperm. (Courtesy of Tammy Dey and Kaylen Silverberg.)

the relative proportions of single-stranded (abnormal) and double-stranded (normal) DNA within the sperm following acid treatment. Data from several studies suggest that infertile men have a significantly greater amount of DNA damage than fertile men (65,67,68). There is also a suggestion that this finding is similarly present in the male partners of couples experiencing recurrent miscarriage. Despite these reports, at the present time, there is no conclusive correlation between the results of sperm DNA integrity testing and pregnancy rates achieved either naturally or with the ARTs. As such, the Practice Committee of the American Society for Reproductive Medicine recommended that the routine testing of sperm DNA integrity should not be included in the evaluation of infertile couples (69).

CONCLUSION

In summary, there have been many recent advances in the diagnostic evaluation of sperm and sperm function. Although many tests of sperm function have been described, there remains a lack of consensus as to the role of testing and the identification of the appropriate test(s) to perform. Owing to the complicated nature of sperm function, it is improbable that a single test will emerge with sufficient sensitivity, specificity, and positive and negative predictive values required of a first-line diagnostic tool for all affected men. A more likely scenario will be similar to that in female infertility, where a battery of tests—each evaluating a specific function—are employed as needed. In light of profound recent advances in gamete micromanipulation, a more germane issue might be the overall relevance of sperm function testing in the contemporary andrology laboratory. Although this issue is quite controversial, it is likely that sperm function testing will continue to play a role in the evaluation of the infertile male. Just as ART is not the treatment of choice for all infertile women, it is not likely that micromanipulation will be the standard treatment for all infertile men. The gold standard of sperm function remains the ability to fertilize an oocyte *in vitro*. Therefore, in order to continue to address the above questions, it is incumbent upon investigators to design appropriate prospective trials to assess these tests thoroughly. Those tests that demonstrate a statistically significant correlation with fertilization *in vitro* must then undergo additional evaluation in order to assess clinical significance if we hope to develop an appropriate diagnostic algorithm.

REFERENCES

1. World Health Organization. *WHO Laboratory Manual for the Examination of Human Semen and Sperm-Cervical Mucus Interaction*, 4th edition. New York, NY: Cambridge University Press, 1999; pp. 60–1.
2. World Health Organization. *WHO Laboratory Manual for the Examination of Human Semen*, 5th edition. Geneva: WHO Press, 2010; pp. 223–5.
3. Cooper TG, Noonan E, von Eckardstein S et al. World Health Organization reference values for human semen characteristics. *Hum Reprod Update* 2010; 16: 231–45.
4. Alexander NJ. Male evaluation and semen analysis. *Clin Obstet Gynecol* 1982; 25: 463–82.
5. Overstreet JW, Katz DF, Hanson FW, Foseca JR. A simple inexpensive method for objective assessment of human sperm movement characteristics. *Fertil Steril* 1979; 31: 162–72.
6. Overstreet JW, Davis RO, Katz DF, Overstreet JW, eds. *Infertility and Reproductive Medicine. Clinics of North America*. Philadelphia, PA: WB Saunders, 1992; pp. 329–40.
7. Koren E, Lukac J. Mechanism of liquefaction of the human ejaculate: I. Changes of the ejaculate proteins. *J Reprod Fertil* 1979; 56: 493–500.
8. Lukac J, Koren E. Mechanism of liquefaction of the human ejaculate: II. Role of collagenase like peptidase and seminal proteinase. *J Reprod Fertil* 1979; 56: 501–10.
9. Cohen J, Aafjes JH. Proteolytic enzymes stimulate human spermatozoal motility and *in vitro* hamster egg penetration. *Life Sci* 1982; 30: 899–904.
10. Van Voorhis BJ, Sparks A. Semen analysis: What tests are clinically useful?. *Clin Obstet Gynecol* 1999; 42: 957–71.
11. Gangi CR, Nagler HM. Clinical evaluation of the subfertile man. In: *Infertility and Reproductive Medicine. Clinics of North America*. Diamond MP, DeCherney AH, Overstreet JW (eds). Philadelphia, PA: WB Saunders, 1992; pp. 299–318.
12. Sathananthan AH, ed. *Visual Atlas of Human Sperm Structure and Function for Assisted Reproductive Technique*. Melbourne: La Trobe and Monash Universities, Singapore: National University, 1996.
13. Kruger TF, Acosta AA, Simmons KF et al. Predictive value of abnormal sperm morphology in *in vitro* fertilization. *Fertil Steril* 1988; 49: 112–17.
14. Kruger TF, Menkveld R, Stander FS et al. Sperm morphologic features as a prognostic factor in *in vitro* fertilization. *Fertil Steril* 1986; 46: 1118–23.
15. Katz DF, Overstreet JW. Sperm motility assessment by videomicrography. *Fertil Steril* 1981; 35: 188–93.
16. Katz DF, Diel L, Overstreet JW. Differences in the movements of morphologically normal and abnormal human seminal spermatozoa. *Biol Reprod* 1982; 26: 566–70.
17. Franken DR, Oehninger S, Burkman LJ et al. The hemizona assay (HZA): A prediction of human sperm fertilizing potential in *in vitro* fertilization (IVF) treatment. *J In Vitro Fert Embryo Transfer* 1989; 6: 44–50.
18. Coetzee K, Kruger TF, Lombard CJ. Predictive value of normal sperm morphology: A structured literature review. *Hum Reprod Update* 1988; 4: 73–82.
19. Enginsu MF, Pieters MGEC, Dumoulin JCM, Evers JLH, Geruedts JPM. Male factor as determinant of *in vitro* fertilization outcome. *Hum Reprod* 1992; 7: 1136–40.
20. Davis R. The promise and pitfalls of computer aided sperm analysis. In: *Infertility and Reproductive Medicine. Clinics of North America*, Diamond MP,

DeCherney AH, Overstreet JW (eds). Philadelphia, PA: WB Saunders, 1992; pp. 341–52.

21. Irvine DS. The computer assisted semen analysis systems: Sperm motility assessment. *Hum Reprod* 1995; 10(Suppl 1): 53–9.
22. Krause W. Computer assisted semen analysis systems: Comparison with routine evaluation and prognostic value in male fertility and assisted reproduction. *Hum Reprod* 1995; 10(Suppl 4): 60–6.
23. Marshburn PB, Kutteh WH. The role of antisperm antibodies in infertility. *Fertil Steril* 1994; 61: 799–811.
24. Golumb J, Vardinon N, Hommonnai ZT et al. Demonstration of antispermotozoal antibodies in varicocelerelated infertility with an enzyme-linked immunosorbent assay (ELISA). *Fertil Steril* 1986; 45: 397–405.
25. Helmerhost FM, Finken MJJ, Erwich JJ. Detection assays for antisperm antibodies: What do they test?. *Hum Reprod* 1999; 14: 1669–71.
26. Bronson R. Detection of antisperm antibodies: An argument against therapeutic nihilism. *Hum Reprod* 1999; 14: 1671–73.
27. World Health Organization. *Manual for Examination of Human Semen and Semen–Cervical Mucus.* Cambridge: Cambridge University Press, 1987; pp. 1–12.
28. Noiles EE, Ruffing NA, Kleinhans FW et al. Critical tonicity determination of sperm using dual fluorescent staining and flow cytometry. In: *Reproduction in Domestic Animals*, (Suppl 1) Boar Semen Preservation II. Proceedings of the Second International Conference on Boar Semen Presentation. Johnson LA, Rath D (eds). Beltsville, MD: Paul Parey, 1991; pp. 359–64.
29. Noiles EE, Mazur, P, Watson PF et al. Determination of water permeability coefficient for human spermatozoa and its activation energy. *Biol Reprod* 1993; 48: 99–109.
30. Jeyendran RS, Van der Ven JJ, Perez-Pelaez M. Development of an assay to assess the functional integrity of the human sperm membrane and its relationship to other semen characteristics. *J Reprod Fertil* 1984; 70: 219–28.
31. Zaneveld LJD, Jeyendran RS. Modern assessment of semen for diagnostic purposes. *Semin Reprod Endocrinol* 1988; 4: 323–37.
32. Chan SYW, Fox EJ, Chan MMC. The relationship between the human sperm hypoosmotic swelling test, routine semen analysis, and the human sperm zona free hamster ovum penetration test. *Fertil Steril* 1985; 44: 688–92.
33. Jeyendran RS, Zaneveld LJD. Human sperm hypoosmotic swelling test. *Fertil Steril* 1986; 46: 151–4.
34. Mladenovic I, Micic S, Genbacev O et al. The hypoosmotic swelling test for quality control of sperm prepared for assisted reproduction. *Arch Androl* 1995; 34: 163–9.
35. Joshi N, Kodwany G, Balaiah D et al. The importance of CASA and sperm function testing in an *in vitro* fertilization program. *Int J Fertil Menopausal Stud* 1996; 41: 46–52.
36. Critser JK, Noiles EE. Bioassays of sperm function. *Semin Reprod Endocrinol* 1993; 11: 1–16.
37. Yanagmachi R. Mammalian fertilization. In: *The Physiology of Reproduction*, 2nd edition. Knobil E, Neill JD (eds). New York, NY: Raven Press; 1994; pp. 189–317.
38. Talbot P, Chacon RS. A triple stain technique for evaluating acrosome reaction of human sperm. *J Exp Zool* 1981; 215: 201–8.
39. Wolf DP, Boldt J, Byrd W et al. Acrosomal status evaluation in human ejaculated sperm with monoclonal antibodies. *Biol Reprod* 1985; 32: 1157–62.
40. Cross N, Morales P, Overstreet JW et al. Two simple methods for detecting acrosome-reacted sperm. *Gamete Res* 1986; 15: 213–6.
41. Holden CA, Hyne RV, Sathananthan AH et al. Assessment of the human sperm acrosome reaction using concanavalin A lectin. *Mol Reprod Dev* 1990;25:247–57.
42. Liu DY, Clarke GN, Martic M et al. Frequency of disordered zona pellucida (ZP)-induced acrosome reaction in infertile men with normal semen analysis and normal spermatozoa-ZP binding. *Hum Reprod* 2001; 16: 1185–90.
43. Oehninger S, Franken DR Sayed E et al. Sperm function assays and their predictive value for fertilization outcome in IVF therapy: A meta analysis. *Hum Reprod Update* 2000; 6: 1160–8.
44. Chan PJ, Corselli JU, Jacobson JD et al. Spermac stain analysis of human sperm acrosomes. *Fertil Steril* 1999; 72: 124–8.
45. Kennedy WP, Kaminski JM, Van der Ven HH et al. A simple clinical assay to evaluate the acrosin activity of human spermatozoa. *J Androl* 1989; 10: 221–31.
46. Mohsenian M, Syner FN, Moghissi KS. A study of sperm acrosin in patients with unexplained infertility. *Fertil Steril* 1982; 37: 223–9.
47. Huszar G, Vigue L, Morshedi M. Sperm creatinine phosphokinaseM-isoform ratios and fertilizing potential of men: A blinded study of 84 couples treated with *in vitro* fertilization. *Fertil Steril* 1992; 57: 882–8.
48. Yanagimachi R, Yanagimachi H, Rogers BJ. The use of zona-free animal ova as a free system for the assessment of their fertilizing capacity of human spermatozoa. *Biol Reprod* 1976; 15: 471–6.
49. Aitken RJ, Thatcher S, Glasier AF et al. Relative ability of modified versions of the hamster oocyte penetration test, incorporating hyperosmotic medium of the ionophore A23187 to predict IVF outcome. *Hum Reprod* 1987; 2: 227–31.
50. Jacobs BR, Caulfield J, Boldt J. Analysis of TEST (TES and tris) yolk buffer effects on human sperm. *Fertil Steril* 1995; 63: 1064–70.
51. Mao C, Grimes DA. The sperm penetration assay: Can it discriminate between fertile and infertile men? *Am J Obstet Gynecol* 1988; 159: 279–86.
52. O'Shea DL, Odem RR, Cholewa C et al. Long-term follow-up of couples after hamster egg penetration testing. *Fertil Steril* 1993; 60: 1040–5.

53. Oehninger S, Franken DR, Sayed E, Barroso G, Kolm P. Sperm function assays and their predictive value for fertilization outcome in IVF therapy: A meta-analysis. *Hum Reprod Update* 2000; 6: 160–8.
54. ESHRE Andrology Special Interest Group. Consensus workshop on advanced diagnostic andrology techniques. *Hum Reprod* 1996; 11: 1463–79.
55. Burkman LJ, Coddington CC, Franken DR et al. The hemizona assay (HZA): Development of a diagnostic test for the binding of human spermatozoa to the human hemizona pellucida to predict fertilization potential. *Fertil Steril* 1988; 49: 688–97.
56. Oehninger S, Acosta AA, Marshedi M et al. Corrective measures and pregnancy outcome in *in vitro* fertilization in patients with severe sperm morphology abnormalities. *Fertil Steril* 1989; 50: 283–7.
57. Liu DY, Baker HW. High frequency of defective sperm–zona pellucida interaction in oligoozospermic infertile men. *Hum Reprod* 2004; 19: 228–33.
58. Coddington CC, Oehninger SC, Olive DL et al. Hemizona index (HZI) demonstrates excellent predictability when evaluating sperm fertilizing capacity in *in vitro* fertilization patients. *J Androl* 1994; 15: 250–4.
59. Arslan M, Morshedi M, Arslan EO et al. Predictive value of the hemi zona assay for pregnancy outcome in patients undergoing controlled ovarian hyperstimulation with intrauterine insemination. *Fertil Steril* 2006; 85: 1697–707.
60. Mori K, Daitoh T, Irahara M et al. Significance of D-mannose as a sperm receptor site on the zona pellucida in human fertilization. *Am J Obstet Gynecol* 1989; 161: 207–11.
61. Mori K, Daitoh T, Kamada M et al. Blocking of human fertilization by carbohydrates. *Hum Reprod* 1993; 8: 1729–32.
62. Tesarik J, Mendoza C, Carreras R. Expression of D-mannose binding sites on human spermatozoa: Comparison of fertile donors and infertile patients. *Fertil Steril* 1991; 56: 113–18.
63. Benoff S, Cooper GW, Hurley I et al. Human sperm fertilizing potential *in vitro* is correlated with differential expression of a head-specific mannose ligand receptor. *Fertil Steril* 1993; 59: 854–62.
64. Silverberg K, Dey T, Witz C et al. D-Mannose binding provides a more objective assessment of male fertility than routine semen analysis: Correlation with *in vitro* fertilization. Presented at the 49th Annual Meeting of the American Fertility Society, October 11–14, 1993, Montreal, Canada.
65. Agarwal A, Said T. Role of sperm chromatin abnormalities and DNA damage in male infertility. *Hum Reprod Update* 2003; 9: 331–45.
66. Evenson DP, Wixon R. Clinical aspects of sperm DNA fragmentation detection and male infertility. *Theriogenology* 2006; 65: 979–91.
67. Zini A, Bielecki R, Phang D et al. Correlations between two markers of sperm DNA integrity, DNA denaturation and DNA fragmentation in fertile and infertile men. *Fertil Steril* 2001; 75: 674–7.
68. Evenson DP, Jost LK, Marshall D et al. Utility of the sperm chromatin assay as a diagnostic and prognostic tool in the human fertility clinic. *Hum Reprod* 1999; 14: 1039–49.
69. The Practice Committee of the American Society for Reproductive Medicine. The clinical utility of sperm DNA integrity testing. *Fertil Steril* 2006; 86(Suppl 4): S35–7.

Sperm preparation techniques

5

HAROLD BOURNE and JANELL ARCHER

OVERVIEW

The aim of sperm preparation for assisted reproduction technology (ART) is to maximize the chances of fertilization to provide as many normally fertilized oocytes as possible for transfer to the uterus or cryopreservation (1). With normal semen it is easy to obtain motile sperm by a variety of techniques. Abnormal semen, which will not yield adequate sperm for standard *in vitro* fertilization (IVF), needs to be recognized so that intracytoplasmic sperm injection (ICSI) can be used. Refinements of the preparation procedures are required to obtain spermatozoa or elongated spermatids with the highest potential for normal fertilization from grossly abnormal semen samples or from samples obtained directly from the male genital tract. Sperm characteristics important for fertilization with standard IVF include normal morphology, normal intact acrosomes, straight-line velocity (VSL) and linearity (LIN), and the ability to bind to the zona pellucida, penetrate the zona pellucida, fuse with the oolemma, activate the oocyte, and form a male pronucleus (1). For ICSI, live sperm with the ability to activate the oocyte and form a pronucleus are necessary but morphology, motility, and acrosome status are generally not important (1–5). It is probably important to remove seminal plasma as it contains decapacitation factors and extraneous cells and degenerating sperm that may produce agents capable of damaging the sperm (6–8). For IVF or gamete intrafallopian transfer (GIFT), the medium should contain protein and buffers that promote sperm capacitation (1). While serum or high-molecular-weight fractions from serum appear to be important for sperm motility, more recently relatively pure preparations of human serum albumin, pasteurized to reduce the risk of transmitting infections, have been found to be adequate for sperm preparation for standard IVF and ICSI (9,10). Purified and appropriately tested human serum albumin preparations are now routinely available from the major IVF media suppliers. The inclusion of protein in the culture medium is required to prevent sperm adhering to surfaces. Although the concentration of albumin in human periovulatory oviductal fluid is reported to be of the order of 30 mg/mL, concentrations of around 4 mg/mL will support normal sperm function in IVF. Bicarbonate ions are required for capacitation of sperm and are normally present at about 25 mmol/L in the medium. Although glucose is utilized as a metabolic substrate by sperm it is not clear whether it is essential for normal function *in vitro*, although glucose is usually included in commercially available media used for fertilization.

Damage to the sperm from dilution, temperature change, centrifugation, and exposure to potentially toxic material must be minimized. Dilution should be performed slowly, especially with cryopreserved sperm. Temperature changes should be gradual. Preparation of the insemination suspension should be performed at or as close as practicable to 37°C. Centrifugal force should be the lowest possible required to bring down the most motile sperm. Minimizing centrifugation, particularly in the absence of seminal plasma, and separating the live motile sperm from the dead sperm and debris early in the procedure should limit oxidative damage caused by free oxygen radicals released from leukocytes or abnormal sperm (6,7,11).

Modifications of sperm preparation may be necessary for the various types of ART. For example, for GIFT or intratubal insemination, suspensions of spermatozoa are to be introduced into the fallopian tubes so debris and bacteria must be removed and no particulate material added that might damage the female genital tract. If cryopreserved donor sperm are to be used, matching and extra care in preparation of the sample is usually required. If the semen is severely abnormal, sperm are prepared for ICSI.

Combinations of gradient centrifugation and swim up may produce higher yields of good-quality sperm (12). In the era of ICSI, the need for special preparation techniques has receded as simple procedures with swim up, washing, or allowing sperm to swim to the medium–oil interface from a centrifuged pellet placed in droplets of medium under oil produce fertilization and pregnancy results as good as those with sperm obtained by more careful and laborious preparation techniques (13). The use of gradient centrifugation may also provide additional safeguards in preparing sperm from men with a chronic viral illness (14,15). The use of tubes specially designed to minimize the risk of carryover of seminal components (e.g., Proinsert™, Nidacon Laboratories AB, Gothenburg, Sweden) may further reduce the risk of cross-infection (16).

The optimal number of sperm for insemination is poorly defined, but several reviews of results of IVF suggest that there is an increase in fertilization rate with insemination of sperm at between 2000 and 500,000/mL (1). There may be some increase in risks of polyspermy with the higher sperm concentrations, thus most groups inseminate oocytes with approximately 100,000 sperm/mL for standard IVF or GIFT. This is more than surround the oocyte *in vivo* and, if better selection of high-quality sperm could be achieved, insemination with lower numbers could be as or more successful. It has been suggested that reduced exposure of the oocyte to sperm may result in improvement in embryo quality and higher implantation rates (17,18). The total volume of sperm suspension added should be minimized to restrict dilution of the oocyte medium.

METHODS

Procedures for preparation of the culture media and sperm isolation are given in Appendices 5.1 through 5.12 and are shown schematically in Figures 5.1 through 5.4.

Collection of semen or sperm

While semen is usually collected by masturbation for ART, sperm may be collected by a variety of methods from several sites in the male genital tract (Figure 5.1). The man should collect semen into a sterile disposable plastic jar in a room adjacent to the IVF laboratory. The sperm should be prepared soon after liquefaction of the seminal plasma. If liquefaction is delayed or the specimen is particularly viscous, syringing the sample through a 21-gauge needle or mixing the specimen 1:1 with medium followed by vigorous shaking may help. If the semen sample is unexpectedly poor, a second sample may provide sufficient sperm. Cryopreserved sperm can also be used, for example, as backup for ICSI for patients with motile sperm present in the semen only intermittently.

The timing of semen collection and preparation does not appear to be critical, especially with good semen samples. In general the oocytes are inseminated four to six hours after collection and the sperm can be prepared during this time. The semen should be placed in a clean area of the laboratory or in a laminar flow hood. The sample must be mixed thoroughly because ejaculation does not result in a homogeneous suspension of sperm in the seminal plasma. The semen sample is examined, any particulate material is allowed to settle, and the supernatant is transferred to another tube if necessary. Following mixing, a small portion (~10 μL) of the sample is taken to check the sperm concentration and motility. With normal semen samples, usually 1 mL of sample is sufficient for preparation of adequate numbers of motile sperm. If the semen sample is mildly to moderately abnormal but judged adequate for standard IVF, then the whole semen volume should be distributed to several tubes for preparation of as many sperm as possible.

Sperm preparation

Initially, IVF involved repeated "washing" of the spermatozoa by dilution of the semen with culture medium supplemented with protein, followed by centrifugation and resuspension of the pellet. This technique has been criticized as it may result in oxidative damage of the sperm by free oxygen radicals (6,7,11,19,20). Sperm for ICSI may be harvested from the oil–medium interface after sperm-containing material is placed in a drop of culture medium under oil (Figure 5.3). Some prepare channels to outlying smaller droplets for this purpose.

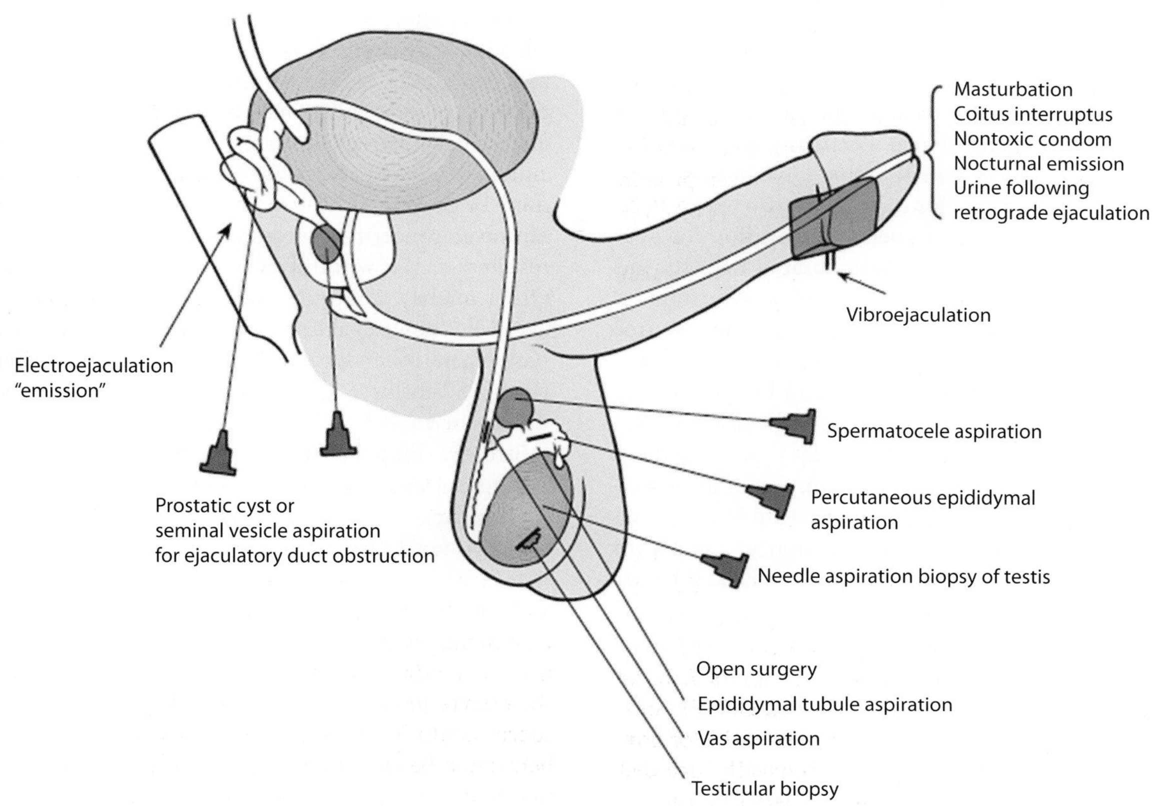

Figure 5.1 Possible sites of collection of sperm or elongated spermatids from the male genital tract for assisted reproduction technology.

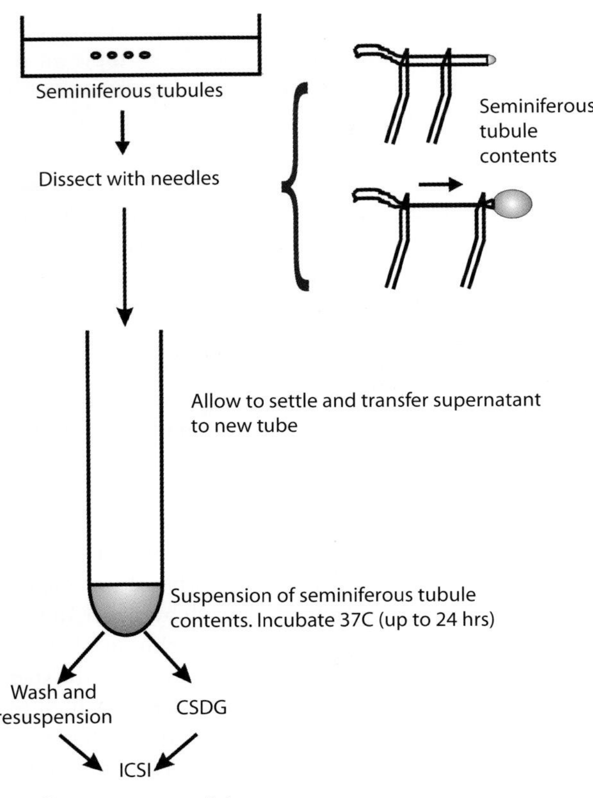

Figure 5.2 Procedure for seminiferous tubules obtained by fine-needle tissue aspiration or open biopsy.

All plastic, glassware and media should be checked for toxicity to sperm or embryos (e.g., sperm may be immobilized by contact with rubber). For many consumables, suppliers have products available that have been specifically tested as appropriate for human *in vitro* use. A variety of media are suitable for sperm preparation for IVF. The medium chosen should be equilibrated with the gas mixture and the temperature maintained constant at 37°C. If not using a commercially available protein source suitable for human ART but preparing a protein source in-house from serum, then this needs to be checked for sperm antibodies and, if pools are used, the donors must be tested for viral illnesses including HIV and hepatitis. However, the use of pooled serum samples is to be discouraged because of the risk of transmitting both known and unknown diseases. Heat inactivation of the serum should not be relied upon to overcome the risk of transmitting infections.

Swim up

Several variations of the swim up procedure are possible. The seminal plasma can be overlaid directly with culture medium and the sperm allowed to swim from the seminal plasma into the culture medium. Following this, the sperm suspension should be washed to ensure adequate removal of seminal plasma constituents. Alternatively, the semen sample may be diluted and centrifuged and the pellet loosened and overlaid or the semen sample may be centrifuged without prior dilution of the seminal plasma and the pellet loosened and overlaid with medium for the swim up procedure. The latter technique may be particularly useful for oligozoospermia as the sperm may be damaged by the dilution procedure. If cryopreserved semen is to be used, dilution of the semen sample should be slow with dropwise addition of culture medium to the thawed sample. If the thawed semen is overlaid directly, the need for slow dilution is eliminated.

After centrifugation, the supernatant is aspirated off the pellet and the pellet gently resuspended in a small volume of liquid. The overlay medium is then gently pipetted onto the surface of the pellet and the tube incubated for 45–60 minutes. Prolonged incubation times may result in a reduced yield of motile sperm from gravitational effects. The use of a conical tube for centrifugation may help maximize yield as the pellet is easier to see and less likely to be disturbed during manipulation. Some recommend that the tubes be placed in the incubator at an angle to increase the surface area of the interface. Following incubation, the upper half to two-thirds of the overlay is aspirated, mixed, and the sperm concentration determined.

Density gradients

Various gradient separation procedures have been introduced. The advantage is that the gradient separation techniques are rapid, requiring 20 minutes of centrifugation compared with an average of 1 hour of incubation for swim up. Shorter times may be utilized for samples with adequate parameters. They are also relatively simple to perform under sterile conditions. The most popular of these is colloidal silica density gradient (CSDG) centrifugation, but other agents have also been used (1,12,21). The colloidal silica particles are coated with polyvinylpyrrolidone (e.g., Percoll™; Pharmacia AB, Uppsala, Sweden). However, concerns regarding the levels of endotoxins have resulted in the withdrawal of Percoll from use in ART. Other media containing silane-coated silica have become available for clinical use from the major IVF media companies and other specialist suppliers, including Isolate™ (Irvine Scientific, Santa Ana, CA), PureSperm™ (Nidacon Laboratories AB, Gothenburg, Sweden), SpermGrad™ (Vitrolife, Englewood, CO), SupraSperm™ (Medicult, Jyllinge, Denmark), PureCeption™ (Sage BioPharma, Bedminster, NJ), Sil-Select™ (FertiPro, Beeman, Belgium), and Sydney IVF sperm gradient medium (William A. Cook, Brisbane, QLD, Australia).

Discontinuous gradients of two or more steps are used. Sperm and other material form distinct bands at the interfaces on the CSDG (Figure 5.4). It has been claimed that abnormal sperm as well as immotile sperm and debris are largely eliminated and a rapid and efficient isolation of motile human sperm, free from contamination with other seminal constituents, is possible. A number of studies have compared CSDG centrifugation with a swim up and occasionally other sperm preparation techniques. The end points of the studies have been recovery of motile sperm,

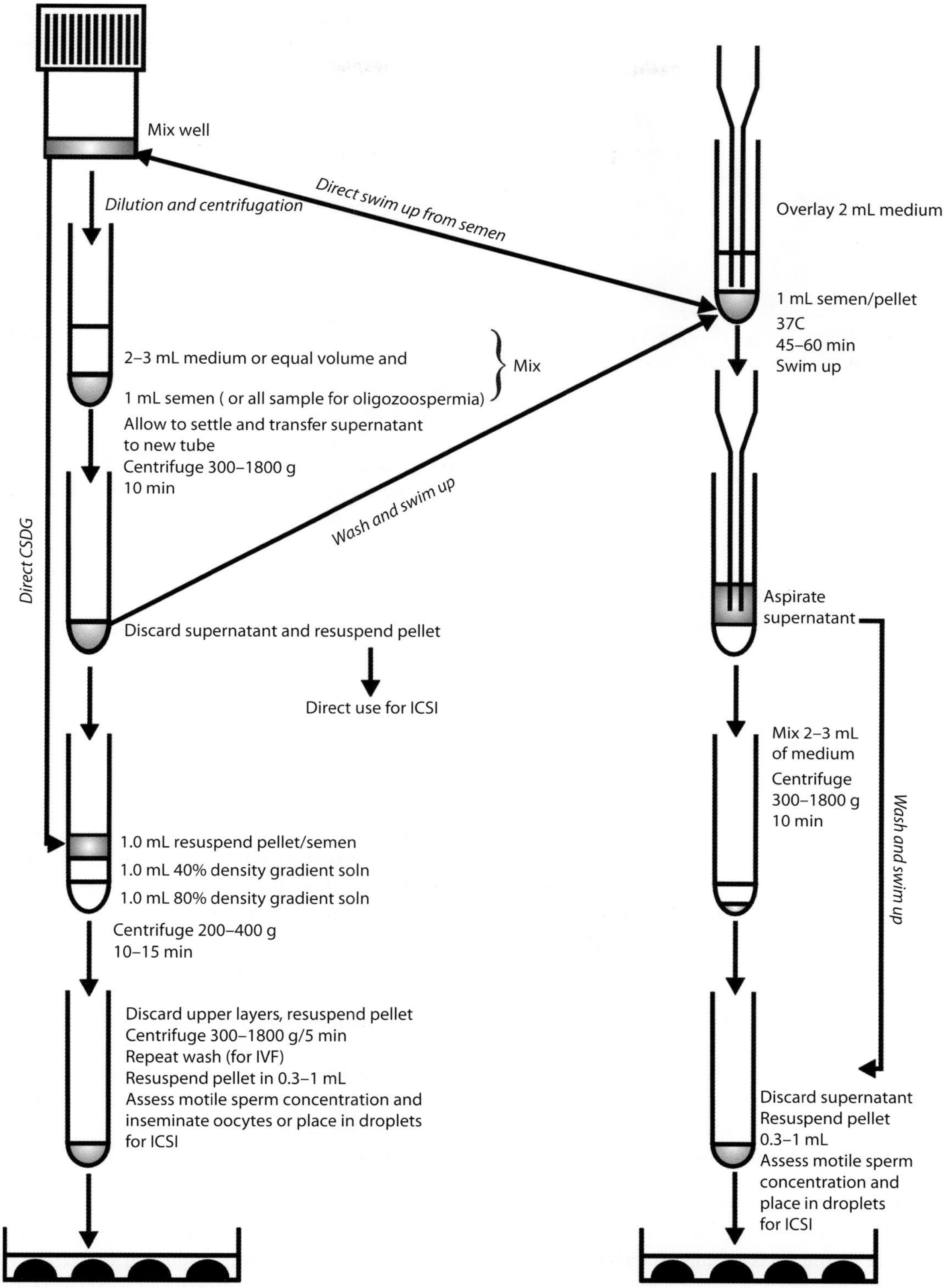

Figure 5.3 Methods of sperm preparation for assisted reproduction technology.

morphology, chromatin structure assessed by the various techniques, and ultrastructure. Generally, the recovery of motile sperm is greater with the gradient techniques, but the percentage of sperm with progressive motility is usually lower and the proportion of sperm with good morphology lower with gradient centrifugation than with swim up (1,8,12,22–24). Some studies suggest that the gradient materials may damage the sperm (25,26). Others indicate gradient preparations produce sperm with less mitochondrial and DNA damage than other procedures

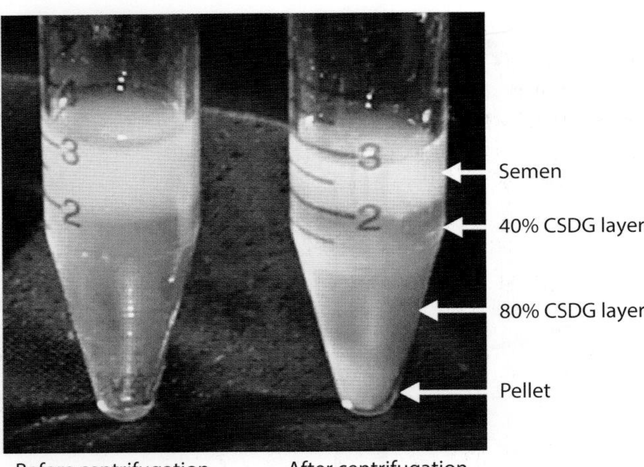

Figure 5.4 Appearance of gradient tubes with overlaid semen prior to and after centrifugation.

(27–30). However, while there are some reports of higher fertilization and pregnancy rates, improved results of IVF and ICSI are not consistently found (27,28). CSDG in combination with swim up has also been reported to reduce the viral load from samples carrying an infectious agent such as HIV (31–35) However, CSDG on its own, or in combination with swim up, should not be relied upon to minimize the risk of infection to the woman or any resulting pregnancy (32,36–40), although modifications to the procedure may further reduce the chance for viral contamination of the final preparation (16,40–42).

Sperm preparation from surgical aspirates or tissue samples

Spermatozoa or elongated spermatids may be obtained for ICSI from the male genital tract by microsurgical epididymal sperm aspiration, percutaneous epididymal sperm aspiration, testicular open biopsy, fine-needle aspiration biopsy, or other techniques (Figure 5.1). Preparing tissue from a fine-needle biopsy can be managed using fine-gauge needles. Processing of large amounts of tissue may be expedited by using bigger implements (e.g., scalpel blades) and/or a sterile mortar and pestle homogenizer in the style of a small conical tube and insert. Methods for preparation are outlined in Appendices 5.7 and 5.8.

Sperm selection from immotile samples

ICSI with immotile sperm is often associated with low fertilization rates, thus every attempt should be made to ensure that live sperm are injected (1–4,43). A variety of agents have been reported to enhance sperm motility (1). Pentoxifylline (POF) has been used for ART. The maximally effective dose of POF is between 0.3 and 0.6 mmol/L and many groups use 3.6 mmol/L (1 mg/mL). POF has been reported to provide greater stimulation of motility and velocity than caffeine or 2-deoxyadenosine. Regulatory authorities are becoming increasingly stringent on appropriate safeguards for the in-house preparation of products for clinical use. Commercial versions of motility stimulants appropriately tested for human use are now available (e.g., SpermMobil®, Gynemed Medizinprodukte GmbH & Co, Lensahn, Germany). Use of an appropriately tested product in preference to an in-house preparation should reduce risk and ensure quality while also complying with regulatory requirements where required.

Exposure of sperm to hypo-osmotic medium is also used to identify potentially viable sperm by detecting membrane integrity. Its use may reveal a higher proportion of viable sperm than utilizing motility stimulants alone; however, it can be technically more difficult in cases where sperm density is high or large amounts of debris or extraneous material are present. The use of a laser pulse applied to the tail tip of an immotile sperm (44) and a mechanical touch technique (45) have also been suggested as useful tools to identify viable sperm for injection, although both of these approaches await verification in a wider setting. In practical terms, the generation of sperm movement from the use of motility stimulants has the added advantage of making live sperm more conspicuous and therefore may be the preferred first choice in identifying viable sperm from an immotile population. Appendices 5.10 and 5.11 give methods for stimulating sperm motility with POF and the use of hypo-osmotic media.

Preparation of semen from HIV-infected men

The use of combination antiretroviral (cARV) therapies has markedly improved the prognosis and life expectancy for men infected with HIV. A population of these men in a discordant relationship (i.e., where the man is seropositive and the women is uninfected) are desiring parenthood using their own gametes. With appropriate medical care and use of ART techniques, safe and effective treatment can now be offered for achieving a pregnancy while minimizing the risk of transmission to either the partner or a resulting baby (14,15,46–53). Most protocols recommend the use of antiretroviral therapies to reduce viral load, subsequent testing of sperm samples for residual viral HIV RNA and DNA using sensitive polymerase chain reaction techniques, and the preparation of cleared samples for clinical use via density gradient centrifugation. Normally, cryopreservation of the sperm is required to allow adequate time for the testing regimens to be completed. Samples with undetectable or sufficiently low viral loads are cleared for use and, depending on the quality of the sperm post-thaw, an attempt at pregnancy is undertaken using intrauterine insemination (IUI), IVF, or ICSI.

More recently, the use of pre-exposure prophylaxis (PrEP) has been reported as a treatment option for discordant couples where the male is seropositive for HIV (54,55). A course of cARV in the male to reduce viral load in blood to an acceptable level is combined with a period of cARV therapy in the woman and unprotected intercourse is timed for the fertile phase of the cycle, thereby bypassing the need for specific *in vitro* procedures. However, this approach is unlikely to be useful in cases with fertility issues in the man or woman. An advantage of PrEP is that it may eliminate the need for further testing of semen samples prior to use in ART. Overall, however, sperm washing is still a recommended approach and studies on the safety and suitability of PrEP and timed intercourse as an alternative to sperm washing and ART are limited.

Sperm selection techniques

A variety of techniques have been reported for the selection of sperm with characteristics that may improve outcome. The quality of sperm DNA packaging, described in terms of DNA damage or fragmentation, has been implicated in poor embryo development and pregnancy loss. Methods to select sperm with reduced levels of damage have been sought in an attempt to improve clinical outcomes following ART.

The use of membrane-based electrophoretic filtration to potentially select sperm with reduced DNA damage has been reported (56). Clinical pregnancies have been achieved; however, sperm recovery, functional parameters, and clinical outcomes were comparable to sperm prepared by CSDG centrifugation, and its benefits may be limited to simplicity of use (57). Other methods utilizing magnetic-activated cell sorting to remove apoptotic sperm, based on the externalization of phosphatidylserine residues, may prove to be more effective in selecting sperm with reduced DNA damage (58,59).

The selection of sperm defined as normal following evaluation under high magnification has been reported as useful for improving outcomes with ICSI (60,61). The approach utilizes live examination of sperm under high-power optics with further virtual magnification via digital imaging. Those motile sperm exhibiting a normal nuclear profile based on shape and absence of vacuolization and lacking neck and tail abnormalities are preferentially selected for injection (62). Improvements in fertilization rate and early embryo development are generally not seen, but significant improvements in implantation rate and reduced pregnancy loss have been reported (60,61). However, the technique is time consuming and requires some specialized equipment, and further prospective randomized controlled trials are still warranted in order to confirm the efficacy of this approach.

Sperm binding to hyaluronic acid has also been described as a sperm selection tool for ICSI, and commercial products are available for clinical use. The ability of sperm to bind to hyaluronic acid is reported as being related to normal morphology, maturity, and DNA integrity (63,64). Sperm are exposed to hyaluronic acid on a coated slide or Petri dish and those that bind are then preferentially used for ICSI (65). However, the ability of hyaluronic binding to identify functional sperm of better quality than by routine techniques may be limited (66). An alternative sperm binding method is to utilize human zonae. The ability of the human zona pellucida to selectively bind sperm with normal morphology and an intact acrosome is well described (67–69). In this approach, immature eggs from the same cohort are incubated for two hours with prepared sperm. Sperm that bind are then removed by aspiration through a fine glass pipette and set aside for ICSI. Preliminary reports show improvements in embryo quality and implantation rate (70–72). However, further trials using sibling oocytes are needed in order to validate any benefits. A method for preparing and selecting sperm by zona pellucida binding is outlined in Appendix 5.12.

RESULTS

Comparisons of normal fertilization and embryo utilization rates for swim up and CSDG, categorized according to male indication, are presented in Table 5.1. Apart from the improvement in the normal fertilization rate with CSDG for IVF with oligozoospermic samples, the results are similar. Results with sperm or elongated spermatids obtained from the genital tract, cryopreserved samples, and following the use of hypo-osmotic swelling have been previously published (4,73–75).

Fertilization results and incidence of poor outcome for different culture conditions and sperm preparation methods are presented in Table 5.2. The normal fertilization rate improved steadily following the introduction of closed mini-incubators (William A. Cook) and the change from a single-stage medium (human tubal fluid, Irvine Scientific, supplemented with 4 mg/mL human serum albumin, Albumex®-20, CSL Ltd, Melbourne, Australia) to a sequential medium formulation containing a different albumin (Quinn's Advantage™ containing 4 mg/mL human albumin, Sage BioPharma). These results were matched by an overall decrease in the incidence of cycles with poor fertilization, indicating that increased fertilization was also achieved in patients with a poor prognosis.

Following the routine introduction of density gradient centrifugation, improvements in fertilization rates and decreases in the incidence of poor fertilization cycles were found for standard IVF inseminations, probably due to a reduced chance for carryover of inhibitory components from seminal plasma following CSDG preparation. No difference in fertilization rate was observed between swim up and CSDG-prepared sperm for ICSI.

Thus, improvements in fertilization results can be achieved by optimizing culture conditions. In preparing sperm for ART, CSDG centrifugation appears to be a more reliable method for standard IVF, while swim up provides a simple alternative approach for ICSI.

Results from the treatment of HIV-discordant couples have been published (52,53). Pregnancy rates following the use of ART with washed sperm are similar to non-infected couples. Overall, the screening and storage of sperm prior to treatment appears to be an effective fertility treatment for couples where the male is HIV positive, with no seroconversions reported in any women or delivered babies to date (76). The role of PrEP as a suitable adjunct or alternative to ART for attempting pregnancy awaits further study.

Table 5.1 Comparison of results with swim up and colloidal silica density gradient (CSDG) preparation of sperm from semen for *in vitro* fertilization (IVF) or intracytoplasmic sperm injection (ICSI) from men with normal semen (sperm concentration ≥20 × 10^6/mL, progressive motility ≥40%, and abnormal morphology ≤85%), abnormal semen (sperm concentration 1–19 × 10^6/mL or progressive motility 1%–39% or abnormal morphology 86%–100%), or oligoasthenoteratozoospermia (sperm concentration 1–19 × 10^6/mL, progressive motility 1%–39%, and abnormal morphology 86%–100%) from 1990 to 1999

	IVF				ICSI			
	Oocytes collected	**IVF**	**Normal fertilization**	**Embryo utilization**	**Oocytes collected**	**ICSI**	**Normal fertilization**	**Embryo utilization**
Normal semen								
Swim up	21,255	21,031	12,286	10,520	1396	1113	665	545
		99	*58*	*49*		*80*	*48*	*39*
CSDG	3319	3298	1833*	1577*	905	685	394	322
		99	*55*	*48*		*76*	*44*	*36*
Abnormal semen								
Swim up	8826	8733	4236	3513	5718	4664	2804	2367
		99	*48*	*40*		*82*	*49*	*41*
CSDG	6126	5943	2720*	2338*	6387	5221	3054	2567
		97	*44*	*38*		*82*	*48*	*40*
Oligoasthenoteratozoospermia								
Swim up	360	354	97	93	1328	1072	610	514
		98	*27*	*26*		*81*	*46*	*39*
CSDG	1183	1158	416*	358	2436	2016	1142	941
		98	*35*	*30*		*83*	*47*	*39*

Note: Men with sperm autoimmunity were excluded. Embryo utilization is the sum of embryos transferred fresh and those frozen for later transfer. Percentages using oocytes collected as the denominator are shown in italics. Asterisks indicate significant differences between results for swim up and CSDG ($p < 0.05$, χ^2 test).

Table 5.2 Comparison of fertilization rate and incidence of cycles with poor fertilization (<20% of eggs fertilized normally) for different culture conditions and sperm preparation methods, introduced sequentially over a three-year period

		ICSI				Standard IVF			
Culture conditions	**Sperm preparation**	**No. of cycles**	**Cycles with <20% fertilization**	**Eggs injected**	**Fertilized normally**	**No. of cycles**	**Cycles with <20% fertilization**	**Eggs inseminated**	**Fertilized normally**
HTF medium/ open incubators	Swim up	1327	106 (8.0%)[a,b]	10,188	6605 (64.8%)[e,f]	1372	254 (18.5%)[g,h]	12174	6455 (53.0%)[k]
Sequential medium/ open incubators	Swim up	330	32 (9.7%)[c,d]	2915	1977 (67.8%)[e]	324	59 (18.2%)[i,j]	3187	1699 (53.3%)[l]
	CSDG	465	24 (5.2%)[a,c]	3829	2597 (67.8%)[f]	392	45 (11.5%)[g,i]	3689	2152 (58.3%)[k,l]
Sequential medium / mini incubators	CSDG	456	17 (3.7%)[b,d]	3921	2848 (72.6%)[e,f]	477	53 (11.1%)[h,j]	4473	2861 (64.0%)[k,l]

[a–l] Results with the same superscript letters are significantly different by χ^2 tests.

Abbreviations: CSDG, colloidal silica density gradient; HTF, human tubal fluid; ICSI, intracytoplasmic sperm injection; IVF, *in vitro* fertilization.

COMPLICATIONS

Although there is potential for semen- or sperm-dependent complications of ART such as infections or allergic reactions, these are very rare. Patients should be tested for serious transmissible infections such as HIV and hepatitis, and standard precautions for handling biological material must be practiced in the embryology laboratory. Transmission of genetic conditions to offspring is possible; suitable counselling and, where possible, screening should be part of the clinical work-up of the couple. Strict laboratory quality control should minimize the risks of loss or errors of identity of gametes or embryos.

With ICSI for primary spermatogenic disorders, an increased frequency of sex chromosomal aneuploidies has been noted in the conceptuses (77). In some clinics there appears to be a higher rate of abnormal fertilization with ICSI using testicular sperm (74,78), although this is not a universal finding,

FUTURE DIRECTIONS AND CONTROVERSIES

The main problems to be solved in the future are the accurate identification of patients who are likely to have problems with fertilization and require ICSI, effective treatment of defective sperm production or function, and improved implantation and pregnancy rates with ART. Improved prediction of results will come from the development of new methods of semen analysis such as automated sperm morphology and simple tests for assessing the ability of sperm to interact with oocytes (1). Effective treatment of most forms of male infertility is only a remote possibility, especially as the pathogenesis remains obscure (79). Further studies should resolve questions about the involvement of free oxygen species in the pathogenesis of sperm defects and whether this may affect the health of the offspring (6,11,19,20,80). New technology may improve the procedures for activation of the oocyte to allow direct injection of a sperm head or nucleus from spermatids or spermatocytes, although there is rarely a need for this clinically (81). The contribution of the sperm to abnormal embryonic development, failure of implantation, and pregnancy wastage will probably become clear as preimplantation genetic diagnosis and other tests of embryos are more widely used. However, advances in sperm selection methods offer some prospect for improved clinical outcome (82). Practical methods for selection of sperm with normal chromosomes or a desired sex chromosome are also likely to be developed (83).

CONCLUSION

The principles of sperm preparation for IVF and ICSI are outlined and practical methods are given.

ACKNOWLEDGEMENTS

The authors thank Associate Professor G.N. Clarke and Dr. D.Y. Liu for advice about cryopreservation procedures, Dr. M. Giles, Dr. A. Mijch, Dr. P. Foster, Professor S. Garland, and Associate Professor S. Tabrizi for assistance with the management and testing of HIV-discordant couples, and Dr. C. Garrett and Ms. P. Sourivong for assistance with the figures.

APPENDICES

Appendix 5.1: Preparation of media

- Suitable culture media are available from a variety of commercial suppliers. The methods in the following have been described using Quinn's Advantage™ (QA) sequential culture media (fertilization medium), QA medium with hydroxyethanepropoxy ethane sulfonate buffer (QA/HEPES) and human albumin from Sage BioPharma (Bedminster, NJ) and PureSperm™ colloidal silica density gradient from Nidacon Laboratories (Gothenburg, Sweden). However, the methods can be followed using other products substituted where required, while taking note of the requirement for equilibration with CO_2 or room atmosphere as appropriate.
- As required, human albumin (ALB) solution (100 mg/mL, Sage BioPharma, pharmaceutical grade) is added (1 part in 25) to give a final concentration of 4 mg/mL.
- Both QA fertilization medium with albumin and QA/HEPES/ALB are prepared and stored refrigerated until required (maximum storage time according to the manufacturer's expiry date: about six weeks).
- Bicarbonate-buffered media requiring CO_2 to attain physiological pH are equilibrated prior to use under a CO_2 atmosphere according to the manufacturer's recommendations.

Appendix 5.2: Choice of method

- Patient and sample identity should be checked with another person and recorded as a quality assurance measure.
- Examine a drop of undiluted semen (hemocytometer or Makler chamber):
  - *For standard in vitro fertilization:*
    - Prepare sperm by density gradient centrifugation.
    - If the sample is unexpectedly poor on the day (e.g., concentration $<10 \times 10^6$/mL, <40% motility, and/or poor forward progression), intracytoplasmic sperm injection should be considered.
  - *For intracytoplasmic sperm injection:*
    - Prepare sperm by density gradient centrifugation or swim up.
    - Even samples with severe oligozoospermia (down to ~10,000/mL) can be prepared using swim up as long as there are some sperm with good forward progression.
    - Alternatively, samples may be concentrated by wash and resuspension and used directly or prepared further by density gradient centrifugation or swim up.
    - Samples with large amounts of debris, extreme oligozoospermia, or severely compromised motility are better prepared by colloidal silica density gradient.
    - Surgical samples obtained from the testis or epididymis and those collected by electro-ejaculation

typically have a low motile sperm concentration and are more suited to colloidal silica density gradient separation to maximize yield and remove tissue debris. Alternatively, surgical samples can be used directly if there is little extraneous cellular material and sufficient progressive motility to allow sperm to migrate to the edge of the drop.

Appendix 5.3: Density gradient

Colloidal silica density gradient stock solutions

- "PureSperm" (to make 50 mL of solution).
  - 40% stock solution: 20 mL "PureSperm," 28 mL Quinn's Advantage (QA)/HEPES, 2 mL of 100 mg/mL human albumin (pharmaceutical grade).
  - 80% stock solution: 40 mL "PureSperm", 8 mL QA/HEPES, 2 mL of 100 mg/mL human albumin (pharmaceutical grade).

Preparation and use of gradients

- Prepare sufficient tubes for each patient:
  - Dispense 1.0 mL of 40% gradient stock solution into a 15-mL conical tube (Falcon 2095, Becton Dickinson, NJ).
  - With a clean Pasteur pipette, underlay 1.0 mL of 80% gradient stock solution.
- Carefully overlay ~1 mL of semen (fresh or thawed) or sperm suspension directly on top of gradient:
  - Ensure gradients are at room temperature before overlaying.
- Prepare multiple gradients if the sperm concentration is low.
- To maximize yield (e.g., for severe oligozoospermia or testicular biopsy samples):
  - Samples may be concentrated by wash and resuspension prior to placing onto gradient.
  - Centrifugation speed and time may be increased, as described below.
  - Additional sperm can also be obtained by wash and resuspension of the upper gradient layers/supernatant that are normally discarded after removal of the bottom gradient layer and pellet.
- Centrifuge at 200–300 g for 10 minutes (braking may be used during deceleration):
  - Increase centrifugation to 400 g for 15 minutes to improve yield of poor intracytoplasmic sperm injection (ICSI) samples.
- Gently remove all but the bottom 0.3–0.5 mL and place in a discard tube.
- With a clean Pasteur pipette, gently aspirate the remaining solution and pellet and transfer to a fresh conical tube containing ~8 mL of medium, in preparation for a single wash:
  - Avoid contact with the sides of the tube to minimize carryover of seminal plasma and debris.
  - For *in vitro* fertilization (IVF), the single large-volume wash may be replaced by two smaller-volume washes (~3–4 mL each) if there are concerns for carryover of seminal components into the final preparation.
- Centrifuge at 300 g for 5 minutes:
  - Use increased centrifugation (up to 1800 g) to maximize yield of poor ICSI samples.
- Remove supernatant and re-suspend in 0.3–1.0 mL of QA/fertilization medium (for IVF) or QA/HEPES/human albumin (for ICSI).
- Assess sperm quality in the final sample (count, motility, and progression) and calculate volume required for insemination as follows:
  - Place ~5 μL of prepared sperm onto a counting chamber (hemocytometer or Makler chamber) and allow to settle (for more than three minutes).
  - Grade forward progression (FP) is as follows: FP0: no movement; FP1: movement but minimal progression; FP2: slow progression; FP3: moderate to rapid progression.
  - Count the number of motile sperm in a minimum of five squares from the central 25 squares (hemocytometer) or a minimum of 10 squares (Makler chamber) to estimate the motile concentration (to improve accuracy, aim to count at least 50 sperm).
  - For IVF: calculate volume of final sperm suspension required for insemination (ideally 10–50 μL) to give a total of 100,000–200,000 FP3 sperm/mL in the medium containing the oocytes.
- Incubate at 37°C under 5% CO_2 (IVF) or room atmosphere (ICSI) until required.

Appendix 5.4: Swim up

- After the semen has liquefied (usually 30 minutes at 37°C), 1-mL aliquots of semen are placed in 5-mL labeled tubes (Falcon 2003) and gently overlaid with 2 mL of medium (Quinn's Advantage/HEPES/human albumin):
  - For samples with poor mucolysis, dilute semen with two to three volumes of appropriate medium and mix vigorously; allow any particulate matter to settle, transfer supernatant to another test tube, and use as described for liquefied semen.
  - Alternatively, samples may be prepared as described for wash and resuspension, or the semen may be centrifuged directly and the seminal plasma removed, prior to overlaying the resulting pellet with medium for swim up.
- Incubate tubes at 37°C for 45–60 minutes to allow progressively motile sperm to swim into the overlaid medium.
- Taking care not to disrupt the interface or collect any seminal plasma, collect the overlaid medium, mix with 2–3 mL of medium, and centrifuge at 300 g for 5–10 minutes (increase centrifugation up to 1800 g to maximize yield of poor intracytoplasmic sperm injection samples).

- Remove the resulting supernatant and re-suspend the pellet in 0.3–1.0 mL of fresh medium.
- Assess sperm quality (count, motility, and velocity) and incubate at 37°C in room atmosphere until required for intracytoplasmic sperm injection.

Appendix 5.5: Wash and resuspension

- Allow semen to liquefy at 37°C for 30 minutes.
- Mix 1 mL of semen with 2–3 mL of appropriate medium.
- Centrifuge for 10 minutes at 300 g (increase centrifugation up to 1800 g to maximize yield of poor intracytoplasmic sperm injection samples).
- Aspirate supernatant and re-suspend pellet in 0.3–1 mL of appropriate medium.
- Assess sperm quality in the final sample (count, motility, and progression) and incubate at 37°C until required, as previously described.

Appendix 5.6: Preparation of slow-frozen sperm

- Double check straw/vial code and patient ID.
- *For standard straws*:
  - Thaw straw in air for 10–20 minutes; check integrity of the straw and discard if damaged.
  - Decontaminate outside of straw by wiping with isopropyl or detergent-impregnated towelettes, or by soaking in hypochlorite solution (~0.5% available chlorine; e.g., 1:1 dilution of Milton antibacterial solution, Milton Australia, Rozelle, Australia) for at least two minutes to disinfect the outside of the straw and reduce chance for cross-infection; rinse in fresh water and wipe excess solution from the straw after soaking.
  - Cut one end and aspirate contents.
- *For vials:*
  - Loosen cap (to prevent the build-up of pressure during thawing) and thaw by placing in a buoyant rack and floating in room temperature water, taking care to keep the water level below the level of the cap; sample should be fully thawed within 10 minutes.
- Assess sperm concentration, motility, and progression.
- Prepare sample by density gradient centrifugation as previously described:
  - Alternatively, samples for intracytoplasmic sperm injection (ICSI) may be prepared by swim up if sufficient motile sperm are present, or via wash and resuspension if the sample has been washed prior to cryopreservation and/or there is minimal extraneous cellular material or debris.
- Assess sperm count, motility, and progression in the final suspension. For *in vitro* fertilization (IVF) samples, calculate the volume required for insemination.
- Incubate at 37°C under 5% CO_2 (IVF) or room atmosphere (ICSI) until required.

Appendix 5.7: Microsurgical epididymal sperm aspiration/percutaneous epididymal sperm aspiration

- Epididymal sperm are obtained either by microsurgery (microsurgical epididymal sperm aspiration) or by percutaneous, fine-needle aspiration (percutaneous epididymal sperm aspiration)
- Expel aspirates into a small Petri dish of warm Quinn's Advantage (QA)/HEPES/human albumin (ALB).
- Pool samples and concentrate if necessary.
- Depending on concentration, motility, and amount of debris, either use directly, prepare by wash and resuspension, or separate on a density gradient.
- Leave sperm to incubate to allow sperm to gain motility:
  - Up to 24 hours in QA fertilization/ALB at 37°C under 5% CO_2.
  - For same-day use, prepare plate for intracytoplasmic sperm injection (ICSI) and leave at 37°C in QA/HEPES/ALB (room atmosphere).
- If extra sperm are available, consider freezing the excess. Samples with >5000 motile sperm/mL should have a sufficient yield of live sperm post-thaw for subsequent ICSI treatments. A method for cryopreservation of such samples is given in Appendix 5.9.

Appendix 5.8: Testicular biopsy

- Testicular tissue is obtained either by open biopsy (testicular sperm extraction) or percutaneous fine-needle aspiration (testicular sperm aspiration).
- Place tissue into a small Petri dish of warm Quinn's Advantage (QA)/HEPES/human albumin (ALB).
- Dissect tubules using fine-gauge needles (Figure 5.2), sterile scalpel blades, and/or macerate using a sterile mortar and pestle-style homogenizer.
- Transfer raw suspension to a test tube.
- Depending on concentration, motility, and amount of debris, either use directly, prepare by wash and resuspension, or separate on a density gradient.
- Leave sperm to incubate to allow sperm to gain motility:
  - Up to 24 hours in QA fertilization/ALB at 37°C under 5% CO_2.
  - For same-day use, prepare plate for intracytoplasmic sperm injection and leave at 37°C in QA/HEPES/ALB (room atmosphere).
- If extra sperm are available, consider freezing the excess (Appendix 5.9).

Appendix 5.9: Freezing protocol for oligozoospermia and washed sperm

- Semen containing only a few motile sperm and sperm suspensions obtained from the genital tract can be stored for subsequent intracytoplasmic sperm injection.
- Epididymal, testicular, and oligozoospermic sperm suspensions are routinely processed by density gradient centrifugation or wash and resuspension.

- Sperm in excess to that required for treatment can be cryopreserved with glucose–citrate–glycine (GCG) glycerol cryoprotectant supplemented with human albumin. Commercial providers also supply preparations suitable for sperm cryopreservation.
- *GCG glycerol cryoprotectant (in-house preparation):*
  - Dissolve glucose (1.0 g) and sodium citrate (1.0 g) in 40 mL of sterile deionized water.
  - Add glycine (1.0 g) (pH ~7.5 and osmolality ~500 mOsm/kg).
  - Add 10 mL of glycerol, mix, and filter (0.2 μm).
  - Store in 2 mL volumes at −70°C.
- *Albumin stock solution:*
  - Dilute albumin (Sage BioPharma, 100 mg/mL) 1:1 with Tyrode buffer to make albumin stock solution (50 mg/mL); filter (0.45 μm) and store at -70°C.
- As required, thaw a vial of GCG glycerol.
- Add an equal volume of albumin stock solution to the sperm sample and mix well.
- Add GCG glycerol solution to sperm/albumin suspension 1:2 (one volume of GCG glycerol to two volumes of sperm/albumin) gradually over about five minutes with mixing.
- Package in cryovials (Nunc A/S, Roskilde, Denmark) and freeze:
  - Freeze gradually by suspending in liquid nitrogen vapor and store similarly.
- Alternatively, samples can be frozen using commercially available freezing media (e.g., QA Sperm Freeze, Sage BioPharma):
  - Add one volume of freezing medium dropwise to an equal volume of sperm suspension (add cold medium slowly over about five minutes and mix well between additions; use cold medium directly from the fridge [4°C] as this can improve post-thaw motility).
  - Place the final sperm/cryoprotectant mixture into a cryovial (~1.5 mL per vial).
  - Freeze and store over liquid nitrogen vapor as described above.

Appendix 5.10: Use of motility stimulants

In-house preparation

- Prepare a 10× concentrated solution of pentoxifylline (POF; Sigma-Aldrich, Sydney, Australia) in protein-free Quinn's Advantage/HEPES (POF MW = 278.3; 10× concentrate = 10 mg/mL).
- Sterilize through a 0.2-μm filter and store at 4°C.
- Dilute 1:9 with sperm suspension to expose sperm to a final concentration of 1 mg/mL POF (3.6 mM).
- Spread the treated sperm suspension adjacent to the holding drops in the injection plate.

Commercial preparation (e.g., SpermMobil)

- Prepare for use according to manufacturer's instructions.
- Add 1.5–2 μL of SpermMobil to prepared sperm suspension (~5 μL) in plate to be used for intracytoplasmic sperm injection (ICSI).

Sperm collection and handling

- Functional sperm should show motility within 10 minutes of exposure to the stimulant.
- Move the motile sperm to clean, stimulant-free medium.
- Expel the treated medium from the injection pipette and rinse with the untreated, clean medium in the holding drop; repeat rinsing of sperm and injection pipette.
- Immobilize the selected sperm and perform ICSI as usual.
- Aim to collect the motile sperm without excessive delay (within about three hours) as the treated sperm may lose motility with time.

Appendix 5.11: Use of hypo-osmotic medium

- Prepare a 100–150-mOsm/kg solution by diluting Quinn's Advantage/HEPES/human albumin 1:1 or 1:2 with purified water.
- Filter and store at 4°C.
- Add a drop of hypo-osmotic medium adjacent to the holding drops in the injection plate.
- Transfer sperm using the injection pipette to the hypo-osmotic medium.
- Immotile sperm with an intact plasma membrane should coil their tails shortly after contacting the hypo-osmotic medium.
- Move the presumptive live sperm to the normo-osmotic oocyte holding drop and leave briefly to equilibrate.
- Expel the hypo-osmotic medium from the injection pipette and rinse with normo-osmotic medium; repeat rinsing of sperm and injection pipette.
- Immobilize the selected sperm and perform intracytoplasmic sperm injection as usual.

Appendix 5.12: Selection of sperm for intracytoplasmic sperm injection following binding to the zona pellucida

- Prepare a sperm suspension as for a standard *in vitro* fertilization insemination, aiming for a final sperm density greater than 1×10^6/mL and motility greater than 50%.
- Select denuded immature egg(s) for exposure to sperm (i.e., germinal vesicle or germinal vesicle breakdown/metaphase I eggs that are not destined to be used clinically).
- Place the selected eggs into the prepared sperm suspension and incubate at 37°C under appropriate CO_2 and O_2 conditions for two hours.
- Transfer the incubated eggs to a clean well of medium using a large-bore Pasteur pipette (>250 μm; i.e., significantly greater than the diameter of the eggs).
- Gently aspirate the eggs using a fresh large-bore pipette to remove unbound sperm and carryover from the insemination drop.

- Transfer the eggs to another clean well of medium and repeat the procedure.
- Repeat the washing step again, before transferring the eggs to a microdrop in the dish to be used for intracytoplasmic sperm injection (ICSI).
- Remove bound sperm from the eggs by repeated aspiration through a fine-bore glass pipette approximating the diameter of the egg (i.e., approximately 120 μm).
- Select and process the isolated motile sperm for ICSI as usual.
- If no or insufficient sperm binding has occurred, perform ICSI using non-bound sperm from the initial sperm suspension.

REFERENCES

1. Baker G, Liu DY, Bourne H. Assessment of the male and preparation of sperm for ARTs. In: *Handbook of in vitro Fertilization*. Trounson AO, Gardner DK (eds.) Boca Raton, FL: CRC Press, 1999; pp. 99–126.
2. Nagy Z, Liu J, Cecile J, Silber S, Devroey P, Van Steirteghem A. Using ejaculated, fresh, and frozen-thawed epididymal and testicular spermatozoa gives rise to comparable results after intracytoplasmic sperm injection. *Fertil Steril* 1995; 63(4): 808–15.
3. Nagy ZP, Verheyen G, Tournaye H, Van Steirteghem AC. Special applications of intracytoplasmic sperm injection: The influence of sperm count, motility, morphology, source and sperm antibody on the outcome of ICSI. *Hum Reprod* 1998; 13(Suppl 1): 143–54.
4. Bourne H, Richings N, Liu DY, Clarke GN, Harari O, Baker HW. Sperm preparation for intracytoplasmic injection: Methods and relationship to fertilization results. *Reprod Fertil Dev* 1995; 7(2): 177–83.
5. Dozortsev D, Rybouchkin A, De Sutter P, Qian C, Dhont M. Human oocyte activation following intracytoplasmic injection: The role of the sperm cell. *Hum Reprod* 1995; 10(2): 403–7.
6. Aitken RJ, Gordon E, Harkiss D et al. Relative impact of oxidative stress on the functional competence and genomic integrity of human spermatozoa. *Biol Reprod* 1998; 59(5): 1037–46.
7. Mortimer D. Sperm preparation techniques and iatrogenic failures of *in-vitro* fertilization. *Hum Reprod* 1991; 6(2): 173–6.
8. Mortimer D. Sperm recovery techniques to maximize fertilizing capacity. *Reprod Fertil Dev* 1994; 6(1): 25–31.
9. Adler A, Reing AM, Bedford JM, Alikani M, Cohen J. Plasmanate as a medium supplement for *in vitro* fertilization. *J Assist Reprod Genet* 1993; 10(1): 67–71.
10. Laverge H, De Sutter P, Desmet R, Van der Elst J, Dhont M. Prospective randomized study comparing human serum albumin with fetal cord serum as protein supplement in culture medium for *in-vitro* fertilization. *Hum Reprod* 1997; 12(10): 2263–6.
11. Aitken RJ, Sawyer D. The human spermatozoon—Not waving but drowning. *Adv Exp Med Biol* 2003; 518: 85–98.
12. Ng FL, Liu DY, Baker HW. Comparison of Percoll, mini-Percoll and swim-up methods for sperm preparation from abnormal semen samples. *Hum Reprod* 1992; 7(2): 261–6.
13. De Vos A, Nagy ZP, Van de Velde H, Joris H, Bocken G, Van Steirteghem A. Percoll gradient centrifugation can be omitted in sperm preparation for intracytoplasmic sperm injection. *Hum Reprod* 1997; 12(9): 1980–4.
14. Savasi V, Ferrazzi E, Lanzani C, Oneta M, Parrilla B, Persico T. Safety of sperm washing and ART outcome in 741 HIV-1-serodiscordant couples. *Hum Reprod* 2007; 22(3): 772–7.
15. Bujan L, Sergerie M, Kiffer N et al. Good efficiency of intrauterine insemination programme for serodiscordant couples with HIV-1 infected male partner: A retrospective comparative study. *Eur J Obstet Gynecol Reprod Biol* 2007; 135(1): 76–82.
16. Fourie JM, Loskutoff N, Huyser C. Semen decontamination for the elimination of seminal HIV-1. *Reprod Biomed Online* 2015; 30(3): 296–302.
17. Gianaroli L, Cristina Magli M, Ferraretti AP et al. Reducing the time of sperm–oocyte interaction in human *in-vitro* fertilization improves the implantation rate. *Hum Reprod* 1996; 11(1): 166–71.
18. Gianaroli L, Fiorentino A, Magli MC, Ferraretti AP, Montanaro N. Prolonged sperm–oocyte exposure and high sperm concentration affect human embryo viability and pregnancy rate. *Hum Reprod* 1996; 11(11): 2507–11.
19. Twigg J, Irvine DS, Houston P, Fulton N, Michael L, Aitken RJ. Iatrogenic DNA damage induced in human spermatozoa during sperm preparation: Protective significance of seminal plasma. *Mol Hum Reprod* 1998; 4(5): 439–45.
20. Twigg JP, Irvine DS, Aitken RJ. Oxidative damage to DNA in human spermatozoa does not preclude pronucleus formation at intracytoplasmic sperm injection. *Hum Reprod* 1998; 13(7): 1864–71.
21. Ord T, Patrizio P, Marello E, Balmaceda JP, Asch RH. Mini-Percoll: A new method of semen preparation for IVF in severe male factor infertility. *Hum Reprod* 1990; 5(8): 987–9.
22. Claassens OE, Menkveld R, Harrison KL. Evaluation of three substitutes for Percoll in sperm isolation by density gradient centrifugation. *Hum Reprod* 1998; 13(11): 3139–43.
23. Carrell DT, Kuneck PH, Peterson CM, Hatasaka HH, Jones KP, Campbell BF. A randomized, prospective analysis of five sperm preparation techniques before intrauterine insemination of husband sperm. *Fertil Steril* 1998; 69(1): 122–6.
24. Centola GM, Herko R, Andolina E, Weisensel S. Comparison of sperm separation methods: Effect on recovery, motility, motion parameters, and hyperactivation. *Fertil Steril* 1998; 70(6): 1173–5.

25. Grab D, Thierauf S, Rosenbusch B, Sterzik K. Scanning electron microscopy of human sperms after preparation of semen for in-vitro fertilization. *Arch Gynecol Obstet* 1993; 252(3): 137–41.
26. Sterzik K, De Santo M, Uhlich S, Gagsteiger F, Strehler E. Glass wool filtration leads to a higher percentage of spermatozoa with intact acrosomes: An ultrastructural analysis. *Hum Reprod* 1998; 13(9): 2506–11.
27. Hammadeh ME, Kuhnen A, Amer AS, Rosenbaum P, Schmidt W. Comparison of sperm preparation methods: Effect on chromatin and morphology recovery rates and their consequences on the clinical outcome after *in vitro* fertilization embryo transfer. *Int J Androl* 2001; 24(6): 360–8.
28. Tomlinson MJ, Moffatt O, Manicardi GC, Bizzaro D, Afnan M, Sakkas D. Interrelationships between seminal parameters and sperm nuclear DNA damage before and after density gradient centrifugation: Implications for assisted conception. *Hum Reprod* 2001; 16(10): 2160–5.
29. Marchetti C, Obert G, Deffosez A, Formstecher P, Marchetti P. Study of mitochondrial membrane potential, reactive oxygen species, DNA fragmentation and cell viability by flow cytometry in human sperm. *Hum Reprod* 2002; 17(5): 1257–65.
30. O'Connell M, McClure N, Powell LA, Steele EK, Lewis SE. Differences in mitochondrial and nuclear DNA status of high-density and low-density sperm fractions after density centrifugation preparation. *Fertil Steril* 2003; 79(Suppl 1): 754–62.
31. Semprini AE, Levi-Setti P, Bozzo M et al. Insemination of HIV-negative women with processed semen of HIV-positive partners. *Lancet* 1992; 340(8831): 1317–9.
32. Marina S, Marina F, Alcolea R et al. Human immunodeficiency virus type 1-serodiscordant couples can bear healthy children after undergoing intrauterine insemination. *Fertil Steril* 1998; 70(1): 35–9.
33. Kim LU, Johnson MR, Barton S et al. Evaluation of sperm washing as a potential method of reducing HIV transmission in HIV-discordant couples wishing to have children. *AIDS* 1999; 13(6): 645–51.
34. Hanabusa H, Kuji N, Kato S et al. An evaluation of semen processing methods for eliminating HIV-1. *AIDS* 2000; 14(11): 1611–6.
35. Pasquier C, Daudin M, Righi L et al. Sperm washing and virus nucleic acid detection to reduce HIV and hepatitis C virus transmission in serodiscordant couples wishing to have children. *AIDS* 2000; 14(14): 2093–9.
36. Chrystie IL, Mullen JE, Braude PR, Rowell P, Williams E, Elkington N, et al. Assisted conception in HIV discordant couples: Evaluation of semen processing techniques in reducing HIV viral load. *J Reprod Immunol* 1998; 41(1-2): 301–6.
37. Leruez-Ville M, de Almeida M, Tachet A et al. Assisted reproduction in HIV-1-serodifferent couples: The need for viral validation of processed semen. *AIDS* 2002; 16(17): 2267–73.
38. Fiore JR, Lorusso F, Vacca M, Ladisa N, Greco P, De Palo R. The efficiency of sperm washing in removing human immunodeficiency virus type 1 varies according to the seminal viral load. *FertilSteril* 2005; 84(1): 232–4.
39. Garrido N, Meseguer M, Bellver J, Remohi J, Simon C, Pellicer A. Report of the results of a 2 year programme of sperm wash and ICSI treatment for human immunodeficiency virus and hepatitis C virus serodiscordant couples. *Hum Reprod* 2004; 19(11): 2581–6.
40. Politch JA, Xu C, Tucker L, Anderson DJ. Separation of human immunodeficiency virus type 1 from motile sperm by the double tube gradient method versus other methods. *Fertil Steril* 2004; 81(2): 440–7.
41. Kato S, Hanabusa H, Kaneko S et al. Complete removal of HIV-1 RNA and proviral DNA from semen by the swim-up method: Assisted reproduction technique using spermatozoa free from HIV-1. *AIDS* 2006; 20(7): 967–73.
42. Loskutoff NM, Huyser C, Singh R et al. Use of a novel washing method combining multiple density gradients and trypsin for removing human immunodeficiency virus-1 and hepatitis C virus from semen. *Fertil Steril* 2005; 84(4): 1001–10.
43. Casper RF, Meriano JS, Jarvi KA, Cowan L, Lucato ML. The hypo-osmotic swelling test for selection of viable sperm for intracytoplasmic sperm injection in men with complete asthenozoospermia. *Fertil Steril* 1996; 65(5): 972–6.
44. Aktan TM, Montag M, Duman S, Gorkemli H, Rink K, Yurdakul T. Use of a laser to detect viable but immotile spermatozoa. *Andrologia* 2004; 36(6): 366–9.
45. de Oliveira NM, Vaca Sanchez R, Rodriguez Fiesta S et al. Pregnancy with frozen–thawed and fresh testicular biopsy after motile and immotile sperm microinjection, using the mechanical touch technique to assess viability. *Hum Reprod* 2004; 19(2): 262–5.
46. Manigart Y, Rozenberg S, Barlow P, Gerard M, Bertrand E, Delvigne A. ART outcome in HIV-infected patients. *Hum Reprod* 2006; 21(11): 2935–40.
47. Gilling-Smith C, Nicopoullos JD, Semprini AE, Frodsham LC. HIV and reproductive care—A review of current practice. *BJOG* 2006; 113(8): 869–78.
48. Terriou P, Auquier P, Chabert-Orsini V et al. Outcome of ICSI in HIV-1-infected women. *Hum Reprod* 2005; 20(10): 2838–43.
49. Semprini AE, Fiore S. HIV and reproduction. *Curr Opin Obstet Gynecol* 2004; 16(3): 257–62.
50. Ohl J, Partisani M, Wittemer C et al. Assisted reproduction techniques for HIV serodiscordant couples: 18 months of experience. *Hum Reprod* 2003; 18(6): 1244–9.

51. Pena JE, Thornton MH, Sauer MV. Assessing the clinical utility of *in vitro* fertilization with intracytoplasmic sperm injection in human immunodeficiency virus type 1 serodiscordant couples: Report of 113 consecutive cycles. *Fertil Steril* 2003; 80(2): 356–62.
52. van Leeuwen E, Repping S, Prins JM, Reiss P, van der Veen F. Assisted reproductive technologies to establish pregnancies in couples with an HIV-1-infected man. *Neth J Med* 2009; 67(8): 322–7.
53. Vitorino RL, Grinsztejn BG, de Andrade CA et al. Systematic review of the effectiveness and safety of assisted reproduction techniques in couples serodiscordant for human immunodeficiency virus where the man is positive. *Fertil Steril* 2011; 95(5): 1684–90.
54. Savasi V, Mandia L, Laoreti A, Cetin I. Reproductive assistance in HIV serodiscordant couples. *Hum Reprod Update* 2013; 19(2): 136–50.
55. Whetham J, Taylor S, Charlwood L et al. Pre-exposure prophylaxis for conception (PrEP-C) as a risk reduction strategy in HIV-positive men and HIV-negative women in the UK. *AIDS Care* 2014; 26(3): 332–6.
56. Ainsworth C, Nixon B, Jansen RP, Aitken RJ. First recorded pregnancy and normal birth after ICSI using electrophoretically isolated spermatozoa. *Hum Reprod* 2007; 22(1): 197–200.
57. Fleming SD, Ilad RS, Griffin AM et al. Prospective controlled trial of an electrophoretic method of sperm preparation for assisted reproduction: Comparison with density gradient centrifugation. *Hum Reprod* 2008; 23: 2646–51.
58. Dirican EK, Ozgun OD, Akarsu S et al. Clinical outcome of magnetic activated cell sorting of non-apoptotic spermatozoa before density gradient centrifugation for assisted reproduction. *J Assist Reprod Genet* 2008; 25(8): 375–81.
59. Said TM, Agarwal A, Zborowski M, Grunewald S, Glander HJ, Paasch U. Utility of magnetic cell separation as a molecular sperm preparation technique. *J Androl* 2008; 29: 134–42.
60. Nadalini M, Tarozzi N, Distratis V, Scaravelli G, Borini A. Impact of intracytoplasmic morphologically selected sperm injection on assisted reproduction outcome: A review. *Reprod Biomed Online* 2009; 19(Suppl 3): 45–55.
61. Souza Setti A, Ferreira RC, Paes de Almeida Ferreira Braga D, de Cassia Savio Figueira R, Iaconelli A, Jr., Borges E, Jr. Intracytoplasmic sperm injection outcome versus intracytoplasmic morphologically selected sperm injection outcome: A meta-analysis. *Reprod Biomed Online* 2010; 21(4): 450–5.
62. Bartoov B, Berkovitz A, Eltes F. Selection of spermatozoa with normal nuclei through improve the pregnancy rate with intracytoplasmic sperm injection. *N Engl J Med* 2001; 345(14): 1067–8.
63. Huszar G, Jakab A, Sakkas D et al. Fertility testing and ICSI sperm selection by hyaluronic acid binding: Clinical and genetic aspects. *Reprod Biomed Online* 2007; 14(5): 650–63.
64. Nasr-Esfahani MH, Razavi S, Vahdati AA, Fathi F, Tavalaee M. Evaluation of sperm selection procedure based on hyaluronic acid binding ability on ICSI outcome. *J Assist Reprod Genet* 2008; 25(5): 197–203.
65. Huszar G, Ozkavukcu S, Jakab A, Celik-Ozenci C, Sati GL, Cayli S. Hyaluronic acid binding ability of human sperm reflects cellular maturity and fertilizing potential: Selection of sperm for intracytoplasmic sperm injection. *Curr Opin Obstet Gynecol* 2006; 18: 260–7.
66. Worrilow KC, Eid S, Woodhouse D et al. Use of hyaluronan in the selection of sperm for intracytoplasmic sperm injection (ICSI): Significant improvement in clinical outcomes—Multicenter, double-blinded and randomized controlled trial. *Hum Reprod* 2013; 28(2): 306–14.
67. Menkveld R, Franken DR, Kruger TF, Oehninger S, Hodgen GD. Sperm selection capacity of the human zona pellucida. *Mol Reprod Dev* 1991; 30(4): 346–52.
68. Liu DY, Baker HW. Acrosome status and morphology of human spermatozoa bound to the zona pellucida and oolemma determined using oocytes that failed to fertilize *in vitro*. *Hum Reprod* 1994; 9(4): 673–9.
69. Liu DY, Baker HW. Human sperm bound to the zona pellucida have normal nuclear chromatin as assessed by acridine orange fluorescence. *Hum Reprod* 2007; 22: 1597–602.
70. Paes Almeida Ferreira de Braga D, Iaconelli A, Jr., Cassia Savio de Figueira R, Madaschi C, Semiao-Francisco L, Borges E, Jr. Outcome of ICSI using zona pellucida-bound spermatozoa and conventionally selected spermatozoa. *Reprod Biomed Online.* 2009; 19(6): 802–7.
71. Black M, Liu de Y, Bourne H, Baker HW. Comparison of outcomes of conventional intracytoplasmic sperm injection and intracytoplasmic sperm injection using sperm bound to the zona pellucida of immature oocytes. *Fertil Steril* 2010; 93: 672–4.
72. Liu F, Qiu Y, Zou Y, Deng ZH, Yang H, Liu de Y. Use of zona pellucida-bound sperm for intracytoplasmic sperm injection produces higher embryo quality and implantation than conventional intracytoplasmic sperm injection. *Fertil Steril* 2011; 95: 815–8.
73. Harari O, Bourne H, McDonald M, Richings N, Speirs AL, Johnston WI et al. Intracytoplasmic sperm injection: A major advance in the management of severe male subfertility. *Fertil Steril* 1995; 64(2): 360–8.
74. Watkins W, Nieto F, Bourne H, Wutthiphan B, Speirs A, Baker HW. Testicular and epididymal sperm in a microinjection program: Methods of retrieval and results. *Fertil Steril* 1997; 67(3): 527–35.
75. Sallam HN, Farrag A, Agameya AF, El-Garem Y, Ezzeldin F. The use of the modified hypo-osmotic swelling test for the selection of immotile testicular spermatozoa in patients treated with ICSI: A randomized controlled study. *Hum Reprod* 2005; 20: 3435–40.

76. Barnes A, Riche D, Mena L et al. Efficacy and safety of intrauterine insemination and assisted reproductive technology in populations serodiscordant for human immunodeficiency virus: A systematic review and meta-analysis. *Fertil Steril* 2014; 102(2): 424–34.
77. Bonduelle M, Wilikens A, Buysse A et al. A follow-up study of children born after intracytoplasmic sperm injection (ICSI) with epididymal and testicular spermatozoa and after replacement of cryopreserved embryos obtained after ICSI. *Hum Reprod* 1998; 13(Suppl 1): 196–207.
78. Anderson AR, Wiemer KE, Weikert ML, Kyslinger ML. Fertilization, embryonic development and pregnancy losses with intracytoplasmic sperm injection for surgically-retrieved spermatozoa. *Reprod Biomed Online* 2002; 5(2): 142–7.
79. De Kretser DM, Baker HW. Infertility in men: Recent advances and continuing controversies. *J Clin Endocrinol Metab* 1999; 84(10): 3443–50.
80. Baker HWG. Marvellous ICSI: The viewpoint of a clinician. *Int J Androl* 1998; 21(5): 249–52.
81. Antinori S, Versaci C, Dani G, Antinori M, Selman HA. Successful fertilization and pregnancy after injection of frozen–thawed round spermatids into human oocytes. *Hum Reprod* 1997; 12(3): 554–6.
82. Said TM, Land JA. Effects of advanced selection methods on sperm quality and ART outcome: A systematic review. *Hum Reprod Update* 2011; 17: 719–33.
83. Fugger EF, Black SH, Keyvanfar K, Schulman JD. Births of normal daughters after MicroSort sperm separation and intrauterine insemination, *in-vitro* fertilization, or intracytoplasmic sperm injection. *Hum Reprod* 1998; 13(9): 2367–70.

Sperm chromatin assessment

6

ASHOK AGARWAL, RAKESH SHARMA, and GULFAM AHMAD

INTRODUCTION

Semen analysis is used routinely to evaluate infertile men. Attempts to introduce quality control within and between laboratories have highlighted the subjectivity and variability of traditional semen parameters. A significant overlap in sperm concentration, motility, and morphology between fertile and infertile men has been demonstrated (1). In addition, standard measurements may not reveal subtle sperm defects such as DNA damage and these defects can affect fertility. New markers are needed to better discriminate infertile men from fertile ones, predict pregnancy outcomes in the female partner, and calculate the risk of adverse reproductive events. In this context, sperm chromatin abnormalities have been studied extensively in past decades as a cause of male infertility (2). Focus on the genomic integrity of the male gamete has been intensified due to growing concerns about transmission of damaged DNA through assisted reproduction technologies (ARTs), especially intracytoplasmic sperm injection (ICSI). It is a particular concern if the amount of sperm DNA damage exceeds the repair capacity of oocytes. There are concerns related to potential chromosomal abnormalities, congenital malformations, and developmental abnormalities in ICSI-born progeny (3–6).

Accumulating evidence suggests that a negative relationship exists between disturbances in the organization of the genomic material in sperm nuclei and the fertility potential of spermatozoa, whether *in vivo* or *in vitro* (2,7–14). Abnormalities in the male genome characterized by damaged sperm DNA may be indicative of male subfertility regardless of normal semen parameters (15,16). Sperm chromatin structure evaluation is an independent measure of sperm quality that provides good diagnostic and prognostic capabilities. Therefore, it may be considered a reliable predictor of a couple's inability to become pregnant (17). This may have an impact on the offspring, resulting in trans-generational infertility (18).

Sperm DNA integrity correlates with pregnancy outcome in *in vitro* fertilization (IVF) (17,19–22). High sperm DNA fragmentation can compromise fertilization rates, embryo quality, and early embryonic growth and result in pregnancy loss (10). In addition, sperm DNA fragmentation may also compromise the progression of pregnancy and result in spontaneous miscarriage or loss of biochemical pregnancy. Sperm DNA fragmentation seems to affect embryo post-implantation development in ICSI procedures (10). Therefore, it is recommended that sperm DNA fragmentation analysis should be included in the evaluation of the infertile male (22).

Many techniques have been described to evaluate the sperm chromatin status. In this chapter, we describe the normal sperm chromatin architecture and the causative factors leading to its aberrations. We also provide the rationale for sperm chromatin assessment and discuss the different methods used to analyze sperm DNA integrity.

HUMAN SPERM CHROMATIN STRUCTURE

In many mammals, spermatogenesis leads to the production of highly homogenous spermatozoa. For example, more than 95% of the nucleoprotein in mouse sperm nuclei is composed of protamines (23). This allows mature sperm nuclei to adopt a volume 40-times less than that of normal somatic nuclei (24). The final, highly compact packaging of the primary sperm DNA filament is produced by DNA–protamine complexes. Contrary to nucleosomal organization in somatic cells, which is provided by histones, these DNA–protamine complexes approach the physical limits of molecular compaction (25,26). Human sperm nuclei, on the other hand, contain considerably fewer protamines (around 85%) than sperm nuclei of the bull, stallion, hamster, and mouse (27,28). Mature human spermatozoa contain some levels of nucleosomes, which are believed to be necessary for organizing higher-order genomic structure through interactions with the nuclear matrix. These regions are non-randomly distributed throughout the sperm genome (29). Human sperm chromatin is therefore less regularly compacted and frequently contains DNA strand breaks (30,31).

To achieve this uniquely condensed state, sperm DNA must be organized in a specific manner that differs substantially from that of somatic cells (24). The fundamental packaging unit of mammalian sperm chromatin is a toroid containing 50–60 kilobases of DNA. Individual toroids represent the DNA loop domains that are highly condensed by protamines and fixed at the nuclear matrix. Toroids are cross-linked by disulfide bonds formed by oxidation of sulfhydryl groups of cysteine present in the protamines (25,32). Thus, each chromosome represents a garland of toroids, while all 23 chromosomes are clustered by centromeres into a compact chromocenter positioned well inside the nucleus; the telomere ends are united into dimers exposed to the nuclear periphery (33,34). This condensed, insoluble, and highly organized nature of sperm chromatin acts to protect the genetic integrity during transport of the paternal genome through the male and female reproductive tracts. It also ensures that the paternal DNA is delivered in the form that sterically allows the proper fusion of two gametic genomes and enables the developing embryo to correctly express the genetic information (34–36).

In comparison with other species (37), human sperm chromatin packaging is exceptionally variable both within and between men. This variability has been mostly attributed to its basic protein component. The retention of 15% histones, which are less basic than protamines, leads to the formation of a less compact chromatin structure (28). Moreover, in contrast to the bull, cat, boar, and ram—whose spermatozoa contain only one type of protamine (P1)—human and mouse spermatozoa contain a second type of protamine called P2, which is deficient in cysteine residues (38). Consequently, the disulfide cross-linking that is responsible for more stable packaging is diminished in human sperm as compared with species containing P1 alone (39). It is interesting to note that altered P1/P2 ratios and the absence of P2 are associated with male fertility problems (40–44). The P1/P2 ratio has been shown to correlate with sperm DNA fragmentation, and significant differences were detected between fertile and infertile men (45). The reference range reported for P1/P2 in a fertile, normozoospermic population ranges from 0.54 to 1.43. Such a wide range of P1/P2 shows that abnormal protamination can be an indicator of other disturbances that occur during spermatogenesis that can cause infertility (46).

ORIGIN OF SPERM CHROMATIN ABNORMALITIES

The susceptibility of male germ cells to DNA damage stems partly from the down-regulation of DNA repair systems during late spermatogenesis. In addition, the cellular machinery that allows these cells to undergo complete apoptosis is progressively lost during spermatogenesis. As a result, the advanced stages of germ cell differentiation cannot be deleted, even though they may have proceeded some way down the apoptotic pathway. As a consequence, the ejaculated gamete may exhibit genetic damage. Such DNA damage will be carried into the zygote by the fertilizing spermatozoon and must be then repaired, preferably prior to the first cleavage division. Several studies have shown that oocytes and early embryos can repair sperm DNA damage (47,48). Consequently, the biological effect of abnormal sperm chromatin structure depends on the combined effects of sperm chromatin damage and the capacity of the oocyte to repair it. Any errors that may occur during this post-fertilization period of DNA repair have the potential to create mutations that can affect fetal development and, ultimately, the health of the child (18,49).

The exact mechanisms by which chromatin abnormalities/DNA damage arise in human spermatozoa are not completely understood. Three main theories have been proposed: defective sperm chromatin packaging, abortive apoptosis, and oxidative stress (OS) (50). Deficiencies in recombination may also play a role.

DEFECTIVE SPERM CHROMATIN PACKAGING

Stage-specific introduction of transient DNA strand breaks during spermiogenesis has been described (50–52). DNA breaks have been found in round and elongating spermatids. Such breaks are necessary for transient relief of torsional stress. During maturation, the nucleosome histone cores in elongating spermatids are cast off and replaced with transitional proteins and protamines (50,52–54). Thus, chromatin repackaging includes a sensitive step necessitating endogenous nuclease activity, which is evidently fulfilled by coordinated loosening of the chromatin by histone hyperacetylation and by topoisomerase II, which can create and ligate breaks (53,54). Although there is little evidence to suggest that spermatid maturation-associated DNA breaks are fully ligated, unrepaired DNA breaks are not allowed (55).

Ligation of DNA breaks is necessary not only to preserve the integrity of the primary DNA structure, but also for reassembly of the important unit of genome expression—the DNA loop domain. Interaction of sperm DNA with protamines results in the coiling of sperm DNA into toroidal subunits known as doughnut loops (56). If these temporary breaks are not repaired because of excessive topoisomerase II activity or a deficiency of topoisomerase II inhibitors (57,58), then DNA fragmentation in ejaculated spermatozoa may result. Similarly, if appropriate disulfide bridge formation does not occur because of inadequate oxidation of thiols during epididymal transit, the DNA will be more vulnerable to damage caused by suboptimal compaction. Recent studies have postulated the hypothesis that large nuclear vacuoles could be an indicator of abnormal chromatin packaging (59,60).

Further, the ratio of P1 to P2 maintained by P2 precursor (pre-P2) has a crucial role in sperm fertilization. Abnormal sperm morphogenesis with reduced motility can also result due to defective pre-P2 mRNA translation (61–63).

ABORTIVE APOPTOSIS

The incidence of apoptosis in ejaculated sperm is still a contentious issue. Until recently, the inability of a mature spermatozoon to synthesize new proteins was believed to make it impossible for such cells to respond to any of the signals that lead to the programmed death cascade. However, a number of recent observations have raised the possibility that abortive apoptosis may contribute to DNA damage in human spermatozoa: (1) the detection of Fas on ejaculated spermatozoa (64); (2) the high proportion of spermatozoa with potentially apoptotic mitochondria (65); and (3) the finding that potential mediators of apoptosis, including endonuclease activity, are present in spermatozoa (66). It has been postulated that OS can interfere with sperm chromatin remodeling. Cells with altered chromatin structure can enter the apoptotic pathway, which is characterized by loss of motility, caspase activation, phosphatidylserine externalization, and the activation of reactive oxygen species (ROS) generation by the mitochondria. ROS causes lipid peroxidation and oxidative DNA damage, which, in turn, leads to DNA fragmentation and eventually cell death (67).

It has been suggested that an early apoptotic pathway, initiated in spermatogonia and spermatocytes, is mediated by Fas protein. Fas is a type I membrane protein that belongs to the tumor necrosis factor–nerve growth factor receptor family (68,69). It has been shown that Sertoli cells express Fas ligand, which by binding to Fas leads to cell death via apoptosis (68,69). This in turn limits the size of the germ cell population to a number that Sertoli cells can support (70). Ligation of Fas ligand to Fas in the cellular membrane triggers the activation of caspases and therefore this pathway is also characterized as a caspase-induced apoptosis (71).

Men exhibiting deficiencies in their semen profile often possess a large number of spermatozoa that bear Fas. This fact prompts the suggestion that these dysfunctional cells are the product of an incomplete apoptotic cascade (30). However, a contribution of aborted apoptosis in the DNA damage seen in the ejaculated spermatozoa is doubtful in cases where this process is initiated at the early stages of spermatogenesis. This is because at the stage of DNA fragmentation, apoptosis is an irreversible process (72), and these cells should be digested by Sertoli cells and removed from the pool of ejaculated sperm. Some studies have not found correlations between DNA damage and Fas expression (73), or, in contrast, have not revealed ultrastructural evidence for the association of apoptosis with DNA damage in sperm (74). Alternatively, if the apoptotic cascade is initiated at the round spermatid phase, where transcription (and mitochondria) is still active, abortive apoptosis might be an origin of the DNA breaks. A Bcl2 anti-apoptotic family gene member called Bclw has been shown to suppress apoptosis in elongating spermatids (75). Although many apoptotic biomarkers have been found in the mature male gamete, particularly in infertile men, their definitive association with DNA fragmentation remains elusive (76–85).

OXIDATIVE STRESS

Normal levels of ROS play an important physiological role, modulating gene and protein activities that are vital for sperm proliferation, differentiation, and function. In semen, the amount of ROS generation is controlled by seminal antioxidants that ensure a balance between ROS and antioxidant capacity. Any imbalance that occurs either by high ROS production or low antioxidant levels leads to OS (86).The human spermatozoon is highly susceptible to OS. This process induces peroxidative damage in the sperm plasma membrane and DNA fragmentation. A number of pro-inflammatory cytokines at physiological levels are responsible for the lipid peroxidation of sperm membrane, which is considered important for the fecundation capacity of the spermatozoa. However, OS may lead to abnormal production of certain interleukin/cytokines such as IL-8 and TNF-α, either alone or in combination with any infection, which may be able to drive the lipid peroxidation to a level that can affect the sperm fertilizing capacity (87). Such stress may arise from a variety of sources. Morphologically abnormal spermatozoa (with residual cytoplasm, in particular) and leukocytes are the main sources of excessive ROS generation in semen (86). Also, a lack of antioxidant protection and the presence of redox cycling xenobiotics may be the cause of OS. Whenever levels of OS in the male germ line are high, the peroxidation of unsaturated fatty acids in the sperm plasma membrane leads to the depressed fertilization rates associated with DNA damage (18).

DEFICIENCIES IN RECOMBINATION

Meiotic crossing-over is associated with the genetically programmed introduction of DNA double-strand breaks (DSBs) by specific nucleases of the SPO11 family (88). These DNA DSBs should be ligated until the end of meiosis I. Normally, a recombination checkpoint in meiotic prophase does not allow meiotic division I to proceed until DNA is fully repaired or defective spermatocytes are ablated (88,89). A defective checkpoint may lead to persistent sperm DNA fragmentation in ejaculated spermatozoa, although direct data for this hypothesis in humans is lacking.

The processes leading to DNA damage in ejaculated sperm are inter-related. For example, a defective spermatid protamination and disulfide bridge formation caused by inadequate oxidation of thiols during epididymal transit, resulting in diminished sperm chromatin packaging, makes sperm cells more vulnerable to ROS-induced DNA fragmentation. A two-step hypothesis has been proposed, suggesting that OS acts on poorly protaminated cells that are generated as a result of defective spermiogenesis (90).

CONTRIBUTING FACTORS

Advanced paternal age, smoking, obesity, radiofrequency, electromagnetic radiation, and xenobiotics are the common factors attributed to sperm DNA damage (91). Advancing age has been associated with an increased percentage of ejaculated spermatozoa with DNA damage (11,92,93). Young men with cancer typically have poor semen quality and sperm DNA damage even before starting therapy. Further damage from radiation or chemotherapy is dependent on both the duration and dose of radiation (94,95). Spermatogenesis may not occur months to years after therapy, but evidence of sperm DNA damage often persists beyond that period (96,97). Data on men with testicular cancer showed that radiation therapy induced transient sperm DNA damage and that this damage was present three to five years later, but three or more cycles of chemotherapy, in turn, decreased the percentage of sperm with DNA damage (97).

Cigarette smoking is associated with a decrease in sperm count and motility and an increase in abnormal sperm forms and sperm DNA damage (98). It is suggested that smoking increases production of leukocyte-derived ROS; the OS may be the underlying reason why sperm DNA from smokers contains more strand breaks than that from non-smokers (98,99). Also, genital tract infections and inflammation result in leukocytospermia and have been associated with OS and subsequent sperm DNA damage (100). Exposure to pesticides (organophosphates), persistent organochlorine pollutants, and air pollution have also been associated with sperm DNA damage (11,101–103). Varicocele has been associated with seminal OS and sperm DNA damage (104–106). Sperm DNA integrity has been shown to improve after varicocele repair (107,108).

A deficiency in gonadotropic hormones such as follicle-stimulating hormone (FSH) can cause sperm chromatin defects. FSH receptor-knockout mice have been found to have higher levels of DNA damage in sperm (109). Febrile illness has been shown to cause an increase in the histone/protamine ratio and DNA damage in ejaculated sperm (110). Direct mild testicular and epididymal hyperthermia has also been shown to cause these effects (111,112). Finally, sperm preparation techniques involving repeated high-speed centrifugation and the isolation of spermatozoa from the seminal plasma, which is a protective antioxidant environment, may contribute to increased sperm DNA damage via mechanisms that are mediated by the enhanced generation of ROS (14,113).

INDICATIONS FOR SPERM CHROMATIN ASSESSMENT

Evaluating sperm chromatin can be challenging for several reasons: it can be difficult to link the results of chromatin integrity tests to known physiological mechanisms; the role that sperm chromatin structure assessment plays in clinical practice (especially in ART) is still controversial; and there is no one standardized method for measuring sperm chromatin integrity. On the other hand, sperm chromatin structure is complex, and several methods may be necessary in order to assess this. In addition, a number of confounding factors can complicate the interpretation of the results, including heterogeneity in the sperm population and the fact that not all DNA damage is lethal (most DNA contains non-coding regions or introns, and oocytes can repair sperm DNA damage). Nevertheless, at the present time, it is clear that sperm chromatin assessment provides good diagnostic and prognostic capabilities for fertility/infertility.

It must be stressed that among all methods employed for sperm chromatin assessment, clinical thresholds so far have been demonstrated only for the sperm chromatin structure assay (SCSA) and terminal deoxynucleotidyl transferase (TdT)-mediated dUTP nick end labeling (TUNEL) assay, and these thresholds have been confirmed by different laboratories for SCSA only. However, a recent study published a detailed step-by-step approach for measuring sperm DNA fragmentation by TUNEL using a benchtop flow cytometer, which is user friendly and facilitates data interpretation (114). Also, the reported biological variability of sperm DNA damage within men over time should be considered, although it is more stable than standard semen parameters (115–117). Indications for sperm DNA evaluation include male infertility diagnosis, recurrent pregnancy loss, unexplained infertility, use of ARTs, and follow-up after oncological treatment such as radiotherapy or chemotherapy.

DIAGNOSIS OF MALE INFERTILITY

Although a spermatozoon with damaged DNA can fertilize an egg, future embryonic growth is compromised, which may ultimately lead to miscarriage or child deformities. Many studies have shown, using a variety of techniques, significant differences in sperm DNA damage levels between fertile and infertile men (118–123). Moreover, spermatozoa from infertile patients are generally more susceptible to the effects of DNA-damaging agents such as H_2O_2, smoking, obesity, and radiation (124). The probability of fertilization *in vivo* reduces drastically if the proportion of sperm cells with DNA damage exceeds 30% as detected by the SCSA (17,125) or 20% as detected by TUNEL (126). However, the latest commentary on the utilization of sperm DNA fragmentation testing in fertility outcomes suggests avoiding this test. The debate argues that several couples have become pregnant even though the threshold of DNA damage was higher than what we consider normal; in addition, some studies failed to find any difference in outcome in men who differ in sperm DNA fragmentation levels (127). In continuation of such investigations, some people support the diagnostic value of sperm DNA integrity and suggest that it may be considered an objective marker of sperm function that serves as a significant prognostic factor for male infertility (7). A significant increase in SCSA-defined DNA damage in sperm from infertile men with normal sperm parameters has been demonstrated (123), indicating that analysis of sperm DNA damage may reveal a hidden sperm abnormality in infertile men classified with idiopathic infertility based on apparently normal standard semen parameters.

ASSISTED REPRODUCTION TECHNOLOGIES

The probability of fertilization by intrauterine insemination (IUI) or IVF is reduced in cases where the proportion of sperm cells with DNA damage exceeds 30% by means of SCSA (12,19,128,129) or 12% by TUNEL (19). As described in the previous section, the controversy as to whether sperm DNA damage negatively affects the results of IVF and ICSI has yet to be resolved. Although no association between sperm DNA damage and IVF/ICSI outcome has been demonstrated in some studies (130), most show a significant negative correlation between sperm DNA damage and embryo quality in IVF cycles (131), blastocyst development following IVF (132), and fertilization rates following IVF (133) and ICSI (134), even though sperm DNA damage may not necessarily preclude fertilization and pronucleus formation during ICSI (135). Two meta-analyses concluded that sperm DNA damage is predictive for reduced pregnancy success using routine IVF but has no significant effect on ICSI outcome (9,136). Thus, assessment of sperm chromatin may help predict the success rates of IUI and IVF. It has been also suggested that in patients with a high proportion of DNA-damaged sperm who are seeking to use ART, ICSI should be the method of choice (12).

EMBRYONAL LOSS

Data on miscarriages as a possible consequence of sperm DNA damage are rather scarce. It has been shown that the proportion of sperm with DNA damage is significantly higher in men from couples with recurrent pregnancy loss than in the general population or fertile donors (137). It

Table 6.1 Various methods for assessing sperm chromatin abnormalities

Assay	Parameter	Method of analysis
Acidic aniline blue (144)	Nuclear maturity (DNA protein composition)	Optical microscopy
Toluidine blue staining (145)	Nuclear maturity (DNA protein composition)	Optical microscopy
Chromomycin A_3 (146)	Nuclear maturity (DNA protein composition)	Fluorescence microscopy
DNA breakage detection–fluorescence *in situ* hybridization (147)	DNA fragmentation (ssDNA)	Fluorescence microscopy
In situ nick translation (148)	DNA fragmentation (ssDNA)	Fluorescence microscopy Flow cytometry
Acridine orange (149)	DNA denaturation (acid)	Fluorescence microscopy Flow cytometry
Sperm chromatin dispersion (150)	DNA fragmentation	Fluorescence microscopy
Comet (neutral) (151)	DNA fragmentation (dsDNA)	Fluorescence microscopy
Comet (alkaline) (152)	DNA fragmentation (ssDNA/dsDNA)	
TUNEL (74,114,153,154)	DNA fragmentation	Fluorescence microscopy Flow cytometry
Sperm chromatin structure assay (17)	DNA denaturation (acid/heat)	Flow cytometry
8-OHdG measurement (155)	8-OHdG	High-performance lipid chromatography

Abbreviations: 8-OHdG, 8-hydroxy-2-deoxyguanosine; dsDNA, double-stranded DNA; ssDNA, single-stranded DNA; TUNEL, terminal deoxynucleotidyl transferase-mediated dUTP nick end labeling.

has also been reported that 39% of miscarriages could be predicted using a combination of selected cutoff values for percentage spermatozoa with denatured (likely fragmented) DNA and/or abnormal chromatin packaging as assessed by SCSA (17). The percentage of spontaneous abortion following IVF/ICSI was increased when sperm with high levels of DNA damage were used (138,139), which highlights the need to assess sperm DNA damage in order to predict possible future miscarriage.

CANCER PATIENTS

Sperm DNA evaluation in patients with cancer requires special attention when future fertility and the health of the baby are considered. The stressful microenvironment that develops during cancer can cause OS, which indirectly can damage sperm DNA. Patients with cancer are often referred to sperm banks before chemotherapy, radiation therapy, or surgery is initiated. Data suggest there is compromised semen quality including DNA integrity before commencement of treatment (140,141) and increased chromosomal aneupoloidy after chemotherapy (142). The extent of DNA damage may help to determine how semen should be cryopreserved before therapy begins. Specimens with high sperm concentrations and motility and low levels of DNA damage should be preserved in relatively large aliquots that are suitable for IUI. If a single specimen of good quality is available, then it should be preserved in multiple small aliquots suitable for IVF or ICSI (143).

METHODS USED IN THE EVALUATION OF SPERM CHROMATIN/DNA INTEGRITY

Different methods can be used to evaluate the status of the sperm chromatin/DNA for the presence of abnormalities or simply immaturity (Table 6.1). These methods include simple staining techniques such as the acidic aniline blue (AAB) and basic toluidine blue (TB), fluorescent staining techniques such as the sperm chromatin dispersion (SCD) test, chromomycin A_3 (CMA_3), DNA breakage detection–fluorescence *in situ* hybridization (DBD–FISH), *in situ* nick translation (NT), and flow cytometric-based SCSA. Some techniques employ more than one method for the analysis of their results. Examples of these include the acridine orange (AO) and TUNEL assays. Other methods less frequently used include measurement of 8-hydroxy-2-deoxyguanosine (8-OHdG) by high-performance liquid chromatography (HPLC).

AAB staining

Principle

Aniline blue is an acidic dye that has more binding affinity with the proteins in decondensed or loose chromatin due to the residual histones. AAB staining differentiates between lysine-rich histones and arginine/cysteine-rich protamines. This technique provides a specific positive reaction for lysine and reveals differences in the basic nuclear protein composition of ejaculated human spermatozoa. Histone-rich nuclei of immature spermatozoa are rich in lysine and will consequently take up the blue stain. On the other hand, protamine-rich nuclei of mature spermatozoa are rich in arginine and cysteine and contain relatively low levels of lysine, which means they will not take up the stain (156).

Technique

Slides are prepared by smearing 5 μL of either a raw or washed semen sample, which is air-dried and fixed for 30 minutes in 3% glutaraldehyde in phosphate-buffered saline

(PBS). The fixed smear is dried and stained in 5% aqueous aniline blue solution (pH 3.5) for five minutes. The staining characteristics depict the status of nuclear maturity. Sperm heads containing immature nuclear chromatin stain blue and those with mature nuclei do not. A total of 200 spermatozoa per slide are counted using bright field microscopy, and the percentage of spermatozoa stained with aniline blue is determined (144).

Modification of the AAB assay with eosin

One of the limitations of AAB staining is poor visualization of unstained sperm cells under ordinary light microscopy. To overcome this issue, counterstaining using eosin-Y is recommended. Sperm smears are fixed in 4% formalin solution for five minutes and rinsed in water. Slides are stained in 5% aniline blue prepared in 4% acetic acid (pH 3.5) solution for five minutes, rinsed in water, and counterstained in 0.5% eosin for one minute followed by rinsing and air drying (157).

Clinical significance

AAB staining has shown a linkage between chromatin immaturity and male infertility. In patients with varicocele, unilateral cryptorchidism, and idiopathic infertility, high sperm nuclear instability with a higher number of AAB-stained spermatozoa was observed (158). However, the correlation between the percentage of aniline blue-stained spermatozoa and other sperm parameters remains controversial. AAB-stained spermatozoa showed normal conventional parameters such as count, motility, and morphology. Immature sperm chromatin may or may not correlate with asthenozoospermic samples and abnormal morphology patterns (155,156). Most important is the finding that chromatin condensation as visualized by aniline blue staining is a good predictor for IVF outcome, although it cannot determine the fertilization potential and the cleavage and pregnancy rates following ICSI (157,158). Evaluation of sperm chromatin using AAB staining could be considered as one of the complementary tests of semen analysis for assessment of male factor infertility (159,160). Counterstaining with eosin can facilitate interpretation of sperm chromatin integrity (157).

Advantages and limitations

The AAB technique is simple and inexpensive and requires only bright field microscopy for analysis. The only drawback is the heterogeneous slide staining.

TB staining

Principle

TB or tolonium chloride is a basic thiazine metachromatic dye that selectively binds the acidic components of the tissue. It partially dissolves in water and alcohol. Alternatively known as methylamine or aminotoluene, the dye represents three isoforms: ortho-toluidine, para-toluidine, and meta-toluidin. It has high binding affinity for phosphate residues of sperm DNA in immature nuclei and provides a metachromatic shift from light blue to a purple–violet color (161). This stain is a sensitive structural probe for DNA structure and packaging.

Technique

TB staining follows the principle of metachromasia in which a dye can absorb light at different wavelengths and can change color without changing chemical structure. Sperm smears are air-dried, fixed in freshly made 96% ethanol–acetone (1:1) at 4°C for at least 30 minutes, hydrolyzed in 0.1 N HCl at 4°C for five minutes, and rinsed three times in distilled water for two minutes each. Smears are stained with 0.05% TB for five minutes. The staining buffer consists of 50% citrate phosphate (McIlvain buffer, pH 3.5). Permanent preparations are dehydrated in tertiary butanol twice for three minutes each at 37°C and in xylene twice for three minutes each; the preparations are embedded in DPX (a mixture of distyrene, a plasticizer, and xylene). Sperm heads with good chromatin integrity stain light blue and those of compromised integrity stain violet (purple) (162). The results of the TB test are visualized using light microscopy. Based on the different optical densities of cells stained with TB, the image analysis cytometry test is elaborated (Figure 6.1a) (144).

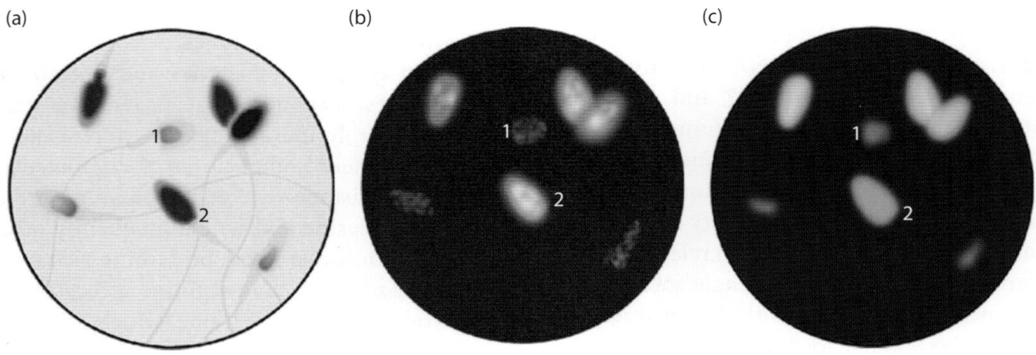

Figure 6.1 (a) Human ejaculate stained with toluidine blue: (1) sperm heads with normal chromatin conformation are light blue; (2) sperm heads with abnormal chromatin conformation are violet. (b) DNA breakage detection–fluorescence *in situ* hybridization labeling with a whole-genome probe (red fluorescence), demonstrating extensive DNA breakage in those nuclei that are intensely labeled. (c) Acridine orange stain to native DNA fluoresces green (1), whereas relaxed/denatured DNA fluoresces red (2).

Clinical significance

TB staining may be considered a fairly reliable method for assessing sperm chromatin. Abnormal nuclei (purple–violet sperm heads) have been shown to be correlated with counts of red–orange sperm heads as revealed by the AO method (161). Significant correlations between the results of the TB, SCSA, and TUNEL tests have been demonstrated (162). Clinical applicability of the TB test for male fertility potential assessment has also been demonstrated, with specificity for infertility diagnosis as high as 92% and sensitivity reaching 42% when the threshold of 45% is used for sperm cells with abnormal nuclei (163). TB staining has been used in several studies for evaluating sperm chromatin quality (164–168), alone and in conjunction with other tests, proving it to be an effective tool for evaluation of chromatin status.

Advantages and limitations

The TB method is simple and inexpensive and has the advantage of providing permanent preparations for use on an ordinary microscope. The stained smears can also be used for morphological assessment of the cells. Also, with the threshold for infertility diagnostics using TB staining having been established, the TB staining method is more advantageous. However, this method may have the inherent limitations of reproducibility dictated by the limited number of cells that can be reasonably scored.

CMA_3 assay

Principle

CMA_3 is a guanine–cytosine-specific fluorochrome that reveals poorly packaged chromatin in spermatozoa and is the indirect measure of protamine deficiency in sperm DNA (169). CMA_3 is specific for GC-rich sequences and is believed to compete with protamines for binding to the minor groove of DNA. Therefore, high CMA_3 fluorescence is a strong indicator of a low protamination state in spermatozoa (145).

Technique

Sperm smears are fixed in methanol–glacial acetic acid 3:1 at 4°C for 20 minutes and are then allowed to air-dry at room temperature for 20 minutes. The slides are treated for 20 minutes with 100 μL CMA_3 solution. The CMA_3 solution consists of 0.25 mg/mL CMA_3 in McIlvain's buffer (pH 7.0) supplemented with 10 mmol/L $MgCl_2$. The slides are rinsed in buffer and mounted with 1:1 v/v PBS–glycerol. The slides are then kept at 4°C overnight. Fluorescence is evaluated using a fluorescent microscope. A total of 200 spermatozoa are randomly evaluated on each slide. CMA_3 staining is evaluated by distinguishing spermatozoa that stain bright yellow (CMA_3 positive) from those that stain a dull yellow (CMA_3 negative) (146,149).

Clinical significance

As a discriminator of IVF success (>50% oocytes fertilized), CMA_3 staining has a sensitivity of 73% and a specificity of 75%. Therefore, it can distinguish between IVF success and failure (170). In cases of ICSI, Sakkas et al. (171) reported that the percentage of CMA_3 positivity does not indicate failure of fertilization entirely and suggested that poor chromatin packaging contributes to a failure in the decondensation process and probably reduced fertility. It appears that semen samples with high CMA_3 positivity (>30%) may have significantly lower fertilization rates if used for ICSI (172), but this observation is not seen in studies (173).

Advantages and limitations

The CMA_3 assay yields reliable results as it is strongly correlated with other assays used in the evaluation of sperm chromatin (145,174). CMA_3 staining results have been reported to have a strong negative correlation with sperm concentration, motility, and especially normal morphology. Men with low scores of morphologically normal spermatozoa tend to have a greater degree of protamine deficiency and DNA damage (59,174). The number of CMA_3-positive sperm was significantly higher in globozoopermic patients than in controls, which indicates high levels of DNA damage (169). In addition, the sensitivity and specificity of the CMA_3 stain are comparable with those of the AAB stain (75% and 82% vs. 60% and 91%, respectively) if used to evaluate the chromatin status in infertile men (146). However, the CMA_3 assay is limited by observer subjectivity.

DBD–FISH assay

Principle

The DBD–FISH is a technique that can detect DNA breaks in single cells, not only in the whole genome, but also in specific sequences of DNA. Cells embedded within an agarose matrix on a slide are exposed to an alkaline unwinding solution, which transforms DNA strand breaks into single-stranded DNA motifs. After neutralization and protein removal, single-stranded DNA becomes accessible to hybridization with whole-genome or specific DNA probes that highlight the chromatin area to be analyzed. As the number of DNA breaks increase, so does production of single-stranded DNA by the alkaline solution, resulting in an increase in fluorescence intensity and the surface area of the FISH signal. Abnormal chromatin packaging in sperm cells greatly increases the accessibility of DNA ligands and the sensitivity of DNA to denaturation by alkali, and this relates to the presence of intense labeling (red fluorescence) by DBD–FISH. Therefore, DBD–FISH allows *in situ* detection and quantification of DNA breaks and reveals structural features in the sperm chromatin (146,175).

Technique

Sperm cells are mixed with 1% low-melting point agarose to a final concentration of 0.7% at 37°C. A volume of 300 μL of the mixture is pipetted onto polystyrene slides and allowed to solidify at 4°C. The slides are immersed into a freshly prepared alkaline denaturation solution

(0.03 mol/L NaOH, 1 mol/L NaCl) for five minutes at 22°C in the dark to generate single-stranded DNA from DNA breaks. The denaturation is then stopped, and proteins are removed by transferring the slides to a tray with neutralizing and lysing solution 1 (0.4 mol/L Tris, 0.8 mol/L dithiothreitol [DTT], 1% sodium dodecylsulfate [SDS], and 50 mmol/L ethylenediaminetetraacetic acid [EDTA], pH 7.5) for 10 minutes at room temperature, which is followed by incubation in a neutralizing and lysing solution 2 (0.4 mol/L Tris, 2 mol/L NaCl, and 1% SDS, pH 7.5) for 20 minutes at room temperature. The slides are thoroughly washed in Tris–borate–EDTA buffer (0.09 mol/L Tris–borate and 0.002 mol/L EDTA, pH 7.5) for 15 minutes, dehydrated in sequential 70%, 90%, and 100% ethanol baths (two minutes each), and air-dried. A human whole-genome probe is hybridized overnight (4.3 ng/μL in 50% formamide/2 × standard saline citrate [SSC], 10% dextran sulfate, and 100 mmol/L calcium phosphate, pH 7.0; 1 × SSC is 0.015 mol/L sodium citrate and 0.15 mol/L sodium chloride, pH 7.0). It is then washed twice in 50% formamide/2 × SSC (pH 7.0) for five minutes and twice in 2 × SSC (pH 7.0) for three minutes at room temperature. The hybridized probe is detected with streptavidin indocarbocyamine (1:200) (Sigma Chemical Co., St Louis, MO), and cells are counterstained with 4',6-diamidino-2-phenylindole (DAPI) (1 μg/mL) and visualized using fluorescence microscopy (Figure 6.1b) (147).

Advantages and limitations

DBD–FISH is used to detect *in situ* DNA breaks as well as to reveal structural features of chromatin. Its major advantage is the possibility to simultaneously detect and discriminate single- and double-strand DNA breaks (176). Nevertheless, it is expensive and time consuming and involves sophisticated laboratory procedures.

In situ NT assay

Principle

The NT assay is a modified version of the TUNEL assay; it quantifies the incorporation of biotinylated dUTP at single-strand DNA breaks in a reaction that is catalyzed by the template-dependent (unlike TUNEL) enzyme DNA polymerase I.

It specifically stains spermatozoa that contain appreciable and variable levels of endogenous DNA damage. The NT assay indicates anomalies that have occurred during remodeling of the nuclear DNA in spermatozoa. In doing so, it is more likely to detect sperm anomalies that are not indicated by morphology.

Technique

To perform the assay, smears containing 500 sperm each should be prepared. The fluorescent staining solution is prepared by mixing 10 μL streptavidin–fluorescein–isothiocyanate, 90 μL Tris buffer, and 900 μL double-distilled water. A total of 100 μL of this solution is added to the slides. The slides are incubated in a moist chamber at 37°C for 30 minutes. After incubation, the slides are rinsed in PBS twice, washed with distilled water, and finally mounted with a 1:1 mixture of PBS and glycerol. The slides are examined using fluorescence microscopy. A total of 100–200 spermatozoa should be counted, and those fluorescing and hence incorporating the dye are classified as having endogenous nicks (148).

Clinical significance

Sperm nuclear integrity as assessed by the NT assay demonstrates a very clear relationship with sperm motility and morphology and, to a lesser extent, sperm concentration (31,131,177). Results of the assay are supported by the strong positive correlations detected with the sensitivity of CMA_3 and TUNEL assays ($r = 0.86$, $p < 0.05$ and $r = 0.87$, $p < 0.05$, respectively) (145). The NT assay can also indicate if there is damage arising from factors such as heat exposure (178) or the generation of ROS following exposure to leukocytes within the male reproductive tract (179).

Advantages and limitations

The advantage of the NT assay is that the reaction is based on direct labeling of the termini of DNA breaks. Thus, the lesions that are measured are identifiable at the molecular level. In addition, if flow cytometry is used to analyze the results, it may be performed on fixed cells, as the duration of cell storage in ethanol may vary (147). However, the NT assay has a lower sensitivity than the other assays and does not correlate with fertilization in *in vivo* studies.

AO assay

Principle

AO is a dye that intercalates with DNA or RNA and fluoresces to emit different colors, making it easy to differentiate cellular organelles. The binding that occurs is the property of electrostatic interactions between acridine molecules and base pairs of nucleic acid. It measures the susceptibility of sperm nuclear DNA to acid-induced denaturation *in situ* by quantifying the metachromatic shift of AO fluorescence from green (native DNA) to red (denatured DNA) (180). The fluorochrome AO intercalates into double-stranded DNA as a monomer and binds to single-stranded DNA as an aggregate. The monomeric AO bound to native DNA fluoresces green whereas the aggregated AO on relaxed or denatured DNA fluoresces red (Figure 6.1c) (181).

Technique

The AO assay can be used for either fluorescence or flow cytometry. For fluorescence microscopy, thick semen smears are fixed in Carnoy's fixative (methanol:acetic acid 1:3) for at least two hours. The slides are stained in AO for five minutes and gently rinsed with deionized water. At least 200 cells should be counted so that the estimates of the numbers of sperm with green and red fluorescence are accurate. Spermatozoa that emit green fluorescence are considered to have normal DNA content, whereas those displaying a spectrum of yellow–orange to red fluorescence are considered to have damaged DNA. The DNA fragmentation index (DFI) can be calculated by the ratio of (yellow to red)/(green + yellow to red) fluorescence (180).

For flow cytometry, aliquots of semen (about 25–100 μL, containing 1 million spermatozoa) are suspended in 1 mL of ice-cold PBS (pH 7.4) and centrifuged at 600 g for five minutes. The pellet is resuspended in ice-cold TNE (0.01 mol/L Tris-HCl, 0.15 mol/L NaCl, and 1 mmol/L EDTA, pH 7.4) and again centrifuged at 600 g for five minutes. The pellet is then resuspended in 200 μL of ice-cold TNE with 10% glycerol and immediately fixed in 70% ethanol for 30 minutes. The fixed samples are treated for 30 seconds with 400 μL of a solution of 0.1% Triton X-100, 0.15 mol/L NaCl, and 0.08 N HCl (pH 1.2). After 30 seconds, 1.2 mL of staining buffer (6 μg/mL AO, 37 mmol/L citric acid, 126 mmol/L Na_2HPO_4, 1 mmol/L disodium EDTA, and 0.15 mol/L NaCl, pH 6.0) is added to the test tube and analyzed by flow cytometry. After excitation by a 488-nm wavelength light source, AO bound to double-stranded DNA fluoresces green (515–530 nm) and AO bound to single-stranded DNA fluoresces red (630 nm or greater). A minimum of 5000 cells are analyzed by fluorescent-activated cell sorting (148).

Clinical significance

The AO technique has shown significantly higher DNA damage in infertile men with and without varicocele as compared to controls (167). Further, a decrease in AO-positive spermatozoa has also been documented after varicocelectomy, which shows its clinical utility in the evaluation of DNA integrity (107). AO-positive cells are likely to have more structural abnormalities than AO-negative cells (182). A negative correlation has been reported between AO staining results and conventional sperm parameters (183). The "cutoff" value set to differentiate between fertile and infertile men varies between 20% and 50% (17,149,184). Studies show that single-stranded DNA that is detected by a low incidence (<50%) of green AO fluorescence negatively affects the fertilization process in a classical IVF program, resulting in lower fertilization and pregnancy rates and a lower proportion of grade A embryos (125,181,185–187). However, no correlation was found with the pregnancy rate and live births achieved by ICSI except in patients having 0% of spermatozoa with single-stranded DNA, in whom the pregnancy rate was significantly higher (125,185–187).

Advantages and limitations

The AO assay is a biologically stable measure of sperm DNA quality. The intra-assay variability is less than 5%, rendering the technique highly reproducible (188). A strong positive correlation exists between the AO assay and other techniques used to evaluate single-stranded DNA (e.g., the TUNEL assay (see the "TUNEL assay" section) (122). Limitations include inter-observer variability in case of fluorescence microscopic analysis and expensive instrumentation for flow cytometric analysis.

SCD test (Halosperm® assay)

Principle

The SCD test produces sperm nucleoids consisting of a central or core and peripheral halo caused by release of DNA loops, signifying the absence of DNA fragmentation. When sperm are treated with an acid solution prior to lysis buffer, a complete absence or a minimal halo is produced in spermatozoa with fragmented DNA. A distinct halo is seen in spermatozoa with intact DNA integrity (150). When spermatozoa with non-fragmented DNA are immersed in an agarose matrix and directly exposed to lysing solutions, the resulting deproteinized nuclei (nucleoids) show extended halos of DNA dispersion, which can be observed either by bright field microscopy or fluorescence microscopy. The presence of DNA breaks promotes the expansion of the halo of the nucleoid (189–195).

Technique

Aliquots of sperm at a concentration of 5–10 million/mL are prepared by diluting in PBS. The samples are mixed with 1% low-melting point aqueous agarose (to obtain a 0.7% final agarose concentration) at 37°C. Aliquots of 50 μL of the mixture are pipetted onto a glass slide precoated with 0.65% standard agarose dried at 80°C, covered with a coverslip, and left to solidify at 4°C for four minutes. The coverslips are then carefully removed, and the slides are immediately immersed horizontally in a tray of freshly prepared acid denaturation solution (0.08 N HCl) for seven minutes at 22°C in the dark, which generates restricted single-stranded DNA motifs from DNA breaks. Denaturation is then stopped, and the proteins are removed by transferring the slides to a tray with neutralizing and lysing solution 1 (0.4 mol/L Tris, 0.8 mol/L DTT, 1% SDS, and 50 mmol/L EDTA, pH 7.5) for 10 minutes at room temperature. The slides are then incubated in neutralizing and lysing solution 2 (0.4 mol/L Tris, 2 mol/L NaCl, and 1% SDS, pH 7.5) for five minutes at room temperature. The slides are thoroughly washed in Tris–borate EDTA buffer (0.09 mol/L Tris–borate and 0.002 mol/L EDTA, pH 7.5) for two minutes, dehydrated in sequential 70%, 90%, and 100% ethanol baths (two minutes each), and air-dried. Cells are stained with DAPI (2 μg/mL) for fluorescence microscopy (Figure 6.2a) (149).

Advantages and limitations

The SCD test is simple, fast, and reproducible, with comparable results to those of the SCSA (190,193) and TUNEL assay (196). The currently available protocol is suitable for bright field microscopy as it significantly reduces equipment cost. The test is successfully used in clinical studies to detect sperm DNA damage (197) and can be simultaneously combined with the FISH (SCD–FISH) assay for detection of aneuploidy in sperm cells (198). This is the only test allowing assessment of sperm DNA fragmentation

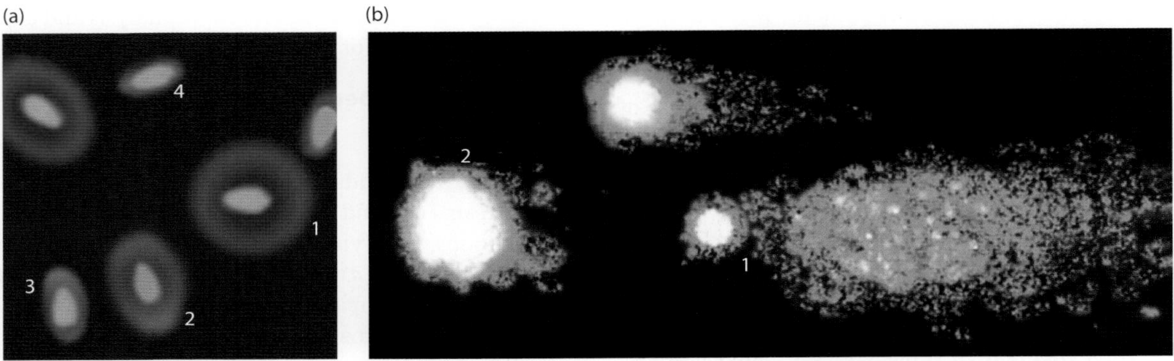

Figure 6.2 (a) Spermatozoa embedded in an agarose microgel stained with 4′,6-diamidino-2-phenylindole staining (blue fluorescence) and showing spermatozoa with different patterns of DNA dispersion: (1) Large-sized halo; (2) medium-sized halo; (3) very small size halo; and (4) no halo. (b) Comet images showing damaged (1) and undamaged DNA (2).

and chromosomal aneuploidy by FISH in the same cell. Oxidative DNA damage also can be simultaneously determined in the same sperm cell by combining the SCD test and incubation with an 8-oxoguanine DNA probe (199). A commercially available Halosperm® kit has been recently developed (200). Reports suggest that sperm DNA fragmentation as reported by the SCD test is negatively correlated with fertilization rates and embryo quality in IVF/ICSI, but not with clinical pregnancy rates or births (191,201).

Comet assay

Principle

The comet assay (single-cell gel electrophoresis) was first introduced by Ostling and Johanson in 1984 (202–206) and is based on the principle of permeabilization and electrophoretic migration of cleaved fragments of DNA. In the beginning, neutral electrophoresis buffer conditions were used to show that the migration of double-stranded DNA loops from a damaged cell in the form of a tail unwinding from the relaxed supercoiled nucleus was proportional to the extent of damage inflicted on the cell. This finding took on the appearance of a comet with a tail when viewed using a fluorescence microscope and DNA stains. Singh et al. modified the comet assay in 1988 (151) by using alkaline electrophoresis buffers to expose alkali-labile sites on the DNA; this modification increased the sensitivity of the assay to detect both single- and double-stranded DNA breaks (151). The routine comet assay lacks the ability to differentiate between single- and double-stranded DNA breaks in the same sperm cell, but a modified two-tailed comet assay can simultaneously evaluate single- and double-stranded DNA breaks (207).

The chromosome comet assay is a new application that detects DNA damage by generating comets in sub-nuclear units, such as the chromosome, based on the chromosome isolation protocols currently used for whole-chromosome mounting in electron microscopy. It has not been used with sperm cells thus far (208).

In the comet assay, DNA damage is quantified by measuring the displacement between the genetic material of the nucleus "comet head" and the resulting tail. The tail lengths are used as an index for the damage. Also, the tail moment—the product of the tail length and intensity (fraction of total DNA in the tails)—has been used as a measuring parameter. The tail moment can be more precisely defined as being equivalent to the torsional moment of the tail (209).

Technique

Sperm cells are cast into miniature agarose gels on microscopic slides and lysed *in situ* to remove DNA-associated proteins in order to allow the compacted sperm DNA to relax. The lysis buffer (Tris 10 mmol/L, 0.5 mol/L EDTA, and 2.5 mol/L NaCl, pH 10) contains 1% Triton X-100, 40 mmol/L DTT, and 100 μg/mL proteinase K. The slide immersion time in alkaline lysis solution ranges between 1 and 20 minutes and does not affect assay results (210). Micro-gels are then electrophoresed (20 minutes at 25 V/0.01 A) in neutral buffer (Tris 10 mmol/L containing 0.08 mol/L boric acid and 0.5 mol/L EDTA, pH 8.2), during which time the damaged DNA migrates from the nucleus toward the anode. The DNA is visualized by staining the slides with the fluorescent DNA binding dye SYBR Green I. Comet measurements are performed manually or by computerized image analysis using fluorescence microscopy (Figure 6.2b) (150).

In the two-tailed comet technique, sperm cells are diluted in PBS to a concentration of 10×10^6 spermatozoa/mL. A 25-μL cell suspension is mixed with 50 μL of 1% low-melting point agarose in distilled water at 37°C. A total of 15 μL of the mixture is placed on the slide, covered with a coverslip, and transferred to an ice-cold plate. As soon as the gel solidifies, the coverslips are removed and the slides are rinsed in two lysing solutions: lysing solution 1 (0.4 mol/L Tris–HCl, 0.8 mol/L DTT, and 1% SDS, pH 7.5) for 30 minutes, followed by lysing solution 2 (0.4 mol/L Tris–HCl, 2 mol/L NaCl, 1% SDS, and 0.05 mol/L EDTA, pH 7.5) for 30 minutes. Then, the slides are rinsed in TBE buffer (0.09 mol/L Tris–borate and 0.002 mol/L EDTA, pH 7.5) for 10 minutes, transferred to an electrophoresis tank, and immersed in fresh TBE electrophoresis buffer. Electrophoresis is performed at 20 V (1 V/cm) and 12 mA for 12.5 minutes. After washing in 0.9% NaCl, nucleoids are unwound in an alkaline solution (0.03 mol/L NaOH and 1 mol/L NaCl) for 2.5 minutes, transferred to an electrophoresis chamber, and oriented at 90° to the first electrophoresis.

The second electrophoresis is performed at 20 V (1 V/cm), and 12 mA for four minutes in 0.03 mol/L NaOH. Then, the slides are rinsed in a neutralization buffer (0.4 mol/L Tris–HCl, pH 7.5) for five minutes, briefly washed in TBE buffer, dehydrated in increasing concentrations of ethanol, and air-dried. DNA is stained with SYBR Green I at a 1:3000 dilution in Vectashield® (Vector Laboratories, Burlingame, CA). Samples are assessed by visual scoring or digitalization and image processing. The frequency of sperm cells with fragmented DNA is established by measuring at least 500 sperm cells per slide. Cells are classified as undamaged or damaged based on the length of the tail, which contains DNA fragment single-stand breaks (up/down migration), DSBs (right/left migration), or both (207).

Clinical significance

The assay has been successfully used to evaluate DNA damage after cryopreservation (211). It may also predict embryo development after IVF and ICSI, especially in couples with unexplained infertility (212,213), and some clinical thresholds were set for infertility diagnostics and IVF outcome prediction (214–217), although some studies failed to demonstrate such an association (218). A modified version of the comet assay protocol is capable of detecting different mutagen impacts on sperm DNA integrity (219).

Advantages and limitations

The comet assay is a well-standardized, simple, versatile, sensitive, and rapid assay that correlates significantly with the TUNEL assay and SCSA (220). It can assess DNA damage qualitatively as well as quantitatively with low intra-assay variation. Two-tailed comet assay can discriminate between single- and double-stranded DNA breaks; for example, the resistance of sperm DNA to oxidative damage can be specifically assessed (221). Because it is based on fluorescence microscopy, the assay requires an experienced observer to analyze the slides and interpret the results.

TUNEL assay

Principle

This single-step staining method labels DNA breaks with fluorescein isothiocyanate (FITC)-dUTP followed by flow cytometric analysis. TUNEL utilizes a template-independent DNA polymerase called TdT, which non-preferentially adds deoxyribonucleotides to 3′-hydroxyl (OH) single- and double-stranded DNA. dUTP is the substrate that is added by the TdT enzyme to the free 3′-OH break-ends of DNA (Figure 6.3) (114,153,154).

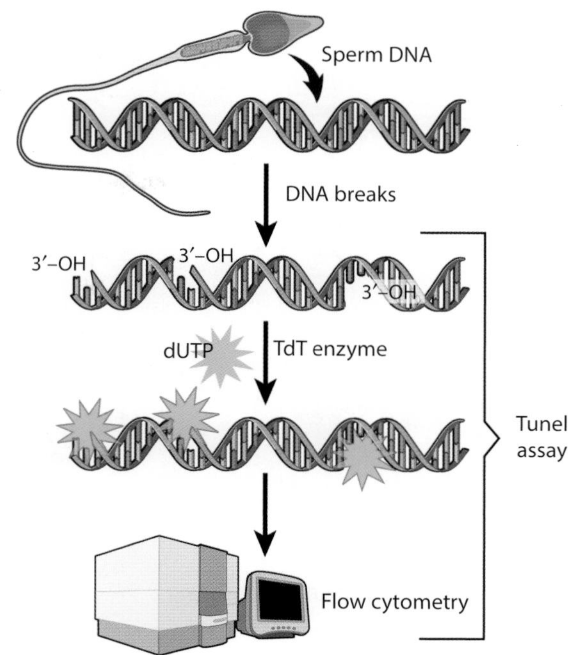

Figure 6.3 Schematic of DNA staining using the terminal deoxynucleotidyl transferase-mediated dUTP nick end labeling assay.

Technique

Strand breaks can be quantified with conventional or the newly introduced benchtop flow cytometry or fluorescence microscopy in which DNA-damaged sperm fluoresce intensely (114). To assess the DNA fragmentation by TUNEL, an APO-DIRECT™ Kit (BD Pharmingen, CA, USA) is used. It contains the reaction buffer, TdT, FITC-dUTP, and propidium iodide/RNase stain. The assay kit also contains negative and the positive controls, which are not sperm cells. About 5×10^6 sperm cells are fixed with 3.7% paraformaldehyde for a minimum of 30 minutes at 4°C. The sample is centrifuged at 300 g for seven minutes. Paraformaldehyde is removed by centrifuging the samples at 300 g for seven minutes. Supernatants are discarded and the pellets resuspended with 1 mL of ice-cold ethanol (70% v/v). The tubes are kept at −20°C for at least 30 minutes. To create negative sperm controls, the enzyme terminal transferase is omitted from the reaction mixture. To create positive sperm controls, the samples are pretreated with 0.1 IU DNase I for 30 minutes at room temperature. A total of 50 μL of the stain is added and incubated for one hour. Following two washes with 1 mL of the "rinse buffer," propidium iodide/RNase stain is added and incubated for 30 minutes. For flow cytometry, two laser detectors are used: FL1 (488) with a standard 533/30 band-pass (BP) that detects green fluorescence; and FL2 with a standard 585/40 BP that detects red or propidium iodide fluorescence. The tubes are analyzed for DNA fragmentation using the BD Accuri™ C6 flow cytometer (BD cytometers, USA) (Figure 6.4). A quality control assay is also run using the eight-peak beads as per the manufacturer's

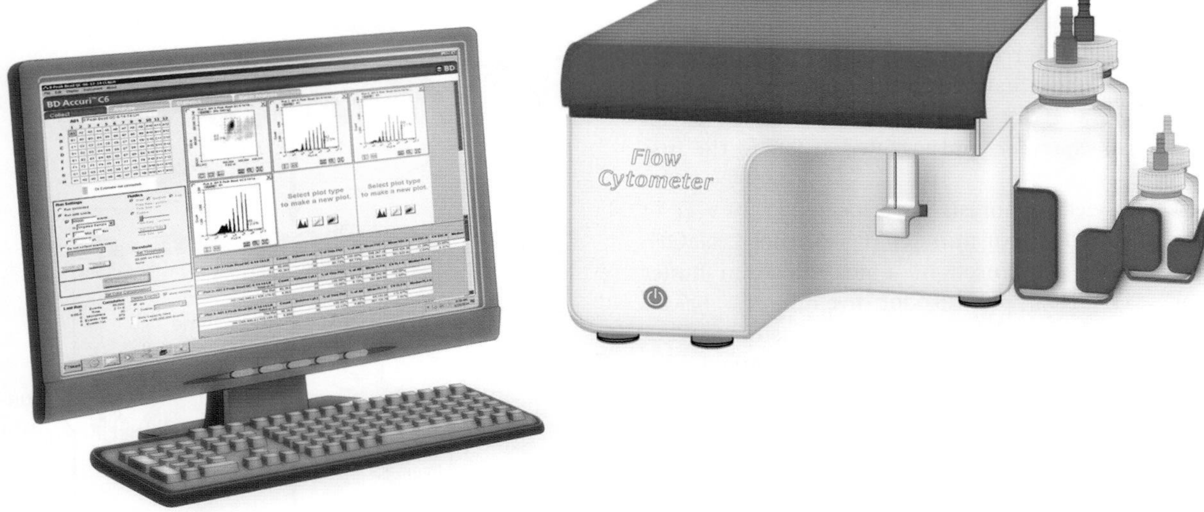

Figure 6.4 BD Accuri C6 flow cytometer.

instructions. Although less accurate, the samples can also be assessed by scoring about 500 sperm cells under fluorescence microscopy (153).

The standard TUNEL assay can be improved to become more sensitive to DNA fragmentation by incubating sperm cells in 2 mm DTT solution for 45 minutes prior to fixation with formaldehyde. This modified version of the TUNEL assay was shown to significantly enhance its sensitivity. Mitchell et al. modified the TUNEL methodology by incubating spermatozoa for 30 minutes at 37°C with LIVE /DEAD™ Fixable Dead Cell Stain (far red) (Molecular Probes, Eugene, OR). The cells were then washed three times with Biggers–Whitten–Whittingham medium (BWW) before incubation with DTT—this allowed both DNA integrity and vitality to be simultaneously assessed (222).

Clinical significance

The TUNEL assay has been widely used in male infertility research related to sperm DNA fragmentation. A negative correlation was found between the percentage of DNA-fragmented sperm and motility, morphology, and concentration in the ejaculate. It also appears to be potentially useful as a predictor for IUI pregnancy rates, IVF embryo cleavage rates, and ICSI fertilization rates. In addition, it provides an explanation for recurrent pregnancy loss (18,19,137,220). A cutoff value of 19.2% has been shown significant differentiation between fertile and infertile men with a sensitivity of 64.9% and a specificity of 100% (126,220). This is higher than that demonstrated for IUI procedures (12%) (19). We have recently reported a very high specificity (91.6%) and positive predictive value (PPV) (90%) at a cutoff point of 16.8%. The high specificity of the TUNEL assay is helpful in correctly identifying infertile patients who do not have sperm DNA fragmentation as a contributory factor (154). Due to its high positive predictive value, the assay is able to confirm that a man who tests positive is likely to be infertile due to elevated sperm DNA fragmentation. A similar specificity (91%) of the TUNEL assay was reported (Figure 6.5a and 6.5b) (223). The calculated cutoff would be ideal as any value above this threshold will be strongly associated with infertility.

Advantages and limitations

The TUNEL assay is relatively expensive and time and labor consuming. Also, a number of factors can significantly affect assay results, including the type and concentration of fixative, fixed sample storage time, the fluorochrome used to label DNA breaks, and the method used to analyze flow cytometric data (224). The flow cytometric method of assessment is generally more accurate and reliable than fluorescence microscopy, but it is also more sophisticated and expensive and it presents limitations in the accuracy and reproducibility of the measures of sperm DNA fragmentation (225). Fairly good-quality control parameters with minimal inter- and intra-observer variation (<8%) have been demonstrated for the fluorescent TUNEL assay using the benchtop flow cytometer (154) with few exceptions (8).

Sperm chromatin structure assay

Principle

The SCSA measures *in situ* DNA susceptibility to the acid-induced conformational helix–coil transition by AO fluorescence staining. The extent of conformational transition *in situ* following acid or heat treatment is determined by measuring the metachromatic shift of AO fluorescence from green (native DNA) to red (denatured or relaxed DNA). This protocol has been divided into $SCSA_{acid}$ and $SCSA_{heat}$ in order to distinguish the physical means of inducing conformational transition. The two methods give essentially the same results, but the $SCSA_{acid}$ method is easier to use. DNA damage that is SCSA-defined is manifested by the DFI (17).

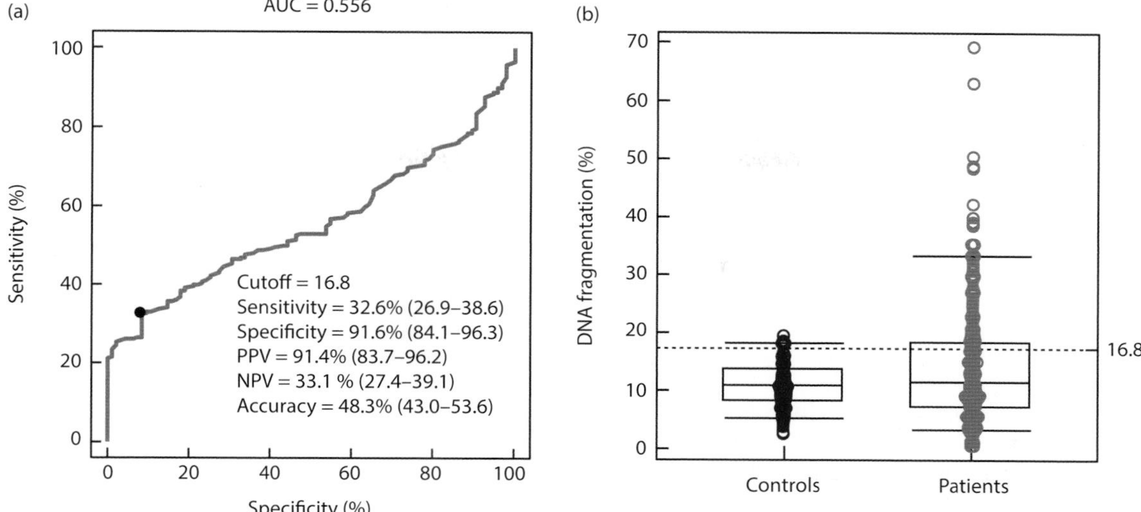

Figure 6.5 (a) Receiver operator characteristic curve showing terminal deoxynucleotidyl transferase-mediated dUTP nick end labeling (TUNEL) cutoff and the area under the curve (AUC). Values within the parentheses represent 95% confidence intervals. (b) Distribution of TUNEL values between controls and infertile men. PPV: positive predictive value; NPV: negative predictive value.

Technique

To perform SCSA, an aliquot of unprocessed semen (about 13–70 μL) is diluted to a concentration of 1–2 × 10^6 sperm/mL with TNE buffer (0.01 M Tris–HCl, 0.15 M NaCl, and 1 mM EDTA, pH 7.4). This cell suspension is treated with an acid detergent solution (pH 1.2) containing 0.1% Triton X-100, 0.15 mol/L NaCl, and 0.08 N HCl for 30 seconds and then stained with 6 mg/L purified AO in a phosphate–citrate buffer (pH 6.0). The stained sample is placed into the flow cytometer sample chamber (17).

Clinical significance

Because the SCSA results are more constant over prolonged periods of time than routine World Health Organization (WHO) semen parameters, it may be used effectively in epidemiological studies of male infertility (226). No significant male age-related increase in DFI has been demonstrated (227). Currently, the SCSA is the only assay that has clearly established clinical thresholds for utility in the human infertility clinic (228). In clinical applications, the SCSA parameters not only distinguish fertile and infertile men, but also are able to classify men according to the level of *in vivo* fertility as high fertility (pregnancy initiated in less than three months), moderate fertility (pregnancy initiated within 4–12 months), and no proven fertility (no pregnancy by 12 months). In addition, a DFI threshold was established that identifies samples that are compatible with *in vivo* pregnancy (<30%) (12,229–232).

The SCSA has been considered a gold standard as a robust assay for measuring DNA damage by flow cytometry and can predict various ART outcomes. However, the ability to predict ART outcomes, including fertilization and implantation rates, is true only for neat semen (9,12,136,233,234). An increased abortion rate in the high-DFI (>27%) group has been reported (218). It has also been suggested that DFI can be used as an independent predictor of fertility in couples undergoing IUI (9), but the association between SCSA results and IVF and ICSI outcomes is not strong enough (235). It has also been proposed that all infertile men should be tested with the SCSA in addition to standard semen analysis (236) and if DFI is higher than 30%, ICSI should recommended (12). The SCSA also measures sperm with high DNA stainability, which is related to the nuclear histones retained in immature sperm. Sperm with high DNA stainability is reported to be predictive of pregnancy failure (237). The current clinical threshold has changed from >30% to 25% DFI. DNA fragmentation above 25% categorizes a patient into the following statistical probabilities: (a) longer time to natural pregnancy; (b) low odds of IUI pregnancy; (c) more miscarriages; or (d) no pregnancy (237). The SCSA is considered to be a precise and repeatable DNA fragmentation test that can reliably identify a man who is at risk for infertility.

Advantages and limitations

The SCSA accurately estimates the percentage of DNA-damaged sperm and has a cutoff point (30% DFI) to differentiate between fertile and infertile samples. This has been recently revised to 25% (9,229,237). However, it requires the presence of expensive instrumentation (flow cytometer) and highly skilled technicians. The SCSA DFI is significantly associated with TUNEL assay results when Spearman's rank correlation is used. However, regression and concordance correlation results showed that these methods are not comparable. The SCSA measures DNA damage in terms of susceptibility to DNA denaturation, whereas TUNEL measures "real" DNA damage (238).

Measurement of 8-OHdG

Principle

This assay measures levels of 8-OHdG, which is a byproduct of oxidative DNA damage, in spermatozoa. It is the most commonly studied biomarker for oxidative DNA damage. Among various oxidative DNA adducts, 8-OHdG has been selected as a representative of oxidative DNA damage owning to its high specificity, potent mutagenicity, and relative abundance in DNA (239).

Technique

Step I

DNA extraction is performed with chloroform–isoamyl alcohol (12:1 v/v) after the sperm cells are washed with sperm wash buffer (10 mmol/L Tris-HCl, 10 mmol/L EDTA, and 1 mol/L NaCl, pH 7.0) and lysed at 55°C for one hour with 0.9% SDS, 0.5 mg/mL proteinase K, and 0.04 mol/L DTT. After ribonuclease A treatment to remove RNA residue, the extracted DNA is dissolved in 10 mmol/L Tris–HCl (pH 7.0) for DNA digestion.

Step II

Enzymatic DNA digestion is performed with three enzymes: DNase I, nuclease P1, and alkaline phosphatase. The final solution is dried under reduced temperature and pressure and is redissolved in distilled and deionized water for HPLC.

Step III

The third step is HPLC analysis. The HPLC system used for 8-OHdG measurements consists of a pump, a Partisphere® 5 C18 column (Hichrom Limited, UK), an electrochemical detector, a UV detector, an autosampler, and an integrator. The mobile phase consists of 20 mmol/L $NH_4H_2PO_4$, 1 mmol/L EDTA, and 4% methanol (pH 4.7). The calibration curves for 8-OHdG are established with standard 8-OHdG, and the results are expressed as 8-OHdG/10^4 dG (152).

Clinical significance

The assay provides the most direct evidence suggesting that oxidative sperm DNA damage is involved in male infertility based on the finding that 8-OHdG levels in sperm are significantly higher in infertile patients than in fertile controls and are inversely correlated with sperm concentration (152). 8-OHdG formation and DNA fragmentation as assessed by TUNEL are highly correlated with each other (240). 8-OHdG levels also are highly correlated with the disruption of chromatin remodeling (90). Levels of 8-OHdG in sperm DNA have been reported to be increased in smokers, and they are inversely correlated with the intake and seminal plasma concentration of vitamin C—the most important antioxidant in sperm. Infertile patients with varicocele have increased 8-OHdG expression in the testis, which is associated with deficient spermatogenesis (241). If not repaired, 8-OHdG modifications in DNA are mutagenic and may cause embryo loss, fetal malformations, or childhood cancer. Moreover, these modifications could be a marker of OS in sperm, which may have negative effects on sperm function (242,243).

Advantages and limitations

Although 8-OHdG is a potential marker for oxidative DNA damage, artificial oxidation of dG can occur during analysis, which can lead to inaccurate results. A fixed number of sperm cells should be analyzed as a precaution. However, the DNA yield cannot be excluded as a potential confounder.

STRATEGIES TO REDUCE SPERM DNA DAMAGE

In view of the impact sperm DNA fragmentation has on reproductive outcomes, it is important to develop and implement appropriate treatment methods, preventive measures, and strategies to minimize DNA damage in the spermatozoa used in assisted reproduction. Some of the strategies include:

1. *Appropriate sperm preparation methods*: Most of the commonly used methods such as density gradient centrifugation, swim up, and glass wool filtration yield sperm with better DNA integrity than native semen (14). Sperm preparation should be aimed at minimizing damage to the spermatozoa and can be accomplished by exercising some simple precautions such as: (i) slow dilution of the samples, especially when using cryopreserved spermatozoa; (ii) gradual changes in temperature and tests performed at 37°C; (iii) minimal use of centrifugation and, when necessary, it being performed at the lowest possible speed; and (iv) controlled exposure to potentially toxic materials. Plastic ware, glassware, media, and gloves should be checked for potential toxicity as the spermatozoa may be immobilized when in contact with any potential toxic substances in these materials. In patients who are unable to produce a semen sample by masturbation, use of non-toxic condoms is important, and when necessary, a second sample should be collected a few hours after the first.
2. *Electrophoretic separation of sperm*: This is based on the principle that high-quality spermatozoa tend to be viable and morphologically normal and have a low degree of DNA fragmentation as measured by TUNEL assay (244).
3. *Antioxidant treatments*: One of the causes of sperm DNA damage is OS. Studies have investigated the ability of antioxidant treatments to manage male subfertility, both *in vivo* and *in vitro*. It is generally accepted that antioxidants may be beneficial for reducing sperm DNA damage, but their exact mechanism of action is still not established, and some studies have reported adverse effects such as increased sperm chromatin decondensation (245,246). Significant improvement in clinical pregnancy and implantation rates have been shown in patients with high sperm DNA damage as assessed by TUNEL assay when treated with antioxidants before assisted reproduction (247,248). Therefore, in patients in whom OS is the cause of sperm DNA damage, adequate oral antioxidant supplementation appears to be a

simple strategy to enhance sperm genome integrity and reproductive outcomes. Standard and reliable oral antioxidant treatment protocols and alternative treatment strategies for non-responders are needed (249).

4. *Magnetic cell separation*: Magnetic cell separation is a useful technique to separate apoptotic and non-apoptotic spermatozoa (250).
5. *High-magnification ICSI for patients with sperm DNA fragmentation*: It is possible to observe spermatozoa with apparently normal morphology and intranuclear vacuoles that appear to be associated with chromatin packaging by using inverted microscopes with Nomarski differential interference contrast optics combined with digitally enhanced secondary magnification (251–254).

CONCLUSION

The importance of assessing sperm chromatin integrity is well established, and the results provide useful information in cases of male idiopathic infertility and in couples pursuing assisted reproduction. Pathologically increased sperm DNA fragmentation is one paternal-derived cause of repeated assisted reproduction failures in the ICSI era. Several studies have demonstrated that sperm DNA integrity correlates with pregnancy outcome in IVF. Therefore, sperm DNA fragmentation should be included in the evaluation of the infertile male. Assessment of sperm DNA damage appears to be a potential tool for evaluating semen samples prior to their use in assisted reproduction. It allows for the selection of spermatozoa with intact DNA or with the least amount of DNA damage for use in assisted conception. It provides better diagnostic and prognostic capabilities than standard sperm parameters for assessing male fertility potential.

There are multiple assays that can be used to evaluate sperm chromatin. Most of these assays have advantages as well as limitations. Choosing the right assay depends on many factors such as the expense, the available laboratory facilities, and the presence of experienced technicians. The establishment of a cutoff point between normal levels in the average fertile population and minimal levels of sperm DNA integrity required for achieving pregnancy still remains to be investigated. Such an average range or value confirmed by different laboratories is still lacking for most of these assays, except for the SCSA. Given the importance of sperm DNA integrity, it is important to determine the real cause of DNA damage and provide proper therapeutic treatment. Methods for selecting sperm with undamaged DNA should be designed, especially in cases where ICSI is strongly recommended.

REFERENCES

1. Guzick DS, Overstreet JW, Factor-Litvak P et al. National cooperative reproductive medicine network. Sperm morphology, motility, and concentration in fertile and infertile men. *N Engl J Med* 2001; 345: 1388–93.
2. Agarwal A, Said TM. Role of sperm chromatin abnormalities and DNA damage in male infertility. *Hum Reprod Update* 2003; 9: 331–45.
3. Hansen M, Kurinczuk JJ, Bower C et al. The risk of major birth defects after intracytoplasmic sperm injection and *in vitro* fertilization. *N Engl J Med* 2002; 346: 725–30.
4. Schieve LA, Meikle SF, Ferre C et al. Low and very low birth weight in infants conceived with use of assisted reproductive technology. *N Engl J Med* 2002; 346: 731–7.
5. Moll AC, Imhof SM, Cruysberg JR et al. Incidence of retinoblastoma in children born after *in-vitro* fertilisation. *Lancet* 2003; 361: 309–10.
6. Orstavik KH, Eiklid K, van der Hagen CB et al. Another case of imprinting defect in a girl with Angelman syndrome who was conceived by intracytoplasmic semen injection. *Am J Hum Genet* 2003; 72: 218–9.
7. Agarwal A, Allamaneni SS. Sperm DNA damage assessment: A test whose time has come. *Fertil Steril* 2005; 84: 850–3.
8. Erenpreiss J, Spano M, Erenpreisa J et al. Sperm chromatin structure and male fertility: Biological and clinical aspects. *Asian J Androl* 2006; 8: 11–29.
9. Evenson D, Wixon R. Meta-analysis of sperm DNA fragmentation using the sperm chromatin structure assay. *Reprod Biomed Online* 2006; 12: 466–72.
10. Borini A, Tarozzi N, Bizzaro D et al. Sperm DNA fragmentation: Paternal effect on early post-implantation embryo development in ART. *Hum Reprod* 2006; 21: 2876–81.
11. Aitken RJ, De Iuliis GN. Origins and consequences of DNA damage in male germ cells. *Reprod Biomed Online* 2007; 14: 727–33.
12. Bungum M, Humaidan P, Axmon A et al. Sperm DNA integrity assessment in prediction of assisted reproduction technology outcome. *Hum Reprod* 2007; 22: 174–9.
13. Ozmen B, Koutlaki N, Youssry M et al. DNA damage of human spermatozoa in assisted reproduction: Origins, diagnosis, impacts and safety. *Reprod Biomed Online* 2007; 14: 384–95.
14. Tarozzi N, Bizzaro D, Flamigni C et al. Clinical relevance of sperm DNA damage in assisted reproduction. *Reprod Biomed Online* 2007; 14: 746–57.
15. Lopes S, Jurisicova A, Sun JG et al. Reactive oxygen species: Potential cause for DNA fragmentation in human spermatozoa. *Hum Reprod* 1998; 13: 896–900.
16. Sakkas D, Tomlinson M. Assessment of sperm competence. *Semin Reprod Med* 2000; 18: 133–9.
17. Evenson DP, Jost LK, Marshall D et al. Utility of the sperm chromatin structure assay as a diagnostic and prognostic tool in the human fertility clinic. *Hum Reprod* 1999; 14: 1039–49.
18. Aitken RJ. The Amoroso Lecture. The human spermatozoon—A cell in crisis? *J Reprod Fertil* 1999; 115: 1–7.

19. Sun JG, Jurisicova A, Casper RF. Detection of deoxyribonucleic acid fragmentation in human sperm: Correlation with fertilization *in vitro*. *Biol Reprod* 1997; 56: 602–7.
20. Duran EH, Morshedi M, Taylor S et al. Sperm DNA quality predicts intrauterine insemination outcome: A prospective cohort study. *Hum Reprod* 2002; 17: 3122–8.
21. Larson KL, DeJonge CJ, Barnes AM et al. Sperm chromatin structure assay parameters as predictors of failed pregnancy following assisted reproductive techniques. *Hum Reprod* 2000; 15: 1717–22.
22. De Jonge C. The clinical value of sperm nuclear DNA assessment. *Hum Fertil* 2002; 5: 51–3.
23. Bellve AR, McKay DJ, Renaux BS et al. Purification and characterization of mouse protamines P1 and P2. Amino acid sequence of P2. *Biochem* 1988; 27: 2890–7.
24. Ward WS, Coffey DS. DNA packaging and organization in mammalian spermatozoa: Comparison with somatic cells. *Biol Reprod* 1991; 44: 569–74.
25. Fuentes-Mascorro G, Serrano H, Rosado A. Sperm chromatin. *Arch Androl* 2000; 45: 215–25.
26. Oliva R, Castillo J. Proteomics and the genetics of sperm chromatin condensation. *Asian J Androl* 2011; 13: 24–30.
27. Gatewood JM, Cook GR, Balhorn R et al. Sequence-specific packaging of DNA in human sperm chromatin. *Science* 1987; 236: 962–4.
28. Bench GS, Friz AM, Corzett MH et al. DNA and total protamine masses in individual sperm from fertile mammalian subjects. *Cytometry* 1996; 23: 263–71.
29. Johnson GD, Lalancette C, Linnemann AK et al. The sperm nucleus: Chromatin, RNA, and the nuclear matrix. *Reproduction* 2011; 141:21–36.
30. Sakkas D, Mariethoz E, Manicardi G et al. Origin of DNA damage in ejaculated human spermatozoa. *Rev Reprod* 1999; 4: 31–7.
31. Irvine DS, Twigg JP, Gordon EL et al. DNA integrity in human spermatozoa: Relationships with semen quality. *J Androl* 2000; 21: 33–44.
32. Ward WS. Deoxyribonucleic acid loop domain tertiary structure in mammalian spermatozoa. *Biol Reprod* 1993; 48: 1193–201.
33. Zalensky AO, Allen MJ, Kobayashi A et al. Well-defined genome architecture in the human sperm nucleus. *Chromosoma* 1995; 103: 577–90.
34. Solov'eva L, Svetlova M, Bodinski D et al. Nature of telomere dimers and chromosome looping in human spermatozoa. *Chromosome Res* 2004; 12: 817–23.
35. Ward WS, Zalensky AO. The unique, complex organization of the transcriptionally silent sperm chromatin. *Crit Rev Eukaryot Gene Expr* 1996; 6: 139–47.
36. De Jonge CJ. Paternal contributions to embryogenesis. *Reprod Med Rev* 2000; 8: 203–14.
37. Lewis JD, Song Y, de Jong ME et al. A walk through vertebrate and invertebrate protamines. *Chromosoma* 1999; 111: 473–82.
38. Corzett M, Mazrimas J, Balhorn R. Protamine 1: Protamine 2 stoichiometry in the sperm of eutherian mammals. *Mol Reprod Dev* 2002; 61: 519–27.
39. Jager S. Sperm nuclear stability and male infertility. *Arch Androl* 1990; 25: 253–9.
40. Balhorn R, Reed S, Tanphaichitr N. Aberrant protamine 1/protamine 2 ratio in sperm of infertile human males. *Experientia* 1988; 44: 52–5.
41. Bench G, Corzett MH, De Yebra L et al. Protein and DNA contents in sperm from an infertile human male possessing protamine defects that vary over time. *Mol Reprod Dev* 1998; 50: 345–53.
42. de Yebra L, Ballesca JL, Vanrell JA et al. Detection of P2 precursors in the sperm cells of infertile patients who have reduced protamine P2 levels. *Fertil Steril* 1998; 69: 755–9.
43. Nasr-Esfahani MH, Salehi M, Razavi S et al. Effect of protamine-2 deficiency on ICSI outcome. *Reprod Biomed Online* 2004; 9: 652–8.
44. Aoki VW, Liu L, Carrell DT. Identification and evaluation of a novel sperm protamine abnormality in a population of infertile males. *Hum Reprod* 2005; 20: 1298–306.
45. García-Peiró A, Martínez-Heredia J, Oliver-Bonet M et al. Protamine 1 to protamine 2 ratio correlates with dynamic aspects of DNA fragmentation in human sperm. *Fertil Steril* 2011; 95: 105–9.
46. Nanassy L, Liu L, Griffin J et al. The clinical utility of the protamine 1/protamine 2 ratio in sperm. *Protein Pept Lett* 2011; 18: 772–7.
47. Matsuda Y, Tobari I. Chromosomal analysis in mouse eggs fertilized *in vitro* with sperm exposed to ultraviolet light (UV) and methyl and ethyl methanesulfonate (MMS and EMS). *Mutat Res* 1988; 198: 131–44.
48. Genesca A, Caballin MR, Miro R et al. Repair of human sperm chromosome aberrations in the hamster egg. *Hum Genet* 1992; 89: 181–6.
49. Aitken RJ, Krausz C. Oxidative stress, DNA damage and the Y chromosome. *Reproduction* 2001; 122: 497–506.
50. Muratori M, Tamburrino L, Marchiani S et al. Investigation on the origin of sperm DNA fragmentation: Role of apoptosis, immaturity and oxidative stress. *Mol Med* 2015; 21: 109–22.
51. Sakkas D, Manicardi G, Bianchi PG et al. Relationship between the presence of endogenous nicks and sperm chromatin packaging in maturing and fertilizing mouse spermatozoa. *Biol Reprod* 1995; 52: 1149–55.
52. Marcon L, Boissonneault G. Transient DNA strand breaks during mouse and human spermiogenesis: New insights in stage specificity and link to chromatin remodeling. *Biol Reprod* 2004; 70: 910–18.
53. McPherson SM, Longo FJ. Localization of DNase I-hypersensitive regions during rat spermatogenesis: Stage-dependent patterns and unique sensitivity of elongating spermatids. *Mol Reprod Dev* 1992; 31: 268–79.

54. Laberge RM, Boissonneault G. On the nature and origin of DNA strand breaks in elongating spermatids. *Biol Reprod* 2005; 73: 289–96.
55. Kierszenbaum AL. Transition nuclear proteins during spermiogenesis: Unrepaired DNA breaks not allowed. *Mol Reprod Dev* 2001; 58: 357–8.
56. Balhorn R, Cosman M, Thornton K et al. Protamine mediated condensation of DNA in mammalian sperm. In: *The Male Gamete: From Basic Knowledge to Clinical Applications*. Gagnon C (ed.). Vienna, IL: Cache River Press, 1999, pp. 55–70.
57. Morse-Gaudio M, Risley MS. Topoisomerase II expression and VM-26 induction of DNA breaks during spermatogenesis in *Xenopus laevis*. *J Cell Sci* 1994; 107: 2887–98.
58. Bizzaro D, Manicardi G, Bianchi PG et al. Sperm decondensation during fertilisation in the mouse: Presence of DNase I hypersensitive sites *in situ* and a putative role for topoisomerase II. *Zygote* 2000; 8: 197–202.
59. Franco JG Jr, Mauri AL, Petersen CG et al. Large nuclear vacuoles are indicative of abnormal chromatin packaging in human spermatozoa. *Int J Androl* 2012; 35: 46–51.
60. Boitrelle F, Ferfouri F, Petit JM et al. Large human sperm vacuoles observed in motile spermatozoa under high magnification: Nuclear thumbprints linked to failure of chromatin condensation. *Hum Reprod* 2011; 26: 1650–8.
61. Aoki VW, Liu L, Jones KP et al. Sperm protamine1/protamine 2 ratios are related to *in vitro* fertilization pregnancy rates and predictive of fertileization ability. *Fertil Steril* 2006; 86: 1408–15.
62. Carrell DT, Emery BR, Hammoud S. Altered protamine expression and diminished spermato-genesis: What is the link? *Hum Reprod Update* 2007; 13: 313–27.
63. Tseden K, Topaloglu O, Meinhardt A et al. Premature translation of transition protein 2 mRNA causes sperm abnormalities and male infertility. *Mol Reprod Dev* 2007; 74: 273–79.
64. Sakkas D, Mariethoz E, St John JC. Abnormal sperm parameters in humans are indicative of an abortive apoptotic mechanism linked to the Fas-mediated pathway. *Exp Cell Res* 1999; 251: 350–5.
65. Donnelly ET, O'Connell M, McClure N et al. Differences in nuclear DNA fragmentation and mitochondrial integrity of semen and prepared human spermatozoa. *Hum Reprod* 2000; 15: 1552–61.
66. Spadafora C. Sperm cells and foreign DNA: A controversial relation. *Bioessays* 1998; 20: 955–64.
67. Aitken RJ, Koppers AJ. Apoptosis and DNA damage in human spermatozoa. *Asian J Androl* 2011; 13: 36–42.
68. Suda T, Takahashi T, Golstein P et al. Molecular cloning and expression of the Fas ligand, a novel member of the tumor necrosis factor family. *Cell* 1993; 75:1169–78.
69. Krammer PH, Behrmann I, Daniel P et al. Regulation of apoptosis in the immune system. *Curr Opin Immunol* 1994; 6: 279–89.
70. Rodriguez I, Ody C, Araki K et al. An early and massive wave of germinal cell apoptosis is required for the development of functional spermatogenesis. *EMBO J* 1997; 16:2262–70.
71. Said TM, Paasch U, Glander HJ et al. Role of caspases in male infertility. *Hum Reprod Update* 2004; 10: 39–51.
72. Zhivotovsky B, Kroemer G. Apoptosis and genomic instability. *Nat Rev Mol Cell Biol* 2004; 5: 752–62.
73. Muratori M, Piomboni P, Baldi E et al. Functional and ultrastructural features of DNA-fragmented human sperm. *J Androl* 2000; 21: 903–12.
74. Barroso G, Morshedi M, Oehninger S. Analysis of DNA fragmentation, plasma membrane translocation of phosphatidylserine and oxidative stress in human spermatozoa. *Hum Reprod* 2000; 15: 1338–44.
75. Ross AJ, Waymire KG, Moss JE et al. Testicular degeneration in Bclw-deficient mice. *Nat Genet* 1998; 18: 251–6.
76. Sakkas D, Moffatt O, Manicardi GC et al. Nature of DNA damage in ejaculated human spermatozoa and the possible involvement of apoptosis. *Biol Reprod* 2002; 66: 1061–7.
77. Sutovsky P, Neuber E, Schatten G. Ubiquitin-dependent sperm quality control mechanism recognizes spermatozoa with DNA defects as revealed by dual ubiquitin–TUNEL assay. *Mol Reprod Dev* 2002; 61: 406–13.
78. Muratori M, Maggi M, Spinelli S et al. Spontaneous DNA fragmentation in swim-up selected human spermatozoa during long term incubation. *J Androl* 2003; 24: 253–62.
79. Sakkas D, Seli E, Bizzaro D et al. Abnormal spermatozoa in the ejaculate: Abortive apoptosis and faulty nuclear remodelling during spermatogenesis. *Reprod Biomed Online* 2003; 7: 428–32.
80. Cayli S, Sakkas D, Vigue L et al. Cellular maturity and apoptosis in human sperm: Creatin kinase, caspase-3 and Bcl-XL levels in mature and diminished maturity sperm. *Mol Hum Reprod* 2004; 10: 365–72.
81. Henkel R, Hajimohammad M, Stalf T et al. Influence of deoxyribonucleic acid damage on fertilization and pregnancy. *Fertil Steril* 2004; 81: 965–72.
82. Lachaud C, Tesarik J, Canadas ML et al. Apoptosis and necrosis in human ejaculated spermatozoa. *Hum Reprod* 2004; 19: 607–10.
83. Moustafa MH, Sharma RK, Thornton J et al. Relationship between ROS production, apoptosis, and DNA denaturation in spermatozoa from patients examined for infertility. *Hum Reprod* 2004; 19: 129–38.
84. Paasch U, Sharma RK, Gupta AK et al. Cryopreservation and thawing is associated with varying extent of activation of apoptotic machinery in subsets of ejaculated human spermatozoa. *Biol Reprod* 2004; 71: 1828–37.

85. Sutovsky P, Hauser R, Sutovsky M. Increased levels of sperm ubiquitin correlate with semen quality in men from an andrology clinic population. *Hum Reprod* 2004; 19: 628–35.
86. Aitken RJ, Buckingham D, West K et al. Differential contribution of leucocytes and spermatozoa to the generation of reactive oxygen species in the ejaculates of oligozoospermic patients and fertile donors. *J Reprod Fertil* 1992; 94: 451–62.
87. Martínez P, Proverbio F, Camejo MI. Sperm lipid peroxidation and pro-inflammatory cytokines. *Asian J Androl* 2007; 9: 102–7.
88. Bannister LA, Schimenti JC. Homologous recombinational repair proteins in mouse meiosis. *Cytogenet Genome Res* 2004; 107: 191–200.
89. Page AW, Orr-Weaver TL. Stopping and starting the meiotic cell cycle. *Curr Opin Genet Dev* 1997; 7: 23–31.
90. De Iuliis GN, Thomson LK, Mitchell LA et al. DNA damage in human spermatozoa is highly correlated with the efficiency of chromatin remodelling and the formation of 8-hydroxy-2'-deoxyguanosine, a marker of oxidative stress. *Biol Reprod* 2009; 81: 517–24.
91. Gavriliouk D, Aitken RJ. Damage to sperm DNA mediated by reactive oxygen species: Its impact on human reproduction and the health trajectory of offspring. *Adv Exp Med Biol* 2015; 868: 23–47.
92. Singh NP, Muller CH, Berger RE. Effects of age on DNA double-strand breaks and apoptosis in human sperm. *Fertil Steril* 2003; 80: 1420–30.
93. Schmid TE, Eskenazi B, Baumgartner A et al. The effects of male age on sperm DNA damage in healthy non-smokers. *Hum Reprod* 2007; 22: 180–7.
94. Morris ID. Sperm DNA damage and cancer treatment. *Int J Androl* 2002; 25: 255–61.
95. Sailer BL, Jost LK, Erickson KR et al. Effects of X-irradiation on mouse testicular cells and sperm chromatin structure. *Environ Mol Mutagen* 1995; 25:23–30.
96. Fossa SD, De Angelis P, Kraggerud SM et al. Prediction of posttreatment spermatogenesis in patients with testicular cancer by flow cytometric sperm chromatin structure assay. *Cytometry* 1997; 30: 192–6.
97. Ståhl O, Eberhard J, Jepson K et al. Sperm DNA integrity in testicular cancer patients. *Hum Reprod* 2006; 21: 3199–205.
98. Potts RJ, Newbury CJ, Smith G et al. Sperm chromatin damage associated with male smoking. *Mutat Res* 1999; 423: 103–11.
99. Saleh RA, Agarwal A, Sharma RK et al. Effect of cigarette smoking on levels of seminal oxidative stress in infertile men: A prospective study. *Fertil Steril* 2002; 78: 491–9.
100. Erenpreiss J, Hlevicka S, Zalkalns J et al. Effect of leukocytospermia on sperm DNA integrity: A negative effect in abnormal semen samples. *J Androl* 2002; 23: 717–23.
101. Stronati A, Manicardi GC, Cecati M et al. Relationships between sperm DNA fragmentation, sperm apoptotic markers and serum levels of CB-153 and p,p'-DDE in European and Inuit populations. *Reproduction* 2006 132:949–58.
102. Rubes J, Selevan SG, Evenson DP et al. Episodic air pollution is associated with increased DNA fragmentation in human sperm without other changes in semen quality. *Hum Reprod* 2005; 20: 2776–83.
103. Sanchez-Pena LC, Reyes BE, Lopez-Carrillo L et al. Organophosphorous pesticide exposure alters sperm chromatin structure in Mexican agricultural workers. *Toxicol Appl Pharmacol* 2004; 196: 108–13.
104. Saleh RA, Agarwal A, Sharma RK et al. Evaluation of nuclear DNA damage in spermatozoa from infertile men with varicocele. *Fertil Steril* 2003; 80: 1431–6.
105. Fischer MA, Willis J, Zini A. Human sperm DNA integrity: Correlation with sperm cytoplasmic droplets. *Urology* 2003; 61: 207–11.
106. Zini A, Defreitas G, Freeman M et al. Varicocele is associated with abnormal retention of cytoplasmic droplets by human spermatozoa. *Fertil Steril* 2000; 74: 461–4.
107. Zini A, Blumenfeld A, Libman J et al. Beneficial effect of microsurgical varicocelectomy on human sperm DNA integrity. *Hum Reprod* 2005; 20: 1018–21.
108. Werthman P, Wixon R, Kasperson K et al. Significant decrease in sperm deoxyribonucleic acid fragmentation after varicocelectomy. *Fertil Steril* 2008; 90: 1800–4.
109. Xing W, Krishnamurthy H, Sairam MR. Role of follitropin receptor signaling in nuclear protein transitions and chromatin condensation during spermatogenesis. *Biochem Biophys Res Commun* 2003; 312: 697–701.
110. Evenson DP, Jost LK, Corzett M et al. Characteristics of human sperm chromatin structure following an episode of influenza and high fever: A case study. *J Androl* 2000; 21: 739–46.
111. Ahmad G, Moinard N, Esquerré-Lamare C et al. Mild induced testicular and epididymal hyperthermia alters sperm chromatin integrity in men. *Fertil Steril* 2012; 97: 546–53.
112. Banks S, King SA, Irvine DS et al. Impact of a mild scrotal heat stress on DNA integrity in murine spermatozoa. *Reproduction* 2005; 129: 505–14.
113. Zalata A, Hafez T, Comhaire F. Evaluation of the role of reactive oxygen species in male infertility. *Hum Reprod* 1995; 10: 1444–51.
114. Sharma R, Ahmad G, Esteves S et al. Terminal deoxynucleotidyl transferase dUTP nick end labeling (TUNEL) assay using bench top flow cytometer for evaluation of sperm DNA fragmentation in fertility laboratories: Protocol, reference values, and quality control. *J Assist Reprod Genet* 2016; 33: 291–300.
115. Sergerie M, Laforest G, Boulanger K et al. Longitudinal study of sperm DNA fragmentation as measured by terminal uridine nick end-labelling assay. *Hum Reprod* 2005; 20: 1921–7.

116. Erenpreiss J, Bungum M, Spano M et al. Intra-individual variation in sperm chromatin structure assay parameters in men from infertile couples: Clinical implications. *Hum Reprod* 2006; 21: 2061–4.
117. Smit M, Dohle GR, Hop WC et al. Clinical correlates of the biological variation of sperm DNA fragmentation in infertile men attending an andrology outpatient clinic. *Int J Androl* 2007; 30: 48–55.
118. Spano M, Bonde JP, Hjollund HI et al. Sperm chromatin damage impairs human fertility. The Danish First Pregnancy Planner Study Team. *Fertil Steril* 2000; 73: 43–50.
119. Larson-Cook KL, Brannian JD, Hansen KA et al. Relationship between the outcomes of assisted reproductive techniques and sperm DNA fragmentation as measured by the sperm chromatin structure assay. *Fertil Steril* 2003; 80: 895–902.
120. Host E, Lindenberg S, Kahn JA et al. DNA strand breaks in human sperm cells: A comparison between men with normal and oligozoospermic sperm samples. *Acta Obstet Gynecol Scand* 1999; 78: 336–9.
121. Gandini L, Lombardo F, Paoli D et al. Study of apoptotic DNA fragmentation in human spermatozoa. *Hum Reprod* 2000; 15: 830–9.
122. Zini A, Bielecki R, Phang D et al. Correlations between two markers of sperm DNA integrity, DNA denaturation and DNA fragmentation, in fertile and infertile men. *Fertil Steril* 2001; 75: 674–7.
123. Saleh RA, Agarwal A, Nelson DR et al. Increased sperm nuclear DNA damage in normozoospermic infertile men: A prospective study. *Fertil Steril* 2002; 78: 313–18.
124. McKelvey-Martin V, Melia N, Walsh I et al. Two potential clinical applications of the alkaline single-cell gel electrophoresis assay: (1). Human bladder washings and transitional cell carcinoma of the bladder; and (2). Human sperm and male infertility. *Mutat Res* 1997; 375: 93–104.
125. Zhang Y, Wang H, Wang L et al. The clinical significance of sperm DNA damage detection combined with routine semen testing in assisted reproduction. *Mol Med Report* 2008; 1: 617–24.
126. Sergerie M, Laforest G, Bujan L et al. Sperm DNA fragmentation: Threshold value in male fertility. *Hum Reprod* 2005; 20: 3446–51.
127. Drobnis EZ, Johnson M. The question of sperm DNA fragmentation testing in the male infertility work-up: A response to Professor Lewis' commentary. *Reprod Biomed Online* 2015; 31: 138–9.
128. Saleh RA, Agarwal A, Nada ES et al. Negative effects of increased sperm DNA damge in relation to seminal oxidative stress in men with idiopathic and male factor infertility. *Fertil Steril* 2003; 79: 1597–605.
129. Bungum M, Humaidan P, Spano M et al. The predictive value of sperm chromatin structure assay (SCSA) parameters for the outcome of intrauterine insemination, IVF and ICSI. *Hum Reprod* 2004; 19: 1401–8.
130. Payne JF, Raburn DJ, Couchman GM et al. Redefining the relationship between sperm deoxyribonucleic acid fragmentation as measured by the sperm chromatin structure assay and outcomes of assisted reproductive techniques. *Fertil Steril* 2005; 84: 356–64.
131. Tomlinson MJ, Moffatt O, Manicardi GC et al. Interrelationships between seminal parameters and sperm nuclear DNA damage before and after density gradient centrifugation: Implications for assisted conception. *Hum Reprod* 2001; 16: 2160–5.
132. Seli E, Gardner DK, Schoolcraft WB et al. Extent of nuclear DNA damage in ejaculated spermatozoa impacts on blastocyst development after *in vitro* fertilization. *Fertil Steril* 2004; 82: 378–83.
133. Hammadeh ME, Stieber M, Haidl G et al. Association between sperm cell chromatin condensation, morphology based on strict criteria, and fertilization, cleavage and pregnancy rates in an IVF program. *Andrologia* 1998; 30: 29–35.
134. Lopes S, Sun JG, Jurisicova A et al. Sperm deoxyribonucleic acid fragmentation is increased in poor-quality semen samples and correlates with failed fertilization in intracytoplasmic sperm injection. *Fertil Steril* 1998; 69: 528–32.
135. Twigg JP, Irvine DS, Aitken RJ. Oxidative damage to DNA in human spermatozoa does not preclude pronucleus formation at intracytoplasmic sperm injection. *Hum Reprod* 1998; 13: 1864–71.
136. Li Z, Wang L, Cai J et al. Correlation of sperm DNA damage with IVF and ICSI outcomes: A systematic review and meta-analysis. *J Assist Reprod Genetics* 2006; 23: 367–76.
137. Carrell DT, Liu L, Peterson CM et al. Sperm DNA fragmentation is increased in couples with unexplained recurrent pregnancy loss. *Arch Androl* 2003; 49: 49–55.
138. Virro MR, Larson-Cook KL, Evenson DP. Sperm chromatin structure assay (SCSA) parameters are related to fertilization, blastocyst development, and ongoing pregnancy in *in vitro* fertilization and intracytoplasmic sperm injection cycles. *Fertil Steril* 2004; 81: 1289–95.
139. Check JH, Graziano V, Cohen R et al. Effect of an abnormal sperm chromatin structural assay (SCSA) on pregnancy outcome following (IVF) with ICSI in previous IVF failures. *Arch Androl* 2005; 51: 121–4.
140. Bujan L, Walschaerts M, Brugnon F et al. Impact of lymphoma treatments on spermatogenesis and sperm deoxyribonucleic acid: A multicenter prospective study from the CECOS network. *Fertil Steril* 2014; 102: 667–74.
141. Daudin M, Rives N, Walschaerts M et al. Sperm cryopreservation in adolescents and young adults with cancer: Results of the French national sperm banking network (CECOS). *Fertil Steril* 2015; 103: 478–86.

142. De Mas P, Daudin M, Vincent MC et al. Increased aneuploidy in spermatozoa from testicular tumour patients after chemotherapy with cisplatin, etoposide and bleomycin. *Hum Reprod* 2001; 16: 1204–8.
143. Kobayashi H, Larson K, Sharma R et al. DNA damage in cancer patients before treatment as measured by the sperm chromatin structure assay. *Fertil Steril* 2001; 75: 469–75.
144. Baker H, Liu D. Assessment of nuclear maturity. In: *Human Spermatozoa in Assisted Reproduction*. Acosta A, Kruger T (eds). London: CRC Press, 1996: pp. 193–203.
145. Erenpreisa J, Erenpreiss J, Freivalds T et al. Toluidine blue test for sperm DNA integrity and elaboration of image cytometry algorithm. *Cytometry* 2003; 52: 19–27.
146. Manicardi GC, Bianchi PG, Pantano S et al. Presence of endogenous nicks in DNA of ejaculated human spermatozoa and its relationship to chromomycin A_3 accessibility. *Biol Reprod* 1995; 52: 864–7.
147. Fernandez JL, Vazquez-Gundin F, Delgado A et al. DNA breakage detection–FISH (DBD–FISH) in human spermatozoa: Technical variants evidence different structural features. *Mutat Res* 2000; 453: 77–82.
148. Gorczyca W, Gong J, Darzynkiewicz Z. Detection of DNA strand breaks in individual apoptotic cells by the *in situ* terminal deoxynucleotidyl transferase and nick translation assays. *Cancer Res* 1993; 53: 1945–51.
149. Zini A, Fischer MA, Sharir S et al. Prevalence of abnormal sperm DNA denaturation in fertile and infertile men. *Urology* 2002; 60: 1069–72.
150. Fernandez JL, Muriel L, Rivero MT et al. The sperm chromatin dispersion test: A simple method for the determination of sperm DNA fragmentation. *J Androl* 2003; 24: 59–66.
151. Singh NP, McCoy MT, Tice RR et al. A simple technique for quantitation of low levels of DNA damage in individual cells. *Exp Cell Res* 1988; 175: 184–91.
152. Singh NP, Danner DB, Tice RR et al. Abundant alkali-sensitive sites in DNA of human and mouse sperm. *Exp Cell Res* 1989; 184: 461–70.
153. Sharma R, Agarwal A. Laboratory evaluation of sperm chromatin: TUNEL assay. In: *Sperm Chromatin—Biological and Clinical Applications in Male Infertility and Assisted Reproduction*. New York, NY: Armand Zini and Ashok Agarwal. Springer Science + Business Media, 2011; pp. 201–16.
154. Sharma RK, Sabanegh E, Mahfouz R et al. TUNEL as a test for sperm DNA damage in the evaluation of male infertility. *Urology* 2010; 76: 1380–6.
155. Kodama H, Yamaguchi R, Fukuda J et al. Increased oxidative deoxyribonucleic acid damage in the spermatozoa of infertile male patients. *Fertil Steril* 1997; 68: 519–24.
156. Hammadeh ME, Zeginiadov T, Rosenbaum P et al. Predictive value of sperm chromatin condensation (aniline blue staining) in the assessment of male fertility. *Arch Androl* 2001; 46: 99–104.
157. Wong A, Chuan SS, Patton WC et al. Addition of eosin to the aniline blue assay to enhance detection of immature sperm histones. *Fertil Steril* 2008; 90: 1999–2002.
158. Foresta C, Zorzi M, Rossato M et al. Sperm nuclear instability and staining with aniline blue: Abnormal persistence of histones in spermatozoa in infertile men. *Int J Androl* 1992; 15: 330–7.
159. Kazerooni T, Asadi N, Jadid L et al. Evaluation of sperm's chromatin quality with acridine orange test, chromomycin A_3 and aniline blue staining in couples with unexplained recurrent abortion. *J Assist Reprod Genet* 2009; 26: 591–6.
160. de Jager C, Aneck-Hahn NH, Bornman MS et al. Sperm chromatin integrity in DDT-exposed young men living in a malaria area in the Limpopo Province, South Africa. *Hum Reprod* 2009; 24: 2429–38.
161. Erenpreiss J, Bars J, Lipatnikova V et al. Comparative study of cytochemical tests for sperm chromatin integrity. *J Androl* 2001; 22: 45–53.
162. Erenpreiss J, Jepson K, Giwercman A et al. Toluidine blue cytometry test for sperm DNA conformation: Comparison with the flow cytometric sperm chromatin structure and TUNEL assays. *Hum Reprod* 2004; 19: 2277–82.
163. Tsarev I, Bungum M, Giwercman A et al. Evaluation of male fertility potential by Toluidine Blue test for sperm chromatin structure assessment. *Hum Reprod* 2009; 24: 1569–74.
164. Sadeghi MR, Lakpour N, Heidari-Vala H et al. Relationship between sperm chromatin status and ICSI outcome in men with obstructive azoospermia and unexplained infertile normozoospermia. *Rom J Morphol Embryol* 2011; 52: 645–51.
165. Carretero MI, Giuliano SM, Casaretto CI et al. Evaluation of the effect of cooling and of the addition of collagenase on llama sperm DNA using toluidine blue. *Andrologia* 2011; 44: 239–47.
166. Rybar R, Kopecka V, Prinosilova P et al. Male obesity and age in relationship to semen parameters and sperm chromatin integrity. *Andrologia* 2001; 43: 286–91.
167. Talebi AR, Moein MR, Tabibnejad N et al. Effect of varicocele on chromatin condensation and DNA integrity of ejaculated spermatozoa using cytochemical tests. *Andrologia* 2008; 40: 245–51.
168. Mahfouz RZ, Sharma RK, Said TM et al. Association of sperm apoptosis and DNA ploidy with sperm chromatin quality in human spermatozoa. *Fertil Steril* 2009; 91: 1110–8.
169. Hosseinifar H, Yazdanikhah S, Modarresi T et al. Correlation between sperm DNA fragmentation index and CMA3 positive spermatozoa in globozoospermic patients. *Andrology* 2015; 3: 526–31.
170. Esterhuizen AD, Franken DR, Lourens JG et al. Sperm chromatin packaging as an indicator of *in-vitro* fertilization rates. *Hum Reprod* 2000; 15: 657–61.

171. Sakkas D, Urner F, Bianchi PG et al. Sperm chromatin anomalies can influence decondensation after intracytoplasmic sperm injection. *Hum Reprod* 1996; 11: 837–43.
172. Sakkas D, Urner F, Bizzaro D et al. Sperm nuclear DNA damage and altered chromatin structure: Effect on fertilization and embryo development. *Hum Reprod* 1998; 13: 11–9.
173. Nijs M, Creemers E, Cox A et al. Chromomycin A_3 staining, sperm chromatin structure assay and hyaluronic acid binding assay as predictors for assisted reproductive outcome. *Reprod Biomed Online* 2009; 19: 671–84.
174. Manochantr S, Chiamchanya C, Sobhon P. Relationship between chromatin condensation, DNA integrity and quality of ejaculated spermatozoa from infertile men. *Andrologia* 2012; 44: 187–99.
175. Fernandez JL, Goyanes VJ, Ramiro-Diaz J et al. Application of FISH for *in situ* detection and quantification of DNA breakage. *Cytogenet Cell Genet* 1998; 82: 251–6.
176. Fernández JL, Cajigal D, Gosálvez J. Simultaneous labeling of single- and double-strand DNA breaks by DNA breakage detection–FISH (DBD–FISH). *Methods Mol Biol* 2011; 682: 133–47.
177. Shamsi MB, Kumar R, Dada R. Evaluation of nuclear DNA damage in human spermatozoa in men opting for assisted reproduction. *Indian J Med Res* 2008; 127: 115–23.
178. Setchell BP, Ekpe G, Zupp JL et al. Transient retardation in embryo growth in normal female mice made pregnant by males whose testes had been heated. *Hum Reprod* 1998; 13: 342–7.
179. Aitken RJ, Irvine DS, Wu FC. Prospective analysis of sperm–oocyte fusion and reactive oxygen species generation as criteria for the diagnosis of infertility. *Am J Obstet Gynecol* 1991; 164: 542–51.
180. Mohammed EE, Mosad E, Zahran AM et al. Acridine orange and flow cytometry: Which is better to measure the effect of varicocele on sperm DNA integrity? *Adv Urol* 2015; 2015: 814150.
181. Hoshi K, Katayose H, Yanagida K et al. The relationship between acridine orange fluorescence of sperm nuclei and the fertilizing ability of human sperm. *Fertil Steril* 1996; 66: 634–9.
182. Skowronek F, Casanova G, Alciaturi J et al. DNA sperm damage correlates with nuclear ultrastructural sperm defects in teratozoospermic men. *Andrologia* 2012; 44: 59–65.
183. Varghese AC, Bragais FM, Mukhopadhyay D et al. Human sperm DNA integrity in normal and abnormal semen samples and its correlation with sperm characteristics. *Andrologia* 2009; 41: 207–15.
184. Gopalkrishnan K, Hurkadli K, Padwal V et al. Use of acridine orange to evaluate chromatin integrity of human spermatozoa in different groups of infertile men. *Andrologia* 1999; 31: 277–82.
185. Virant-Klun I, Tomazevic T, Meden-Vrtovec H. Sperm single-stranded DNA, detected by acridine orange staining, reduces fertilization and quality of ICSI-derived embryos. *J Assist Reprod Genet* 2002; 19: 319–28.
186. Katayose H, Yanagida K, Hashimoto S et al. Use of diamide-acridine orange fluorescence staining to detect aberrant protamination of human-ejaculated sperm nuclei. *Fertil Steril* 2003; 79: 670–6.
187. Lazaros LA, Vartholomatos GA, Hatzi EG et al. Assessment of sperm chromatin condensation and ploidy status using flow cytometry correlates to fertilization, embryo quality and pregnancy following *in vitro* fertilization. *J Assist Reprod Genet* 2011; 28: 885–91.
188. Zini A, Kamal K, Phang D et al. Biologic variability of sperm DNA denaturation in infertile men. *Urology* 2001; 58: 258–61.
189. Ankem MK, Mayer E, Ward WS et al. Novel assay for determining DNA organization in human spermatozoa: Implications for male factor infertility. *Urology* 2002; 59: 575–8.
190. Muriel L, Meseguer M, Fernandez JL et al. Value of the sperm chromatin dispersion test in predicting pregnancy outcome in intrauterine insemination: A blind prospective study. *Hum Reprod* 2006; 21: 738–44.
191. Muriel L, Garrido N, Fernandez JL et al. Value of the sperm deoxyribonucleic acid fragmentation level, as measured by the sperm chromatin dispersion test, in the outcome of *in vitro* fertilization and intracytoplasmic sperm injection. *Fertil Steril* 2006; 85: 371–83.
192. Muriel L, Goyanes V, Segrelles E et al. Increased aneuploidy rate in sperm with fragmented DNA as determined by the sperm chromatin dispersion (SCD) test and FISH analysis. *J Androl* 2007; 28: 38–49.
193. Fernandez JL, Muriel L, Goyanes V et al. Halosperm is an easy, available, and cost-effective alternative for determining sperm DNA fragmentation. *Fertil Steril* 2005; 84: 860.
194. Gosálvez J, Rodríguez-Predreira M, Mosquera A et al. Characterisation of a subpopulation of sperm with massive nuclear damage, as recognised with the sperm chromatin dispersion test. *Andrologia* 2014; 46: 602–9.
195. Feijó CM, Esteves SC. Diagnostic accuracy of sperm chromatin dispersion test to evaluate sperm deoxyribonucleic acid damage in men with unexplained infertility. *Fertil Steril* 2014; 101: 58–63.e3.
196. Zhang LH, Qiu Y, Wang KH et al. Measurement of sperm DNA fragmentation using bright-field microscopy: Comparison between sperm chromatin dispersion test and terminal uridine nick-end labeling assay. *Fertil Steril* 2010; 94: 1027–32.
197. Meseguer M, Santiso R, Garrido N et al. Sperm DNA fragmentation levels in testicular sperm samples from azoospermic males as assessed by the sperm chromatin dispersion (SCD) test. *Fertil Steril* 2009; 92: 1638–45.

198. Balasuriya A, Speyer B, Serhal P et al. Sperm chromatin dispersion test in the assessment of DNA fragmentation and aneuploidy in human spermatozoa. *Reprod Biomed Online* 2011; 22: 428–36.
199. Santiso R, Tamayo M, Gosálvez J et al. Simultaneous determination *in situ* of DNA fragmentation and 8-oxoguanine in human sperm. *Fertil Steril* 2010; 93: 314–8.
200. Fernández JL, Cajigal D, López-Fernández C et al. Assessing sperm DNA fragmentation with the sperm chromatin dispersion test. *Methods Mol Biol* 2011; 682: 291–301.
201. Velez de la Calle JF, Muller A, Walschaerts M et al. Sperm deoxyribonucleic acid fragmentation as assessed by the sperm chromatindispersion test in assisted reproductive technology programs: Results of a large prospective multicenter study. *Fertil Steril* 2008; 90: 1792–9.
202. Ostling O, Johanson KJ. Microelectrophoretic study of radiation-induced DNA damages in individual mammalian cells. *Biochem Biophys Res Commun* 1984; 123: 291–8.
203. Ribas-Maynou J, García-Peiró A, Fernández-Encinas A et al. Comprehensive analysis of sperm DNA fragmentation by five different assays: TUNEL assay, SCSA, SCD test and alkaline and neutral comet assay. *Andrology* 2013; 1: 715–22.
204. Simon L, Carrell DT. Sperm DNA damage measured by comet assay. *Methods Mol Biol* 2013; 927: 137–46.
205. Baumgartner A, Cemeli E, Anderson D. The comet assay in male reproductive toxicology. *Cell Biol Toxicol.* 2009; 25: 81–98.
206. Hughes CM, Lewis SE, McKelvey-Martin VJ et al. A comparison of baseline and induced DNA damage in human spermatozoa from fertile and infertile men, using a modified comet assay. *Mol Hum Reprod* 1996; 2(8): 613–9.
207. Enciso M, Sarasa J, Agarwal A et al. A two-tailed comet assay for assessing DNA damage in spermatozoa. *Reprod Biomed Online* 2009; 18: 609–16.
208. Cortés-Gutiérrez EI, Dávila-Rodríguez MI, Fernández JL et al. New application of the comet assay: Chromosome-comet assay. *J Histochem Cytochem* 2011; 59: 655–60.
209. Hellman B, Vaghef H, Bostrom B. The concepts of tail moment and tail inertia in the single cell gel electrophoresis assay. *Mutat Res* 1995; 336: 123–31.
210. Kusakabe H, Tateno H. Shortening of alkaline DNA unwinding time does not interfere with detecting DNA damage to mouse and human spermatozoa in the comet assay. *Asian J Androl* 2011; 13: 172–4.
211. Duty SM, Singh NP, Ryan L et al. Reliability of the comet assay in cryopreserved human sperm. *Hum Reprod* 2002; 17: 1274–80.
212. Morris ID, Ilott S, Dixon L et al. The spectrum of DNA damage in human sperm assessed by single cell gel electrophoresis (comet assay) and its relationship to fertilization and embryo development. *Hum Reprod* 2002; 17: 990–8.
213. Tomsu M, Sharma V, Miller D. Embryo quality and IVF treatment outcomes may correlate with different sperm comet assay parameters. *Hum Reprod* 2002; 17: 1856–62.
214. Lewis SE, Agbaje IM. Using the alkaline comet assay in prognostic tests for male infertility and assisted reproductive technology outcomes. *Mutagenesis* 2008; 23: 163–70.
215. Shamsi MB, Venkatesh S, Tanwar M et al. Comet assay: A prognostic tool for DNA integrity assessment in infertile men opting for assisted reproduction. *Indian J Med Res* 2010; 131: 675–81.
216. Simon L, Lutton D, McManus J et al. Sperm DNA damage measured by the alkaline comet assay as an independent predictor of male infertility and *in vitro* fertilization success. *Fertil Steril* 2011; 95: 652–7.
217. Lewis SE, Simon L. Clinical implications of sperm DNA damage. *Hum Fertil (Camb)* 2010; 13: 201–7.
218. Abu-Hassan D, Koester F, Shoepper B et al. Comet assay of cumulus cells and spermatozoa DNA status, and the relationship to oocyte fertilization and embryo quality following ICSI. *Reprod Biomed Online* 2006; 12: 447–52.
219. Villani P, Spanò M, Pacchierotti F et al. Evaluation of a modified comet assay to detect DNA damage in mammalian sperm exposed *in vitro* to different mutagenic compounds. *Reprod Toxicol* 2010; 30: 44–9.
220. Benchaib M, Braun V, Lornage J et al. Sperm DNA fragmentation decreases the pregnancy rate in an assisted reproductive technique. *Hum Reprod* 2003; 18: 1023–8.
221. Enciso M, Johnston SD, Gosálvez J. Differential resistance of mammalian sperm chromatin to oxidative stress as assessed by a two-tailed comet assay. These cells from the genotoxic effects of adverse environments. *Reprod Fertil Dev* 2011; 23: 633–7.
222. Mitchell LA, De Iuliis GN, Aitken RJ. The TUNEL assay consistently underestimates DNA damage in human spermatozoa and is influenced by DNA compaction and cell vitality: Development of an improved methodology. *Int J Androl* 2011; 34: 2–13.
223. Cui ZL, Zheng DZ, Liu YH et al. Diagnostic accuracies of the TUNEL, SCD, and comet based sperm DNA fragmentation assays for male infertility: A meta-analysis study. *Clin Lab* 2015; 61: 525–35.
224. Muratori M, Tamburrino L, Tocci V et al. Small variations in crucial steps of TUNEL assay coupled to flow cytometry greatly affect measures of sperm DNA fragmentation. *J Androl* 2010; 31: 336–45.
225. Muratori M, Tamburrino L, Marchiani S et al. Critical aspects of detection of sperm DNA fragmentation by TUNEL/flow cytometry. *Syst Biol Reprod Med* 2010; 56: 277–85.
226. Spano M, Kolstad AH, Larsen SB et al. The applicability of the flow cytometric sperm chromatin structure assay in epidemiological studies. *Hum Reprod* 1998; 13: 2495–505.

227. Nijs M, De Jonge C, Cox A et al. Correlation between male age, WHO sperm parameters, DNA fragmentation, chromatin packaging and outcome in assisted reproduction technology. *Andrologia* 2011; 43: 174–9.
228. Evenson DP, Kasperson K, Wixon RL. Analysis of sperm DNA fragmentation using flow cytometry and other techniques. *Soc Reprod Fertil* 2007; 65: 93–113.
229. Evenson DP, Larson KL, Jost LK. Sperm chromatin structure assay: Its clinical use for detecting sperm DNA fragmentation in male infertility and comparisons with other techniques. *J Androl* 2002; 23: 25–43.
230. Bungum M, Bungum L, Giwercman A. Sperm chromatin structure assay (SCSA): A tool in diagnosis and treatment of infertility. *Asian J Androl* 2011; 13: 69–75.
231. Castilla JA, Zamora S, Gonzalvo MC et al. Sperm chromatin structure assay and classical semen parameters: Systematic review. *Reprod Biomed Online* 2010; 20: 114–24.
232. Giwercman A, Lindstedt L, Larsson M et al. Sperm chromatin structure assay as an independent predictor of fertility *in vivo*: A case–control study. *Int J Androl* 2010; 33: e221–7.
233. Bungum M, Spanò M, Humaidan P et al. Sperm chromatin structure assay parameters measured after density gradient centrifugation are not predictive for the outcome of ART. *Hum Reprod* 2008; 23: 4–10.
234. Miciński P, Pawlicki K, Wielgus E et al. The sperm chromatin structure assay (SCSA) as prognostic factor in IVF/ICSI program. *Reprod Biol* 2009; 9: 65–70.
235. Collins JA, Barnhart KT, Schlegel PN. Do sperm DNA integrity tests predict pregnancy with *in vitro* fertilization? *Fertil Steril* 2008; 89: 823–31.
236. Lewis SE, Agbaje I, Alvarez J. Sperm DNA tests as useful adjuncts to semen analysis. *Syst Biol Reprod Med* 2008; 54: 111–25.
237. Evenson DP. Sperm chromatin structure assay (SCSA®). *Methods Mol Biol* 2013; 927: 147–64.
238. Henkel R, Hoogendijk CF, Bouic PJ et al. TUNEL assay and SCSA determine different aspects of sperm DNA damage. *Andrologia* 2010; 42: 305–13.
239. Shen H, Ong C. Detection of oxidative DNA damage in human sperm and its association with sperm function and male infertility. *Free Radic Biol Med* 2000; 28: 529–36.
240. Aitken RJ, De Iuliis GN, Finnie JM et al. Analysis of the relationships between oxidative stress, DNA damage and sperm vitality in a patient population: Development of diagnostic criteria. *Hum Reprod* 2010; 25: 2415–26.
241. Ishikawa T, Fujioka H, Ishimura T et al. Increased testicular 8-hydroxy-2'-deoxyguanosine in patients with varicocele. *BJU Int* 2007; 100: 863–6.
242. Loft S, Kold-Jensen T, Hjollund NH et al. Oxidative DNA damage in human sperm influences time to pregnancy. *Hum Reprod* 2003; 18: 1265–72.
243. Agarwal A, Varghese AC, Sharma RK. Markers of oxidative stress and sperm chromatin integrity. *Methods Mol Biol* 2009; 590: 377–402.
244. Ainsworth C, Nixon B, Aitken RJ. Development of a novel electrophoretic system for the isolation of human spermatozoa. *Hum Reprod* 2005; 20: 2261–70.
245. Zini A, San Gabriel M, Baazeem A. Antioxidants and sperm DNA damage: A clinical perspective. *J Assist Reprod Genet* 2009; 26: 427–32.
246. Ménézo YJ, Hazout A, Panteix G et al. Antioxidants to reduce sperm DNA fragmentation: An unexpected adverse effect. *Reprod Biomed Online* 2007; 14: 418–21.
247. Agarwal A, Nallella KP, Allamaneni SS et al. Role of antioxidants in treatment of male infertility: An overview of the literature. *Reprod Biomed Online* 2004; 8: 616–27.
248. Greco E, Romano S, Iacobelli M et al. ICSI in cases of sperm DNA damage: Beneficial effect of oral antioxidant treatment. *Hum Reprod* 2005; 20: 2590–4.
249. Rolf C, Cooper TG, Yeung CH et al. Antioxidant treatment of patients with asthenozoospermia or moderate oligoasthenozoospermia with high-dose vitamin C and vitamin E: A randomized, placebo-controlled, double-blind study. *Hum Reprod* 1999; 14: 1028–33.
250. Said T, Agarwal A, Grunewald S et al. Selection of nonapoptotic spermatozoa as a new tool for enhancing assisted reproduction outcomes: An *in vitro* model. *Biol Reprod* 2006; 74: 530–37.
251. Berkovitz A, Eltes F, Lederman H et al. How to improve IVF–ICSI outcome by sperm selection. *Reprod Biomed Online* 2006; 12: 634–8.
252. Hazout A, Dumont-Hassan M, Junca AM et al. High-magnification ICSI overcomes paternal effect resistant to conventional ICSI. *Reprod Biomed Online* 2006; 12: 19–25.
253. Lin MH, Kuo-Kuang Lee R et al. Sperm chromatin structure assay parameters are not related to fertilization rates, embryo quality, and pregnancy rates in *in vitro* fertilization and intracytoplasmic sperm injection, but might be related to spontaneous abortion rates. *Fertil Steril* 2008; 90: 352–9.
254. McPherson SM, Longo FJ. Nicking of rat spermatid and spermatozoa DNA: Possible involvement of DNA topoisomerase II. *Dev Biol* 1993; 158: 122–30.

Oocyte retrieval and selection

7

LAURA F. RIENZI and FILIPPO M. UBALDI

INTRODUCTION

Several factors can affect oocyte quality and a controlled ovarian stimulation (COS) protocol is one of the most important. To better understand the treatment strategies, their application, and their potential impact on oocyte quality, it is of utmost importance to understand the physiology of ovarian function.

The demise of the corpus luteum at the end of the luteal phase of the menstrual cycle is responsible for the sudden fall of 17β-estradiol (E2), inhibin A, and progesterone, which induces an increased frequency of pulsatile gonadotropin-releasing hormone (GnRH) secretion and rising serum follicle-stimulating hormone (FSH) levels (1). When serum FSH concentration reaches a critical "threshold" level for ovarian stimulation, class 5 follicles departing from the resting pool are recruited and start a well-characterized growth trajectory (2,3). In the early follicular phase, the increased production of estrogens resulting from FSH-dependent granulosa cell (GC) aromatase activity, together with the increase of inhibin B, is responsible for the falling circulating levels of FSH (4,5), which restricts the time when FSH levels remain above the "threshold" (6,7). As a result, one (dominant) follicle continues its growth, probably due to up-regulation by intraovarian factors that may increase sensitivity for FSH stimulation (8,9), whereas other (non-dominant) follicles (of the same cohort) enter atresia due to diminished sensitivity to FSH and estrogen biosynthesis (as well as elevated intrafollicular androgen levels) (9–11).

On the basis of these findings, the "FSH window" concept has been introduced, suggesting the importance of the duration of FSH elevation above the threshold level rather than the height of the elevation of FSH for single dominant follicle selection (6,7,12). The different stimulation protocols used for controlled ovarian hyperstimulation are based on the concept of widening the FSH window with the use of exogenous gonadotropins from the early follicular phase to the day of human chorionic gonadotropin (hCG) administration. Over the last 25 years different stimulation protocols have been proposed. Easier stimulation regimens such as clomiphene citrate (CC) alone or in combination with human menopausal gonadotropin (hMG) and urinary FSH were gradually abandoned in favor of protocols where GnRH agonists (GnRHas) are used in combination with gonadotropins. These lengthy protocols, which have been for decades the most widely used treatments for ovarian stimulation, allowed us to manage the activity of *in vitro* fertilization (IVF) centers more easily, enabled lower cancellation rates, and raised the number of preovulatory follicles, the number of oocytes retrieved, and the number of good-quality embryos for transfer, thus leading to increased pregnancy rates (13). However, these regimens are not free from complications and costs for the patients. The clinical introduction of GnRH antagonists in IVF (14–16), with their immediate suppression of pituitary function, allows the administration of low doses of gonadotropins from the mid-follicular phase, resulting in more "patient-friendly" stimulation protocols (17,18) with fewer days of stimulation, lower amounts of gonadotropins administered, and fewer oocytes retrieved. However, if these milder protocols may improve patients compliance, reducing the burden of IVF on the couple, the question that remains to be answered is whether the reduced number of oocytes obtained after mild protocols may impair the clinical outcome when calculated cumulatively (including cryopreservation cycles).

Whatever stimulation regimen is used for COS, once the correct follicular and hormonal parameters are reached, ovulation is triggered, normally through the administration of a bolus of hCG. However, it is important to underline that, in order to avoid ovarian hyperstimulation syndrome (OHSS), nowadays it is possible to combine a GnRH antagonist protocol with GnRHa ovulation triggering, taking advantage from the different half-life between luteinizing hormone (60 minutes) and hCG (>24 hours). This approach has made it possible to significantly reduce the risk of OHSS (19). However, the induction of early luteolysis after the GnRHa trigger requires the use of aggressive steroidal luteal support or low-dose hCG to allow successful fresh embryo transfer (20). On the other hand, the enhanced effectiveness of vitrification allows the introduction of cycle segmentation in the GnRHa-triggered approach, resulting in freezing all the obtained embryos for a subsequent cryo-transfer (21–23).

After ovulation triggering, oocyte meiosis (blocked at the prophase of the first meiotic division) is reinitiated, going through germinal vesicle (GV) breakdown and the formation and extrusion of the first polar body (IPB). After entering the second meiotic division, a second arrest occurs at metaphase stage II (MII). Oocyte retrieval is performed 34–36 hours following hCG administration.

Once in the laboratory, oocyte quality is assessed. This evaluation is based on the aspect of the cumulus–corona cells and, if denudation is performed, also on the basis of the morphology of the oocyte cytoplasm and on the aspect of the extracytoplasmic structures (such as zona pellucida [ZP], IPB, and perivitelline space [PVS]). Oocyte selection prior to insemination has been considered a key point of IVF/intracytoplasmic sperm injection (ICSI) programs because of the following:

- It may provide important information with regard to the subsequent developmental ability of the deriving embryo.
- It helps to reduce the number of inseminated oocytes and thus the amount of supernumerary embryos.
- It helps to avoid inseminating "bad-quality oocytes" potentially at risk of carrying chromosomal abnormalities.
- It helps with choosing the appropriate number of oocytes in egg donation programs.

However, the current literature on oocyte assessment is controversial and the selection methods proposed are still largely ineffective. The presence of cumulus and corona cells makes the morphological oocyte evaluation difficult to perform prior to standard IVF. Moreover, the quality and the degree of expansion of these cells seem to be poor markers of oocyte maturity and mostly depend on the type of ovarian stimulation protocol used (24–27). The oocyte can be easily observed only after cumulus–corona cell removal. The presence of the IPB is normally considered to be a marker of oocyte nuclear maturity. However, recent studies using polarized light microscopy have shown that oocytes displaying the IPB may still be immature (28–30). Moreover, nuclear maturity alone is not enough to determine the quality of an oocyte. In fact, nuclear and cytoplasmic maturation should be completed in a coordinated manner to ensure optimal conditions for subsequent fertilization. However, cytoplasmic maturation assessment is still unclear. It has been suggested that disturbances or asynchrony of these two maturation processes may result in a variety of oocyte morphological abnormalities (31–34). Abnormal ZP, large PVS, vacuoles, refractile bodies, increased cytoplasmic granularity, smooth endoplasmic reticulum (sER) clusters, and abnormal, fragmented, or degenerated IPB can be observed after oocyte denudation. The correlation between these abnormal morphotypes and oocyte developmental ability is discussed in this chapter.

OVARIAN STIMULATION PROTOCOLS

Prediction of ovarian response

One of the greatest challenges in human assisted reproduction is to individualize COS according to the specific characteristics of each single patient, in order to optimize the number of oocytes to be obtained and to protect women from iatrogenic damage. Nowadays, different stimulants of multifollicular growth have been suggested, including recombinant or urinary gonadotropins, GnRH analogs (agonists or antagonists), steroid hormones, and other drugs such as aromatase inhibitors or growth hormones. The choice of the most suitable COS regimen is based on the prediction of ovarian response in order to tailor an individualized COS to obtain an ideal number of oocytes, which is suggested to maximize live birth rate per fresh embryo transfer (35). A number of predictors of ovarian reserve have been identified including patient age, biochemical parameters (FSH and anti-Mullerian hormone [AMH]), morphological parameters (antral follicular count [AFC]), and some clinical conditions such as polycystic ovary syndrome and low body mass index (36).

It is well known that the number of germ cells in ovaries declines sharply by as early as around the fifth month of fetal life, and the process continues after birth. The process accelerates again after 30 years of age, reaches critical level after 40, and conception with own eggs is exceptional after 45, both by natural and assisted reproductive techniques. Although ovarian reserve declines with age (37), it does not represent an optimal predictor of ovarian response (38).

Basal serum FSH has been considered for many years the most important and reliable marker to predict ovarian response to stimulation in IVF/ICSI cycles. Basal serum FSH concentration begins to rise on average a decade or more before the menopause. Although the basal FSH level is widely used as a predictor of ovarian response, its accuracy is low, and it is only suggested for counselling purposes (39). The correlation between different groups of patients and basal FSH values is in fact statistically poor and does not allow exact classification. More recently it has been demonstrated that basal serum FSH is a good predictor of ovarian response only at very high threshold levels (>FSH 12 mIU/mL), symptomatic of a very compromised ovarian reserve (39).

AMH is produced by preantral follicles and small antral follicles of up to 7–8 mm in size. It inhibits FSH-mediated GC proliferation, follicular growth, and aromatase activity (40). AMH provides a quantitative evaluation of the amount of follicles available in the ovary (41,42). AMH level has a very low inter- and intra-cycle variability, remaining stable during menstrual cycles (43). AMH level has been demonstrated to predict a number of IVF outcomes. It correlates with oocyte yield (44–46), and the time interval between serum AMH and the beginning of the ovarian stimulation of up to 12 months does not seem to modify the capacity of the marker to identify patients with low or high ovarian response (47). AMH can be performed at any point during a menstrual cycle and has low intra- and inter-cycle variability and good inter-operator and inter-center consistency (43). However, improper storage and handling of blood samples, delayed centrifugation, or storage at room temperature may have a great influence on the result of the assay (48). For these reasons different authors have suggested caution in the interpretation of AMH levels if not performed in a standardized way (49,50). AMH level may also predict embryo quality (51) and several authors suggest that this marker could be used to predict pregnancy outcomes (52–55). However, to date, the association between AMH level and pregnancy rates or live births could not be confirmed by several studies (56–59), including two separate meta-analyses (60,61). The antral follicle count has also been suggested as a predictor of several important IVF outcomes. A linear relationship between AFC and the number of retrieved oocytes has been clearly shown (46,62–64). Moreover, this marker can predict cycle cancellations as a result of poor ovarian response (65,66). AFC is easy to perform, fairly noninvasive, and provides immediate results. On the other hand, it has inter-observer variation due to the subjective determination of follicular number and differences in technology used and training performed. Recently, data have emerged to support the combination of AFC and AMH level as the preferred method for predicting ovarian reserve with a varied degree of precision (41,49,67,68). Receiver operating characteristic curve studies within single centers and meta-analyses have shown that both AFC and AMH levels can identify patients likely to respond to exogenous gonadotrophins with poor, normal, or hyper-response (41,47,67,68).

Individualized stimulating regimens

The main objective of an ideal stimulation protocol is to offer every single woman the best treatment tailored to her own unique characteristics in order to fully exploit the ovarian reserve. The number of oocyte retrieved, in fact, is a key factor for maximizing cumulative birth rates. Several papers have suggested about 15 oocytes retrieved as an ideal number for maximizing the live birth rate in fresh embryo transfer cycles (35). However, when we consider the cumulative live birth rate (fresh + cryo embryo transfers), both clinical pregnancy and live birth rates continue to increase as the number of collected oocytes increases (69,70). Notwithstanding, some authors suggested that excessive ovarian stimulation has a detrimental effect on oocyte quality (71–73), resulting in embryos with a higher rate of aneuploidy (73,74). This finding is not confirmed by our experience where, performing comprehensive chromosomal screening (preimplantation genetic screening) at the blastocyst stage, we observed a clear positive relationship between number of retrieved oocytes, number of blastocysts, and euploid blastocysts available per patient (75). Moreover, the euploidy rate was not related to the number of oocytes retrieved as also reported by Ata and colleagues (76).

Although the first successful pregnancy after IVF and embryo transfer was performed in the natural unstimulated cycle of an infertile woman with a tubal factor (77), it was soon observed that pregnancy rates per IVF attempt increase when more than one embryo is available for transfer (78). Over the last 30 years, different stimulation protocols have been proposed.

At the beginning of the 1990s, short-term treatments with GnRHas combined with gonadotropins were abandoned in favor of long-term GnRHa stimulation protocols that allowed the retrieval of more oocytes (79,80). About 15 years ago, GnRH antagonists were introduced in IVF (14–16). These GnRH analogs induce an immediate suppression of the pituitary function, which allows the administration of gonadotropins without pituitary suppression, resulting in shorter and more "patient-friendly" stimulation protocols (17,18). This approach also allows us to obtain similar ongoing pregnancy and live birth rates compared with the standard long-term GnRHa protocols (81,82), but provides important advantages. In particular, it is possible to trigger ovulation with GnRHa while avoiding the onset of the OHSS in almost all cycles at risk of the syndrome (20,21). These benefits have justified a radical change worldwide from the standard long-term agonist protocol in favor of antagonist regimens.

Over the past few years, particular attention has been also paid to the development of simplified ovarian stimulation regimens in order to identify novel, more convenient approaches as valid alternatives to existing protocols. In this context, the quite recent introduction of a long-acting FSH, corifollitropin alfa, is notable. This new therapeutic option, consisting of a chimeric recombinant molecule composed of FSH and the carboxy-terminal peptide of hCG, functions as a long-acting FSH agonist. Corifollitropin alfa has a longer half-life compared to recombinant FSH (rFSH) and therefore a single injected dose is sufficient to effectively induce and sustain multifollicular growth (83–86). The effectiveness and safety of the treatment have been shown by the absence of any registered difference in clinical pregnancy rate, ongoing pregnancy rate, multiple pregnancy rate, miscarriage rate, ectopic pregnancy rate, and congenital malformation rate (major or minor) (86).

PERIFOLLICULAR VASCULARIZATION EVALUATION

Besides stimulation protocols and gonadotropin preparations, oocyte quality might be influenced by perifollicular vascularization. It has been suggested that insufficient perifollicular vascularization measured using color Doppler ultrasonography correlates with intrafollicular hypoxia (87–89), inducing oocyte cytoplasmic defects, disorganized chromosomes, reduced fertilization, and embryos with multinucleated blastomeres (88,90,91). Embryos with high implantation potential originate from well-vascularized and oxygenated follicles (90). According to these data, several studies have also shown higher pregnancy and implantation rates when embryos resulting from the fertilization of oocytes from better-perfused follicles are transferred (92–96). Unfortunately, other studies were not able to confirm the clinical value of the association between perifollicular vascularization and oocyte competence to improve the reproductive outcomes in young infertile patients who undergo either intrauterine insemination cycles (97) or IVF cycles (98–101). Moreover, it is not technically easy to assess perifollicular vascularity during the oocyte retrieval procedure and to perform the aspiration and flushing of the selected follicle until the oocytes are retrieved. For these reasons, further prospective randomized studies are needed to verify whether a relationship exists between the perifollicular vascularization of selected follicles measured using color Doppler ultrasonography and their reproductive competence.

OOCYTE–CORONA–CUMULUS COMPLEX EVALUATION

Cumulus cells are Graafian follicular cells that surround and nourish the oocyte during its development in the ovary. The innermost layer of cumulus cells, immediately adjacent to the ZP, is called corona radiata. Cells of the corona radiata extend their cytoplasm toward the oocyte through the ZP. Communication (either paracrine interaction or gap junction) occurs between the oocyte and the cumulus–corona cells. Such interactions allow oocyte nutrition and maturation during its preovulatory growth from the diplotene to the MII stage (102,103). Corona radiata and cumulus cells maintain their contact with the oocyte at the time of ovulation, during a normal menstrual cycle, or after withdrawal by aspiration, in hormonally stimulated assisted reproduction cycles.

In mature oocytes, the cumulus–corona mass appears as an expanded and mucified layer, due to the active secretion of hyaluronic acid. This extracellular component interposes among the cells and separates them, conferring on the cumulus–corona mass a fluffy appearance. During unstimulated cycles, the stage of oocyte nuclear maturation is coupled with an increased expansion and mucification of the cumulus layer (24). However, stimulated cycles may be characterized by an asynchrony of these two processes (25). This can be due to a different sensitivity of the oocyte and the cumulus–corona mass to the stimulants (25,104).

Studies from Rattanachaiyanont et al. (27), performed on oocytes scheduled for denudation and insemination by ICSI, reported no correlation between oocyte–corona–cumulus complex (OCCC) morphology and nuclear maturity, fertilization rate, and embryo cleavage. Ebner et al. (105) performed similar grading and drew a similar conclusion; however, they found that the presence of blood clots (but not that of amorphous clumps) was associated with dense central granulation of oocytes and had a negative effect on fertilization and blastocyst rates. Both studies have found a correlation between a very dense corona radiata layer and decreased maturity of oocytes. On the other hand, other authors reported that OCCC scoring was related to fertilization and pregnancy rates (106), as well as to blastocyst quality and development (107).

Lin and colleagues proposed a grading system of OCCCs based on the morphology of the oocyte cytoplasm, cumulus mass, corona cells, and membrana GCs for oocytes prior to insemination by conventional IVF (107). Five grades (mature group, approximately mature, immature, post-mature, and atretic) were described, as shown in Table 7.1 (107). The authors reported higher fertilization rates for the oocytes belonging to the mature group compared with those belonging to the other groups. Moreover, the immature group was characterized by a higher incidence of poor-morphology day 3 embryos as compared with the mature group.

In support of a positive effect of cumulus–corona cells on oocyte development, it was shown that the partial removal of this layer prior to ICSI improved embryo quality and development (108). It has been suggested that the presence of cumulus–corona cells may help embryonic metabolism, by either stimulating gene expression (109) or reducing oxidative stress (110). However, to date there is little evidence to clearly support the role of OCCC morphological analysis in the prediction of oocyte maturity and competence (111). Nevertheless, recently the Alpha Scientists in Reproductive Medicine and the European Society of

Table 7.1 Oocyte–corona–cumulus complex evaluation scheme

Groups	OCCC morphology
Mature	Expanded cumulus Radiant corona Distinct zona pellucida, clear ooplasm Expanded well-aggregated membrane granulosa cells
Approximately mature	Expanded cumulus mass Slightly compact corona radiata Expanded, well-aggregated membrana granulosa cells
Immature	Dense compact cumulus if present Adherent compact layer of corona cells Ooplasm if visible with the presence of germinal vesicle Compact and nonaggregated membrana granulosa cells
Postmature	Expanded cumulus with clumps Radiant corona radiata, yet often clumped, irregular, or incomplete Visible zona, slightly granular or dark ooplasm Small and relatively nonaggregated membrana granulosa cells
Atretic	Rarely with associated cumulus mass Clumped and very irregular corona radiata if present Visible zona, dark and frequently misshapen ooplasm Membrana granulosa cells with very small clumps of cells

Source: Adapted from Lin YC, Chang SY, Lan KC et al. *J Assist Reprod Genet* 2003; 20: 506–12.

Human Reproduction and Embryology (ESHRE) Special Group of Embryology stated that it is reasonable to use a more simple binary score in order to recognize compacted cumulus cells (score 0) or expanded cumulus cells and radiating corona (score 1) (111). In fact, as suggested by Canipari et al. (112), it is reasonable to assume that there is a higher probability of obtaining a better-quality mature oocyte in a normally expanded cumulus than in a non-expanded one.

Although cumulus–corona mass observation is not sufficient to evaluate oocyte maturity and competence, it is reasonable to hypothesize that ooplasm development is influenced by the action of these cells. In accordance with this hypothesis, it has been suggested that cumulus–corona cells play an important role in the *in vitro* maturation of oocytes that were immature at the time of retrieval (113,114).

Recently, more interesting approaches have been developed in order to better understand oocyte quality on the basis of cumulus cells and GCs RNA/protein content and metabolite production (the so-called "omics technology";

that is: genomic, transcriptomic, proteomic, and metabolomic). In fact, given that folliculogenesis and oogenesis, as already mentioned, rely on the bidirectional communication between the oocyte and the surrounding cells, it is conceivable that the study of GCs and cumulus cells function may provide valuable additional information about oocyte competence (115,116). Moreover, since GCs and cumulus cells are usually discarded in ICSI treatments, these new molecular alternatives to standard morphological assessment offer a completely noninvasive tool in the egg selection process.

Transcriptomics (the assessment of the cell total RNA content) (117) enables both quantitative and qualitative analysis of differentially expressed genes under physiologic or pathologic conditions. In the "candidate gene approach," it is possible to study the differential expression of individual already-defined genes, whereas microarrays are used to obtain whole-genome transcriptomic profiling with the creation of a similarly exhaustive list of genes differentially expressed in GCs and cumulus cells surrounding healthy oocytes versus non-viable ones (116). To date, many genes involved in different cellular pathways and processes have been investigated. Unfortunately, the obtained data are still not uniform and conclusive, and there is limited consensus on the identified markers (116). In fact, a lot of information has been generated that we are not yet able to correctly understand, mainly because of the extreme difficulty in the determination of a true threshold value for physiologic inter- and intra-samples variance. Moreover, the studies published so far differ considerably in terms of size of study population, technology employed, treatment protocol, maternal age, culture conditions, transfer policy, and referred outcomes, so that the conclusions appear to be strongly biased (115,116).

Beyond transcriptomics, proteomics (the study of the cell total protein content) (117) is gathering increasing consideration, since it is believed that protein content is more directly linked to a given phenotype (117). Unfortunately, very few articles have been published on the subject and even partial pattern profiling is still lacking (116).

Finally, metabolomics (the study of the complete content of small non-proteinaceous molecules in a given biological fluid, resulting from the action of different proteins and gene expression pathways) (118,119) may provide additional useful information about the immediate functional status of a certain biological system (i.e., OCCC function) (118,119), but this approach is currently under investigation and more studies are needed (116).

OOCYTE NUCLEAR MATURITY EVALUATION

Direct observation of oocyte morphology, including the extracytoplasmic components, is possible only after the denudation of its cumulus and corona layers. The use of hyaluronidase enzyme and mechanical pipetting facilitates the breaking down of the cumulus–corona extracellular matrix. This method is normally used when insemination by ICSI is going to be performed. A meiotically mature oocyte is blocked at the MII stage. Completion of meiotic maturation occurs only after sperm entry and consequent oocyte activation. Currently, oocyte nuclear maturity is determined by the presence of an extruded IPB in the PVS and by the absence of a GV. Nonsynchronous oocyte maturation is often observed after ovarian hyperstimulation. Approximately 85% of the denuded oocytes display the IPB and are classified as MII. In about 10% a GV is present in the oocyte cytoplasm; approximately 5% of the oocytes are in the metaphase of the first meiotic division (MI) with no visible GV and IPB (120). Immature oocytes (GV and MI) can potentially be matured *in vitro* (121–123). However, a high incidence of genetic abnormalities has been observed in the embryos derived from *in vitro*-matured oocytes (124). Similarly, the implantation and pregnancy rates of embryos obtained with *in vitro*-matured oocytes are significantly lower than those observed with *in vivo*-matured counterparts (125). Although a comparable obstetric and neonatal outcome is reported between children conceived with *in vitro*-matured oocytes and those born after traditional IVF (126–128), the low number of children conceived after in vitro maturation (IVM) does not allow for an accurate evaluation of malformation rates. Therefore, immature oocytes obtained by ovarian hyperstimulation should not be selected for insemination.

At the MII stage, the oocyte chromosomes are aligned at the equatorial region of the meiotic spindle (MS). This structure plays a crucial role in the sequence of events leading to the correct completion of meiosis and fertilization and thus is a key determinant of oocyte developmental potential. However, the MS microtubules, which are responsible for proper chromosomal segregation, are highly sensitive to the chemical and physical changes that may occur during oocyte retrieval and handling. It has been shown that oocyte exposure to slight temperature fluctuations dramatically affects microtubular structure, with deleterious consequences on chromosomal organization (129–133). Other parameters, such as increased maternal age (134,135) and oocyte *in vitro* aging (136), are also associated with the disruption of MS architecture. The most potentially dramatic consequences of MS alteration are the unbalanced disjunction and/or non-disjunction of chromatids, chromosome scattering, and the formation of aneuploid embryos (134,137,138). The introduction of an orientation-independent polarized light microscopy system (Spindle View PolScope system, CRI, Woburn, MA), coupled with an image processing software, allowed the visualization of MS in living oocytes (139–141). Parallel-aligned MS microtubules are birefringent and able to shift the plane of polarized light, inducing retardance. These properties enable the system to generate contrast and to image the MS structure. Moreover, digital processing enhances signal sensitivity. Unlike conventional methods of MS imaging, the Spindle View system does not require oocyte fixation and staining. In this way the MS can be visualized in a noninvasive fashion, preserving oocyte viability. Using the Spindle View system, additional information about human oocyte maturity and developmental potentiality has been produced. Several studies (142–149) indicate the importance of the presence of a detectable MS in the oocyte cytoplasm prior to ICSI. A clear positive correlation between MS visualization, fertilization rate, and/or embryo development and/or blastocyst progression was described in these studies (Table 7.2). The absence of a detectable MS and the consequent oocyte developmental impairment may be primarily ascribed to oocyte immaturity (138). It has been hypothesized that the lack of MS formation could be the result of aberrant signaling pathways or low energy supply during oocyte growth, resulting in both nuclear and cytoplasmic immaturity (12,138). Moreover, some oocytes were found to be clearly immature at the stage of telophase I (Figure 7.1) when observed with the Spindle View system (28–30). At this stage there is continuity between the ooplasm and the cytoplasm of the forming IPB, and the MS is interposed between the two separating cells. These oocytes would have been classified as "mature" MII with light microscopy, based on the presence of an IPB (Figure 7.1a). Therefore, the use of the Spindle View system allows an accurate determination of oocyte nuclear maturity and selection of fully mature eggs. However, it must be underlined that unfavorable culture conditions may also induce MS disassembly (11,142,143). In this case the lack of MS should be ascribed to environmental stress and not to oocyte incompetence to reach maturity. The percentage of oocytes displaying a detectable MS varies between 60% and 90% in different studies (Table 7.2) (142,144,145,147). This difference seems to be related to some important laboratory and clinical parameters: (i) the thermal control during oocytes handling (133,150); (ii) the technique of MS visualization (145,147,148); and (iii) the time elapsed from hCG administration (147). Because of the high sensitivity of the MS to temperature variations, thermal stability is

Table 7.2 Relationship between the presence of a detectable meiotic spindle in fresh metaphase stage II oocytes and the intracytoplasmic sperm injection outcome

	Meiotic spindle presence							
	Yes				No			
	Wang et al. (142)	Moon et al. (144)	Rienzi et al. (145)	Cohen et al. (147)	Wang et al. (142)	Moon et al. (144)	Rienzi et al. (145)	Cohen et al. (147)
Injected oocytes (%)	1266 (82.0)	523 (83.5)	484 (91.0)	585 (76.0)	278 (18.0)	103 (16.5)	48 (9.0)	185 (24.0)
Fertilized oocytes (%)	879 (69.4)[a]	430 (82.2)	362 (74.8)[b]	412 (70.4)[c]	175 (62.9)[d]	79 (75.7)	16 (33.3)[e]	115 (62.2)[f]
Good-quality embryos (%)	583 (46.0)[g]	276 (52.8)[h]	268 (55.4)[i]	169 (47.2)	97 (34.9)[j]	28 (27.2)[k]	9 (18.7)[l]	32 (35.6)

[a,d]$p < 0.05$; [b,e]$p < 0.01$; [c,f]$p < 0.035$; [g,j]$p < 0.01$; [h,k]$p < 0.01$; [i,l]$p < 0.01$.

Source: Adapted from Wang WH, Meng L, Hackett RJ et al. *Hum Reprod* 2001; 16: 1464–8; Moon JH, Hyun CS, Lee SW et al. *Hum Reprod* 2003; 18: 817–20; Rienzi L, Ubaldi F, Martinez F et al. *Hum Reprod* 2003; 18: 1289–93; Cohen Y, Malcov M, Schwartz T et al. *Hum Reprod* 2004; 19: 649–54.

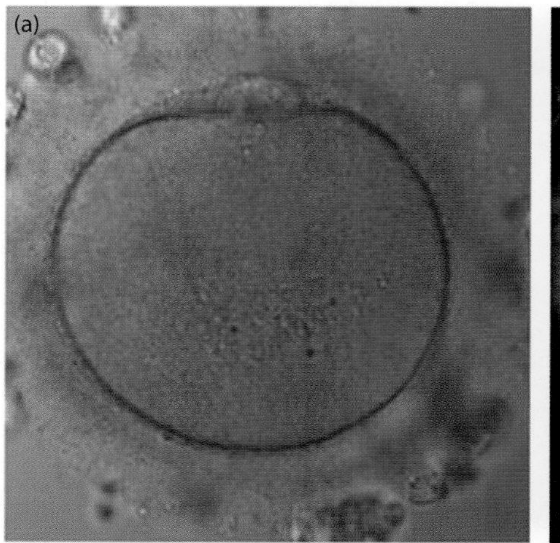

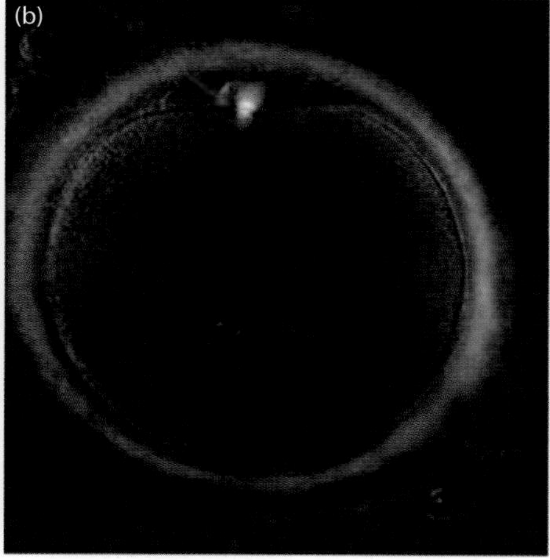

Figure 7.1 (a) Telophase I oocyte observed with light microscopy (Hoffman contrast) and (b) with polarized light microscopy (Spindle View system). Only with this latter system is it possible to observe the immature meiotic spindle (arrow) and to assess the maturation stage of this oocyte. (Magnification 400×.)

necessary during oocyte observation and manipulation. In addition, oocyte rotation, by means of a micropipette, allows correct orientation of the MS structure, which therefore becomes more favorable to visualization under polarized light (145,146). Finally, Cohen and co-authors (147) found that the percentage of oocytes with detectable MS was positively related to the time elapsed from hCG administration. For this reason it was recommended to postpone ICSI to 38–42 hours after hCG injection in order to allow complete oocyte maturation prior to insemination. Besides its role in chromosome segregation, the MS is also a key organelle in the creation of the IPB. Its position at the very periphery of the cell, attached to the oolemma cortex (151), dictates the orientation of the cleavage furrow and thus the IPB extrusion site. However, IPB has been found to be frequently dislocated from the MS location after the denudation procedure (144,145). Artefactual displacement of the IPB from its original extrusion place adjacent to the MS position is believed to be due to the manipulation required for cumulus–corona cell removal (145). No relationship between moderate degree of IPB/MS deviation and ICSI outcomes has been described in these studies. However, we found that the mechanical stress that induces IPB dislocation more than 90° from the MS position correlates with lower fertilization ability (145). Another possible drawback of IPB displacement is the potential injury to the MS during microinsemination. In fact, the ICSI procedure is performed with the IPB at 90° from the injection pipette entry site. Displaced IPB may thus expose the MS to the injection pipette passageway during oocyte microinsemination and therefore to mechanical damage (Figure 7.2). As a consequence, the Spindle View system has been proposed as a useful tool to safely perform ICSI, since it allows the correct orientation of the oocyte with the MS (and not the IPB) as far as possible from the injection needle. The Spindle View system also produced quantitative information about the MS. In fact, the degree of birefringence is directly proportional to the molecular organization of the structure (Figure 7.3). A possible correlation between MS birefringence, oocyte quality, and embryo development has been suggested (30,148,152). Moreover, a negative correlation between female age and MS retardance has been found (Figure 7.4) (30,148), suggesting that older women have a lower MS microtubular density, which could explain their higher risk of producing aneuploid embryos. These results are in agreement with observations by confocal microscopy that MS architecture is strictly related to female age (134). Nevertheless, MS mean retardance, area, and length are not statistically significantly different in conception and non-conception cycles. Thus, it seems that polarization microscopy cannot be used as a noninvasive marker to predict IVF outcome (153,154).

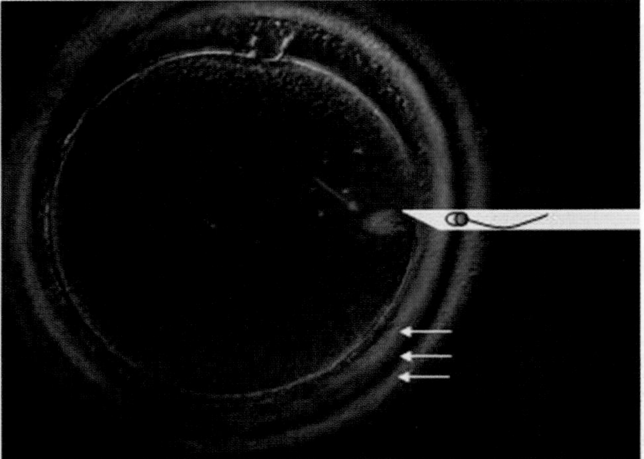

Figure 7.2 Metaphase II oocyte with a meiotic spindle located at three o'clock (red arrow) in the way of the injection pipette. The three different layers of the zona pellucida (ZP) are clearly visible (white arrows). (Magnification 400×.)

As described above, the completion of meiotic maturation occurs only after sperm entry and the extrusion of the second polar body. This event is generally unidentified, occurring before the conventional first pronuclear assessment performed at 16–22 hours post-insemination. Recently, the introduction of time-lapse technology has allowed the observation of the entire progression of embryo development, overcoming the limitations of the traditional static observations. Aguilar et al. (155) have described the whole dynamics of the first cell cycle in human zygotes. Most of the oocytes extruded the second polar body adjacent to the IPB, although a small percentage (10%) extruded it on the opposite side; however, the extrusion location does not seem to have a significant relationship with embryo implantation. Instead, the evaluation of the optimal timing shows that oocytes extruding the second polar body at 1.0–3.2 hours post-ICSI had a lower implantation rate than those taking a longer time (3.3–10.6 hours). Different observations have been reported by Azzarello et al. (156), suggesting a comparable timing of second polar body extrusion in implanted and non-implanted embryos.

MII OOCYTE MORPHOLOGICAL EVALUATION

It is generally recognized that a "normal" human MII oocyte should have a round, clear ZP, a small PVS containing a single, non-fragmented IPB, and a pale, moderately granular cytoplasm with no inclusions (108,157–162). However, the majority of the oocytes retrieved after ovarian hyperstimulation exhibit one or more morphological abnormalities involving the cytoplasm aspect and/or the extracytoplasmic structures (108,158–163). The actual negative impact of the different oocyte "abnormalities" on IVF and ICSI outcomes is unclear (108,161,164). Some authors have suggested that oocytes can be fertilized by ICSI regardless of their morphological appearance (158,160). Furthermore, embryo quality seems not to be affected by oocyte morphology. Similar clinical pregnancy and implantation rates were also obtained after transferring embryos derived from "abnormal" oocytes as compared with those obtained with embryos derived from "normal"-appearing oocytes (27,158–160,165–168). On the other hand, different authors have reported a correlation between oocyte morphology and embryo developmental potential. Regarding the

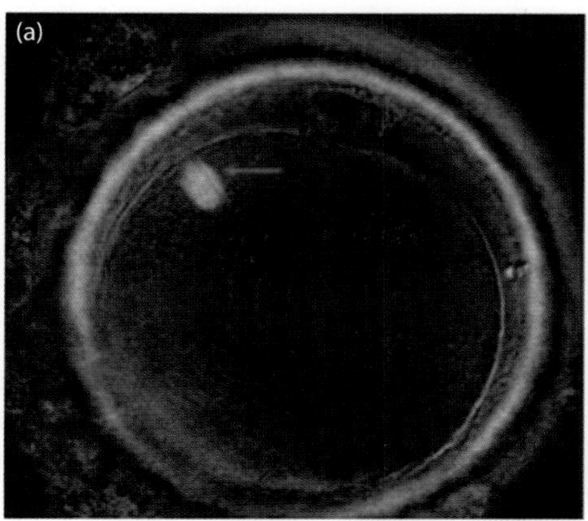

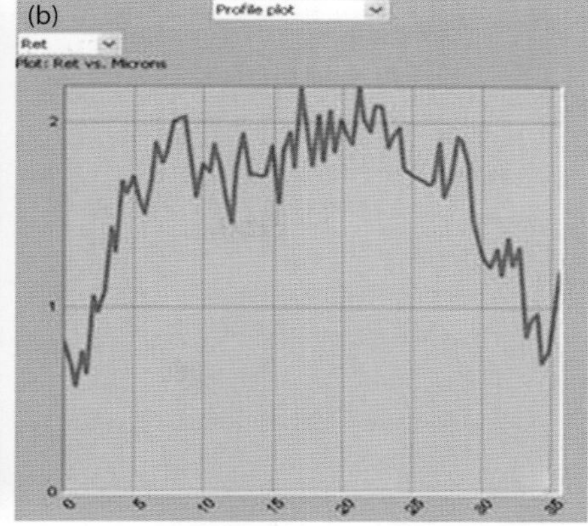

Figure 7.3 (a) Metaphase II oocyte observed with the Spindle View system. (b) Retardance profile of the meiotic spindle. (Magnification 400×.)

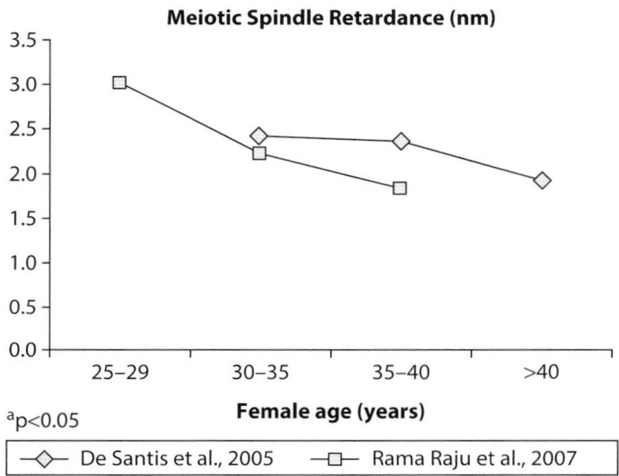

Figure 7.4 Relationship between meiotic spindle retardance and female age. (Adapted from De Santis L, Cino I, Rabellotti E. *Reprod Biomed Online* 2005; 11: 36–42; Rama Raju GA, Prakash GJ, Krishna KM et al. *Reprod Biomed Online* 2007; 14: 166–74.)

cumulative effect of multiple morphological features, Xia (159) showed that oocyte grading based on IPB morphology, size of PVS, and cytoplasmic inclusions was correlated with its developmental potential after ICSI. In the study of Chamayou et al. (167), the cumulative effect of morphological features including cytoplasmic texture, inclusions, vacuoles, refractile bodies, and central granulation was found to be related to impaired embryo quality, but did not influence pregnancy rates. A completely different conclusion has been obtained by Serhal and co-authors (169), who found that similar features did not influence *in vitro* developmental parameters, but implantation and pregnancy rates were lower when embryos were derived from oocytes with cytoplasmic abnormalities. IPB morphology has also been suggested as a possible predictor of oocyte fertilization and embryo quality after ICSI by other authors (30,162,170,171).

Transferring embryos selected according to IPB morphology leads to an increase in implantation and pregnancy rates (170). According to Rienzi and co-authors (172), abnormal (large or degenerated) IPB was related to decreased fertilization rates, but did not show any correlation with pronuclear morphology or embryo quality, while fragmentation was not associated with any of these outcomes. Moreover, embryos derived from oocytes with an intact IPB were more prone to develop into a blastocyst than embryos derived from oocytes with fragmented IPB (173). Navarro et al. (174) found a correlation between large IPB and decreased fertilization, cleavage rates, and compromised embryo quality. Surprisingly, fragmentation or degeneration of IPBs was found to be related to higher fertilization rates and lower levels of fragmentation of embryos by Fancsovits and co-authors (175), while large IPBs were associated with compromised fertilization and low embryo quality. Nevertheless, other studies have failed to demonstrate a relationship between IPB fragmentation and embryo development (30,161,166,176). Moreover, the aneuploidy rate in MII oocytes is reported to be unrelated to the status of the IPB (177). It must be underlined that the frequency of IPB fragmentation is associated with the time elapsed from denudation and ICSI (161,171). This morphological trait seems to be a marker of postovulatory age of the oocyte (32) and thus to be a consequence of *in vitro* aging instead of being a proper marker of oocyte quality. In our experience (172), only the presence of degenerated or large IPBs (Figure 7.5) (but not fragmented) was associated with a reduced fertilization rate after ICSI.

The presence of a degenerated IPB may reflect an asynchrony between nuclear and cytoplasmic maturation (32), which would explain the lower developmental potential of the oocyte (30,159,170). On the other hand, the emission of an abnormally large IPB may be ascribed to the inability of the MS to migrate correctly at the very periphery of the cell (30,178). In these cases, IPB morphology may be considered to be a marker of oocyte maturation disturbance (30,178). Additional information about oocyte quality may be derived by IPB biopsy and chromosomal analysis. This particular aspect is discussed in Chapter 26 by Montag.

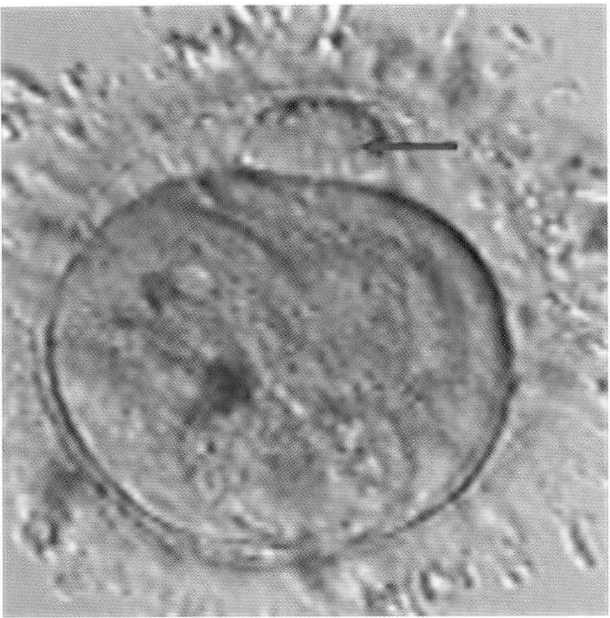

Figure 7.5 Metaphase II oocyte with a giant first polar body (arrow) and abnormal cytoplasm. (Magnification 400×.)

Another factor that may affect oocyte survival (179,180) and fertilization rate (172) after insemination by ICSI is the presence of a large PVS. This feature seems to reflect an over-maturity of the oocytes at the time of ICSI (163). However, different studies have failed to find a correlation between the size and shape of the PVS and fertilization rate and embryo development (158,160,161). Curiously, Ten et al. (176) reported increased embryo quality after fertilization of oocytes with increased PVS. On the other hand, Rienzi and co-authors (172) found a large PVS to be correlated with low fertilization rates and compromised pronuclear morphology, but not with compromised embryo quality. The negative effect of this morphotype may be related to its degree of extension and to the simultaneous presence of other abnormalities, such as enucleated fragments (Figure 7.6).

The aspect of the ZP observed with light microscopy seems not to correlate with normal fertilization and embryo development (33,160,165,172,181). However, the thickness and retardance of the ZP observed with polarized light microscopy have been recently proposed as markers of oocyte quality. Increased ZP thickness variation was associated with increased embryo quality (182). The ZP is composed of three different layers, each characterized by different molecular arrangements and exhibiting different birefringence patterns (Figure 7.2). The external and central layers seem to be of no predictive value, whereas the retardance of the inner layer has been attributed to blastocyst formation (148) and/or to implantation (149,183).

It is generally reported that the cytoplasmic texture is a very important characteristic for oocyte selection (34,158,164,165,184–187). Cytoplasmic alteration, such as granularity and presence of inclusions (Figure 7.7), may be a sign of cytoplasmic incompetence. Some authors have suggested that despite normal fertilization and early embryo development being achieved in oocytes with abnormal cytoplasmic morphology, the resulting embryos have a lower implantation potential (157,184).

Particular cytoplasmic defects (such as centrally located granular area, sER clusters, and vacuoles) have been associated with poorer fertilization and/or embryo developmental potential (34,169,172,180–187). Furthermore, no fertilization has been observed when vacuoles >14 μm in size were present in the injected oocyte (108,187). Conversely, other studies (33,160,169) have shown that slight deviations from the normal cytoplasmic texture were not associated with unfavorable oocyte development. According to Wilding and co-authors (188), any type of cytoplasmic granulation was associated with reduced fertilization rates than in oocytes with a total absence

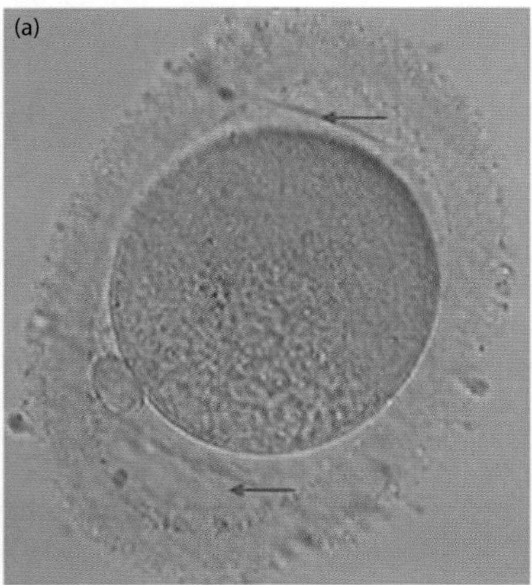

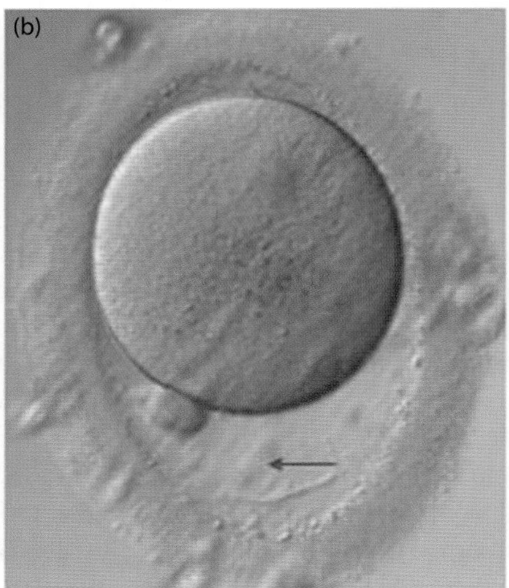

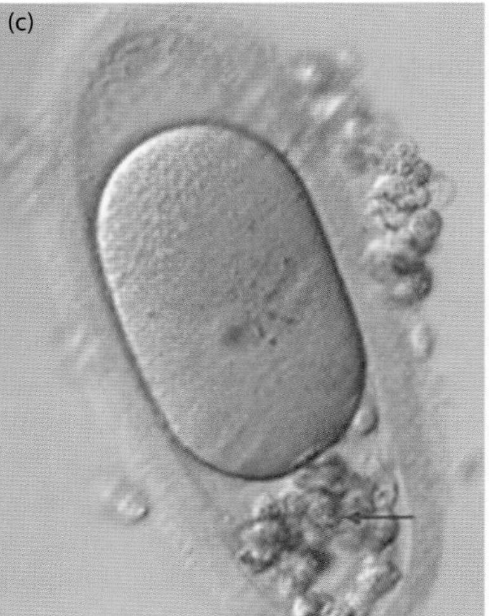

Figure 7.6 Different degrees of perivitelline space (PVS) abnormalities. (a) Enlarged PVS in two areas and with sets (arrows). (b) Enlarged PVS in one area (arrow). (c) Oval oocyte with enlarged PVS containing fragments (arrows). (Magnification 400×.)

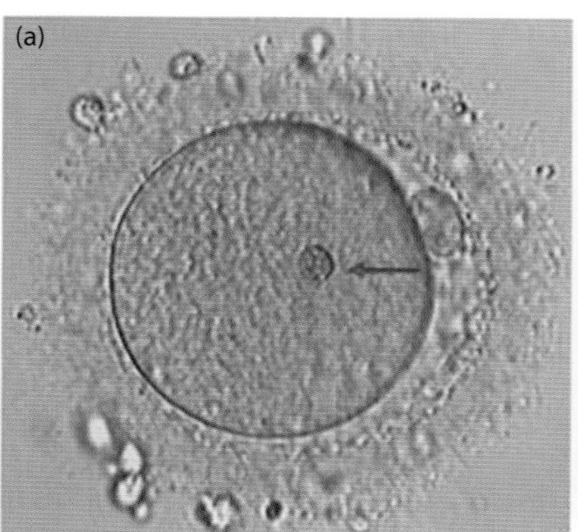

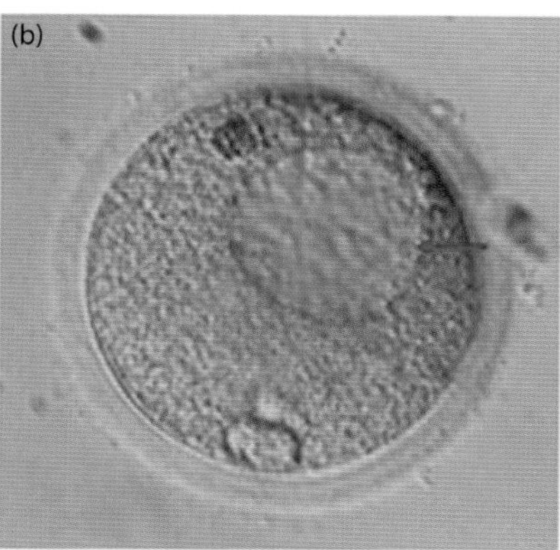

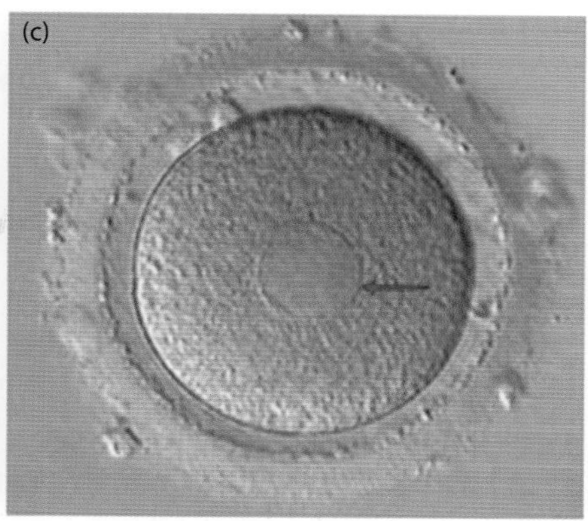

Figure 7.7 Different types of cytoplasmic inclusions. (a) Refractile body (arrow), (b) vacuole (arrow), and (c) smooth endoplasmic reticulum cluster (arrow). (Magnification 400×.)

of granularity. It may thus be hypothesized that not the type but the severity of cytoplasmic defects correlates with oocyte developmental impairment (33,161).

The predictive value of several morphological features according to selected publications is summarized in Table 7.3.

A systematic review of all the papers published between 1996 and 2009 aiming to evaluate the predictive value of oocyte morphology suggested that the influence of oocyte dysmorphisms in terms of IVF success is still controversial (164). Moreover, the employment of different criteria for oocyte evaluation may be responsible for the discrepancies found in different studies. The Alpha Executive and the ESHRE Special Interest Group of Embryology have proposed a common terminology for oocyte morphology assessment in order to simplify inter-laboratory comparison (111). According to the Instanbul Consensus (111), only two oocyte morphological anomalies should be handled with caution: "giant" oocytes because of their likely abnormal genetic constitution (Figure 7.8); and oocytes showing clustering of the sER.

Giant oocytes contain one additional set of chromosomes and display two different MSs when observed under polarized light. The occurrence of these oocytes is relatively rare after ovarian hyperstimulation (it has been estimated that 0.2% of these oocytes have a failure of meiosis) (189). However, the use of these cells for IVF is rather threatening. It has been described that all the embryos generated from giant oocytes are chromosomally abnormal, but they may have normal cleavage and development to the blastocyst stage (190). The transfer of these embryos could thus increase the risk of undesired miscarriages (190).

The potential association between sER aggregation and certain imprinting disorders (e.g., Beckwith–Wiedemann syndrome, diaphragmatic hernia, and multiple malformations) (191–194) has led embryologists to discard these oocytes. However, more recent literature evidence has suggested that embryos derived from sER oocytes may have a normal development, resulting in healthy newborns (195).

According to a recent systematic review (196), 183 babies have been born from sER-positive cycles: 171 were healthy, 8 live births presented malformations, 3 were neonatal deaths, and 1 was stillborn, and 4 additional terminations of pregnancy occurred. Therefore, a continuous follow-up of children born after transfers with embryos originating from sER-positive oocytes should be encouraged in order to investigate the origin and possible effect of sER on the molecular status of oocytes and embryos.

CONCLUSIONS

Useful, effective, and noninvasive grading tools are available for pronuclear, embryo, and blastocyst stage scoring, each of which has been individually shown to be predictive of embryo competence (197–216). However, in addition to morphological assessment, other features of the human embryo may be useful for more accurate selection: embryo physiology, for instance, evaluated by measurements of metabolic activity and normality, may help to determine embryonic "health" (118,217–223). Moreover, preimplantation genetic screening at the blastocyst stage of trophoectoderm chromosomal constitution may give important information about embryonic developmental potential (224–226). With the current trend being toward limiting the number of embryos to be transferred, and thus the occurrence of multiple pregnancies, the ability of the embryologist to identify the embryo with the highest implantation potential is crucial. Nowadays, limited noninvasive tools exist to permit classification of human oocyte quality prior to fertilization.

The stimulation protocols, different pharmacological preparations, and perifollicular vascularization might influence human oocyte quality. In addition, oocyte observation under light microscopy provides assessments of several morphological characteristics. It seems, however, that slight deviations from morphological normality should not be considered as abnormal phenotypes. Only few oocyte morphological anomalies are truly associated with embryo developmental competence (giant

Table 7.3 Morphological features of oocytes with ("Yes") or without ("No") predictive value on *in vitro* or *in vivo* outcome in selected publications

	COCs	Zona	Perivit	PBshape	Oshape	Darkdifg	VacRB	Cgran	Spind	Multiple	Remark
Balaban et al. 1998 (160)	–	No	No	–	No	No	No	–	–	No	
Balakier et al. 2002 (190)	–	–	–	–	Yes	–	–	–	–	–	Giant oocytes
Chamayou et al. 2006 (167)	–	–	Yes	Yes	No	+	+	+	No	Yes	
Ciotti et al. 2004 (171)	–	–	–	No	–	–	–	–	–	–	
Cohen et al. 2004 (147)	–	–	–	–	–	–	–	–	Yes	–	Presence
Cookeet et al. 2003 (146)	–	–	–	–	–	–	–	–	Yes		Presence
De sutter et al. 1996 (158)	–	No	No	–	No	No	No	–	–	–	
Ebner et al. 2000 (162)	–	–	–	Yes	–	–	–	–	–	–	
Ebner et al. 2008 (105)	Yes	–	–	–	–	–	–	Yes	–	–	Blood clots in cum
Fancsovits et al. 2006 (175)	–	–	–	Yes	–	–	–	–	–	–	Fragmented better
											Large impaired
Host et al. 2002 (182)	–	Yes	–	–	–	–	–	–	–	–	Thickness variation
Kahraman et al. 2000 (34)	–	–	–	–	–	–	–	Yes	–	–	
La Sala et al. 2009 (168)	+	+	+	+	–	+	+	–	–	No	
Lin et al. 2003 (107)	Yes	–	–	–	–	–	–	–	–	–	
Loutradis et al. 1999 (33)	–	No	–	–	–	Yes	Yes	–	–	–	
Madaschi et al. 2009 (149)	–	Yes	–	–	–	–	–	–	Yes	–	Retardation
											Presence
Moon et al. 2003 (144)	–	–	–	–	–	–	–	–	Yes	–	Presence+angle
Navarro et al. 2009 (174)	–	–	–	Yes	–	–	–	–	–	–	Large polar body
Ng et al. 1999 (106)	Yes	–	–	–	–	–	–	–	–	–	
Otsuki et al. 2004 (186)	–	–	–	–	–	–	Yes	–	–	–	Smoother cluster
Rama Raju et al. 2007 (148)	–	Yes	–	–	–	–	–	–	Yes	–	Retardation, thickness
											Presence, retard
Rattana et al. 1999 (27)	No	–	–	–	–	–	–	–	–	–	
R ienzi et al. 2003 (145)	–	–	–	–	–	–	–	–	Yes	–	Presence, position
R ienzi et al. 2008 (172)	–	No	Yes	Yes	No	Yes	Yes	Yes	–	Yes	
Shen et al. 2005 (183)	–	–	–	–	–	–	–	–	Yes	–	Retardation
Ten et al. 2007 (176)	No	Yes	No	No	Yes	No		–	–	–	
Verlinsky et al. 2003 (166)	–	–	–	No	–	–	–	–	–	–	
Wang et al. 2001 (142)	–	–	–	–	–	–	–	–	Yes	–	Presence
Wilding et al. 2007 (188)	–	–	–	–	(m)Yes	Yes	Yes	No	–	Yes	(M)membr.
											Properties
Xia et al. 1997 (159)	–	–	+	+	–	–	Yes	–	–	Yes	

Source: Simplified version of the comprehensive table from Rienzi L, Vajta G, Ubaldi F. *Hum Reprod Update* 2011; 17: 34–45.

Abbreviations: COC, cumulus–oocyte complex; Zona, zona pellucida; Perivit, perivitelline space; PBshape, shape of the first polar body; Oshape, shape of the oocyte; Darkdifg, dark ooplasm or diffuse granulation; VacRB, vacuoles, inclusions, and refractile bodies; Cgran, central granulation; Spind, meiotic spindle; Multiple, multiple features evaluated together (by using a scoring system).

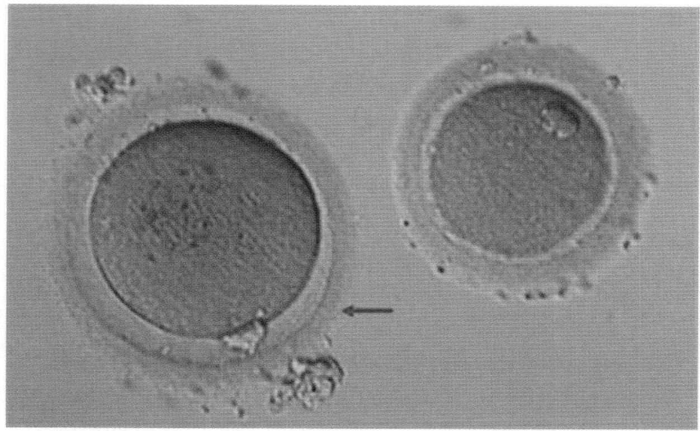

Figure 7.8 Giant oocyte (arrow) and normally sized oocyte. (Magnification 400×.)

oocytes)—the remaining should be ascribed to phenotypic variance (111).

The analysis of MSs in living oocytes with the Spindle View system has shown that detectable MSs are functionally superior to non-detectable ones (133,142,143). Furthermore, embryos derived from oocytes with functionally poor MSs have impaired cell development (144,145,147). However, it must be underlined that more than 90% of MII oocytes not exposed to unfavorable laboratory conditions display a detectable MS when observed with the Spindle View system. Therefore, while having ascertained that the absence of a signal is an important negative prognostic factor, the presence of MSs, which involves the majority of the MII oocytes subjected to this evaluation, is of limited value for oocyte selection (30).

In addition to the above-mentioned evaluation criteria, other methods could be able to provide additional information on oocyte quality, such as (227):

- Assessment of GC and cumulus cell apoptosis status
- Evaluation of oxidative stress in follicular fluid and GCs
- Follicular cell gene expression profiles by real-time polymerase chain reaction or DNA microarray
- Measurement of follicular fluid molecular content
- Ultramicrofluorimetric quantitation of oocyte carbohydrate consumption and metabolite release in the culture medium

Although potentially useful, further investigation is needed to ensure the consistency, reliability, and sensitivity of these methods. In addition, some of these methods are characterized by time-consuming protocols that imply *in vitro* oocyte aging.

On the basis of the above-mentioned potentialities of oocyte selection tools, future perspectives for the betterment of assisted reproductive techniques reside in creating a direct connection between IVF laboratories and research units. The so-called "omics technologies" (transcriptomic, proteomic, and metabolomic) is gaining increased interest from the scientific community. The results obtained so far are intriguing and encouraging, but it would be wise to raise some concerns. In fact, the high costs, difficulty of the techniques, and time required for testing are currently limiting their routine applicability. Moreover, it is of the utmost importance to provide definitive evidence of the bio-safety of these techniques, and more studies are required in order to determine their predictive power (115,117).

REFERENCES

1. Le Nestour E, Marraoui J, Lahlou N et al. Role of estradiol in the rise in follicle stimulation hormone levels during the luteal-follicular transition. *J Clin Endocrinol Metab* 1993; 77: 439–42.
2. Hodgen GD. The dominant ovarian follicle. *Fertil Steril* 1982; 38: 281–300.
3. Goungeon A, Testart J. Influence of human menopausal gonadotropin on the recruitment of human ovarian follicles. *Fertil Steril* 1990; 54: 848–52.
4. Messinis IE, Templeton AA. The importance of follicle-stimulating hormone increase for folliculogenesis. *Hum Reprod* 1990; 5: 153–6.
5. Van Der Meer M, Hompes PGA, Scheele F et al. Follicle stimulating hormone (FSH) dynamics of low dose step-up ovulation induction with FSH in patients with polycystic ovary syndrome. *Hum Reprod* 1994; 9: 1612–7.
6. Baird DT. A model for follicular selection and ovulation: Lessons from superovulation. *J Steroid Biochem* 1987; 27: 15–23.
7. Brown JB. Pituitary control of ovarian function: Concepts derived from gonadotropin therapy. *Aust NZ J Obstet Gynaecol* 1978; 18: 46–54.
8. Erickson GF, Danforth DR. Ovarian control of follicle development. *Am J Obstet Gynecol* 1995; 172: 736–47.
9. Fauser BC, Van Heusden AM. Manipulation of human ovarian function: Physiological concepts and clinical consequences. *Endocr Rev* 1997; 18: 71–106.
10. Zelenzik AJ, Kubik CJ. Ovarian responses in macaques to pulsatile infusion of follicle-stimulating hormone (FSH) and luteinizing hormone: Increased sensitivity of the maturing follicle to FSH. *Endocrinology* 1986; 119: 2025–32.
11. Van Santbrink EJ, Hop WC, Van Dessel TJ et al. Decremental follicle-stimulating hormone and dominant follicle development during the normal menstrual cycle. *Fertil Steril* 1995; 64: 37–43.
12. Fauser BC. Step-down follicle-stimulating hormone regimens in polycystic ovary syndrome. In: *Ovulation Induction: Basic Science and Clinical Advances*. Filicori M, Flamigni C (eds). Amsterdam: Elsevier, 1994; pp. 153–62.
13. Hughes EG, Fedorkow DM, Daya S et al. The routine use of gonadotropin-releasing hormone agonists prior to *in vitro* fertilization and gamete intrafallopian transfer: A meta-analysis of randomized controlled trials. *Fertil Steril* 1992; 58: 888–96.
14. Albano C, Felberbaum RE, Smitz J et al. Ovarian stimulation with HMG: Results of a prospective randomized phase III European study comparing the

luteinizing hormone-Releasing hormone (LHRH)-antagonist cetrorelix and the LHRH-agonist buserelin. *Hum Reprod* 2000; 15: 526–31.
15. Olivennes F, Belaisch-Allart J, Emperaire JC et al. Prospective, randomized, controlled study of *in vitro* fertilization-embryo transfer with a single dose of a luteinizing hormone-releasing hormone (LH-RH) antagonist (cetrorelix) or a depot formula of an LH-RH antagonist (triptorelin). *Fertil Steril* 2000; 73: 314–20.
16. Fluker M, Grifo J, Leader A et al. Efficacy and safety of ganirelix acetate versus leuprolide acetate in women undergoing controlled ovarian hyperstimulation. *Fertil Steril* 2001; 75: 38–45.
17. De Jong D, Macklon NS, Fauser BC. A pilot study involving minimal ovarian stimulation for *in vitro* fertilization: Extending the "follicle-stimulating hormone window" combined with gonadotropinreleasing hormone antagonist cetrorelix. *Fertil Steril* 2000; 73: 1051–4.
18. Hohmann FP, Macklon NS, Fauser BC. A randomized comparison of two ovarian stimulation protocols with gonadotropin-releasing hormone (GnRH) antagonist cotreatment for *in vitro* fertilization commencing recombinant follicle stimulating hormone on cycle day 2 or 5 with the standard long GnRH agonist protocol. *J Clin Endocrinol Metab* 2003; 88: 166–73.
19. Youssef MA, Van der Veen F, Al-Inany HG et al. Gonadotropin-releasing hormone agonist versus HCG for oocyte triggering in antagonist-assisted reproductive technology. *Cochrane Database Syst Rev* 2014; 10: CD008046.
20. Humaidan P, Engmann L, Benadiva C. Luteal phase supplementation after gonadotropin-releasing hormone agonist trigger in fresh embryo transfer: The American versus European approaches. *Fertil Steril* 2015; 103: 879–85.
21. Devroey P, Polyzos NP, Blockeel C. An OHSS-free clinic by segmentation of IVF treatment. *Hum Reprod* 2011; 26: 2593–7.
22. Garcia-Velasco JA. Agonist trigger: What is the best approach? Agonist trigger with vitrification of oocytes or embryos. *Fertil Steril* 2012; 97: 527–8.
23. Engmann L, Benadiva C. Agonist trigger: What is the best approach? Agonist trigger with aggressive luteal support. *Fertil Steril* 2012; 97: 531–3.
24. Testart J, Lassalle B, Frydman R et al. A study of factors affecting the success of human fertilization *in vitro*. II. Influence of semen quality and oocyte maturity on fertilization and cleavage. *Biol Reprod* 1983; 28: 425–31.
25. Laufer N, Tarlatzis BC, DeCherney AH et al. Asynchrony between human cumulus–corona cell complex and oocyte maturation after human menopausal gonadotropin treatment for *in vitro* fertilization. *Fertil Steril* 1984; 42: 366–72.
26. Khamsi F, Roberge S, Lacanna IC et al. Effects of granulosa cells, cumulus cells, and oocyte density on *in vitro* fertilization in women. *Endocrine* 1999; 10: 161–6.
27. Rattanachaiyanont M, Leader A, Leveille MC. Lack of correlation between oocyte–corona–cumulus complex morphology and nuclear maturity of oocytes collected in stimulated cycles for intracytoplasmic sperm injection. *Fertil Steril* 1999; 71: 937–40.
28. Rienzi L, Ubaldi F, Iacobelli M et al. Significance of morphological attributes of the early embryo. *Reprod Biomed Online* 2005; 10: 669–81.
29. Montag M, Schimming T, van der Ven H. Spindle imaging in human oocytes: The impact of the meiotic cell cycle. *Reprod Biomed Online* 2006; 12: 442–6.
30. De Santis L, Cino I, Rabellotti E. Polar body morphology and spindle imaging as predictors of oocyte quality. *Reprod Biomed Online* 2005; 11: 36–42.
31. Hassan-Ali H, Hisham-Saleh A, El-Gezeiry D et al. Perivitelline space granularity: A sign of human menopausal gonadotrophin overdose in intracytoplasmic sperm injection. *Hum Reprod* 1998; 13: 3425–30.
32. Eichenlaub-Ritter U, Schmiady H, Kentenich H et al. Recurrent failure in polar body formation and premature chromosome condensation in oocytes from a human patient: Indicators of asynchrony in nuclear and cytoplasmic maturation. *Hum Reprod* 1995;10:2343–9.
33. Loutradis D, Drakakis P, Kallianidis K et al. Oocyte morphology correlates with embryo quality and pregnancy rate after intracytoplasmic sperm injection. *Fertil Steril* 1999; 72: 240–4.
34. Kahraman S, Yakin K, Donmez E et al. Relationship between granular cytoplasm of oocytes and pregnancy outcome following intracytoplasmic sperm injection. *Hum Reprod* 2000; 15: 2390–3.
35. Sunkara SK, Rittenberg V, Raine-Fenning N et al. Association between the number of eggs and live birth in IVF treatment: An analysis of 400135 treatment cycles. *Hum Reprod* 2011; 26: 1768–74.
36. Ubaldi F, Vaiarelli A, D'Anna R et al. Management of poor responders in IVF: Is there anything new? *Biomed Res Int* 2014; 2014: 352098.
37. Faddy MJ, Gosden RG, Gougeon A et al. Accelerated disappearance of ovarian follicles in mid-life: Implications for forecasting menopause. *Hum Reprod* 1992; 7: 1342–6.
38. Al-Azemi M, Killick SR, Duffy S et al. Multi-marker assessment of ovarian reserve predicts oocyte yield after ovulation induction. *Hum Reprod* 2011; 26: 414–22.
39. Broekmans FJ, Kwee J, Hendriks DJ et al. A systematic review of tests predicting ovarian reserve and IVF outcome. *Hum Reprod Update* 2006; 12: 685–718.
40. La Marca A, Stabile G, Artenisio AC et al. Serum anti-Mullerian hormone throughout the human menstrual cycle. *Hum Reprod* 2006; 21: 3103–7.
41. La Marca A, Sighinolfi G, Radi D et al. Anti-Mullerian hormone (AMH) as a predictive marker in assisted reproductive technology (ART). *Hum Reprod Update* 2010; 16: 113–30.

42. Amer SA, Mahran A, Abdelmaged A et al. The influence of circulating anti-Müllerian hormone on ovarian responsiveness to ovulation induction with gonadotrophins in women with polycystic ovarian syndrome: A pilot study. *Reprod Biol Endocrinol* 2013; 11: 115.
43. Fleming R, Seifer DB, Frattarelli JL et al. Assessing ovarian response: Antral follicle count versus anti-Müllerian hormone. *Reprod Biomed Online* 2015; 31: 486–96.
44. Nardo LG, Gelbaya TA, Wilkinson H et al. Circulating basal anti-Müllerian hormone levels as predictor of ovarian response in women undergoing ovarian stimulation for *in vitro* fertilization. *Fertil Steril* 2009; 92: 1586–93.
45. Blazar AS, Lambert-Messerlian G, Hackett R et al. Use of in-cycle antimüllerian hormone levels to predict cycle outcome. *Am J Obstet Gynecol* 2011; 205: 223.e1–5.
46. Tsakos E, Tolikas A, Daniilidis A et al. Predictive value of anti-Müllerian hormone, follicle-stimulating hormone and antral follicle count on the outcome of ovarian stimulation in women following GnRH-antagonist protocol for IVF/ET. *Arch Gynecol Obstet* 2014; 290: 1249–53.
47. Polyzos NP, Nelson SM, Stoop D et al. Does the time interval between antimüllerian hormone serum sampling and initiation of ovarian stimulation affect its predictive ability in *in vitro* fertilization-intracytoplasmic sperm injection cycles with a gonadotropin-releasing hormone antagonist? A retrospective single-center study. *Fertil Steril* 2013; 100: 438–44.
48. Nelson SM, Broekmans FJ. The relationship between anti-Müllerian hormone in women receiving fertility assessments and age at menopause in subfertile women: Evidence from large population studies. *J Clin Endocrinol Metab* 2013; 98: 1946–53.
49. Iliodromiti S, Anderson RA, Nelson SM. Technical and performance characteristics of anti-Müllerian hormone and antral follicle count as biomarkers of ovarian response. *Hum Reprod Update* 2015; 21: 698–710.
50. Rustamov O, Smith A, Roberts SA et al. The measurement of anti-Müllerian hormone: A critical appraisal. *J Clin Endocrinol Metab* 2014; 99: 723–32.
51. Irez T, Ocal P, Guralp O et al. Different serum anti-Müllerian hormone concentrations are associated with oocyte quality, embryo development parameters and IVF–ICSI outcomes. *Arch Gynecol Obstet* 2011; 284: 1295–301.
52. Arce JC, La Marca A, Mirner Klein B et al. Antimüllerian hormone in gonadotropin releasing-hormone antagonist cycles: Prediction of ovarian response and cumulative treatment outcome in good-prognosis patients. *Fertil Steril* 2013; 99: 1644–53.
53. Khader A, Lloyd SM, McConnachie A et al. External validation of anti-Müllerian hormone based prediction of live birth in assisted conception. *J Ovarian Res* 2013; 6: 3.
54. Li HW, Lee VC, Lau EY et al. Role of baseline antral follicle count and anti-Mullerian hormone in prediction of cumulative live birth in the first *in vitro* fertilisation cycle: A retrospective cohort analysis. *PLoS One* 2013; 8(4): e61095.
55. Lukaszuk K, Liss J, Kunicki M et al. Anti-Müllerian hormone (AMH) is a strong predictor of live birth in women undergoing assisted reproductive technology. *Reprod Biol* 2014; 14: 176–81.
56. Kedem A, Haas J, Geva LL et al. Ongoing pregnancy rates in women with low and extremely low AMH levels. A multivariate analysis of 769 cycles. *PLoS One* 2013; 8(12): e81629.
57. Lin WQ, Yao LN, Zhang DX et al. The predictive value of anti-Mullerian hormone on embryo quality, blastocyst development, and pregnancy rate following *in vitro* fertilization–embryo transfer (IVF–ET). *J Assist Reprod Genet* 2013; 30: 649–55.
58. Mutlu MF, Erdem M, Erdem A et al. Antral follicle count determines poor ovarian response better than anti-Müllerian hormone but age is the only predictor for live birth in *in vitro* fertilization cycles. *J Assist Reprod Genet* 2013; 30: 657–65.
59. Reichman DE, Goldschlag D, Rosenwaks Z. Value of antimüllerian hormone as a prognostic indicator of *in vitro* fertilization outcome. *Fertil Steril* 2014; 101: 1012–8.
60. Broer SL, Dólleman M, Van Disseldorp J et al.; IPD-EXPORT Study Group. Prediction of an excessive response in *in vitro* fertilization from patient characteristics and ovarian reserve tests and comparison in subgroups: An individual patient data meta-analysis. *Fertil Steril* 2013; 100: 420–9.
61. Iliodromiti S, Kelsey TW, Wu O et al. The predictive accuracy of anti-Müllerian hormone for live birth after assisted conception: A systematic review and meta-analysis of the literature. *Hum Reprod Update* 2014; 20: 560–70.
62. Chang MY, Chiang CH, Hsieh TT et al. Use of the antral follicle count to predict the outcome of assisted reproductive technologies. *Fertil Steril* 1998; 69: 505–10.
63. Himabindu Y, Sriharibabu M, Gopinathan K et al. Anti-Mullerian hormone and antral follicle count as predictors of ovarian response in assisted reproduction. *J Hum Reprod Sci* 2013;6:27–31.
64. Hsu A, Arny M, Knee AB et al. Antral follicle count in clinical practice: Analyzing clinical relevance. *Fertil Steril* 2011; 95: 474–9.
65. Frattarelli JL, Lauria-Costab DF, Miller BT et al. Basal antral follicle number and mean ovarian diameter predict cycle cancellation and ovarian responsiveness in assisted reproductive technology cycles. *Fertil Steril* 2000; 74: 512–7.
66. Tomas C, Nuojua-Huttunen S, Martikainen H. Pretreatment transvaginal ultrasound examination predicts ovarian responsiveness to gonadotrophins in *in-vitro* fertilization. *Hum Reprod* 1997; 12: 220–3.

67. Hendriks DJ, Mol BW, Bancsi LF et al. Antral follicle count in the prediction of poor ovarian response and pregnancy after *in vitro* fertilization: A meta-analysis and comparison with basal follicle-stimulating hormone level. *Fertil Steril* 2005; 83: 291–301.
68. Lukaszuk K, Kunicki M, Liss J et al. Use of ovarian reserve parameters for predicting live births in women undergoing *in vitro* fertilization. *Eur J Obstet Gynecol Reprod Biol* 2013; 168: 173–7.
69. Ji J, Liu Y, Tong XH et al. The optimum number of oocytes in IVF treatment: An analysis of 2455 cycles in China. *Hum Reprod* 2013; 28: 2728–34.
70. Briggs R, Kovacs G, MacLachlan V et al. Can you ever collect too many oocytes? *Hum Reprod* 2015; 30: 81–87.
71. Pena JE, Chang PL, Chan LK et al. Supraphysiological estradiol levels do not affect oocyte and embryo quality in oocyte donation cycles. *Hum Reprod* 2002; 17: 83–7.
72. Greb RR, Behre HM, Simoni M. Pharmacogenetics in ovarian stimulation—Current concepts and future options. *Reprod Biomed Online* 2005; 11: 589–600.
73. Baart EB, Martini E, Eijkemans MJ et al. Milder ovarian stimulation for *in-vitro* fertilization reduces aneuploidy in the human preimplantation embryo: A randomized controlled trial. *Hum Reprod* 2007; 22: 980–8.
74. Kirkegaard K, Sundvall L, Erlandsen M et al. Timing of human preimplantation embryonic development is confounded by embryo origin. *Hum Reprod* 2016; 31: 324–31.
75. Colamaria S. Female age, number of mature eggs and biopsied blastocysts effectively define the chance for obtaining at least one euploid embryo: Implication for counselling and decision-making during blastocyst stage preimplantation genetic screening cycles. Oral Presentation at the ESHRE 2015 Annual Meeting. Lisbon, Portugal, Session 35, June 16, 2015.
76. Ata B, Kaplan B, Danzer H et al. Array CGH analysis shows that aneuploidy is not related to the number of embryos generated. *Reprod Biomed Online* 2012; 24: 614–20.
77. Steptoe P, Edwards R. Birth after the reimplantation of a human embryo. *Lancet* 1978; 12: 366.
78. Laufer N, DeCherney AH, Haseltine FP et al. The use of high-dose human menopausal gonadotropin in an *in vitro* fertilization program. *Fertil Steril* 1983; 40: 734–41.
79. Edwards RG, Lobo R, Bouchard P. Time to revolutionize ovarian stimulation. *Hum Reprod* 1996; 11: 917–9.
80. Fauser BC, Devroey P, Yen SS et al. Minimal ovarian stimulation for IVF: Appraisal of potential benefits and drawbacks. *Hum Reprod* 1999; 14: 2681–6.
81. Al-Inany HG, Youssef MA, Aboulghar et al. GnRH antagonists are safer than agonists: An update of a Cochrane review. *Hum Reprod Update* 2011; 17: 435.
82. Xiao JS, Su CM, Zeng XT. Comparisons of GnRH antagonist versus GnRH agonist protocol in supposed normal ovarian responders undergoing IVF: A systematic review and meta-analysis. *PLoS One* 2014; 9(9): e106854.
83. Loutradis D, Drakakis P, Vlismas A et al. Corifollitropin alfa, a long-acting follicle-stimulating hormone agonist for the treatment of infertility. *Curr Opin Investig Drugs* 2009; 10: 372–80.
84. Fauser BC, Mannaerts BM, Devroey P et al. Advances in recombinant DNA technology: Corifollitropin alfa, a hybrid molecule with sustained follicle-stimulating activity and reduced injection frequency. *Hum Reprod Update* 2009; 15: 309–21.
85. Fauser BC, Alper MM, Ledger W et al. Pharmacokinetics and follicular dynamics of corifollitropin alfa versus recombinant FSH during ovarian stimulation for IVF. *Reprod Biomed Online* 2010; 21: 593–601.
86. Pouwer AW, Farquhar C, Kremer JA. Long-acting FSH versus daily FSH for women undergoing assisted reproduction. *Cochrane Database Syst Rev* 2015; 7: CD009577.
87. Van Blerkom J. The influence of intrinsic and extrinsic factors on the developmental potential and chromosomal normality of the human oocyte. *J Soc Gynecol Investig* 1996; 3: 3–11.
88. Van Blerkom J, Antezak M, Schrader R. The developmental potential of human oocyte is related to the dissolved oxygen content of follicular fluid: Association with vascular endothelial growth factor levels and perifollicular blood flow characteristics. *Hum Reprod* 1997; 12: 1047–55.
89. Battaglia C, Genazzani AD, Regnani G et al. Perifollicular Doppler flow and follicular fluid vascular endothelial growth factor concentrations in poor responders. *Fertil Steril* 2000; 74: 809–12.
90. Van Blerkom J. Epigenetic influences on oocyte developmental competence: Perifollicular vascularity and intrafollicular oxygen. *J Assist Reprod Genet* 1998; 15: 226–34.
91. Coulam CB, Goodman C, Rinehart JS. Colour Doppler indices of follicular blood flow as predictors of pregnancy after *in-vitro* fertilization and embryo transfer. *Hum Reprod* 1999; 14: 1979–82.
92. Chui DK, Pugh ND, Walker SM et al. Follicular vascularity—The predictive value of transvaginal power Doppler ultrasonography in an *in-vitro* fertilization programme: A preliminary study. *Hum Reprod* 1997; 12: 191–6.
93. Bhal PS, Pugh ND, Chui DK et al. The use of transvaginal power Doppler ultrasonography to evaluate the relationship between perifollicular vascularity and outcome in *in-vitro* fertilization treatment cycles. *Hum Reprod* 1999; 14: 939–45.
94. Bhal PS, Pugh ND, Gregory L et al. Perifollicular vascularity as a potential variable affecting outcome in stimulated intrauterine insemination treatment cycles: A study using transvaginal power Doppler. *Hum Reprod* 2001; 16: 1682–9.

95. Borini A, Maccolini A, Tallarini A et al. Perifollicular vascularity and its relationship with oocyte maturity and IVF outcome. *Ann NY Acad Sci* 2001; 943: 64–7.
96. Costello MF, Sjoblom P, Shrestha SM. Use of Doppler ultrasound imaging of the ovary during IVF treatment as a predictor of success. In: *The Infertility Manual.* Rao KA, Brinsdon PR, Sathananthan H (eds). New Delhi, India: JAYPEE Brothers Medical, 2004: pp. 344–9.
97. Ragni G, Anselmino M, Nicolosi AE et al. Follicular vascularity is not predictive of pregnancy outcome in mild controlled ovarian stimulation and IUI cycles. *Hum Reprod* 2007; 22: 210–4.
98. Huey S, Abuhamad A, Barroso G et al. Perifollicular blood flow Doppler indices, but not follicular pO_2, pCO_2, or pH, predict oocyte developmental competence *in vitro* fertilization. *Fertil Steril* 1999; 72: 707–12.
99. Kan A, Ng EH, Yeung WS et al. Perifollicular vascularity in poor ovarian responders during IVF. *Hum Reprod* 2006; 21: 1539–44.
100. Ng EH, Tang OS, Chan CC et al. Ovarian stromal vascularity is not predictive of ovarian response and pregnancy. *Reprod Biomed Online* 2006; 12: 43–9.
101. Palomba S, Russo T, Falbo A. Clinical use of the perifollicular vascularity assessment in IVF cycles: A pilot study. *Hum Reprod* 2006; 21: 1055–61.
102. Dong J, Albertini DF, Nishimori K et al. Growth differentiation factor-9 is required during early ovarian folliculogenesis. *Nature* 1996; 383: 531–5.
103. Albertini DF, Combelles CM, Benecchi E et al. Cellular basis for paracrine regulation of ovarian follicle development. *Reproduction* 2001; 121: 647–53.
104. Bar-Ami S, Gitay-Goren H, Brandes JM. Different morphological and steroidogenic patterns in oocyte/cumulus–corona cell complexes aspirated at *in vitro* fertilization. *Biol Reprod* 1989; 41: 761–70.
105. Ebner T, Moser M, Shebl O et al. Blood clots in the cumulus-oocyte complex predict poor oocyte quality and post-fertilization development. *Reprod Biomed Online* 2008; 16: 801–7.
106. Ng ST, Chang TH, Wu TC. Prediction of the rates of fertilization, cleavage, and pregnancy success by cumulus–coronal morphology in an *in vitro* fertilization program. *Fertil Steril* 1999; 72: 412–7.
107. Lin YC, Chang SY, Lan KC et al. Human oocyte maturity *in vivo* determines the outcome of blastocyst development *in vitro*. *J Assist Reprod Genet* 2003; 20: 506–12.
108. Ebner T, Moser M, Tews G. Is oocyte morphology prognostic of embryo developmental potential after ICSI? *Reprod Biomed Online* 2006; 12: 507–12.
109. McKenzie LJ, Pangas SA, Carson SA et al. Human cumulus granulosa cell gene expression: A predictor of fertilization and embryo selection in women under- going IVF. *Hum Reprod* 2004; 19: 2869–74.
110. Fatehi AN, Roelen BA, Colenbrander B et al. Presence of cumulus cells during *in vitro* fertilization protects the bovine oocyte against oxidative stress and improves first cleavage but does not affect further development. *Zygote* 2005; 13: 177–85.
111. Alpha Scientists in Reproductive Medicine and ESHRE Special Interest Group of Embryology. The Istanbul consensus workshop on embryo assessment: Proceedings of an expert meeting. *Hum Reprod* 2011; 26: 1270–83.
112. Canipari R, Camaioni A, Scarchilli L et al. Oocyte maturation and ovulation: Mechanism of control. *2PN Attual Scient Biol Ripr* 2004; 1: 62–8.
113. Goud PT, Goud AP, Qian C et al. *In-vitro* maturation of human germinal vesicle stage oocytes: Role of cumulus cells and epidermal growth factor in the culture medium. *Hum Reprod* 1998; 13: 1638–44.
114. Yamazaki Y, Wakayama T, Yanagimachi R. Contribution of cumulus cells and serum to the maturation of oocyte cytoplasm as revealed by intracytoplasmic sperm injection (ICSI). *Zygote* 2001; 9: 277–82.
115. Huang Z, Wells D. The human oocyte and cumulus cells relationship: New insights from the cumulus cell transcriptome. *Mol Hum Reprod* 2010; 16: 715–25.
116. Uyar A, Torrealday S, Seli E. Cumulus and granulosa cell markers of oocyte and embryo quality. *Fertil Steril* 2013; 99: 979–97.
117. Seli E, Robert C, Sirard MA. OMICS in assisted reproduction: Possibilities and pitfalls. *Mol Hum Reprod* 2010; 16: 513–30.
118. Nagy ZP, Sakkas D, Behr B. Symposium: Innovative techniques in human embryo viability assessment. Non-invasive assessment of embryo viability by metabolomic profiling of culture media ('metabolomics'). *Reprod Biomed Online* 2008; 17: 502–7.
119. Revelli A, Delle Piane L, Casano S et al. Follicular fluid content and oocyte quality: From single biochemical markers to metabolomics. *Reprod Biol Endocrinol* 2009; 7: 40.
120. Ubaldi F, Rienzi L. Micromanipulation techniques in human infertility: PZD, SUZI, ICSI, MESA, PESA, FNA and TESE. In: *Biotechnology of Human Reproduction*. Revelli A, Tur-Kaspa I, Holte JG, Massobrio M (eds). Oxford, U.K.: Parthenon Publishing, 2003: pp. 315–36.
121. Nagy ZP, Cecile J, Liu J et al. Pregnancy and birth after intracytoplasmic sperm injection of *in vitro* matured germinal-vesicle stage oocytes: Case report. *Fertil Steril* 1996; 65: 1047–50.
122. De Vos A, Van de Velde H, Joris H et al. *In-vitro* matured metaphase-I oocytes have a lower fertilization rate but similar embryo quality as mature metaphase-II oocytes after intracytoplasmic sperm injection. *Hum Reprod* 1999; 14: 1859–63.
123. Edirisinghe WR, Junk SM, Matson PL et al. Birth from cryopreserved embryos following *in vitro*

maturation of oocytes and intracytoplasmic sperm injection. *Hum Reprod* 1997; 12: 1056–8.
124. Nogueira D, Staessen C, Van de Velde H et al. Nuclear status and cytogenetics of embryos derived from *in vitro*-matured oocytes. *Fertil Steril* 2000; 74: 295–8.
125. Sauerbrun-Cutler MT, Vega M, Keltz M et al. *In vitro* maturation and its role in clinical assisted reproductive technology. *Obstet Gynecol Surv* 2015; 70: 45–57.
126. Practice Committees of the American Society for Reproductive Medicine the Society for Assisted Reproductive Technology. *In vitro* maturation: A committee opinion. *Fertil Steril* 2013; 99: 663–6.
127. Buckett WM, Chian RC, Holzer H et al. Obstetric outcomes and congenital abnormalities after *in vitro* maturation, *in vitro* fertilization, and intracytoplasmic sperm injection. *Obstet Gynecol* 2007; 110: 885–91.
128. Soderstrom-Antilla V, Salokorpi T, Pihlaja M et al. Obstetric and perinatal outcome and preliminary results of development of children born after *in vitro* maturation of oocytes. *Hum Reprod* 2006; 21: 1508–13.
129. Sathananthan AH, Trounson A, Freemann L et al. The effects of cooling human oocytes. *Hum Reprod* 1988; 3: 968–77.
130. Pickering SJ, Braude PR, Johnson MH et al. Transient cooling to room temperature can cause irreversible disruption of the meiotic spindle in the human oocyte. *Fertil Steril* 1990; 54: 102–8.
131. Almeida PA, Bolton VN. The effect of temperature fluctuations on the cytoskeletal organisation and chromosomal constitution of the human oocyte. *Zygote* 1995; 3: 357–65.
132. Zenzes MT, Bielecki R, Casper RF et al. Effects of chilling to 0°C on the morphology of meiotic spindles in human metaphase II oocytes. *Fertil Steril* 2001; 75: 769–77.
133. Wang WH, Meng L, Hackett RJ et al. Limited recovery of meiotic spindles in living human oocytes after cooling–rewarming observed using polarized light microscopy. *Hum Reprod* 2001; 16: 2374–8.
134. Battaglia DE, Goodwin P, Klein NA et al. Influence of maternal age on meiotic spindle assembly in oocytes from naturally cycling women. *Hum Reprod* 1996; 11: 2217–22.
135. Volarcik K, Sheean L, Goldfarb J et al. The meiotic competence of *in-vitro* matured human oocytes is influenced by donor age: Evidence that folliculogenesis is compromised in the reproductively aged ovary. *Hum Reprod* 1998; 13: 154–60.
136. Eichenlaub-Ritter U, Vogt E, Yin H et al. Spindles, mitochondria and redox potential in ageing oocytes. *Reprod Biomed Online* 2004; 8: 45–58.
137. Bernard A, Fuller BJ. Cryopreservation of human oocytes: A review of current problems and perspectives. *Hum Reprod Update* 1996; 2: 193–207.
138. Eichenlaub-Ritter U, Shen Y, Tinneberg HR. Manipulation of the oocyte: Possible damage to the spindle apparatus. *Reprod Biomed Online* 2002; 5: 117–24.
139. Oldenbourg R, Mei G. New polarized light microscope with precision universal compensator. *J Microsc* 1995; 180: 140–7.
140. Oldenbourg R. Polarized light microscopy of spindles. *Methods Cell Biol* 1999; 61: 175–208.
141. Liu L, Trimarchi JR, Oldenbourg R et al. Increased birefringence in the meiotic spindle provides a new marker for the onset of activation in living oocytes. *Biol Reprod* 2000; 63: 251–8.
142. Wang WH, Meng L, Hackett RJ et al. Developmental ability of human oocytes with or without birefringent spindles imaged by Polscope before insemination. *Hum Reprod* 2001; 16: 1464–8.
143. Wang WH, Meng L, Hackett RJ et al. The spindle observation and its relationship with fertilization after intracytoplasmicsperm injection in living human oocytes. *Fertil Steril* 2001; 75: 348–53.
144. Moon JH, Hyun CS, Lee SW et al. Visualization of the metaphase II meiotic spindle in living human oocytes using the PolScope enables the prediction of embryonic developmental competence after ICSI. *Hum Reprod* 2003; 18: 817–20.
145. Rienzi L, Ubaldi F, Martinez F et al. Relationship between meiotic spindle location with regard to the polar body position and oocyte developmental potential after ICSI. *Hum Reprod* 2003; 18: 1289–93.
146. Cooke S, Tyler JP, Driscoll GL. Meiotic spindle location and identification and its effect on embryonic cleavage plane and early development. *Hum Reprod* 2003; 18: 2397–405.
147. Cohen Y, Malcov M, Schwartz T et al. Spindle imaging: A new marker for optimal timing of ICSI? *Hum Reprod* 2004; 19: 649–54.
148. Rama Raju GA, Prakash GJ, Krishna KM et al. Meiotic spindle and zona pellucida characteristics as predictors of embryonic development: A preliminary study using PolScope imaging. *Reprod Biomed Online* 2007; 14: 166–74.
149. Madaschi C, Aoki T, de Almeida Ferreira Braga DP et al. Zona pellucida birefringence score and meiotic spindle visualization in relation to embryo development and ICSI outcomes. *Reprod Biomed Online* 2009; 18: 681–6.
150. Wang WH, Meng L, Hackett RJ et al. Rigorous thermal control during intracytoplasmic sperm injection stabilizes the meiotic spindle and improves fertilization and pregnancy rates. *Fertil Steril* 2002; 77: 1274–7.
151. Maro B, Verlhac MH. Polar body formation: New rules for asymmetric divisions. *Nat Cell Biol* 2002; 4: E281–3.
152. Trimarchi JR, Karin RA, Keefe DL. Average spindle retardance observed using the PolScope predicts cell number in day 3 embryos. *Fertil Steril* 2004; 82: S268.
153. Swiatecka J, Bielawski T, Anchim T et al. Oocyte zona pellucida and meiotic spindle birefringence as a biomarker of pregnancy rate outcome in IVF–ICSI treatment. *Ginekol Pol* 2014; 85: 264–71.

154. Korkmaz C, Sakinci M, Bayoglu Tekin Y et al. Do quantitative birefringence characteristics of meiotic spindle and zona pellucida have an impact on implantation in single embryo transfer cycles? *Arch Gynecol Obstet* 2014; 289: 433–8.
155. Aguilar J, Motato Y, Escriba MJ et al. The human first cell cycle: Impact on implantation. *Reprod Biomed Online* 2014; 28: 475–84.
156. Azzarello, A, Hoest, T, Mikkelsen AL et al. The impact of pronuclei morphology and dynamicity on live birth outcome after time-lapse culture. *Hum Reprod* 2012; 27: 2649–57.
157. Alikani M, Palermo G, Adler A et al. Intracytoplasmic sperm injection in dysmorphic human oocytes. *Zygote* 1995; 3: 283–8.
158. De Sutter P, Dozortsev D, Qian C et al. Oocyte morphology does not correlate with fertilization rate and embryo quality after intracytoplasmic sperm injection. *Hum Reprod* 1996; 11: 595–7.
159. Xia P. Intracytoplasmic sperm injection: Correlation of oocyte grade based on polar body, perivitelline space and cytoplasmic inclusions with fertilization rate and embryo quality. *Hum Reprod* 1997; 12: 1750–5.
160. Balaban B, Urman B, Sertac A et al. Oocyte morphology does not affect fertilization rate, embryo quality and implantation rate after intracytoplasmic sperm injection. *Hum Reprod* 1998; 13: 3431–3.
161. Balaban B, Urman B. Effect of oocyte morphology on embryo development and implantation. *Reprod Biomed Online* 2006; 12: 608–15.
162. Ebner T, Yaman C, Moser M et al. Prognostic value of first polar body morphology on fertilization rate and embryo quality in intracytoplasmic sperm injection. *Hum Reprod* 2000; 15: 427–30.
163. Mikkelsen AL, Lindenberg S. Morphology of *in-vitro* matured oocytes: Impact on fertility potential and embryo quality. *Hum Reprod* 2001; 16: 1714–8.
164. Rienzi L, Vajta G, Ubaldi F. Predictive value of oocyte morphology in human IVF: A systematic review of the literature. *Hum Reprod Update* 2011; 17: 34–45.
165. Esfandiari N, Burjaq H, Gotlieb L et al. Brown oocytes: Implications for assisted reproductive technique. *Fertil Steril* 2006; 86: 1522–5.
166. Verlinsky Y, Lerner S, Illkevitch N et al. Is there any predictive value of first polar body morphology for embryo genotype or developmental potential? *Reprod Biomed Online* 2003; 7: 336–41.
167. Chamayou S, Ragolia C, Alecci C et al. Meiotic spindle presence and oocyte morphology do not predict clinical ICSI outcomes: A study of 967 transferred embryos. *Reprod Biomed Online* 2006; 13: 661–7.
168. La Sala GB, Nicoli A, Villani MT et al. The effect of selecting oocytes for insemination and transferring all resultant embryos without selection on outcomes of assisted. *Fertil Steril* 2009; 91: 96–100.
169. Serhal PF, Ranieri DM, Kinis A et al. Oocyte morphology predicts outcome of intracytoplasmic sperm injection. *Hum Reprod* 1997; 12: 1267–70.
170. Ebner T, Moser M, Yaman C et al. Elective transfer of embryos selected on the basis of first polar body morphology is associated with increased rates of implantation and pregnancy. *Fertil Steril* 1999; 72: 599–603.
171. Ciotti PM, Notarangelo L, Morselli-Labate AM et al. First polar body morphology before ICSI is not related to embryo quality or pregnancy rate. *Hum Reprod* 2004; 19: 2334–9.
172. Rienzi L, Ubaldi FM, Iacobelli M et al. Significance of metaphase II human oocyte morphology on ICSI outcome. *Fertil Steril* 2008; 90: 1692–700.
173. Ebner T, Moser M, Sommergruber M et al. First polar body morphology and blastocyst formation rate in ICSI patients. *Hum Reprod* 2002; 17: 2415–8.
174. Navarro PA, de Araujo MM, de Araujo CM et al. Relationship between first polar body morphology before intracytoplasmic sperm injection and fertilization rate, cleavage rate, and embryo quality. *Int J Gynaecol Obstet* 2009; 104: 226–9.
175. Fancsovits P, Tothne ZG, Murber A et al. Correlation between first polar body morphology and further embryo development. *Acta Biol Hung* 2006; 57: 331–8.
176. Ten J, Mendiola J, Vioque J et al. Donor oocyte dysmorphisms and their influence on fertilization and embryo quality. *Reprod Biomed Online* 2007; 14: 40–8.
177. Verlinsky Y, Lerner S, Illkevitch N et al. Is there any predictive value of first polar body morphology for embryo genotype or developmental potential? *Reprod Biomed Online* 2003; 7: 336–41.
178. Verlhac MH, Lefebvre C, Guillaud P et al. Asymmetric division in mouse oocytes: With or without Mos. *Curr Biol* 2000; 10: 1303–6.
179. Ebner T, Yaman C, Moser M et al. A prospective study on oocyte survival rate after ICSI: Influence of injection technique and morphological features. *J Assist Reprod Genet* 2001; 18: 623–8.
180. Plachot M, Selva J, Wolf JP et al. Consequences of oocyte dysmorphy on the fertilization rate and embryo development after intracytoplasmic sperm injection. A prospective multicenter study. *Gynecol Obstet Fertil* 2002; 30: 772–9.
181. Balaban B, Urman B. Embryo culture as a diagnostic tool. *Reprod Biomed Online* 2003; 7: 671–82.
182. Høst E, Gabrielsen A, Lindenberg S et al. Apoptosis in human cumulus cells in relation to zona pellucida thickness variation, maturation stage, and cleavage of the corresponding oocyte after intracytoplasmic sperm injection. *Fertil Steril* 2002; 77: 511–5.
183. Shen Y, Stalf T, Mehnert C et al. High magnitude of light retardation by the zona pellucida is associated with conception cycles. *Hum Reprod* 2005; 20: 1596–606.
184. Serhal PF, Ranieri DM, Kinis A et al. Oocyte morphology predicts outcome of intracytoplasmic sperm injection. *Hum Reprod* 1997;12:1267–70.

185. Meriano JS, Alexis J, Visram-Zaver S et al. Tracking of oocyte dysmorphisms for ICSI patients may prove relevant to the outcome in subsequent patient cycles. *Hum Reprod* 2001; 16: 2118–23.
186. Otsuki J, Okada A, Morimoto K, Nagai Y, Kubo H. The relationship between pregnancy outcome and smooth endoplasmic reticulum clusters in MII human oocytes. *Hum Reprod* 2004; 19: 1591–7.
187. Ebner T, Moser M, Sommergruber M et al. Occurrence and developmental consequences of vacuoles throughout preimplantation development. *Fertil Steril* 2005; 83: 1635–40.
188. Wilding M, Di ML, D'Andretti S et al. An oocyte score for use in assisted reproduction. *J Assist Reprod Genet* 2007; 24: 350–8.
189. Pergament E, Confino E, Zhang JX et al. Recurrent triploidy of maternal origin. *Prenat Diagn* 2000;20:561–3.
190. Balakier H, Bouman D, Sojecki A et al. Morphological and cytogenetic analysis of human giant oocytes and giant embryos. *Hum Reprod* 2002; 17: 2394–401.
191. Otsuki J, Okada A, Morimoto K et al. The relationship between pregnancy outcome and smooth endoplasmic reticulum clusters in MII human oocytes. *Hum Reprod* 2004; 19: 1591–7.
192. Ebner T, Moser M, Shebl O et al. Prognosis of oocytes showing aggregation of smooth endoplasmic reticulum. *Reprod Biomed Online* 2008; 16: 113–8.
193. Akarsu C, Cağlar G, Vicdan K et al. Smooth endoplasmic reticulum aggregations in all retrieved oocytes causing recurrent multiple anomalies: Case report. *Fertil Steril* 2009; 92: 1496–8.
194. Sa′ R, Cunha M, Silva J et al. Ultrastructure of smooth endoplasmic reticulum aggregates in human metaphase II oocytes and clinical implications. *Fertil Steril* 2011; 96: 143–9.
195. Mateizel I, Van Landuyt L, Tournaye H et al. Deliveries of normal healthy babies from embryos originating from oocytes showing the presence of smooth endoplasmic reticulum aggregates. *Hum Reprod* 2013; 28: 2111–7.
196. Shaw-Jackson C, van Beirs N, Thomas A et al. Can healthy babies originate from oocytes with smooth endoplasmic reticulum aggregates? A systematic mini-review. *Hum Reprod* 2014; 29: 1380–6.
197. Scott L, Smith S. The successful use of pronuclear embryo transfers the day following oocyte retrieval. *Hum Reprod* 1998; 13: 1003–13.
198. Tesarik J, Greco E. The probability of abnormal preimplantation development can be predicted by a single static observation on pronuclear stage morphology. *Hum Reprod* 1999; 14: 1318–23.
199. Tesarik J, Junca AM, Hazout A et al. Embryos with high implantation potential after intracytoplasmic sperm injection can be recognized by simple, noninvasive examination of pronuclear morphology. *Hum Reprod* 2000; 15: 1396–9.
200. Scott L, Alvero R, Leondires M et al. The morphology of human pronuclear embryos is positively related to blastocyst development and implantation. *Hum Reprod* 2000; 15: 2394–403.
201. Lukaszuk K, Liss J, Bialobrzeska D et al. Prognostic value of the pronuclear morphology pattern of zygotes for implantation rate. *Ginekol Pol* 2003; 74: 508–13.
202. Senn A, Urner F, Chanson A et al. Morphological scoring of human pronuclear zygotes for prediction of pregnancy outcome. *Hum Reprod* 2006; 21: 234–9.
203. Depa-Martynow M, Jedrzejczak P, Pawelczyk L. Pronuclear scoring as a predictor of embryo quality in *in vitro* fertilization program. *Folia Histochem Cytobiol* 2007; 45(Suppl 1): S85–9.
204. Veeck LL. Preembryo grading and degree of cytoplasmic fragmentation. In: *An Atlas of Human Gametes and Conceptuses*. Veeck LL (ed.). New York, NY and London, U.K.: Parthenon Publishing Group, 1999, pp. 46–50.
205. Fisch JD, Rodriguez H, Ross R et al. The Graduated Embryo Score (GES) predicts blastocyst formation and pregnancy rate from cleavage-stage embryos. *Hum Reprod* 2001; 16: 1970–5.
206. Rienzi L, Ubaldi F, Iacobelli M et al. Significance of morphological attributes of the early embryo. *Reprod Biomed Online* 2005; 10: 669–81.
207. Cutting R, Morrol D, Roberts SA et al. Elective single embryo transfer: Guidelines for practice British Fertility Society and Association of Clinical Embryologists. *Hum Fertil* 2008; 11: 131–46.
208. Pelinck M, Hoek A, Simons AH et al. Embryo quality and impact of specific embryo characteristics on ongoing implantation in unselected embryos derived from modified natural cycle *in vitro* fertilization. *Fertil Steril* 2010; 94: 527–34.
209. Herrero J, Tejera A, Albert C et al. A time to look back: Analysis of morphokinetic characteristics of human embryo development. *Fertil Steril* 2013; 100: 1602–9.
210. Advanced Fertility Center of Chicago. IVF embryo quality and day 3 embryos grading after *in vitro* fertilization, cleavage stage embryo grading. www.advancedfertility.com/embryoquality.htm (2 February, 2014).
211. Gardner DK, Schoolcraft WB. *In vitro* culture of human blastocysts. In: *Toward Reproductive Certainty: Fertility and Genetics Beyond 1999*. Jansen R, Mortimer D (eds). London, U.K.: Parthenon Publishing, 1999: pp. 378–88.
212. Gardner DK, Schoolcraft WB. Culture and transfer of human blastocysts. *Curr Opin Obstet Gynecol* 1999; 11: 307–11.
213. Gardner DK, Surrey E, Minjarez D et al. Single blastocyst transfer: A prospective randomized trial. *Fertil Steril* 2004; 81: 551–5.

214. Santos Filho E, Noble JA, Poli M et al. A method for semi-automatic grading of human blastocyst microscope images. *Hum Reprod* 2012; 27: 2641–8.
215. Richardson A, Brearley S, Ahitan S et al. A clinically useful simplified blastocyst grading system. *Reprod Biomed Online* 2015; 31: 523–30.
216. Nasiri N, Eftekhari-Yazdi P. An overview of the available methods for morphological scoring of preimplantation embryos in *in vitro* fertilization. *Cell J* 2015; 16: 392–405.
217. Lane M, Gardner DK. Selection of viable mouse blastocysts prior to transfer using a metabolic criterion. *Hum Reprod* 1996; 11: 1975–8.
218. Gardner DK. Changes in requirements and utilization of nutrients during mammalian preimplantation embryo development and their significance in embryo culture. *Theriogenology* 1998; 49: 83–102.
219. Conaghan J, Hardy K, Handyside AH et al. Selection criteria for human embryo transfer: A comparison of pyruvate uptake and morphology. *J Assist Reprod Genet* 1993; 10: 21–30.
220. Jones GM, Trounson AO, Vella PJ et al. Glucose metabolism of human morula and blastocyst-stage embryos and its relationship to viability after transfer. *Reprod Biomed Online* 2001; 3: 124–32.
221. Houghton FD, Hawkhead JA, Humpherson PG et al. Non-invasive amino acid turnover predicts human embryo developmental capacity. *Hum Reprod* 2002; 17: 999–1005.
222. Sakkas D, Gardner DK. Noninvasive methods to assess embryo quality. *Curr Opin Obstet Gynecol* 2005; 17: 283–8.
223. Nel-Themaat L, Nagy ZP. A review of the promises and pitfalls of oocyte and embryo metabolomics. *Placenta* 2011; 32(Suppl 3): S257–63.
224. Scott RT, Upham KM, Forman EJ et al. Cleavage-stage biopsy significantly impairs human embryonic implantation potential while blastocyst biopsy does not: A randomized and paired clinical trial. *Fertil Steril* 2013; 100: 624–30.
225. Capalbo A, Rienzi L, Cimadomo D et al. Correlation between standard blastocyst morphology, euploidy and implantation: An observational study in two centers involving 956 screened blastocysts. *Hum Reprod* 2014; 29: 1173–81.
226. Ubaldi FM, Capalbo A, Colamaria S et al. Reduction of multiple pregnancies in the advanced maternal age population after implementation of an elective single embryo transfer policy coupled with enhanced embryo selection: Pre- and post-intervention study. *Hum Reprod* 2015; 30: 2097–106.
227. Wang Q, Sun QY. Evaluation of oocyte quality: Morphological, cellular and molecular predictors. *Reprod Fertil Dev* 2007; 19: 1–12.

Preparation and evaluation of oocytes for intracytoplasmic sperm injection

8

IRIT GRANOT and NAVA DEKEL

INTRODUCTION

Resumption of meiosis in the oocyte is an essential prelude to successful fertilization. The meiotic division of the mammalian oocyte is initiated during fetal life, proceeds up to the diplotene stage of the first prophase, and arrests at birth. Meiotic arrest persists throughout childhood until the onset of puberty. In a sexually mature female, at each cycle one or more oocytes, according to the species, reinitiate the meiotic division. The chromatin in the meiotically arrested oocytes is encapsulated by a nuclear structure known as the germinal vesicle (GV; Figure 8.1a). The GV in oocytes resuming meiosis disappears (Figure 8.1b), the condensed chromosomes align on the newly formed meiotic spindle, and the pairs of homologous chromosomes segregate between the oocyte and the first polar body (Figure 8.1c). Emission of the first polar body, which represents the completion of the first round of meiotic division, is immediately followed by the formation of the second meiotic spindle with the remaining set of homologous chromosomes aligned on its equatorial plate. The whole series of events, initiated by GV breakdown (GVB) and completed at the metaphase of the second round of meiosis (MII), leads to the production of a mature fertilizable oocyte, also known as an egg. The egg is arrested at MII and will complete the meiotic division only after the penetration of the spermatozoon (1). The physiological stimulus for re-initiation of meiosis is provided by the preovulatory surge of luteinizing hormone (LH) (2). Once oocyte maturation is completed, LH further induces ovulation, during which the follicle releases the mature oocyte that is picked up by the infundibular fimbria of the oviduct.

The egg released from the ovarian follicle is accompanied by the cumulus cells. Prior to ovulation, in concomitance with oocyte maturation, the cumulus undergoes characteristic transformations that are also stimulated by LH. In response to this gonadotropin, the cumulus cells produce specific glycosaminoglycans, the secretion of which results in cumulus mucification and its expansion. The major component of the extracellular matrix secreted by the cumulus cells is hyaluronic acid (3–7). The mucified cumulus mass that encapsulates the ovulated egg is penetrated by the spermatozoon that uses enzymes localized on its surface membrane to accomplish this mission. Sperm membrane protein PH-20, which is present on the plasma membrane of sperm cells of many species, such as guinea pigs, mice, macaques, and humans, exhibits hyaluronidase-like activity that facilitates this action (8–11). Furthermore, a later study has demonstrated that a plasma membrane-associated hyaluronidase is localized to the posterior acrosomal region of equine sperm (12).

Having traversed the cumulus, the spermatozoon undergoes acrosome reaction and binds to the zona pellucida. Sperm–zona pellucida binding is mediated by specific sperm surface receptors. The primary ligand on the zona pellucida, ZP3, specifically binds to the plasma membrane of the acrosomal cap of the intact sperm. The secondary zona ligand, ZP2, binds to the inner acrosomal membrane of the spermatozoon (13–15). One of the inner acrosomal membrane sperm receptors was identified as acrosin (16–18). In order to penetrate the zona pellucida, the spermatozoon utilizes enzymatic as well as mechanical mechanisms. Specific enzymes that are released by the acrosome-reacted spermatozoon allow the invasion of the zona pellucida by local degradation of its components (19,20). This enzymatic action is assisted by mechanical force generated by vigorous tail beatings that facilitate the penetration of the sharp sperm head (18–22).

Having penetrated the zona pellucida, the sperm crosses the perivitelline space and its head attaches to the egg's plasma membrane (oolemma). Sperm head attachment to the oolemma is followed by its incorporation into the egg cytoplasm (ooplasm). Sperm incorporation is initiated by phagocytosis of the anterior region of its head followed by fusion of the head's posterior region as well as the tail with the egg membrane (23–25). The scientific efforts that have been invested by reproductive biologists in studying the process of gametogenesis and fertilization in animal models laid the groundwork for the design of *in vitro* procedures for assisted reproduction. These procedures that are successfully practiced at present in human patients essentially attempted to mimic the biological processes *in vivo*.

In vitro fertilization (IVF) regimens of treatment, which are continuously being improved, have allowed the birth of over a million babies all over the world. One such improvement, which represents a major breakthrough in this area, is intracytoplasmic sperm injection (ICSI). Until 1992, most infertility failures originating from a severe male factor were untreatable. Micromanipulation techniques such as partial zona dissection (26–29) and subzonal sperm injection (28,30–34), designed to overcome the poor performance of sperm cells, did not result in a substantial improvement of the rate of success of *in vivo* fertilization. However, ICSI, which was established by the team led by Professor Van Steirteghen at the Free University in Brussels, Belgium, and initially reported by Palermo

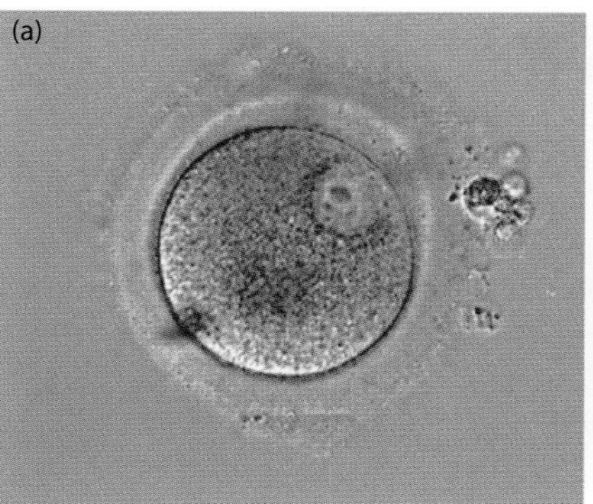

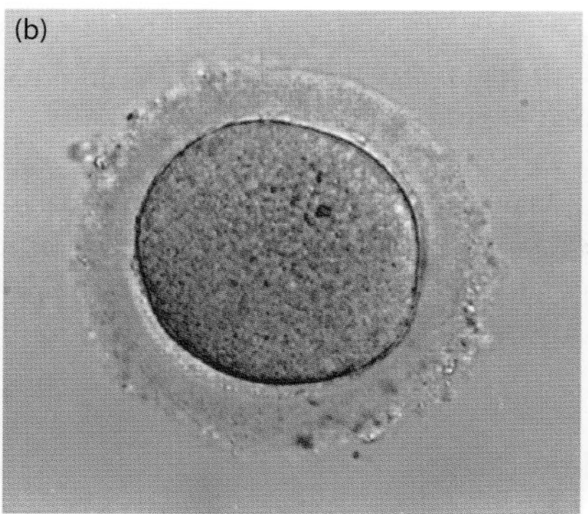

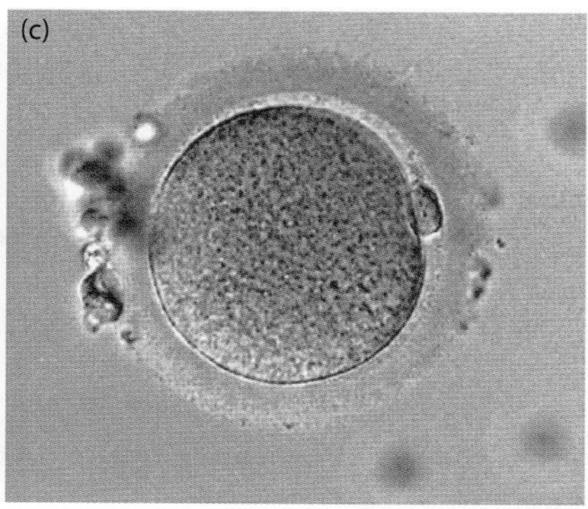

Figure 8.1 Morphological markers characterizing the meiotic status of oocytes. (a) Immature germinal vesicle (GV) oocyte: meiosis has not been reinitiated and the typical nuclear structure is visible. (b) Immature GV breakdown oocyte (metaphase I [MI]): meiosis has been reinitiated, the GV has disappeared, but the first polar body is still absent. (c) Mature oocyte (MII): the GV has disappeared and the first polar body has been extruded.

et al. (34), has generated dramatic progress (35–38). The ICSI procedure involves the injection of a single sperm cell intracytoplasmically into an egg. Fertility failures associated with an extremely low sperm count were found to be successfully treated by this technique. Furthermore, as the sperm is microinjected into the ooplasma, it bypasses the passage through the zona pellucida and is not required to interact with the oolemma. Therefore, infertility problems that originate from faulty sperm–egg interaction may also be resolved by this IVF protocol of treatment.

HANDLING OF OOCYTES

Similar to conventional IVF, patients for ICSI undergo programmed induction of superovulation followed by scheduled oocyte retrieval (Chapter 7). Under all protocols of treatment, identification of the cumulus–oocyte complexes and evaluation of their maturity are carried out immediately after follicle aspiration, as described in Chapter 7. However, unlike conventional IVF, in which intact mature cumulus–oocyte complexes are inseminated, cumulus cells that surround the eggs are removed before microinjection.

Denudation of the mature oocytes is an essential prerequisite for ICSI. Cumulus cells may block the injecting needle, thus interfering with oocyte microinjection. Furthermore, in the presence of the cumulus, visualization of the egg is very limited. Since only mature oocytes that have reached MII are suitable for ICSI, optimal optical conditions that allow the assessment of the meiotic status of the oocytes are required. Oocyte maturation is determined morphologically by the absence of the GV and the presence of the first polar body. Good optical conditions are also necessary for the positioning of the mature oocyte in the right orientation for injection (Chapter 13). Preparation of the retrieved mature oocytes for ICSI should be carried out under conditions of constant pH of 7.3 and a stable temperature of 37°C. In order to maintain the appropriate pH, 4-(2-hydroxyet4hyl)-1-piperazineethane sulfonic acid (HEPES)-buffered culture media are used. The correct temperature is maintained during egg handling by the use of a microscope equipped with a heated stage. Most of the procedures are performed under Earle's balanced salts solution-treated and CO_2-equilibrated paraffin/mineral oil that prevents evaporation of the medium and minimizes the fluctuations of both the pH and the temperature.

Temperature fluctuations that are likely to accompany the handling of eggs have been shown to be specifically detrimental for the microtubular system. Changes in spindle organization were observed in human mature oocytes cooled to room temperature for only 10 minutes. These changes included a reduction in spindle size, disorganization of microtubules within the spindle, and, in some cases, even a complete absence of microtubules (39,40). The susceptibility of the microtubules to temperature variations has been also shown in mature mouse oocytes (41). Interference with spindle organization can disturb the faithful segregation of the chromosomes, resulting in aneuploidy.

LABORATORY PROCEDURES

Removal of the surrounding cumulus cells is accomplished by combined enzymatic and mechanical treatment carried out under a stereoscopic dissecting microscope. A preincubation period of at least three hours between oocyte retrieval and removal of the cumulus cells was recommended by one study (42). This recommendation was challenged by other studies, which did not demonstrate differences in ICSI outcomes that correlated with the time interval between egg aspiration and microinjection (43,44). On the other hand, preincubation time that exceeded nine hours resulted in embryos of lower quality (43). Garor et al. (45) have recently demonstrated that it is not the time of oocyte denudation and injection that determines the ICSI outcome, but in fact the time interval between human chorionic gonadotropin (hCG) administration and oocyte pickup (OPU). Specifically, fertilization as well as pregnancy rates were significantly higher in

IVF cycles in which the hCG–OPU interval exceeded 36 hours, regardless of the time of oocyte handling (45). Since oocyte denudation cannot be carried out before some preliminary laboratory preparations that are described below are completed, a preincubation period of at least one hour is unavoidable. During this period, the retrieved mature cumulus–oocyte complexes are kept in the incubator at 37°C with 5%–6% CO_2 according to the recommendations of the culture media manufacturer.

Preliminary preparations for oocyte denudation

Injecting dish

A special shallow Falcon dish (type 1006) is used for placing the denuded eggs. Nine small droplets of MOPS (3-(*N*-morpholino)propanesulfonic acid)-HEPES-buffered human tubal fluid culture media (MHM, Irvine Scientific, CA, USA), containing 10% synthetic serum, 5 μL each, are arranged in a square of 3 × 3 within this dish. An additional 10th droplet serves for orientation. The middle droplet, in which the sperm will be placed, contains 7%–10% polyvinylpyrrolidone (PVP). The droplets are then covered with either paraffin or mineral oil, and the dish is placed on the heated area in the hood to warm up before removal of the cumulus cells.

Enzymatic solution

Since hyaluronic acid is a major component of the mucified cumulus mass that surrounds the mature oocyte, hyaluronidase is employed for enzymatic removal of these cells (80 IU/mL; Sage In-Vitro Fertilization, Inc., Trumbull, CT). The high concentration of 760 IU/mL of hyaluronidase that was used initially (46) was found to induce parthenogenetic activation of the mature oocytes. A lower concentration of the enzyme, such as 80 IU/mL, which is commonly used, significantly decreased the rate of parthenogenesis (47). According to our experience, hyaluronidase at a concentration of 60 IU/mL effectively denudes the oocytes. Further reduction of the enzyme concentration to as low as 10 IU/mL was also found to be sufficient (48).

Denuding dish

A drop of 100 μL of hyaluronidase solution and five 100 μL drops of MHM containing 10% serum covered with oil are placed in a culture dish and placed on the heated area in the hood to warm up. In order to maintain the drops at 37°C, the temperature in the working areas (hood and microscope) must be calibrated to a higher temperature (around 38°C).

Removal of the cumulus cells

Cumulus–oocyte complexes are transferred into the drop of hyaluronidase solution and repeatedly aspirated through a Pasteur pipette for up to 30–40 seconds. At this time, dissociation of the cells is initially observed. Further mechanical denudation is carried out in the enzyme-free MHM drops by repeated aspiration through commercially prepared stripper tips with decreasing inner diameters of 170–140 μM and, when necessary, 135 μM. The oocytes are then transferred through the drops of medium, until all coronal cells have been finally removed and all traces of enzyme have been washed off. This procedure is carried out very gently in order to avoid mechanical damage to the oocytes. Pricking of the oocyte has been shown to induce parthenogenetic activation (49,50). Finally, the denuded oocytes are placed in the droplets of the injecting dish and their morphology and meiotic status are evaluated. These procedures are performed on the heated area in the hood.

In cases of extremely low sperm count or testicular sperm injection, oocytes must be kept in the incubator in CO_2-equilibrated culture medium until a sufficient number of sperm cells have been collected.

Evaluation of denuded oocytes for ICSI

Oocytes are assessed for their maturation and for their morphology under an inverted microscope equipped with Nomarski differential interference contrast optics at 200× magnification. It is commonly accepted that only mature oocytes that resume their first meiotic division, reaching MII, are appropriate for ICSI. Evaluation of the meiotic status of the oocyte is based on morphological markers. In mature oocytes, the GV has disappeared and the first polar body is present and localized in the perivitelline space (Figure 8.1c).

Several studies have reported that 10%–12% of the retrieved oocytes have not resumed their meiotic division (51–54). These oocytes can be divided into two categories: first, GV oocytes in which meiosis has not been reinitiated and the typical nuclear structure is visible (Figure 8.1a); and second, GVB oocytes in which meiosis has been reinitiated but did not proceed beyond the first metaphase (MI). In these oocytes, the GV has disappeared but the first polar body has not been extruded (Figure 8.1b). Oocytes in both of these categories are separated from the MII oocytes. MI oocytes are further incubated and those that extrude the first polar body within two to four hours are inseminated by ICSI (55). It has been reported that 74% of the MI oocytes completed meiosis *in vitro* within 20 hours after retrieval. This report did not find differences in the rates of fertilization and embryo development between these oocytes and other oocytes retrieved at MII. However, only sporadic pregnancies were achieved following the transfer of embryos obtained from fertilized MI oocytes that had matured *in vitro* (56,57). Another study demonstrated that 26.7% of MI oocytes extruded the first polar body *in vitro* within four hours. These oocytes were injected on the same day of follicle aspiration in parallel to the oocytes retrieved at MII. In this study, however, the MI oocytes that completed their maturation *in vitro* exhibited a lower fertilization rate, but again no differences were observed in embryo quality between oocytes that underwent maturation *in vitro* and those retrieved at MII. Similarly to the previous study, only sporadic pregnancies were obtained following transfer of embryos developed from MI oocytes that had matured *in vitro* (57,58). More recent studies support these observations, showing that although *in vitro*-matured (IVM) MI oocytes can be normally fertilized, the embryos derived from these oocytes rarely provide pregnancies (59,60). This is compatible with the findings that these embryos exhibit low morphological quality and a high rate of chromosomal abnormalities (54). In patients with few MII oocytes, rescue of MI oocytes may increase the number of embryos for transfer; however, the chance of improving pregnancy rates by this procedure is minimal. Oocytes with GV require an overnight (30-hour) incubation in order to reach the MII stage. Only sporadic pregnancies were reported from oocytes that were at the GV stage when retrieved during standard IVF treatment with controlled ovarian hyperstimulation (58,59,61). Because of the poor results, these GV oocytes are usually discarded. Only in cases in which very few or no MII oocytes are retrieved are the GV oocytes rescued for fertilization, provided they complete their maturation. Immature GV oocytes can also be retrieved from the small (3–13 mm) ovarian follicles present in unstimulated patients (62–65). Although these oocytes were not exposed to LH *in vivo*, they are apparently meiotically competent and can be expected to mature spontaneously *in vitro* and produce normal eggs. In 1998, Goud et al. showed a fertilization rate of 46% by ICSI of such IVM GV oocytes (65), resulting in a few pregnancies. However, as more experience is gained in handling immature oocytes, success rates are increasing worldwide (66,67). Recent studies demonstrated that hCG administration before oocyte retrieval from the small follicles accelerates their *in vitro* maturation, resulting in better embryonic development and leading to higher pregnancy rates. It was further demonstrated that administration of low doses of follicle-stimulating hormone (FSH) before hCG priming enables the retrieval of IVM oocytes (MII) from the small follicles (<10 mm). Such oocytes have a higher potential to develop into good-quality embryos than IVM oocytes, achieving even higher pregnancy rates (68). In addition to the meiotic status, the morphology of the oocytes is also evaluated before ICSI. The various morphological defects may be manifested by an amorphic shape of the oocyte, enlargement of or granularity in the perivitelline space, inclusions, vacuolization, granularity, and dark color of the cytoplasm, changes in the color and construction of the zona pellucida, and changes in the shape and size of the polar body (Figure 8.2). Most defective oocytes exhibit more than one of the above-mentioned abnormalities. All these observations should be recorded and may help in later analysis of the fertilization rate, embryo development, and pregnancy outcomes after ICSI. The correlations between egg morphology and the rates of fertilization, embryo quality, and pregnancy after ICSI have been extensively studied. Most of the studies reported that abnormal egg morphologies of patients undergoing ICSI are associated with a lower rate of fertilization, embryos of poor quality, and, consequently, a lower rate of successful pregnancy (69–71). Other studies demonstrated successful

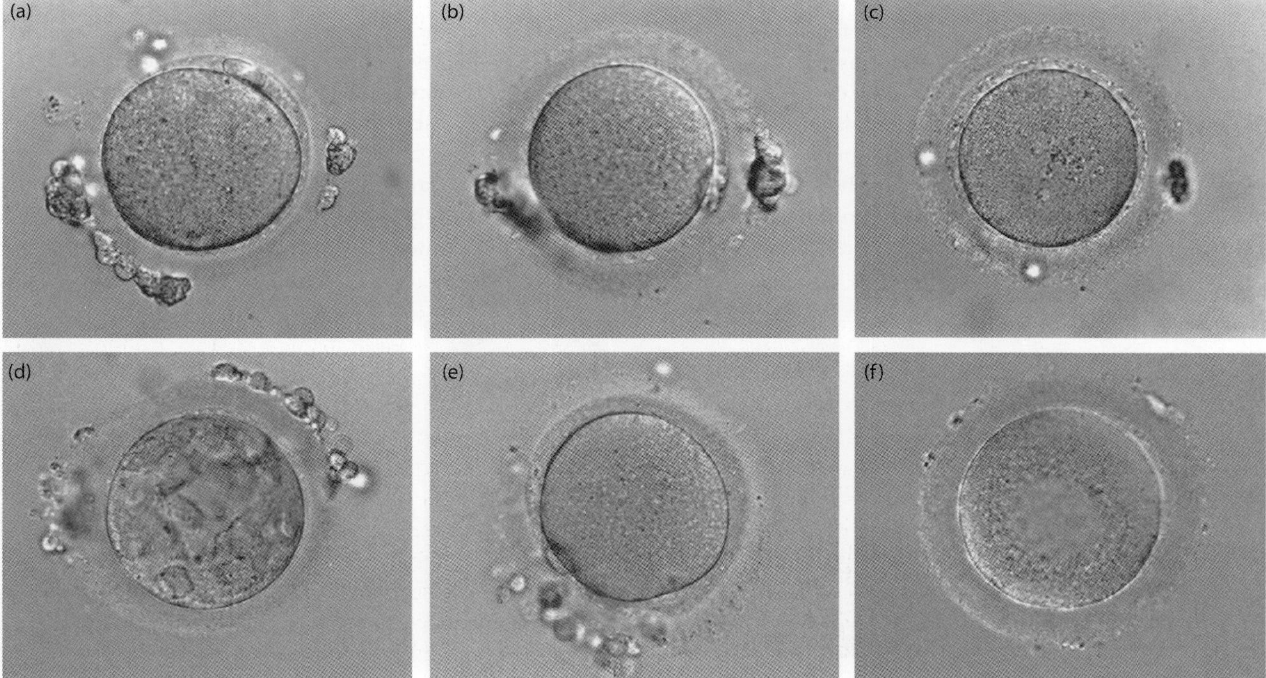

Figure 8.2 Various morphological abnormalities exhibited by oocytes. (a) Granulated perivitelline space; (b) a fragmented polar body; (c) thickened and dark-colored zona pellucida; (d) cytoplasmic inclusions; (e) enlarged and granulated perivitelline space; and (f) a large cytoplasmic vacuole.

fertilization and normal early embryo development in microinjected eggs with defective morphologies, such as large perivitelline space, cytoplasmic vacuoles, or a fragmented polar body (72–75). However, the transfer of these seemingly normal embryos resulted in a poor implantation rate (71) and a high incidence of early pregnancy loss (73). This controversy may be partially attributed to the absence of standard criteria for evaluation of oocyte morphology. To overcome this confusion, the use of triple markers, namely polar body, size of the perivitelline space, and cytoplasmic inclusions, has been suggested by Xia for human oocyte grading (70). This laboratory reported that the evaluation of oocyte quality based on these criteria correlated well with the rate of fertilization and with embryo quality after ICSI.

As mentioned previously in this chapter, the integrity of the meiotic spindle in MII oocytes is crucial for fertilization capacity and embryo development. Therefore, in addition to the above-mentioned features of the oocyte, the morphology of the spindle may serve as a reliable marker for predicting its potential for normal fertilization and embryonic development (76). A modification of the polarized light microscope, "PolScope" equipped with novel image-processing software (77) has emerged as a noninvasive tool to view the meiotic spindle in living oocytes and is being used in several IVF units worldwide (40,76,78,79). The image of the spindle is based on the highly birefringent characteristic of the microtubule filaments under a polarization microscope. The obvious advantage of the PolScope over conventional techniques such as immunocytochemistry and electron microscopy is that through a PolScope one can view the spindle in a living oocyte. Use of the PolScope for examination of human oocytes has indeed demonstrated that the absence or abnormal morphology of the spindle is highly correlated with lower fertilization rates and impaired embryonic development (78–80). Furthermore, spindle assessment with the PolScope has been shown to facilitate the selection of embryos with high implantation potential for transfer (76). In most MII oocytes, the second meiotic spindle is adjacent to the first polar body (Figure 8.3b), making the first polar body a marker for appropriate orientation of the ICSI micropipette to avoid interference with chromosome alignment. However, observations by Silva et al. (78) and ourselves that the meiotic spindle is not always adjacent to the polar body (Figure 8.3c) have made use of the PolScope even more valuable. Furthermore, in those oocytes that have not yet completed the formation of the first polar body, the PolScope can detect the presence of microtubules in the mid-body, suggesting that the second meiotic spindle has not yet been fully organized (Figure 8.3a). These oocytes are considered suitable for ICSI, having high potential for developing into an embryo. Appropriate ovarian stimulation protocols normally provide functional, fertilizable mature oocytes, while oocytes of poor quality may represent a disturbed hormonal balance. For example, exposure to high dosage of human menopausal gonadotropin (hMG) has been shown to be associated with granularity of the perivitelline space (53). Moreover, an extended exposure to high doses of this hormone may lead to the senescence of the mature oocyte before retrieval. As previously mentioned, oocyte maturation and ovulation are both stimulated by LH. However, studies have shown that the ovulatory response is less sensitive to this gonadotropin, requiring higher concentrations of the hormone (81). Therefore, the relatively high concentration of LH in hMG effectively promotes oocyte maturation, but is insufficient to stimulate ovulation. Delayed administration of hCG in these patients entraps the mature oocytes in the follicle, leading to oocyte aging. One notable morphological marker in this case is the fragmentation of the first polar body (82). The presence of aged oocytes can also explain the decreased quality of oocytes and lower fertilization rate in polycystic ovarian syndrome patients (83) who exhibit relatively high serum concentrations of LH throughout their menstrual cycle (84). Nowadays, pure FSH preparations (recombinant FSH) are widely used for the stimulation of follicular growth and development. However, it has been demonstrated that introducing low concentrations

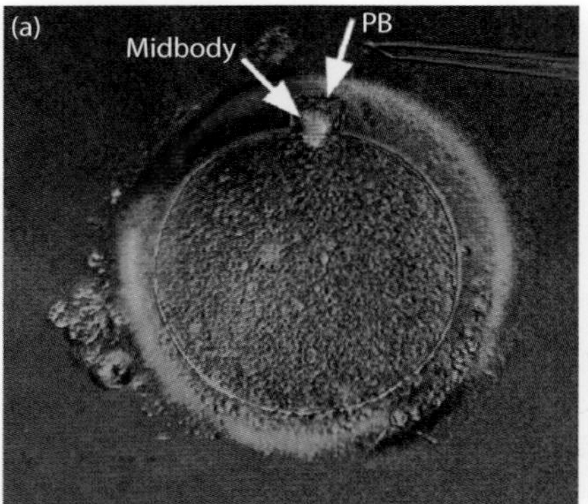

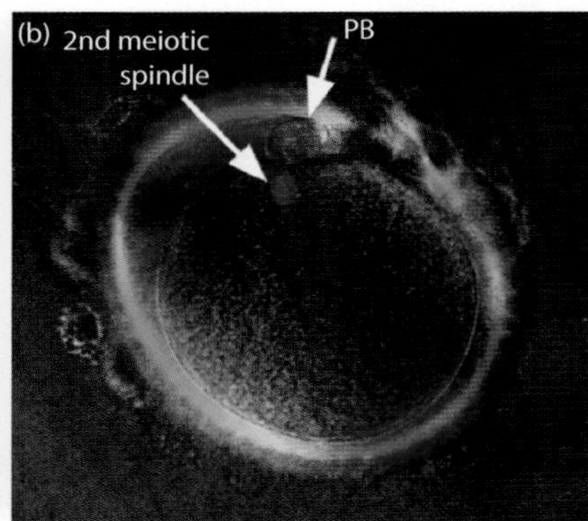

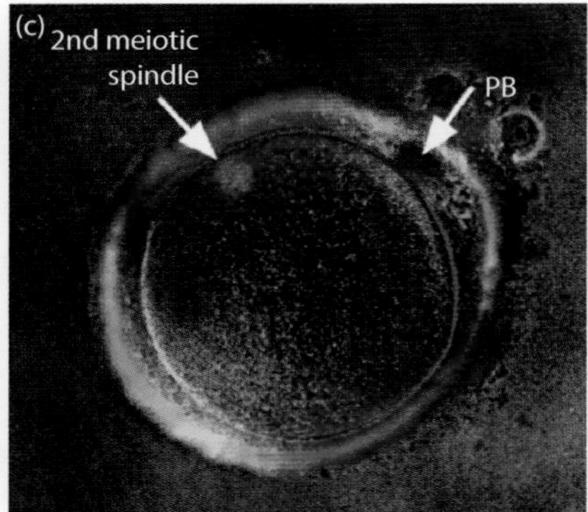

Figure 8.3 Microtubule images in metaphase II (MII) human oocytes. (a) Microtubules of the mid-body extending from the cytoplasm into the first polar body (PB). (b) Microtubules of the second meiotic spindle located adjacent to the PB. (c) Microtubules of the second meiotic spindle at a distal location from the PB.

of LH (recombinant LH) in addition to FSH significantly improves IVF outcomes (85).

EPILOGUE

A baby girl is born with her ovaries containing about 2 million oocytes, all of which arrested at the prophase of the first meiotic division. This pool of oocytes remains dormant throughout childhood until the onset of puberty. In sexually mature females, at each cycle, one such "sleeping beauty" is kissed by the LH "prince" and awakened to continue its meiotic division. Once maturation has been completed, the oocyte is released from the ovarian follicle into the fallopian tube, a site at which it will eventually meet the spermatozoon and undergo fertilization. Hormonal stimulation protocols are designed to mimic the natural events that lead to the production of mature oocytes. In IVF patients, these oocytes are aspirated from the ovarian follicles prior to ovulation and allowed to meet the sperm cells in the Petri dish. A higher scale of assistance, designed to overcome the poor performance of spermatozoa, is offered by ICSI. The information regarding oocyte handling for this later modification of the classical IVF protocol has been summarized in this chapter.

APPENDIX

Laboratory protocol

The following protocol is used in our laboratory.

Preliminary preparations for oocyte denudation

1. Injecting dish: the droplets may be placed on the dish in any arrangement the laboratory prefers. Our laboratory recommends the following layout. Place nine droplets, 5 μL each, of MHM containing 10% serum, arranged in a 3 × 3 square within a shallow Falcon dish (type 1006). Place one additional droplet for orientation. Cover with oil. Replace 4 μL of the middle droplet with a solution of 7%–10% PVP where the sperm will be placed. Place the dish on the heated area in the hood to warm up. In cases of extremely low sperm counts, MHM as well as more than one PVP droplet can be used for sperm.
2. Enzymatic solution: dilute hyaluronidase solution of 80 IU/mL (Sage) with MHM containing 10% serum to obtain a final concentration of 60 IU/mL and warm to 37°C.
3. Denuding dish: place a drop of 100 μL of the above hyaluronidase solution and five 100 μL drops of enzyme-free MHM containing 10% serum in a culture dish. Cover with oil and place on the heated area in the hood to warm up.
4. Prepare stripper tips with inner diameters of 170 and 140 μM.

Removal of the cumulus cells

1. Place the cumulus–oocyte complexes into the drop of the hyaluronidase solution (up to five complexes at a time) and aspirate repeatedly through a Pasteur pipette for up to 40 seconds.
2. Transfer the cumulus–oocyte complexes to a drop of enzyme-free MHM containing 10% serum and aspirate repeatedly through a 170 μM diameter stripper tip. Continue aspirating with a 140 μM tip while passing the oocytes through the other four drops of the medium, until all coronal cells have been totally removed.
3. Transfer the denuded oocytes to the MHM droplets in the injecting dish, one in each droplet.

Microscopic evaluation

1. Place the injecting dish containing the oocytes on the heated stage of an inverted microscope equipped with differential interference contrast.
2. Evaluate oocyte morphology and meiotic status at 200× magnification.

REFERENCES

1. Dekel N, Aberdam E, Goren S, Feldman B, Shalgi R. Mechanism of action of GnRH-induced oocyte maturation. *J Reprod Fert* 1989; 37: 319–27.
2. Lindner HR, Tsafriri A, Lieberman ME et al. Gonadotropin action on cultured Graafian follicles: Induction of maturation division of the mammalian oocyte and differentiation of the luteal cell. *Recent Prog Horm Res* 1974; 30: 79–138.
3. Dekel N. Hormonal control of ovulation. In: *Biochemical Action of Hormones*. Litwack G (ed.). Orlando, FL: Academic Press, 1986; pp. 57–90.
4. Buccione R, Vanderhyden BC, Caron PJ, Eppig JJ. FSH induced expansion of the mouse cumulus oophorus *in vitro* is dependent upon a specific factor(s) secreted by the oocyte. *Dev Biol* 1990; 138: 16–25.
5. Salustri A, Yanagishita M, Hascall VC. Mouse oocytes regulate hyaluronic acid synthesis and mucification by FSH-stimulated cumulus cells. *Dev Biol* 1990; 138: 26–32.
6. Vanderhyden BC, Caron PJ, Buccione R, Eppig JJ. Developmental pattern of the secretion of cumulus expansion-enabling factor by mouse oocytes and the role of oocytes in promoting granulosa cell differentiation. *Dev Biol* 1990; 140: 307–17.
7. Vanderhyden BC. Species differences in the regulation of cumulus expansion by an oocyte secreted factor(s). *J Reprod Fertil* 1993; 98: 219–27.
8. Lin Y, Mahan K, Lathorp W, Myles D, Primakoff P. A hyaluronidase activity of the sperm plasma membrane protein PH-20 enables sperm to penetrate the cumulus cell layer surrounding the egg. *J Cell Biol* 1994; 125: 1157–63.
9. Cherr G, Meyers S, Yudin A et al. The PH-20 protein in cynomologus macaque spermatozoa: Identification of two different forms exhibiting hyaluronidase activity. *Dev Biol* 1996; 175: 142–53.
10. Oversreet J, Lin Y, Yudin A et al. Location of the PH-20 protein on acrosome-intact and acrosome-reacted spermatozoa of cynomologus macaques. *Biol Reprod* 1995; 52: 105–14.

11. Sabeur K, Cherr G, Yudin A et al. The PH-20 protein in human spermatozoa. *J Androl* 1997; 18: 151–8.
12. Meyers SA, Rosenberger AE. A plasma membrane-associated hyaluronidase is localized to the posterior acrosomal region of stallion sperm and is associated with spermatozoal function. *Biol Reprod* 1999; 61: 444–51.
13. Bleil JD, Wasserman PM. Autoradiographic visualization of the mouse egg's sperm receptor bound to sperm. *J Cell Biol* 1986; 102: 1363–71.
14. Beaver EL, Friend DS. Morphology of mammalian sperm membranes during differentiation, maturation, and capacitation. *J Electr Microscop Tech* 1990; 16: 281–97.
15. Mortillo S, Wasserman PM. Differential binding of gold-labeled zona pellucid glycoproteins mZP2 and mZP3 to mouse sperm membrane compartments. *Development* 1991; 113: 141–9.
16. Jones R. Interaction of zona pellucida glycoproteins, sulphated carbohydrates and synthetic polymers with proacrosin, the putative egg-binding protein from mammalian spermatozoa. *Development* 1991; 111: 1155–63.
17. Urch UA, Patel H. The interaction of boar sperm proacrosin with its natural substrate, the zona pellucida, and with polysulphated polysaccharides. *Development* 1991; 111: 1165–72.
18. Yanagimachi R. *Fertilization and Embryonic Development In Vitro*. New York, NY: Plenum Press, 1981.
19. Brown CR, Cheng WTK. Limited proteolysis of the porcine zona pellucida by homologous sperm acrosin. *J Reprod Fertil* 1985; 74: 257–60.
20. Dunbar BS, Prasad SV, Timmons TM. *Comparative Overview of Mammalian Fertilization*. New York, NY: Plenum Press, 1991.
21. Dunbar BS, Budkiewicz AB, Bundman DS. Proteolysis of specific porcine zona pellucida glycoproteins by boar acrosin. *Biol Reprod* 1985; 32: 619–30.
22. Yanagimachi R. Time and process of sperm penetration into hamster ova *in vivo* and *in vitro*. *J Reprod Fertil* 1966; 11: 359–70.
23. Phillips DM, Shalgi RM. Sperm penetration into rat ova fertilized *in vivo*. *J Exp Zool* 1982; 221: 373–8.
24. Shalgi R, Phillips D. Mechanics of sperm entry in cycling hamsters. *J Ultrastruct Res* 1980; 71: 154–61.
25. Shalgi R, Phillips DM, Jones R. Status of the rat acrosome during sperm–zona pellucida interactions. *Gamete Res* 1989; 22: 1–13.
26. Cohen J, Malter H, Fehilly C et al. Implantation of embryos after partial opening of oocyte zonal pellucid to facilitate sperm penetration. *Lancet* 1988; 2: 162.
27. Cohen J, Malter H, Wright G et al. Partial zona dissection of human oocytes when failure of zona pellucida is anticipated. *Hum Reprod* 1989; 4: 435–42.
28. Cohen J, Talanski BE, Malter HM et al. Microsurgical fertilization and teratozoospermia. *Hum Reprod* 1991; 6: 118–23.
29. Tucker MJ, Bishop FM, Cohen J et al. Routine application of partial zona dissection for male factor infertility. *Hum Reprod* 1991; 6: 676–81.
30. Laws-King A, Trounson A, Sathananthan H et al. Fertilization of human oocytes by microinjection of single spermatozoon under zona pellucida. *Fertil Steril* 1987; 48: 637–42.
31. Ng SC, Bongso A, Ratnam SS et al. Pregnancy after transfer sperm under zona. *Lancet* 1988; 2: 790.
32. Bongso TA, Sathananthan AH, Wong C et al. Human fertilization by microinjection of immotile spermatozoa. *Hum Reprod* 1989; 4: 175–9.
33. Palermo G, Joris H, Devoroey P et al. Induction of acrosome reaction in human spermatozoa used subzonal insemination. *Hum Reprod* 1992; 7: 248–54.
34. Palermo G, Joris H, Devoroey P et al. Pregnancies after intracytoplasmic injection of a single spermatozoon into an oocyte. *Lancet* 1992; 340: 17–8.
35. Palermo G, Joris H, Devoroey P et al. Sperm characteristics and outcome of human assisted fertilization by subzonal insemination and intracytoplasmic sperm injection. *Fertil Steril* 1993; 59: 826–35.
36. Van Steirteghem AC, Liu J, Nagy Z et al. Use of assisted fertilization. *Hum Reprod* 1993; 8: 1784–5.
37. Van Steirteghem AC, Liu J, Joris H et al. Higher success rate by intracytoplasmic sperm injection than by subzonal insemination. Report of second series of 300 consecutive treatment cycles. *Hum Reprod* 1993; 8: 1055–60.
38. Van Steirteghem AC, Nagy Z, Joris H et al. High fertilization and implantation rates after intracytoplasmic sperm injection. *Hum Reprod* 1993; 8: 1061–6.
39. Pickering SJ, Braude PR, Johnson MH, Cant A, Currie J. Transient cooling to room temperature can cause irreversible disruption of the meiotic spindle in the human oocyte. *Fertil Steril* 1990; 54: 102–8.
40. Wang WH, Meng L, Hackett RJ, Odenbourg R, Keefe DL. Limited recovery of meiotic spindle in living human oocytes after cooling–rewarming observed using polarized microscopy. *Hum Reprod* 2001; 16: 2374–8.
41. Magistrini M, Szollosi D. Effects of cold and isopropyl-N-phenylcarbamate on the second meiotic spindle of mouse oocytes. *Eur J Cell Biol* 1980; 22: 699–707.
42. Rienzi L, Ubaldi F, Anniballo R, Cerulo G, Greco E. Preincubation of human oocytes may improve fertilization and embryo quality after intracytoplasmic sperm injection. *Hum Reprod* 1998; 13: 1014–9.
43. Yanagida K, Yazawa H, Katayose H et al. Influence of preincubation time on fertilization after intracytoplasmic sperm injection. *Hum Reprod* 1998; 13: 2223–6.
44. Van de Velde H, De Vos A, Joris H, Nagy ZP, Van Steirteghem AC. Effect of timing of oocyte denudation and micro-injection on survival, fertilization and embryo quality after intracytoplasmic sperm injection. *Hum Reprod* 1998; 13: 3160–4.

45. Garor R, Shufaro Y, Kotler N, Shefer, D, Krasilnikov N, Ben-Haroush A, Pinkas H, Fisch B, Sapir O. Prolonging oocyte *in vitro* culture and handling time does not compensate for a shorter interval from human chorionic gonadotropin administration to oocyte pickup. *Fertil Steril* 2015; 103: 72–5.
46. Palermo G, Joris H, Derde MP et al. Sperm characteristics and outcome of human assisted fertilization by subzonal insemination and intracytoplasmic sperm injection. *Fertil Steril* 1993; 59: 826–35.
47. Joris H, Nagy Z, Van de Velde H, De Vos A, Van Steirteghem A. Intracytoplasmic sperm injection: Laboratory set-up and injection procedure. *Hum Reprod* 1998; 13(Suppl 1): 76–86.
48. Van de Velde H, Nagy ZP, Joris H, De Vos A, Van Steirteghem AC. Effects of different hyaluronidase concentrations and mechanical procedures for cumulus cell removal on the outcome of intracytoplasmic sperm injection. *Hum Reprod* 1997; 12: 2246–50.
49. Iritani A. Micromanipulation of gametes for *in vitro* assisted fertilization. *Mol Reprod Dev* 1991; 28: 199–207.
50. Flaherty SP, Payne D, Swann NG et al. Aetiology of failed and abnormal fertilization after intracytoplasmic sperm injection. *Hum Reprod* 1995; 10: 2629–32.
51. Junca AM, Mandelbaum J, Belaisch-Allert J et al. Oocyte maturity and quality: Value of intracytoplasmic sperm injection. Fertility of microinjected oocytes after *in vitro* maturation. *Contracept Fertil Sex* 1995; 23: 463–645.
52. Mandelbaum J, Junca AM, Balaisch-Allert J et al. Oocyte maturation and intracytoplasmic sperm injection. *Contracept Fertil Sex* 1996; 24: 534–8.
53. Hassan-Ali H, Hisham-Saleh A, El-Gezeiry D et al. Perivitelline space granularity: A sign of human menopausal gonadotropin overdose in intracytoplasmic sperm injection. *Hum Reprod* 1998; 13: 4325–30.
54. De Vos A, Van de Velde H, Joris H, Van Steirteghem A. In-vitro matured metaphase-I oocytes have a lower fertilization rate but similar embryo quality as mature metaphase-II oocytes after intracytoplasmic sperm injection. *Hum Reprod* 1999; 14: 1859–63.
55. Strassburger D, Goldstein A, Friedler S et al. The cytogenetic constitution of embryos derived from immature (metaphase I) oocytes obtained after ovarian hyperstimulation. *Fertil Steril* 2010; 94: 971–8.
56. Coetzee K, Windt ML. Fertilization and pregnancy using metaphase I oocytes in an intracytoplasmic sperm injection program. *J Assist Reprod Genet* 1996; 13: 768–71.
57. Strassburger D, Friedler S, Raziel A et al. The outcome of ICSI of immature MI oocytes and rescued *in vitro* matured MII oocytes. *Hum Reprod* 2004; 19: 1587–90.
58. Nagy ZP, Cecile J, Liu J et al. Pregnancy and birth after intracytoplasmic sperm injection of *in vitro* matured germinal-vesicle stage oocytes: Case report. *Fertil Steril* 1996; 65: 1047–50.
59. Jaroudi KA, Hollanders JMG, Sieck UV et al. Pregnancy after transfer of embryos which were generated from *in-vitro* matured oocytes. *Hum Reprod* 1997; 12: 857–9.
60. Liu J, Katz E, Garcia JE et al. Successful *in vitro* maturation of human oocytes not exposed to human chorionic gonadotropin during ovulation induction, resulting in pregnancy. *Fertil Steril* 1997; 67: 566–8.
61. Menezo YJ, Nicollet B, Rollet J, Hazout A. Pregnancy and delivery after *in vitro* maturation of naked ICSI-GV oocytes with GH and transfer of a frozen thawed blastocyst: Case report. *J Assist Reprod Genet* 2006; 23: 47–9.
62. Edrishinghe WR, Junk SM, Matson PL, Yovich JL. Birth from cryopreserved embryos following *in-vitro* maturation of oocytes and intracytoplasmic sperm injection. *Hum Reprod* 1997; 12: 1056–8.
63. Trounson A, Anderiesz C, Jones GM et al. Oocyte maturation. *Hum Reprod* 1998; 13(Suppl 3): 52–62; discussion 71–5.
64. Russel JB. Immature oocyte retrieval with *in-vitro* maturation. *Curr Opin Obstet Gynecol* 1999; 11: 289–96.
65. Goud PT, Goud AP, Qian C et al. *In-vitro* maturation of human germinal vesicle stage oocytes: Role of cumulus cells and epidermal growth factor in the culture medium. *Hum Reprod* 1998; 13: 1638–44.
66. Mikkelsen AL. Strategies in human *in-vitro* maturation and their clinical outcome. *Reprod Biomed Online* 2005; 10: 593–9.
67. Al-Sunaidi M, Tulandi T, Holzer H et al. Repeated pregnancies and live births after *in vitro* maturation treatment. *Fertil Steril* 2007; 87: 1212.e9-12.
68. Weon-Young S, Seang LT. Laboratory and embryological aspect of hCG-primed *in vitro* maturation cycles for patients with polycystic ovaries. *Hum Reprod* 2010; 6: 675–89.
69. Sousa M, Tesarik J. Ultrastructural analysis of fertilization failure after intracytoplasmic sperm injection. *Hum Reprod* 1994; 9: 2374–80.
70. Xia P. Intracytoplasmic sperm injection: Correlation of oocyte grade based on polar body, perivitelline space and cytoplasmic inclusions with fertilization rate and embryo quality. *Hum Reprod* 1997; 12: 1750–5.
71. Loutradis D, Drakakis P, Kallianidis K et al. Oocyte morphology correlates with embryo quality and pregnancy rate after intracytoplasmic sperm injection. *Fertil Steril* 1999; 72: 240–4.
72. De Sutter P, Dozortsev D, Qian C, Dhont M. Oocyte morphology does not correlate with fertilization rate and embryo quality after intracytoplasmic sperm injection. *Hum Reprod* 1996; 11: 595–7.
73. Alikani M, Palermo G, Adler A et al. Intracytoplasmic sperm injection in dismorphic human oocytes. *Zygote* 1995; 3: 283–8.
74. Serhal PF, Ranieri DM, Kinis A et al. Oocyte morphology predicts outcome of intracytoplasmic sperm injection. *Hum Reprod* 1997; 12: 1267–70.

75. Balaban B, Urman B, Sertac A et al. Oocyte morphology does not affect fertilization rate, embryo quality and implantation rate after intracytoplasmic sperm injection. *Hum Reprod* 1998; 13: 3431–3.
76. Kilani S, Cooke S, Tilia L, Chapman M. Does meiotic spindle normality predict improved blastocyst development, implantation and live birth rates? *Fertil Steril* 2011; 96: 389–93.
77. Oldenbourg R, Mei G. New polarized light microscope with precision universal compensator. *J Microsc* 1995; 180: 140–7.
78. Silva CP, Kommineni K, Oldenbourg R, Keefe DL. The first polar body does not predict accurately the location of the metaphase II meiotic spindle in mammalian oocytes. *Fertil Steril* 1999; 71: 719–21.
79. Wang WH. Spindle observation and its relationship with fertilization after ICSI in living human oocytes. *Fertil Steril* 2001; 75: 348–53.
80. Moon JH, Hyun CS, Lee SW et al. Visualization of the metaphase II meiotic spindle in living human oocytes using the PolScope enables the prediction of embryonic developmental competence after ICSI. *Hum Reprod* 2003; 18: 817–20.
81. Dekel N, Ayalon D, Lewysohn O et al. Experimental extension of the time interval between oocyte maturation and ovulation: Effect on fertilization and first cleavage. *Fertil Steril* 1995; 64: 1023–8.
82. Eichenlaub-Ritter U, Schmiady H, Kentenich H et al. Recurrent failure in polar body formation and premature chromosome condensation in oocytes from a human patient: Indicators of asynchrony in nuclear and cytoplasmic maturation. *Hum Reprod* 1995; 10: 2343–9.
83. Aboulghar MA, Mansour RT, Serour GI, Ramzy AM, Amin YM. Oocyte quality in patients with severe ovarian hyperstimulation syndrome. *Fertil Steril* 1997; 68: 1017–21.
84. Shoham Z, Jacobs HS, Insler V. Luteinizing hormone: Its role, mechanism of action, and detrimental effects when hypersecreted during the follicular phase. *Fertil Steril* 1993; 59: 1153–61.
85. Franco JC Jr, Baruffi RLR, Oliveira JBA et al. Effects of recombinant LH supplementation to recombinant FSH during induced ovarian stimulation in the GnRH agonist protocol: A matched case-control study. *Reprod Biol Endocrinol* 2010; 94: 971–8.

Advanced sperm selection techniques for intracytoplasmic sperm injection

9

TAMER M. SAID, REDA Z. MAHFOUZ, and ALFONSO P. DEL VALLE

INTRODUCTION

Intracytoplasmic sperm injection (ICSI) was initially introduced in the early 1990s as a treatment for male factor infertility. Nowadays, ICSI is considered one of the gold standards for fertility treatment and is offered to a significant portion of couples in need of assisted reproduction. One of the advantages of ICSI is that only a single spermatozoon is required to fertilize each retrieved oocyte. This, however, presents a unique challenge since the single spermatozoon used during ICSI does not always reflect the overall quality seen in the whole ejaculate. Therefore, traditional methods for assessment of male fertility would be of lesser value in determining ICSI outcomes. In support, the routine semen analysis, which is the main pillar for male fertility workup, has been labeled as a test that possesses limited predictive ability, even when conducted under appropriate controls (1).

In general, it is challenging to identify a set of factors in the ejaculate that will reliably predict the outcome of male fertility. The human ejaculate includes a very heterogeneous group of spermatozoa that vary widely in terms of their fertility potential and their ability to produce a high-quality embryo following ICSI (2). Spermatozoa are highly specialized cells that act as vehicles that deliver the paternal genome to the oocytes. Although both sperm and oocyte genomes contribute equally to the developing embryo, it has been hypothesized that the extent of the sperm contribution to a successful live birth is a mere 10%–15% (3). While this percentage appears to be limited, if an abnormal spermatozoa is used during ICSI, it could cause a significant impediment to embryo development. Therefore, it is safe to assume that ICSI outcomes and success rates will be dependent on sperm quality, among other factors. In support, embryo aneuploidies seen after assisted reproduction were significantly correlated with teratozoospermia (4). The status of the paternal genome and sperm DNA fragmentation also appear to influence pregnancy rates and the risk of pregnancy loss following ICSI (5,6). Similarly, it is important to note that poor *in vivo* reproductive outcomes including recurrent pregnancy loss have been associated with abnormal sperm parameters, including aneuploidies and poor DNA integrity (7).

During ICSI, the raw seminal ejaculate is processed to select spermatozoa that are presumed to have the highest fertilization potential. The processing also aims at excluding immotile, non-viable, morphologically abnormal spermatozoa, as well as other extraneous components of the ejaculate such as blood cells, debris, and seminal plasma. There are different technical protocols that are currently routinely used for processing the seminal ejaculate during ICSI. Often referred to as sperm preparation techniques, these protocols mainly use the concepts of sperm migration and differential density separation to provide a cellular population enriched with spermatozoa that are motile, morphologically normal, and carrying intact DNA.

The concept of sperm migration can be seen at work while performing the swim up protocol. This relies on the active movement of normal motile spermatozoa upwards away from a pellet and towards an environment of clean culture media. On the other hand, the protocol of density gradient centrifugation (DGC) allows for sperm separation using increasingly dense medium layers. In comparison with DGC, swim up yields much more limited numbers of spermatozoa. DGC also appears to be superior to swim up in providing spermatozoa with normal morphology and DNA integrity (8,9).

During ICSI, embryologists subjectively select spermatozoa showing the best morphological criteria and motility (if present) for oocyte injection. The assessment is routinely performed using 400× inverted phase contrast microscopy. Many of the sperm parameters that affect its fertilization and embryo development potential, such as apoptosis and DNA fragmentation, cannot be evaluated under these conditions. Routine sperm preparation techniques such as swim up and DGC, which are currently in use during ICSI, are established as reliable methods. However, they lack the ability to specifically target these critical sperm parameters. Thus, it is very likely that apoptosis/DNA fragmentation will be significantly present in a normal-shaped, motile spermatozoa. The inclusion of such sperm may be the reason behind failed ICSI treatments. It is currently expected that only an extremely limited number of fertilized oocytes actually result in a live birth, even when proven-fertile healthy donors are acting as gamete providers (10,11).

In light of the above, there is an obvious need for a different approach to the sperm selection procedures during ICSI. Due to the complete absence of natural selection processes during ICSI, it is imperative that every effort should be made to ensure that only spermatozoa with the highest quality and fertilization potential are used for ICSI. Noninvasive techniques that use a detailed assessment of spermatozoa are required to achieve sperm selection according to more physiological criteria. In this chapter, we describe the recent advances in molecular/ultrastructural-based sperm selection techniques that could be of benefit if implemented during ICSI. The currently available advanced techniques include sperm selection according to its surface charge, hyaluronic acid (HA) binding, apoptosis, and high-magnification morphology. The rationale and technical description will be described for each method and the question of whether they offer any advantages compared to routine ICSI will be addressed.

SPERM SURFACE CHARGE

Rationale

An electrokinetic movement can be initiated whenever the surface charge of a cell interacts with an external electric force. Depending on whether the surface charge is net negative or net positive, the end outcome can be either repulsion or attraction (12). Mature spermatozoa carry an electronegative surface charge, which is attributed to sialic acid residues including the CD52 found in the sperm plasma membrane (13). Spermatozoa acquire CD52 mainly during epididymal maturation. The presence of CD52 has been correlated with normal sperm morphology and capacitation; therefore, it can be considered as an indication of sperm maturity and quality (14).

There are two different techniques that rely on the sperm negative surface charge as the basis for sperm selection. First, the electrophoresis technique (i.e., motion of a particle in liquid medium) entails the application of an external electric current. The end result would be the movement of the negatively charged spermatozoa towards the positive electrode of an electrophoresis device (15). Second, the sperm ζ-potential (electrokinetic potential) technique relies on the electric potential between the sperm membrane and its surroundings measuring −16 to −20 mV in mature sperm (16). Since the ζ-potential further decreases with capacitation (17), sperm selection can be performed as negatively charged spermatozoa will move towards and adhere to a positively charged surface (18).

Technique

An electrophoresis device has been designed to select spermatozoa based on their electronegative surface charge (SpermSep Cell Sorter-10 [CS-10], Nusep Ltd, Frenchs Forest, Australia). The device also considers cellular size, which ensures the exclusion of leukocytes and immature germ cells (Figure 9.1a,b). The CS-10 device was successfully used in oligozoospermic samples, testicular sperm, and frozen spermatozoa (15). CS-10 is simple to operate: it entails exposing the ejaculate to an electric field of an applied constant current measuring 75 mA with a variable voltage of between 18 and 21 V for five minutes. Thereafter, mature sperm suspended in HEPES buffer is collected in a 400 μL chamber. Even with the addition of time used for sample loading and preparation, CS-10 is less time consuming compared to all other routine sperm preparation techniques such as DGC (19). However, the need to procure an additional device may be cost prohibitive in some laboratory settings.

On the other hand, sperm selection using the ζ-potential approach requires merely a simple centrifuge tube, which has been positively charged by rotation a few times in a latex glove. Spermatozoa that have been washed by DGC are incubated in the positively charged tube for one minute; thereafter, centrifugation takes place and the supernatant is discarded. The negatively charged (mature) sperm are expected to adhere to the tube's surface (Figure 9.1c,d). This mature sperm population can be collected by rinsing the tube with serum-supplemented media to be used for ICSI (20). Due to the extremely limited amount of time and resources required, the ζ-potential method offers a unique advantage, especially for less equipped andrology laboratories.

Results

In comparison with other routine sperm preparation techniques, spermatozoa selected using CS-10 are expected to

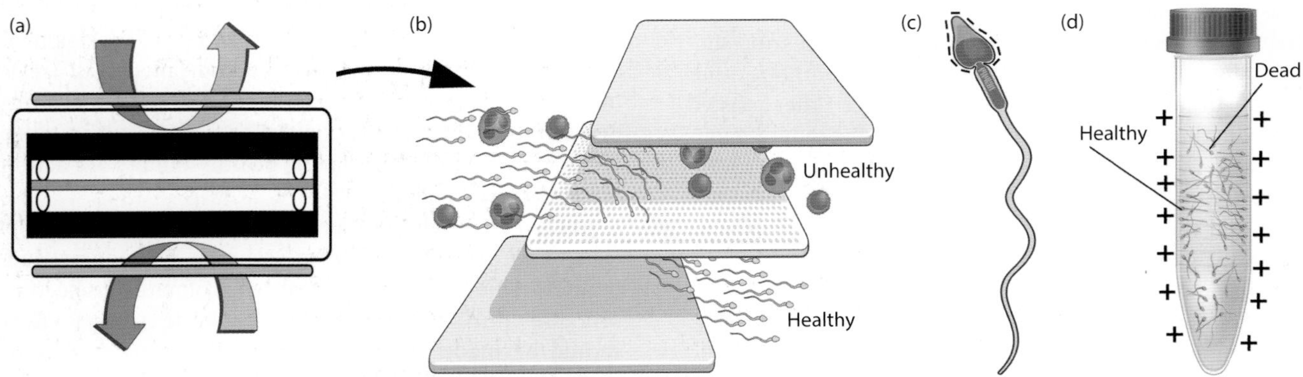

Figure 9.1 (a,b) A special electrophoretic chamber is constructed to force cells passing through a 5 μm polycarbonate membrane from the inoculation side towards the collection part through a unidirectional flow buffering system while restriction membranes isolate cells from both anodes and cathodes. Healthy sperm are separated from non-sperm or unhealthy sperm. (c) Sorting is based upon the presence of negative charges on mature human spermatozoa. (d) The same sorting principle works for positively charged tubes that attract and adhere mature spermatozoa.

have lower number of morphological abnormalities and DNA fragmentation (15,21). In addition, the electrophoresis system is capable of excluding a significant number of leukocytes that are normally present in the ejaculate (15). Electrophoresis can have negative effect on sperm motility; therefore, careful consideration should be given as to which cases would be good candidates for this sperm selection approach (22). To date, electrophoresis has been mainly suggested for sperm selection in ejaculates characterized by a high level of sperm DNA fragmentation (15).

The benefits of using the ζ-potential method for sperm selection have been documented to a certain extent. A combined protocol of DGC + ζ-potential resulted in a sperm population that is characterized by lower DNA fragmentation, protamine deficiency, and morphological abnormalities (23). It is important to note that while the ζ-potential selection method has a similar capacity to select higher-quality spermatozoa in terms of morphology and DNA integrity, it does not display the same negative effects on motility reported with CS-10 (18,20,24,25). Since the ζ-potential method does not include using high-voltage electricity, it could be considered safer than electrophoresis. However, it is not suitable for ejaculates with low sperm counts, since sperm recovery rates are limited (18).

The use of electronegative spermatozoa selected by electrophoresis during ICSI had a positive association with fertilization and blastocyst development rates (21). However, research on ICSI of sibling oocytes showed no clear benefits for using CS-10 compared to DGC as regards fertilization and embryo cleavage rates (19). Conversely, ICSI of sibling oocytes following ζ-potential sperm selection was characterized by higher fertilization rates compared to DGC (24). Finally, a case report of a patient presenting with repeated failed ICSI cycles and high levels of sperm DNA fragmentation documented a healthy live birth following the use of CS-10, which supports the limited indication for this electrophoresis system (26).

HA BINDING

Rationale

During late spermatogenesis, remodeling of the sperm plasma membrane occurs, leading to the formation of HA binding sites. Therefore, the presence of HA binding sites on the sperm plasma membrane can be considered as a sign of sperm maturity. In support of this, several indicators of sperm maturity such as creatine kinase, heat shock-related protein 2, and aniline blue staining were significantly identified on spermatozoa with HA binding properties (27). HA is the main component of the cumulus oophorus; it plays a role in the natural selection of mature spermatozoa during *in vivo* fertilization. Therefore, the sperm's ability to bind to HA and subsequently to the zona pellucida can be used as the basis for *in vitro* sperm selection (28). Since HA is a physiological component of the cervix, cumulus cells, and follicular fluid, it should pose no additional safety risks when used for sperm selection (29).

Technique

A hyaluronate-rich preparation medium is currently available to select mature spermatozoa that have HA binding ability (SpermSlow™, Origio, MediCult, Målov, Denmark). A drop of semen that has been washed using a routine sperm preparation technique (e.g., DGC) is placed close to a SpermSlow drop and a junction is created between both drops using an ICSI pipette. Incubation at 37°C takes place for 15 minutes; thereafter, the "slowed" spermatozoa found in the junction between both drops can be collected and used for ICSI (Figure 9.2a,b).

A modified Petri dish that includes four powdered HA drops has been designed as a sperm selection device (PICSI®, MidAtlantic Diagnostics, Inc., Mt Laurel, NJ). Prior to the use of the PICSI dishes, HA drops are rehydrated using a culture medium. For sperm selection, one drop of washed spermatozoa is placed at the edge of each HA drop. The mature, HA-bound spermatozoa can be identified by having absolutely no progressive motion despite vigorous tail movement. After 15 minutes of incubation at 37°C, HA-bound sperm can be retrieved by a pipette and used for ICSI (Figure 9.2c,d) (30).

Results

SpermSlow and PICSI dishes deliver comparable outcomes following ICSI; however, SpermSlow has two advantages: (1) it requires significantly less time to perform; and (2) it can be combined with other advanced sperm selection techniques such as intracytoplasmic morphologically selected sperm injection (IMSI) (31). Spermatozoa selected by HA binding display a higher percentage of normal morphology and a lower frequency of autosomal disomy, diploidy, and sex chromosome disomy (30,32). HA-bound

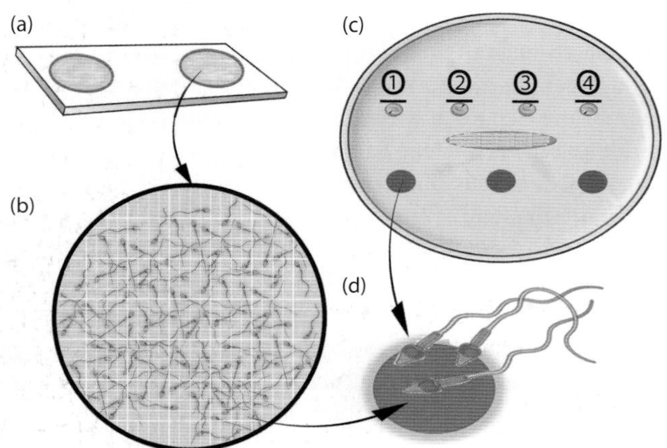

Figure 9.2 (a,b) Hyaluronic acid (HA)-rich preparation medium may be used to identify a mature and healthy spermatozoon through adding the semen specimen into pre-coated HA slide. (c,d) HA-rich medium slows down mature sperm to facilitate sorting and immobilization and then moving them to a new polyvinylpyrrolidone droplet to be ready for injecting the oocytes (O1 to O4) into an intracytoplasmic sperm injection Petri dish.

sperm also have lower apoptosis manifestations such as caspase-3 activation and DNA fragmentation compared to spermatozoa in raw semen and those selected by DGC (33,34). However, in comparison with other advanced sperm selection techniques, HA binding failed to deliver better-quality spermatozoa in terms of DNA fragmentation compared to the ζ-potential selection method (25).

There are contradictory reports that describe the impact of HA sperm selection on ICSI outcomes. At present, there is insufficient evidence to document an improvement in live birth or pregnancy outcomes following ICSI as a result of using HA-selected sperm (35). A limited number of studies showed that spermatozoa selected by HA binding can result in significantly higher fertilization and implantation rates following ICSI (36,37). However, this was not consistent with other studies showing a lack of improvement in fertilization, embryo quality, and cleavage rates (38,39). The benefits of using HA binding for sperm selection have been repeatedly discredited by various reports including studies conducted on sibling oocytes. It was reported that the use of HA-bound sperm does not result in any better cleavage rates, embryo development (Z-scores), or miscarriage and pregnancy rates following ICSI (34,40,41). The only consistent potential benefit for using HA-bound sperm could be a decrease in pregnancy loss rate following ICSI, especially in samples characterized by lower HA binding ability (42,43).

APOPTOTIC SPERM BINDING

Rationale

Programmed cell death (apoptosis) is a physiological phenomenon that entails a series of morphological and biochemical changes that ultimately result in cellular death (44). Apoptosis-related features have been reported in human spermatozoa. They are indicative of abnormalities associated with the regulation of testicular apoptosis (45). It has been postulated that damage to the plasma cellular membrane occurs at an early stage of apoptosis that precedes extensive nuclear damage and irreversible apoptosis (46,47). The extrusion of phosphatidylserine (PS), which is normally present in the inner leaflet of the plasma membrane, to the outer surface has been identified as one of the early apoptotic changes in human spermatozoa (48). Externalization of PS (EPS), mitochondrial dysfunction, and nuclear DNA damage are all markers of sperm apoptosis that were detected at significantly higher levels in infertile men and those with varicoceles (49).

In vivo and *in vitro* male fertility decline whenever apoptosis markers are increased in human spermatozoa (50–52). Although routine sperm preparation techniques such as swim up or DGC can isolate motile, morphologically normal sperm (53), they lack the ability to specifically target sperm based on apoptosis manifestations. Therefore, it is possible that spermatozoa selected following swim up or DGC may be apoptotic and may have fragmented DNA (54). Since DNA fragmentation has been recognized as a late apoptosis event, oocytes could be fertilized with an apoptotic sperm during ICSI, which will result in poor outcomes. In support, sperm DNA fragmentation was positively correlated with increased miscarriage rates following ICSI (55). Targeting the selection of non-apoptotic spermatozoa prior to ICSI can prevent similar negative outcomes and should increase the possibility of using a DNA-intact sperm during ICSI.

Technique

Magnetic-activated cell sorting (MACS) has been proposed as a noninvasive and feasible approach for the selection of non-apoptotic spermatozoa (56). The technique employs paramagnetic microbeads (∼50 nm) conjugated with annexin V, a 35–36 kDa phospholipid binding protein, which has a selective affinity to bind with PS (57). As one of the early manifestations of apoptosis, EPS allows for binding with annexin V microbeads and separation of spermatozoa using a MACS system (Miltenyi Biotec GmbH, Bergisch Gladbach, Germany). The magnet included in the system retains the apoptotic sperm labeled with microbeads. The unlabeled spermatozoa can be considered as non-apoptotic and collected for use in ICSI (Figure 9.3a–d).

The human ejaculate normally includes several elements such as white blood cells, immature germ cells, and seminal plasma that should be excluded in preparation for ICSI. As much as the MACS technique has been proven to be effective at excluding apoptotic sperm, it does not

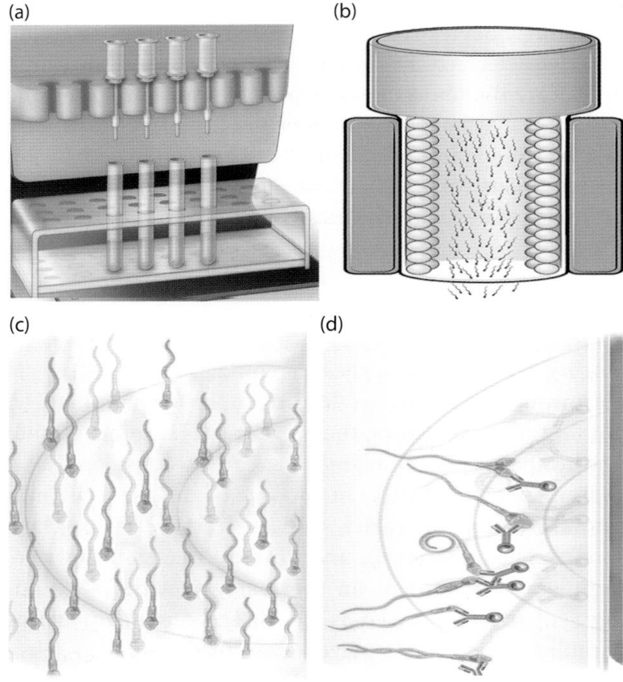

Figure 9.3 (a) Magnetic-activated cell sorting apparatus. (b,c) Sperm samples mixed with beads pass through an iron-laden column placed in a strong magnet with gravity. (d) Non-apoptotic spermatozoa will pass through and can be collected, while apoptotic sperm will bind to the column.

address any of these elements. Therefore, two-layer DGC has been recommended to precede MACS in order to yield a clean sperm suspension (56).

Results

A combined protocol of DGC and MACS for sperm selection can be completed in less than one hour using limited technical resources (58). The protocol results in a sperm population characterized by higher motility and viability as well as lower acrosomal damage, cytoplasmic droplets, and sperm deformity index compared to other routine sperm preparation techniques (56,59). Ample evidence suggests that the technique can yield spermatozoa that exhibit significantly lesser apoptosis manifestations. Specifically, lower caspase-3 and DNA fragmentation and higher mitochondrial membrane potential were seen in annexin-negative spermatozoa selected by MACS (60–63).

Using the hamster oocyte penetration assay to assess sperm function, spermatozoa prepared by DGC + MACS showed a higher ability to penetrate oocytes, which could be considered a sign for increased fertilization potential (62). Also in infertile men, sperm chromatin decondensation following 18 hours of hamster oocyte ICSI was significantly improved following the application of DGC + MACS (64). In comparison with other advanced sperm selection techniques, DGC + MACS has proved to be more effective at selecting spermatozoa with normal sperm morphology, DNA integrity, and lower protamine deficiency compared to the DGC + ζ-potential method (65).

Numerous reports have documented the benefits of using MACS in the context of assisted reproduction resulting in healthy live births (66,67). Fertilization rates, embryo cleavage rates, and pregnancy rates were all reported to be significantly higher following ICSI when sperm selection was conducted using DGC + MACS (68,69). A comprehensive meta-analysis described the results of 499 patients that were pooled from five prospective controlled studies. The concluding results showed that pregnancy rates after ICSI significantly improve with the use of sperm selected by MACS (70). The combined DGC + MACS protocol can be used in various patient indications. While it is recognized that this approach may not be routinely warranted (71), there appears to be a specific group of indications where subtle benefits have been demonstrated. These would include patients presenting with repeated failed ICSI cycles and those with exceptionally high levels of caspase-3 and DNA fragmentation (67,72,73). In support, pregnancy rates were skewed significantly higher following ICSI with MACS-selected sperm (64.9% vs. 36.6% in controls) in patients with moderate DNA fragmentation (22.6%) in the raw ejaculate (74).

HIGH-MAGNIFICATION REAL-TIME MICROSCOPY

Rationale

The impact of sperm morphology on male *in vivo* and *in vitro* fertility has been well established (75,76). Nevertheless, routine sperm morphology assessment using stained smears and 1000× magnification does not equate to the sperm selection during ICSI, which takes place using low-power (400×) inverted phase contrast microscopy (77). Any sperm ultrastructural abnormalities that affect fertilization and embryo development, if present, will not be detected using such low magnification. To address this issue, a real-time sperm selection method has been developed based on the motile sperm organelle morphology examination (MSOME) at a magnification of >6000× (77).

Different sperm organelles can be visualized using MSOME (nucleus, acrosome, post-acrosomal lamina, neck, tail, and mitochondria) (Figure 9.4a,b). The detailed organelle assessment allows the identification of specific abnormalities such as the lack of acrosomes in globozoospermia cases (78). The integration of MSOME with ICSI has led to the development of IMSI, which entails sperm selection using MSOME (79). IMSI has been suggested as a useful tool in specific indications: (1) male patients presenting with high levels of DNA fragmentation and aneuploidies; (2) abnormal semen parameters; and (3) repeated implantation failure following ICSI (80,81).

Technique

To perform MSOME, a routine sperm preparation technique is initially performed to isolate a motile sperm population. Thereafter, examination of the prepared sperm

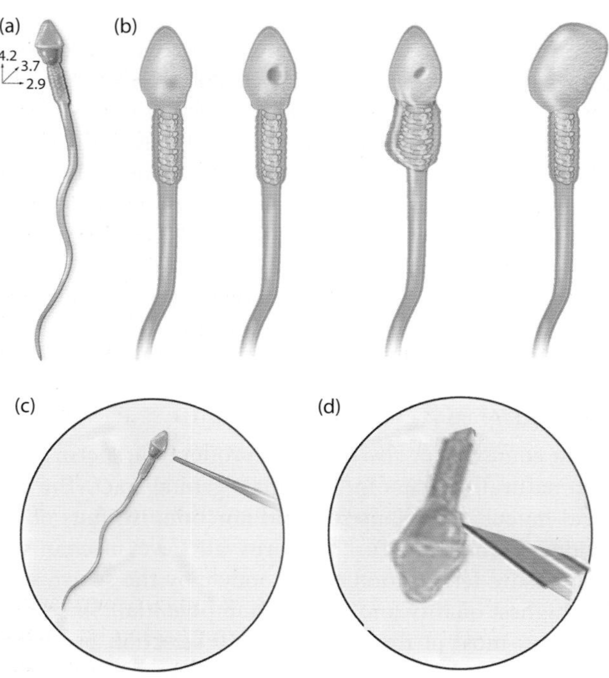

Figure 9.4 (a,b) Sperm sorting depends upon using selection criteria for morphologically normal (a) versus abnormal spermatozoon (b). (c,d) Differences in sperm details with magnification between intracytoplasmic sperm injection (c) and intracytoplasmic morphologically selected sperm injection (d).

population takes place under oil immersion using an inverted microscope equipped with high-power Nomarski optics and digital enhancement resulting in >6000× magnification (Figure 9.4c,d) (77). MSOME followed by IMSI is laborious and time consuming, adding hours of processing time to the already complex routine ICSI procedures. The expense associated with additional instrumentation is also a disadvantage (82).

Since the assessment of the sperm nucleus appears to have the most significant impact on ICSI results, a grading system has been developed to identify the spermatozoa most likely to result in a successful outcome. During IMSI, preference is given to the selection and use of grade I spermatozoa (normal shape and no vacuoles) followed by grade II spermatozoa (normal shape and ≤2 small vacuoles) (83).

Results

Spermatozoa selected via MSOME are expected to show lower incidence of DNA fragmentation and aneuploidies and higher mitochondrial membrane potential compared to unselected ones (84,85). Nuclear vacuoles as identified by MSOME have the strongest association with sperm DNA fragmentation (85,86). MSOME also appears to be slightly superior compared to the HA binding method as regards the selection of DNA-intact spermatozoa (87).

Fertilization, implantation, embryo quality, and pregnancy and live birth rates were significantly improved following IMSI compared to routine ICSI (77,88). Also, the incidences of miscarriages and birth defects were lower following IMSI (89–92). Patients seeking fertility treatment due to advanced maternal age (≥37 years old) were identified as a group that would benefit from IMSI application (93). Despite the reported benefits of IMSI, there is no current consensus that advocates the use of IMSI on a wide scale. A multicenter randomized controlled trial, a randomized sibling oocyte trial, and the Cochrane Database Systematic Reviews all report lack of evidence for the advantages of using IMSI over ICSI (94–96). Yet, cases presenting with teratozoospermia or extensive sperm DNA fragmentation may be further evaluated as regards the potential beneficial effects of IMSI (95).

SUMMARY

In the context of *in vivo* human reproduction, sperm selection naturally occurs in the female genital tract. The cervical mucus, uterus, utero-tubal junction, isthmus of the oviducts, and cumulus oophorus all have mechanisms that ensure fertilization of the oocyte by the sperm with the highest quality and fertilization potential. Since ICSI bypasses most of the sperm natural selection processes, not only are the treatment success rates of concern, but also the health and well-being of the offspring. Selecting the most mature, DNA-intact spermatozoa for inclusion in ICSI alleviates, at least in part, the concern of using a dysfunctional paternal genome. Routine sperm preparation techniques that are currently used during ICSI select spermatozoa based on their motility and density. They do lack the ability to specifically target other important aspects of the sperm quality and function. Sperm DNA integrity is one of those parameters that could have a significant impact on ICSI outcomes and the health of the offspring.

Several advanced sperm selection techniques have been recently proposed for integration with ICSI. The concepts of advanced sperm selection techniques include selection according to the sperm negative surface charges, HA binding, exclusion of apoptotic sperm, and high-magnification real-time morphology. These advanced sperm selection techniques have been successfully used in clinical ICSI settings. Other additional techniques that have been described as potential candidates for sperm selection include microfluidic sorters, Raman spectroscopy, polarizing microscopy, and confocal light absorption and scattering spectroscopic microscopy. In the future, these methods may prove to be of potential benefit in the context of ICSI.

Selection according to the sperm surface charge is the least time consuming, and the ζ-potential method requires the least instrumentation. On the other hand, IMSI requires the most time to perform and entails the most expensive instrumentation. Advanced sperm selection methods have a proven ability to yield a sperm population with higher quality in terms of motility, viability, and morphology and lesser apoptosis manifestations, including DNA fragmentation. Nevertheless, at present, there is not a single sperm selection method that possesses all the criteria of an ideal technique. Those should include: (1) a documented ability to select spermatozoa with the highest quality (motile, normal morphology, DNA integrity, etc.) and fertilization potential; (2) deselecting the seminal plasma and other extraneous components of the ejaculate; (3) not inflicting any iatrogenic damage on spermatozoa; (4) quick and feasible; and (5) non-cost prohibitive.

Sperm selection using the electrophoresis CS-10 device can be performed on the neat ejaculate—no initial or subsequent processing is required. All other described advanced sperm selection techniques require combination with a routine sperm preparation method. Performing a combination of two different technical protocols (e.g., DGC + ζ or DGC + MACS) will result in added technical steps that will require additional human resources, skills, instrumentation, and time commitment. With the exception of electrophoresis, iatrogenic damage was not consistently reported as a result of using one of the advanced sperm selection methods, whether alone or in combination with other routine sperm preparation techniques. However, such damage can never be ruled out, especially when spermatozoa are exposed to excessive manipulation (centrifugation/resuspension), extended incubation periods, and temperature fluctuations. Also, significant sperm loss and low recovery rates following extensive processing should be considered and would exclude samples with limited sperm counts from being potential candidates for advanced sperm selection techniques.

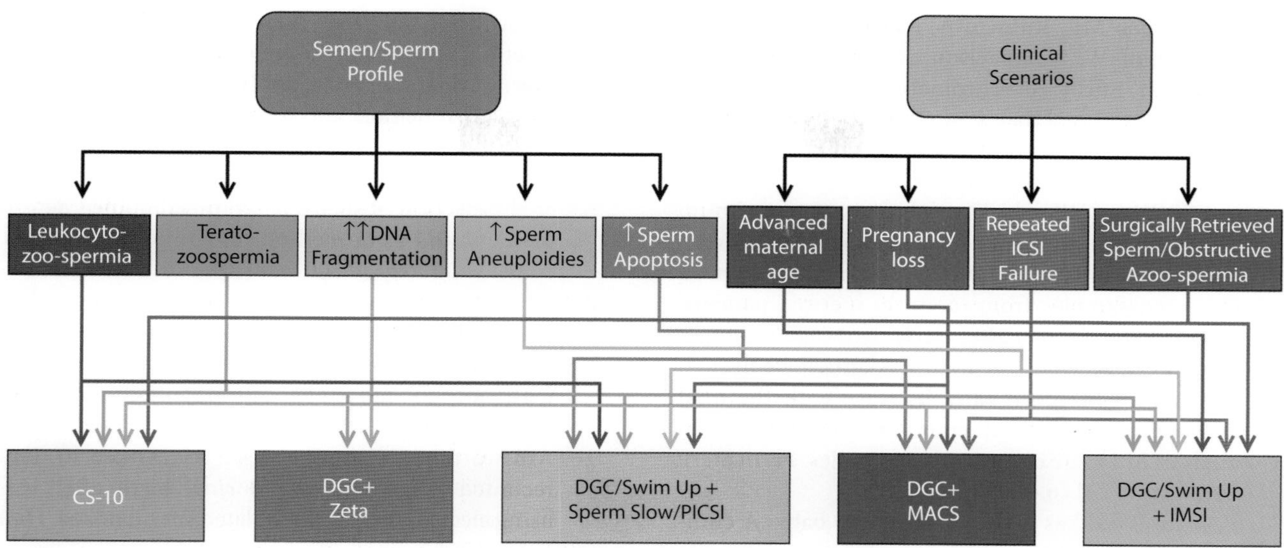

Figure 9.5 Summary of the potential applications of advanced sperm selection technologies that are currently available. The left column depicts various semen/sperm abnormalities that could be seen in diagnostic laboratories. The right column represents some common clinical conditions that may be seen by fertility practitioners.

Appropriate safety data should be generated for the proposed advanced sperm selection techniques. Although healthy live births have been reported following the application of most advanced sperm selection methods, there has not been a long-term follow-up study of the health and development of the offspring. It should also be noted that unintentional gender selection could be experienced in some cases at a higher incidence compared to routine sperm preparation methods. For example, the ζ-potential technique, which selects spermatozoa based on their surface charge, may be more prone to deliver X-bearing sperm since such sperm presents with a higher net negative charge compared to Y-bearing sperm.

Additional research is required to properly evaluate the benefits of integrating advanced sperm selection techniques in routine ICSI. Despite the reporting of promising data on ICSI outcomes following the use of all of the discussed advanced sperm selection techniques, well-designed prospective randomized controlled research is scarce. Systematic reviews of the currently available randomized controlled studies reveal no added benefit for using any of the advanced sperm selection techniques during ICSI (35,96). Thus, it is evidently clear that these advanced sperm selection techniques should not be considered routinely for all cases undergoing ICSI. Alternatively, further research should focus on identifying which seminal profiles and clinical scenarios would benefit the most from the application of the advanced sperm selection technologies. A summary of the potential indications for advanced sperm selection techniques is presented in Figure 9.5. At present, preliminary data limit the benefits of advanced sperm selection methods to cases presenting with increased apoptosis markers and DNA fragmentation in spermatozoa. Also, patients with repeated failed ICSI cycles and advanced maternal age may benefit from a similar approach.

REFERENCES

1. De Jonge C. Semen analysis: Looking for an upgrade in class. *Fertil Steril* 2012; 97(2): 260–6.
2. Wang J, Fan HC, Behr B, Quake SR. Genome-wide single-cell analysis of recombination activity and *de novo* mutation rates in human sperm. *Cell* 2012; 150(2): 402–12.
3. Sakkas D, Ramalingam M, Garrido N, Barratt CL. Sperm selection in natural conception: What can we learn from Mother Nature to improve assisted reproduction outcomes? *Hum Reprod Update* 2015; 21(6): 711–26.
4. Kahraman S, Findikli N, Biricik A et al. Preliminary FISH studies on spermatozoa and embryos in patients with variable degrees of teratozoospermia and a history of poor prognosis. *Reprod Biomed Online* 2006; 12(6): 752–61.
5. Borini A, Tarozzi N, Bizzaro D et al. Sperm DNA fragmentation: Paternal effect on early post-implantation embryo development in ART. *Hum Reprod* 2006; 21(11): 2876–81.
6. Zini A, Boman JM, Belzile E, Ciampi A. Sperm DNA damage is associated with an increased risk of pregnancy loss after IVF and ICSI: Systematic review and meta-analysis. *Hum Reprod* 2008; 23(12): 2663–8.
7. Zidi-Jrah I, Hajlaoui A, Mougou-Zerelli S et al. Relationship between sperm aneuploidy, sperm DNA integrity, chromatin packaging, traditional semen parameters, and recurrent pregnancy loss. *Fertil Steril* 2016; 105(1): 58–64.

8. Hammadeh ME, Kuhnen A, Amer AS, Rosenbaum P, Schmidt W. Comparison of sperm preparation methods: Effect on chromatin and morphology recovery rates and their consequences on the clinical outcome after *in vitro* fertilization embryo transfer. *Int J Androl* 2001; 24(6): 360–8.
9. Xue X, Wang WS, Shi JZ et al. Efficacy of swim-up versus density gradient centrifugation in improving sperm deformity rate and DNA fragmentation index in semen samples from teratozoospermic patients. *J Assist Reprod Genet* 2014; 31(9): 1161–6.
10. Garrido N, Bellver J, Remohi J, Alama P, Pellicer A. Cumulative newborn rates increase with the total number of transferred embryos according to an analysis of 15,792 ovum donation cycles. *Fertil Steril* 2012; 98(2): 341–6.e1–2.
11. Patrizio P, Sakkas D. From oocyte to baby: A clinical evaluation of the biological efficiency of *in vitro* fertilization. *Fertil Steril* 2009; 91(4): 1061–6.
12. Simon L, Ge SQ, Carrell DT. Sperm selection based on electrostatic charge. *Methods Mol Biol* 2013; 927: 269–78.
13. Schroter S, Derr P, Conradt HS, Nimtz M, Hale G, Kirchhoff C. Male-specific modification of human CD52. *J Biol Chem* 1999; 274(42): 29862–73.
14. Giuliani V, Pandolfi C, Santucci R et al. Expression of gp20, a human sperm antigen of epididymal origin, is reduced in spermatozoa from subfertile men. *Mol Reprod Dev* 2004; 69(2): 235–40.
15. Ainsworth C, Nixon B, Aitken RJ. Development of a novel electrophoretic system for the isolation of human spermatozoa. *Hum Reprod* 2005; 20(8): 2261–70.
16. Ishijima SA, Okuno M, Mohri H. Zeta potential of human X- and Y-bearing sperm. *Int J Androl* 1991; 14(5): 340–7.
17. Focarelli R, Rosati F, Terrana B. Sialyglycoconjugates release during in vitro capacitation of human spermatozoa. *J Androl* 1990; 11(2): 97–104.
18. Chan PJ, Jacobson JD, Corselli JU, Patton WC. A simple zeta method for sperm selection based on membrane charge. *Fertil Steril* 2006; 85(2): 481–6.
19. Fleming SD, Ilad RS, Griffin AM et al. Prospective controlled trial of an electrophoretic method of sperm preparation for assisted reproduction: Comparison with density gradient centrifugation. *Hum Reprod* 2008; 23(12): 2646–51.
20. Kam TL, Jacobson JD, Patton WC, Corselli JU, Chan PJ. Retention of membrane charge attributes by cryopreserved–thawed sperm and zeta selection. *J Assist Reprod Genet* 2007; 24(9): 429–34.
21. Simon L, Murphy K, Aston KI, Emery BR, Hotaling JM, Carrell DT. Micro-electrophoresis: A noninvasive method of sperm selection based on membrane charge. *Fertil Steril* 2015; 103(2): 361–6.e3.
22. Engelmann U, Krassnigg F, Schatz H, Schill WB. Separation of human X and Y spermatozoa by free-flow electrophoresis. *Gamete Res* 1988; 19(2): 151–60.
23. Zarei-Kheirabadi M, Shayegan Nia E, Tavalaee M et al. Evaluation of ubiquitin and annexin V in sperm population selected based on density gradient centrifugation and zeta potential (DGC-zeta). *J Assist Reprod Genet* 2012; 29(4): 365–71.
24. Kheirollahi-Kouhestani M, Razavi S, Tavalaee M et al. Selection of sperm based on combined density gradient and Zeta method may improve ICSI outcome. *Hum Reprod* 2009; 24(10): 2409–16.
25. Razavi SH, Nasr-Esfahani MH, Deemeh MR, Shayesteh M, Tavalaee M. Evaluation of zeta and HA-binding methods for selection of spermatozoa with normal morphology, protamine content and DNA integrity. *Andrologia* 2010; 42(1): 13–9.
26. Ainsworth C, Nixon B, Jansen RP, Aitken RJ. First recorded pregnancy and normal birth after ICSI using electrophoretically isolated spermatozoa. *Hum Reprod* 2007; 22(1): 197–200.
27. Huszar G, Ozenci CC, Cayli S, Zavaczki Z, Hansch E, Vigue L. Hyaluronic acid binding by human sperm indicates cellular maturity, viability, and unreacted acrosomal status. *Fertil Steril* 2003; 79(Suppl 3): 1616–24.
28. Huszar G, Sbarcia M, Vigue L, Miller D, Shur B. Sperm plasma membrane remodeling during spermiogenetic maturation in men: Relationship among plasma membrane beta 1,4-galactosyltransferase, cytoplasmic creatine phosphokinase, and creatine phosphokinase isoform ratios. *Biol Reprod* 1997; 56: 1020–4.
29. Cayli S, Jakab A, Ovari L et al. Biochemical markers of sperm function: Male fertility and sperm selection for ICSI. *Reprod Biomed Online* 2003; 7(4): 462–8.
30. Jakab A, Sakkas D, Delpiano E et al. Intracytoplasmic sperm injection: A novel selection method for sperm with normal frequency of chromosomal aneuploidies. *Fertil Steril* 2005; 84(6): 1665–73.
31. Parmegiani L, Cognigni GE, Bernardi S et al. Comparison of two ready-to-use systems designed for sperm–hyaluronic acid binding selection before intracytoplasmic sperm injection: PICSI vs. Sperm Slow: A prospective, randomized trial. *Fertil Steril* 2012; 98(3): 632–7.
32. Prinosilova P, Kruger T, Sati L et al. Selectivity of hyaluronic acid binding for spermatozoa with normal Tygerberg strict morphology. *Reprod Biomed Online* 2009; 18(2): 177–83.
33. Cayli S, Sakkas D, Vigue L, Demir R, Huszar G. Cellular maturity and apoptosis in human sperm: Creatine kinase, caspase-3 and Bcl-XL levels in mature and diminished maturity sperm. *Mol Hum Reprod* 2004; 10(5): 365–72.
34. Tarozzi N, Nadalini M, Bizzaro D et al. Sperm-hyaluronan-binding assay: Clinical value in conventional IVF under Italian law. *Reprod Biomed Online* 2009; 19(Suppl 3): 35–43.

35. McDowell S, Kroon B, Ford E, Hook Y, Glujovsky D, Yazdani A. Advanced sperm selection techniques for assisted reproduction. *Cochrane Database Syst Rev* 2014; 10: CD010461.
36. Mokanszki A, Tothne EV, Bodnar B et al. Is sperm hyaluronic acid binding ability predictive for clinical success of intracytoplasmic sperm injection: PICSI vs. ICSI? *Syst Biol Reprod Med* 2014; 60(6): 348–54.
37. Nasr-Esfahani MH, Razavi S, Vahdati AA, Fathi F, Tavalaee M. Evaluation of sperm selection procedure based on hyaluronic acid binding ability on ICSI outcome. *J Assist Reprod Genet* 2008; 25(5): 197–203.
38. Parmegiani L, Cognigni GE, Ciampaglia W, Pocognoli P, Marchi F, Filicori M. Efficiency of hyaluronic acid (HA) sperm selection. *J Assist Reprod Genet* 2010; 27: 13–6.
39. Parmegiani L, Cognigni GE, Bernardi S, Troilo E, Ciampaglia W, Filicori M. "Physiologic ICSI": Hyaluronic acid (HA) favors selection of spermatozoa without DNA fragmentation and with normal nucleus, resulting in improvement of embryo quality. *Fertil Steril* 2010; 93(2): 598–604.
40. Choe SA, Tae JC, Shin MY et al. Application of sperm selection using hyaluronic acid binding in intracytoplasmic sperm injection cycles: A sibling oocyte study. *J Korean Med Sci* 2012; 27(12): 1569–73.
41. Van Den Bergh MJ, Fahy-Deshe M, Hohl MK. Pronuclear zygote score following intracytoplasmic injection of hyaluronan-bound spermatozoa: A prospective randomized study. *Reprod Biomed Online* 2009; 19(6): 796–801.
42. Majumdar G, Majumdar A. A prospective randomized study to evaluate the effect of hyaluronic acid sperm selection on the intracytoplasmic sperm injection outcome of patients with unexplained infertility having normal semen parameters. *J Assist Reprod Genet* 2013; 30(11): 1471–5.
43. Worrilow KC, Eid S, Woodhouse D et al. Use of hyaluronan in the selection of sperm for intracytoplasmic sperm injection (ICSI): Significant improvement in clinical outcomes—Multicenter, double-blinded and randomized controlled trial. *Hum Reprod* 2013; 28(2): 306–14.
44. Vaux D, Korsmeyer S. Cell death in development. *Cell* 1999; 96: 245–54.
45. Taylor SL, Weng SL, Fox P et al. Somatic cell apoptosis markers and pathways in human ejaculated sperm: Potential utility as indicators of sperm quality. *Mol Hum Reprod* 2004; 10(11): 825–34.
46. Scabini M, Stellari F, Cappella P, Rizzitano S, Texido G, Pesenti E. *In vivo* imaging of early stage apoptosis by measuring real-time caspase-3/7 activation. *Apoptosis* 2011; 16(2): 198–207.
47. Martinez MM, Reif RD, Pappas D. Early detection of apoptosis in living cells by fluorescence correlation spectroscopy. *Anal Bioanal Chem* 2010; 396(3): 1177–85.
48. Oosterhuis GJ, Mulder AB, Kalsbeek-Batenburg E, Lambalk CB, Schoemaker J, Vermes I. Measuring apoptosis in human spermatozoa: A biological assay for semen quality? *Fertil Steril* 2000; 74(2): 245–50.
49. Wu GJ, Chang FW, Lee SS, Cheng YY, Chen CH, Chen IC. Apoptosis-related phenotype of ejaculated spermatozoa in patients with varicocele. *Fertil Steril* 2009; 91(3): 831–7.
50. Barroso G, Taylor S, Morshedi M, Manzur F, Gavino F, Oehninger S. Mitochondrial membrane potential integrity and plasma membrane translocation of phosphatidylserine as early apoptotic markers: A comparison of two different sperm subpopulations. *Fertil Steril* 2006; 85(1): 149–54.
51. Carrell D, Wilcox A, Lowy L et al. Elevated sperm chromosome aneuploidy and apoptosis in patients with unexplained recurrent pregnancy loss. *Obstet Gynecol* 2003; 101(6): 1229–35.
52. Seli E, Gardner DK, Schoolcraft WB, Moffatt O, Sakkas D. Extent of nuclear DNA damage in ejaculated spermatozoa impacts on blastocyst development after *in vitro* fertilization. *Fertil Steril* 2004; 82(2): 378–83.
53. Le Lannou D, Blanchard Y. Nuclear maturity and morphology of human spermatozoa selected by Percoll density gradient centrifugation or swim-up procedure. *J Reprod Fertil* 1988; 84: 551–6.
54. Barroso G, Valdespin C, Vega E et al. Developmental sperm contributions: Fertilization and beyond. *Fertil Steril* 2009; 92(3): 835–48.
55. Robinson L, Gallos ID, Conner SJ et al. The effect of sperm DNA fragmentation on miscarriage rates: A systematic review and meta-analysis. *Hum Reprod* 2012; 27(10): 2908–17.
56. Said TM, Grunewald S, Paasch U et al. Advantage of combining magnetic cell separation with sperm preparation techniques. *Reprod Biomed Online* 2005; 10: 740–6.
57. Grunewald S, Paasch U, Glander HJ. Enrichment of non-apoptotic human spermatozoa after cryopreservation by immunomagnetic cell sorting. *Cell Tissue Bank* 2001; 2(3): 127–33.
58. Said TM, Agarwal A, Zborowski M, Grunewald S, Glander HJ, Paasch U. Utility of magnetic cell separation as a molecular sperm preparation technique. *J Androl* 2008; 29(2): 134–42.
59. Aziz N, Said T, Paasch U, Agarwal A. The relationship between human sperm apoptosis, morphology and the sperm deformity index. *Hum Reprod* 2007; 22: 1413–9.
60. de Vantery Arrighi C, Lucas H, Chardonnens D, de Agostini A. Removal of spermatozoa with externalized phosphatidylserine from sperm preparation in human assisted medical procreation: Effects on viability, motility and mitochondrial membrane potential. *Reprod Biol Endocrinol* 2009; 7: 1.

61. Grunewald S, Paasch U, Said TM, Rasch M, Agarwal A, Glander HJ. Magnetic-activated cell sorting before cryopreservation preserves mitochondrial integrity in human spermatozoa. *Cell Tissue Bank* 2006; 7(2): 99–104.
62. Said TM, Agarwal A, Grunewald S et al. Selection of non-apoptotic spermatozoa as a new tool for enhancing assisted reproduction outcomes: An *in-vitro* model. *Biol Reprod* 2006; 74: 530–7.
63. Said TM, Grunewald S, Paasch U, Rasch M, Agarwal A, Glander HJ. Effects of magnetic-activated cell sorting on sperm motility and cryosurvival rates. *Fertil Steril* 2005; 83(5): 1442–6.
64. Grunewald S, Reinhardt M, Blumenauer V et al. Increased sperm chromatin decondensation in selected nonapoptotic spermatozoa of patients with male infertility. *Fertil Steril* 2009; 92(2): 572–7.
65. Zahedi A, Tavalaee M, Deemeh MR, Azadi L, Fazilati M, Nasr-Esfahani MH. Zeta potential vs apoptotic marker: Which is more suitable for ICSI sperm selection? *J Assist Reprod Genet* 2013; 30(9): 1181–6.
66. Polak de Fried E, Denaday F. Single and twin ongoing pregnancies in two cases of previous ART failure after ICSI performed with sperm sorted using annexin V microbeads. *Fertil Steril.* 2010; 94(1): 351.e15–8.
67. Rawe VY, Boudri HU, Sedo CA, Carro M, Papier S, Nodar F. Healthy baby born after reduction of sperm DNA fragmentation using cell sorting before ICSI. *Reprod Biomed Online* 2010; 20(3): 320–3.
68. Dirican EK, Ozgun OD, Akarsu S et al. Clinical outcome of magnetic activated cell sorting of non-apoptotic spermatozoa before density gradient centrifugation for assisted reproduction. *J Assist Reprod Genet* 2008; 25(8): 375–81.
69. Sheikhi A, Jalali M, Gholamian M, Jafarzadeh A, Jannati S, Mousavifar N. Elimination of apoptotic spermatozoa by magnetic-activated cell sorting improves the fertilization rate of couples treated with ICSI procedure. *Andrology* 2013; 1(6): 845–9.
70. Gil M, Sar-Shalom V, Melendez Sivira Y, Carreras R, Checa MA. Sperm selection using magnetic activated cell sorting (MACS) in assisted reproduction: A systematic review and meta-analysis. *J Assist Reprod Genet* 2013; 30(4): 479–85.
71. Romany L, Garrido N, Motato Y, Aparicio B, Remohi J, Meseguer M. Removal of annexin V-positive sperm cells for intracytoplasmic sperm injection in ovum donation cycles does not improve reproductive outcome: A controlled and randomized trial in unselected males. *Fertil Steril.* 2014; 102(6): 1567–75.e1.
72. Alvarez Sedo C, Uriondo H, Lavolpe M, Noblia F, Papier S, Nodar F. Clinical outcome using non-apoptotic sperm selection for ICSI procedures: Report of 1 year experience. *Fertil Steril* 2010; 94(4): S232.
73. Herrero MB, Delbes G, Chung JT et al. Case report: The use of annexin V coupled with magnetic activated cell sorting in cryopreserved spermatozoa from a male cancer survivor: Healthy twin newborns after two previous ICSI failures. *J Assist Reprod Genet* 2013; 30(11): 1415–9.
74. Carchenilla MSC, Agudo D, Rubio S et al. Magnetic activated cell sorting (MACS) is a useful technique to improved pregnancy rate in patients with high level of sperm DNA fragmentation. *Hum Reprod* 2013; 28: i118–37.
75. Kruger TF, Coetzee K. The role of sperm morphology in assisted reproduction. *Hum Reprod Update* 1999; 5(2): 172–8.
76. van der Merwe FH, Kruger TF, Oehninger SC, Lombard CJ. The use of semen parameters to identify the subfertile male in the general population. *Gynecol Obstet Invest* 2005; 59(2): 86–91.
77. Bartoov B, Berkovitz A, Eltes F, Kogosowski A, Menezo Y, Barak Y. Real-time fine morphology of motile human sperm cells is associated with IVF–ICSI outcome. *J Androl* 2002; 23(1): 1–8.
78. Check JH, Levito MC, Summers-Chase D, Marmar J, Barci H. A comparison of the efficacy of intracytoplasmic sperm injection (ICSI) using ejaculated sperm selected by high magnification versus ICSI with testicular sperm both followed by oocyte activation with calcium ionophore. *Clin Exp Obstet Gynecol* 2007; 34(2): 111–2.
79. Bartoov B, Berkovitz A, Eltes F et al. Pregnancy rates are higher with intracytoplasmic morphologically selected sperm injection than with conventional intracytoplasmic injection. *Fertil Steril* 2003; 80(6): 1413–9.
80. Boitrelle F, Guthauser B, Alter L et al. High-magnification selection of spermatozoa prior to oocyte injection: Confirmed and potential indications. *Reprod Biomed Online* 2014; 28(1): 6–13.
81. Lo Monte G, Murisier F, Piva I, Germond M, Marci R. Focus on intracytoplasmic morphologically selected sperm injection (IMSI): A mini-review. *Asian J Androl* 2013; 15(5): 608–15.
82. Berkovitz A, Eltes F, Yaari S et al. The morphological normalcy of the sperm nucleus and pregnancy rate of intracytoplasmic injection with morphologically selected sperm. *Hum Reprod* 2005; 20(1): 185–90.
83. Vanderzwalmen P, Hiemer A, Rubner P et al. Blastocyst development after sperm selection at high magnification is associated with size and number of nuclear vacuoles. *Reprod Biomed Online* 2008; 17(5): 617–27.
84. Garolla A, Fortini D, Menegazzo M et al. High-power microscopy for selecting spermatozoa for ICSI by physiological status. *Reprod Biomed Online* 2008; 17(5): 610–6.
85. Hammoud I, Boitrelle F, Ferfouri F et al. Selection of normal spermatozoa with a vacuole-free head (x6300) improves selection of spermatozoa with intact DNA in patients with high sperm DNA fragmentation rates. *Andrologia* 2013; 45(3): 163–70.

86. Franco JG, Jr., Baruffi RL, Mauri AL, Petersen CG, Oliveira JB, Vagnini L. Significance of large nuclear vacuoles in human spermatozoa: Implications for ICSI. *Reprod Biomed Online* 2008; 17(1): 42–5.
87. Mongkolchaipak S, Vutyavanich T. No difference in high-magnification morphology and hyaluronic acid binding in the selection of euploid spermatozoa with intact DNA. *Asian J Androl* 2013; 15(3): 421–4.
88. Wilding M, Coppola G, di Matteo L, Palagiano A, Fusco E, Dale B. Intracytoplasmic injection of morphologically selected spermatozoa (IMSI) improves outcome after assisted reproduction by deselecting physiologically poor quality spermatozoa. *J Assist Reprod Genet* 2011; 28(3): 253–62.
89. Antinori M, Licata E, Dani G et al. Intracytoplasmic morphologically selected sperm injection: A prospective randomized trial. *Reprod Biomed Online* 2008; 16(6): 835–41.
90. Cassuto NG, Hazout A, Bouret D et al. Low birth defects by deselecting abnormal spermatozoa before ICSI. *Reprod Biomed Online.* 2014; 28(1): 47–53.
91. Hazout A, Dumont-Hassan M, Junca AM, Cohen Bacrie P, Tesarik J. High-magnification ICSI overcomes paternal effect resistant to conventional ICSI. *Reprod Biomed Online* 2006; 12(1): 19–25.
92. Souza Setti A, Ferreira RC, Paes de Almeida Ferreira Braga D, de Cassia Savio Figueira R, Iaconelli A, Jr, Borges E, Jr. Intracytoplasmic sperm injection outcome versus intracytoplasmic morphologically selected sperm injection outcome: A meta-analysis. *Reprod Biomed Online* 2010; 21(4): 450–5.
93. Setti AS, Figueira RC, Braga DP, Aoki T, Iaconelli A, Jr, Borges E, Jr. Intracytoplasmic morphologically selected sperm injection is beneficial in cases of advanced maternal age: A prospective randomized study. *Eur J Obstet Gynecol Reprod Biol* 2013; 171(2): 286–90.
94. De Vos A, Van de Velde H, Bocken G et al. Does intracytoplasmic morphologically selected sperm injection improve embryo development? A randomized sibling-oocyte study. *Hum Reprod* 2013; 28(3): 617–26.
95. Leandri RD, Gachet A, Pfeffer J et al. Is intracytoplasmic morphologically selected sperm injection (IMSI) beneficial in the first ART cycle? A multicentric randomized controlled trial. *Andrology* 2013; 1(5): 692–7.
96. Teixeira DM, Barbosa MA, Ferriani RA et al. Regular (ICSI) versus ultra-high magnification (IMSI) sperm selection for assisted reproduction. *Cochrane Database Syst Rev* 2013; 7: CD010167.

Use of *in vitro* maturation in a clinical setting

Patient populations and outcomes

10

YOSHIHARU MORIMOTO, AISAKU FUKUDA, and MANABU SATOU

HISTORY OF IVM

In vitro maturation (IVM) is not a new technology. Its use was first reported by Pincus and Enzmann (1) in mammals in 1935. Preclinical studies were continued in animals by Edwards (2), and Edwards et al. (3) reported clinical application in humans, obtaining immature oocytes from cases with ovarian stimulation. Veeck et al. (4) achieved the first successful birth from immature oocytes produced during an *in vitro* fertilization (IVF) program. Thereafter, Cha et al. (5) initiated the use of immature oocytes from unstimulated ovaries of patients in a donation program. Following this, Trounson et al. (6) achieved another breakthrough in the development of IVM. They chose immature oocytes aspirated from patients with polycystic ovary syndrome (PCOS) as a source for the procedure. Gonadotropins, estradiol, and fetal calf serum were supplemented in the medium and a 65% maturation rate was achieved within 43–47 hours of culture. Then, the maturation rate was acceptable, but the pregnancy success rate was only 11.1%. However, IVM has become a mainstream choice for PCOS treatment. Patients with PCOS are hypersensitive to stimulating drugs, and ovarian stimulation for conventional IVF in PCOS patients carries the risk of severe ovarian hyperstimulation syndrome (OHSS), causing some patients to quit treatment. Use of IVM is the only method that can completely prevent OHSS.

INDICATIONS OF IVM

IVM was originally applied in patients with PCOS without gonadotropin stimulation to avoid OHSS caused by controlled ovarian hyperstimulation (COH) (5,6). IVM is indicated not only for patients with PCOS, but also for women with polycystic ovaries (PCOs) who are at higher risk of OHSS by standard COH compared to regular-cycling women. IVM should also be considered in patients who are anxious about the long-term side effects of gonadotropin, since some patients worry about not only the stimulating effect of gonadotropins, but also prospective events after aging (7,8). Regular-cycling women are also successfully treated with IVM with or without gonadotropin administration, but its indication for regular-cycling women remains controversial due to the lower number of oocytes available (9–18). The clinical benefits of follicle-stimulating hormone (FSH) administration to regular-cycling women are yet to be determined (19,20). Poor embryo quality or repeated failures by conventional IVF are other proposed indications for IVM. Women with the so-called egg factor in which no mature eggs are found in repeated cycles (germinal vesicles only), recurrent fertilization failure, or very poor-quality embryos are also IVM targets (21). Patients who repeatedly failed IVF without distinct causes are also IVM candidates (22,23).

We have achieved 88 clinical pregnancies by IVM from 1999 to 2008. Twenty-one pregnancies (24%) resulted after repeated IVF failures. Eight of these 21 pregnancies (38%) were treated by IVM due to poor-quality embryos generated by IVF. Figure 10.1 shows the number of failed IVF cycles and IVM cycles to achieve pregnancy in 18 ongoing cases. They failed 4.9 times with IVF and needed IVM 2.3 times to achieve pregnancy. In conclusion, the primary indication for IVM is PCOS or PCOs with a high risk of OHSS. Other indications are patients who desire not to undergo gonadotropin administration, and repeated IVF failure due to impaired oocyte or embryo qualities. IVM is an alternative to conventional assisted reproduction technology (ART).

FSH PRIMING

With the target follicles in IVM being only 5–10 mm, beginners find it quite difficult to puncture these small follicles. Therefore, it is more practical to stimulate and prepare rather easier conditions by using bigger follicles. FSH priming prior to IVM has been tried from the initial stage of IVM development, and FSH is usually administered from day 3 or 5 at a dose of 150–300 IU. Several studies have reported the effectiveness and ineffectiveness of FSH priming. Wynn et al. (19) added recombinant FSH on days 2, 4, and 6 and achieved significant numbers of retrieved oocytes and an increased maturation rate. On the other hand, Mikkelsen et al. (10) found no difference between the two groups of primed and non-primed patients after three days of addition of FSH from day 3. Moreover, the combination of FSH and human chorionic gonadotropin (hCG) at the same time was reported by Lin et al. (24), and no significant effectiveness was shown in the literature.

The advantage for FSH priming can be described as easier follicular preparation; however, we need to consider its disadvantages. After immature follicles are recruited from the cohort, the dominant follicles start to grow and differentiate. At this moment, apoptosis of follicles and oocytes starts to be atretic in follicles and degenerative in oocytes. This phenomenon may affect both the quality and

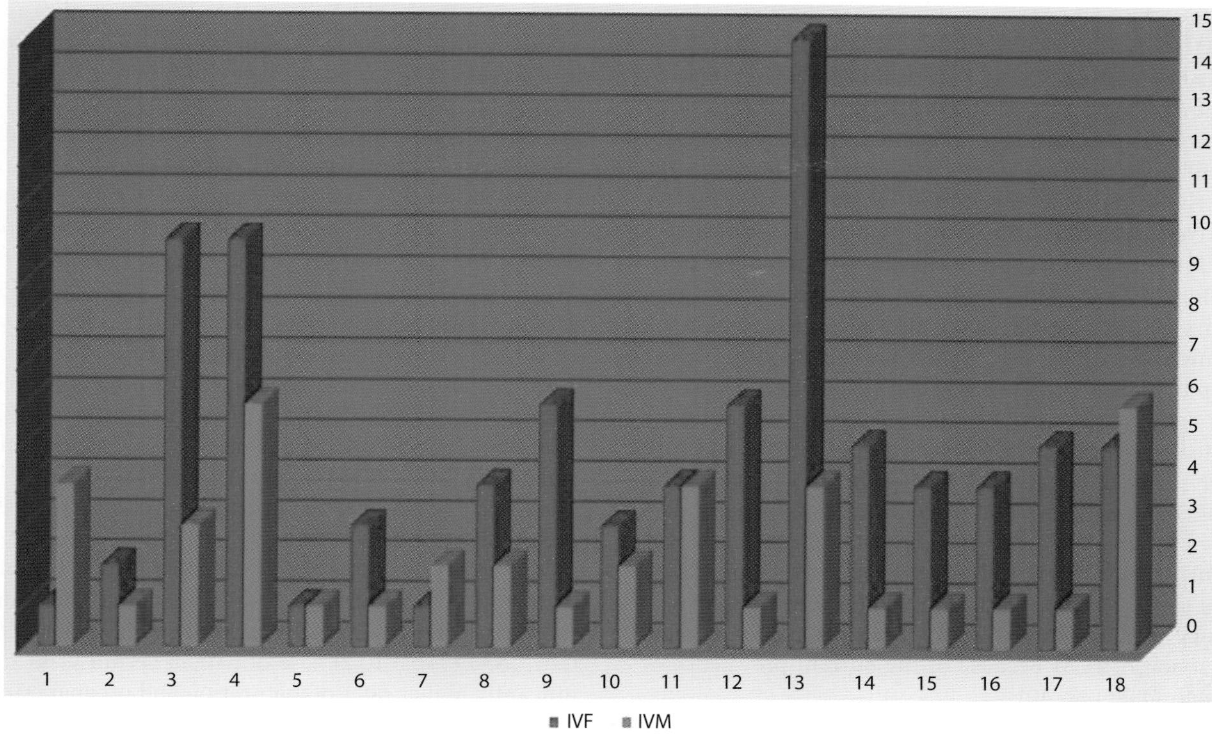

Figure 10.1 The number of failed *in vitro* fertilization cycles (red bar) and *in vitro* maturation cycles (green bar) to achieve pregnancy in 18 ongoing cases.

the developmental competence of oocytes for fertilization and embryogenesis. FSH priming may accelerate the speed of folliculogenesis; that is, the follicles proceed to be atretic in an unusual manner. Therefore, it would be difficult to estimate optimal timing for ovum pickup (OPU) in IVM.

hCG PRIMING

Chian et al. (25) reported the efficacy of hCG administration 36 hours prior to OPU in patients with PCOS. A total of 10,000 U of hCG was used for priming. The mean number of oocytes retrieved was equivalent for the hCG-primed and -non-primed groups, but the oocyte maturation rate was significantly improved in the hCG-primed group. The time course changed between the hCG-primed and -non-primed groups. There were no differences in the rates of fertilization and cleavage. The possible presence of luteinizing hormone (LH) or hCG receptors has been described in small follicles. LH induces the rupture of mature follicles, and surges in its level offer the optimal basis for ovulation. Thus, it is obvious that mature follicles possess LH receptors. However, LH receptors are not proven to exist in immature oocytes; rather, they mainly exists in the cumulus–oocyte complexes (COCs). Ge et al. (26) investigated the effect of hCG addition to IVM medium in patients undergoing IVM. Patients with PCOs were non-primed with hCG, and the patients were allocated to one of three groups according to the medium used, namely the hCG-containing medium, initially non-hCG followed by hCG-containing medium, and non-hCG medium groups. No differences were observed between the three groups in terms of the numbers of retrieved oocytes, maturation rates, fertilization rates, or implantation rates. Surprisingly, high maturation rates of over 60% were obtained without using hCG. Further investigations and clinical data are needed to clarify the effectiveness of hCG priming.

APPLICATION OF CRYOPRESERVATION OF EMBRYOS IN IVM

IVM has been applied not only for PCOS or PCOs, but also for repeated IVF failures for more than a decade. However, the overall pregnancy rate achieved by IVM is still inferior to that by conventional IVF due to its lower implantation rate (27,28). Therefore, many infertility specialists hesitate to adopt IVM as a routine ART procedure. The major causes of its inferiority to IVF come from the discrepancy of synchronization between not only nuclear and cytoplasmic maturation in the oocytes but also between the developmental speed of the embryos and the endometrial lining. Endometrial development synchronized with embryonic growth is essential in any ART procedure, but a dominant follicle or corpus luteum does not routinely exist in IVM. Therefore, the contribution of the follicular and luteal sex steroids to the endometrium is possibly compromised. We achieved the first IVM pregnancy and birth in Japan (29), but the success rate was far beyond that of IVF at our institution. To improve IVM pregnancy rates, we included frozen–thawed transfer in the IVM protocol to adjust the embryonics and endometrial development (30,31). Our protocol is illustrated in Figure 10.2. Briefly, the scan is started on day 6–8 of the menstrual cycle to measure endometrial thickness and the number and size of the antral follicles, and to exclude the presence of dominant follicles >14 mm. Pretreatment with metformin for more than a month and low-dose FSH administration are selectively performed. A second evaluation is performed a few days later to determine a suitable day of hCG administration. hCG is given when more than two follicles grow to a size >8 mm. On the day of hCG administration, if the endometrial thickness is ≥8 mm, the transfer of fresh day 2/3 embryo or blastocyst is usually scheduled. However, if the endometrium thickness is <8 mm, two-pronuclear oocytes or cleaved embryos are cryopreserved for future frozen–thawed embryo transfer as shown in Figure 10.2 (31–34). Frozen–thawed embryo transfer is usually performed under a hormone-supplemented cycle. The medication after transfer was identical in both fresh and frozen cycles (Figure 10.2). Vitrification of the embryos derived from IVM oocytes is a routine procedure in the clinical application of IVM because of the current prevalence of the techniques (35–40).

IVM MEDIUM

Retrieved COCs were transferred to IVM culture medium, cultured for 24–26 hours, and assessed for maturity after removal of cumulus cells (CCs) (Figure 10.3). All IVM cases undergo intracytoplasmic sperm injection (ICSI). IVM culture should be completed without the use of mineral oil to avoid absorption of the steroids secreted by CCs (41).

We compared the MediCult IVM® system (MediCult, Origio, Måløv, Denmark) and tissue culture medium 199 (TCM199, Invitrogen, Carlsbad, CA) (Table 10.1). Both IVM media were supplemented with FSH, hCG, and patient serum. The rates of maturation and pregnancy were significantly increased by changing from TCM199 to MediCult (49.1% versus 53.3% and 15.9% versus 30.0%, respectively). Some studies have compared IVM outcomes using different culture media. Söderström-Anttila et al. and Filali et al. reported similar clinical outcomes between MediCult and TCM199 culturing (42,43). However, de Araujo et al reported that TCM199 is more suited for human IVM than human tubal fluid (HTF) (44). Therefore, TCM199 or commercialized IVM media are preferred for human IVM.

We have also compared different protein sources: patient's own serum, donor's follicular fluid, and serum substitute supplement (SSS; Irvine Scientific, Santa Ana, CA, USA) (Table 10.2). Use of patient serum yielded significantly higher rates of maturation and pregnancy compared to the use of donor's follicular fluid and SSS. Human IVM medium is usually supplemented with patient serum (5,6,45,46). Mikkelsen et al. reported the use of patient serum to be more effective than human serum albumin for human IVM (47). Serum may contain factors preferable for oocyte maturation such as epidermal growth factor

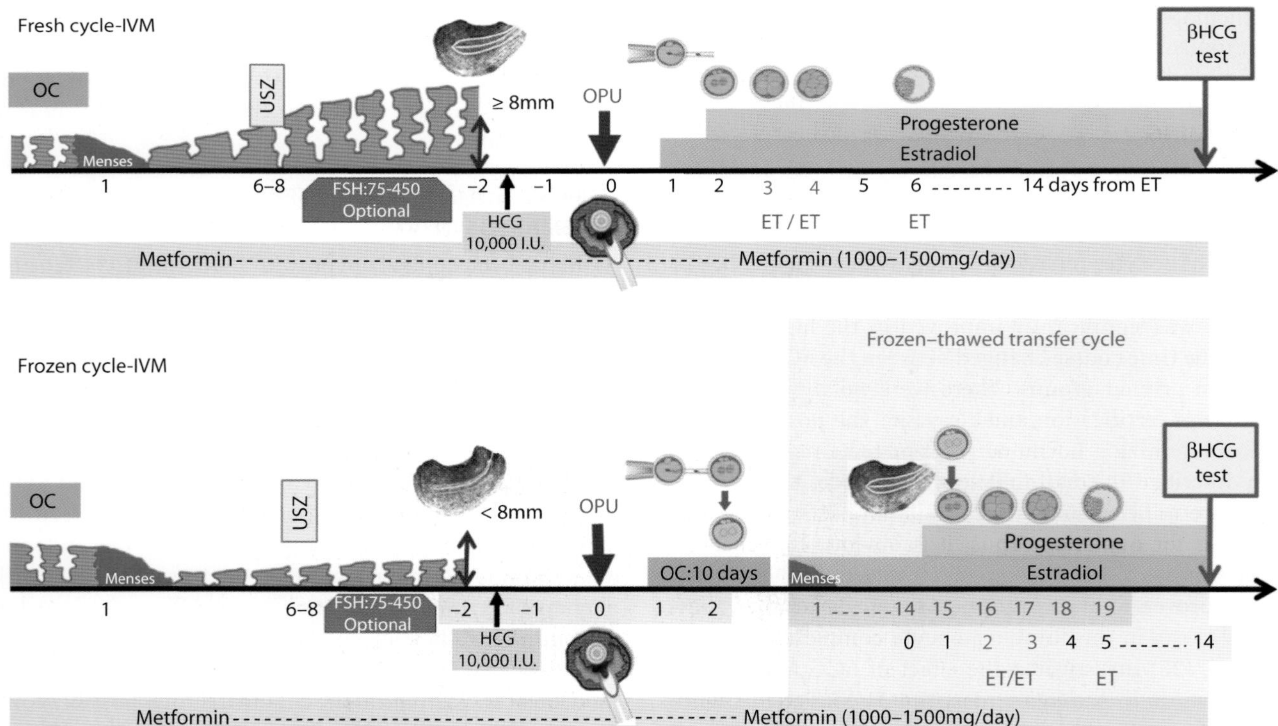

Figure 10.2 This illustration shows how to choose fresh or frozen *in vitro* maturation cycles by the thickness of the endometrial lining on the day of human chorionic gonadotropin administration.

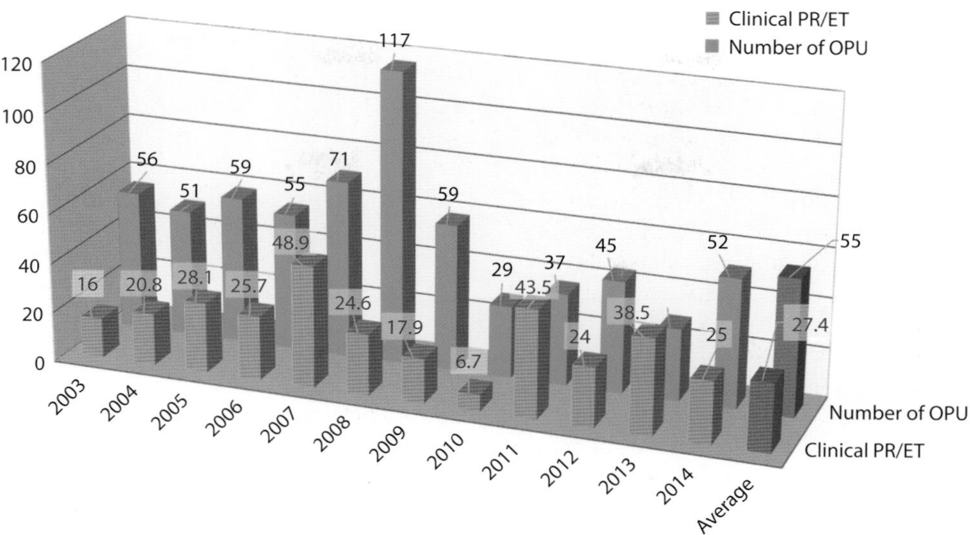

Figure 10.3 The number of *in vitro* maturation cases and clinical pregnancy rates from 2003 through to 2014 at our institution.

(EGF), and EGF-like growth factor improves the maturation of human immature oocytes (48). Further, patient serum is easily available and is not contaminated with foreign viruses or factors.

OOCYTE IDENTIFICATION

The follicular aspirate is collected in collection tubes containing 4-(2-hydroxyet4hyl)-1-piperazineethane sulfonic acid (HEPES)-buffered HTF with 0.4% heparin to prevent blood clot formation during oocyte retrieval. There are two ways to identify COCs in the follicular aspirates. First, a small volume of follicular aspirate is poured directly into a Petri dish and examined for COCs under a stereomicroscope (25,49). COCs aspirated from IVM cycles have only small amounts of CCs compared to those from COH cycles, and denuded oocytes are sometimes included (Figure 10.4). Because of the low number of CCs and partially denuded oocytes, it is difficult to identify COCs aspirated from the IVM cycles in a large amount of follicular fluids in a Petri dish. In particular, in the hCG-primed IVM cycles, CC expansion is induced by a high-dose hCG signal, thus making COC identification easier.

Another method of COC identification is to the use of a cell strainer (70 μm nylon mesh, Becton Dickinson, Franklin Lakes, NJ, USA) (50,51). The follicular aspirates in the collection tubes are filtered with the cell strainer (Figure 10.5), and the collected aspirates are washed with HEPES-buffered HTF containing SSS and 0.4% heparin to remove red blood cells and small cells. The cell strainer is then transferred upside down to a Petri dish, and the collected aspirates are flushed with HTF from the backside of the cell strainer and observed for COCs under a stereomicroscope. The COCs with dispersed CCs are sticky and sometimes block the pores of the cell strainer. It is hard to flush the cell strainer and time consuming to search for the COCs. Therefore, at our center, after identifying the oocytes

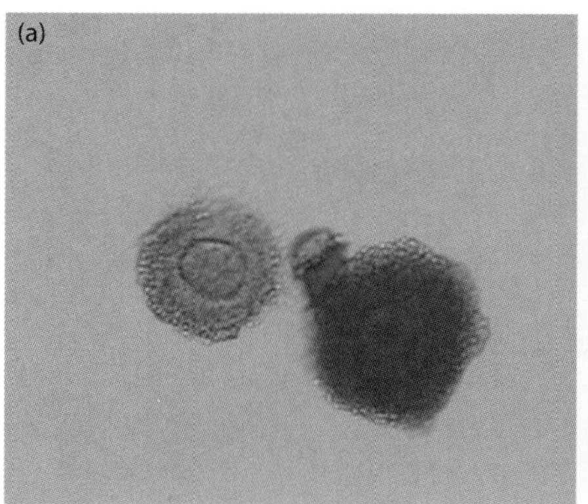

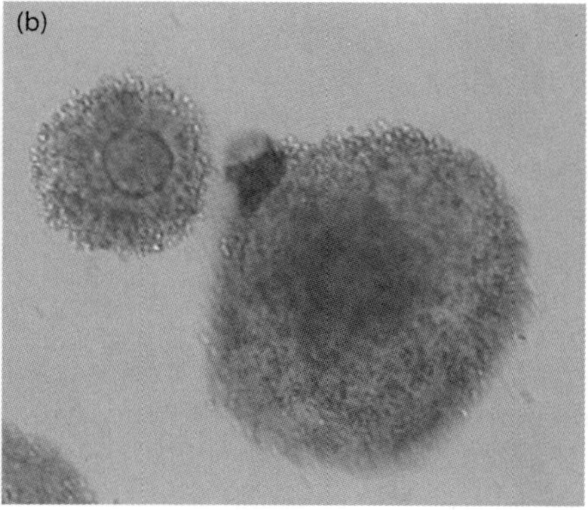

Figure 10.4 Morphological changes of COCs before and after culture in the IVM medium. (a) The immature COCs after oocyte retrieval. (b) The same COCs 26 hours after culture in the IVM medium. The CCs has expanded, and COCs volume increased to approximately 2 or 3 times as before culture. Original magnification ×200.

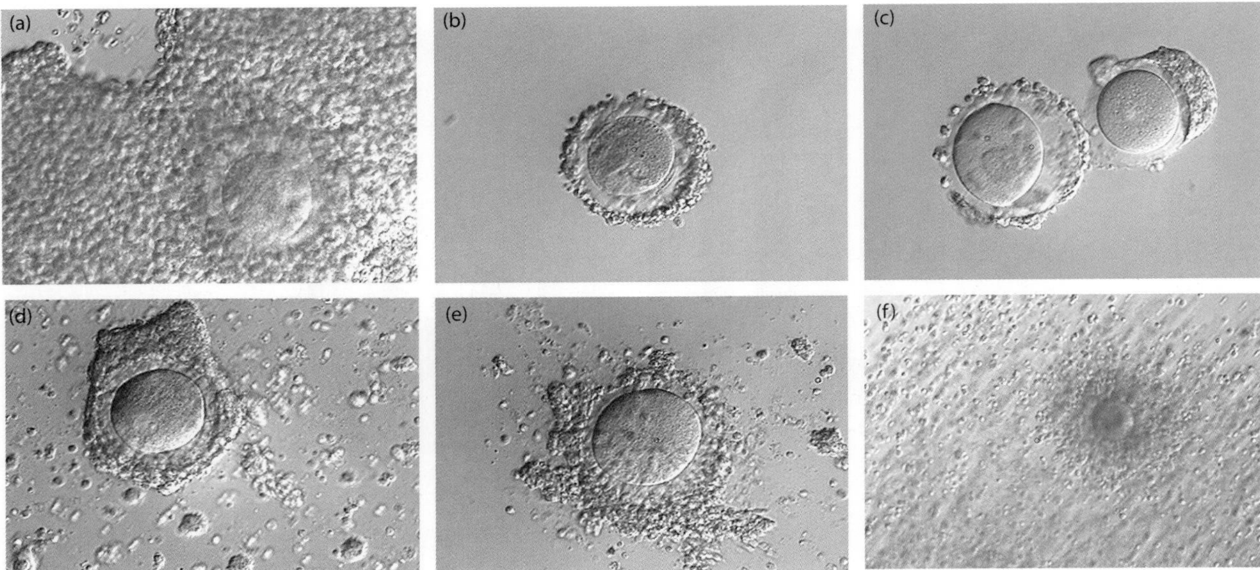

Figure 10.5 Various morphologies of the cumulus–oocyte complexes (COCs) observed at the time of oocyte collection. (a) The oocyte with compacted, rich cumulus cells (CCs). (b) Germinal vesicle (GV)-stage oocyte with less than two to three CC layers. (c) Metaphase I-stage oocyte showing small-volume CCs and is partially denuded. (d) GV-stage oocyte with partially dispersed CCs. (e) Metaphase I-stage oocyte with dispersed CCs. (f) COCs with fully expanded CCs retrieved in controlled ovarian hyperstimulation cycles. Original magnification (a–e) 200×, (f) 100×.

with dispersed CCs under a stereomicroscope, the remaining aspirates are filtered through a cell strainer to facilitate identification of the oocytes with a lower number of CCs.

There are various morphologies of retrieved COCs in hCG-primed IVM cycles (Figure 10.4a–e). Son et al. revealed that *in vivo*-matured oocytes are included on the day of oocyte retrieval. It has been also reported that *in vivo*-matured oocytes have high developmental potential (46), which suggests that it is necessary to perform ICSI is adapted to oocyte maturation conditions. To observe oocyte maturation without removing CCs, it stretches thin the COCs on the Petri dish. If no identify GV by stretching the COC, it has been confirmed by removing of CCs in our center.

OPU FOR IVM

The application of IVM has been limited since its development due to the difficulty in puncturing small follicles. Unstimulated follicles are mobile and therefore it is not easy to puncture at the correct point of the ovary. The needles for IVM usually range from 21 to 19 gauge. Before the procedure, positioning of the large pelvic vessels by the color Doppler method is recommended. A careful ultrasonography beforehand makes OPU easier and safer. A complete record of the size and numbers of follicles is an important resource for further improvement of the procedure.

To facilitate easier puncturing of small follicles, we developed a newly designed needle (IVF OSAKA IVM Needle, Kitazato Medical Co. Ltd, Tokyo, Japan). The needle is composed of two needles, one for puncturing (21 G) and one for holding (17 G) (Figure 10.6). The puncture needle is located inside the holding needle. First, the vaginal skin is penetrated without anesthesia and the needle is inserted and reaches 1 cm into the ovary to hold it. Second, the puncture needle is smoothly inserted into the holding needle without any resistance from hard skin. Small follicles are sequentially punctured by rotating the needle (Figure 10.7).

The aspiration pressure used for puncturing in IVM is an important issue. We compared 180 and 300 mmHg as the puncture pressures for oocyte retrieval (52). The rate of transferable embryos of retrieved oocyte number was significantly higher in the lower-pressure group (low, 23.8%; high, 12.8%). The ongoing pregnancy rate was also better in the group used low pressure at puncture (low, 30.0%; high, 4.3%). This finding indicates that high-pressure aspiration may impair oocyte quality and developmental competence for embryogenesis.

METFORMIN APPLICATION IN IVM

Metformin, an oral biguanide insulin-sensitizing agent used in type 2 diabetes mellitus, can reduce the hyperinsulinemia and hyperandrogenemia associated with PCOS and aid in ovulation (53–58). We have tried several approaches, including new needle systems, aspiration pressure changes, and frozen–thawed cycles, to improve the clinical outcomes compared to conventional IVF (30,31); however, pregnancy rates did not improve as per expectations. The quality of either the oocyte that matured *in vitro* or the resulting embryos was an integral factor for achieving this goal. We then evaluated serum levels of insulin and homeostasis model assessment for insulin

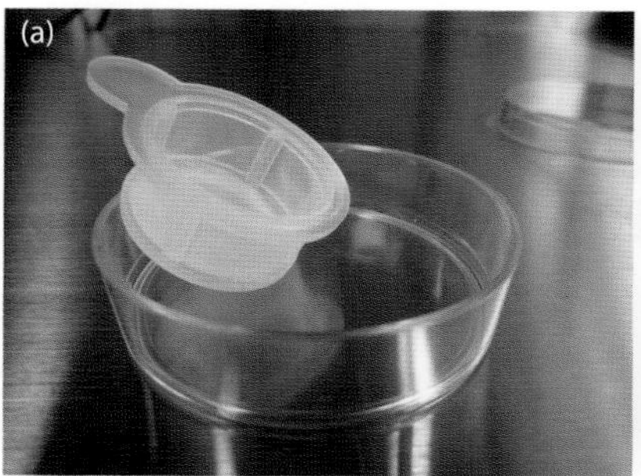

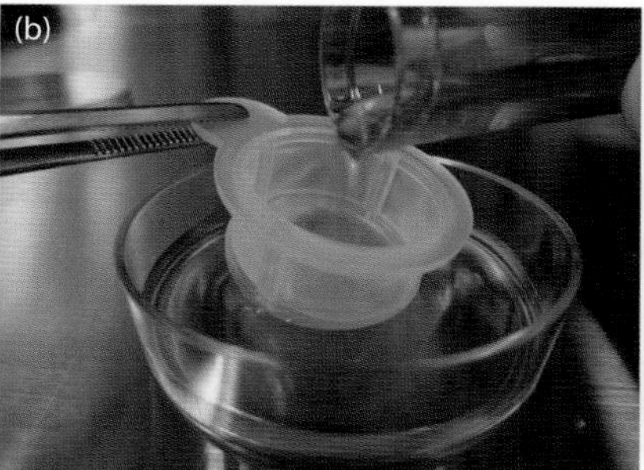

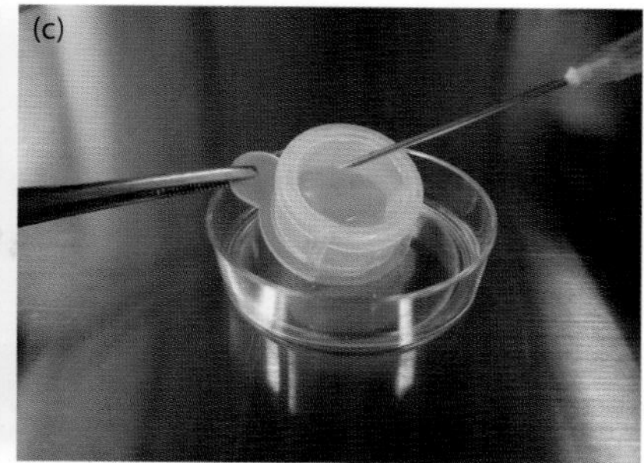

Figure 10.6 The schematic procedure of oocyte collection using a cell strainer. (a) The cell strainer is kept in a Petri dish (Falcon, 60 × 15 mm). (b) Follicular aspirates containing human tubal fluid with heparin are filtered with a cell strainer. (c) After filtering, the collected aspirates are rinsed and transferred into another Petri dish for identification of COCs under a stereomicroscope.

resistance (HOMA-R). When HOMA-R was >1.25, metformin (1500 mg/day) was administrated at least one month before IVM. If the patient was unable to tolerate the side effects such as diarrhea and nausea, the dose was reduced to 750–1000 mg/day. We applied metformin in an IVM protocol as shown in Figure 10.2, because metformin improves not only the environment of the intrafollicular milieu, but also endometrial condition (32,33). Following the initiation of routine metformin use in 2007, the clinical outcomes improved significantly as shown in Figure 10.8. We analyzed the effect of metformin on IVM results (Table 10.1). In the metformin-treated group, the number of oocytes retrieved was significantly higher and the pregnancy rate was also significantly improved in fresh IVM cycles. However, the clinical outcomes of frozen–thawed cycles did not show any significant improvements. Metformin may improve oocytes quality by reducing hyperinsulinemia and by modulating local insulin and insulin-like growth factor levels, but we could not prove this suspicion (59). Although an efficacious implantation in human reproduction is the result of endometrial factors or oocyte and embryonic features (60), our data suggest a beneficial effect of metformin on endometrial development and receptivity as shown by some studies (61–63). In conclusion, metformin pretreatment of patients with PCOs before IVM has a positive effect on the clinical outcome of IVM.

IVM is a relatively new ART compared to IVF (64). Although IVM was invented 13 years after IVF and clinically applied two years later (5,6), 20 years have passed since the first IVM baby was born. The clinical outcome of IVM varies not only by institution, but also by patient type. The pregnancy rate per IVM transfer for either PCOS or PCO patients is in the range of 21.5%–52.9% (15,24,25,42,49,65–70). The major reason for this difference might be the different pretreatments such as FSH and hCG used in different patients. Women with normal ovaries or regular cycles experience less success with IVM. Pregnancy rates are as low as 4%–33.3% per transfer (10,15,17,20,42,50,71,72). To date, FSH priming with hCG administration seems to be a common pretreatment for the IVM procedure. However, we recommend metformin pretreatment and use of frozen–thawed cycles for patients with poor endometrium development (31–33).

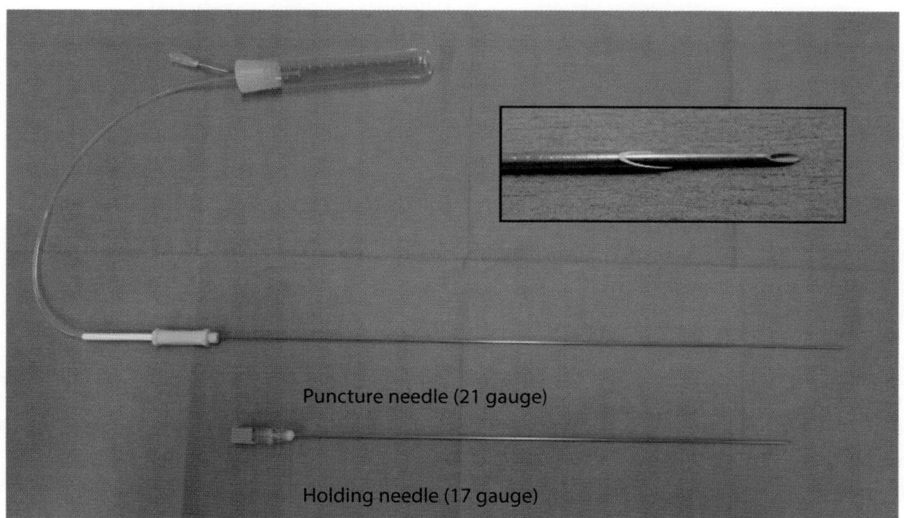

Figure 10.7 The IVF-OSAKA IVM needle is composed of a puncture needle (21 gauge) and a holding needle (17 gauge).

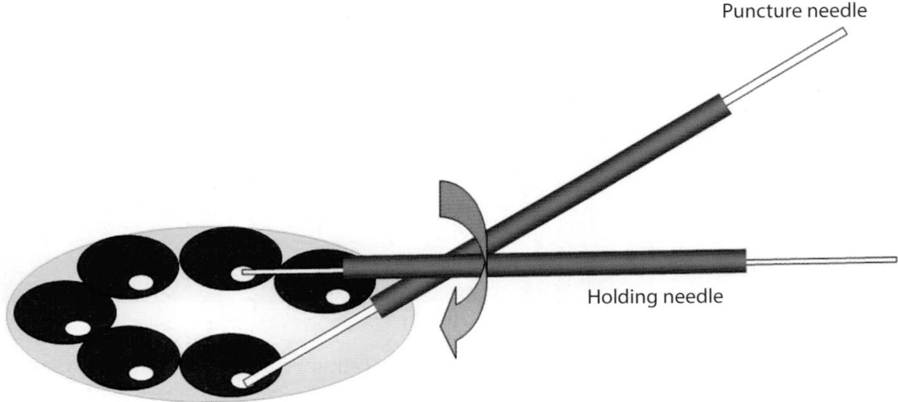

Figure 10.8 After the ovary was fixed by the holding needle, every follicle can be easily punctured by rotation of the puncture needle.

We started IVM from 1999 and spent a few years improving its methodology. The latest data of our IVM results are shown in Figure 10.9. We performed 660 IVM cycles (387 fresh and 273 frozen cycles); from 2003 to 2014, the pregnancy rate per transfer was 27.4%, while the miscarriage rate was 21.6%. However, the average pregnancy rate over the last three years was >30%. Various attempts have been made to improve the clinical outcome. Several authors have reported a significant increase in malformations in IVM babies (42,67,68,73). No differences were observed in the perinatal morbidity, birth weight, gestational age at delivery, APGAR scores (the score for evaluation of the newborn infant), umbilical cord pH, or congenital abnormalities among IVM, IVF, and ICSI treatment outcomes (74). Our data also did not show any increase in the malformation rate for IVM treatment using either fresh or frozen cycles.

FOLLOW-UP OF IVM CHILDREN

It is estimated that globally >1300 IVM babies have been born, in contrast to an estimated 3 million babies conceived by standard IVF/ICSI over the last 33 years (75). However, there may not be much information available about these children in terms of published or unpublished data (67,76,77). In animal models, there have been rising concerns about IVM and its influences on epigenetic disorders (78–81). These theoretical concerns must be recognized in humans as well, but such effects have not been confirmed in IVM babies until now. As the importance of epigenetics in IVF is still controversial after millions of babies have been born via IVF, it will take some time to collect the IVM data that are required for meaningful analysis. We have completed 945 IVM cycles between 1999 and 2012 and achieved 116 pregnancies (76 deliveries and

Table 10.1 Comparison of clinical outcomes between the TCM199 and MediCult *in vitro* maturation systems

Culture medium	No. of cycles	Mean number of oocytes retrieved	Culture time (hours)	*In vitro* maturation rate (%)	Pregnancy rate per embryo transfer (%)
TCM199	447	8.4	24	49.1^{a}	15.9^{A}
MediCult *in vitro* maturation system	591	8.7	26	53.3^{b}	30.0^{B}

Significant differences between the different superscript characters ($p < 0.01$: a–b, A–B).

Table 10.2 Comparison of clinical outcomes between three protein supplementation in the MediCult *in vitro* maturation system

Protein supplementation	No. of cycles	Mean number of oocytes retrieved	Culture time (hours)	*In vitro* maturation rate (%)	Pregnancy rate per embryo transfer (%)
Donor's follicular fluid	154	9.2	26	49.6^{a}	28.1
Patient's own serum	271	8.9	26	57.7^{b}	38.8^{A}
Serum substitute supplement (Irvine Scientific)	166	7.9	26	52.7^{c}	23.1^{B}

Significant differences between the different superscript character ($p < 0.01$: a–b, a–c, A–B; $p < 0.05$: b–c).

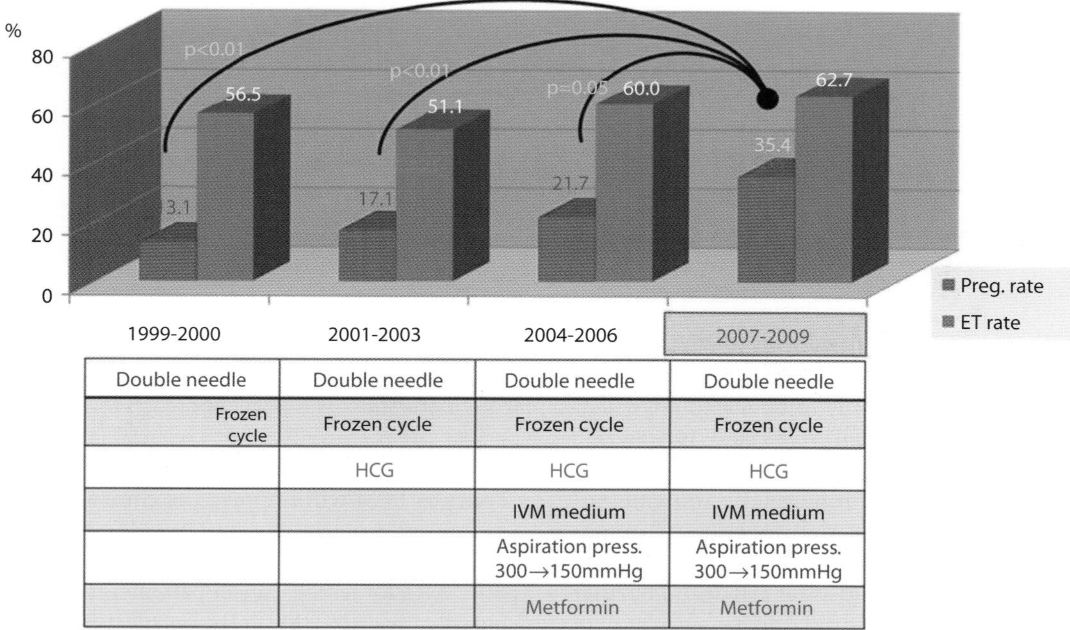

Figure 10.9 Clinical outcomes of fresh transfer cycles in *in vitro* maturation at IVF Osaka Clinic (a) from 1999 to 2009 and various changes of procedure performed in the meantime (b).

86 babies born). To date, 54 children born via IVM (37 fresh cycles and 17 frozen cycles) were followed until seven years of age by parental questionnaire sheets for their parents. The congenital major malformation rate was 1.8% (1/54), which did not differ from Japanese data of natural conception (NC). The physical and mental development of IVM babies was identical to NC babies, as determined on the basis of statistical data cited in the statistics from the Japan Ministry of Health, Labour and Welfare (2010 edition). Although other reports are retrospective and limited in size, they suggest that the perinatal outcomes of births from IVM cycles are similar to those of conventional ART, also considering the incidence of major and minor abnormalities (77). However, one child was normal at birth, but appeared to have Asperger's syndrome later, and long-term follow-up of IVM babies is warranted.

OOCYTE MATURATION, ULTRASTRUCTURE, AND MITOCHONDRIAL DISTRIBUTION

The IVM procedure has developed and is now used worldwide. Although its simplicity appeals to patients, it is not yet an alternative to conventional IVF because of its low or unstable success rates, caused by low maturation rates. To improve the maturation and success rates, it is essential to elucidate the human oocyte maturation process. The oocytes mature in the zona pellucida, cytoplasm, and nucleus; it is also necessary to maintain the harmony of each maturation factor in order to achieve maturation. The nuclear maturation process has been well investigated, but in contrast, the mechanism and manner of maturation in the cytoplasm remains unclear. Nuclear maturation is identified by germinal vesicle breakdown and the extrusion of polar bodies on light microscopy, unlike cytoplasmic maturation.

Ultrastructural investigation can be used to study the process of cytoplasmic maturation. We observed oocytes during IVM using electron microscopy. In the germinal vesicle stage of unstimulated oocytes, the mitochondria were dense and scattered in the cytoplasm. The volume of smooth endoplasmic reticulum (sER) was small. Microvilli were not yet developed at this stage. Within 6–12 hours of culture, the germinal vesicles underwent breakdown and the appearance of the cytoplasm changed dramatically. The mitochondria enlarged and sER ballooned. At this stage of metaphase I, the communication between the CCs and the oolemma was remarkably activated. The processes from the CC surface reached the oolemma through the zona pellucida. In metaphase II, the mitochondria increased in number and aggregated in the center of the cytoplasm. The microvilli on the surface of the oolemma developed and elongated, extending into the perivitelline space. At this stage, the first and second lysosomes were seen, and the sER increased in quantity and ballooned. Mitochondria play an essential role in oocyte maturation. A low oocyte respiration rate indicates that ATP production resulted in maturation failure and atresia in IVF (82). The ATP content is related not only to oocyte maturation, but also to fertilization, embryogenesis, and implantation (83).

Mitochondria migrate and are distributed in each stage of maturation. The mitochondria distribution pattern was found to be homogenous in the germinal vesicles and heterogonous in metaphase I and II (84–86). Wilding et al. (87) described that the mitochondrial distribution pattern was homogenous in poor-quality embryos. The mitochondria distribution is controlled by the microtubule network. Inappropriate network formation may cause abnormal mitochondrial distribution, which indicates the shortage

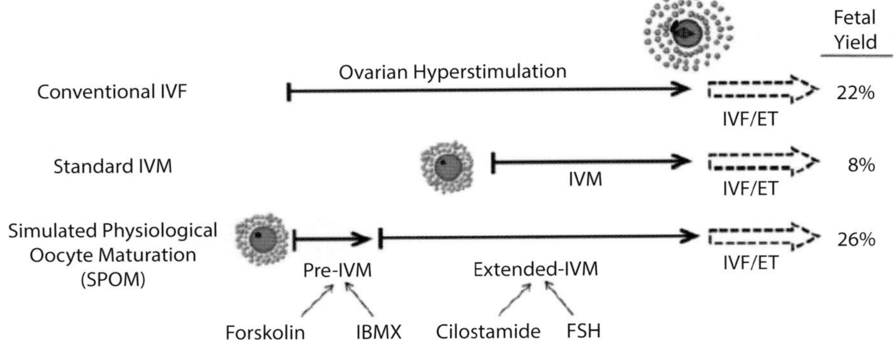

Figure 10.10 The methodology of simulated physiological oocyte maturation as a novel approach for *in vitro* maturation. (Adapted from Wilding M et al. *Hum Reprod* 2001; 16: 909–17.)

of an energy source to maintain oogenesis and embryogenesis (87). Mitochondria are multifunctioning organelles. They not only create energy, but also transiently store calcium ions and regulate apoptosis for cell death. Further investigation of the mitochondrial function in human oocytes do benefit the improvement in the embryo quality and better clinical IVM outcome.

There have been advances in efforts to improve maturation and oocyte quality in animal biology. Albuz et al. (89) proposed a new method for IVM and named it simulated physiological oocyte maturation (SPOM) (Figure 10.10). This is a method for arranging the basic signaling molecule and the level of the gonadotropin second messenger cyclic AMP (cAMP) in oocytes. High levels of cAMP induce meiotic arrest. SPOM enables the cytoplasm to enhance maturation during arrest of nuclear maturation. They settled one to two pre-IVM term using forskolin that increases cAMP and 3-isobutyl-1-methylxanthine (IBMX), which is one of the phosphodiesterase (PDE) inhibitors. At the next extended IVM term using FSH that acts as final maturation mediator and cilostamide that is a PDE were used. Improvements in blastocyst rates, implantation rates, and fetus yield rates in bovines and mice were demonstrated by this method. This could be a novel method for overcoming the disadvantage of current clinical IVM, which is the diminished rate of oocyte maturation and pregnancy outcomes.

FURTHER APPLICATIONS OF IVM PREIMPLANTATION GENETIC DIAGNOSIS AND DONOR OOCYTE SOURCES

Although at present it may be premature to offer IVM to all types of patients, IVM is definitely a safer option than IVF in patients who are extremely sensitive to gonadotropins, because it completely avoids the risk of OHSS. From the point of view of safety, IVM should be applied for any male factor-related infertility such as testicular sperm extraction and ICSI cases without female disorders such as PCOS/PCOs (15,24,25,42,49,65–69,71) or normal ovaries/regular-cycling women (10,17,20,50,71,72). Vitrification of human embryos has become a routine ART method. Not only cleaved embryos, but also oocytes have been successfully vitrified (38,39,88,89). Application of frozen cycles in IVM will improve the clinical outcome because of improved uterine receptivity. Moreover, cryopreservation of either immature oocytes or mature oocytes is a safer ART for female cancer patients, especially those with breast cancer (90). Recently, oncofertility is a hot topic in reproductive medicine. IVM is an indispensable technology for frozen ovarian tissues from cancer patients or is suitable for urgent retrieval of multiple oocytes without stimulation when patients have short time before emergency chemotherapy or surgery (91).

In vitro follicular growth (92) is used with IVM because it is a necessary step for IVM when ovarian tissue cryopreservation is clinically applied. Other than routine therapeutic ART procedures, IVM benefits oocyte donors by avoiding the risks of both OHSS and unknown long-term side effects (8). Recurrent pregnancy loss patients are also good candidates for IVM, since many of them need several trials in order to acquire a healthy baby. These patients are usually reluctant to undergo ART treatment because of the high cost and the complicated procedure of the ART itself. If patients have sufficient antral follicle counts, IVM is a preferable option for performing a safer preimplantation genetic diagnosis procedure (93). IVM is also a strong treatment tool for repeated IVF failure for many reasons such as premature ovarian failure or insufficiency, poor response, poor embryo quality, abnormal oocytes, and empty follicle syndrome, among others. IVM is not only indicated for PCOS/PCO patients in order to avoid the risk of OHSS, but will also play an integral role in the development of future ARTs.

REFERENCES

1. Pincus G, Enzmann EV. The comparative behavior of mammalian eggs *in vivo* and *in vitro*: I. The activation of ovarian eggs. *J Exp Med* 1935; 62: 655–75.
2. Edwards R. Maturation *in vitro* of mouse, sheep, cow, pig, rhesus monkey and human ovarian oocytes. *Nature* 1965; 20: 349–51.
3. Edwards R, Bavister B, Steptoe P. Early stages of fertilization *in vitro* of human oocytes matured *in vitro*. *Nature* 1969; 221: 632–5.

4. Veeck LL, Wortham JW, Jr, Witmyer J et al. Maturation and fertilization of morphologically immature human oocytes in a program of *in vitro* fertilization. *Fertil Steril* 1983; 39: 594–602.
5. Cha KY, Koo JJ, Ko JJ et al. Pregnancy after *in vitro* fertilization of human follicular oocytes collected from nonstimulated cycles, their culture *in vitro* and their transfer in a donor oocyte program. *Fertil Steril* 1991; 55: 109–13.
6. Trounson A, Wood C, Kaushe A. *In vitro* maturation and the fertilization and developmental competence of oocytes recovered from untreated polycystic ovarian patients. *Fertil Steril* 1994; 62: 353–62.
7. Whittemore AS, Harris R, Itnyre J et al. Characteristics relating to ovarian cancer risk: Collaborative analysis of 12 US case–control studies. *Am J Epidemiol* 1992; 136: 1184–203.
8. Whittemore AS. The risk of ovarian cancer after treatment for infertility. *N Engl J Med* 1994; 331: 805–6.
9. Barnes FL, Crombie A, Gardner DK et al. Blastocyst development and birth after *in vitro* maturation of human primary oocytes, intracytoplasmic sperm injection and assisted hatching. *Hum Reprod* 1995; 10: 3243–7.
10. Mikkelsen AL, Smith SD, Lindenberg S. *In-vitro* maturation of human oocytes from regularly menstruating women may be successful without follicle stimulating hormone priming. *Hum Reprod* 1999; 14: 1847–51.
11. Son WY, Park SJ, Hyun CS et al. Successful birth after transfer of blastocysts derived from oocytes of unstimulated women with regular menstrual cycle after IVM approach. *J Assist Reprod Genet* 2002; 19: 541–3.
12. Papanicolaou EG, Platteau P, Albano C et al. Immature oocyte *in-vitro* maturation: Clinical aspects. *Reprod Biomed Online* 2005; 10: 587–92.
13. Loutradis D, Kiapekou E, Zapanti E et al. Oocyte maturation in assisted reproductive technologies. *Ann NY Acad Sci* 2006; 1092: 235–46.
14. Cobo AC, Requena A, Neuspiller F et al. Maturation *in vitro* of human oocytes from unstimulated cycles: Selection of the optimal day for ovum retrieval based on follicular size. *Hum Reprod* 1999; 14: 1864–8.
15. Child TJ, Abdul-Jalil AK, Gulekli B et al. *In vitro* maturation of oocytes from unstimulated normal ovaries, polycystic ovaries, and women with polycystic ovary syndrome. *Fertil Steril* 2001; 76: 936–42.
16. Dal Canto MB, Miginini Renzini M, Brambillasca F et al. IVM—The first choice for IVF in Italy. *Reprod Biomed Online* 2006; 13: 159–65.
17. Yoon HG, Yoon SH, Son WY et al. Pregnancies resulting from *in vitro* matured oocytes collected from women with regular menstrual cycle. *J Assist Reprod Genet* 2001; 18: 325–9.
18. Bos-Mikich A, Ferreira M, Höher M et al. Fertilization outcome, embryo development and birth after unstimulated IVM. *J Assist Reprod Geneti* 2011; 28: 107–10.
19. Wynn P, Picton HM, Krapez JA et al. Pretreatment with follicle stimulating hormone promotes the numbers of human oocytes reaching metaphase II by *in vitro* maturation. *Hum Reprod* 1998; 13: 3132–8.
20. Fadini R, Dal Canto MB, Miginini Renzini M et al. Effect of different gonadotrophin priming on IVM of oocytes from women with normal ovaries: A prospective randomized study. *Reprod Biomed Online* 2009; 19: 343–51.
21. Hourvitz A, Maman E, Brengauz M et al. *In vitro* maturation for patients with repeated *in vitro* fertilization failure due to "oocyte maturation abnormalities". *Fertil Steril* 2010; 94: 496–501.
22. Gulekli B, Kovali M, Aydiner F et al. IVM is an alternative for patients with PCO after failed conventional IVF attempt. *J Assist Reprod Genet* 2011; 28: 495–9.
23. Fukuda A, Kanaya H, Sugihara K et al. Clinical outcomes of IVM–IVF (*in vitro* maturation, *in vitro* fertilization and embryo transfer) as a routine ART treatment and follow up study of IVM–IVF pregnancies in PCO patients. *Fertil Steril* 2007; 88: S261.
24. Lin YH, Hwang JL, Huang LW et al. Combination of FSH priming and hCG priming for *in-vitro* maturation of human oocytes. *Hum Reprod* 2003; 18: 1632–6.
25. Chian RC, Buckett WM, Tulandi T et al. Prospective randomized study of human chorionic gonadotrophin priming before immature oocyte retrieval from unstimulated women with polycystic ovarian syndrome. *Hum Reprod* 2000; 15: 165–70.
26. Ge HS, Huang XF, Zhang W et al. Exposure to human chorionic gonadotropin during *in vitro* maturation does not improve the maturation rate and developmental potential of immature oocytes from patients with polycystic ovary syndrome. *Fertil Steril* 2008; 89: 98–103.
27. Edwards RG. IVF, IVM, natural cycle IVF, minimal stimulation IVF—Time for a rethink. *Reprod Biomed Online* 2007; 15: 106–19.
28. Son WY, Chung JT, Herrero B et al. Selection of the optimal day for oocyte retrieval based on the diameter of the dominant follicle in hCG primed *in vitro* maturation cycles. *Hum Reprod* 2008; 23: 2680–5.
29. Fukuda A, Kawata A, Tohnaka M et al. Successful pregnancies by intracytoplasmic sperm injection (ICI) of *in vitro* matured oocytes from non-stimulated women. *J Fertil Implant* 2001; 18: 1–4.
30. Fukuda A, Tohnaka M, Yamasaki M et al. Improved pregnancy rate of IVM–IVF by selecting either fresh or frozen–thawed embryo transfer on endometrial thickness in unstimulated cycles. *J Fertil Implant* 2002; 19: 32–5.

31. Fukuda AI, Nakaoka Y, Tohnaka M et al. Establishment of *in vitro* maturation system (IVM–IVF) as a routine ART procedure by combination of hCG administration and frozen–thawed embryo transfer. *Fertil Steril* 2002; 78: S232.
32. Fukuda AI, Kanaya H, Oku H et al. Pretreatment of polycystic ovarian syndrome (PCOS) patients with Metformin optimizes results from the clinical application of *in vitro* maturation, *in vitro* fertilization and embryo transfer (IVM–IVF). *Fertil Steril* 2004; 82: S49–50.
33. Fukuda AI, Kanaya H, Sugihara K et al. Low dose FSH administration over Metformin pretreatment on polycystic ovarian syndrome (PCOS) patients improves the clinical outcome of *in vitro* maturation, *in vitro* fertilization and embryo transfer (IVM–IVF) treatment. *Fertil Steril* 2004; 84: S83–4.
34. Fukuda AI, Sato M, Sugihara K et al. *In vitro* maturation, *in vitro* fertilization and embryo transfer (IVM–IVF) combined with low dose FSH administration over Metformin pretreatment and frozen-thawed cycles should be a routine ART option for polycystic ovarian syndrome (PCOS) patients. *Fertil Steril* 2006; 86: S128–9.
35. Hashimoto S. Application of *in vitro* maturation to assisted reproductive technology. *J Reprod Dev* 2009; 55: 1–5.
36. Hashimoto S, Murata Y, Kikkawa M et al. Successful delivery after transfer of twice-vitrified embryos derived from in-vitro matured oocytes: A case study. *Hum Reprod* 2007; 22: 221–3.
37. Godin PA, Gaspard O, Thonon F et al. Twin pregnancy obtained with frozen thawed embryos after *in vitro* maturation in a patient with polycystic ovarian syndrome. *J Assist Reprod Genet* 2003; 20: 347–50.
38. Yang SH, Qin SL, Xu Y et al. Healthy live birth from vitrified blastocysts produced from natural cycle IVF/IVM. *Reprod Biomed Online* 2010; 20: 656–9.
39. Vanderzwalmen P, Ectors F, Grobet L et al. Aseptic vitrification of blastocysts from infertile patients, egg donors and after IVM. *Reprod Biomed Online* 2009; 19: 700–7.
40. Dowling-Lacey D, Jones E, Bocca S et al. Two singleton live birth after the transfer of cryopreserved–thawed day-3 embryos following an unstimulated *in-vitro* oocyte maturation cycle. *Reprod Biomed Online* 2010; 20: 387–90.
41. Shimada M, Kawano N, Terada T. Delay of nuclear maturation and reduction in developmental competence of pig oocytes after mineral oil overlay of *in vitro* maturation media. *Reproduction* 2002; 124: 557–64.
42. Söderström-Anttila V, Mäkinen S, Tuuri T et al. Favourable pregnancy results with insemination of *in vitro* matured oocytes from unstimulated patients. *Hum Reprod* 2005; 20: 1534–40.
43. Filali M, Hesters L, Fanchin R et al. Retrospective comparison of two media for *in-vitro* maturation of oocytes. *Reprod Biomed Online* 2008; 16: 250–6.
44. de Araujo CH, Nogueira D, de Araujo MC et al. Supplemented tissue culture medium 199 is a better medium for *in vitro* maturation of oocytes from women with polycystic ovary syndrome women than human tubal fluid. *Fertil Steril* 2009; 91: 509–13.
45. Park SE, Son WY, Lee SH et al. Chromosome and spindle configurations of human oocytes matured *in vitro* after cryopreservation at the germinal vesicle stage. *Fertil Steril* 1997; 68: 920–6.
46. Son WY, Tan SL. Laboratory and embryological aspects of hCG-primed *in vitro* maturation cycles for patients with polycystic ovaries. *Hum Reprod Update* 2010; 16: 675–89.
47. Mikkelsen AL, Høst E, Blaabjerg J et al. Maternal serum supplementation in culture medium benefits maturation of immature human oocytes. *Reprod Biomed Online* 2001; 3: 112–6.
48. Ben-Ami I, Komsky A, Bern O et al. *In vitro* maturation of human germinal vesicle-stage oocytes: Role of epidermal growth factor-like growth factors in the culture medium. *Hum Reprod* 2011; 26: 76–81.
49. Cha KY, Han SY, Chung HM et al. Pregnancies and deliveries after *in vitro* maturation culture followed by *in vitro* fertilization and embryo transfer without stimulation in women with polycystic ovary syndrome. *Fertil Steril* 2000; 73: 978–83.
50. Mikkelsen AL, Smith S, Lindenberg S. Impact of oestradiol and inhibin A concentrations on pregnancy rate in *in-vitro* oocyte maturation. *Hum Reprod* 2000; 15: 1685–90.
51. Son WY, Yoon SH, Park SJ et al. Ongoing twin pregnancy after vitrification of blastocysts produced by *in-vitro* matured oocytes retrieved from a woman with polycystic ovary syndrome: Case report. *Hum Reprod* 2002; 17: 2963–6.
52. Hashimoto S, Fukuda A, Murata Y et al. Effect of aspiration vacuum on the developmental competence of immature human oocytes retrieved using a 20-gauge needle. *Reprod Biomed Online* 2007; 14: 444–9.
53. Velázquez E, Acosta A, Mendoza SG. Menstrual cyclicity after metformin therapy in polycystic ovary syndrome. *Obstet Gynecol* 1997; 90: 392–5.
54. Nestler JE, Jakubowicz DJ, Evans WS et al. Effects of metformin on spontaneous and clomiphene-induced ovulation in the polycycstic ovary syndrome. *N Engl J Med* 1998; 338: 1876–80.
55. Ehrmann DA, Cavaghan MK, Imperial J et al. Effects of metformin on insulin secretion, insulin action, and ovarian steroidogenesis in women with polycystic ovary syndrome. *J Clin Endocrinol Metab* 1997; 82: 524–30.
56. Morin-Papunen LC, Koivunen RM, Ruokonen A et al. Metformin therapy improves the menstrual pattern with minimal endocrine and metabolic effects in women with polycystic ovary syndrome. *Fertil Steril* 1998; 69: 691–6.
57. Sattar N, Hopkinson ZE, Greer IA. Insulin-sensitising agents in polycystic-ovary syndrome. *Lancet* 1998; 351: 305–7.

58. Boomsma CM, Eijkemans MJ, Hughes EG et al. A meta-analysis of pregnancy outcomes in women with polycystic ovary syndrome. *Hum Reprod Update* 2006; 12: 673–83.
59. Franks S, Gilling-Smith C, Watson H et al. Insulin action in the normal and polycystic ovary. *Endocrinol Metab Clin North Am* 1999; 28: 361–78.
60. Schwarz LB, Chiu AS, Courtney M et al. The embryo versus endometrium controversy revisited as it relates to predicting pregnancy outcome in *in-vitro* fertilization–embryo transfer cycles. *Hum Reprod* 1997; 12: 45–50.
61. Jakubowicz DJ, Seppälä M, Jakubowicz S et al. Insulin reduction with metformin increases luteal phase serum glycodelin and insulin-like growth factor-binding protein 1 concentration and enhances uterine vascularity and blood flow in the polycystic ovary syndrome. *J Clin Endocrinol Metab* 2001; 86: 1126–33.
62. Kocak M, Caliskan E, Simsir C et al. Metformin therapy improves ovulatory rates, cervical scores, and pregnancy rates in clomiphene citrate-resistant women with polycystic ovary syndrome. *Fertil Steril* 2002; 77: 101–6.
63. Palomba S, Russo T, Orio F, Jr et al. Uterine effects of metformin administration in anovulatory cycle women with polycystic ovary syndrome. *Hum Reprod* 2006; 21: 457–65.
64. Steptoe PC, Edwards RG. Birth after the implantation of a human embryo. *Lancet* 1978; 2: 366.
65. Son WY, Chung JT, Demirtas E et al. Comparison of *in-vitro* maturation cycles with and without *in-vivo* matured oocytes retrieved. *Reprod Biomed Online* 2008; 17: 59–67.
66. Lim JH, Yang SH, Xu Y et al. Selection of patients for natural cycle *in vitro* fertilization combined with *in vitro* maturation of immature oocytes. *Fertil Steril* 2009; 91: 1050–5.
67. Cha KY, Chung HM, Lee DR et al. Obstetric outcome of patients with polycystic ovary syndrome treated by *in vitro* maturation and *in vitro* fertilization-embryo transfer. *Fertil Steril* 2005; 83: 1461–5.
68. Mikkelsen AL, Lindenberg S. Benefit of FSH priming of women with PCOS to the *in vitro* maturation procedure and outcome: A randomized prospective study. *Reproduction* 2001; 122: 587–92.
69. Child TJ, Phillips SJ, Abdul-Jalil AK et al. A comparison of *in vitro* maturation and *in vitro* fertilization for women with polycystic ovaries. *Obstet Gynecol* 2002; 100: 665–70.
70. Le Du A, Kodach IJ, Bourcigaux N et al. *In vitro* oocyte maturation for the treatment of infertility associated with polycystic ovarian syndrome. *Human Reprod* 2005; 20: 420–4.
71. Mikkelsen AL, Andersson AM, Skakkebeak NE et al. Basal concentrations of oestradiol may predict the outcome of *in-vitro* maturation in regularly menstruating women. *Hum Reprod* 2001; 16: 862–7.
72. Fadini R, Dal Canto MB, Miginini Renzini M et al. Predictive factors in *in-vitro* maturation in unstimulated women with normal ovaries. *Reprod Biomed Online* 2009; 18: 251–61.
73. Suikkari AM, Salokorpi T, Pihlaja M et al. Healthy children born after *in vitro* maturation of oocytes. *Hum Reprod* 2005; 20: i105.
74. Buckett WM, Chian RC, Holzer H et al. Congenital abnormalities and perinatal outcome in pregnancies following IVM, IVF and ICSI delivered in a single center. *Fertil Steril* 2005; 84: S80–1.
75. Suikkari AM. *In vitro* maturation: Its role in fertility treatment. *Curr Opin Obstet Gynecol* 2008; 20: 242–8.
76. Söderström-Anttila V, Salokorpi T, Pihlaja M et al. Obstetric and perinatal outcome and preliminary results of development of children born after *in-vitro* maturation of oocytes. *Hum Reprod* 2006; 21: 1508–13.
77. Fadini R, Mignini Renzini M, Guamieri T et al. Comparison of the obstetric and perinatal outcomes of children conceived from *in vitro* maturation treatments with birth from conventional ICSI cycles. *Human Reprod* 2012; 27: 3601–8.
78. Mikkelsen AL. Strategies in human *in-vitro* maturation and their clinical outcome. *Reprod Biomed Online* 2005; 10: 593–9.
79. Albertini DF, Sanfins A, Combelles CM. Origins and manifestations of oocyte maturation competencies. *Reprod Biomed Online* 2003; 6: 410–5.
80. Fauser BC, Bouchard P, Coelingh-Bennink HJ et al. Alternative approaches in IVF. *Hum Reprod Update* 2002; 8: 1–9.
81. Young LE, Fernandes K, McEvoy TG et al. Epigenetic change in IGF2R is associated with fetal overgrowth after sheep embryo culture. *Nat Genet* 2001; 27: 153–4.
82. Kerjean A, Couvert P, Heams T et al. *In vitro* follicular growth affects oocyte imprinting establishment in mice. *Eur J Hum Genet* 2003; 11: 493–6.
83. Scott L, Berntsen J, Davies D et al. Symposium: Innovative techniques in human embryo viability assessment. Human oocyte respiration-rate measurement—Potential to improve oocyte and embryo selection? *Reprod Biomed Online* 2008; 17: 461–9.
84. Van Blerkom J, Davis PW, Lee J. ATP content of human oocytes and developmental potential and outcome after *in-vitro* fertilization and embryo transfer. *Hum Reprod* 1995; 10: 415–24.
85. Nishi Y, Takeshita T, Sato K, Araki T. Change of the mitochondrial distribution in mouse ooplasm during *in vitro* maturation. *J Nippon Med Sch* 2003; 70: 408–15.
86. Torner H, Brüssow KP, Alm H et al. Mitochondrial aggregation patterns and activity in porcine oocytes and apoptosis in surrounding cumulus cells depends on the stage of pre-ovulatory maturation. *Theriogenology* 2004; 61: 1675–89.

87. Wilding M, Dale B, Marino M et al. Mitochondrial aggregation patterns and activity in human oocytes and preimplantation embryos. *Hum Reprod* 2001; 16: 909–17.
88. Wang LY, Wang DH, Zou XY et al. Mitochondrial functions on oocytes and preimplantation embryos. *J Zhejiang Univ Sci B* 2009; 10: 483–92.
89. Albuz FK, Sasseville M, Lane M, Armstrong DT, Thompson JG, Gilchrist RB. Simulated physiological oocyte maturation (SPOM): A novel *in vitro* maturation system that substantially improves embryo yield and pregnancy outcomes. *Hum Reprod* 2010; 25: 2999–3011.
90. Asimakopoulos B, Kotanidis L, Nikolettos N. *In vitro* maturation and fertilization of vitrified immature human oocytes, subsequent vitrification of produced embryos, and embryo transfer after thawing. *Fertil Steril* 2011; 95: 2123.e1–2.
91. Chung K, Donnez J, Ginsburg E, Meirow D. Emergency IVF versus ovarian tissue cryopreservation: Decision making in fertility preservation for female cancer patients. *Fertil Steril* 2013; 99: 1534–42.
92. Chian RC, Gilbert L, Huang JYC et al. Live birth after vitrification of *in vitro* matured human oocytes. *Fertil Steril* 2009; 91: 372–6.
93. Oktay K, Buyuk E, Rodrigues-Wallberg KA et al. *In vitro* maturation improves oocyte or embryo cryopreservation outcome in breast cancer patients undergoing ovarian stimulation for fertility preservation. *Reprod Biomed Online* 2010; 20: 634–8.

Intracytoplasmic sperm injection

Technical aspects

11

QUEENIE V. NERI, NIGEL PEREIRA, TYLER COZZUBBO, ZEV ROSENWAKS, and GIANPIERO D. PALERMO

BACKGROUND

The use of assisted reproduction technology (ART) to overcome infertility has increased steadily in the U.S.A. and worldwide (1). Based on 2012 estimates, approximately 456 ART clinics in the U.S.A. performed 157,635 ART procedures resulting in 51,261 live deliveries and 65,151 infants (1). In 2012, ART contributed to 1.5% of all infants born in the U.S.A. (1). ART generally includes treatments such as *in vitro* fertilization (IVF), gamete intrafallopian transfer and zygote intrafallopian transfer, with IVF accounting for approximately 99% of all ART procedures (1). Soon after the establishment of IVF, it became clear that as many as 40% of conventional IVF cycles were affected by fertilization failure or by an extremely low fertilization rate, even though spermatozoa were placed in close proximity to oocytes (2). This was particularly problematic in patients with diminished sperm motility and/or poor morphology (i.e., it presented a complex obstacle for spermatozoa to penetrate the zona pellucida [ZP], a thick glycoprotein layer surrounding the oocyte) (2). In such cases, gamete micromanipulation was thought to be the only way to overcome this problem. The different techniques developed in this regard focused on assisting the spermatozoon to penetrate the ZP by "softening" it enzymatically with trypsin or pronase, or penetrating it chemically via localized or "pinpoint" exposure to acidified Tyrode's solution prior to sperm exposure (3). The placing of the spermatozoon beneath the ZP yielded consistent results, achieving a fertilization rate of ~20% (4). However, these techniques were abandoned because of limiting factors such as the need for many functional spermatozoa with good progressive motility, and complications like polyspermy (5). These initial efforts to assist sperm penetration soon became obsolete with the introduction of a microsurgical method for insertion of spermatozoa directly into the oocyte.

INTRACYTOPLASMIC SPERM INJECTION

Intracytoplasmic sperm injection (ICSI) involves the injection of a single spermatozoon directly into the cytoplasm of an oocyte. ICSI bypasses both the ZP barrier and sperm defects in the male gamete that compromise its ability to fertilize. The ability of ICSI to achieve higher fertilization and pregnancy rates regardless of sperm characteristics makes it the most powerful micromanipulation procedure yet for treating male factor infertility (6). In fact, the therapeutic possibilities of ICSI range from cases in which, after sperm selection, the spermatozoa show poor progressive motility, to its application in azoospermic men where spermatozoa are microsurgically retrieved from the epididymis and the testis (7–9). Retrieval of a low number of oocytes represents a further indication for this procedure. In fact, the availability of ICSI has been instrumental in some European countries (e.g., Italy and Germany) to circumvent restrictive legislation that limits the number of oocytes inseminated or embryos to be replaced (10,11). ICSI has also made the consistent fertilization of cryopreserved oocytes possible (12) since freezing can lead to premature exocytosis of cortical granules and ZP hardening that inhibit natural sperm penetration (13–16). When preimplantation genetic screening is to be performed on oocytes, the removal of the polar body requires the stripping of cumulus corona cells, thus supporting ICSI as the only insemination method to avoid polyspermy. When embryos need to be analyzed for gene defects, the avoidance of contaminating spermatozoa on the ZP reduces the chance of false amplification by polymerase chain reaction. ICSI is the preferred method of insemination by several groups for HIV-discordant couples because it virtually avoids the interaction of oocytes with semen, thereby reducing the risk of viral exposure (17–19). Advantages of ICSI over intrauterine insemination for HIV-discordant couples also include the considerably higher success rate (17), requiring fewer attempts to achieve a pregnancy with obviously reduced chances of viral exposure (18) for the unaffected partner. Reassuringly, no seroconversions have been reported following ART use for HIV-discordant couples (20).

In this chapter, we describe the quintessential technical details involved in the proper execution of ICSI. We also present the clinical outcomes associated with ICSI and appraise its safety.

SEMEN COLLECTION

Semen samples are collected by masturbation after 3–5 days of abstinence and allowed to liquefy for at least 20 minutes at 37°C before analysis. When the semen has high viscosity, this can be reduced within three to five minutes usually by adding it to 2–3 mL of 4-(2 hydroxyethyl)-1-piperazine-ethanesulfonic acid (HEPES)-buffered human tubal fluid (HTF) containing 200–300 IU of chymotrypsin (Sigma Chemical Co., St Louis, MO). The use of limited proteolytic enzyme with chymotrypsin was shown to effectively disperse hyperviscous samples for semen preparation (21,22). Electroejaculation is applied in cases of spinal cord injury or psychogenic anejaculation (23).

In cases of irreparable obstructive azoospermia, a condition often caused by congenital bilateral absence of the vas deferens and associated with a cystic fibrosis gene mutation, spermatozoa are retrieved by percutaneous epididymal sperm aspiration or microsurgical epididymal sperm aspiration (24–26). Variable volumes of fluid (1–500 μL) are collected from the epididymal lumen by a glass micropipette or a metal needle. Since spermatozoa are highly concentrated, only microliter quantities are needed. Alternatively, azoospermic patients undergo testicular sperm retrieval when the epididymal approach is not feasible because of scarring or due to impaired sperm production as in non-obstructive situations. An open biopsy or the more recent fine-needle aspiration technique is used for testicular sampling (27). The biopsy specimen of approximately 500 mg is rinsed in medium to remove red blood cells and is divided into small pieces with sterile tweezers under a stereomicroscope (28). Testicular sperm extraction (TESE) and the now refined micro-TESE procedures retrieve seminiferous tubules with residual spermatogenesis, granting a higher probability of sperm retrieval while maintaining greater anatomical integrity of the testicle (29,30). Motility in place or twitching is then assessed on a microscope at 100–200×, and a second biopsy specimen is obtained if spermatozoa are not found. After the micro-TESE procedure, the testicular samples are maintained overnight in medium at 37°C. Testicular tissue is exposed to collagenase type IV (1000 IU/mL) combined with 25 mg/mL of DNase I (31). The tissue is incubated with collagenase for one hour, and the suspension is mixed every 10–15 minutes to enhance enzymatic digestion. Large portions of undigested tissue such as tubular walls and connective tissue are removed, and the digested suspension is centrifuged twice at 500 g for five minutes. When no spermatozoa are identified in the pellet, the supernatant is further centrifuged at 1500–3000 g for five minutes. The pellet from this fraction is also examined. Both pellets are resuspended in a medium with a volume ranging from 20 to 200 μL. Sperm presence, viability, and motility characteristics together with the presence of other germ cells are noted. If no spermatozoa are seen, the resuspended sample is placed in individual 8 μL drops under oil and assessed under an inverted microscope at 400×.

SEMEN PROCESSING: ANALYSIS AND SELECTION

Semen concentration and motility are assessed in a Makler® counting chamber (Sefi Medical Instruments, Haifa, Israel). Morphologic characterization of sperm has a significant correlation with male infertility, and is performed using Kruger's strict criteria (32). Evaluation is usually made after spreading 5 μL of semen or sperm suspension on pre-stained slides (Testsimplets®; Boehringer, Munster, Germany), which can allow rapid assessment. The specimen is examined microscopically, and at least 100–200 spermatozoa are categorized. Semen parameters are considered to be impaired when the sperm concentration is $<15 \times 10^6$/mL, the progressive motility is <40%, or a normal morphology is exhibited by <4% of the spermatozoa (33). For selection of spermatozoa, the sample is washed by centrifugation at 500 g for five minutes in HTF medium supplemented with 6% (v/v) human serum albumin (HSA; Vitrolife, Englewood, CO). Semen samples with $<5 \times 10^6$/mL spermatozoa or <20% motile spermatozoa are washed in HTF medium by a single centrifugation at 500–1800 g for five minutes. The resuspended pellet is layered on a discontinuous ISolate® gradient (Irvine Scientific, Irvine, CA) on two layers (90% and 45%) and centrifuged at 300 g for 10 minutes. A one-layer ISolate gradient (90%) is used when samples have a sperm density $<5 \times 10^6$/mL spermatozoa and <20% motile spermatozoa. The sperm-rich ISolate fraction is washed by adding 4 mL of HTF medium and centrifuged at 600–800 g for 5–10 minutes to remove the silica gel particles. For spermatozoa with poor kinetic characteristics, the sperm suspension is exposed to a 3 mmol/L solution of pentoxifylline and is centrifuged again. The concentration of the assessed sperm suspension is adjusted to $1–1.5 \times 10^6$/mL, when necessary, by the addition of HTF medium, and subsequently incubated at 37°C in a gas atmosphere of 5% CO_2 in air until utilization for ICSI.

SPERM CRYOPRESERVATION

The sperm suspension (adjusted to a concentration of $\sim 30 \times 10^6$/mL) is diluted with at least an equal amount of cryopreservation medium (Freezing Medium-Test Yolk Buffer with Glycerol; Irvine Scientific), and up to 1 mL aliquots of the final solution are placed in 1 mL cryogenic vials (Nalgene Brand Products, Rochester, NY). The vials are exposed to liquid nitrogen vapor at -70°C for 15 minutes, and then plunged into liquid nitrogen at -196°C. Vials are thawed at 37°C for 15 minutes when spermatozoa are needed for injection. When in excess, epididymal spermatozoa and testicular tissue are cryopreserved for later use (34). Surgically retrieved samples are cryopreserved similarly to fresh semen with an excess of cryoprotectant and, when appropriate, exposed to a motility enhancer (3 mmol/L pentoxifylline) to facilitate the identification of viable spermatozoa (8).

COLLECTION AND PREPARATION OF OOCYTES

Baseline blood work and pelvic ultrasound are performed on menstrual cycle day 2 for patients treated with gonadotropin-releasing hormone (GnRH) antagonist protocols and on menstrual cycle day 3 for patients treated with the long GnRH agonist protocol (35). Normal baseline parameters include follicle-stimulating hormone (FSH) <12 mIU/mL, estradiol <75 pg/mL, and progesterone <1 ng/mL. Pelvic ultrasound is performed to evaluate endometrial thickness and to assess the antral follicle count and the presence of ovarian cysts.

Controlled ovarian superovulation (COS), human chorionic gonadotropin (hCG) trigger, and oocyte retrieval are performed per standard protocols (35,36). COS is carried out to maximize follicular response while minimizing the risk of ovarian hyperstimulation syndrome. In general, the hCG trigger is given when the two lead follicles attain a mean diameter of 17 mm. Oocyte retrieval is performed under conscious sedation using transvaginal ultrasound guidance approximately 35–36 hours after hCG administration. Under the inverted microscope at 100×, the cumulus–corona cell complexes are scored as mature, slightly immature, completely immature, or slightly hypermature. Thereafter, the oocytes are incubated for about four hours. Immediately prior to micromanipulation, the cumulus–corona cells are removed by exposure to HTF-HEPES-buffered medium containing 40 IU/mL of Cumulase® (Halozyme Therapeutics, Inc., San Diego, CA). A good and timely cumulus removal (37) is necessary for observation of the oocyte and effective use of the holding and/or injecting pipette during micromanipulation. For final removal of the residual corona cells, the oocytes are repeatedly aspirated in and out of an EZ-Tip® 290–135 μm (Research Instruments Ltd, Bickland Industrial Park, U.K.) locked on a STRIPPER® (ORIGIO, Knardrupvej, Denmark). Each oocyte is then examined under the microscope to assess nuclear maturity and morphology; metaphase II (MII) is assessed according to the absence of the germinal vesicle and the presence of an extruded polar body. ICSI is performed only in oocytes that have reached this level of maturity.

SETTING FOR THE MICROINJECTION

The holding pipette (HP-120-30; 120 μm outer diameter [OD]) and injecting pipette (IC-C1; 5–7 μm inner diameter [ID]) are both made from glass capillary tubes (Vitrolife AB, Göteborg, Sweden). Both pipettes are bent to an angle of approximately 30° at 1 mm from the tip, to be able to perform the injection procedure with the tips of the tools horizontally positioned in a plastic Petri dish (model 351006, Falcon; Becton and Dickinson, Lincoln Park, NJ). Immediately before injection, 1 μL of the sperm suspension is diluted with 4 μL of a 7% polyvinylpyrrolidone (PVP) solution with HSA (90121, Irvine Scientific) in HTF-HEPES medium placed in the middle of a plastic Petri dish. It is necessary to use the viscous solution during the procedure in order to slow down the aspiration and prevent the sperm from sticking to the wall of the injection pipette. When there are <100,000 spermatozoa per sample, the sperm suspension is concentrated to approximately 3 μL and transferred directly in drop #8 (Figure 11.1) where each oocyte is placed in the remaining 8 μL drops of G-MOPS™ (Vitrolife) supplemented with 6% G-MM™ (Vitrolife). These drops are covered with light-weight oil (Sage Medical, Trumbull, CT). Following immobilization, an individual spermatozoon is aspirated at the three o'clock edge of the PVP drop. For low concentration, a spermatozoon is retrieved by the injection tool from drop #8 and moved to the viscous medium central drop in order to remove debris, to gain better aspiration control, and to carry out immobilization. The procedure is carried out on a custom-designed heated stage (Eastech Laboratory, Centereach, NY) fitted on a Nikon TE2000U inverted microscope at 400× using Nikon Modulation contrast optics. This microscope is equipped with a customized micromanipulation

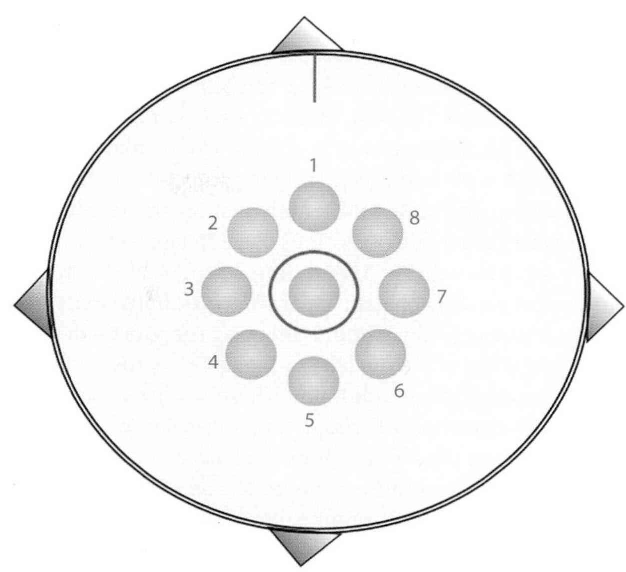

Figure 11.1 An intracytoplasmic sperm injection (ICSI) dish is made of 8 μL drops of ICSI medium plus one central drop overlaid with paraffin oil. The drops are labeled with a red pencil that is not embryo toxic. The central drop is marked with a circle while the surrounding drops are numbered 1–8 in a counterclockwise fashion. The central drop is removed and with replaced polyvinylpyrrolidone while drops 1–8 will contain a single oocyte each. Specimens with very few spermatozoa are concentrated to a very small volume and placed on drop #8.

set-up (NAI-20P, Narishige Co. Ltd, Tokyo, Japan) consisting of two motor-driven coarse control manipulators and two hydraulic micromanipulators. These custom manipulators have a modified low-position microscope mounting adaptor, a single power supply for the motor-drive coarse unit, and a tubing-free joystick. The micro-tools are controlled by two micro-injectors, one air control (IM-9B) for the holding pipette and the other IM-6 is oil operated and fitted with a metal syringe for the injection tool.

SELECTION OF THE SPERMATOZOON AND IMMOBILIZATION

Normally, at a magnification of 400×, it is not easy to select spermatozoa according to morphologic characteristics while they are in motion in medium. However, selection of a normal spermatozoon can be accomplished by observing its shape, its light refraction, and its motion pattern in viscous medium (7). When 1 μL of sperm suspension was added to the drop containing PVP, motile spermatozoa progress into the viscous medium while debris, other cells, bacteria, and immotile spermatozoa remain at the PVP–paraffin oil interface. The viscous medium, by decelerating the spermatozoon, allows evaluation of its tridimensional motion pattern, permitting morphological assessment as well as favoring aspiration into the pipette.

Although ICSI does not require any specific spermatozoon pretreatment, gentle immobilization achieved through mechanical pressure is needed to permeabilize the membrane, which allows the release of a sperm cytosolic factor, resulting in oocyte activation and improved fertilization rates (38–40). Human spermatozoa undergo important modifications in the nuclear chromatin where sperm DNA is packed very tightly to protect it during transition within the male and female genital tracts. Shaping of the male gamete nucleus takes place in late spermiogenesis as its chromatin is undergoing a remarkable condensation that renders the sperm transcriptionally inert and highly resistant to digestion. Following the morphological transformation of the nucleus in the testis, as spermatozoa transit through the epididymis, there occurs a stabilization of the chromatin through establishment of disulfide bonds between the thiol-rich protamines (41). Qualitative and quantitative modifications of the plasma membrane occurring in the lipidic composition (42) and the absorption of specific proteins secreted by the epididymal epithelium result in changes of its electric charge (43,44). The lack of all these changes is associated with a decreased ability of epididymal spermatozoa to bind and penetrate the oocyte (45). Owing to physiologic differences in their membrane characteristics, a more aggressive immobilization technique is necessary when using epididymal and/or testicular spermatozoa.

When the immobilization procedure is performed in a standard fashion, a spermatozoon is positioned at 90° to the tip of the pipette, which is then lowered gently to compress the sperm flagellum. The spermatozoon immobilized in this manner should maintain the shape of its tail. If during the process the latter is damaged or kinked, that spermatozoon is discarded and the procedure repeated with another sperm. An alternative and more effective procedure is aggressive immobilization, where the sperm tail is rolled over the bottom of the Petri dish in a location posterior to the mid-piece. This induces a permanent crimp in the tail section, making it kinked, looped, or convoluted (Figure 11.2). When these two distinct immobilization methods were applied to immature spermatozoa and the fertilization rates after ICSI were compared, the more extensive sperm tail disruption prior to oocyte injection appeared to improve the outcome. When the fertilization rate was compared within ejaculated spermatozoa, the difference was less remarkable (46–48). The findings were clarified in a later study where spermatozoa were mechanically immobilized and inserted into the perivitelline space of mouse oocytes (47) to allow ultrathin transmission electron microscopy (TEM) sections that revealed consistent alterations in the acrosomal region, including disruption of the plasma membrane, vesiculation, or even loss of the acrosome. All of the sperm that were assessed had undergone some membrane disorganization of the head, in contrast to the majority of control sperm. Immobilization of sperm immediately prior to the ICSI procedure is fundamental for its consistent success (47–52). A possible explanation of the variation in fertilization rate after aggressive immobilization may lie in the structural membrane differences between mature and immature spermatozoa. Immature gametes probably require additional manipulation to promote membrane permeabilization, which enhances the post-injection events involved in sperm nuclear decondensation.

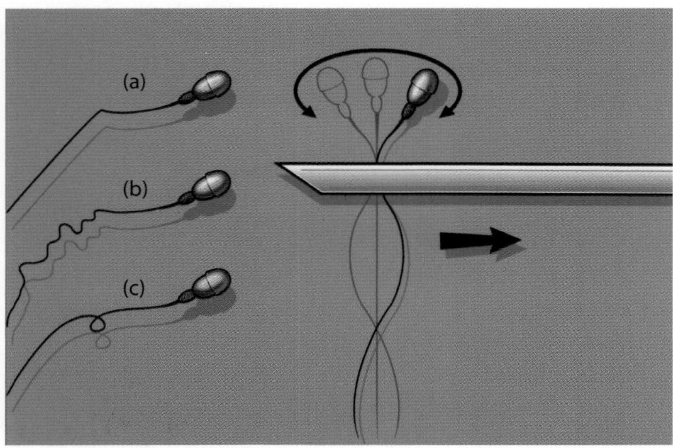

Figure 11.2 Aggressive immobilization of the spermatozoon for intracytoplasmic sperm injection. The correctly immobilized spermatozoon has its tail permanently kinked (a), convoluted (b), or looped (c).

Several studies have shown that suboptimal sperm morphology is often associated with aneuploidy, nuclear DNA damage, and, at times, impaired ICSI outcome (53–55). Some of the available methods for detecting sperm DNA integrity include the sperm chromatin structure assay, the terminal deoxynucleotidyl transferase dUTP nick-end labeling assay, and the comet assay. All of these require fixation and thus destruction of the sperm being assessed (56). It has been postulated that infertile men have compromised DNA integrity as measured by these methods without, however, a correlation with sperm concentration and morphology (57,58). However, by systematic observation performed in our laboratory, we identified an inverse relationship of a correlation between DNA fragmentation and motility (59). Perhaps the reason why there is a lack of predictability between DNA integrity and pregnancy outcome with ICSI inseminations may be explained by the fact that only motile spermatozoa are utilized for injection.

OOPLASMIC INJECTION

The oocyte is held in place by the suction applied to the holding pipette. The inferior pole of the oocyte touching the bottom of the dish allows a better grip of the oocyte during the injection procedure. The injection pipette is lowered and focused in accordance with the outer right border of the oolemma on the equatorial plane at three o'clock. The spermatozoon is then brought into proximity with the beveled opening of the injection pipette (Figure 11.3). The latter is pushed against the ZP, permitting its penetration to the inner surface of the oolemma. As the point of the pipette reaching the approximate center of the oocyte, a break in the membrane should occur. This is reflected by a sudden quivering of the convexities (at the site of invagination) of the oolemma

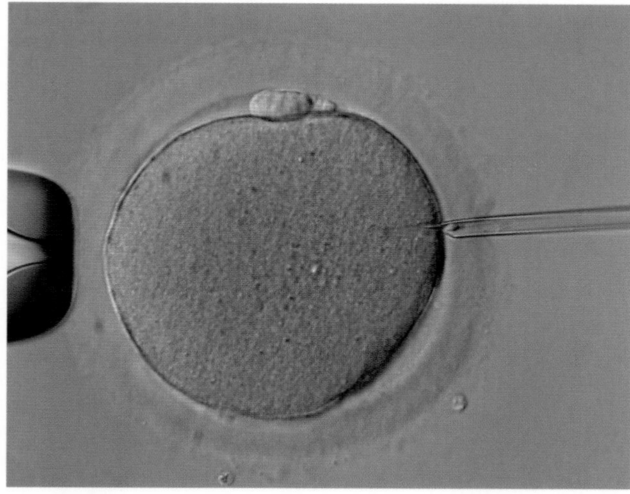

Figure 11.3 Intracytoplasmic sperm injection procedure. Prior to penetrating the oolemma, the spermatozoon is brought into proximity with the beveled opening of the injection pipette.

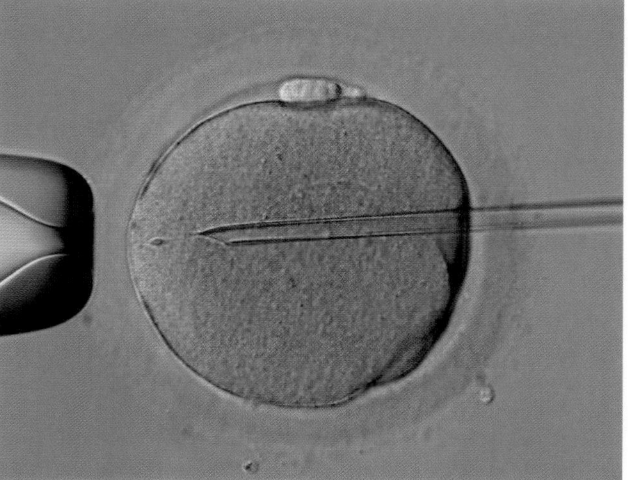

Figure 11.4 Intracytoplasmic sperm injection procedure. After the injection pipette has reached the approximate center of the oocyte, a break in the oolemma is visible as a quivering of the convexities of the membrane above and below the site of penetration.

above and below the penetration point, as well as the proximal flow of the cytoplasmic organelles and the spermatozoon moving upward into the pipette (Figure 11.4). These are then slowly ejected back into the cytoplasm, where the aspiration of the cytoplasm becomes an additional stimulus for activating the oocyte. To optimize the interaction with the ooplasm, the sperm cell should be ejected past the tip of the pipette to ensure an intimate position among the organelles that will help to maintain the sperm in place while withdrawing the pipette. When the pipette is approximately at the center of the oocyte, eventual surplus medium is re-aspirated, with the result that the cytoplasmic organelles tighten around the sperm, thereby reducing the size of the breach produced during injection. Once the pipette is removed, the breach area is observed, and the order of the opening should maintain a funnel shape with a vertex into the oocyte (Figure 11.5). If the border of the oolemma becomes inverted, ooplasmic organelles can leak out (46). Interestingly, the introduction of sequential media, fashioned by glucose and protein starvation, can result in complications during the execution of ICSI, resulting in increased oocyte damage. This phenomenon can be so severe that ICSI operators have to somewhat retrain themselves in performing the procedure, paying attention so as to avoid the eversion of the oolemma due to the adhesion to the injection tool as a consequence of the poor protein content (60). In addition, low-protein content media have also been adopted for sperm incubation with a consequential decreased ability of the male gamete to undergo capacitation and related membrane changes. Therefore, when performing ICSI, it is necessary to have multiple sequential strikes of the sperm flagellum to obtain effective immobilization and consequent membrane permeabilization (60).

EVALUATION OF FERTILIZATION, EMBRYO DEVELOPMENT, CULTURE CONDITIONS, AND EMBRYO REPLACEMENT

Around 12–17 hours after injection, oocytes are analyzed with regard to the integrity of the cytoplasm as well as the number and size of pronuclei. First-day cleavage is assessed 24 hours after fertilization, and the number and size of blastomeres are recorded for each embryo. At 72 hours after microinjection (the afternoon of day 3), those with good morphology are transferred into the uterine cavity.

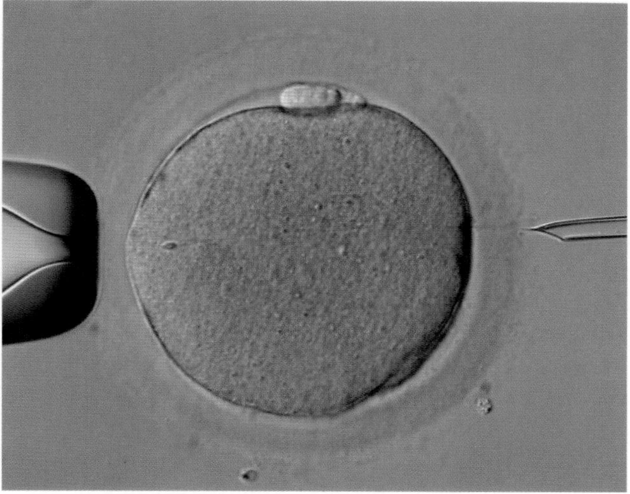

Figure 11.5 Intracytoplasmic sperm injection procedure. After the needle is withdrawn from the oocyte, the breach in the oolemma should be observed as a cone-shaped opening with its vertex toward the center of the oocyte.

The number of embryos transferred depends on embryo quality, availability, and maternal age. The association between the increased incidence of multiple pregnancies after IVF and the occurrence of maternal and neonatal complications is well documented (61,62). Blastocyst culture and transfer has recently been embraced as a strategy to overcome this problem due to the introduction of more sophisticated culture media. The extended culture of embryos to the blastocyst stage allows a "self-embryo selection," indicating the fast cleaving of embryos, and thus permitting the transfer of a lower number of them (63), moving toward a single embryo transfer. Studies have suggested that delaying transfer of embryos to the blastocyst stage (day 4/5) rather than the traditional cleavage stage (day 3) allows for better selection of the best conceptus to maximize pregnancy rates following a single embryo transfer (64).

Patients who are considered candidates for blastocyst culture are young women (<35 years old) with a good ovarian reserve, or older patients with an adequate number of pronuclear embryos. The number of embryos observed on day 3 and the capacity for embryo cleavage are also important criteria for selecting cases suitable for this procedure. Sequential culture media that meet the changing physiologic requirements of the embryos are used, thus supporting the viability of the blastocyst. Injected oocytes are rinsed and placed in a culture medium that is a variation of G1 medium previously described by Barnes et al. and Gardner et al. until assessment of fertilization (65,66). On day 3, after evaluation of embryo cell number and morphology, all embryos are transferred to a modified G2 medium and cultured for 48 hours (63,65). Thereafter, blastocyst formation is assessed and blastocysts are selected according to the established criteria for subsequent transfer (67).

EXTENDED SPERM SEARCH

In cases where no spermatozoa are identified at the initial analysis and after high-speed centrifugation still no sperm cells are found, an extensive search is performed. A dish is made in the same manner as an injection dish, with PVP solution placed in the central drop. The surrounding droplets of medium can be replaced with the actual specimen and pentoxifylline is added to each drop to help augment sperm motility. Each drop is browsed and motile spermatozoa that are identified should be picked up and transferred to the PVP drop. The same procedure is performed for surgically retrieved specimens that have been freshly retrieved or recently thawed. Several dishes may have to be made and thoroughly searched for TESE patients until enough spermatozoa are found for injection.

In TESE specimens, sperm may be extremely rare, if not totally absent. In such cases, the extended searches may take greater than three hours to complete, depending on the number of oocytes awaiting injection (68). Unsurprisingly, the level of difficulty in finding and acquiring sperm is negatively related to the clinical outcome. About 60% of testicular biopsies done on non-obstructive azoospermic (NOA) men are successful in retrieving spermatozoa

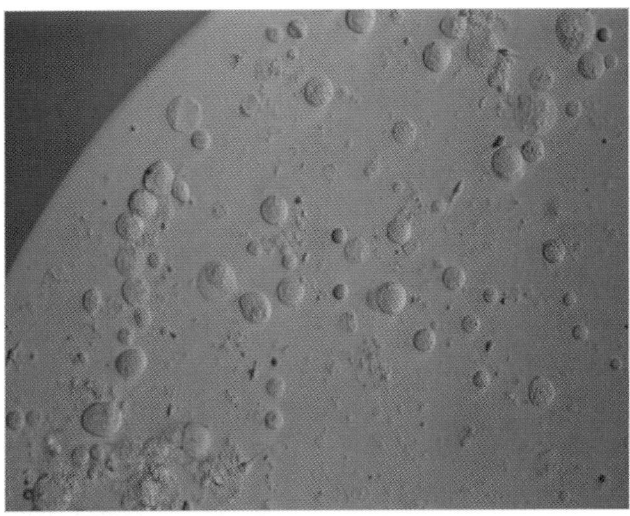

Figure 11.6 An example of a testicular sample for an extensive sperm search that has yielded spermatozoa for pickup and injection.

(Figure 11.6). At our center, when an extended search time is used as a parameter and categorized into 30 minutes to one hour, one to two hours, two to three hours, and more than three hours, the fertilization rates (54.2%, 46.3%, 28.0%, and 25.4%, respectively; $p < 0.001$) of the oocytes, the overall clinical pregnancy rates (44.1%, 37.8%, 31.8%, and 23.8%, respectively; $p < 0.0001$), and the overall live birth rates (32.4%, 23.5%, 18.2%, and 9.5%, respectively; $p < 0.0001$) declined as search time increased (Figure 11.7). Although there is a pronounced decrease in pregnancy outcome as extensive search time increases, the search is still an important and valuable tool overall, as it represents the best opportunity for a male patient with NOA to bear their own biological child. In fact, even in the search of more than three hours, achieving pregnancy is still attainable as long as a spermatozoon is identified.

OPTIONAL SPERM SELECTION TECHNIQUES

While ICSI has been the gold standard for most IVF centers for more than 15 years with no proven significant or attributable side effects, some researchers still question the possible deleterious effects of a process that bypasses the natural gamete selecting processes of *in vivo* human reproduction. Toward that end, several methods have been introduced that expound upon the procedures of ICSI with additional protocols aimed at finding the optimal spermatozoon to inject into an oocyte.

Intracytoplasmic morphologically selected sperm injection (IMSI) is a procedure where high-power magnification is adopted to morphologically screen for optimal spermatozoa (69). This technique, referred to as motile sperm organelle morphology examination (MSOME), uses an inverted light microscope with high-resolution Nomarski optics followed by computer-assisted magnification up to 6300× or even higher. When using MSOME, the criteria for sperm selection include a normal nuclear shape with

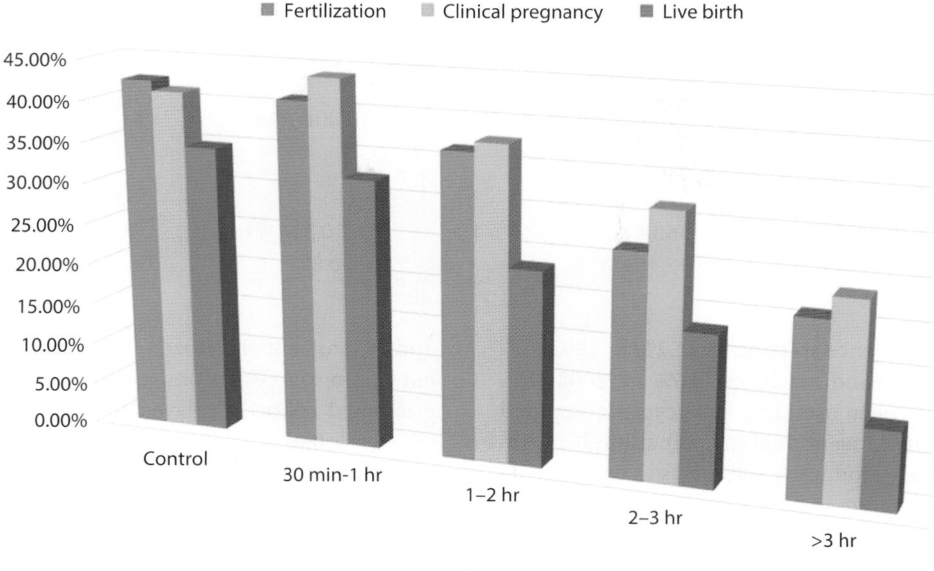

Figure 11.7 Pregnancy outcomes according to the amount of time spent searching for spermatozoa.

lengths and widths no greater than two standard deviations away from the average measurements of 4.75 μm by 3.28 μm. A spermatozoon with normal nuclear content is identified, meaning that no greater than one vacuole (taking up to <4% of the nuclear area) can be present in the nucleus. Since searching for normal sperm under high magnification and strict criteria takes more time, the sperm sample must be kept at a lower temperature of 21°C to reduce sperm cell metabolism (69). Pregnancy outcomes in trials comparing IMSI and conventional ICSI have showed controversial results. Some studies have shown an increase in pregnancy outcomes and a decrease in pregnancy losses with IMSI, while other centers have seen no difference between the two methods (70). IMSI has shown possible clinical promise; however, some of the inherent characteristics of the procedure may prevent it from being used more routinely in many clinics. With this technique, finding the necessary number of spermatozoa to inject all retrieved oocytes may take hours to complete as compared to standard ICSI. Complicating matters further is the expensive new equipment that is necessary for such searching, as well as the additional time and costs. Finally, the whole concept of IMSI is best suited for cases where selection of morphologically normal spermatozoa is feasible, but it cannot practically be employed in severe oligozoospermic cases such as cryptozoospermia and NOA, where only scarce viable cells are present. More recently, three-dimensional sperm surface reconstruction has been utilized for *in vitro* assessment of sperm surface morphology, though its functional capabilities are yet to be evaluated (71).

Physiologic ICSI (PICSI) makes use of hyaluronic acid (HA), a substance naturally present in the human body (72). HA can be found in the cumulus oophorus around the oocyte and represents a barrier to the immature gametes by only relenting to "mature" spermatozoa. These so-called "mature" spermatozoa that have undergone the complete process of plasma membrane remodeling, cytoplasmic extrusion, and nuclear maturity will have a significantly higher number of HA receptors and binding sites. Two methods have been proposed for performing PICSI. In the first method, a special dish is used in which microdots of HA hydrogel have been attached to the bottom of the dish. When spermatozoa are added, this allows examination of bound spermatozoa. At this point, only HA-bound sperm are recovered using a standard ICSI injection pipette (73). The other method is to use a viscous medium composed partially of HA (72), which would fully replace PVP. Some studies have also shown that spermatozoa capable of HA binding have lower DNA fragmentation rates than simple post-swim up spermatozoa. In addition, the nucleus normalcy rate (according to MSOME criteria) has been shown to be higher in spermatozoa bound to HA as compared with sperm in PVP (72). Moreover, PICSI correlations to overall results such as pregnancy rate, delivery rate, or malformation proportion have been inconsistent. Ultimately, PICSI is still affected by the same major drawbacks as IMSI.

CLINICAL RESULTS WITH ICSI

In a cross-sectional survey of ART procedures performed in 55 countries during 2007, the International Committee for Monitoring Assisted Reproductive Technologies reported that 65.2% (400,617 of 614,540) of all cycles utilized ICSI (74). However, there was considerable variation in ICSI rates, ranging from 49.1% in Asia to 97.8% in the Middle East (74). In another recent publication analyzing the trends in ICSI use between 1996 and 2012 in the U.S.A., ICSI use increased from 36.4% in 1996 to 76.2% in 2012 (75). At our center, there has been a steady and progressive

Table 11.1 Intracytoplasmic sperm injection outcomes using ejaculated, epididymal, and testicular spermatozoa.

Parameter	Ejaculated	Epididymal	Testicular
Maternal age (years)	37.9 ± 5	35.2 ± 5	33.3 ± 6
Cycles	27,284	1083	1631
Fertilization rate (%)	168,411/224,247 (75.1)	7326/10,314 (71.0)	8466/16,188(52.3)
Clinical pregnancy (%)	12,469 (45.7)	550 (50.8)	661 (40.5)

increase in ICSI prevalence starting at 32.2% in 1993, rising to 48.8% in 1995, and reaching 73.6% by 2002 (76). Since 1993, ICSI has been used in 29,998 cycles compared to 13,454 cycles with conventional insemination. ICSI has yielded comparable reproductive outcomes in comparison to conventional IVF, but is also capable of consistently overcoming unforeseen sperm cell dysfunction (76). The overall fertilization rates (1993–2015) after ICSI and conventional IVF were 74.4% (161,842/217,449) and 60.6% (74,741/123,316), respectively. However, with standard IVF, the two-pronucleus formation rate is calculated over the total number of oocytes retrieved, so once corrected for ICSI, the fertilization rate is comparable between the two insemination methods (58.5% ICSI vs. 60.6% IVF). Clinical pregnancy rate as defined by the presence of a fetal heartbeat on ultrasound was 45.7% (12,066/26,429) for ICSI compared to 40.0% (4473/11,189) for IVF. Thus far, 16,511 babies have been born by the two ART procedures, of which 10,199 were conceived with ICSI.

Between September 1993 and June 2015, we performed 29,998 ICSI cycles. Of these, approximately 91% (n = 27,284) of all ICSI cycles were performed using ejaculated spermatozoa and the remainder involved specimens that were surgically retrieved from the epididymis or testis at out center. In cycles utilizing ejaculated spermatozoa, a total of 224,247 MII oocytes were injected, resulting in a survival rate of 97.3%. Of those that survived, 75.1% of oocytes fertilized normally, with only one pronucleus and three pronuclei in 2.4% and 3.5% of oocytes, respectively. No fertilization was noted in 16.3% of oocytes.

Table 11.1 summarizes the fertilization and clinical pregnancy rates in ICSI cycles using ejaculated, epididymal, and testicular spermatozoa. When examining three different sperm sources encompassing all maternal ages, and the ejaculated cohort displayed the highest fertilization rates despite containing older women ($p < 0.001$). Epididymal spermatozoa achieved a somewhat lower fertilization rate but reported the highest clinical pregnancies as defined by the presence of a least one fetal heartbeat. Cycles using testicular spermatozoa had the lowest fertilization rates despite containing the youngest women ($p < 0.001$). The pregnancy rates were somewhat lower compared to the other groups. It must be noted that this analysis is purely academic, because the surgically retrieved spermatozoa address different clinical indications.

Table 11.2 Intracytoplasmic sperm injection outcomes in men with severe oligospermia (<1 × 10^6/mL of spermatozoa).

Parameter	Value
Cycles	1820
Mean concentration (10^6 per mL ± SD)	0.3 ± 0.3
Mean motility (% ± SD)	19.1 ± 24.0
Mean morphology (% ± SD)	0.9 ± 1
Fertilization (%)	11,082/17,360 (63.8%)
Clinical pregnancy (%)	748 (41.1%)

Our center also treats severely oligozoospermic men with a concentration of <1 × 10^6/mL of spermatozoa. Outcomes of ICSI cycles in these men are highlighted in Table 11.2. If the initial semen specimen examination showed no spermatozoa, then high-speed centrifugation is used. In 311 cycles, after high-speed centrifugation, a mean density of 0.60 ± 1.1 × 10^6/mL and motility of 39.2 ± 34% was reached. In this cohort, a fertilization rate of 59.7% (1881/3150) and a clinical pregnancy rate of 37.6% (117/311) were achieved (76).

A total of 1013 cycles were performed with epididymal spermatozoa and 1395 cycles were performed with testicular samples. When the fertilization and pregnancy characteristics were analyzed according to whether the sample was cryopreserved, we observed that after cryopreservation, epididymal samples had lower motility parameters ($p < 0.0001$) as well as pregnancy outcomes ($p < 0.0001$), though without affecting fertilization rate. When testicular samples were used for ICSI, the situation was reversed, with zygote formation being higher in the fresh specimens ($p = 0.02$) while the ability of the embryo to implant was unaffected Table 11.3.

The pregnancy outcomes of 20,629 ICSI cycles are described in Table 11.4.

Of the 10,783 patients presenting with positive β-hCG (52.3%), 1681 were biochemical (8.1%) and 701 were blighted ova (3.4%). Among 8293 patients in whom a viable fetal heartbeat was observed, 750 had a miscarriage or were therapeutically aborted. The clinical pregnancy rate was 40.2% per retrieval (8293/20,629) and 43.1% per replacement (8293/19,226). A total of 9717 neonates were born from 7543 deliveries, with 4732 being female and 4985 being male, with an overall frequency of multiple deliveries of 28.8% (2175/7543): 1962 twins (26.0%), 209

Table 11.3 Spermatozoal parameters and intracytoplasmic sperm injection outcomes according to retrieval sites and specimen condition.

	Spermatozoa			
	Epididymal		Testicular	
Outcome	Fresh	Frozen/thawed	Fresh	Frozen/thawed
Cycles	339	674	1031	364
Density (10^6/mL ± SD)	47.5 ± 44	20.3 ± 25	0.5 ± 4	0.2 ± 0.7
Motility (% ± SD)	19.5 ± 16†	4.1 ± 9†	1.8 ± 7	0.9 ± 5
Morphology (% ± SD)	1.8 ± 2	1.5 ± 2	0	0
Fertilization (%)	2484/3437 (71.2)	4387/6212(70.6)	5590/10221 (54.7)‡	1652/3153 (52.4)‡
Clinical pregnancies (%)	209 (61.7)§	306 (45.4)§	433 (42.0)	132 (36.3)

† Student's t-test, two independent samples, effect of epididymal cryopreservation on sperm motility, $p < 0.0001$.
‡ χ^2, 2 · 2, 1 df, effect of testicular cryopreservation on fertilization rate, $p = 0.02$.
§ χ^2, 2 · 2, 1 df, effect of epididymal cryopreservation on clinical pregnancy rate, $p = 0.0001$.

Table 11.4 Evolution of intracytoplasmic sperm injection (ICSI) pregnancies in 20,629 cycles.

No. of		Positive outcomes	
ICSI cycles	20,629		
Embryo replacements	19,226		
Positive human chorionic gonadotropin	10,783	Pregnancy	52.3% (10,783/20,629)
Biochemical pregnancies	1681		
Blighted ova	701		
Ectopic pregnancies	108		
Positive fetal heartbeats	8293	Clinical pregnancy	40.2% (8293/20,629)
Miscarriages/therapeutic abortions	750		
Deliveries	7543	Delivery rate	36.6% (7543/20,629)

triplets (2.8%), and four quadruplets (0.05%). Of these deliveries, a total of 9150 ICSI were live-born infants, and 330 (3.6%) of them exhibited congenital abnormalities, a rate that was comparable to IVF babies at 3.6% (187/5183) (Figure 11.8).

SAFETY OF ICSI

At present, 1%–3% of children born in developed countries are conceived via ART (77,78). It is well established that assisted reproduction is associated with adverse perinatal outcomes, including increased risks of preterm delivery, low birth weight, and neonatal mortality (79–81). In recent years, there has been considerable work investigating health outcomes in IVF and ICSI children beyond the neonatal period (82,83). Follow-up of children following ART use is highly recommended and is being increasingly applied (83–85), but this is extremely time consuming and costly for the family.

ICSI's safety has often been criticized because the fertilizing spermatozoon neither binds to the ZP nor fuses with the oolemma (86). Bypassing these physiologic steps together with the arbitrary selection of the spermatozoon has been a reason for concern (87–89). Thus far, ICSI offspring undergoing adolescence and beyond have provided sufficient information to allay these qualms. Follow-up studies of ICSI children beginning in the mid-1990s have revealed an incidence of malformations within the expected range for the general population of New

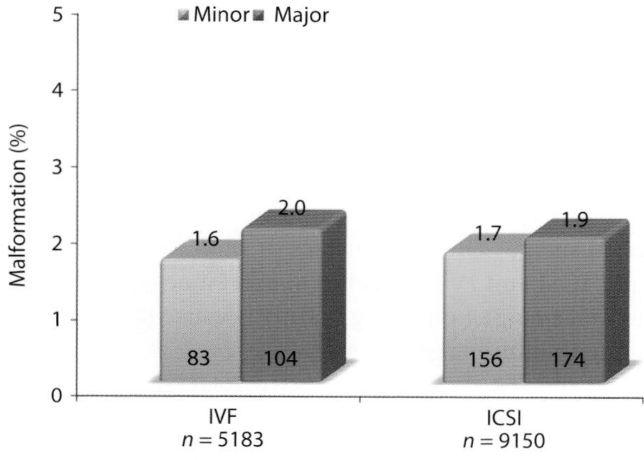

Figure 11.8 Congenital malformation rates of live-born IVF and ICSI neonates. *Abbreviations*: ICSI, intracytoplasmic sperm injection; IVF, *in vitro* fertilization.

York State (89). Another series investigating the outcomes of neonates generated by different assisted conception procedures—ICSI versus IVF with conventional fertilization—provided further confirmation of the expected rate of malformation (90). In one study evaluating the medical and developmental state of one-year-old children born after ICSI or IVF as well as after natural conceptions, the authors found that most one-year-old ICSI children were healthy and were developing normally, as measured by the Bayley Scales of Infant Development (91). However, about 17% displayed an increase in learning difficulties compared with those conceived by IVF or naturally. A later report dismissed this concern in two-year-old ICSI toddlers (92). In a different follow-up of 10-year-old children, it was found that ICSI children and their naturally conceived counterparts had similar motor skills and IQ scores (93).

Our center has compared the pregnancy outcomes and the developmental well-being of children conceived from 12,866 ICSI cycles to naturally conceived singleton pregnancies (87). From a total of 3277 couples delivering 5891 neonates, the incidence of low birth weight and gestational length were comparable with their naturally conceived counterparts, after controlling for maternal age. Rates of malformation in ICSI offspring ranged from 3.5% to 6.2% compared to 6.5% in the natural conception group. In the ICSI group, the major malformations included two neonates with a cardiac disease (ventricular septal defect and severe tricuspid regurgitation), one with talipes, and one with trisomy 7 mosaicism. Among the naturally conceived pregnancies, there were two neonates with cardiac defects (ventricular septal defect and patent foramen ovale/atrial septal defect), one with encephalopathy, one polydactyly, and one severe mid-shaft hypospadias with penile angulation. At three years of age ($n = 811$), the proportion of children "at risk" for developmental delay was 10.4% in ICSI and 10.7% in IVF singletons. However, high-order gestations were characterized by 19.4% of the children having compromised development. To study the long-term effects of ICSI, the physical and psychological outcomes of five-year-old ICSI children were compared to those conceived naturally. The average maternal age was higher in the ICSI group than their naturally conceived counterparts (35.6 ± 4 years versus 31.6 ± 6 years; $p < 0.001$). No overall differences were found in the IQ assessments between ICSI and naturally conceived children. No differences were found between ICSI and control children in regard to general health such as chronic illnesses or physical development. Thus, ICSI and IVF appeared to exert a negative effect on the well-being of offspring mainly because of the association with multiple gestations (87).

The specific concerns in regard to ICSI, whether real or theoretical (94–97), involve the insemination method, the use of spermatozoa with genetic or structural defects, and the possible introduction of foreign genes. Several epidemiological studies of assisted reproduction children report a two-fold increase in infant malformations (98), a recurrent reduction in birth weight (99), certain rare syndromes related to imprinting errors (100–105), and even a higher frequency of some cancers (106). However, current evidence does not prove that there is an increased risk of imprinting disorders and even less so childhood cancers in ICSI children (97). Epigenetic imbalances have been similarly linked to the exposure of the embryos to long-term culture (107). Thus far, Beckwith–Wiedemann syndrome is the only epigenetic disorder that has been clearly associated with ART procedures (108) and has been found to be equally distributed among the *in vitro* conception methods. At present, there is no evidence that the ICSI insemination itself is responsible for any increase in epigenetic disorders, findings that have been confirmed in animal studies (109).

CONCLUSIONS

ICSI has established itself as the most reliable technique to overcome fertilization failure. By pinpointing the beginning of fertilization, it has helped us to better understand some important aspects of early gamete interaction. The observed high performance of aggressively immobilized spermatozoa suggests a more efficient destabilization and consequent permeabilization of the sperm membrane, which is responsible for a more prompt release of the oocyte-activating factor (110). These profound physiologic changes induced on the sperm membrane by the action of the injection needle seem to be critically important for immature, surgically retrieved spermatozoa (9). It has been demonstrated that the positive outcome of ICSI is largely independent of the basic sperm parameters such as concentration, motility, and morphology. This is particularly evident with cryptozoospermia or when no spermatozoa are present in the ejaculate (7). It is in these azoospermic men that the surgical isolation of spermatozoa together with ICSI is able to yield fertilization and support embryo development. The possibility of bypassing the steps of testicular and epididymal sperm maturation, acrosome reaction, binding to the ZP, and fusion with the oolemma now permits infertility due to various forms of male factor to be addressed successfully. In fact, in cases of men diagnosed as NOA, as long as a viable spermatozoon is isolated, there is a chance of generating a conceptus. However, we should be cautious about the acquired evidence that subfertile men have a higher frequency of genetic abnormalities that may be passed on through their gametes (9,111). Therefore, the earlier concern focused on ICSI insemination itself has shifted to the screening of the subfertile man who may transmit his genetic defects to the offspring, specifically boys (112). A large, worldwide experience suggested that men with extreme male factor conditions caused by a direct genetic component such as Klinefelter's syndrome or Yq micro-deletions can be successfully treated by ICSI and still generate healthy offspring (9). The practice of ICSI has promoted a more careful quest for the ideal spermatozoon to inject. Higher-magnification screening of sperm surface irregularities by MSOME is an example of this attempt, even though its claimed benefits remain unproven (70). The potential effects of ART on child development should always be kept in mind and the monitoring of child health can be accomplished by a parent-administered questionnaire that provides a cost- and time-effective approach to measuring the child's physical and psychological well-being. In recent years, a large number of studies have provided information on the health of children born after ART, and therefore, current evidence shows that the outcomes of singletons born at term following ART are generally reassuring (113). The increased awareness of the risks related to multiple gestations has supported measures aimed at obtaining singleton births, with obvious benefits for the long-term welfare of the offspring.

In the evaluation of the infertile male we still rely on the basic semen analysis measures that are capable of indicating a compromised cellular program that is altered during spermatogenesis. However, it is still unclear whether semen analysis data provide information on an individual sperm's real potential to generate offspring, rather than reflecting the real etiology underlying spermatogenesis. Spermatozoa are not just a vehicle that delivers the male genomic contribution to the oocyte. Upon fertilization, the spermatozoon provides a complete, highly structured, and epigenetically marked genome that, together with a defined complement of RNAs and proteins, plays a distinct role in early embryonic development. Often the origin of these abnormalities has been associated with specific gene alterations and most of the time the cause remains idiopathic. Future research will be focused on exploring the effects of genetic variants such as single-nucleotide polymorphisms, copy number variants, differential genome packaging, differential methylation, proteomic changes, and differential sperm RNAs in order to enlighten the conundrum represented by what we generally define as male infertility.

ACKNOWLEDGEMENTS

We thank the clinicians, embryologists, and scientists of The Ronald O. Perelman and Claudia Cohen Center for Reproductive Medicine. We also thank Dr. Peter Schlegel and Dr. Marc Goldstein from the Urology Department, Weill Cornell Medical College, New York. We are thankful to Stephanie Cheung, Stephen Chow, and Claire O'Neill for their assistance with ICSI.

REFERENCES

1. Sunderam S, Kissin DM, Crawford SB et al. Assisted reproductive technology surveillance—United States, 2012. *MMWR Surveill Summ* 2015; 64(Suppl 6): 1–29.
2. Cohen J, Edwards RG, Fehilly CB et al. Treatment of male infertility by *in vitro* fertilization: Factors affecting fertilization and pregnancy. *Acta Eur Fertil* 1984; 15(6): 455–65.
3. Malter HE, Cohen J. Partial zona dissection of the human oocyte: A nontraumatic method using micro-manipulation to assist zona pellucida penetration. *Fertil Steril* 1989; 51: 139–48.
4. Palermo G, Joris H, Devroey P, Van Steirteghem AC. Induction of acrosome reaction in human spermatozoa used for subzonal insemination. *Hum Reprod* 1992; 7: 248–54.
5. Cohen J, Alikani M, Malter HE et al. Partial zona dissection or subzonal sperm insertion: Microsurgical fertilization alternatives based on evaluation of sperm and embryo morphology. *Fertil Steril* 1991; 56: 696–706.
6. Pereira N, Neri QV, Lekovich JP, Spandorfer SD, Palermo GD, Rosenwaks Z. Outcomes of intracytoplasmic sperm injection cycles for complete teratozoospermia: A case–control study using paired sibling oocytes. *Biomed Res Int* 2015; 2015: 470819.
7. Palermo GD, Cohen J, Alikani M, Adler A, Rosenwaks Z. Intracytoplasmic sperm injection: A novel treatment for all forms of male factor infertility. *Fertil Steril* 1995; 63: 1231–40.
8. Palermo GD, Cohen J, Rosenwaks Z. Intracytoplasmic sperm injection: A powerful tool to overcome fertilization failure. *Fertil Steril* 1996; 65: 899–908.
9. Palermo GD, Schlegel PN, Hariprashad JJ et al. Fertilization and pregnancy outcome with intracytoplasmic sperm injection for azoospermic men. *Hum Reprod* 1999; 14: 741–8.
10. Benagiano G, Gianaroli L. The new Italian IVF legislation. *Reprod Biomed Online* 2004; 9: 117–25.
11. Ludwig M, Diedrich K. Regulation of assisted reproductive technology: The German experience. In: *Regulation of Assisted Reproductive Technology: The German Experience*. Brinsden PR (ed.). New York, NY: Parthenon Publishing Group, Inc., 1999, pp. 431–4.
12. Porcu E, Fabbri R, Seracchioli R et al. Birth of a healthy female after intracytoplasmic sperm injection of cryopreserved human oocytes. *Fertil Steril* 1997; 68: 724–6.
13. Johnson MH. The effect on fertilization of exposure of mouse oocytes to dimethyl sulfoxide: An optimal protocol. *J In Vitro Fert Embryo Transf* 1989; 6: 168–75.
14. Schalkoff ME, Oskowitz SP, Powers RD. Ultrastructural observations of human and mouse oocytes treated with cryopreservatives. *Biol Reprod* 1989; 40: 379–93.
15. Van Blerkom J, Davis PW. Cytogenetic, cellular, and developmental consequences of cryopreservation of immature and mature mouse and human oocytes. *Microsc Res Tech* 1994; 27: 165–93.
16. Vincent C, Pickering SJ, Johnson MH. The hardening effect of dimethylsulphoxide on the mouse zona pellucida requires the presence of an oocyte and is associated with a reduction in the number of cortical granules present. *J Reprod Fertil* 1990; 89: 253–9.
17. Mencaglia L, Falcone P, Lentini GM et al. ICSI for treatment of human immunodeficiency virus and hepatitis C virus-serodiscordant couples with infected male partner. *Hum Reprod* 2005; 20: 2242–6.

18. Pena JE, Klein J, Thornton M, Chang PL, Sauer MV. Successive pregnancies with delivery of two healthy infants in a couple who was discordant for human immunodeficiency virus infection. *Fertil Steril* 2002; 78: 421–3.
19. Sauer MV, Chang PL. Establishing a clinical program for human immunodeficiency virus 1-seropositive men to father seronegative children by means of *in vitro* fertilization with intracytoplasmic sperm injection. *Am J Obstet Gynecol* 2002; 186: 627–33.
20. van Leeuwen E, Repping S, Prins JM, Reiss P, van der Veen F. Assisted reproductive technologies to establish pregnancies in couples with an HIV-1-infected man. *Neth J Med* 2009; 67: 322–7.
21. Daw C, Neri QV, Monahan D et al. Semen hyperviscosity treatment and IUI outcome. *Fertil Steril* 2011; 96(3 Suppl 1): S266–7.
22. Mortimer D. Sperm recovery techniques to maximize fertilizing capacity. *Reprod Fertil Dev* 1994; 6: 25–31.
23. Bennett CJ, Seager SW, Vasher EA, McGuire EJ. Sexual dysfunction and electroejaculation in men with spinal cord injury: Review. *J Urol* 1988; 139: 453–7.
24. Schlegel PN, Berkeley AS, Goldstein M et al. Epididymal micropuncture with *in vitro* fertilization and oocyte micromanipulation for the treatment of unreconstructable obstructive azoospermia. *Fertil Steril* 1994; 61: 895–901.
25. Schlegel PN, Cohen J, Goldstein M et al. Cystic fibrosis gene mutations do not affect sperm function during *in vitro* fertilization with micromanipulation for men with bilateral congenital absence of vas deferens. *Fertil Steril* 1995; 64: 421–6.
26. Tsirigotis M, Pelekanos M, Yazdani N et al. Simplified sperm retrieval and intracytoplasmic sperm injection in patients with azoospermia. *Br J Urol* 1995; 76: 765–8.
27. Friedler S, Raziel A, Strassburger D et al. Testicular sperm retrieval by percutaneous fine needle sperm aspiration compared with testicular sperm extraction by open biopsy in men with non-obstructive azoospermia. *Hum Reprod* 1997; 12: 1488–93.
28. Silber SJ, Van Steirteghem AC, Liu J et al. High fertilization and pregnancy rate after intracytoplasmic sperm injection with spermatozoa obtained from testicle biopsy. *Hum Reprod* 1995; 10: 148–52.
29. Ramasamy R, Reifsnyder JE, Bryson C et al. Role of tissue digestion and extensive sperm search after microdissection testicular sperm extraction. *Fertil Steril* 2011; 96: 299–302.
30. Schlegel PN. Nonobstructive azoospermia: A revolutionary surgical approach and results. *Semin Reprod Med* 2009; 27: 165–70.
31. Reis MM, Tsai MC, Schlegel PN et al. Xenogeneic transplantation of human spermatogonia. *Zygote* 2000; 8: 97–105.
32. Kruger TF, Menkveld R, Stander FS et al. Sperm morphologic features as a prognostic factor in *in vitro* fertilization. *Fertil Steril* 1986; 46: 1118–23.
33. WHO. *WHO Laboratory Manual for the Examination and Processing of Human Semen*, 5th edition. Cambridge, U.K.: Cambridge University Press, 2010.
34. Verheyen GI, Pletincx I, Van Steirteghem A. Effect of freezing method, thawing temperature and post-thaw dilution/washing on motility (CASA) and morphology characteristics of high-quality human sperm. *Hum Reprod* 1993; 8: 1678–84.
35. Huang JY, Kang HJ, Rosenwaks Z. How to monitor for best results. In: *Cup Book: How to Improve IVF Success Rates*. 1st edition. Kovacs G (ed.). Cambridge, U.K.: Cambridge University Press, 2011 , pp. 120–126.
36. Zarek SM, Muasher SJ. Mild/minimal stimulation for *in vitro* fertilization: An old idea that needs to be revisited. *Fertil Steril* 2011; 95: 2449–55.
37. Pereira N, Neri QV, Lekovich JP, Palermo GD, Rosenwaks Z. The role of *in-vivo* and *in-vitro* maturation time on ooplasmic dysmaturity. *Reprod Biomed Online* 2016; 32: 401–6.
38. Dozortsev D, Rybouchkin A, De Sutter P, Qian C, Dhont M. Human oocyte activation following intracytoplasmic injection: The role of the sperm cell. *Hum Reprod* 1995; 10: 403–7.
39. Fishel S, Lisi F, Rinaldi L et al. Systematic examination of immobilizing spermatozoa before intracytoplasmic sperm injection in the human. *Hum Reprod* 1995; 10: 497–500.
40. Palermo G, Joris H, Derde MP et al. Sperm characteristics and outcome of human assisted fertilization by subzonal insemination and intracytoplasmic sperm injection. *Fertil Steril* 1993; 59: 826–35.
41. Calvin HI, Bedford JM. Formation of disulphide bonds in the nucleus and accessory structures of mammalian spermatozoa during maturation in the epididymis. *J Reprod Fertil Suppl* 1971; 13(Suppl 13): 65–75.
42. Neri QV, Hu J, Rosenwaks Z, Palermo GD. Understanding the spermatozoon. *Methods Mol Biol* 2014; 1154: 91–119.
43. Bedford JM, Calvin H, Cooper GW. The maturation of spermatozoa in the human epididymis. *J Reprod Fertil Suppl* 1973; 18: 199–213.
44. Kirchhoff C, Osterhoff C, Habben I, Ivell R, Kirchloff C. Cloning and analysis of mRNAs expressed specifically in the human epididymis. *Int J Androl* 1990; 13: 155–67.
45. Moore HD, Hartman TD, Pryor JP. Development of the oocyte-penetrating capacity of spermatozoa in the human epididymis. *Int J Androl* 1983; 6: 310–8.
46. Palermo GD, Alikani M, Bertoli M et al. Oolemma characteristics in relation to survival and fertilization patterns of oocytes treated by intracytoplasmic sperm injection. *Hum Reprod* 1996; 11: 172–6.

47. Takeuchi T, Colombero LT, Neri QV, Rosenwaks Z, Palermo GD. Does ICSI require acrosomal disruption? An ultrastructural study. *Hum Reprod* 2004; 19: 114–7.
48. Palermo GD, Schlegel PN, Colombero LT et al. Aggressive sperm immobilization prior to intracytoplasmic sperm injection with immature spermatozoa improves fertilization and pregnancy rates. *Hum Reprod* 1996; 11: 1023–9.
49. Fishel S, Lisi F, Rinaldi L et al. Intracytoplasmic sperm injection (ICSI) versus high insemination concentration (HIC) for human conception *in vitro*. *Reprod Fertil Dev* 1995; 7: 169–174; discussion 174–5.
50. Gerris J, Mangelschots K, Van Royen E et al. ICSI and severe male-factor infertility: Breaking the sperm tail prior to injection. *Hum Reprod* 1995; 10: 484–86.
51. Katayama M, Sutovsky P, Yang BS et al. Increased disruption of sperm plasma membrane at sperm immobilization promotes dissociation of perinuclear theca from sperm chromatin after intracytoplasmic sperm injection in pigs. *Reproduction* 2005; 130: 907–16.
52. Van den Bergh M, Bertrand E, Englert Y. Second polar body extrusion is highly predictive for oocyte fertilization as soon as 3 hr after intracytoplasmic sperm injection (ICSI). *J Assist Reprod Genet* 1995; 12: 258–62.
53. Tang SS, Gao H, Zhao Y, Ma S. Aneuploidy and DNA fragmentation in morphologically abnormal sperm. *Int J Androl* 2010; 33: 163–79.
54. Tasdemir I, Tasdemir M, Tavukcuoglu S, Kahraman S, Biberoglu K. Effect of abnormal sperm head morphology on the outcome of intracytoplasmic sperm injection in humans. *Hum Reprod* 1997; 12: 1214–7.
55. Templado C, Hoang T, Greene C et al. Aneuploid spermatozoa in infertile men: Teratozoospermia. *Mol Reprod Dev* 2002; 61: 200–4.
56. Zini A, Sigman M. Are tests of sperm DNA damage clinically useful? Pros and cons. *J Androl* 2009; 30: 219–29.
57. Zini A, Bielecki R, Phang D, Zenzes MT. Correlations between two markers of sperm DNA integrity, DNA denaturation and DNA fragmentation, in fertile and infertile men. *Fertil Steril* 2001; 75: 674–7.
58. Spano M, Bonde JP, Hjøllund HI et al. Sperm chromatin damage impairs human fertility. The Danish First Pregnancy Planner Study Team. *Fertil Steril* 2000; 73: 43–50.
59. Palermo GD, Neri QV, Cozzubbo T, Rosenwaks Z. Perspectives on the assessment of human sperm chromatin integrity. *Fertil Steril* 2014; 102: 1508–17.
60. Palermo GD, Neri QV, Monahan D, Kocent J, Rosenwaks Z. Development and current applications of assisted fertilization. *Fertil Steril* 2012; 97: 248–59.
61. Society for Assisted Reproductive Technology, American Society for Reproductive Medicine. Assisted reproductive technology in the United States and Canada: 1995 results generated from the American Society for Reproductive Medicine/Society for Assisted Reproductive Technology Registry. *Fertil Steril* 1998; 69: 389–98.
62. Gardner DK, Schoolcraft WB. *Elimination of High Order Multiple Gestations by Blastocyst Culture and Transfer. Female Infertility Therapy: Current Practice.* London, U.K.: Martin Dunitz, 1998.
63. Gardner DK, Lane M. Towards a single embryo transfer. *Reprod Biomed Online* 2003; 6: 470–81.
64. Zander-Fox DL, Tremellen K, Lane M. Single blastocyst embryo transfer maintains comparable pregnancy rates to double cleavage-stage embryo transfer but results in healthier pregnancy outcomes. *Aust NZ J Obstet Gynaecol* 2011; 51: 406–10.
65. Barnes FL, Crombie A, Gardner DK et al. Blastocyst development and birth after *in-vitro* maturation of human primary oocytes, intracytoplasmic sperm injection and assisted hatching. *Hum Reprod* 1995; 10: 3243–7.
66. Gardner DK, Vella P, Lane M et al. Culture and transfer of human blastocysts increases implantation rates and reduces the need for multiple embryo transfers. *Fertil Steril* 1998; 69: 84–8.
67. Schoolcraft WB, Gardner DK, Lane M et al. Blastocyst culture and transfer: Analysis of results and parameters affecting outcome in two *in vitro* fertilization programs. *Fertil Steril* 1999; 72: 604–9.
68. Palermo GD, Neri QV, Schlegel PN, Rosenwaks Z. Intracytoplasmic sperm injection (ICSI) in extreme cases of male infertility. *PLoS One* 2014; 9(12): e113671.
69. Berkovitz A, Eltes F, Yaari S et al. The morphological normalcy of the sperm nucleus and pregnancy rate of intracytoplasmic injection with morphologically selected sperm. *Hum Reprod* 2005; 20: 185–90.
70. Palermo GD, Hu JCY, Rienzi L, Maggiulli R, Takeuchi T. Thoughts on IMSI. In: *Biennial Review of Infertility*. Racowsky C and Schlegel PN (eds). New York, NY: Springer, 2011; 2: pp. 277–289.
71. Levine BA, Feinstein J, Neri QV, Goldschlag D, Rosenwaks Z, Belongie S, Palermo GD. Three-dimensional sperm surface reconstruction: A novel approach to assessing sperm morphology. *Fertil Steril* 2015; 104: e14–5.
72. Parmegiani L, Cognigni GE, Bernardi S et al. "Physiologic ICSI": Hyaluronic acid (HA) favors selection of spermatozoa without DNA fragmentation and with normal nucleus, resulting in improvement of embryo quality. *Fertil Steril* 2010; 93: 598–604.
73. Yagci A, Murk W, Stronk J, Huszar G. Spermatozoa bound to solid state hyaluronic acid show chromatin structure with high DNA chain integrity: An acridine orange fluorescence study. *J Androl* 2010; 31: 566–72.
74. Ishihara O, Adamson GD, Dyer S et al. International committee for monitoring assisted reproductive technologies: World report on assisted reproductive technologies, 2007. *Fertil Steril* 2015; 103: 402–13.e11.

75. Boulet SL, Mehta A, Kissin DM, Warner L, Kawwass JF, Jamieson DJ. Trends in use of and reproductive outcomes associated with intracytoplasmic sperm injection. *JAMA* 2015; 313: 255–63.
76. Palermo GD, Neri QV, Rosenwaks Z. To ICSI or Not to ICSI. *Semin Reprod Med* 2015; 33: 92–102.
77. Andersen AN, Goossens V, Ferraretti AP et al. Assisted reproductive technology in Europe, 2004: Results generated from European registers by ESHRE. *Hum Reprod* 2008; 23: 756–71.
78. Wright VC, Chang J, Jeng G, Macaluso M. Assisted reproductive technology surveillance—United States, 2005. *MMWR Surveill Summ* 2008; 57: 1–23.
79. Helmerhorst FM, Perquin DA, Donker D, Keirse MJ. Perinatal outcome of singletons and twins after assisted conception: A systematic review of controlled studies. *BMJ* 2004; 328: 261.
80. Jackson RA, Gibson KA, Wu YW, Croughan MS. Perinatal outcomes in singletons following *in vitro* fertilization: A meta-analysis. *Obstet Gynecol* 2004; 103: 551–63.
81. McDonald SD, Murphy K, Beyene J, Ohlsson A. Perinatal outcomes of singleton pregnancies achieved by *in vitro* fertilization: A systematic review and meta- analysis. *J Obstet Gynaecol Can* 2005; 27: 449–59.
82. Basatemur E, Sutcliffe A. Follow-up of children born after ART. *Placenta* 2008; 29(Suppl B): 135–40.
83. Sutcliffe AG, Ludwig M. Outcome of assisted reproduction. *Lancet* 2007; 370: 351–9.
84. Bonduelle M, Bergh C, Niklasson A, Palermo GD, Wennerholm UB. Medical follow-up study of 5-year-old ICSI children. *Reprod Biomed Online* 2004; 9: 91–101.
85. Leunens L, Celestin-Westreich S, Bonduelle M, Liebaers I, Ponjaert-Kristoffersen I. Cognitive and motor development of 8-year-old children born after ICSI compared to spontaneously conceived children. *Hum Reprod* 2006; 21: 2922–9.
86. Ombelet W, Peeraer K, De Sutter P et al. Perinatal outcome of ICSI pregnancies compared with a matched group of natural conception pregnancies in Flanders (Belgium): A cohort study. *Reprod Biomed Online* 2005; 11: 244–53.
87. Palermo GD, Neri QV, Takeuchi T, Squires J, Moy F, Rosenwaks Z. Genetic and epigenetic characteristics of ICSI children. *Reprod Biomed Online* 2008; 17: 820–33.
88. Palermo GD, Neri QV, Rosenwaks Z. Safety of intracytoplasmic sperm injection. *Methods Mol Biol* 2014; 1154: 549–62.
89. Palermo GD, Colombero LT, Schattman GL, Davis OK, Rosenwaks Z. Evolution of pregnancies and initial follow-up of newborns delivered after intracytoplasmic sperm injection. *JAMA* 1996; 276: 1893–7.
90. Neri QV, Takeuchi T, Kang HJ, Lin K, Wang A, Palermo GD. Genetic assessment and development of children that result from assisted reproductive technology. *Clin Obstet Gynecol* 2006; 49: 134–7.
91. Bowen JR, Gibson FL, Leslie GI, Saunders DM. Medical and developmental outcome at 1 year for children conceived by intracytoplasmic sperm injection. *Lancet* 1998; 351: 1529–34.
92. Bonduelle M, Joris H, Hofmans K, Liebaers I, Van Steirteghem A. Mental development of 201 ICSI children at 2 years of age. *Lancet* 1998; 351: 1553.
93. Leunens L, Celestin-Westreich S, Bonduelle M, Liebaers I, Ponjaert-Kristoffersen I. Follow-up of cognitive and motor development of 10-year-old singleton children born after ICSI compared with spontaneously conceived children. *Hum Reprod* 2008; 23: 105–11.
94. Cummins JM, Jequier AM. Treating male infertility needs more clinical andrology, not less. *Hum Reprod* 1994; 9: 1214–9.
95. de Kretser DM. The potential of intracytoplasmic sperm injection (ICSI) to transmit genetic defects causing male infertility. *Reprod Fertil Dev* 1995; 7: 137–141; discussion 141–2.
96. De Rycke M, Liebaers I, Van Steirteghem A. Epigenetic risks related to assisted reproductive technologies: Risk analysis and epigenetic inheritance. *Hum Reprod* 2002; 17: 2487–94.
97. Edwards RG, Ludwig M. Are major defects in children conceived *in vitro* due to innate problems in patients or to induced genetic damage? *Reprod Biomed Online* 2003; 7: 131–8.
98. Hansen M, Kurinczuk J, Bower C, Webb S. The risk of major birth defects after intracytoplasmic sperm injection and *in vitro* fertilization. *N Engl J Med* 2002; 346: 725–30.
99. Schieve LA, Meikle SF, Ferre C et al. Low and very low birth weight in infants conceived with use of assisted reproductive technology. *N Engl J Med* 2002; 346: 731–7.
100. Cox GF, Burger J, Lip V et al. Intracytoplasmic sperm injection may increase the risk of imprinting defects. *Am J Hum Genet* 2002; 71: 162–4.
101. DeBaun MR, Niemitz EL, Feinberg AP. Association of *in vitro* fertilization with Beckwith–Wiedemann syndrome and epigenetic alterations of LIT1 and H19. *Am J Hum Genet* 2003; 72: 156–60.
102. Gicquel C, Gaston V, Mandelbaum J et al. *In vitro* fertilization may increase the risk of Beckwith–Wiedemann syndrome related to the abnormal imprinting of the *KCN1OT* gene. *Am J Hum Genet* 2003; 72: 1338–41.
103. Halliday J, Oke K, Breheny S, Algar E, J Amor D. Beckwith–Wiedemann syndrome and IVF: A case–control study. *Am J Hum Genet* 2004; 75: 526–8.
104. Maher ER, Brueton LA, Bowdin SC et al. Beckwith–Wiedemann syndrome and assisted reproduction technology (ART). *J Med Genet* 2003; 40: 62–4.

105. Orstavik KH. Intracytoplasmic sperm injection and congenital syndromes because of imprinting defects. *Tidsskr Nor Laegeforen* 2003; 123: 177.
106. Moll AC, Imhof SM, Schouten-van Meeteren AY, van Leeuwen FE. *In-vitro* fertilisation and retinoblastoma. *Lancet* 2003; 361: 1392.
107. Rivera RM, Stein P, Weaver JR et al. Manipulations of mouse embryos prior to implantation result in aberrant expression of imprinted genes on day 9.5 of development. *Hum Mol Genet* 2008; 17: 1–14.
108. Sutcliffe AG, Peters CJ, Bowdin S et al. Assisted reproductive therapies and imprinting disorders—A preliminary British survey. *Hum Reprod* 2006; 21: 1009–11.
109. Wilson TJ, Lacham-Kaplan O, Gould J et al. Comparison of mice born after intracytoplasmic sperm injection with *in vitro* fertilization and natural mating. *Mol Reprod Dev* 2007; 74: 512–9.
110. Wolny YM, Fissore RA, Wu H et al. Human glucosamine-6-phosphate isomerase, a homologue of hamster oscillin, does not appear to be involved in Ca^{2+} release in mammalian oocytes. *Mol Reprod Dev* 1999; 52: 277–87.
111. De Kretser DM, Burger HG, Fortune D et al. Hormonal, histological and chromosomal studies in adult males with testicular disorders. *J Clin Endocrinol Metab* 1972; 35: 392–401.
112. Katagiri Y, Neri QV, Takeuchi T et al. Y chromosome assessment and its implications for the development of ICSI children. *Reprod Biomed Online* 2004; 8: 307–18.
113. Steel AJ, Sutcliffe A. Long-term health implications for children conceived by IVF/ICSI. *Hum Fertil (Camb)* 2009; 12: 21–7.

Assisted hatching

12

ANNA VEIGA and ITZIAR BELIL

INTRODUCTION

The zona pellucida

The zona pellucida (ZP) of mammalian eggs and embryos is an acellular matrix composed of sulfated glycoproteins with different roles during fertilization and embryo development (1).

Three distinct glycoproteins have been described both in mice and in humans (ZP1, ZP2, and ZP3) (2). Acrosome-reacted spermatozoa bind to ZP receptors, and biochemical changes have been observed after fertilization (3) that are responsible for the prevention of polyspermic fertilization.

The main function of the ZP after fertilization is protection of the embryo and maintenance of its integrity (4). It has been postulated that blastomeres may be weakly connected, and that the ZP is needed during the migration of embryos through the reproductive tract to maintain the embryo structure. Implantation has been observed after replacement of zona-free mouse morulae or blastocysts, while the transfer of zona-free precompacted embryos results in the adherence of transferred embryos to the oviductal walls or to one another. A possible protective role against hostile uterine factors has also been described (4). Degeneration of sheep eggs after complete or partial ZP removal that could be ascribed to an immune response was described by Trounson and Moore (5).

Hatching

Once in the uterus, the blastocysts must get out of the ZP (hatching) so that the trophectoderm cells can interact with endometrial cells and implantation can occur. The loss of the ZP *in utero* is the result of embryonic and uterine functions.

ZP hardening after ZP reaction subsequent to fertilization occurs, and is evidenced by an increased resistance to dissolution by different chemical agents. A loss of elasticity is also observed. This physiological phenomenon is essential for polyspermy block and for embryo protection during transport through the reproductive tract.

It has been postulated that additional ZP hardening may occur in both mice and humans as a consequence of *in vitro* culture (4–7). Hatching could be inhibited in some *in vitro*-cultured human embryos owing to the inability of the blastocysts to escape from a thick or hardened ZP (8).

Schiewe et al. performed a study to characterize ZP hardening in unfertilized and abnormal embryos and to correlate it with culture duration, patient age, and ZP thickness (9). Dispersion of ZP glycoproteins and the time needed for complete digestion after α-chymotrypsin treatment were assessed. The results obtained proved that ZP hardening of fertilized eggs was increased compared with inseminated unfertilized eggs. Wide patient-to-patient variation in ZP hardness was observed, but no correlation was established between ZP hardness or thickness and patient age. Furthermore, the data obtained did not support the concept that additional ZP hardening occurred during extended culture.

Expansion and ZP thinning occur in mammalian blastocysts prior to hatching.

Cycles of contraction and expansion have been described in mice, sheep, cattle, and human blastocysts *in vitro* prior to ZP hatching. As a result of several cycles of contraction and expansion and because of its elasticity, the ZP thins. Contraction–expansion cycles as well as cytoplasmic extensions of trophectoderm (trophectoderm projections [TEPs]) have been documented by time-lapse video recording (10) in human blastocysts. TEPs could be a component of ZP escape in cultured embryos. It is not clear whether TEPs are needed *in vivo* for ZP hatching, but they seem to have a role in attachment, implantation, and possibly embryo locomotion (11).

Lysins of embryonic and/or uterine origin are involved in ZP thinning and hatching. Gordon and Dapunt showed that, in mice, hatching is predominantly the result of ZP lysis, and that the pressure exerted against the ZP by the expanding blastocyst plays little or no part in the escape of the embryo from the ZP (12).

Schiewe et al. demonstrated with the use of a mouse anti-hatching model the involvement of ZP lysins in the mechanism of hatching (13); physical expansion of the blastocyst, even though involved in hatching, does not seem to be the primary mechanism. Their results also show that trophectoderm cells are responsible for secreting the ZP lysins required for hatching. On the other hand, two observational studies demonstrated that a natural hatching site usually develops in close proximity to the inner cell mass (ICM) of blastocysts in humans, whereas that of the mouse is at the opposite side to the ICM (14,15).

A study on mouse blastocysts indicated that hatching *in vitro* is dependent on a sufficient number of cells constituting the embryo. Hatching *in vivo* must be different from that *in vitro*, with the difference involving uterine and/or uterine-induced trophectoderm lytic factors (16).

ASSISTED HATCHING

The first report of the use of assisted hatching (AH) in human embryos was published by Cohen et al. in 1990 (7). These authors documented an important increase in implantation rates with mechanical AH in embryos from unselected *in vitro* fertilization (IVF) patients.

Why perform AH?

The ratio of lysin production to ZP thickness could determine whether the embryo will lyse the ZP and undergo hatching. Embryos with thick ZPs or those that present extensive fragmentation or cell death after freezing and thawing may benefit from AH (17).

Both quantitative and qualitative deficiencies in lysin secretion could result in hatching impairment. Suboptimal culture conditions may cause such deficiencies. The trophectoderm of some embryos may not be able to secrete the "hatching factor," and lysin production could be influenced by a patient's age (8,13). Uterine lysin action could also be impaired in some patients or cycles (18).

It is believed that ZP hardening may be exacerbated at any stage of embryo development after long-term *in vitro* culture and cryopreservation of embryos (19). Furthermore, experiments on mouse embryos have demonstrated that damaged blastomeres have a toxic effect, reducing dramatically the rate of hatching (20). However, embryo viability was restored after microsurgical removal of the degenerating material (21). Removal of necrotic blastomeres from frozen–thawed, partially damaged human embryos significantly increased the implantation rate (22). It has been stated that overall ZP thickness varies between age groups and types of infertility (23). The variability of ZP thickness in the same embryo is one of the most significant morphologic predictive factors of implantation (24). Palmstierna et al. demonstrated that human embryos with a ZP thickness variation of >20% resulted in a 76% pregnancy rate with two embryos transferred (25). ZP-assisted thinning of a substantial area may favor complete hatching in embryos with invariable ZP thickness (26). Khalifa et al. have shown that ZP thinning significantly increases the complete hatching of mouse embryos (27). Gordon and Dapunt demonstrated the usefulness of ZP thinning with acid Tyrode's (AT) solution for improved hatching in hatching-defective mouse embryos created by the destruction of a quarter of the blastomeres (17). They reported normal implantation rates in pseudopregnant female mice after the transfer of assisted-hatched embryos that had cell numbers reduced.

The mechanism by which AH promotes embryo implantation remains unclear. The implantation window is the critical period when the endometrium reaches its ideal receptive state for implantation. Precise synchronization between the embryo and the endometrium is essential. In a randomized study, Liu et al. demonstrated that implantation occurred significantly earlier in patients whose embryos were submitted to AH when compared with the control group, possibly by allowing an earlier embryo–endometrium contact (28). Furthermore, although most molecules are able to cross the ZP, the rate of transport may be related to ZP thickness. The presence of an artificial gap may alter the two-way transport of metabolites and growth factors across the ZP, permitting earlier exposure of the embryo to vital growth factors (8).

It has been also reported that the location of herniation of fresh, human-hatched blastocysts can predict their implantation behavior (29). Significantly higher clinical pregnancy rates were observed if blastocysts that hatched close to the ICM were transferred (72%) as compared with those that herniated from the mural trophectoderm (51%). Another study suggested the existence of polarity in the hatching process of vitrified–thawed human blastocysts. Laser AH performed close to the ICM improved complete hatching rates, whereas AH at the anembryonic site caused embryo trapping within the ZP (30). It is likely that in vitrified and warmed blastocysts the complete opening of the ZP by means of laser pulses changes the pressure conditions would be one of the prerequisites for optimal hatching (31). Applying AH at a specific site of the ZP may enhance vitrified blastocyst implantation.

METHODS

Embryos at the six- to eight-cell stage at day 3 after insemination or at the blastocyst stage at day 5 or 6 after insemination can be manipulated with different methods for the performance of AH. When breaches are made in the ZP of early-cleavage IVF embryos, embryonic cell loss may occur through the ZP as a result of uterine contractions after replacement of the embryos. It is advisable to manipulate embryos for AH after the adherence between blastomeres has increased, just before compaction (32). Artificial opening of the ZP of blastocysts can also be performed to promote complete blastocyst hatching (33,34).

Microtools for AH can be made by means of a pipette puller and microforge, but are also commercially available. Micropipettes are mounted on micromanipulators. It is very important to minimize the time that the embryo is out of the incubator and to optimize methodologies to reduce pH and temperature variations that can be detrimental for embryo development.

To reduce environmental variations, AH has to be performed in microdrops of 4-(2-hydroxyethyl)-1-piperazineethanesulfonic acid (HEPES) or equivalent buffered medium covered with oil, under an inverted microscope with Nomarski or Hoffman optics, on a heated microscope stage at 37°C.

It is important that the size of the hole created in the ZP is large enough to avoid trapping of the embryo during hatching, but not so large that it permits blastomere loss (35–38). Monozygotic twinning has been described as a consequence of AH (39). The adequate size of the hole seems to be 30–40 μm when AH is performed on day-3 embryos. Nevertheless, AH applied to cryopreserved blastocysts seems to give better results when ≥50% of the ZP is opened or the ZP is totally removed (40,41). Half thinning of the ZP in early-stage vitrified embryos seems to be associated with higher pregnancy rates than quarter thinning (42).

Different protocols have been described, but a minimum 30-minute culture period seems to be sufficient before the transfer of the manipulated embryos.

Embryo transfer to the uterus has to be performed as non-traumatically as possible to avoid damage to the ZP-manipulated embryos.

Treatment over four days, starting on the day of oocyte retrieval, with broad-spectrum antibiotics and corticosteroids (methyl prednisolone, 16 mg daily) has been postulated. Cohen et al. suggested that such treatment may be useful for patients whose embryos have been assisted-hatched in order to avoid infection and immune cell invasion of the embryos (7).

Partial ZP dissection

Partial ZP dissection (PZD) is a mechanical AH procedure similar to that described for oocytes to assist ZP penetration by spermatozoa (43). The denuded embryo is held with a holding pipette, and the ZP is tangentially pierced with a microneedle from the 1 o'clock to the 11 o'clock position. The embryo is released from the holding pipette, and the part of the ZP between the two points is rubbed against the holding pipette until a slit is made in the ZP. The embryo is washed twice in a fresh culture medium and placed in the transfer dish.

A 3D-PZD in the shape of a cross has been described (38). The procedure starts as conventional PZD and a second cut is made in the ZP under the first slit. A cross-shaped cut can be seen on the surface of the ZP. This method allows the creation of larger openings while permitting protection of the embryo by the ZP flaps during embryo transfer.

A new technique called "controlled ZP dissection" has been described as a variation of PZD (34). The embryo is held at the eight o'clock position by a bevel-opened holding pipette, and a thin, angled hatching needle with a blunted tip pierces the ZP at the five o'clock position. The hatching needle is inserted deeply into the holding pipette until the embryo is pushed to the angle of the hatching needle. The curve of the needle is then pressed against the bottom of the dish to cut the pierced ZP. A large slit (two-thirds of the embryo's diameter) created by controlled ZP dissection significantly enhances the rate of complete *in vitro* hatching of blastocysts compared with 3D-PZD. Long ZP dissection has been also applied using intracytoplasmic sperm injection (ICSI) pipettes. A large split created on the ZP of vitrified–thawed blastocyst embryo transfer (ET) cycles significantly improves implantation and pregnancy rates compared to PZD (44).

AT solution AH

It has been described that ZP hardening and the increase in volume of the perivitelline space in zygotes and embryos allow a more efficient and safe use of AT solution in human embryos for ZP drilling compared with oocytes. Nevertheless, it has to be taken into account that the use of acidic solutions for AH may be detrimental for the blastomere(s) adjacent to the drilled portion of the ZP. Limiting embryo exposure to AT by adequate and quick manipulation is necessary to avoid harmful effects on embryo development.

AT solution can be prepared in the laboratory based on the protocol of Hogan et al. (45) and adjusted to a pH of 2.5, or can be purchased commercially.

One advantage of AT drilling compared with PZD is the possibility of increasing the size of the hole in the ZP. Large holes have proved to be more efficient for enhancing hatching and avoiding embryo entrapment (7,37,46). The embryo is held with a holding pipette in such a way that the micropipette containing AT solution (internal diameter 3–5 μm) at the three o'clock position faces a large perivitelline space or an area with cytoplasmic fragments of the embryo. The acidic solution is gently delivered with the help of a microinjector over a small area of the ZP, with the tip of the pipette positioned very close to the ZP. Accumulation of AT solution in a single area must be avoided. Extracellular fragments can also be removed during the procedure (8). As soon as a hole is created in the ZP, suction is applied to avoid excess AT solution entering the perivitelline space. If the inner region of the ZP is difficult to breach, creation of the hole can be facilitated by pushing the AT micropipette against the ZP (47).

It is necessary to rinse the embryo several times in fresh culture medium.

Laser-assisted hatching

The use of laser techniques in the field of assisted reproduction for application in gametes or embryos was first described by Tadir et al. (48,49). For a fast and an efficient clinical use of laser systems in AH, it is important that the laser is accurately controlled and produces precise ZP openings without thermal or mutagenic effects. The application of a laser on the ZP for AH results in the photoablation of the ZP.

Contact lasers

The procedure is performed on a microscope slide, and the embryo is placed on a drop of the medium covered with paraffin oil. The embryo is held with a holding pipette, and the laser is delivered through a microscopic laser glass fiber, fitted to the manipulator by a pipette holder, in direct contact with the ZP. Several pulses are necessary to penetrate the ZP. Because each laser pulse removes only small portions of the ZP, the fiber tip has to be continuously readjusted to guarantee that the laser is in close contact with the remaining zona.

The first use of a laser for ZP drilling was reported by Palanker et al. with an argon fluoride (ArF) excimer laser (UV region, 193 nm wavelength) (50). This laser system makes it necessary to touch the ZP with the laser-delivering pipette (contact mode laser). The erbium:yttrium–aluminum–garnet (Er:YAG) laser (2940 nm radiation), also working in contact mode, has been used for ZP AH and thinning, and its safety and efficacy have been demonstrated in clinical practice (51,52). Obruca et al. performed a study to evaluate the ultrastructural effects of the Er:YAG laser on the ZP and membrane of oocytes and embryos (53). No degenerative alterations were observed using light and scanning electron microscopy after ZP drilling with such a system. Antinori et al. (54) described the method for ZP thinning with the use of an Er:YAG laser. Five to eight pulses were needed to ablate 50% of the ZP thickness over a length of 20 μm. The necessity of sterile micropipettes and optical fibers to deliver the laser beam to the target is the main disadvantage of contact mode lasers (55).

Noncontact lasers

Noncontact laser systems allow microscope objective-delivered accessibility of laser light to the target. Laser propagation is made through water, and as it avoids the UV absorption peak of DNA, no mutagenic effect on the oocyte or embryo is expected. Blanchet et al. first reported the use of a noncontact laser system (248 nm krypton fluoride [KrF] excimer) for mouse ZP drilling (56). Neev et al. described the use of a noncontact holmium:yttrium–scandium–gallium–garnet laser (2.1 μm wavelength) for AH in mice (57). The study showed a lack of embryotoxic effects as well as improved blastocyst hatching. Similar results were reported by Schiewe et al. (58).

Rink et al. designed and introduced a noncontact infrared diode laser (1.48 μm wavelength) that delivers laser light through the microscope objective (59). The drilling mechanism is explained by a thermal effect induced at the focal point by absorption of the laser energy by water and/or ZP macromolecules, leading to the thermolysis of the ZP matrix. Laser absorption by the culture dish and medium is minimal. The effect on the ZP is greatly localized, and the holes are cylindrical and precise. Exposure time (1–40 ms) can be minimized. The safety and usefulness of the system was demonstrated in mice and humans (60–62). Its use for polar body as well as blastomere and blastocyst biopsy has also been reported (63–65). The system is compact and easily adapted to all kinds of microscopes. The size of the hole is related to the laser exposure time, and thus the system is simple, quick, and easy to use. Figure 12.1 shows an eight-cell embryo in which laser AH has been performed.

Antinori et al. have reported the use of a compact, noncontact UV (337 nm wavelength) laser microbeam system to create holes in the ZP of human embryos (66,67). This equipment requires the manipulation of the oocytes and embryos in Petri dishes with a membrane bottom.

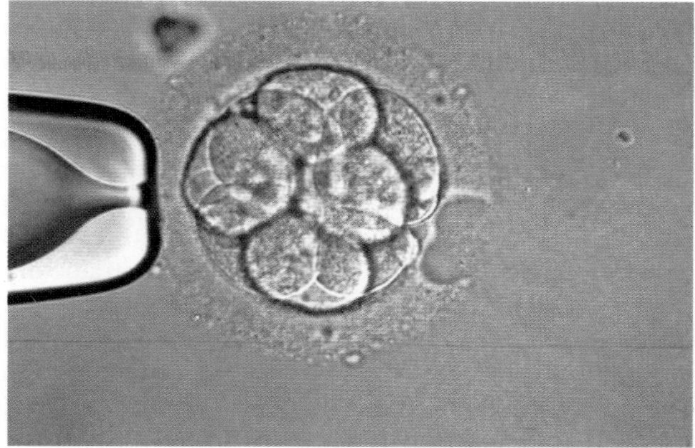

Figure 12.1 Day-3 embryo in which the zona pellucida has been drilled with two laser shots (courtesy of Fertilase®, MTM, Montreaux, Switzerland).

Depending on the laser equipment, different methods are used, varying in energy, time, and number of pulses needed to open the ZP. Two studies have reported the immediate effects of localized heating after the use of noncontact infrared lasers in animal models (68,69). The diode laser beam produces superheated water approaching 200°C on the beam axis. The action of the laser must be strictly limited to the targeted region of the ZP, since focused laser irradiation on a specific cell will cause damage and probably be lethal to that cell. Following irradiation, the heat is conducted away from the target and is dissipated into the surrounding medium. The potential to damage blastomeres adjacent to the hole created by the laser is minimized by using pulse durations of $\leq$5 ms and laser powers of $\sim$100 mW at a safe distance from the blastomeres.

In a study of a murine model to determine the optimal technical settings for laser AH—changing laser intensity, pulse duration, number of pulses, and depth of disruptions—the highest hatching rate seemed to be achieved when laser intensity was reduced (70).

There are studies that compared laser AH with other AH methods (71,72). Sister embryos of patients undergoing preimplantation genetic diagnosis, randomly assigned on day 3 to AT solution ZP drilling or to laser ZP drilling, showed similar blastocyst development rates (71). However, implantation rates of laser ZP-drilled embryos were significantly higher than those of mechanically treated embryos, when the embryos of women of advanced age (39 years) underwent AH (72).

ZP thinning

The aim of ZP thinning is to thin the ZP without complete lysis and perforation. By not breaching the ZP, the potential risk of blastomere loss and embryonic infection is minimized.

ZP thinning with AT has been described in mice and humans (27,73). It involves bidirectional thinning of a cross-shaped area of the ZP over about a quarter of the embryo's circumference. Care has to be taken not to rupture the ZP completely. Embryos are washed in fresh droplets of the medium and cultured before transfer. This methodology has proved useful for hatching enhancement in mice but not in humans, probably because of differences observed in both the morphologic and the biophysical characteristics of the ZP between the two species. The mouse ZP has a monolayer structure whereas the human ZP, as shown by electron microscopy, is composed of a less dense, easily digestible, thick outer layer and a more compact but resilient inner layer (73).

The use of laser technology for ZP thinning at the cleavage stage seems to be beneficial for embryo implantation for certain authors (26,54,74–76). Antinori et al. demonstrated a significant increase in implantation and pregnancy rates when 50% of the ZP thickness from two-day-old embryos was thinned to a length of 20 μm using a

YAG contact laser (w). Diode laser ZP thinning enhances the variation of ZP thickness in human embryos, allows natural ZP thinning, and significantly increases the rate of blastocyst hatching (26). Acceptable clinical pregnancy rates were obtained after transfer of frozen–thawed blastocysts that underwent laser-assisted thinning at the day-3 cleaving stage before freezing (74). Laser partial ZP thinning has also been associated with higher implantation and pregnancy rates than total laser AH, especially in women who suffer from recurrent implantation failure (76,77). However, recent time-lapse studies in a mouse model suggest that laser ZP thinning procedures may not only fail to facilitate hatching, but may induce abnormal forms of hatching and prevent escape of the embryo from the ZP altogether (78).

The enzymatic action of pronase to thin the ZP of human early-cleaving embryos yields similar benefits to other AH methods (79). Nevertheless, ZP thinning for cryopreserved–thawed embryos using pronase action or laser methodology has failed to show an improvement in the implantation rate (80–83).

A new method for mechanical AH, inspired by the natural expanding effects of blastocysts on the ZP, has been described (84). This mechanical AH method expands/stretches the ZP by injecting hydrostatic pressure into the perivitelline space using an ICSI injection needle and culture medium, inducing a short-term (≤30-second) ZP thinning. Mechanically expanding the ZP of frozen–thawed day-3 human embryos with injected hydrostatic pressure has been shown to increase implantation and clinical pregnancy rates when compared with control embryos (84).

Blastocyst AH

Even though AH has been initially performed on early-cleavage embryos (day 3, six- to eight-cell stage), it can also be applied to blastocysts to increase implantation rates. A monozygotic twin pregnancy was achieved after transfer of a frozen–thawed human blastocyst on which ZP rubbing was applied with a microneedle (85). The size of the hole made on the human blastocyst's ZP during AH seems to be important to final hatching development. A large slit created on the ZP of human blastocysts after mechanical AH with long zona dissection (LZD) significantly enhanced total blastocyst hatching *in vitro* compared to a moderately sized slit (two-fifths of the ZP diameter) (34). A ZP opening of small or moderate size induced the hatching blastocyst into a "figure of eight" shape and often trapped the ICM.

Fong et al. described a method for enzymatic treatment with pronase of the ZP of blastocysts (86). Just before complete disappearance of the ZP, the blastocysts were placed in a fresh medium and washed twice. The ZP-manipulated blastocysts have shown a high implantation rate (33%), and therefore there is a need to limit the number of AH blastocysts to be transferred to one or two in order to reduce multiple pregnancies.

Park et al. reported the use of a 1.48 μm noncontact diode laser for AH of *in vitro*-matured/*in vitro*-fertilized/*in vitro*-cultured bovine blastocysts (87). Short irradiation exposure times (3–5 ms) were applied, and a significant increase in the hatching rate was observed.

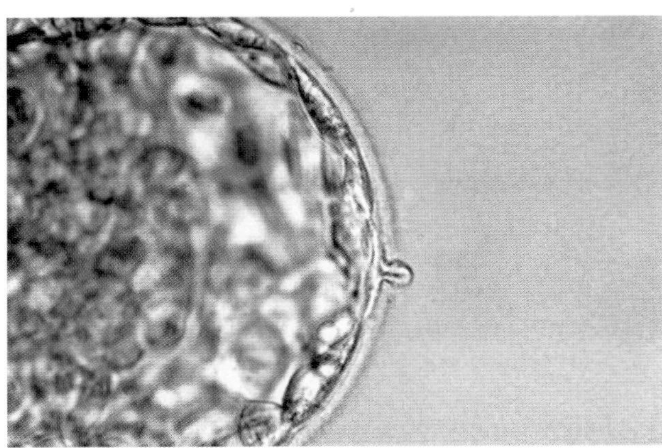

Figure 12.2 Laser-assisted hatching (Fertilase®, MTM, Montreaux, Switzerland) in an expanded blastocyst. A trophectoderm cell is protruding through the thin zona pellucida.

We have described the use of a 1.48 μm diode laser for AH in human blastocysts (88). Even though no statistically significant differences were observed, a trend toward higher pregnancy and implantation rates was obtained when laser-drilled AH blastocysts were replaced, compared with non-drilled blastocysts (44.4% vs. 23.8% and 30.6% vs. 11.6%) (Figure 12.2).

Artificial opening of the ZP by 3D-PZD or by laser and total ZP removal after the warming of vitrified blastocysts significantly improved implantation and pregnancy rates (33,40,41). A recent study suggests that quarter ZP opening by laser AH significantly improves the clinical outcomes of vitrified–warmed blastocysts, especially of day-6 vitrified blastocysts, developed from low-grade cleavage-stage embryos (89). Conversely, a study performed on vitrified–warmed blastocyst transfer has shown that the site of AH has no influence on implantation, pregnancy, and live birth rates (90).

CONSIDERATIONS AND CONCLUSIONS

Several studies have been performed to demonstrate the usefulness and efficacy of AH in different groups of patients using the various methods described. Most of the studies have been done in patients with poor prognosis, including advanced-age patients, patients with elevated concentrations of follicle-stimulating hormone (FSH), patients with previous implantation failures, or patients with embryos with thick ZPs, some of them showing contradictory results. One study included women with endometriosis not showing improvement after AH (91). AH has been applied to fresh, early cleavage-stage embryos and blastocysts and also to frozen–thawed embryos and vitrified–warmed blastocysts. Removal of necrotic blastomeres from partially damaged cryopreserved–thawed embryos may help to maintain their development potential (22,92).

Tables 12.1 and 12.2 show the results reported by different authors.

The variability of methodologies, study designs, and groups of patients described in the published AH studies makes it very difficult to come to a definitive conclusion on the possible effect of AH on clinical outcomes. The last Cochrane review of this area concludes that even though live birth should be considered the primary outcome, the available data do not show any positive effect of AH on live birth rates (93). On the other hand, a recent systematic review and meta-analysis of the medical literature evaluating the effect of AH on assisted reproduction outcomes concluded that AH was related to increased clinical pregnancy and multiple pregnancy rates in women with previous repeated failure or in frozen–thawed embryo transfer (94). Further, a retrospective study of children born after single

Table 12.1 Assisted hatching results reported by different authors (1992–1999)

First author, year	Study method	Population	Randomized	Pregnancy rate increase
Cohen, 1992 (8)	AT	Normal FSH	Yes	Yes, NS
		≥15 μm ZP	Yes	Yes, sig.
Tucker, 1993 (73)	AT	All IVF	Yes	No
	ZP thinning			
Olivennes, 1994 (96)	PZD	Impl. failures	No (no control)	—
		Day 3, FSH >15 mIU/mL	Yes	Yes, sig.
Obruca, 1994 (52)	Er:YAG laser	Impl. failures	No	Yes, sig.
Tucker, 1994 (97)	AT, CC	Age ≥38 years, impl. failures	Yes (control: AT)	Yes, sig.
Schoolcraft, 1994 (47)	AT	Elevated FSH, age ≥39 years	No	Yes, sig.
		Impl. failures		
Schoolcraft, 1995 (98)	AT	Age ≥40 years	No, retrosp.	Yes, sig.
Stein, 1995 (99)	PZD	≥3 impl. failures	Yes	Yes, sig. age >38 years
Hellebaut, 1996 (75)	PZD	First cycle	Yes	No
Antinori, 1996 (54)	UV laser	Impl. failures	No	Yes, sig.
Check, 1996 (100)	AT	Frozen ET	No	Yes, NS
Antinori, 1996 (66)	Er:YAG laser	First cycle	Yes	Yes, sig.
		Impl. failures	Yes	Yes, sig.
Tucker, 1996 (101)	AT	ICSI, age ≥35 years	No	Yes, sig.
Bider, 1997 (102)	AT	Age ≥38 years	No	No
Chao, 1997 (103)	PZD	Impl. failures	Yes	Yes, IVF
				No, TET
Hurst, 1998 (104)	AT	First cycle	Yes	No
Magli, 1998 (105)	AT	Age ≥38 years	No	Yes, sig.
		≥3 impl. failures		Yes, sig.
		Both	Yes	No
Lanzendorf, 1998 (106)	AT	Age ≥36 years	Yes	No
Meldrum, 1998 (107)	AT	Age ≥35 years	No	Yes, NS
	Er:YAG laser	First cycle	Yes	Yes (?)
Antinori, 1999 (67)	PZD	≥6 impl. failures	Yes	Yes (?)
Edirisinghe, 1999 (108)		Age ≥38 years, ZP ≥15, ≥1 μm impl. failure	No	No
Baruffi, 1999 (62)	Diode laser, ZP thinning	Age <37 years, first cycle	Yes	No
Veiga, 1999 (88)	Diode laser	Impl. failure, CC	Yes	Yes, NS
		First cycle	Yes	No (unpubl.)
Cieslak, 1999 (38)	3D-PZD	All IVF	Yes (control: conv. PZD)	Yes, NS
Alikani, 1999 (109)	PZD + frag. removal	≥6% frag.	No, retrosp.	Yes, sig.
Nakayama, 1999 (110)	Piezomicromanipulator	≥2 impl. failures	Yes	Yes, sig.

Abbreviations: AT, acid Tyrode's; blast., blastomere; CC, co-culture; conv., conventional; Er:YAG, erbium:yttrium–aluminum–garnet; ET, embryo transfer; frag., fragmented; FSH, follicle-stimulating hormone; ICSI, intracytoplasmic sperm injection; impl. implantation; IVF, *in vitro* fertilization; NS, not significant; PZD, partial zona pellucida dissection; retrosp., retrospective; sig., significant; TET, thawed embryo transfer; unpubl., unpublished; ZP, zona pellucida.

Table 12.2 Assisted hatching results reported by different authors (2000–2010)

First author, year	Study method	Population	Randomized	Pregnancy rate increase
Mansour, 2000 (111)	ZP removal, AT	First cycle	Yes	No
		Age ≥40 years ≥2 impl. failures	Yes	Yes, sig.
Mantoudis, 2001 (112)	Diode laser	Poor responders aged ≥38 years, ≥2	No	Yes, sig.
	Total AH, partial AH, ZP	Impl. failures, frozen ET		(for ZP thinning)
Malter, 2001 (113)	Diode laser versus AT	All IVF/ICSI	Yes (control: AT)	No
Balaban, 2002 (79)	PZD	All IVF/ICSI	No, retrosp.	No
	AT			No
	Diode laser			No
	Pronase thinning			No
Rienzi, 2002 (22)	Diode laser	Frozen ET	Yes	Yes, sig.
	Necrotic blast. removal			
Hsieh, 2002 (114)	Diode laser versus AT	Age ≥38 years	Yes	Yes, sig. (for laser)
Milki, 2002 (115)	AH D + 3 versus CC	Age 40–43 years	No, retrosp.	No
Vanderzwalmen, 2003 (33)	PZD blastocysts	Frozen (vitrif.) ET	No, retrosp	Yes, sig.
Gabrielsen, 2004 (116)	AT	Frozen ET	Yes	No
Petersen, 2005 (76)	Diode laser, ZP thinning	≥2 impl. failures	Yes	Yes, NS
Ng, 2005 (81)	Diode laser, ZP thinning	Frozen ET	Yes	No
Nadir, 2005 (91)	Diode laser, ZP thinning	Endometriosis	Yes	No
Frydman, 2006 (117)	Diode laser, ZP thinning	Age ≥37 years	Yes	No
Balaban, 2006 (118)	Diode laser	Frozen ET	Yes	Yes, sig.
Sifer, 2006 (80)	Pronase, ZP thinning	Frozen ET	Yes	No
Petersen, 2006 (82)	Diode laser, ZP thinning	Frozen ET	Yes	Yes, NS
		From OHSS IVF cycles		
Sagoskin, 2007 (119)	Diode laser	Good prognosis	Yes	No
Hiraoka, 2007 (41)	Diode laser versus AT	≥2 impl. failures	No, retrosp.	Yes, sig. (for total removal)
	Total ZP removal versus partial drilling	Frozen ET		
	Blastocyst AH			
Hiraoka, 2008 (40)	Diode laser	≥2 impl. failures	No, retrosp.	Yes, sig. (for 50%)
	ZP drilling	Frozen ET		
	ET 50% versus 40 μm			
Hiraoka, 2009 (42)	Diode laser, ZP thinning	Frozen ET	Yes	Yes, sig. (for 50%)
	D + 3 50% versus 25%			
Valojerdi, 2010 (83)	Diode laser, ZP thinning	Frozen ET	Yes	No (sig. decrease)
	D + 3 vitrified			
Fang, 2010 (84)	Mechanical expansion D + 3	Frozen ET	Yes	Yes, sig.

Abbreviations: AT, acid Tyrode's; AH, assisted hatching; blast., blastomere; CC, co-culture; D, day; ET, embryo transfer; FSH, follicle-stimulating hormone; ICSI, intracytoplasmic sperm injection; impl. implantation; IVF, *in vitro* fertilization; PZD, partial zona pellucida dissection; retrosp., retrospective; NS, not significant; sig., significant; OHSS, ovarian hyperstimulation syndrome; vitrif., vitrification; ZP, zona pellucida.

assisted-hatched embryo transfer suggest that AH alone does not increase the risk of major congenital abnormalities (95).

From the published results and taking into account the variability in methods and study designs, the conclusions concerning AH's benefits are as follows:

1. AH does not increase pregnancy and implantation rates in patients in their first IVF attempt.
2. There is some evidence that AH increases pregnancy and implantation rates in patients with previous implantation failures.

3. It is not clear whether AH enhance embryo implantation and pregnancy rates in patients undergoing frozen–thawed embryo transfer, patients of an advanced age, or patients with thick ZP embryos.
4. There is clear evidence that AH increase multiple pregnancy rates.
5. Currently, there is insufficient evidence to recommend AH as a routine technique in patients undergoing assisted reproductive techniques.

The potential of AH in assisted conception makes it imperative that studies of adequate methodological quality (preferably multicenter trials with appropriate design, adequate power, and appropriate duration of follow-up) are undertaken to investigate the role of the various methods of AH when applied at different development stages and sites of the embryo and in different subgroups of the population—women undergoing frozen embryo transfers, women in older age groups, women following repeated implantation failure, women with high early proliferative phase serum FSH levels, and women with embryos with thick or hardened ZPs or poor-quality embryos—in order to provide urgently needed answers.

It is questionable whether different methods of AH yield similar outcomes. Large randomized studies comparing AH methods with regard to embryo implantation and live birth rates are needed, and follow-up of obstetric and post-natal outcomes is recommended. Mechanical hatching by PZD is limited by the difficulty of creating a hole of consistent size. The variability and possible embryotoxicity are potential problems with the use of AT for ZP drilling. Enzymatic methods to dissolve or thin the ZP seem to be effective and safe. Although the equipment may be expensive, the use of a 1.48 μm diode infrared laser system for ZP drilling offers low potential risk, is quick and relatively simple to perform with high consistency between operators, and appears to be the most suitable method for AH in the IVF laboratory.

REFERENCES

1. Dean J. Biology of mammalian fertilization: the role of the zona pellucida. *J Clin Invest* 1992; 89: 1055–59.
2. Shabanowitz RB, O'Rand MG. Characterization of the human zona pellucida from fertilized and unfertilized eggs. *J Reprod Fert* 1988; 82: 151–61.
3. Ducibella T, Kurasawa S, Ramgarajan S, Kopf GS, Schultz RM. Precocious loss of cortical granules during oocyte meiotic maturation and correlation with an egg-induced modification of the zona pellucida. *Dev Biol* 1990; 137: 46–55.
4. Cohen J. Assisted hatching of human embryos. *J In Vitro Fert Embryo Transfer* 1991; 8: 179–90.
5. Trounson AO, Moore NW. The survival and development of sheep eggs following complete or partial removal of the zona pellucida. *J Reprod Fert* 1974; 41: 97–105.
6. De Felici M, Siracusa G. Spontaneous hardening of the zona pellucida of mouse oocytes during *in vitro* culture. *Gamete Res* 1982; 6: 107–13.
7. Cohen J, Elsner C, Kort H et al. Impairment of the hatching process following IVF in the human and improvement of implantation by assisted hatching using micromanipulation. *Hum Reprod* 1990; 5: 7–13.
8. Cohen J, Alikani M, Trowbridge J, Rosenwaks Z. Implantation enhancement by selective assisted hatching using zona drilling of human embryos with poor prognosis. *Hum Reprod* 1992; 7: 685–91.
9. Schiewe MC, Araujo JR, Asch RH, Balmaceda JP. Enzymatic characterization of zona pellucida hardening in human eggs and embryos. *J Assist Reprod Genet* 1995; 12: 2–7.
10. Gonzales D, Bavister B. Zona pellucida escape by hamster blastocysts *in vitro* is delayed and morphologically different compared with zona escape *in vivo*. *Biol Reprod* 1995; 52: 470–80.
11. Gonzales DS, Jones JM, Pinyopumintr P et al. Trophectoderm projections: A potential means for locomotion, attachment and implantation of bovine, equine and human blastocysts. *Hum Reprod* 1996; 11: 2739–45.
12. Gordon J, Dapunt U. A new mouse model for embryos with a hatching deficiency and its use to elucidate the mechanism of blastocyst hatching. *Fertil Steril* 1993; 59: 1296–301.
13. Schiewe MC, Hazeleger NL, Sclimenti C, Balmaceda JP. Physiological characterization of blastocyst hatching mechanisms by use of a mouse antihatching model. *Fertil Steril* 1995; 63: 288–94.
14. Veeck LL, Zaninovic N. Blastocyst hatching. In: *An Atlas of Human Blastocysts*. Veeck LL, Zaninovic N (eds). London, U.K.: Informa Healthcare, 2003, pp. 159–71.
15. Gonzales DS, Jones JM, Pinyopummintr T et al. Trophectoderm projections: A potential means for locomotion, attachment and implantation of bovine, equine and human blastocysts. *Hum Reprod* 1996; 11: 2739–45.
16. Montag M, Koll B, Holmes P, Van der Ven H. Significance of the number of embryonic cells and the state of the zona pellucida for hatching of mouse blastocysts *in vitro* versus *in vivo*. *Biol Reprod* 2000; 62: 1738–44.
17. Gordon J, Dapunt U. Restoration of normal implantation rates in mouse embryos with a hatching impairment by use of a new method of assisted hatching. *Fertil Steril* 1993; 59: 1302–7.
18. Mandelbaum J. The effects of assisted hatching on the hatching process and implantation. *Hum Reprod* 1996; 11: 43–50.
19. Ludwig M, Al-Hasani S, Felderbaum DK. New aspects of cryopreservation of oocytes and embryos in assisted reproduction and future perspectives. *Hum Reprod* 1999; 14(Suppl 1): 162–85.
20. Alikani M, Oliviennes F, Cohen J. Microsurgical correction of partially degenerate mouse embryos promotes hatching and restores their viability. *Hum Reprod* 1993; 8: 1723–8.

21. Elliot TA, Colturato LFA, Taylor TA et al. Lysed cell removal promotes frozen–thawed embryo development. *Fertil Steril* 2007; 87: 1444–9.
22. Rienzi L, Nagy ZP, Ubaldi F et al. Laser-assisted removal of necrotic blastomeres from cryopreserved embryos that were partially damaged. *Fertil Steril* 2002; 77: 1196–201.
23. Loret de Mola JR, Garside WT, Bucci J et al. Analysis of the human zona pellucida during culture; Correlation with diagnosis and the preovulatory hormonal environment. *Assist Reprod Genet* 1997; 14: 332–6.
24. Cohen J, Wiker SR, Inge KL et al. Videocinematography of fresh and cryopreserved embryos: A retrospective analysis of embryonic morphology and implantation. *Fertil Steril* 1989; 51: 821–7.
25. Palmstierna M, Murkes D, Csemiczdy G et al. Zona pellucida thickness variation and occurrence of visible mononucleated blastomeres in pre-embryos are associated with a high pregnancy rate in IVF treatments. *J Assist Reprod Genet* 1998; 15: 70–5.
26. Blake DA, Forsberg AS, Johansson BR, Wikland M. Laser zona pellucida thinning—An alternative approach to assisted hatching. *Hum Reprod* 2001; 16: 1959–64.
27. Khalifa EAM, Tucker MJ, Hunt P. Cruciate thinning of the zona pellucida for more successful enhancement of blastocyst hatching in the mouse. *Hum Reprod* 1992; 7: 532–6.
28. Liu HC, Cohen J, Alikani M, Noyes N, Rosenwaks Z. Assisted hatching facilitates earlier implantation. *Fertil Steril* 1993; 60: 871–5.
29. Ebner T, Gruber I, Moser M. Location of herniation predicts implantation behavior of hatching blastocysts. *J. Turkish German Gynecol Assoc* 2007; 8: 184–8.
30. Miyata H, Matsubayashi H, Fukutomi N et al. Relevance of the site of assisted hatching in thawed human blastocysts: A preliminary report. *Fertil Steril* 2010; 94: 2444–7.
31. Ebner T, Shebl O, Mayer RB et al. Relevance of the site of assisted hatching in thawed human blastocysts (Letter to the editor). *Fertil Steril* 2010; 94: e65.
32. Dale B, Talevi R, Gualtieri R et al. Intercellular communication in the early human embryo. *Mol Reprod Dev* 1991; 29: 22–8.
33. Vanderzwalmen P, Bertin G, Debauche Ch et al. Vitrification of human blastocysts with the Hemi-Straw carrier: Application of assisted hatching after thawing. *Hum Reprod* 2003; 18: 1504–11.
34. Lyu QF, Wu LQ, Li YP et al. An improved mechanical technique for assisted hatching. *Hum Reprod* 2005; 20: 1619–23.
35. Talansky BE, Gordon JW. Cleavage characteristics of mouse embryos inseminated and cultures after zona pellucida drilling. *Gamete Res* 1998; 21: 277–8.
36. Nichols J, Garner RL. Effect of damage of the zona pellucida on development of preimplantation embryos in the mouse. *Hum Reprod* 1989; 4: 180–7.
37. Cohen J, Feldberg D. Effects of the size and number of zona pellucida openings on hatching and trophoblast outgrowth in the mouse embryo. *Mol Reprod Dev* 1991; 30: 70–8.
38. Cieslak J, Ivakhnenko V, Wolf G, Sheleg S, Verlinsky Y. Three dimensional partial zona dissection for preimplantation genetic diagnosis and assisted hatching. *Fertil Steril* 1999; 71: 308–13.
39. Alikani M, Noyes N, Cohen J, Rosenwaks Z. Monozygotic twinning in the human is associated with the zona pellucida architecture. *Hum Reprod* 1994; 9: 1318–21.
40. Hiraoka K, Fuchiwaki M, Horaoka K et al. Effect of the size of zona pellucida outcome of frozen cleaved embryos that were cultured to blastocyst after thawing in women with multiple implantation failures of embryo transfer: A retrospective study. *J Assist Reprod Genet* 2008; 25: 129–35.
41. Hiraoka K, Fuchiwaki M, Horaoka K et al. Zona pellucida removal and vitrified blastocyst transfer outcome: A preliminary study. *Reprod Biomed Online* 2007; 15: 68–75.
42. Hiraoka K, Hiraoka K, Horiuchi T et al. Impact of the size of zona pellucida on vitrified-warmed cleavage-stage embryo transfers: A prospective, randomized study. *J Assist Reprod Genet* 2009; 26: 515–21.
43. Malter HE, Cohen J. Partial zona dissection of the human oocyte: A no traumatic method using micromanipulation to assist zona pellucida penetration. *Fertil Steril* 1989; 51: 139–48.
44. Sun S-T, Choi J-R, Son J-B et al. The effect of long zona dissection using ICSI pipettes for mechanical assisted hatching in vitrified-thawed blastocyst transfers. *J Assist Reprod Genet* 2012; 29: 1431–4.
45. Hogan B, Constantini F, Lacy E. *Manipulating the Mouse Embryo: a Laboratory Manual.* New York, NY: Cold Spring Harbor Laboratory Press, 1986.
46. Malter H, Cohen J. Blastocyst formation and hatching *in vitro* following zona drilling of mouse and human embryos. *Gamete Res* 1989; 24: 67–80.
47. Schoolcraft W, Schenker T, Gee M, Jones GS, Jones HW. Assisted hatching in the treatment of poor prognosis *in vitro* fertilization candidates. *Fertil Steril* 1994; 62: 551–4.
48. Tadir Y, Wright WH, Vafa O et al. Micromanipulation of sperm by a laser generated optical trap. *Fertil Steril* 1989; 52: 870–3.
49. Tadir Y, Wright WH, Vafa O et al. Micromanipulation of gametes using laser microbeams. *Hum Reprod* 1991; 6: 1011–16.
50. Palanker D, Ohad S, Lewis A, Simon A, Shenkar J, Penchas S, Laufer N. Technique for cellular microsurgery using the 193 nm excimer laser. *Laser Surg Med* 1991; 11(6): 580–6.
51. Strohmer H, Feichtinger W. Successful clinical application of laser for micromanipulation in an *in vitro* fertilization program. *Fertil Steril* 1992; 58: 212–4.

52. Obruca A, Strohmer H, Sakkas D et al. Use of lasers in assisted fertilization and hatching. *Hum Reprod* 1994; 9: 1723–6.
53. Obruca A, Strohmer H, Blaschitz A et al. Ultrastuctural observations in human oocytes and preimplantation embryos after zona opening using an Er:YAG laser. *Hum Reprod* 1997; 12: 2242–5.
54. Antinori S, Panci C, Selman HA et al. Zona thinning with the use of laser: A new approach to assisted hatching in humans. *Hum Reprod* 1996; 11: 590–4.
55. Neev J, Tadir Y, Ho P et al. Microscope-delivered ultraviolet laser zona dissection: Principles and practices. *J Assist Reprod Genet* 1992; 9: 513–23.
56. Blanchet GB, Russell JB, Fincher CR, Portman M. Laser micromanipulation in the mouse embryo: A novel approach to zona drilling. *Fertil Steril* 1992; 57: 1337–41.
57. Neev J, Schiewe M, Sung VW et al. Assisted hatching in mouse embryos using a noncontact Ho:YSGG laser system. *J Assist Reprod Genet* 1995; 12: 288–93.
58. Schiewe M, Neev J, Hazeleger NL et al. Developmental competence of mouse embryos following zona drilling using a non-contact Ho:YSGG laser system. *Hum Reprod* 1995; 10: 1821–4.
59. Rink K, Delacretaz G, Salathe RP et al. Non-contact microdrilling of mouse zona pellucida with an objective-delivered 1.48-microns diode laser. *Laser Surg Med* 1996; 18: 52–62.
60. Germond M, Nocera D, Senn A et al. Microdissection of mouse and human zona pellucida using a 1.48 μm diode laser beam: Efficacy and safety of the procedure. *Fertil Steril* 1995; 64: 604–11.
61. Germond M, Nocera D, Senn A et al. Improved fertilization and implantation rates after non touch zona pellucida microdrilling of mouse oocytes with a 1.48 μm diode laser beam. *Hum Reprod* 1996; 11: 1043–8.
62. Baruffi R, Mauri AL, Petersen C et al. Assisted hatching with a laser diode in patients $<$37 years old with no previous failure of implantation: a prospective ran- domized study [Abstracts of the 15th Annual meeting of the ESHRE, Tours, France]. *Hum Reprod* 1999; 14: abstr book 1.
63. Montag M, Van der Ven K, Delacretaz G et al. Laser assisted microdissection of the zona pellucida facilitates polar body biopsy. *Fertil Steril* 1998; 69: 539–42.
64. Boada M, Carrera M, de la Iglesia C et al. Successful use of a laser for human embryo biopsy in preimplantation genetic diagnosis: report of two cases. *J Assist Reprod Genet* 1998; 15: 302–7.
65. Veiga A, Sandalinas M, Benkhalifa M et al. Laser blastocyst biopsy for preimplantation diagnosis in the human. *Zygote* 1997; 5: 351–4.
66. Antinori S, Selman HA, Caffa B et al. Zona opening of human embryos using a non contact UV laser for assisted hatching in patients with poor prognosis of pregnancy. *Hum Reprod* 1996; 11: 2488–92.
67. Antinori S, Versaci C, Dani L et al. Laser assisted hatching at the extremes of the IVF spectrum: first cycle and after 6 cycles: a randomized prospective trial [Abstracts of the 15th Annual Meeting of the ESHRE, Tours, France]. *Hum Reprod* 1999; 14: abstr book 1.
68. Douglas-Hamilton DH, Conia J. Thermal effects in laser-assisted pre-embryo zona drilling. *J Biomed Optics* 2001; 6: 205–13.
69. Chatzimeletiou K, Picton HM, Handyside AH. Use of a non-contact, infrared laser for zona drilling of mouse embryos: Assessment of immediate effects on blastomere viability. *Reprod Biomed Online* 2001; 2: 178–87.
70. Tinney GM, Windt ML, Kruger TF, Lombard CJ. Use of a zona laser treatment system in assisted hatching: optimal laser utilization parameters. *Fertil Steril* 2005; 84: 1737–41.
71. Jones AE, Wright G, Kort HI et al. Comparison of laser-assisted hatching and acidified Tyrode's hatching by evaluation of blastocyst development rates in sibling embryos: A prospective randomized trial. *Fertil Steril* 2006; 85: 487–91.
72. Makrakis E, Angeli I, Agapitou K et al. Laser versus mechanical assisted hatching: A prospective study of clinical outcomes. *Fertil Steril* 2006; 86: 1596–600.
73. Tucker MJ, Luecke NM, Wiker SR, Wright G. Chemical removal of the outside of the zona pellucida of day 3 human embryos has no impact on implantation rate. *J Assist Reprod Genet* 1993; 10: 187–91.
74. Kung FT, Lin YC, Tseng YJ et al. Transfer of frozen–thawed blastocysts that underwent quarter laser-assisted hatching at the day 3 cleaving stage before freezing. *Fertil Steril* 2003; 79: 893–9.
75. Hellebaut S, De Sutter P, Dozortsev D et al. Does assisted hatching improve implantation rates after *in vitro* fertilization or intracytoplasmic sperm injection in all patients? A prospective randomized study. *J Assist Reprod Genet* 1996; 13: 19–22.
76. Petersen CG, Mauri AL, Baruffi RL et al. Implantation failures: success of assisted hatching with quarter-laser zona thinning. *Reprod Biomed Online* 2005; 10: 224–9.
77. Ghobara TS, Cahill DJ, Ford WCL et al. Effects of assisted hatching method and age on implantation rates of IVF and ICSI. *Reprod Biomed Online* 2006; 13: 261–7.
78. Schimmel T, Cohen J, Saunders H, Alikani M. Laser-assisted zona pellucida thinning does not facilitate hatching and may disrupt the *in vitro* hatching process: A morphokinetic study in the mouse. *Hum Reprod* 2014; 29: 2670–9.
79. Balaban B, Urman B, Alatas C et al. A comparison of four different techniques of assisted hatching. *Hum Reprod* 2002; 17: 1239–43.
80. Sifer C, Sellami A, Poncelet C et al. A prospective randomized study to assess the benefit of partial zona pellucida digestion before frozen–thawed embryo. *Hum Reprod* 2006; 21: 2384–9.

81. Ng EHY, Naveed F, Lau EYL et al. A randomized double-blind controlled study of the efficacy of laser-assisted hatching on implantation and pregnancy rates of frozen–thawed embryo transfer at the cleavage stage. *Hum Reprod* 2005; 20: 979–85.
82. Petersen CG, Mauri AL, Baruffi RL et al. Laser-assisted hatching of cryopreserved–thawed embryos by thinning one quarter of the zona. *Reprod Biomed Online* 2006; 13: 668–75.
83. Valojerdi MR, Eftekhari-Yazdi P, Karimian L et al. Effect of laser zona thinning on vitrified-warmed embryo transfer at the cleavage stage: A prospective, randomized study. *Reprod Biomed Online* 2010; 20: 234–42.
84. Fang C, Li T, Miao BY et al. Mechanically expanding the zona pellucida of human frozen thawed embryos: A new method of assisted hatching. *Fertil Steril* 2010; 94: 1302–7.
85. Nijs M, Vanderzwalmen P, Segal-Berti G et al. A monozygotic twin pregnancy after application of zona rubbing on a frozen–thawed blastocyst. *Hum Reprod* 1993; 8: 127–9.
86. Fong CY, Bongso A, Ng SC et al. Blastocyst transfer after enzymatic treatment of the zona pellucida: Improving *in vitro* fertilization and understanding implantation. *Hum Reprod* 1998; 13: 2926–32.
87. Park S, Kim EY, Yoon SH, Chung KS, Lim JH. Enhanced hatching rate of bovine IVM/IVF/IVC blastocysts using a 1.48 μm diode laser beam. *J Assist Reprod Genet* 1999; 16: 97–101.
88. Veiga A, Torelló MJ, Ménézo Y et al. Use of co-culture of human embryos on Vero cells to improve clinical implantation rate. *Hum Reprod* 1999; 14: 112–20.
89. Wan C-Y, Song C, Diao L-H et al. Laser-assisted hatching improves clinical outcomes of vitrified-warmed blastocysts developed from low-grade cleavage-stage embryos: A prospective randomized study. *Reprod Biomed Online* 2014; 28: 582–9.
90. Ren X, Liu Q, Chen W, Zhu G. Effect of the site of assisted hatching on vitrified-warmed blastocyst transfer cycles: A prospective randomized study. *J Assist Reprod Genet* 2013; 30: 691–7.
91. Nadir H, Bener F, Karagenc L et al. Impact of assisted hatching on ART outcome in women with endometriosis. *Hum Reprod* 2005; 20: 2546–9.
92. Rienzi L, Ubaldi F, Iacobelli M et al. Developmental potential of fully intact and partially damaged cryopreserved embryos after laser-assisted removal of necrotic blastomeres and post-thaw culture selection. *Fertil Steril* 2005; 84: 888–94.
93. Carney SK, Das S, Blake D, Farquhar C et al. Assisted hatching on assisted conception (IVF and ICSI). *Cochrane Database Syst Rev* 2012: 2: CD001894.
94. Martins WP, Rocha IA, Ferriani RA et al. Assisted hatching of human embryos: A systematic review and meta-analysis of randomized controlled trials. *Hum Reprod Update* 2011; 17: 438–53.
95. Jwa J, Jwa SC, Kuwahara A et al. Risk of major congenital anomalies after assisted hatching: Analysis of three-year data from the national assisted reproduction registry in Japan. *Fertil Steril* 2015; 104: 71–8.
96. Oliviennes F, Bergere M, Fanchin R et al. L'éclosion embryonnaire assistée. *Contracept Fertil Sex* 1994; 22: 493–7.
97. Tucker M, Ingargiola P, Massey JB et al. Assisted hatching with or without bovine oviductal epithelial cell co-culture for poor prognosis *in vitro* fertilization patients. *Hum Reprod* 1994; 9: 1528–31.
98. Schoolcraft WB, Schlenker T, Jones GS, Jones HW. *In vitro* fertilization in women age 40 and older: The impact of assisted hatching. *J Assist Reprod Genet* 1995; 12: 581–4.
99. Stein A, Rufas O, Amit S et al. Assisted hatching by partial zona dissection of human pre-embryos in patients with recurrent implantation failure after *in vitro* fertilization. *Fertil Steril* 1995; 63: 838–41.
100. Check JH, Hoover L, Nazari A, O'Shaughnessy A, Summers D. The effect of assisted hatching on pregnancy rates after frozen embryo transfer. *Fertil Steril* 1996; 65: 254–7.
101. Tucker MJ, Morton PC, Wright G et al. Enhancement of outcome from intracytoplasmic sperm injection: Does co-culture or assisted hatching improve implantation rates? *Hum Reprod* 1996; 11: 2434–7.
102. Bider D, Livshits A, Yonish M et al. Assisted hatching by zona drilling of human embryos in women of advanced age. *Hum Reprod* 1997; 12: 317–20.
103. Chao KH, Chen SU, Chen HF et al. Assisted hatching increases the implantation and pregnancy rate of *in vitro* fertilization (IVF)–embryo transfer (ET), but not that of IVF–tubal ET in patients with repeated IVF failures. *Fertil Steril* 1997; 67: 904–8.
104. Hurst BS, Tucker KE, Awoniyi CA, Schlaff WD. Assisted hatching does not enhance IVF success in good-prognosis patients. *J Assist Reprod Genet* 1998; 15: 62–4.
105. Magli MC, Gianaroli L, Ferraretti AP et al. Rescue of implantation potential in embryos with poor prognosis by assisted zona hatching. *Hum Reprod* 1998; 13: 1331–5.
106. Lanzendorf SE, Nehchiri F, Mayer JF, Oehninger S, Muasher SJ. A prospective, randomized, double-blind study for the evaluation of assisted hatching in patients with advanced maternal age. *Hum Reprod* 1998; 13: 409–13.
107. Meldrum DR, Wisot A, Yee B et al. Assisted hatching reduces the age-related decline in IVF outcome in women younger than age 43 without increasing miscarriage or monozygotic twinning. *J Assist Reprod Genet* 1998; 15: 418–21.
108. Edirisinghe WR, Ahnonkitpanit V, Promviengchai S et al. A study failing to determine significant benefits from assisted hatching: patients selected for advanced age, zonal thickness of embryos, and previous failed attempts. *J Assist Reprod Genet* 1999; 16: 294–301.

109. Alikani M, Cohen J, Tomkin G et al. Human embryo fragmentation *in vitro* and its implications for pregnancy and implantation. *Fertil Steril* 1999; 71: 836–42.
110. Nakayama T, Fujiwara H, Yamada S et al. Clinical application of a new assisted hatching method using a piezo-micromanipulator for morphologically low-quality embryos in poor-prognosis infertile patients. *Fertil Steril* 1999; 71: 1014–8.
111. Mansour RT, Rhodes CA, Aboulghar MA, Serour GI, Kamal A. Transfer of zona-free embryos improves outcome in poor prognosis patients: a prospective randomized controlled study. *Hum Reprod* 2000; 15: 1061–4.
112. Mantoudis E, Podsiadly BT, Gorgy A, Venkat G, Craft IL. A comparison between quarter, partial and total laser assisted hatching in selected infertility patients. *Hum Reprod* 2001; 16: 2182–6.
113. Malter H, Schimmel T, Cohen J. Zona dissection by infrared laser: Developmental consequences in the mouse, technical considerations, and controlled clinical trial. *Reprod Biomed Online* 2001; 3: 117–23.
114. Hsieh YY, Huang CC, Cheng TC et al. Laser-assisted hatching of embryos is better than the chemical method for enhancing the pregnancy rate in women with advanced age. *Fertil Steril* 2002; 78: 179–82.
115. Milki AA, Hinckley MD, Behr B. Comparison of blastocyst transfer to day 3 transfer with assisted hatching in the older patient. *Fertil Steril* 2002; 78: 1244–7.
116. Gabrielsen A, Agerholm I, Toft B et al. Assisted hatching improves implantation rates on cryopreserved–thawed embryos. A randomized prospective study. *Hum Reprod* 2004; 19: 2258–62.
117. Frydman N, Madoux S, Hesters L et al. A randomized double-blind controlled study on the efficacy of laser zona pellucida thinning on live birth rates in cases of advanced female age. *Hum Reprod* 2006; 21: 2131–5.
118. Balaban B, Urman B, Yakin K, Isiklar F. Laser-assisted hatching increases pregnancy and implantation rates in cryopreserved embryos that were allowed to cleave *in vitro* after thawing: A prospective randomized study. *Hum Reprod* 2006; 21: 2136–40.
119. Sagoskin AW, Levy MJ, Tucker MJ et al. Laser assisted hatching in good prognosis patients undergoing *in vitro* fertilization–embryo transfer: A randomized controlled trial. *Fertil Steril* 2007; 87: 283–7.

Human embryo biopsy procedures

13

JASON KOFINAS, CAROLINE McCAFFREY, and JAMES GRIFO

INTRODUCTION AND HISTORY OF EMBRYO BIOPSY

Embryo biopsy (EB) was developed out of the necessity for single-gene disorder testing and for the potential of sexing embryos. In 1967, Edwards and Gardner published their report on rabbit EB and sexing (1). Two decades passed before EB research began to lend itself to clinical application and interest for human embryos. In 1989, Wilton et al. reported successful single-cell biopsy and cryopreservation in the mouse (2). That same year, Handyside et al. reported the biopsy of human preimplantation embryos and sexing by DNA amplification for couples at risk of transmitting recessive X-linked diseases, as well as DNA analysis of human oocytes for cystic fibrosis diagnosis (3,4). The feasibility of single-cell polymerase chain reaction (PCR) for the diagnosis of single-gene disorders was demonstrated by Coutelle et al. in 1989, where unfertilized oocytes were used as an example for single-cell PCR (3). The first pregnancies were reported in 1990 by Handyside et al., while Grifo et al. reported the first pregnancy after human EB and sexing in the U.S.A. in 1992 (5,6).

The plethora of data and the development of EB procedures since these initial reports have been staggering. The development of various methodologies for the biopsy procedures at different stages of preimplantation development has been of significant interest in the last two decades. Different biopsy techniques have been investigated in animal and human studies and these include polar body biopsy, blastomere biopsy, trophectoderm (TE; blastocyst) biopsy, and, most recently, blastocoel fluid aspiration. In 1988, TE biopsy was first reported in the marmoset monkey and remarkably showed normal *in vivo* development of these embryos (7).

The different biopsy techniques, their safety profiles, the actual performance of these techniques, and their current clinical applications will be the subjects of discussion of this chapter. Emphasis on safety and clinical outcome will be a unifying theme.

PRINCIPLES

The primary aim of EB is to remove a cell or sample of cells (i.e., genetic material) from the preimplantation embryo to allow for diagnosis of the chromosomal complement of the embryo. It is imperative that the procedure is carried out in such a way as to effect the least possible detriment to the developing embryo, that the diagnosis is accurate and representative of the entire embryo, and that analysis for monogenic diseases can be combined with aneuploidy screening.

TYPES OF BIOPSY

Polar body biopsy

Polar body biopsy in humans was first described in 1990 (8). The procedure was developed in an effort to decrease the invasive nature of EB since the polar body(ies) is already separated from the embryo and will not contribute to the developing embryo. Removal of the first polar body (PB1) or both the first (PB1) and the second polar body (PB2) requires creating a hole in the zona pellucida (ZP) and removing the PB1 possibly prior to fertilization or the removal of both polar bodies after fertilization. The genetic material in PB1 is only representative of the DNA in the oocyte (maternal contributions) and specifically only maternal DNA that is not included in the embryo. For this reason, polar body biopsy is particularly useful for detecting maternally inherited monogenic diseases and for numerical/structural chromosomal aberrations in the oocyte (9).

Single-cell biopsy, such as polar body biopsy, however, raises legitimate concerns of reliability. Specifically, allele dropout (ADO) involving the biopsy of PB1 is of concern. The accuracy of polar body biopsy is improved if both PB1 and PB2 are analyzed (10). Ideally, sequential biopsy on different days should be completed in order to be certain that you are obtaining and correctly identifying each polar body (11).

Polar body biopsy has gained increased interest recently due to the growing problem of mosaicism in embryos. Investigators have suggested that sequential polar body biopsy and subsequent analysis will allow the identification of maternally derived mosaicism (12), and since more than 90% of human aneuploids are maternally derived, this is a means to detect a significant number of these without biopsying the embryo. However, the major limitation of the analysis of PB1 is that it focuses on only the maternal genome, whereas other forms of EB provide information on both the maternal and paternal genome. Many errors of meiosis are due to premature separation of sister chromatids as opposed to nondisjunction, and in fact abnormal polar bodies may represent a normal embryo (11).

To date, there has been very little direct evaluation regarding the safety of polar body biopsy and the subsequent developmental capacity of embryos derived from these oocytes. In the small number of studies reported, methodologies were different and these were not randomized controlled trials. However, it seems intuitive that biopsy of the polar bodies should be less invasive than blastomere or TE biopsy, since the polar bodies are by-products of the meiotic division and not part of the embryo per se. Verlinsky et al. in 1990 showed that removal and analysis of the polar bodies did not affect subsequent fertilization rates and embryonic development to the blastocyst stage (8). Hammoud et al. in 2010 compared ZP drilling of oocytes, ZP drilling, and polar body biopsy versus no intervention and found no difference between the three groups in respect to oocyte activation (achieved with calcium ionophor) and *in vitro* development to the cleavage stage. However, these authors described the risk of cell lysis and found a 2% lysis rate with ZP drilling alone and a 4% lysis risk with drilling plus polar body biopsy (13). Another study found higher rates of cleavage arrest, fragmentation on day 2, lower rates of good-quality cleavage embryos, and lower blastomere cell numbers in embryos that had undergone polar body biopsy as opposed to a control group (14). As with any procedure, the benefits should be weighed against the risks and although in highly skilled hands polar body biopsy has been shown to have no deleterious effect on the developing embryo, it has been reported that the information obtained from polar body biopsy, even sequential biopsy of PB1 and PB2, is of limited value in identifying aneuploidies at later stages of development (15–17).

Day-3 cleavage-stage (blastomere) biopsy

The intent of day-3 biopsy is to remove one blastomere from the embryo at the cleavage stage of development as a representative sample of the entire embryo. As with all other biopsy procedures, this requires creating a hole in the ZP followed by removal of one or possibly two blastomeres from the embryo. The question as to whether a single cell is sufficient to obtain reliable test results and whether it is representative of the entire embryo and resulting fetus still remains. Does the removal of one cell or more cells from the cleavage-stage embryo affect the development of that embryo?

Single-cell PCR in human gametes was demonstrated by Coutelle et al. in 1988 with the use of unfertilized oocytes (3), although it was not until 1989 that a single blastomere was removed from a cleavage-stage embryo. The technology available at that time allowed for specific base pairs to match with a 3–4 kb repeat sequence within the Y chromosome. This allowed for the identification of the Y chromosome within the biopsied embryos and thus the ability to sex the embryos. This was a significant step forward for reducing the need for late-trimester abortions of X-linked recessive-affected male embryos (4).

There are, however, concerns with the biopsy of day-3 embryos. Given that typically only one blastomere is removed for analysis, the problem of ADO leading to misdiagnosis in approximately 10% of cases is one that cannot be ignored (9). ADO occurs if only one of the two alleles is successfully amplified in a heterozygous cell (18). Van de Velde et al. in 2000 considered the problem of ADO and compared one-cell versus two-cell blastomere biopsy and found that implantation rates and ongoing pregnancy rates were not significantly different between the two groups (19). The ability to compare the results of two blastomeres and ensure the accuracy of the results decreased the incidence of ADO (19). Although this study reported no adverse effect on implantation rates of removing two cells versus one cell, the study was subject to criticism in that the group with two blastomeres removed had significantly better and more advanced embryos based on morphologic criteria prior to biopsy. In 2008, Goossens et al. reported that removal of two blastomeres from a cleavage-stage embryo negatively impacted subsequent embryo development by day 5 (20). It stands to reason that removal of a considerable fraction of a cleavage-stage embryo on day 3 will compromise the developmental potential of that embryo and limit its ability for continued development, implantation, and pregnancy establishment.

Interestingly, the cavitation and hatching rates of embryos have not been shown to be significantly affected by micromanipulation of the embryo (21). However, recent data demonstrate that biopsied embryos show a significant decrease in implantation potential when biopsied on day 3 versus biopsy at the blastocyst stage (22). However, despite the inherent concerns with day-3 biopsy, according to the 13th annual European Society of Human Reproduction and Embryology (ESHRE) PGD consortium data compiled from 2010 data, 80% (4526/5651) of EB cycles from 62 centers were still being conducted at the cleavage stage (23).

It is now widely accepted that day-3 biopsy can compromise the implantation potential of biopsied embryos as compared to day-5 biopsy (22,24). As discussed above, the problems with ADO seen with day-3 EB can be mitigated by removal of two cells. However, Goossens et al. showed that blastocyst formation was decreased with removal of two cells as opposed to one cell, although that same study reported that the implantation rates were not significantly different for two-cell versus one-cell cleavage-stage biopsy (20). Many cleavage-stage embryos lack the developmental competence to reach the blastocyst stage, irrespective of any impact of the biopsy. Unfortunately, there is a lack of randomized controlled data to compare one- and two-cell blastomere biopsy techniques. However, a very elegant study in 2013 presented convincing data about the safety profile of day-3 versus day-5 biopsy (22), and these findings have helped push the standard of care for EB to be exclusively day 5.

Blastocyst (TE) biopsy

The intent of TE biopsy is to remove and test 5–10 cells from the TE layer (a portion of the embryo that is destined to become placental tissue) as a representative sample of the entire embryo and the resulting fetus. Again, the biopsy is facilitated by means of an opening created in the ZP through which cells are removed from the TE. The question as to whether these cells are sufficient to perform genetic testing and whether they are representative of the fetus that will form must be considered. Analysis of multiple cells is advantageous in ensuring that the DNA obtained is sufficient to obtain a diagnosis and to avoid the problem of ADO. However, in some instances, cells from a single biopsy specimen may yield different genetic results as a result of mosaicism (25), which is caused by the presence of a mix of normal and abnormal cells or a mix of different abnormalities with no normal cells present. In addition, the question of whether the removal of multiple cells from the TE affects the further development or ability of the blastocyst to implant and establish a pregnancy needs to be considered.

In 1990, Dokras et al. reported the successful biopsy of 47 human embryos at the blastocyst stage. The report examined the size of the slit and degree of herniation necessary to achieve optimal biopsy conditions. They showed that development of the manipulated embryos did not appear to be impaired. Notably, they biopsied ~10–30 cells on average, significantly more cells than would be considered standard today (26). One of the distinct benefits associated with blastocyst biopsy is the ability to biopsy only those embryos that have demonstrated the potential for continued embryonic development. In this way it reduces the probability of selecting an aneuploid embryo since many of these embryos will arrest before they ever reach the blastocyst stage (27,28). Embryos arrested in development at the cleavage stage showed increased aneuploidy involving chromosomes X, Y, 16, 18, and 21. In one study, TE biopsy of four to five cells led to a complete genotype in 94.3% of cases (29).

Table 13.1 provides a summary of the pros and cons of the different biopsy methods available.

Given the data we have available to date, it is clear that day-5 biopsy provides more cells for genetic analysis while decreasing the invasiveness of the biopsy technique (as evidenced by the non-significant difference in implantation rates between biopsied embryos and non-biopsied controls). In our center, we currently perform EB at the blastocyst stage.

Blastocoel fluid aspiration

The objective of blastocoel fluid aspiration is to collect samples of the fluid that accumulates in the blastocoel cavity. Fragments of DNA shed from the embryo accumulate in this fluid. Removal of this fluid thereby could allow for the collection and analysis of these DNA fragments. If these fragments are determined to be a reliable and sufficient source of DNA for analysis and are found to be representative of the embryo and resulting fetus, this will obviate the need to physically separate cells from the embryo proper. Already, collapsing of the blastocyst and removal of the blastocoel fluid prior to vitrification has been shown to improve survival rates of cryopreserved embryos, indicating that removal of this fluid does not harm the developmental capacity of the blastocyst.

More recently, there have been efforts to determine if analysis of the fluid that accumulates inside the cavity of the developing blastocyst could offer a less invasive means to obtain ploidy information on the embryo. Following differentiation of the cells of the blastocyst into inner cell mass (ICM) and TE cells, sodium ions begin to accumulate, creating an osmotic gradient that pulls fluid in between these cell lineages, creating what is known as the blastocoel cavity. This fluid accumulation is facilitated by tight junctions between the adjoining cells in the TE that form a seal and prevent fluid leakage (30,31). Initial analysis of the blastocoel fluid involved metabolomic profiling in an effort to ascertain if the fluid could reveal information about the implantation potential of the embryo (32). The blastocoel fluid is sampled by means of inserting an intracytoplasmic sperm injection (ICSI) needle through the mural wall and into the cavity on the opposite side of the ICM to aspirate fluid. In 2013, the first report of the existence of embryonic DNA in the blastocoel fluid was published (33). DNA was isolated from blastocoel fluid from as many as 76.5% of the samples analyzed. Another study reported concordance rates per chromosome of 93.5%, 94%, and 96.6% in polar bodies, blastomeres, and TE, respectively, when compared to blastocoel fluid (34). However, in another recent study involving array comparative genomic hybridization of blastocoel fluid, DNA was obtained in only 63% of blastocoel fluid samples. Discordancy rates were found to be 52% between blastocoel fluid and ICM–TE samples. Interestingly, blastomere analysis revealed that 70% of aneuploid cleavage-stage embryos normalized by day 5, and of these embryos, 86% had aneuploid nuclei within the blastocoel fluid cavity. The authors concluded that blastocoel fluid may be a mechanism by which the embryo partitions abnormal cells (35,36). Given the inconsistencies reported in studies looking at blastocoel fluid analysis in predicting embryo ploidy, blastocoel fluid analysis for the purposes of genetic evaluation of a preimplantation embryo should still be considered experimental. Further studies are warranted to validate this methodology and confirm if it is sufficient for diagnostic purposes.

EQUIPMENT SET-UP FOR EB

The set-up and procedures described will focus on TE biopsy since this has become the standard of care for all EB procedures at our center unless there are extenuating circumstances or special cases requiring polar body biopsy or blastomere biopsy. For details of how to conduct a polar body biopsy, blastomere biopsy or aspiration, and analysis of blastocoel fluid, readers should refer to the papers referenced in this chapter.

EB is a micromanipulation technique that requires a precise set-up and reliable equipment similar to an ICSI set-up. Micromanipulation techniques used in EB have evolved over the years as EB procedures have changed and improved. A variety of techniques for breaching the ZP and removing of a cell or cells from the egg, zygote, cleavage-stage embryo, or blastocyst have been employed and will be described. Special focus will be devoted to the use of laser technology and blastocyst biopsy since these techniques have shown significantly superior results in terms of reducing impact on embryo development and clinical outcome (11,22). However, all egg or EB procedures have some common needs: (a) an inverted microscope that provides optimal magnification and optics to visualize

Table 13.1 Advantages and disadvantage of various embryo biopsy techniques

Type of embryo biopsy	Advantages	Disadvantages
Polar body biopsy	1. Significantly less invasive 2. Provides early information on egg genetic make-up 3. Potential applications for monitoring egg quality in oocyte cryopreservation cycles	1. Requires both polar bodies for accurate diagnosis 2. Targets meiotic errors only and only considers the maternal genome 3. Suffers from significant allele dropout 4. Requires significant technical expertise 5. Lack of randomized controlled trials to determine its potential use 6. May falsely label an embryo aneuploid
Cleavage-stage biopsy	1. Has been in use for >20 years and technically feasible for many *in vitro* fertilization centers 2. Provides information on the whole embryo (maternal and paternal genome) 3. There are studies suggesting its safety and universal applicability	1. Most invasive form of embryo biopsy 2. A randomized controlled trial has called into question the safety profile of removing an embryonic cell at this stage of development 3. Requires significant technical skill 4. Has significant non-detection and error rates 5. Allele dropout is a consideration
Blastocyst-stage biopsy	1. Current standard of care 2. Technically feasible 3. Provides information on the whole embryo (maternal and paternal genome) 4. Safety profile has been proven	1. Requires extended culture 2. Requires investment in a laser system 3. Technically challenging 4. Lack of randomized controlled trials showing clinical benefit in younger population (although these studies are ongoing at this time)
Blastocoel fluid aspiration	1. Significantly less invasive than direct embryonic cell biopsy 2. Provides further information about the embryo 3. May have use in discerning mosaicism	1. May not provide accurate representation of embryonic ploidy status 2. Has a low concordance rate with standard of care day-5 biopsy 3. Lack of randomized controlled trials to determine its efficacy and safety 4. As yet experimental

the egg or embryo being biopsied; (b) micromanipulation controls and mechanics to allow for smooth manipulation; (c) appropriate microtools; (d) a suitable workstation with dissecting microscope to handle eggs, embryos, and biopsy samples; (e) an anti-vibration surface on which to support the microscope and micromanipulator, particularly if TE biopsy is being performed; and (f) a laser system integrated into the inverted microscope (37–40).

Many IVF laboratories use an Olympus or Nikon inverted microscope with 4×, 10×, 20×, and 40× objectives. There are a number of micromanipulation systems available including the Narishige, Research Instruments, or Eppendorf. The Narishige has traditionally been the most commonly used micromanipulation set-up in IVF labs. This system consists of coarse and fine manipulators allowing for a wide range of movement, yet precise control when working at the micrometer scale with eggs and embryos. The coarse manipulator may be driven either electrically or mechanically, while the fine manipulator is hydraulically driven. The joystick allows for comfortable hand movements of the embryologist while performing laser-assisted ZP ablation or TE biopsy.

Biopsy involves a two-step process:

1. Breaching of the ZP
2. Removal of genetic material (a cell, a number of cells, or DNA fragments) to test as a representative fraction of the entire embryo

Breaching of the ZP has been achieved in a number of ways, including mechanical means, chemical means, or by means of a laser. The earliest methods used to create an opening in the ZP were performed by mechanical means of partial ZP dissection in which the egg/embryo was held in place by suction on a holding pipette and the ZP tangentially pierced through using a fine needle. The egg or embryo is then released from the holding pipette while still held on the needle and the ZP is breached by gently rubbing the holding pipette and needle together. Mechanical means of ZP breaching were subsequently replaced in most centers by chemical means using acid Tyrode's solution (pH 2.2–2.4) to dissolve the ZP glycoproteins. The embryo is held in place using a holding pipette and an "assisted hatching" pipette attached to the manipulator on the right-hand side of the set-up filled with acid Tyrode's solution and lowered into the drop close to the embryo. When positioned at an appropriate position close to the ZP but with the maximum perivitelline space between the ZP and the blastomeres, acid Tyrode's solution is released so that a localized area of the ZP is dissolved. However, the use of acid Tyrode's solution is not appropriate for breaching the ZP prior to polar body biopsy since exposure of the oocyte to acid Tyrode's solution has been shown to have an inhibitory effect on embryonic development.

The introduction of laser-assisted opening of the ZP has now largely replaced all other means of ZP breaching for EB procedures. This dramatic shift is most likely due to ease of use, speed, reproducibility, and the advent of TE biopsy, which necessitates the use of a laser to separate the cells of the TE. The laser in use in IVF labs is the near-infrared solid-state compact diode 1.48 μm laser. The most common systems in use include systems from Hamilton Thorne (ZILOS-tk® and the LYKOS®), Research Instruments (Saturn™), and MTG (OCTAX™). All of these laser systems use high-energy light and consequently heat to dissolve the targeted area of the ZP. When the laser beam comes into contact with the culture droplet, heat is dissipated through the medium, creating temperature gradients in concentric circles from the laser beam (41,42).

A laser has three different properties that determine its performance: (a) power (energy per unit time), which is measured in milliwatts (mW) and can range from <20 mW to 400 mW; (b) wavelength—all lasers used in IVF utilize near-infrared wavelengths (750–2500 nm); and (c) pulse duration, which is the length of time the laser beam is activated for. Pulse duration can range from 10 μs to >10 ms. Longer pulse durations result in increased power and consequently increased temperature gradients within the medium. To illustrate, a laser with low energy and long pulse lengths will produce greater temperature gradients than a laser with high energy and shorter pulse lengths. Since smaller temperature gradients are less risky for embryos, lasers employed in IVF should use multiple pulses of short duration in preference to long-duration pulses. Care should always be taken to ensure that the laser is used properly.

When choosing a laser system for your lab, it is advisable to review the options available to ensure the best choice in your setting. The best-known systems are the ZILOS and LYKOS from Hamilton Thorne (http://hamiltonthorne.com/index.php/products/clinical-lasers), the Saturn from Research Instruments (https://www.nikoninstruments.com/Products/Light-Sources/Saturn-5-Lasers), and the OCTAX from MTG (http://www.mtg-de.com/products_overview/#octax-lasers-imaging-systems/octax-laser-shot-navilase-laser-systems). All companies provide installation and training. Factors to consider when choosing a system include adaptability for the microscope in use, access to technical support, simplicity and ease of use, and cost. Some systems have features such as having the laser fully integrated into the objective with no additional cables or interfering wires. Others include features such as the laser beam being movable, allowing the laser to be positioned on the target rather than the target positioned in the laser beam.

ZP breaching procedure

The ZP breaching procedure may be performed on day 3, day 4, or even day 5/6 once it has been determined that the embryos will be biopsied. At our center, we routinely perform the ablation procedure on day 4. All of the embryos are assessed and each developing embryo is then subjected to ZP ablation using laser treatment. The procedure is performed on the embryos in their original culture dish and does not require the transfer of the embryos to a separate dish. The procedure employed at our lab using the Research Instruments Saturn laser is as follows:

1. The dish containing the embryos to be subjected to ZP ablation is positioned so that the drop containing the first embryo is in the center of the field of view.
2. The inner layer of the ZP is brought into focus at an area of the embryo where there is maximum perivitelline space. It is important not to subject any of the cells of the embryo to the laser energy. The desired laser settings are selected based on the size of the opening the operator desires. We currently employ a setting of a "6.4 μm" opening for ZP breaching. Breaching is conducted from the outside layer of the ZP to the inside using multiple pulses of short duration, taking care to minimize the number of pulses to confirm that the ZP is breached.
3. This procedure is repeated for each developing embryo in numerical order.
4. Following ZP breaching, the embryos are returned to the incubator to resume culture.

Day 5: Assessment for biopsy readiness and biopsy procedure

1. On day 5, all embryos are assessed and graded as per routine day-5 assessment.
2. Each embryo is assessed for readiness for TE biopsy based on its developmental stage. TE biopsy can only be performed on blastocysts showing clear differentiation of the ICM and TE cells and must be of a quality grade that is suitable for cryopreservation. For example, we grade blastocysts on a modified Gardner scale where "A" denotes excellent-quality ICM or TE, "B" denotes good-quality ICM or TE, "C" denotes moderate ICM or TE and "D" denotes non-viable cells. We require a grade C or better for both the ICM and TE cells to proceed with biopsy. Any embryo that does not meet these criteria is replaced in the incubator for re-assessment later on during day 5 and again on day 6 if necessary. Day-7 biopsy is generally not performed as the implantation potential of these embryos is significantly impaired, but consideration for day 7 biopsy is made if there are no blastocysts available for biopsy on days 5 or 6.

Biopsy dishes are prepared once it has been determined how many embryos are suitable for biopsy. Of utmost importance is embryo tracking and identification at every step of the procedure. Care must be taken to ensure that the biopsy dishes are labeled with the patient name and the number of the embryo to be biopsied. The biopsy dish is prepared with a 10 μl drop of polyvinylpyrrolidone (circled) and a 10 μl drop of buffered culture media for each embryo to be biopsied. At most, each dish will contain sufficient drops to perform biopsy on two embryos only. The drops are covered with pre-equilibrated paraffin oil.

Setting up the micromanipulator

1. Before starting biopsy, the manipulators are set so that the X, Y, and Z axes of both manipulators are at the middle ranges and have the maximum range of movement in all direction.
2. If hydraulic manipulators are being used, it is important to ensure that that oil levels in the holding syringe are at the top of the microtool holders by removing the collar and moving the oil with the syringes until it is at the top and free of bubbles.
3. The holding pipette is set up on the microtool holder and checked to ensure that the level of oil and is allowing for precise control of movement. The biopsy pipette is placed on the second tool holder. Using the 4× objective center, both microtools are brought into focus.

Once the set-up is complete, the laser objective is engaged.

TE biopsy (see Figures 13.1 through 13.3)

1. At our facility, two embryologists are required to witness any procedure involving the transfer of gametes or embryos between dishes. As such, for all biopsy procedures, one embryologist performs the biopsy procedure and a second embryologist witnesses the transfer of each individual embryo from one dish to a second dish. The second embryologist also performs the vitrification procedure of the blastocyst immediately following biopsy.
2. Avoidance of contamination is of crucial importance in any EB procedure, but is of even more importance when the analysis if for a genetic disease. To prevent contamination, all embryologists must wear personal protective equipment such as scrubs, gloves, a head cover, and a facemask. Gloves should be changed frequently and always if there is a possibility of contaminants being introduced. If a contaminating cell from another individual is inadvertently introduced, this cell may be amplified and analyzed in place of the cells from the embryo.
3. Each blastocyst is handled individually at all times. The blastocyst is placed into a HEPES-buffered medium culture drop in the biopsy dish and the bottom of the dish is labeled with the embryo number and the cryo-letter assigned to that specific embryo number.
4. The biopsy dish is placed on the heated stage of the inverted microscope and the blastocyst is brought into focus.
5. Blastocysts that are already showing expansion may have cells herniating out through the hole created during ZP breaching. If the protruding cells are TE cells, the biopsy procedure may proceed. The blastocyst is held in position so that the protruding TE cells are at the three o' clock position. The laser beam and the TE cells to be separated are aligned so that the beam will target the junctions of the TE cells to be separated. Gentle suction on the TE cells is applied and, at the same time, two to three pulses of laser beam deliver are delivered to the target area to separate the cells. Sometimes more pulses are required. It is important not to hit the same area over and over as the cells will become hardened and will not separate.

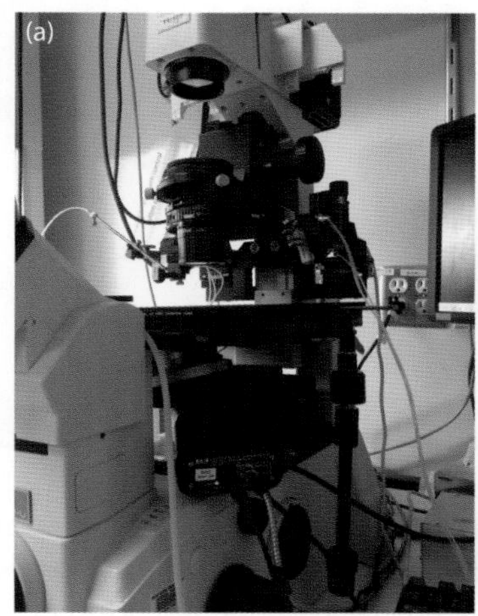

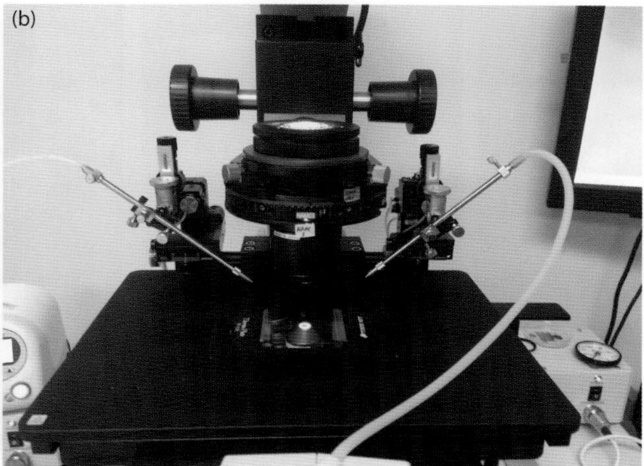

Figure 13.1 (a) Microscope fitted with Saturn laser (Research Instruments) system. (b) Microscope set-up showing laser objective in place.

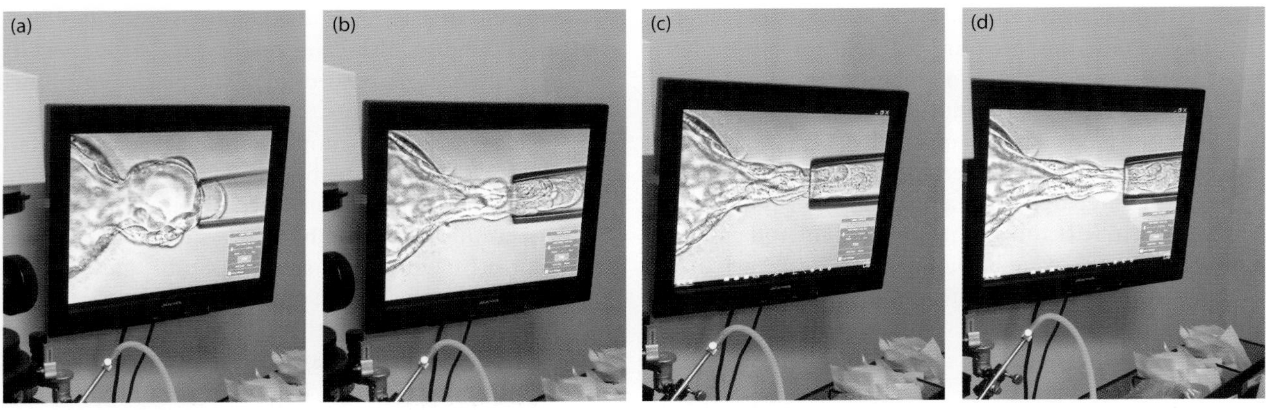

Figure 13.2 (a) Initial positioning of the biopsy pipette on the extruding trophectoderm cells. (b) Trophectoderm cells gently aspirated into the biopsy pipette and laser targeted at junctions between cells. (c) A total of 5–10 trophectoderm cells are separated from the remainder using gentle suction on the cells and laser pulses. (d) Cells are separated and aspirated into the biopsy pipette.

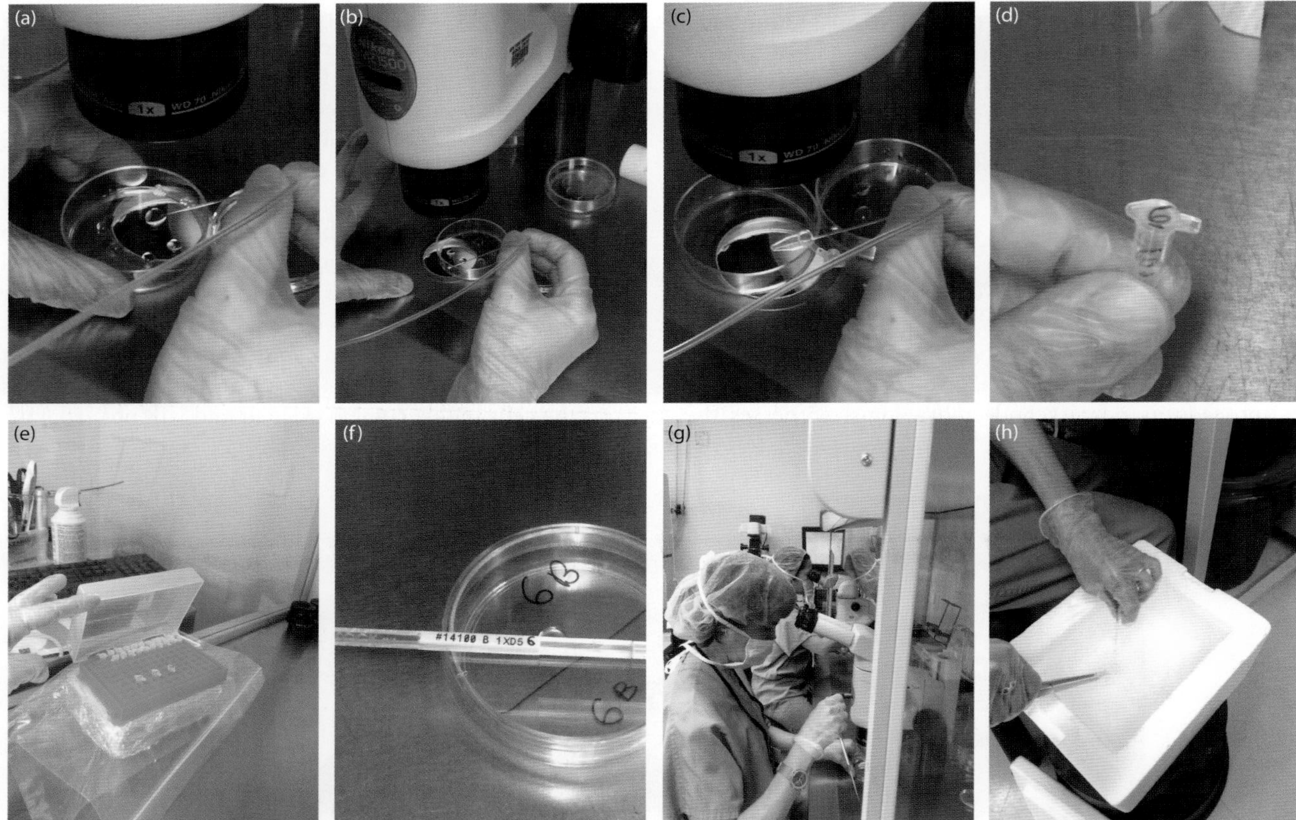

Figure 13.3 (a,b) Biopsied cells are washed through buffer drops and (c) loaded into a polymerase chain reaction (PCR) tube under the dissecting microscope. (d) The PCR tube containing the biopsied cells is clearly labeled with the embryo number on the top and side of the tube. (e) The PCR tubes containing the biopsied cells are placed in a rack for transport to the genetics lab. (f) Preparation for vitrification of the biopsied blastocyst requires accurate tracking and labeling of the cryo-device to ensure it is linked to the biopsied sample. (g) Two embryologists verify accurate tracking of every step of the procedure. (h) The biopsied blastocyst is vitrified immediately after the biopsy procedure and placed in cryostorage pending receipt of results.

The protruding cells are aspirated until separation of about five to six TE cells is achieved.

6. The cells that have been biopsied are expelled from the biopsy pipette and the blastocyst is moved to a location in the drop away from the cells.
7. Procedures provided by the genetics lab for handling the biopsied cells should be followed. These instructions usually involve washing the biopsied TE cells through several drops of non-stick wash buffer provided by the genetics lab.
8. The biopsied cells are loaded into a PCR tube that must clearly be labeled top and side with the embryo number from which the TE cells were biopsied. The cells are placed into the bottom of the PCR tube in 2.5 μl of buffer using a 100 μl pipette or stripper tip. Accurate labeling of the PCR tube is verified by two embryologists prior to placing in the provided kit. At a minimum, the kit must be clearly labeled with the patient's name, a secondary identifier such as date of birth, the genetic test type, the date of procedure, and the embryo stage.
9. Following TE biopsy, each blastocyst is individually vitrified by the second embryologist, taking extreme care to maintain embryo identification throughout all steps. This vitrification step is performed while the blastocyst remains collapsed following its biopsy procedure. The cryo-device should be appropriately labeled with patient name, date of birth, cryo-number, embryo stage, and, very importantly, embryo number. This device is again identified and verified by both embryologists working on the case. Once vitrified, the embryos are placed in cryostorage pending receipt of the genetic analyses.
10. The biopsy procedure is repeated for each suitable embryo. All documentation is verified and the biopsy samples are transported per provided instructions to the genetics lab unless analysis is to be performed in-house.
11. On day 6, all remaining embryos are reassessed for possible biopsy and any suitable embryos are biopsied at that stage.
12. For those blastocysts that are of good quality on day 6 but have not yet shown extrusion of cells through the ZP breach, TE biopsy may still be performed. In these instances, it is necessary to try to locate the existing breach in the ZP. If not possible, it may be necessary to create another breach in the ZP using the laser. Having located the opening or created a new one, the biopsy pipette is placed through the opening and gentle suction is applied to the TE in order to aspirate a few cells out of the ZP while at the same time using the laser to detach the cells from the blastocyst.

Receipt of results from the genetics laboratory

Once the genetic results are received from the laboratory, verify that all samples are reported upon and that the interpretation of the result is clear.

ACKNOWLEDGEMENTS

The authors wish to thank the following individuals for assistance in obtaining information for this chapter: Diarmaid H. Douglas-Hamilton, Chief Technical Officer, Hamilton Thorne, Inc.; Joel Lopez (Hamilton Thorne); Tim Schimmel (Embryos.net); and Dave McCulloh (NYU Fertility Center).

REFERENCES

1. Edwards R, Gardner R. Sexing of live rabbit blastocysts. *Nature* 1967; 214: 576–7.
2. Wilton L, Shaw J, Trounson A. Successful single-cell biopsy and cryopreservation of preimplantation mouse embryos. *Fertil Steril* 1989; 51(3): 513–7.
3. Coutelle C et al. Genetic analysis of DNA from single human oocytes: a model for preimplantation diagnosis of cystic fibrosis. *BMJ* 1989; 299(6690): 22–4.
4. Handyside A et al. Biopsy of human preimplantation embryos and sexing by DNA amplification. *Lancet* 1989; 333(8634): 347–9.
5. Handyside AH et al. Pregnancies from biopsied human preimplantation embryos sexed by Y-specific DNA amplification. *Nature* 1990; 344(6268): 768–70.
6. Grifo JA et al. Pregnancy after embryo biopsy and coamplification of DNA from X and Y chromosomes. *JAMA* 1992; 268(6): 727–9.
7. Summers P, Campbell J, Miller M. Normal *in-vivo* development of marmoset monkey embryos after trophectoderm biopsy. *Hum Reprod* 1988; 3(3): 389–93.
8. Verlinsky Y et al. Analysis of the first polar body: preconception genetic diagnosis. *Hum Reprod* 1990; 5(7): 826–9.
9. Montag M et al. Polar body biopsy: A viable alternative to preimplantation genetic diagnosis and screening. *Reprod Biomed Online* 2009; 18: 6–11.
10. Strom CM et al. Three births after preimplantation genetic diagnosis for cystic fibrosis with sequential first and second polar body analysis. *Am J Obstet Gynecol* 1998; 178(6): 1298–306.
11. Scott KL, Hong KH, Scott RT. Selecting the optimal time to perform biopsy for preimplantation genetic testing. *Fertil Steril* 2013; 100(3): 608–14.
12. Geraedts J et al. What next for preimplantation genetic screening? A polar body approach! *Hum Reprod* 2010; 25(3): 575–7.
13. Hammoud I et al. Are zona pellucida laser drilling and polar body biopsy safe for *in vitro* matured oocytes? *J Assist Reprod Genet* 2010; 27(7): 423–7.
14. Levin I et al. Effects of laser polar-body biopsy on embryo quality. *Fertil Steril* 2012; 97(5): 1085–8.
15. Treff NR et al. Characterization of the source of human embryonic aneuploidy using microarray-based 24 chromosome preimplantation genetic diagnosis (mPGD) and aneuploid chromosome fingerprinting. *Fertil Steril* 2008; 90: S37.

16. Northrop LE et al. SNP microarray-based 24 chromosome aneuploidy screening demonstrates that cleavage-stage FISH poorly predicts aneuploidy in embryos that develop to morphologically normal blastocysts. *Mpl Hum Reprod* 2010; 6: 590–600.
17. Capalbo A et al. Sequential comprehensive chromosome analysis on polar bodies, blastomeres and trophoblast: insight into female meiotic errors and chromosomal segregation in the preimplantation window of embryos development. *Hum Reprod* 2013; 28: 509–18.
18. Grifo JA et al. Healthy deliveries from biopsied human embryos. *Hum Reprod* 1994; 9(5): 912–6.
19. Van de Velde H et al. Embryo implantation after biopsy of one or two cells from cleavage-stage embryos with a view to preimplantation genetic diagnosis. *Prenat Diagn* 2000; 20(13): 1030–7.
20. Goossens V et al. Diagnostic efficiency, embryonic development and clinical outcome after the biopsy of one or two blastomeres for preimplantation genetic diagnosis. *Hum Reprod* 2008; 23(3): 481–92.
21. Malter HE, Cohen J. Blastocyst formation and hatching *in vitro* following zona drilling of mouse and human embryos. *Gamete Res* 1989; 24(1): 67–80.
22. Scott RT et al. Cleavage-stage biopsy significantly impairs human embryonic implantation potential while blastocyst biopsy does not: A randomized and paired clinical trial. *Fertil Steril* 2013; 100(3): 624–30.
23. De Rycke M et al. ESHRE PGD Consortium data collection XIII: Cycles from January to December 2010 with pregnancy follow-up to October 2011. *Hum Reprod* 2015; 30(8): 1763–89.
24. Mastenbroek S et al. *In vitro* fertilization with preimplantation genetic screening. *N Engl J Med* 2007; 357: 9–17.
25. Munne S et al. Chromosome mosaicism in human embryos. *Biol Reprod* 1994; 51: 373–9.
26. Dokras A et al. Trophectoderm biopsy in human blastocysts. *Hum Reprod* 1990; 5(7): 821–5.
27. Adler A et al. Blastocyst culture selects for euploid embryos: Comparison of blastomere and trophectoderm biopsies. *Reprod Biomed Online* 2014; 28(4): 485–91.
28. Demko ZP et al. Effects of maternal age on euploidy rates in a large cohort of embryos analyzed with 24-chromosome single-nucleotide polymorphism-based preimplantation genetic screening. *Fertil Steril* 2016; 105(5): 1307–13.
29. Kokkali G et al. Blastocyst biopsy versus cleavage stage biopsy and blastocyst transfer for preimplantation genetic diagnosis of β-thalassaemia: A pilot study. *Hum Reprod* 2007; 22(5): 1443–9.
30. Barcroft LC et al. Aquaporin proteins in murine trophectoderm mediate transepithelial water movements during cavitation. *Dev Biol* 2003; 256(2): 342–54.
31. Watson A, Natale D, Barcroft L. Molecular regulation of blastocyst formation. *Anim Reprod Sci* 2004; 82: 583–92.
32. D'Alessandro A et al. A mass spectrometry-based targeted metabolomics strategy of human blastocoele fluid: A promising tool in fertility research. *Mol Biosyst* 2012; 8(4): 953–8.
33. Palini S et al. Genomic DNA in human blastocoele fluid. *Reprod Biomed Online* 2013; 26(6): 603–10.
34. Gianaroli L et al. Blastocentesis: A source of DNA for preimplantation genetic testing. Results from a pilot study. *Fertil Steril* 2014; 102(6): 1692–9.e6.
35. Tobler KJ et al. Blastocoel fluid from differentiated blastocysts harbors embryonic genomic material capable of a whole-genome deoxyribonucleic acid amplification and comprehensive chromosome microarray analysis. *Fertil Steril* 2015; 104(2): 418–25.
36. Tobler K et al. The potential use of blastocoel fluid (BF) from expanded blastocysts as a less invasive form of embryo biopsy for preimplantation genetic testing. *Fertil Steril* 2014; 3(102): e183–4.
37. Tadi Y, Douglas-Hamilton DH. Laser effects in the manipulation of human eggs and embryos for *in vitro* fertilization. *Methods Cell Biol* 2007; 82: 409–31.
38. Thornhill AR, Ottolini C, Handyside AH. Human embryo biopsy procedures. In: *Textbook of Assisted Reproductive Techniques: Laboratory Perspectives*, Fourth edition, 2012; 1: 197–211.
39. Joris H. Hydraulic manipulators for ICSI. In: *Practical manual of In vitro Fertilization. Advanced Methods and Novel Devices*. 2012, pp. 329–34.
40. Montag MHM et al. Application of non-contact laser technology in assisted reproduction. *Sci Direct* 2009; 24: 57–64.
41. Douglas-Hamilton DH, Conia J. Thermal effects in laser-assisted pre-embryo zona drilling. *J Biomed Optics* 2001; 6(2): 205–13.
42. Montag M et al. Laser-assisted microdissection of the zona pellucida facilitates polar body biopsy. *Fertil Steril* 1998; 69(3): 539–42.

Assisted oocyte activation

Current understanding, practice, and future perspectives

14

JUNAID KASHIR and KARL SWANN

INTRODUCTION

A key technique in assisted reproductive technology (ART) is intracytoplasmic sperm injection (ICSI), whereby a sperm is microinjected directly into the oocyte cytosol. Predominantly used to treat male factor infertility following the failure of conventional *in vitro* fertilization (IVF), ICSI remains a successful technique that results in normal fertilization in 70% of injected oocytes. However, a noted phenomenon associated with male infertility is the failure of some oocytes to activate, with embryos failing either to protrude the second polar body or to successfully proceed past the first cell division, even following ICSI. One approach to cases of failed oocyte activation after ICSI is to stimulate the oocyte artificially. So-called artificial oocyte activation (AOA) has already been attempted in many different clinics, to varying degrees of success. Herein, we discuss oocyte activation at mammalian fertilization and relate this fundamental biological process with the clinical phenomenon of oocyte activation deficiency. We also discuss the science behind the stimuli used to induce AOA, alongside future directions for treatment.

OOCYTE ACTIVATION AND THE ROLE OF Ca^{2+} AND PHOSPHOLIPASE C ZETA

IVF involves a series of concurrent events required to ensure that the mature sperm and oocyte are able to successfully combine to produce a new individual. For competent fertilization to occur, it is essential to alleviate meiotic arrest (at the second metaphase of meiosis [MII]) of the unfertilized oocyte. The most obvious indications of such meiotic resumption are second polar body extrusion and formation of the male and female pronuclei (1). Fertilization also involves cortical granule exocytosis and the initiation of the first cell cycle (1–5). These early biochemical and morphological events in the oocyte are collectively termed "oocyte activation." It is important to appreciate that oocyte activation is a distinct and separable part of the fertilization process, in that oocyte activation can occur without sperm entry, and that sperm entry can occur without oocyte activation. It is this second scenario, where a sperm is clearly within the oocyte without the occurrence of activation events, which suggests one can induce activation via artificial means. Such methods have generally been based upon our fluctuating understanding of how the sperm causes physiological oocyte activation at fertilization.

The universal trigger for oocyte activation at fertilization in all animals studied is an increase in cytosolic concentrations of free calcium (Ca^{2+}) (6,7). Mammalian oocytes undergo a series of these Ca^{2+} transients, termed Ca^{2+} oscillations (4,5). Figure 14.1 shows the type of Ca^{2+} oscillations (also called repetitive Ca^{2+} spikes) that occur during fertilization in mouse oocytes, and are typical of the response in mammals. Ca^{2+} oscillations in mammalian oocytes are direct consequences of inositol trisphosphate (IP_3)-mediated Ca^{2+} release (5,8–12). The significance of Ca^{2+} and IP_3 in oocyte activation is illustrated by the fact that blocking Ca^{2+} transients by introducing Ca^{2+} chelators into the oocyte blocks cortical granule exocytosis and meiotic resumption (2). Blocking or down-regulating IP_3 receptors that mediate Ca^{2+} release also eliminates Ca^{2+} oscillations in fertilized mouse oocytes (13–18). Increasing Ca^{2+} concentrations within the oocyte can lead to activation of development as judged by events such as second polar body protrusion and pronuclear formation (5,19). Increases in Ca^{2+} can also be induced within oocytes by treatment with Ca^{2+} ionophores, by electroporation, or by direct Ca^{2+} microinjection. In each case, oocytes were activated, supporting parthenogenetic development to the blastocyst stage (19–21).

Transients in intracellular Ca^{2+} stimulate meiotic resumption by stimulating calmodulin-dependent protein kinase II, inactivating a protein termed Emi2, leading to loss of a maturation protein factor (MPF) composed of cyclin B1 and cyclin-dependent kinase 1. Hence, Ca^{2+} is both necessary and sufficient for sperm-induced oocyte activation, and is mechanistically linked to key events of meiotic resumption at oocyte activation. Consequently, the Ca^{2+} increases during fertilization are not just an event accompanying oocyte activation, but are the root cause of physiological activation. In mammals, Ca^{2+} transients initiate during or immediately after sperm–oocyte membrane fusion (22), suggesting that the sperm introduces a factor into the oolemma to cause Ca^{2+} release. Evidence for such a factor emerged from studies in hamsters and mice, where cytosolic sperm extract injection caused the same pattern of Ca^{2+} oscillations observed at fertilization (23). The sperm factor was eventually shown to be a protein that mediates its effects via IP_3 generation. Intriguingly, the sperm extracts themselves exhibited high phospholipase C (PLC) activity (24,25), collectively suggesting that mammalian sperm introduces a sperm-specific PLC, generating

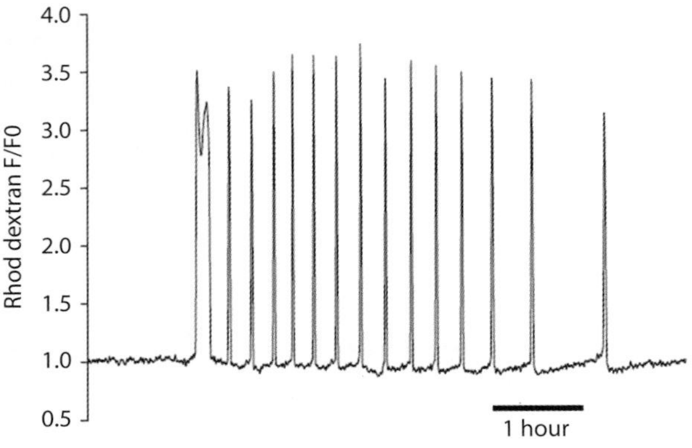

Figure 14.1 Ca^{2+} oscillations at fertilization in a mouse oocyte. The sperm was added (before the start of the trace) to an oocyte previously injected with a Ca^{2+}-sensitive dye (Rhod dextran). The Ca^{2+} increases are seen as sharp spikes in the trace as monitored by the fluorescence of Rhod dextran. The F/FO is the fluorescence divided by the resting fluorescence value. Further details on methods can be found in Saunders et al. (25) and Nomikos et al. (37).

IP_3 and Ca^{2+} release within the oocyte. The specific PLC isozyme responsible for Ca^{2+}-releasing activity in oocytes was first identified using mouse express sequence tag databases to describe a novel, testis-specific PLC, termed PLCζ, an approximately 74 kDa protein. Immunodepletion of PLCζ from soluble sperm extracts suppressed their ability to release Ca^{2+} in mouse oocytes or sea urchin egg homogenates (25). Most significantly, injection of recombinant PLCζ protein or cRNA into mouse oocytes causes Ca^{2+} oscillations that are similar in character to those observed at fertilization, supporting embryonic development to the blastocyst stage (25,26).

Quantification of PLCζ protein expressed in mouse oocytes following cRNA injection indicated that the pattern of Ca^{2+} oscillations observed corresponded to the same range as the amount of PLCζ found in a single sperm (25–35). Finally, transgenic mice with disrupted PLCζ expression in the testis through RNA interference exhibited sperm that induced prematurely ending Ca^{2+} oscillations. While these mice were not infertile, mating experiments yielded significantly reduced litter sizes (36). These data all provide very strong support for the idea that PLCζ is responsible for the Ca^{2+} oscillations that activate the oocyte at fertilization (Figures 14.1 and 14.2). This is particularly relevant as numerous studies have presented biochemical and physiological evidence to support PLCζ as the mammalian sperm factor (for more detailed reviews, see References 34,35,36).

Numerous cases of failed fertilization following the application of ART have been reported in humans, particularly following ICSI (whereby a single sperm in directly injected into the oolemma), which in turn is suggested to be due to a lack of an oocyte-activating sperm factor in many cases (39–41). Indeed, sperm involved in such cases of ICSI failure exhibit a reduced or absent capacity to cause Ca^{2+} oscillations, and are deficient with regards to PLCζ (31,42–45). Interestingly, the levels of PLCζ in sperm and the proportions of sperm exhibiting detectable PLCζ levels have recently been suggested to strongly correlate to failed fertilization following ICSI (45,46).

Whilst we have focused on the role of PLCζ in oocyte activation, it is worth noting that another protein termed post-acrosomal WW binding protein (PAWP) has been suggested to be a sperm-borne oocyte-activating factor, and has been reported to cause Ca^{2+} oscillations in mouse and human oocytes (47). However, none of the data in this paper can be reproduced (48,49). We have tried injecting mouse or human PAWP, as protein or RNA, into mouse oocytes over a wide range of concentrations and failed to detect any Ca^{2+} increases (37). Furthermore, transgenic PAWP-knockout male mice, in which the PAWP gene is deleted, produced normal sperm completely lacking PAWP. These sperm were able to generate normal Ca^{2+} oscillations and oocyte activation following ICSI and IVF (50). Consequently, it seems unlikely that sperm-derived PAWP has any role in eliciting Ca^{2+} oscillations at oocyte activation.

FAILURE OF OOCYTE ACTIVATION AFTER ICSI

ICSI, an effective method for assisting reproduction in men with suboptimal semen parameters such as abnormal sperm concentration, motility, or morphology, is a sophisticated technique involving the injection of a single sperm directly into the ooplasm via micromanipulation. Such methodology is also applied in cases experiencing low fertilization success or complete fertilization failure following conventional IVF. Following the occurrence of the first pregnancies using ICSI in the early 1990s (51), ICSI is now used to treat cases of almost any type of sperm abnormality, making it the most successful and widely used treatment for male factor infertility.

However, despite relatively high rates of ICSI success, total fertilization failure, of all oocytes collected in a cycle, still occurs in 1%–5% of all ICSI cycles. This is referred to as total fertilization failure as all oocytes collected in a cycle fail to fertilize, and can be a recurring phenomenon in subsequent cycles (52,53). It is currently estimated that total fertilization failure following ICSI would affect ~1500 cases per year in the U.K. Furthermore, considering that ICSI is now widely used in conjunction with other ART methodologies and is rapidly becoming the dominant technique used worldwide, a significant number of patients would be affected. In addition to total fertilization failure, there is a more insidious problem with fertilization after ICSI. Even in cases where the sperm and oocyte appear normal (e.g., in many cases where treatment is for tubal blockage), the success rate of fertilization is still only around 70% (54). Hence, between one in three to one in four oocytes fail to fertilize despite being injected with a sperm. This may not be a major issue when there are ~10 oocytes, but becomes a concern with lighter ovulation protocols where lower oocyte numbers are obtained, or more obviously with natural ovulation treatment cycles (55). There are many possible reasons

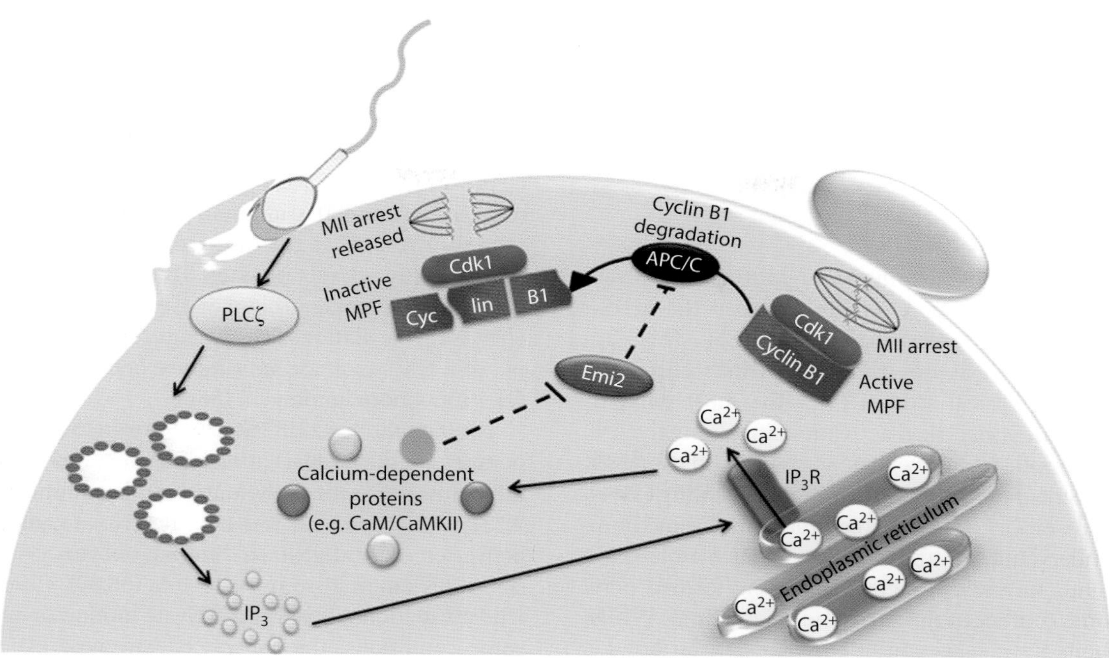

Figure 14.2 Schematic representation of the signaling mechanism downstream of Ca^{2+} release at fertilization following PLCζ release into the oolemma, leading to subsequent embryogenesis. PLCζ targets intracellular vesicle-bound phosphatidylinositol 4,5-bisphosphate (PIP_2), resulting in the generation of IP_3. IP_3 targets specific receptors on intracellular Ca^{2+} stores such as the endoplasmic reticulum, resulting in Ca^{2+} release. The alleviation of MII arrest in mammalian oocytes is thought to occur through the degradation of cyclin B1, mediated by ubiquitin/proteasome activation via Ca^{2+} oscillations. Binding of Ca^{2+} to Ca^{2+}-dependent proteins such as CaM or CAMKII, a repetitive process that reoccurs coincident with each Ca^{2+} peak in fertilized mouse oocytes, leads to cyclin B1 polyubiquitination by APC/C, an E3 ubiquitin ligase, resulting in cyclin B1 degradation. This process is prevented in unfertilized oocytes by Emi2, which assists MPF (a complex between cdk1 and cyclin B1) in maintaining MII arrest. *Abbreviations*: PLC, phospholipase C; IP_3: inositol trisphosphate; MPF, M-phase promoting factor; U, ubiquitination; CaM, calmodulin; CaMKII, calmodulin-dependent kinase II; APC/C, anaphase-promoting complex/cyclosome; CSF, cytostatic factor; MAPK, mitogen-associated protein kinase; MII, metaphase II.

underlying failed fertilization, including failed sperm head decondensation, premature sperm chromatin condensation, oocyte spindle defects, and sperm aster defects (41,56). It is also possible to have the incorrect injection or expulsion of sperm, or low gamete quality (57,58). However, such factors are only considered to be causative in a minority of cases, with a failure of the oocyte activation mechanism considered the main contributory factor (39,41,52,59–61).

Ooplasmic component defects may also contribute to failed activation at fertilization (62,63). Indeed, human oocytes ovulated for ART purposes occasionally exhibit a significant lack of cytoplasmic maturity, despite synchrony in nuclear maturity (64). Apart from meiotic progression failure, sperm centrosomal dysfunction and a concomitant lack of sperm aster formation may also lead to pronuclear arrest of human zygotes (65,66,67). However, while such cases are considered clinically as failed fertilization after ICSI, these should be distinguished from activation failure and MII arrest. Moreover, while some ooplasmic factors may represent occasional causative factors behind oocyte activation deficiency, they may only represent a minority of cases, as defects in such basic parameters as protein synthesis or metabolism would probably render an oocyte incapable of maturing to the MII-arrested stage. It seems to us more likely that sperm-related defects are the main causative factors behind oocyte activation deficiency (41,68), as factors required by the sperm to activate the oocyte, such as PLCζ, do not seem essential for basic sperm function. In fact, PLCζ may need to be held inactive in the sperm prior to fertilization (38).

The mouse oocyte activation test (MOAT) was first used to examine the activation capacity of morphologically abnormal sperm, or sperm from patients experiencing recurrent failed ICSI, examining the ability of such sperm to cause pronuclear protrusion and early cell division (42,61,69–72). This test involves injecting patient sperm into mouse oocytes, in what is effectively a bioassay of the activation function of the sperm. Alongside previous indications of failed activation in human oocytes, such studies have shown that sperm that fails in clinical procedures is often poor in ability to activate mouse oocytes. Intriguingly, even morphologically normal sperm from several patients fails to activate mouse oocytes (42,61), indicating that perhaps such a phenomenon relates to the molecular players involved in Ca^{2+} release at oocyte activation. Indeed, examination of the Ca^{2+} oscillation profiles elicited by mouse oocytes following infertile human sperm injection indicated a lack of Ca^{2+} oscillatory ability of such sperm in mouse oocytes (31,42). Intriguingly, artificial mechanisms of causing Ca^{2+} transients through AOA were able to "rescue" such cases, indicating that the underlying mechanism behind ICSI failure in the majority of cases relates to a defect in Ca^{2+} oscillatory ability.

AOA USING PHYSICAL STIMULI

At present, cases of ICSI failure are routinely resolved in the clinic through AOA, which involves the artificial induction of Ca^{2+} release following ICSI. This can be achieved through a wide range of various chemical, mechanical, or physical stimuli (73). The most popular physical stimulus is electrical activation, involving the use of a directly applied high voltage across the lipid bilayer proteins that form pores in the membrane, enabling extracellular influx of Ca^{2+} into the oolemma from the medium (74–77). Understandably, the efficiency of such a methodology depends on various factors including formed pore size and ionic content of the surrounding medium. While such methods have successfully been applied on bovine and human oocytes (75,78), these procedures may induce reactive oxygen species within oocytes (79). Furthermore, a single electroporation pulse will only induce a single Ca^{2+} transient, with Ca^{2+} levels returning to basal limits without the induction of oscillations (3). Some studies in mouse and rabbit oocytes have used multiple electrical pulses to generate a series of Ca^{2+} increases that can mimic those seen at fertilization (21,80). However, such protocols require specialist equipment to allow rapid washing of oocytes after electrical stimulation to ensure their survival. Such specialized equipment is not readily available for either clinics, or even most research laboratories.

Another physical method of activation is the so-called "mechanical activation" of oocytes, relying on the principle of oolemma piercing using micromanipulations to elicit a Ca^{2+} influx, following which ICSI is performed (68,81). This method of AOA includes the manual disruption of the plasma membrane, followed by vigorous cytoplasmic aspiration using a modified ICSI procedure (70,82), increasing oocyte Ca^{2+} load during injection and leading to higher fertilization rates. Such a methodology has also been suggested to establish closer contact of the injected sperm with oocyte intracellular Ca^{2+} stores, enabling a more rapid diffusion of the physiological signaling pathway (83). These ideas have no real support, and it is more likely that mechanical damage of internal organelles leads to Ca^{2+} leakage. Another related physical method for mechanical oocyte activation is the direct microinjection of Ca^{2+} into the oocyte (61,68). However, all these mechanical methods are likely to be difficult to standardize, and as with most other physical methods they will only induce a single Ca^{2+} increase (41).

OOCYTE ACTIVATION WITH Ca^{2+} IONOPHORES

Ca^{2+} ionophores are usually lipid-soluble molecules that transport Ca^{2+} across cell membranes by increasing Ca^{2+} permeability. They can cause extracellular Ca^{2+} influx and also act on intracellular Ca^{2+} stores to release stored Ca^{2+} (84,85). Such agents have been shown to activate oocytes from all animals examined in studies dating back to the 1970s. Examples of well-used Ca^{2+} ionophores include ionomycin and A23187 (Figure 14.3). Ionomycin is the most specific Ca^{2+} ionophore and has value for some experimental studies in that it is non-fluorescent. However, A23187 is the most commonly used ionophore to artificially activate oocytes. These agents both result in a similar and single prolonged Ca^{2+} rise, and they do not elicit Ca^{2+} oscillations (41,85). Figure 14.4 shows an example of a Ca^{2+} increase in a mouse oocyte exposed to the Ca^{2+} ionophore ionomycin (86).

The ionophore A23187 was first shown to activate human oocytes in the 1990s with activation rates of 50%–60% (87). However, some subsequent studies found that either A23187 or ionomycin was not effective at causing oocyte activation in unfertilized human oocytes, with activation rates ranging from 0% to 16% (88,89). Consequently, whilst Ca^{2+} ionophores can activate human oocytes under some conditions, the general effectiveness of ionomycin or A23187 in activating "unfertilized" human oocytes is unclear. In fact, those working on animal oocytes do not generally use ionophores alone to induce oocyte activation. Instead, most such studies use agents that cause Ca^{2+} oscillations, or else a combination of an ionophore and another chemicals agent that we discuss later (3,90).

Despite inconsistencies in their effectiveness, there is little doubt that ionophores such as A23187 can cause a large intracellular Ca^{2+} increase and are also relatively simple to apply to oocytes. Thus, it is perhaps unsurprising to find that the earliest attempts at promoting oocyte activation after failed fertilization used such ionophores. One of the first reports on ICSI couples characterized by poor fertilization rates utilized Ca^{2+} ionophore treatment post-ICSI and resulted in moderate proportions of zygote formation (83). A subsequent report involving patients with a history of inconsistent fertilization due to severe sperm morphological abnormalities used ionomycin to enhance fertilization, but failed to generate good-quality embryos (91). Separate studies examining cases of sperm defects and failed fertilization used oocytes that were treated with $CaCl_2$ injection concurrent with ICSI, followed by sequential Ca^{2+} ionophore treatments. These showed increased fertilization rates and clinical pregnancies and births (61,68,92,93). Numerous case reports now exist demonstrating that ICSI combined with AOA greatly increases fertilization and subsequent pregnancy rates (43,61,70–72,94–97).

Collectively, such studies may indicate that fertilization and pregnancy rates following AOA are markedly improved in cases of previous fertilization failure (41). However, this is not necessarily true across the board for such patients, with many AOA studies indicating either small or no marked improvements in fertilization and pregnancy rates (68,98). Indeed, this corresponds with observations that sperm defective in morphology, motility, and overall concentration are at a significantly greater

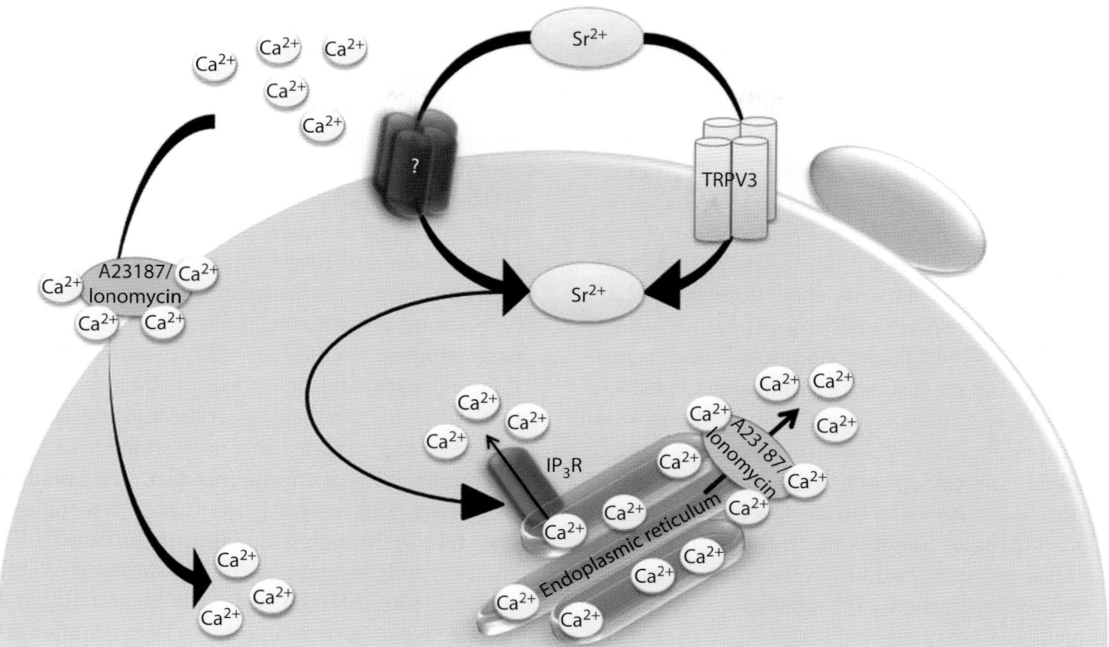

Figure 14.3 Schematic representation of metaphase II arrest alleviation in mammalian oocytes mediated via Ca^{2+} ionophores. Agents such as A23187 or ionomycin exert effect by facilitating transport of Ca^{2+} across membranes. This may include transport of extracellular Ca^{2+} into the oolemma or by facilitating Ca^{2+} transport across membranes of intracellular Ca^{2+} stores such as the endoplasmic reticulum. Sr^{2+} acts by entering the oocyte via membrane channels such as TRPV3 alongside and potentially via other channels. Sr^{2+} is currently considered to subsequently modulate inositol trisphosphate receptors on intracellular Ca^{2+} stores such as the endoplasmic reticulum, modulating Ca^{2+} release.

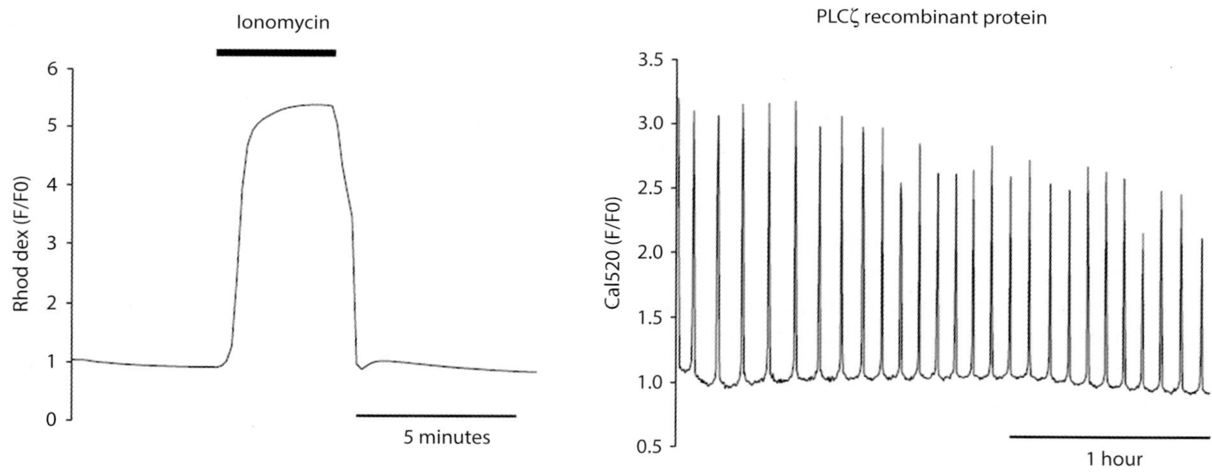

Figure 14.4 Artificially induced Ca^{2+} transients in mouse oocytes. Mouse oocytes were loaded with Ca^{2+}-sensitive dyes (Rhod dextran or Cal520) and fluorescence was plotted against time (F/F0 is fluorescence divided by resting fluorescence) as a measure of intracellular Ca^{2+} levels. In the left-hand panel, oocytes were exposed to 5 μM ionomycin for the period of time indicated by the bar. In the right-hand panel, the oocytes were microinjected with NusA–PLCζ recombinant protein just prior to the start of the recording. Please note the different timescales. Further details can be found in Sanusi et al. (86). *Abbreviation*: PLC, phospholipase C.

risk of oocyte activation deficiency comparative to normozoospermic sperm (41). One such sperm defect is that of globozoospermia, a condition affecting 0.1% of nfertile men in which acrosome formation is abnormal (56).

Sermondade et al. (99) recently demonstrated a successful pregnancy and birth in the absence of AOA using sperm from a globozoospermic male exhibiting an acrosomal bud using motile sperm organelle morphology evaluation

(MSOME), a technique for classifying sperm morphology at high magnification. Furthermore, Vanden Meerschaut et al. (100) indicated that AOA may not be beneficial for all patients experiencing oocyte activation deficiency, with fertilization history and sperm parameters seemingly playing an important role (68,100,101). Furthermore, Vanden Meerschaut et al. (101) recently applied the MOAT to study the Ca^{2+} responses of sperm from a wide range of ICSI patients, and indicated that not only do sperm from various groups of ICSI-failed patients elicit differential Ca^{2+} responses, but also that sperm cells from the same patient possess differential Ca^{2+} oscillatory abilities. Thus, it is prudent to say that it is not yet clear what group of patients AOA would be most likely to benefit, apart from severe cases of oocyte activation deficiency, without further clinical investigations. Indeed, current opinion with regards to this is split within the literature. A recent prospective multicenter study concluded that Ca^{2+} ionophore treatment successfully increased clinical pregnancy and live birth rates in patients with low or failed fertilization (102). However, a systematic review and meta-analysis suggested that ICSI-AOA may not significantly improve fertilization rates in such patients (103).

In the published literature, reported fertilization and pregnancy rates following AOA are highly variable, most likely due to the heterogenic and low number of patients recruited in the vast majority of studies. Furthermore, differences in patient baseline characteristics coupled with the fact that different activating agents have been used make it hard to compare different reports (85,101). Remarkably, even AOA protocols used throughout the published literature diverge in the ionophore concentration used, duration of ionophore exposure, time of ionophore exposure following ICSI, and number of ionophore exposures (85). Thus, it appears likely that while AOA is a significantly effective method with which to resolve cases of extreme oocyte activation deficiency, current AOA protocols may not necessarily be effective for all groups of patients. Indeed, Ebner et al. (102) suggested that success following ionophore treatment is related to fertilization rates in previous cycles, with AOA presenting with the best results in patients with a history of less than 30% fertilization in a previous ICSI cycle and with earlier studies providing a similar outlook (100,102).

It should be noted that ionophore use post-ICSI may not result in the same response in oocytes as when ionophore is applied to an "unfertilized" oocyte that has not been injected with a sperm. Studies injecting human sperm into mouse oocytes suggest that sperm from both fertile control men, as well as from men with poor ICSI outcomes, exhibit a wide variation in Ca^{2+} oscillatory ability. This implies that some sperm may contain a small amount of PLCζ, and that many cases of failed fertilization after ICSI may have occurred following sperm delivery of some PLCζ to the oocyte, but not enough to activate it. In these cases, the addition of Ca^{2+} ionophore may effectively enhance the activity of the suboptimal PLCζ already in the oocyte. In fact, addition of A23187 to some human oocytes that failed to activate after ICSI resulted in small high-frequency Ca^{2+} oscillations (104). Although these oscillations did not resemble those seen at normal fertilization, they do suggest a synergy between Ca^{2+} and small amounts of PLCζ, which is consistent with the Ca^{2+}-sensitive IP_3 production observed with PLCζ in biochemical assays (28).

OTHER CHEMICAL MEANS OF OOCYTE ACTIVATION

One of the few chemical agents reported to produce oscillations instead of single transients is strontium-containing medium (Sr^{2+}). Sr^{2+} treatment of mouse oocytes leads to Ca^{2+} oscillations, accompanied by oocyte activation and efficient parthenogenesis (105,106). Sr^{2+} is widely used to activate mouse oocytes and rat oocytes, and has proved more effective at causing parthenogenetic activation than other Ca^{2+} ionophores. It is also a relatively simple matter to incubate oocytes in Sr^{2+}-containing (but Ca^{2+}-free) media for one or two hours. Figure 14.3 shows that Sr^{2+} is thought to cause Ca^{2+} release through stimulating the oocyte IP_3R1 receptors and Sr^{2+} probably gains entry into the oocyte via the TRPV3 channel (15,16,107). Early reports suggested that Sr^{2+} might be effective at activating human oocytes after failed fertilization in ICSI (108). However, such studies lacked control groups, making it unclear whether Sr^{2+} was effective. There have been no further reports of the use of Sr^{2+} for activating human oocytes, which is surprising given the simplicity of the protocols. We have tried using Sr^{2+} to activate human oocytes using the same protocols and media that work highly effectively in mouse oocytes (109), but were unable to observe any Ca^{2+} oscillations or indication of oocyte activation. This lack of effect has been observed in two different laboratories using oocytes from separate clinics. Such lack of effect may not be specific to human oocytes since there are no reports of Sr^{2+} media causing Ca^{2+} oscillations in oocytes of domestic animals (cows, pigs, and sheep). The reasons underlying Sr^{2+} effectiveness in rodent oocytes but not those of other species are unclear, but it could involve influx mechanisms. All mammalian oocytes express the same type 1 IP_3 receptor, so there is no intrinsic reason why Sr^{2+} could not trigger Ca^{2+} release in all oocytes. However, the Ca^{2+} influx and hence Sr^{2+} influx pathways may vary between oocyte species (110), potentially causing Sr^{2+} entry to be less effective in human oocytes.

Some other activating agents that have been reported to cause monotonic or oscillatory Ca^{2+} increases in mammalian oocytes include 7% ethanol, phorbol esters, or thimerosal (3,111–113). Phorbol esters or ethanol have not proved to be effective in human oocyte activation (88). Thimerosal does trigger Ca^{2+} oscillations in human oocytes, probably by stimulating $InsP_3$ receptors (114), but it is a sulfhydryl reagent and is probably not suitable for triggering embryo development since it is non-specific. However, it has been used in an activation protocol in pig oocytes where it is applied first and then a reducing agent such as dithiothreitol is added to reverse thimerosal's effects (115). While this allows for subsequent development, the addition of reducing agents is applied just 10 minutes following thimerosal, stopping Ca^{2+} release, resulting in only one large Ca^{2+} transient rather than oscillations (113,115).

Alternative AOA approaches have also been suggested by incubation of oocytes with inhibitors to reduce the level of MPF as opposed to eliciting Ca^{2+} transients in the oolemma (Figure 14.5). Such examples include protein synthesis or kinase inhibitors such as puromycin or 6-dimethylaminopurine that block the synthesis of cyclin B or inhibit CDK1 activity, respectively (116). Another approach involves incubation of oocytes with N,N,N′,N′-tetrakis(2-pyridylmethyl)ethane-1,2-diamine, a chemical that targets zinc ions (Zn^{2+}) required for Emi2 activity, which inhibits destruction of cylcin B and hence MPF activity (117,118). However, such inhibitors are generally not very specific towards MPF, and although they do result in MPF degradation, they may also impact upon downstream signaling pathways. Furthermore, the highest rates of efficiency seem to be reached in conjunction with other methods of AOA. In fact, standard protocols for oocyte activation in domestic animals, particularly after nuclear transfer for cloning experiments, is to use a combination of Ca^{2+} ionophore followed by either a protein synthesis inhibitor or a protein kinases inhibitor (90,116). This double treatment protocol is more effective than ionophore alone and is thought to work by providing a Ca^{2+} stimulus to initiate a decrease in MPF activity, and then keeping MPF activity low by inhibiting either its protein kinase activity or by stopping the re-synthesis of cyclin B (119). Puromycin, a similar chemical agent, is able to activate human oocytes (88,120), but has not been used as a clinical treatment, possibly due to a high proportion of second polar body retention in human oocytes (121). Studies in cattle have also shown that activation protocols based on ionophore and protein synthesis or kinase inhibitors increase the rates of aneuploidy compared to IVF (90).

SAFETY OF AOA

Collectively, it is apparent that the advent of technologies such as ICSI combined with AOA has given much hope for the treatment of specific groups of patients presenting with severe forms of oocyte activation deficiency, particularly those with sperm abnormalities such as globozoospermia or oligoasthenozoospermia (41). However, despite such assertions, concerns have been raised with regards to the clinical safety of AOA use.

One concern is the non-physiological manner in which Ca^{2+} transients are induced within the oocyte. As previously detailed, mammalian oocyte activation involves a concerted profile of Ca^{2+} oscillations, with characteristic frequencies and amplitudes of each transient (38), released in an IP_3-dependant manner. The main issue with most clinically used Ca^{2+} ionophores is that these agents cause a single large transient. Several studies in animals demonstrated that the number and amplitude of Ca^{2+} transients not only affect activation efficiency, but can also influence subsequent embryonic development (80,122,123), blastocyst quality (124), and the implantation potential of rabbit parthenogenotes (125) and mouse zygotes (80), resulting in altered embryonic gene expression (80). Nevertheless, some of these studies demonstrating post-implantation effects have involved extreme differences in Ca^{2+} pulses, comparing zygotes that underwent two to three sperm-induced Ca^{2+} transients versus ones that received an

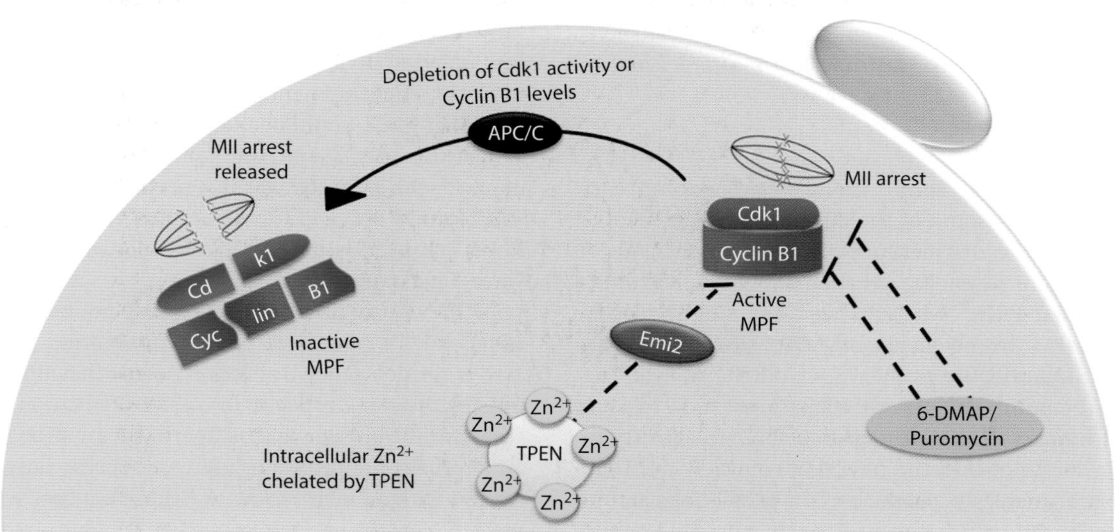

Figure 14.5 Schematic representation of MII arrest alleviation in mammalian oocytes mediated via chemical agents that do not induce Ca^{2+} release. Agents such as 6-DMAP or puromycin act by inhibiting either cdk1 activity or replenishing cyclin B1 levels in the MII-arrested oocyte. Such action results in increased instability of MPF, resulting in sufficient progression of MII. On the other hand, TPEN is an intracellular Zn^{2+} chelator that exerts effect by sequestering Zn^{2+} away from Emi2, which requires Zn^{2+} for its activity. Such chelation results in the inability of Emi2 to prevent cyclin B1 degradation, resulting in alleviation of MII arrest. *Abbreviations*: 6-DMAP, 6-dimethylaminopurine; APC/C, anaphase-promoting complex/cyclosome; MII, metaphase II; MPF, maturation protein factor; TPEN, N,N,N′,N′-tetrakis(2-pyridylmethyl)ethane-1,2-diamine.

additional 20 large electric field-induced Ca^{2+} transients (80). This is a more dramatic difference than with ionophore use. In fact, controlled studies in mice have suggested that ionomycin treatment does not have any clear detrimental effect. For example, mouse zygotes treated with ionomycin shortly after fertilization exhibited normal pre- and post-implantation development, resulting in normal development of fertile pups (126). A subsequent report showed no adverse effects following the application of ionomycin, electrical pulses, or Sr^{2+} in an activation-deficient mouse model, resulting in normal development and fertile pups (101). These data suggest that the Ca^{2+} increase provided by ionophore does not have any clear detrimental effects upon later development.

More recent studies have also been performed in an attempt to examine the potential effects of AOA upon resultant children. Vanden Meerschaut et al. (77) examined 21 children aged 3–10 years born following ICSI combined with AOA, looking at the obstetric, neonatal, neurodevelopmental, and behavioral outcomes of such children, and did not observe any serious adverse effects. Similar observations have also been reported, albeit as posters at scientific meetings, with no observable differences in developmental characteristics in babies born as a result of treatment with or without AOA, also showing that AOA did not seemingly adversely affect the growth or health of babies (127–129). A further study reported no significant alteration in the language development capacity of children born as a result of ICSI-AOA as indicated by general language scores (130), suggesting that development of cognitive abilities remain comparable to normal conception. However, the sample sizes of these studies were quite small, ranging from 10–25 children being examined. Thus, it would be helpful to repeat such studies in larger cohorts in order to obtain definitive conclusions.

FUTURE PROSPECTS

Considering concerns about the effectiveness or the long-term effects of some of the current AOA protocols, it is prudent to consider methods of AOA that elicit Ca^{2+} release in a more physiological manner. Thus, it would make sense that PLCζ is targeted as a potential replacement for most current agents of AOA, since a lack of PLCζ may underlie the problems of oocyte activation. An increasing number of clinical reports have now linked defects in human PLCζ with cases of oocyte activation deficiency. Sperm of infertile men that routinely fail IVF and ICSI are unable to produce Ca^{2+} oscillations upon microinjection into mouse oocytes, or they produce those that are uncharacteristic of oscillations observed from microinjection of sperm from fertile men, being reduced in both frequency and amplitude (31,42). Importantly, immunofluorescence and immunoblot analysis indicated that sperm from such ICSI-failed patients exhibited reduced/absent levels of PLCζ within the sperm head (31,42,44). Identification of mutations from an ICSI-failed patient indicates that PLCζ may be contributing not only to male infertility, but also perhaps cases of male subfertility (42,131). Furthermore, Yelumalai et al. (46) suggested that levels of PLCζ in sperm and the proportion of sperm exhibiting detectable PLCζ positively correlated with ICSI success rates. Thus, the clinical potential of PLCζ is apparent, both as a therapeutic intervention and as a prognostic indicator of oocyte activation deficiency.

Yoon et al. (31) demonstrated that abnormalities in sperm PLCζ could be counteracted by co-injection with mouse PLCζ mRNA, while Rogers et al. (109) showed the parthenogenetic generation of blastocysts by injection of PLCζ cRNA into human oocytes. However, the therapeutic use of PLCζ cRNA is not likely, as the amount of PLCζ expression is variable in human oocytes, with overexpression being detrimental to preimplantation development (109,132). Injecting RNA can also be considered to be introducing genetic material into the oocyte. Consequently, the use a purified and enzymatically active recombinant form of PLCζ is likely to be effective and acceptable. Significantly, Nomikos et al. (133) were able to demonstrate the production of stable, purified recombinant human PLCζ protein that can induce Ca^{2+} oscillations within a physiological range. This study also demonstrated that deleterious effects of mutant PLCζ may be efficiently overcome by utilization of purified recombinant PLCζ protein. Figure 14.4 shows an example of a mouse oocyte injected with recombinant PLCζ and it can be seen that it triggers a prolonged series of Ca^{2+} oscillations.

A recent study utilizing a mouse model of ICSI failure, which used gentle heat treatment to inactivate the ability of sperm to cause Ca^{2+} oscillations, found that recombinant PLCζ injection after ICSI failure was able to recuse embryo development to the blastocyst stage (86). The same study also found that if PLCζ protein was injected into oocytes after ICSI, with normal sperm this also lead to normal development to the blastocyst stage. This suggests that PLCζ could be injected in a way that can rescue activation defects and yet not inhibit normal development if such a rescue was not needed because the sperm still retained some PLCζ (86). However, further studies of PLCζ may be advisable in a clinical setting before its widespread use in fertility clinics.

As previously discussed, AOA may not be entirely beneficial for all groups of patients presenting with oocyte activation deficiency. Indeed, it seems that not all sperm possess the same capacity for oocyte activation, or not all cases would present with a sperm factor problem. Thus, an alternative approach to increase success rates for cases treated with AOA is to identify those patients who would most benefit from such protocols. To that extent, PLCζ may represent a powerful biomarker with which to examine sperm functional competency (131,134,135). Indeed, Kashir et al. (136) examined the effects of cryopreservation upon sperm PLCζ from fertile males, showing that cryopreservation led to a decrease in total levels of PLCζ in such sperm. A further study utilizing PLCζ as a biomarker indicated that the MSOME methodology, relying on high-powered magnification analysis of human sperm before a modified version of ICSI is applied (intracytoplasmic morphologically selected sperm injection), may select sperm with higher total levels of PLCζ, as well as selecting a higher proportion of sperm exhibiting the presence of PLCζ (135).

A diagnostic test based on human sperm microinjection into mouse oocytes (known as the MOAT) has previously been developed as a heterologous model to evaluate the activation capacity of human sperm (41,61,69,71). However, considering that human PLCζ is thought to be more potent in its activity compared to mouse PLCζ (9), the MOAT may only detect extreme cases of PLCζ deficiency, where PLCζ is completely absent from sperm, and not where a more subtle reduction is present in a clinical setting. Coupled with animal facility requirements and specialized equipment and skills, the MOAT may not be considered a viable diagnostic assessment of oocyte activation capability (41). Indeed, the MOAT perhaps represents a procedure to identify the most probable underlying reason for low or failed fertilization following ICSI (101), and may thus represent a more of a specialized research tool. Perhaps a more attractive option is direct examination of sperm PLCζ. Indeed, previous immunofluorescence studies of human sperm have demonstrated a pattern of PLCζ localization in the sperm head that is consistent with fertile sperm (42,137), with abnormal patterns being evident in ICSI-failed sperm (31,42,44).

CONCLUSIONS

Oocyte activation is a fundamental component of mammalian fertilization and determines the efficacy of subsequent elements of early embryogenesis. It is therefore prudent to suggest that alterations or aberrations in this process may profoundly influence the new embryo following already-invasive procedures such as ART use. Indeed, reports increasingly suggest that alterations or aberrations experienced by embryos during the initial phases of development correlate with an amplified risk of chronic disease, including obesity, diabetes, and cardiovascular disease (77,138). Considering such alarming implications, it is only common sense that ART should move towards minimal impact, but also that further technologies such as AOA should follow in line with such shifts.

It is evident that the current AOA protocols need continued monitoring to establish whether the non-physiological manner of elicited Ca^{2+} increases is effective as well as having any longer-term effects upon the developing embryo and subsequent progeny. This is not to say that such treatment should be stopped outright. Indeed, the studies published thus far attempting to examine any obvious changes in offspring resultant from AOA seem encouraging, and it would not be prudent to dash all hopes of the groups of patients who stand to benefit from such treatment. Nevertheless, we suggest that alternative methods of AOA that mimic physiological patterns of Ca^{2+} oscillation events should be considered the priority. It seems likely to us that agents mimicking the sperm's ability to cause Ca^{2+} oscillations will prove to be both more effective and reliable than current activation protocols (17,139–198).

REFERENCES

1. Miyazaki S, Ito M. Calcium signals for egg activation in mammals. *J Pharmacol Sci* 2006; 100: 545–52.
2. Kline D, Kline JT. Repetitive calcium transients and the role of calcium in exocytosis and cell cycle activation in the mouse egg. *Dev Biol* 1992; 149: 80–9.
3. Swann K, Ozil JP. Dynamics of the calcium signal that triggers mammalian egg activation. *Int Rev Cytol* 1994; 152: 183–222.
4. Publicover S, Harper CV, Barratt C. $[Ca^{2+}]_i$ signalling in sperm—Making the most of what you've got. *Nat Cell Biol* 2007; 9: 235–42.
5. Swann K, Yu Y. The dynamics of calcium oscillations that activate mammalian eggs. *Int J Dev Biol* 2008; 52: 585–94.
6. Stricker SA. Comparative biology of calcium signalling during fertilisation and egg activation in mammals. *Dev Biol* 1999; 211: 157–76.
7. Horner VL, Wolfner MF. Transitioning from egg to embryo: Triggers and mechanisms of egg activation. *Dev Dyn* 2008; 237: 527–44.
8. Parrington J. Does a soluble sperm factor trigger calcium release in the egg at fertilization? *J Androl* 2001; 22: 1–11.
9. Swann K, Saunders CM, Rogers NT, Lai FA. PLCzeta (zeta): A sperm protein that triggers Ca^{2+} oscillations and egg activation in mammals. *Semin Cell Dev Biol* 2006; 17: 264–73.
10. Whitaker M. Calcium at fertilization and in early development. *Physiol Rev* 2006; 86: 25–88.
11. Saunders CM, Swann K, Lai FA. PLC zeta, a sperm-specific PLC and its potential role in fertilization. *Biochem Soc Symp* 2007; 74: 23–36.
12. Parrington J, Davis LC, Galione A, Wessel G. Flipping the switch: How a sperm activates the egg at fertilization. *Dev Dyn* 2007; 236: 2027–38.
13. Miyazaki S, Yuzaki M, Nakada K, Shirakawa H, Nakanishi S, Nakade S, Mikoshiba K. Block of Ca^{2+} wave and Ca^{2+} oscillation by antibody to the inositol 1,4,5-trisphosphate receptor in fertilized hamster eggs. *Science* 1992; 257: 251–5.
14. Miyazaki S, Shirakawa H, Nakada K, Honda Y. Essential role of the inositol 1,4,5-trisphosphate receptor/Ca^{2+} release channel in Ca^{2+} waves and Ca^{2+} oscillations at fertilization of mammalian eggs. *Dev Biol* 1993; 158: 62–78.
15. Brind S, Swann K, Carroll J. Inositol 1,4,5-trisphosphate receptors are downregulated in mouse oocytes in response to sperm or adenophostin A but not to increases in intracellular Ca^{2+} or egg activation. *Dev Biol* 2000; 223: 251–65.
16. Jellerette T, He CL, Wu H, Parys JB, Fissore RA. Down-regulation of the inositol 1,4,5-trisphosphate receptor in mouse eggs following fertilization or parthenogenetic activation. *Dev Biol* 2000; 223: 238–50.

17. Xu Z, Williams CJ, Kopf GS, Schutlz RM. Maturation-associated increase in IP3 receptor type 1: Role in conferring increased IP3 sensitivity and Ca^{2+} oscillatory behavior in mouse eggs. *Dev Biol* 2003; 254: 163–71.
18. Swann K. Ca^{2+} oscillations and sensitization of Ca^{2+} release in unfertilized mouse eggs injected with a sperm factor. *Cell Calcium* 1994; 15: 331–339.
19. Fulton BP, Whittingham DG. Activation of mammalian oocytes by intracellular injection of calcium. *Nature* 1978; 273: 149–51.
20. Steinhardt RA, Epel D. Activation of sea-urchin eggs by a calcium ionophore. *Proc Natl Acad Sci USA* 1974; 71: 1915–9.
21. Ozil JP. The parthenogenetic development of rabbit oocytes after repetitive pulsatile electrical stimulation. *Development* 1990; 109: 117–27.
22. Lawrence Y, Whitaker M, Swann K. Sperm-egg fusion is the prelude to the initial Ca^{2+} increase at fertilization in the mouse. *Development* 1997; 124: 233–41.
23. Swann K. A cytosolic sperm factor stimulates repetitive calcium increases and mimics fertilization in hamster eggs. *Development* 1990; 110: 1295–302.
24. Jones KT, Matsuda M, Parrington J, Katan M, Swann K. Different Ca^{2+}-releasing abilities of sperm extracts compared with tissue extracts and phospholipase C isoforms in sea urchin egg homogenate and mouse eggs. *Biochem J* 2000; 346(Pt 3): 743–9.
25. Saunders CM, Larman MG, Parrington J, Cox LJ, Royse J, Blayney LM, Swann K, Lai FA. PLC zeta: A sperm-specific trigger of Ca^{2+} oscillations in eggs and embryo development. *Development* 2002; 129: 3533–44.
26. Kouchi Z, Fukami K, Shikano T, Oda S, Nakamura Y, Takenawa T, Miyazaki S. Recombinant phospholipase Czeta has high Ca^{2+} sensitivity and induces Ca^{2+} oscillations in mouse eggs. *J Biol Chem* 2004; 279: 10408–12.
27. Cox LJ, Larman MG, Saunders CM, Hashimoto K, Swann K, Lai FA. Sperm phospholipase C zeta from humans and cynomolgus monkeys triggers Ca^{2+} oscillations, activation and development of mouse oocytes. *Reproduction* 2002; 124: 611–23.
28. Nomikos M, Blayney LM, Larman MG, Campbell K, Rossbach A, Saunders CM, Swann K, Lai FA. Role of phospholipase C-zeta domains in Ca^{2+}-dependent phosphatidylinositol 4,5-bisphosphate hydrolysis and cytoplasmic Ca^{2+} oscillations. *J Biol Chem* 2005; 280: 31011–8.
29. Yoneda A, Kashima M, Yoshida S, Terada K, Nakagawa S, Sakamoto A, Hayakawa K, Suzuki K, Ueda J, Watanabe T. Molecular cloning, testicular postnatal expression, and oocyte-activating potential of porcine phospholipase C zeta. *Reproduction* 2006; 132: 393–401.
30. Suh PG, Park JI, Manzoli L, Cocco L, Peak JC, Katan M, Fukami K, Kataoka T, Yun S, Ryu SH. Multiple roles of phosphoinositide-specific phospholipase C isozymes. *BMB Rep* 2008; 41: 415–34.
31. Yoon SY, Jellerette T, Salicioni AM, Lee HC, Yoo MS, Coward K, Parrington J, Grow D, Cibelli JB, Visconti PE et al. Human sperm devoid of PLC, zeta 1 fail to induce Ca^{2+} release and are unable to initiate the first step of embryo development. *J Clin Invest* 2008; 118: 3671–81.
32. Young C, Grasa P, Coward K, Davis LC, Parrington J. Phospholipase C zeta undergoes dynamic changes in its pattern of localization in sperm during capacitation and the acrosome reaction. *Fertil Steril* 2009; 91: 2230–42.
33. Bedford-Guaus SJ, McPartlin LA, Xie J, Westmiller SL, Buffone MG, Roberson MS. Molecular cloning and characterization of phospholipase C zeta in equine sperm and testis reveals species-specific differences in expression of catalytically active protein. *Biol Reprod* 2011; 85: 78–88.
34. Swann K, Lai FA. PLCζ and the initiation of Ca^{2+} oscillations in fertilizing mammalian eggs. *Cell Calcium* 2013; 53: 55–62.
35. Nomikos M. Novel signalling mechanism and clinical applications of sperm-specific PLCζ. *Biochem Soc Trans* 2015; 43: 371–6.
36. Knott JG, Kurokawa M, Fissore RA, Schultz RM, Williams CJ. Transgenic RNA interference reveals role for mouse sperm phospholipase Czeta in triggering Ca^{2+} oscillations during fertilization. *Biol Reprod* 2005; 72: 992–6.
37. Nomikos M, Sanders JR, Theodoridou M, Kashir J, Matthews E, Nounesis G, Lai FA, Swann K. Sperm-specific post-acrosomal WW-domain binding protein (PAWP) does not cause Ca^{2+} release in mouse oocytes. *Mol Hum Reprod* 2014; 20: 938–47.
38. Kashir J, Nomikos M, Lai FA, Swann K. Sperm-induced Ca^{2+} release during egg activation in mammals. *Biochem Biophys Res Commun* 2014; 450: 1204–11.
39. Sousa M, Tesarik J. Ultrastructural analysis of fertilization failure after intracytoplasmic sperm injection. *Hum Reprod* 1994; 9: 2374–80.
40. Mahutte NG, Arici A. Failed Fertilization: Is it possible? *Curr Opin Obstet Gynecol* 2003; 15: 211–8.
41. Kashir J, Heindryckx B, Jones C, De Sutter P, Parrington J, Coward K. Oocyte activation, phospholipase C zeta and human infertility. *Hum Reprod Update* 2010; 16: 690–703.
42. Heytens E, Parrington J, Coward K et al. Reduced amounts and abnormal forms of phospholipase C zeta in spermatozoa from infertile men. *Hum Reprod* 2009; 24: 2417–28.
43. Taylor SL, Yoon SY, Morshedi MS, Lacey DR, Jellerette T, Fissore RA, Oehninger S. Complete globozoospermia associated with PLCzeta deficiency treated with calcium ionophore and ICSI results in pregnancy. *Reprod Biomed Online* 2010; 20: 559–64.
44. Kashir J, Jones C, Lee HC, Rietdorf K, Nikiforaki D, Durrans C, Ruas M, Tee ST, Heindryckx B, Galione A, De Sutter P, Fissore RA, Parrington J, Coward K. Loss of activity mutations in phospholipase C zeta

(PLCzeta) abolishes calcium oscillatory ability of human recombinant protein in mouse oocytes. *Hum Reprod* 2011; 26: 3372–87.

45. Kashir J, Jones C, Mounce G, Ramadan WM, Lemmon B, Heindryckx B, De Sutter P, Parrington J, Turner K, Child T, McVeigh E, Coward K. Variance in total levels of phospholipase C zeta (PLC-zeta) in human sperm may limit the applicability of quantitative immunofluorescent analysis as a diagnostic indicator of oocyte activation capability. *Fertil Steril* 2013; 99: 107–17.
46. Yelumalai S, Yeste M, Jones C, Amdani SN, Kashir J, Mounce G, Da Silva SJ, Barratt CL, McVeigh E, Coward K. Total levels, localization patterns, and proportions of sperm exhibiting phospholipase C zeta are significantly correlated with fertilization rates after intracytoplasmic sperm injection. *Fertil Steril* 2015; 104: 561–8.e4.
47. Aarabi M, Balakier H, Bashar S, Moskovtsev SI, Sutovsky P, Librach CL, Oko R. Sperm-derived WW domain-binding protein, PAWP, elicits calcium oscillations and oocyte activation in humans and mice. *FASEB J* 2014; 28: 4434–40.
48. Kashir J, Nomikos M, Swann K, Lai FA. PLCζ or PAWP: revisiting the putative mammalian sperm factor that triggers egg activation and embryogenesis. *Mol Hum Reprod* 2015; 21: 383–8.
49. Nomikos M, Swann K, Lai FA. Is PAWP the "real" sperm factor? *Asian J Androl* 2015; 17: 444–6.
50. Satouh Y, Nozawa K, Ikawa M. Sperm postacrosomal WW domain-binding protein is not required for mouse egg activation. *Biol Reprod* 2015; 93: 94.
51. Palermo G, Joris H, Devroey P, Van Steirteghem AC. Pregnancies after intracytoplasmic injection of single spermatozoon into an oocyte. *Lancet* 1992; 340: 17–8.
52. Flaherty SP, Payne D, Matthews CD. Fertilization failures and abnormal fertilization after intracytoplasmic sperm injection. *Hum Reprod* 1998; 13(Suppl 1): 155–64.
53. Esfandiari N, Javed MH, Gotlieb L, Casper RF. Complete failed fertilization after intracytoplasmic sperm injection—Analysis of 10 years' data. *Int J Fertil Womens Med* 2005; 50: 187–92.
54. Bukulmez O, Yarali H, Yucel A, Sari T, Gurgan T. Intracytoplasmic sperm injection versus *in vitro* fertilization for patients with a tubal factor as their sole cause of infertility: A prospective, randomized trial. *Fertil Steril* 2000; 73: 38–42.
55. Mahutte NG, Arici A. Role of gonadotropin-releasing hormone antagonists in poor responders. *Fertil Steril* 2007; 87: 241–9.
56. Swain JE, Pool TB. ART failure: Oocyte contributions to unsuccessful fertilization. *Hum Reprod Update* 2008; 14: 431–46.
57. Dam AH, Feenstra I, Westphal JR, Ramos L, van Golde RJ, Kremer JA. Globozoospermia revisited. *Hum Reprod Update* 2007; 13: 63–75.
58. Yanagida K. Complete fertilization failure in ICSI. *Hum Cell* 2004; 17: 187–93.
59. Liu J, Nagy Z, Joris H, Tournaye H, Devroey P, Van Steirteghem A. Successful fertilization and establishment of pregnancies after intracytoplasmic sperm injection in patients with globozoospermia. *Hum Reprod* 1995; 10: 626–9.
60. Rawe VY, Olmedo SB, Nodar FN, Doncel GD, Acosta AA, Vitullo AD. Cytoskeletal organization defects and abortive activation in human oocytes after IVF and ICSI failure. *Mol Hum Reprod* 2000; 6: 510–6.
61. Heindryckx B, De Gheselle S, Gerris J, Dhont M, De Sutter P. Efficiency of assisted oocyte activation as a solution for failed intracytoplasmic sperm injection. *Reprod Biomed Online* 2008; 17: 662–8.
62. Eichenlaub-Ritter U, Schmiady H, Kentenich H, Soewarto D. Recurrent failure in polar body formation and premature chromosome condensation in oocytes from a human patient: Indicators of asynchrony in nuclear and cytoplasmic maturation. *Hum Reprod* 1995; 10: 2343–9.
63. Miyara F, Aubriot FX, Glissant A, Nathan C, Douard S, Stanovici A, Herve F, Dumont-Hassan M, LeMeur A, Cohen-Bacrie P, Debey P. Multiparameter analysis of human oocytes at metaphase II stage after IVF failure in non-male infertility. *Hum Reprod* 2003; 18: 1494–503.
64. Dale B, Menezo Y, Coppola G. Trends, fads and ART! *J Assist Reprod Genet* 2015; 32: 489–93.
65. Van Blerkom J. Sperm centrosome dysfunction: A possible new class of male factor infertility in the human. *Mol Hum Reprod* 1996; 2: 349–54.
66. Rawe VY, Terada Y, Nakamura S, Chillik CF, Olmedo SB, Chemes HE. A pathology of the sperm centriole responsible for defective sperm aster formation, syngamy and cleavage. *Hum Reprod* 2002; 17: 2344–9.
67. Rawe VY, Díaz ES, Abdelmassih R, Wójcik C, Morales P, Sutovsky P, Chemes HE. The role of sperm proteasomes during sperm aster formation and early zygote development: Implications for fertilization failure in humans. *Hum Reprod* 2008; 23: 573–80.
68. Neri QV, Lee B, Rosenwaks Z, Machaca K, Palermo GD. Understanding fertilization through intracytoplasmic sperm injection (ICSI). *Cell Calcium* 2014; 55: 24–37.
69. Rybouchkin A, Dozortsev D, Pelinck MJ, De Sutter P, Dhont M. Analysis of the oocyte activation capacity and chromosomal complement of round-headed human spermatozoa by their injection into mouse oocytes. *Hum Reprod* 1996; 11: 2170–5.
70. Tesarik J, Rienzi L, Ubaldi F, Mendoza C, Greco E. Use of a modified intracytoplasmic sperm injection technique to overcome sperm-borne oocyte activation failures. *Fertil Steril* 2002; 78: 619–24.
71. Heindryckx B, Van der Elst J, De Sutter P, Dhont M. Treatment option for sperm- or oocyte-related fertilization failure: Assisted oocyte activation following diagnostic heterologous ICSI. *Hum Reprod* 2005; 20: 2237–41.

72. Kyono K, Nakajo Y, Nishinaka C, Hattori H, Kyoya T, Ishikawa T, Abe H, Araki Y. A birth from the transfer of a single vitrified-warmed blastocyst using intracytoplasmic sperm injection with calcium ionophore oocyte activation in a globozoospermic patient. *Fertil Steril* 2009; 91: 931.e7–11.
73. Alberio R, Zakhartchenko V, Motlik J, Wolf E. Mammalian oocyte activation: Lessons from the sperm and implications for nuclear transfer. *Int J Dev Biol* 2001; 45: 797–809.
74. Egashira A, Murakami M, Haigo K, Horiuchi T, Kuramoto T. A successful pregnancy and live birth after intracytoplasmic sperm injection with globozoospermic sperm andelectrical oocyte activation. *Fertil Steril* 2009; 92: 2037.e5–9.
75. Yanagida K, Katayose H, Yazawa H, Kimura Y, Sato A, Yanagimachi H, Yanagimachi R. Successful fertilization and pregnancy following ICSI and electrical oocyte activation. *Hum Reprod* 1999; 14: 1307–11.
76. Yanagida K, Fujikura Y, Katayose H. The present status of artificial oocyte activation in assisted reproductive technology. *Reprod Med Biol* 2008; 7: 133–42.
77. Vanden Meerschaut F, Nikiforaki D, Heindryckx B, De Sutter P. Assisted oocyte activation following ICSI fertilization failure. *Reprod Biomed Online* 2014; 28: 560–71.
78. Zhang J, Wang CW, Blaszcyzk A, Grifo JA, Ozil J, Haberman E, Adler A, Krey LC. Electrical activation and *in vitro* development of human oocytes that fail to fertilize after intracytoplasmic sperm injection. *Fertil Steril* 1999; 72: 509–12.
79. Koo OJ, Jang G, Kwon DK, Kang JT, Kwon OS, Park HJ, Kang SK, Lee BC. Electrical activation induces reactive oxygen species in porcine embryos. *Theriogenology* 2008; 70: 1111–8.
80. Ozil JP, Banrezes B, Tóth S, Pan H, Schultz RM. Ca^{2+} oscillatory pattern in fertilized mouse eggs affects gene expression and development to term. *Dev Biol* 2006; 300: 534–44.
81. Tesarik J, Sousa M, Testart J. Human oocyte activation after intracytoplasmic sperm injection. *Hum Reprod* 1994; 9: 511–8.
82. Ebner T, Moser M, Sommergruber M, Jesacher K, Tews G. Complete oocyte activation failure after ICSI can be overcome by a modified injection technique. *Hum Reprod* 2004; 19: 1837–41.
83. Tesarik J, Sousa M. Key elements of a highly efficient intracytoplasmic sperm injection technique: Ca^{2+} fluxes and oocyte cytoplasmic dislocation. *Fertil Steril* 1995; 64: 770–6.
84. Yoshida S, Plant S. Mechanism of release of Ca^{2+} from intracellular stores in response to ionomycin in oocytes of the frog *Xenopus laevis*. *J Physiol* 1992; 458: 307–18.
85. Vanden Meerschaut F, Nikiforaki D, De Roo C, Lierman S, Qian C, Schmitt-John T, De Sutter P, Heindryckx B. Comparison of pre- and post-implantation development following the application of three artificial activating stimuli in a mouse model with round-headed sperm cells deficient for oocyte activation. *Hum Reprod* 2013; 28: 1190–8.
86. Sanusi R, Yu Y, Nomikos M, Lai FA, Swann K. Rescue of failed oocyte activation after ICSI in a mouse model of male factor infertility by recombinant phospholipase Cζ. *Mol Hum Reprod* 2015; 21: 783–91.
87. Winston N, Johnson M, Pickering S, Braude P. Parthenogenetic activation and development of fresh and aged human oocytes. *Fertil Steril* 1991; 56: 904–12.
88. Balakier H, Casper RF. Experimentally induced parthenogenetic activation of human oocytes. *Hum Reprod* 1993; 8: 740–3.
89. Rinaudo P, Pepperell JR, Buradgunta S, Massobrio M, Keefe DL. Dissociation between intracellular calcium elevation and development of human oocytes treated with calcium ionophore. *Fertil Steril* 1997; 68: 1086–92.
90. Ross PJ, Beyhan Z, Iager AE, Yoon SY, Malcuit C, Schellander K, Fissore RA, Cibelli JB. Parthenogenetic activation of bovine oocytes using bovine and murine phospholipase C zeta. *BMC Dev Biol* 2008; 8: 16.
91. Moaz MN, Khattab S, Foutouh IA, Mohsen EA. Chemical activation of oocytes in different types of sperm abnormalities in cases of low or failed fertilization after ICSI: A prospective pilot study. *Reprod Biomed Online* 2006; 13: 791–4.
92. Nasr-Esfahani MH, Razavi S, Javdan Z, Tavalaee M. Artificial oocyte activation in severe teratozoospermia undergoing intracytoplasmic sperm injection. *Fertil Steril* 2008; 90: 2231–7.
93. Mansour R, Fahmy I, Tawab NA, Kamal A, El-Demery Y, Aboulghar M, Serour G. Electrical activation of oocytes after intracytoplasmic sperm injection: A controlled randomized study. *Fertil Steril* 2009; 91: 133–9.
94. Rybouchkin AV, Van der Straeten F, Quatacker J, De Sutter P, Dhont M. Fertilization and pregnancy after assisted oocyte activation and intracytoplasmic sperm injection in a case of round-headed sperm associated with deficient oocyte activation capacity. *Fertil Steril* 1997; 68: 1144–7.
95. Kim ST, Cha YB, Park JM, Gye MC. Successful pregnancy and delivery from frozen–thawed embryos after intracytoplasmic sperm injection using round-headed spermatozoa and assisted oocyte activation in a globozoospermic patient with mosaic Down syndrome. *Fertil Steril* 2001; 75: 445–7.
96. Dirican EK, Isik A, Vicdan K, Sozen E, Suludere Z. Clinical pregnancies and livebirths achieved by intracytoplasmic injection of round headed acrosomeless spermatozoa with and without oocyte activation in familial globozoospermia: Case report. *Asian J Androl* 2008; 10: 332–6.

97. Tejara A, Mollá M, Muriel L, Remohi J, Pellicer A, De Pablo JL. Successful pregnancy and childbirth after intracytoplasmic sperm injection with calcium ionophore oocyte activation in a globozoospermic patient. *Fertil Steril* 2008; 90: 1202.e1–5.
98. Check JH, Levito MC, Summers-Chase D, Marmar J, Barci H. A comparison of the efficacy of intracytoplasmic sperm injection (ICSI) using ejaculated sperm selected by high magnification versus ICSI with testicular sperm both followed by oocyte activation with calcium ionophore. *Clin Exp Obstet Gynecol* 2007; 34: 111–2.
99. Sermondade N, Hafhouf E, Dupont C, Bechoua S, Palacios C, Eustache F, Poncelet C, Benzacken B, Lévy R, Sifer C. Successful childbirth after intracytoplasmic morphologically selected sperm injection without assisted oocyte activation in a patient with globozoospermia. *Hum Reprod* 2011; 26: 2944–9.
100. Vanden Meerschaut F, Nikiforaki D, De Gheselle S, Dullaerts V, Van den Abbeel E, Gerris J, Heindryckx B, De Sutter P. Assisted oocyte activation is not beneficial for all patients with a suspected oocyte-related activation deficiency. *Hum Reprod* 2012; 27: 1977–84.
101. Vanden Meerschaut F, Leybaert L, Nikiforaki D, Qian C, Heindryckx B, De Sutter P. Diagnostic and prognostic value of calcium oscillatory pattern analysis for patients with ICSI fertilization failure. *Hum Reprod* 2013; 28: 87–98.
102. Ebner T, Montag M; Oocyte Activation Study Group, Montag M, Van der Ven K, Van der Ven H, Ebner T, Shebl O, Oppelt P, Hirchenhain J, Krüssel J, Maxrath B, Gnoth C, Friol K, Tigges J, Wünsch E, Luckhaus J, Beerkotte A, Weiss D, Grunwald K, Struller D, Etien C. Live birth after artificial oocyte activation using a ready-to-use ionophore: A prospective multicentre study. *Reprod Biomed Online* 2015; 30: 359–65.
103. Sfontouris IA, Nastri CO, Lima ML, Tahmasbpourmarzouni E, Raine-Fenning N, Martins WP. Artificial oocyte activation to improve reproductive outcomes in women with previous fertilization failure: A systematic review and meta-analysis of RCTs. *Hum Reprod* 2015; 30: 1831–41.
104. Tesarik J, Testart J. Treatment of sperm-injected human oocytes with Ca^{2+} ionophore supports the development of Ca^{2+} oscillations. *Biol Reprod* 1994; 51: 385–91.
105. Bos-Mikich A, Swann K, Whittingham DG. Calcium oscillations and protein synthesis inhibition synergistically activate mouse oocytes. *Mol Reprod Dev* 1995; 41: 84–90.
106. Ma SF, Liu XY, Miao DQ, Han ZB, Zhang X, Miao YL, Yanagimachi R, Tan JH. Parthenogenetic activation of mouse oocytes by strontium chloride: A search for the best conditions. *Theriogenology* 2005; 64: 1142–57.
107. Carvacho I, Lee HC, Fissore RA, Clapham DE. TRPV3 channels mediate strontium-induced mouse-egg activation. *Cell Rep* 2013; 5: 1375–86.
108. Yanagida K, Morozumi K, Katayose H, Hayashi S, Sato A. Successful pregnancy after ICSI with strontium oocyte activation in low rates of fertilization. *Reprod Biomed Online* 2006; 13: 801–6.
109. Rogers NT, Hobson E, Pickering S, Lai FA, Braude P, Swann K. Phospholipase Czeta causes Ca^{2+} oscillations and parthenogenetic activation of human oocytes. *Reproduction* 2004; 128: 697–702.
110. Machaty Z. Signal transduction in mammalian oocytes during fertilization. *Cell Tissue Res* 2016; 363: 169–83.
111. Cuthbertson KS, Cobbold PH. Phorbol ester and sperm activate mouse oocytes by inducing sustained oscillations in cell Ca^{2+}. *Nature* 1985; 316: 541–2.
112. Swann K. Thimerosal causes calcium oscillaitons and sensitizes calcium-induced calcium release in unfertilized hamster oocytes. *FEBS Lett* 1992; 278: 175–8.
113. Fissore RA, Pinto-Correia C, Robl JM. Inositol trisphosphate-induced calcium release in the generation of calcium oscillations in bovine eggs. *Biol Reprod* 1995; 53: 766–74.
114. Homa ST and Swann K. A cytosolic sperm factor triggers calcium oscillations and membrane hyperpolarizations in human oocytes. *Hum Reprod* 2009; 9: 2356–61.
115. Macháty Z, Wang WH, Day BN, Prather RS. Complete activation of porcine oocytes induced by the sulfhydryl reagent, thimerosal. *Biol Reprod* 1997; 57: 1123–7.
116. Heindryckx B, De Sutter P, Gerris J. Somatic nuclear transfer to *in vitro*-matured human germinal vesicle oocytes. In: *Stem Cells in Human Reproduction. Simon C, Pellicer A* (eds). 2009, pp. 226–42.
117. Suzuki T, Yoshida N, Suzuki E, Okuda E, Perry AC. Full-term mouse development by abolishing Zn^{2+}-dependent metaphase II arrest without Ca^{2+} release. *Development* 2010; 137: 2659–69.
118. Lee K, Davis A, Zhang L, Ryu J, Spate LD, Park KW, Samuel MS, Walters EM, Murphy CN, Machaty Z, Prather RS. Pig oocyte activation using a Zn^{2+} chelator, TPEN. *Theriogenology* 2015; 84: 1024–32.
119. Ducibella T, Fissore R. The roles of Ca^{2+}, downstream protein kinases, and oscillatory signaling in regulating fertilization and the activation of development. *Dev Biol* 2008; 315: 257–79.
120. De Sutter P, Dozortsev D, Cieslak J, Wolf G, Verlinsky Y, Dyban A. Parthenogenetic activation of human oocytes by puromycin. *J Assist Reprod Genet* 1992; 9: 328–37.
121. De Sutter P, Dozortsev D, Vrijens P, Desmet R, Dhont M. Cytogenetic analysis of human oocytes parthenogenetically activated by puromycin. *J Assist Reprod Genet* 1994; 11: 382–8.
122. Ducibella T, Huneau D, Angelichio E, Xu Z, Schultz RM, Kopf GS, Fissore R, Madoux S, Ozil JP. Egg-to-embryo transition is driven by differential responses to Ca^{2+} oscillation number. *Dev Biol* 2002; 250: 280–91.

123. Kim BY, Yoon SY, Cha SK, Kwak KH, Fissore RA, Parys JB, Yoon TK, Lee DR. Alterations in calcium oscillatory activity in vitrified mouse eggs impact on egg quality and subsequent embryonic development. *Pflugers Arch* 2011; 461: 515–26.
124. Bos-Mikich A, Whittingham D, Jones KT. Meiotic and mitotic Ca^{2+} oscillations affect cell composition in resulting blastocysts. *Dev Biol* 1997; 182: 172–9.
125. Ozil JP, Huneau D. Activation of rabbit oocytes: The impact of the Ca^{2+} signal regime on development. *Development* 2001; 128: 917–28.
126. Heytens E, Soleimani R, Lierman S, De Meester S, Gerris J, Dhont M, Van der Elst J, De Sutter P. Effect of ionomycin on oocyte activation and embryo development in mouse. *Reprod Biomed Online* 2008; 17: 764–71.
127. Sato Y, Nakamura Y, Sakamoto E, Tasaka A, Usui K, Hattori H, Ito Y, Nakajo Y, Doshida M, Kyono K. Follow up of children following new technology: TESE, IVM, and oocyte activation. *Hum Reprod* 2011; 26: I274.
128. Takisawa T, Doshida M, Hattori H, Nakamura Y, Kyoya T, Shibuya Y, Nakajo Y, Tasaka A, Toya M, Kyono K. Effect of oocyte activation by calcium ionophore A23187 or strontium chloride in patients with low fertilization rates and follow-up of babies. *Hum Reprod* 2011; 26: I178–9.
129. Takisawa T, Sato Y, Tasaka A, Ito Y, Nakamura Y, Hattori H. Effect of oocyte activation by calcium ionophore A23187 or strontium chloride in patients with low fertilization rates and follow-up of babies. *Fertil Steril* 2011; 96: S162.
130. D'haeseleer E, Vanden Meerschaut F, Bettens K, Luyten A, Gysels H, Thienpont Y, De Witte G, Heindryckx B, Oostra A, Roeyers H, Sutter PD, van Lierde K. Language development of children born following intracytoplasmic sperm injection (ICSI) combined with assisted oocyte activation (AOA). *Int J Lang Commun Disord* 2014; 49: 702–9.
131. Kashir J, Konstantinidis M, Jones C, Heindryckx B, De Sutter P, Parrington J, Wells D, Coward K. Characterization of two heterozygous mutations of the oocyte activation factor phospholipase C zeta (PLCζ) from an infertile man by use of minisequencing of individual sperm and expression in somatic cells. *Fertil Steril* 2012; 98: 423–31.
132. Yu, Y, Saunders CM, Lai FA, Swann K. Preimplantation development of mouse oocytes activated by different levels of human phospholipase Czeta. *Human Reprod* 2008; 23: 365–73.
133. Nomikos M, Yu Y, Elgmati K, Theodoridou M, Campbell K, Vassilakopoulou V, Zikos C, Livaniou E, Amso N, Nounesis G, Swann K, Lai FA. Phospholipase Cζ rescues failed oocyte activation in a prototype of male factor infertility. *Fertil Steril* 2013; 99: 76–85.
134. Kashir J, Konstantinidis M, Jones C, Lemmon B, Lee HC, Hamer R, Heindryckx B, Deane CM, De Sutter P, Fissore RA, Parrington J, Wells D, Coward K. A maternally inherited autosomal point mutation in human phospholipase C zeta (PLCζ) leads to male infertility. *Hum Reprod* 2012; 27: 222–31.
135. Kashir J, Sermondade N, Sifer C, Oo SL, Jones C, Mounce G, Turner K, Child T, McVeigh E, Coward K. Motile sperm organelle morphology evaluation-selected globozoospermic human sperm with an acrosomal bud exhibits novel patterns and higher levels of phospholipase C zeta. *Hum Reprod* 2012; 27: 3150–60.
136. Kashir J, Heynen A, Jones C, Durrans C, Craig J, Gadea J, Turner K, Parrington J, Coward K. Effects of cryopreservation and density-gradient washing on phospholipase C zeta concentrations in human spermatozoa. *Reprod Biomed Online* 2011; 23: 263–7.
137. Grasa P, Coward K, Young C, Parrington J. The pattern of localization of the putative oocyte activation factor, phospholipase C zeta, in uncapacitated, capacitated, and ionophore-treated human spermatozoa. *Hum Reprod* 2008; 23: 2513–22.
138. Silveira PP, Portella AK, Goldani MZ, Barbieri MA. Developmental origins of health and disease (DOHaD). *J Pediatr (Rio J)* 2007; 83: 494–504.
139. Ajduk A, Małagocki A, Maleszewski M. Cytoplasmic maturation of mammalian oocytes: Development of a mechanism responsible for sperm-induced Ca^{2+} oscillations. *Reprod Biol* 2008; 8: 3–22.
140. Backs J, Stein P, Backs T, Duncan FE, Grueter CE, McAnally J, Qi X, Schultz RM, Olson EN. The gamma isoform of CaM kinase II controls mouse egg activation by regulating cell cycle resumption. *Proc Natl Acad Sci USA* 2010; 107: 81–6.
141. Coward K, Campos-Mendoza A, Larman M, Hibbitt O, McAndrew B, Bromage N, Parrington J. Teleost fish spermatozoa contain a cytosolic protein factor that induces calcium release in sea urchin egg homogenates and triggers calcium oscillations when injected into mouse oocytes. *Biochem Biophys Res Commun* 2003; 305: 299–304.
142. Dale B. Primary and secondary messengers in the activation of Ascidian eggs. *Exp Cell Res* 1988; 177: 205–11.
143. Dale B, DeFelice LJ, Ehrenstein G. Injection of a soluble sperm fraction into sea-urchin eggs triggers the cortical reaction. *Experientia* 1985; 41: 1068–70.
144. Dong JB, Tang TS, Sun FZ. *Xenopus* and chicken sperm contain a cytosolic soluble protein factor which can trigger calcium oscillations in mouse eggs. *Biochem Biophys Res Commun* 2000; 268: 947–51.
145. Ducibella T, Schultz RM, Ozil JP. Role of calcium signals in early development. *Semin Cell Dev Biol* 2006; 17: 324–32.
146. Ebner T, Köster M, Shebl O, Moser M, Van der Ven H, Tews G, Montag M. Application of a ready-to-use calcium ionophore increases rates of fertilization and pregnancy in severe male factor infertility. *Fertil Steril* 2012; 98: 1432–7.

147. Evans JP, Kopf GS. Molecular mechanisms of sperm–egg interactions and egg activation. *Andrologia* 1998; 30: 297–307.
148. Goud PT, Goud AP, Van Oostveldt P, Dhont M. Presence and dynamic redistribution of type I inositol 1,4,5-trisphosphate receptors in human oocytes and embryos during *in-vitro* maturation, fertilization and early cleavage divisions. *Mol Hum Reprod* 1999; 5: 441–51.
149. Hwang JI, Oh YS, Shin KJ, Kim H, Ryu SH, Suh PG. Molecular cloning and characterization of a novel phospholipase C, PLC-eta. *Biochem J* 2005; 389: 181–6.
150. Hyslop LA, Nixon VL, Levasseur M, Chapman F, Chiba K, McDougall A. Ca^{2+}-promoted cyclin B1 degradation in mouse oocytes requires the establishment of a metaphase arrest. *Dev Biol* 2004; 269: 206–19.
151. International Committee for Monitoring Assisted Reproductive Technology (ICMART); de Mouzon J, Lancaster P, Nygren KG, Sullivan E, Zegers-Hochschild F, Mansour R, Ishihara O, Adamson D. World Collaborative Report on Assisted Reproductive Technology, 2002. *Hum Reprod* 2009; 24: 2310–20.
152. Isom SC, Stevens JR, Li R, Spollen WG, Cox L, Spate LD, Murphy CN, Prather RS. Transcriptional profiling by RNA-Seq of peri-attachment porcine embryos generated by a variety of assisted reproductive technologies. *Physiol Genomics* 2013; 45: 577–89.
153. Iwao Y. Egg activation in physiological polyspermy. *Reproduction* 2012; 144: 11–22.
154. Jaffe LF. Sources of calcium in egg activation: A review and hypothesis. *Dev Biol* 1983; 99: 265–76.
155. Jaffe LA. First messengers at fertilization. *J Reprod Fertil Suppl* 1990; 42: 107–16.
156. Jaffe LF. The path of calcium in cytosolic calcium oscillations: A unifying hypothesis. *Proc Natl Acad Sci USA* 1991; 88: 9883–7.
157. Jones KT. Turning it on and off: M-phase promoting factor during meiotic maturation and fertilization. *Mol Hum Reprod* 2004; 10: 1–5.
158. Jones KT. Mammalian egg activation: from Ca^{2+} spiking to cell cycle progression. *Reproduction* 2005; 130: 813–23.
159. Jones KT. Intracellular calcium in the fertilization and development of mammalian eggs. *Clin Exp Pharmacol Physiol* 2007; 34: 1084–9.
160. Jones KT, Soeller C, Cannell MB. The passage of Ca^{2+} and fluorescent markers between the sperm and egg after fusion in the mouse. *Development* 1998; 125: 4627–35.
161. Kashir J, Deguchi R, Jones C, Coward K, Stricker SA. Comparative biology of sperm factors and fertilization-induced calcium signals across the animal kingdom. *Mol Reprod Dev* 2013; 80: 787–815.
162. Kauffman RF, Taylor RW, Pfeiffer DR. Cation transport and specificity of ionomycin. Comparison with ionophore A23187 in rat liver mitochondria. *J Biol Chem* 1980; 255: 2735–9.
163. Kelley GG, Reks SE, Ondrako JM, Smrcka AV. Phospholipase Cε: A novel Ras effector. *EMBO J* 2001; 20: 743–54.
164. Kennedy CE, Krieger KB, Sutovsky M, Xu W, Vargovič P, Didion BA, Ellersieck MR, Hennessy ME, Verstegen J, Oko R, Sutovsky P. Protein expression pattern of PAWP in bull spermatozoa is associated with sperm quality and fertility following artificial insemination. *Mol Reprod Dev* 2014; 81: 436–49.
165. Kishikawa H, Wakayama T, Yanagimachi R. Comparison of oocyte-activating agents for mouse cloning. *Cloning* 1999; 1: 153–9.
166. Krauchunas AR, Wolfner MF. Molecular changes during egg activation. *Curr Top Dev Biol* 2013; 102: 267–92.
167. Kyozuka K, Deguchi R, Mohri T, Miyazaki S. Injection of sperm extract mimics spatiotemporal dynamics of Ca^{2+} responses and progression of meiosis at fertilization of ascidian oocytes. *Development* 1998; 125: 4099–105.
168. Lorca T, Cruzalegui FH, Fesquet D, Cavadore JC, Méry J, Means A, Dorée M. Calmodulin-dependent kinase II mediates inactivation of MPF and CSF upon fertilization of *Xenopus* eggs. *Nature* 1993; 366: 270–3.
169. Malcuit C, Kurokawa M, Fissore RA. Calcium oscillations and mammalian egg activation. *J Cell Physiol* 2006; 206: 565–73.
170. Markoulaki S, Matson S, Ducibella T. Fertilization stimulates long-lasting oscillations of CaMKII activity in mouse eggs. *Dev Biol* 2004; 272: 15–25.
171. Nakahara M, Shimozawa M, Nakamura Y, Irino Y, Morita M, Kudo Y, Fukami K. A novel phospholipase C, PLC(eta)2, is a neuron-specific isozyme. *J Biol Chem* 2005; 280: 29128–34.
172. Nasr-Esfahani MH, Deemeh MR, Tavalaee M. Artificial oocyte activation and intracytoplasmic sperm injection. *Fertil Steril* 2009; 94: 520–6.
173. Nomikos M, Kashir J, Swann K, Lai FA. Sperm PLCζ: from structure to Ca^{2+} oscillations, egg activation and therapeutic potential. *FEBS Lett* 2013; 587: 3609–16.
174. Nomikos M, Sanders JR, Kashir J, Sanusi R, Buntwal L, Love D, Ashley P, Sanders D, Knaggs P, Bunkheila A, Swann K, Lai FA. Functional disparity between human PAWP and PLCζ in the generation of Ca^{2+} oscillations for oocyte activation. *Mol Hum Reprod* 2015; 21: 702–10.
175. Parrington J, Swann K, Shevchenko VI, Sesay AK, Lai FA. Calcium oscillations in mammalian eggs triggered by a soluble sperm protein. *Nature* 1996; 25: 364–8.
176. Parrington J, Jones KT, Lai FA, Swann K. The soluble sperm factor that causes Ca^{2+} release from sea urchin egg homogenates also triggers Ca^{2+} oscillations after injection into mouse eggs. *Biochem J* 1999; 341: 1–4.
177. Racowsky C, Kaufman ML, Dermer RA, Homa ST, Gunnala S. Chromosomal analysis of meiotic stages of human oocytes matured *in vitro*: Benefits of

protease treatment before fixation. *Fertil Steril* 1992; 57: 1026–33.
178. Reed PW, Lardy HA. A23187: A divalent cation ionophore. *J Biol Chem* 1972; 247: 6970–7.
179. Rhee SG. Regulation of phosphoinositide-specific phospholipase C. *Annu Rev Biochem* 2001; 70: 281–312.
180. Rosenbusch BE. Frequency and patterns of premature sperm chromosome condensation in oocytes failing to fertilize after intracytoplasmic sperm injection. *J Assist Reprod Genet* 2000; 17: 253–9.
181. Santella L, Dale B. Assisted yes, but where do we draw the line? *Reprod Biomed Online* 2015; 31: 476–8.
182. Schultz RM, Kopf GS. Molecular basis of mammalian egg activation. *Curr Top Dev Biol* 1995; 30: 21–62.
183. Sette C, Bevilacqua A, Bianchini A, Mangia F, Geremia R, Rossi P. Parthenogenetic activation of mouse eggs by microinjection of a truncated c-kit tyrosine kinase present in spermatozoa. *Development* 1997; 124: 2267–74.
184. Sette C, Bevilacqua A, Geremia R, Rossi P. Involvement of phospholipase Cgamma1 in mouse egg activation induced by a truncated form of the C-kit tyrosine kinase present in spermatozoa. *J Cell Biol* 1998; 142: 1063–74.
185. Sette C, Paronetto MP, Barchi M, Bevilacqua A, Geremia R, Rossi P. Tr-kit-induced resumption of the cell cycle in mouse eggs requires activation of a Src-like kinase. *EMBO J* 2002; 21: 5386–95.
186. Song C, Hu CD, Masago M, Kariyai K, Yamawaki-Kataoka Y, Shibatohge M, Wu D, Satoh T, Kataoka T. Regulation of a novel human phospholipase C, PLCepsilon, through membrane targeting by Ras. *J Biol Chem* 2001; 276: 2752–7.
187. Stitzel ML, Seydoux G. Regulation of the oocyte-to-zygote transition. *Science* 2007; 316: 407–8.
188. Swain JE, Ding J, Wu J, Smith GD. Regulation of spindle and chromatin dynamics during early and late stages of oocyte maturation by aurora kinases. *Mol Hum Reprod* 2008; 14: 291–9.
189. Swann K, Larman MG, Saunders CM, Lai FA. The cytosolic sperm factor that triggers Ca^{2+} oscillations and egg activation in mammals is a novelphospholipase C: PLCzeta. *Reproduction* 2004; 127: 431–9.
190. van Blerkom J, Cohen J, Johnson M. A plea for caution and more research in the 'experimental' use of ionophores in ICSI. *Reprod Biomed Online* 2015; 30: 323–4.
191. Vanderheyden V, Wakai T, Bultynck G, De Smedt H, Parys JB, Fissore RA. Regulation of inositol 1,4,5-trisphosphate receptor type 1 function during oocyte maturation by MPM-2 phosphorylation. *Cell Calcium* 2009; 46: 56–64.
192. Van Wissen B, Eisenberg C, Debey P, Pennehouat G, Auger J, Bomsel-Helmreich O. *In vitro* DNA fluorescence after *in vitro* fertilization (IVF) failure. *J Assist Reprod Genet* 1992; 9: 564–71.
193. Vasilev F, Chun JT, Gragnaniello G, Garante E, Santella L. Effects of ionomycin on egg activation and early development in starfish. *PLoS One* 2012; 7: e39231.
194. Wolosker H, Kline D, Bian Y, Blackshaw S, Cameron AM, Fralich TJ, Schnaar RL, Snyder SH. Molecularly cloned mammalian glucosamine-6-phosphate deaminase localizes to transporting epithelium and lacks oscillin activity. *FASEB J* 1998; 12: 91–9.
195. Wu H, He CL, Fissore RA. Injection of a porcine sperm factor triggers calcium oscillations in mouse oocytes and bovine eggs. *Mol Reprod Dev* 1997; 46: 176–89.
196. Wu AT, Sutovsky P, Manandhar G, Xu W, Katayama M, Day BN, Park KW, Yi YJ, Xi YW, Prather RS, Oko R. PAWP, a sperm-specific WW domain-binding protein, promotes meiotic resumption and pronuclear development during fertilization. *J Biol Chem* 2007; 282: 12164–75.
197. Yamano S, Nakagawa K, Nakasaka H, Aono T. Fertilization failure and oocyte activation. *J Med Invest* 2000; 47: 1–8.
198. Zhou Y, Wing MR, Sondek J, Harden TK. Molecular cloning and characterization of PLCeta2. *Biochem J* 2005; 391: 667–76.

15

Analysis of fertilization

THOMAS EBNER

INTRODUCTION

In vitro fertilization (IVF) and intracytoplasmic sperm injection (ICSI) cycles have shown that women have only a finite number of gametes out of a pool of collected oocytes that are viable for generating a term pregnancy. This demonstrates the need for simple methods of preimplantation embryo assessment in the prediction of pregnancy rates. In this respect, intensive research has been done at the zygote stage on day 1 of preimplantation development.

Independently of the mode of fertilization, a sperm-borne enzyme called phospholipase C-ζ enters the oocyte and activates it via the inositol-3-phosphate pathway. In detail, this molecule binds to the corresponding receptor at the endoplasmic reticulum where it causes Ca^{2+} release in the form of oscillations. This Ca^{2+} response drives the extrusion of the second polar body and the formation of both pronuclei.

While conventional IVF more or less mimics natural fertilization, ICSI is a rather invasive procedure circumventing some of the major steps in the process of oocyte activation and fertilization. Consequently, the ICSI schedule differs slightly from the IVF one (1). This delay is attributed to the time needed for the sperm to pass through the oocyte outer complex, particularly the cumulus and corona cells, as well as the zona pellucida. Fusion of the spermatozoon with the oolemma and incorporation into the oocyte plasma, on the other hand, seem to occur very rapidly (2). In ICSI, fertilization usually has to be assessed approximately two hours earlier (e.g., 16–18 hours post-insemination) than in IVF (18–20 hours post-insemination) in order to find identical developmental stages (3).

TIMING OF FERTILIZATION EVENTS

Either active propulsion (conventional IVF) or direct deposition (ICSI) ensures presence of a spermatozoon in the cytoplasm. Original time-lapse video cinematography of ICSI gametes has proven that regular fertilization follows a definite course of events, though the timing of these events may vary between eggs (4). In the era of time-lapse imaging, additional information comes from morphokinetic analysis of developmental events.

Following an international consensus meeting, a time-lapse user group proposed guidelines on the nomenclature of human embryo development, including the dynamic fertilization process (5). Per the definition, the time at which insemination occurs (IVF or ICSI) is called t0. Consequently, tPB2 marks the time at which the second polar body is extruded and tPN marks the time at which the fertilization status is confirmed. For proper analysis of the time period in which the two pronuclei are visible (VP), their appearance (tPNa) and fading (tPNf) should be documented. It is important to note the time of time-lapse pronuclear assessment (tZ) since the pronuclear pattern is a dynamic event and its morphology can change between tPNa and tPNf (6).

Approximately 90% of the oocytes showed circular waves of granulation within the cytoplasm after ICSI (periodicity of 20–53 minutes). During this granulation phase, the head of the spermatozoon decondensed. Subsequently, the second polar body was extruded, which was followed by the central formation of the male pronucleus. At about the same time, the female counterpart formed and was drawn towards the male pronucleus until the two abutted. Data from the literature suggest (7) that during this process the male pronucleus rotates onto the female one, in which the chromatin condensates on the side facing the center of the egg, in order to also align its chromatin towards the spindle forming between both pronuclei. Both pronuclei then increase in size, and their nucleoli move around and arrange themselves near the common junction (4).

Within both nuclei, nucleoli form at sites on the DNA known as the "nucleolar organizing regions" located on the chromosomes where the ribosomal genes are situated (8). This means that the nucleoli are the active sites of rRNA synthesis. During the course of development, nucleoli tend to fuse due to an increase in protein synthesis (4,9). It should be emphasized once again that IVF zygotes reach the final stage of nucleolar organization at a later time than ICSI zygotes.

The size and distribution patterns of the nucleoli may serve as prognostic parameters of the events of fertilization, the completion of meiosis, and the cell cycle, leading to the first mitotic division, the normality of the chromatin complement in the two nuclei, and the formation with chromosome attachment of the mitotic spindle (8).

In particular, asynchrony in formation and polarization of nucleoli (Figure 15.1a) may severely impair further development of the preimplantation embryo (10–14). Consequently, good-quality embryos can arise from oocytes that had more uniform timing from injection to pronuclear abuttal (4).

PRONUCLEAR GRADING

According to the above-mentioned agreement (5), pronuclear pattern assessment should be done immediately

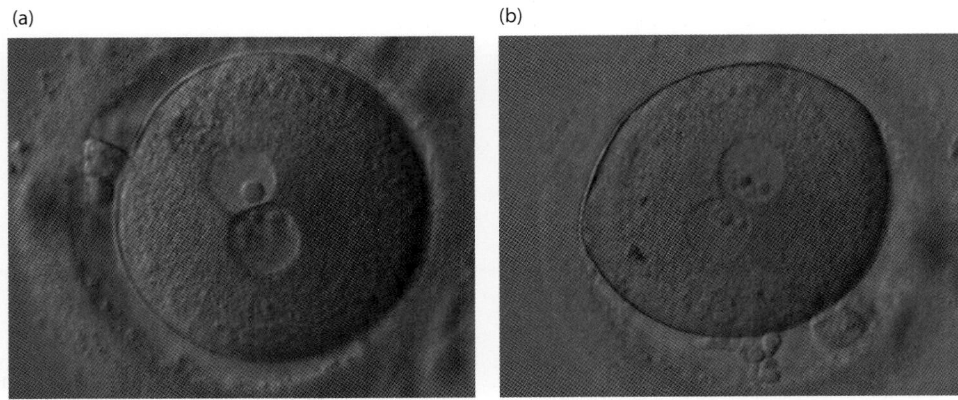

Figure 15.1 (a) Bad-prognosis zygote with an asymmetric pronuclear pattern corresponding to pattern 4 (12) or Z3 (14). (b) Zygote showing optimal pronuclear pattern 0B (12) or Z1 (14) and a clear halo.

before tPBf, particularly if time-lapse techniques are available. However, embryologists are faced with several pronuclear patterns at the time of fertilization assessment. Based on original data from Wright et al. (15), Scott and Smith (11) were the first to attribute zygote morphology with a certain prognostic value for subsequent implantation. In particular, the alignment of nucleoli at the junction of the two pronuclei was found to be a selection criterion for embryo transfer. Since this zygote score did not exclusively rely on the pronuclear pattern but also comprised multiple other parameters, including the appearance of cytoplasm and timing of nuclear membrane breakdown, the actual impact of pronuclear morphology on further outcomes remained unclear.

Thus, Tesarik and Greco (12) were the pioneers in predicting preimplantation development by focusing exclusively on the number and distribution of nucleoli (nucleolar precursor bodies [NPBs]) in each pronucleus. They considered inter-pronuclear synchrony, evaluated 12–20 hours post-IVF/ICSI, as being more important than the actual NPB polarity at the site of pronuclear apposition since they presumed that polarization of nucleoli is not evident from the beginning of pronuclei formation, but rather appears progressively with time (9). According to Tesarik and Greco (12), the optimal synchronized pattern 0 yields 37.3% good-quality embryos compared to all other patterns (27.8%). In addition, the frequency of developmental arrest of pattern 0 zygotes was only 8.5% as compared with 25.6% in the other patterns.

Since all these previous reports were of retrospective character, particular importance must be assigned to a prospective multicenter study of Montag and Van der Ven (3). These authors highlighted that cycles with transfer of at least one embryo derived from pattern 0B (Figure 15.1b), but not pattern 0A, resulted in significantly higher rates of pregnancy (37.9%) and implantation (20.5%) than non-pattern 0B cycles (26.4% and 15.7%). Similar results have been published by others (13) who found significantly increased pregnancy rates (44.8% vs. 30.2%) if embryos derived from zygotes with pattern 0 were transferred. Obviously, NPB polarization at the area of pronuclear contact outdoes pronuclear symmetry.

Recently, Scott et al. (14,16) further refined their score by also creating a single observation zygote score. This so-called Z-score was comparable with the score introduced by Tesarik and Greco (12), since patterns Z1 and Z2 resemble patterns 0B and 0A. Several other authors successfully used the zygote scores of Scott et al. (11,13) and Tesarik and Greco (12) for prognostic purposes (3,13,17–20). Though the grading systems differ slightly in some of these papers, the conclusion is a common one. Zygotes showing pronuclei with approximately the same number and alignment of NPBs in the furrow between the nuclei had the best prognosis in terms of subsequent implantation.

It is noteworthy that Salumets et al. (21) failed to show any correlation between zygote score and pregnancy rate. This is of particular interest because this group only analyzed single-embryo transfers and, consequently, the actual implantation potential could be accurately estimated. Though two different scores were applied (11,12), no correlation to treatment outcome could be demonstrated. This discrepancy in literature results may be explained by the use of different culture media and stimulation protocols and differences in timing of fertilization assessments (e.g., the inclusion of early cleavage in the Scott and Smith [11] scoring system).

An increased incidence of subsequent blastocyst formation in zygotes with optimal patterns of the pronuclei (14,19,22) seems to be consistent with the reported increase in terms of pregnancy rate. Theoretically, a lower blastocyst formation rate in abnormal zygotes could be related to their chromosomal status since there is information from the literature that several pronuclear patterns seem to be associated with aneuploidy (23–26).

In detail, Kahraman and colleagues (25) found a 52.2% rate of chromosomal abnormality in biopsied embryos derived from suspicious zygotes (showing an asymmetric distribution of NPBs), which was significantly lower than the observed 37.6% in the normal control zygotes. Others (26) also confirmed that the position of pronuclei within the cytoplasm, the size and distribution of nucleoli, and the orientation of polar bodies with respect to pronuclei were highly predictive of the presence of chromosomal abnormalities in the corresponding embryos. In this study (26), zygotes with abutted pronuclei, large-sized nucleoli, and polar bodies with small angles subtended by pronuclei and polar bodies were the configurations associated with the highest rates of euploidy. Using the Z-score, it could be shown (24) that Z1 patterns had a significantly higher rate of euploidy (71%) as compared to Z3 (35%) and Z4 (36%) patterns. The same also holds true for the score of Tesarik and Greco (12), since pattern 0 was associated with a minimal rate of aneuploidy (26%), whereas patterns with poor prognosis showed higher rates of up to 83% (23).

It is important to note that not all studies published to date suggest complete reliance on zygote morphology (21,27). One problem is that overall up to 14 different zygote scoring systems have been published so far. On the basis of those papers that made their way into a recent meta-analysis (28), it can be concluded that there is a lack of conclusive data on the clinical efficacy of zygote scoring.

Further evidence on the limited potential of pronuclear scoring comes from time-lapse imaging since none of the tested scoring systems (16,29) were shown to predict the live birth outcome (6). On the other hand, tPNf occurred significantly later in embryos resulting in live birth and was never observed earlier than at 20 hours and 45 minutes (6).

A definite difference between IVF and ICSI cycles with regard to the frequency of good patterns (pattern 0 according to Tesarik and Greco [12]) was reported (3). In particular, superior pronuclear patterns were observed in ICSI cycles. This phenomenon may be due to the above-mentioned accelerated course of development in ICSI (1,30). Zygotes showing this most advanced stage of nuclear polarization seem to reach that stage earlier after ICSI than after conventional IVF (3).

However, the study did not evaluate the position of the pronuclei relative to the presumed polar axis. This arrangement has been reported to relate to embryo quality (31,32). Edwards and Beard (33) suggested that the oocyte may establish this polarity by either ooplasmic or pronuclear rotation towards the second polar body. Such a resetting of a new axis after fertilization is governed by cytoplasmic contraction waves organized by the sperm centrosome (33). Embryos unable to achieve optimal pronuclear orientation, possibly due to shorter cytoplasmic waves (4), may exhibit poor morphology (e.g., uneven cleavage or fragmentation) (31).

ABNORMAL PRONUCLEAR FORMATION AND PATTERNS

Single-pronucleate (1PNs) zygotes can be obtained following IVF and ICSI at frequencies ranging from 2% to 5% (34). They were reported to show a trend towards higher frequency in ICSI (34).

Karyotyping indicated that following IVF more than half of 1PN embryos are in fact diploid, but these studies (35,36) did not differentiate between diploidy produced by fusion of both pronuclei or fertilization by parthenogenetic activation. However, in further studies it could be demonstrated that when embryos were diploid, approximately half of them were fertilized (37,38). Two mechanisms could be responsible for this observation: asynchronous appearance or fusion of both pronuclei (39). If there is no other choice, such IVF embryos could be considered for transfer, particularly if the single pronucleus is larger than regular size.

Both studies dealing with 1PN zygotes generated by ICSI indicated that the vast majority of these were activated but not fertilized (38,39). Such embryos should not be replaced into the patient.

The presence of 3PN zygotes after IVF is the most common fertilization anomaly in humans. This is mostly caused by dispermy (3PN, two polar bodies), and the majority of the corresponding embryos will cleave but stop development at later stages (34). In ICSI, some 4% (34) of zygotes show digynic triploidy, meaning that a single sperm is present in the egg but the second polar body was not extruded (non-disjunction). In this case, the chromosomes of the three pronuclei are organized in a single bipolar spindle at syngamy, indicating that only one centrosome deriving from one sperm is active.

Within 3PN zygotes, a special case is the presence of 2PNs with a third additional small nucleus (Figure 15.2). Since it was shown that this smaller nucleus may contain chromosomal material (unpublished data), it is particularly important not to transfer embryos or blastocysts stemming from such abnormal zygotes. Due to the sometimes small size of these additional nuclei, there is of course a high risk of missing them during routine fertilization checks, especially when using objectives of lower magnification.

Peripheral positioning of pronuclei

Regardless of the pronuclear pattern that the oocyte reflects, it is generally accepted that both pronuclei should be located in the center of the female gamete. Cytoplasmic inclusions,

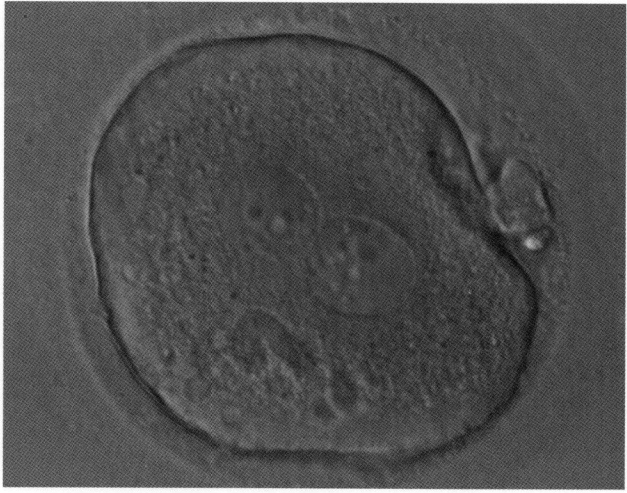

Figure 15.2 Zygote showing two pronuclei with an additional smaller nucleus (2 o'clock position) possibly containing chromosomal material.

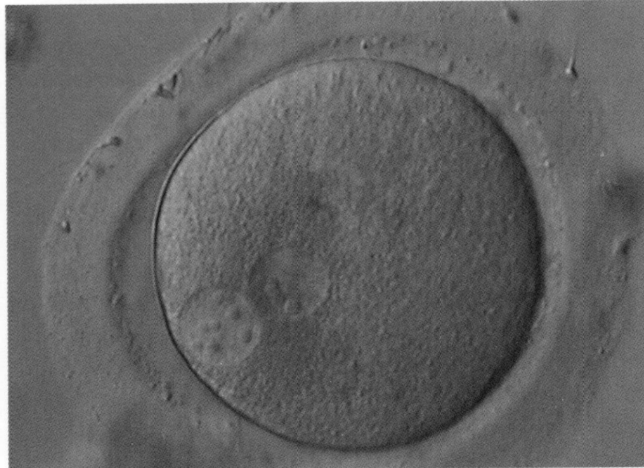

Figure 15.3 *In vitro* fertilization zygote showing peripheral apposition of both pronuclei.

such as dense granularity, large refractile bodies, and/or vacuoles, may displace both pronuclei. However, this scenario can also happen in zygotes with normal homogeneous ooplasm. Any deviation from the presumed optimal central arrangement (e.g., peripheral apposition of both pronuclei) (Figure 15.3) is most likely associated with reduced developmental capacity (31). Considering the fact that the first cleavage plane runs through the contact zone of both pronuclei, it is a frequent phenomenon that the corresponding embryo will show uneven cleavage. This scenario is more frequent in conventional IVF than in ICSI (3.3% vs. 11.8%), probably due to varying sites of sperm entrance in IVF (32) (e.g., near-spindle penetration of the zona, which in turn could force eccentric formation of pronuclei [7]).

Missing alignment of pronuclei

Another problem occasionally arising during fertilization is a failure in alignment of both pronuclei (Figure 15.4), which is caused by an intrinsic defect of the cytoskeleton, or the parental centrosome may cause a complete failure in alignment (11). While it is quite uncommon in assisted reproduction technologies (approximately 1%), it is rather detrimental since the vast majority of zygotes with unaligned pronuclei fail to cleave or show developmental arrest at early stages (12) if not resulting in chromosomal aberrations at all (26).

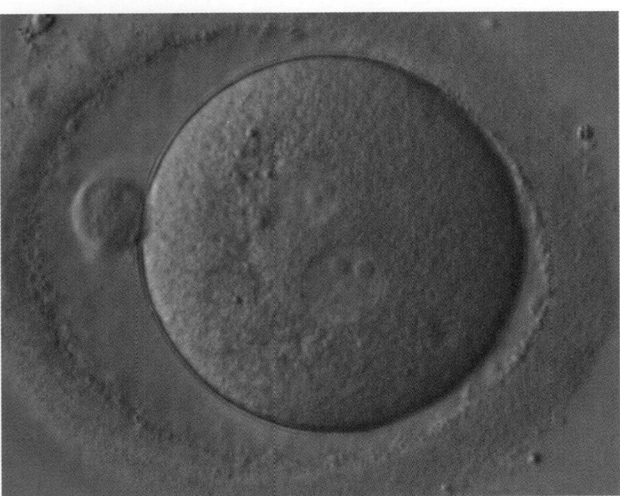

Figure 15.4 Zygote with failure in alignment of both pronuclei.

Uneven size of pronuclei

Though the female pronucleus usually is smaller than its male counterpart (4), more extensive differences in size (>4 μm) may be observed *in vitro* (Figure 15.5). This divergence most likely is the result of problems arising during male pronucleus formation, since *in vitro*-matured oocytes from ICSI with labeled spermatozoa showed proximity of the fluorescent sperm mid-piece remnant to the smaller pronucleus (40). Uneven pronuclear size severely affects the viability of the corresponding embryos since more than 87% were found to be aneuploid, mostly mosaics (41,42). This fact probably led them to arrest at a significantly higher rate than zygotes with pronuclear diameters showing no excessive differences. In addition, a higher incidence of day-2 multinucleation was observed (41).

Undocumented zygotes

Interestingly, 1% of all zygotes do not show pronuclei at all (34). Manor et al. (42) demonstrated that 57% of such undocumented zygotes are normal diploid. If two polar bodies were present on day 1, corresponding embryos may be considered for transfer in case insufficient bipronucleated embryos are available. The most probable reason for this failure in detection is an abnormal developmental speed and/or inaccurate timing of fertilization control. It has also been reported that pronuclei may be hidden to extensive cytoplasmic granularity (34).

CYTOPLASMIC HALO

Immediately prior to pronuclear growth, a microtubule-mediated withdrawal of mitochondria and other

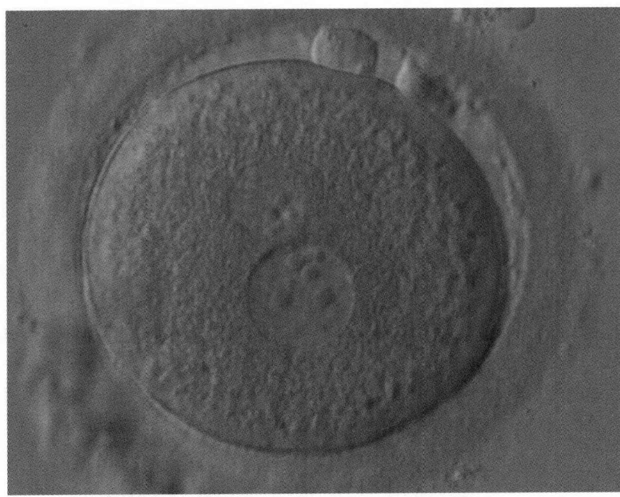

Figure 15.5 Zygote with uneven pronuclear size.

cytoplasmic components contracts from the cortex towards the center of the oocyte, leaving a clear halo around the cortex (4). Since the presence of a halo effect (Figure 15.1b) within the ooplasm may be recognized in 65%–85% of all zygotes (19,21,43), it is less applicable for scoring purposes than the pronuclear pattern. Nevertheless, this particular morphism was found to be correlated with better embryo quality (16,21), increased blastocyst formation on day 5 (44), and a higher pregnancy rate (43).

The physiological role of mitochondrial redistribution in zygotes is still unknown, but it has been speculated that clustering of mitochondria to perinuclear regions may be involved in cell cycle regulation (45–47) (e.g., by means of calcium mobilization and ATP liberation [48–50]). In addition, location of mitochondria next to the pronuclei would allow immature mitochondria, as seen in zygotes (51), to complete maturation, presuming that some input from the nucleus is needed (47).

There is a certain disagreement between most of the studies dealing with cytoplasmic appearance at zygote stage. Some did not distinguish between several types of haloes, thus pooling symmetrical and polar haloes (11,21), whereas others presuppose that symmetrical (43) or extreme haloes (44) are abnormal. In view of this lack of uniformity, our working group (19) set up a prospective trial to investigate the actual influence of certain subtypes of haloes on the preimplantation development of IVF and ICSI embryos. In this paper, haloes were measured accurately in order to see if a light or extreme halo effect would have any impact on subsequent developmental stages. Based on our findings, it was concluded that any halo effect, irrespective of its grade and dimension, is of positive predictive power in terms of blastocyst quality and, consequently, clinical pregnancy rate (19). Neither the method used for insemination (IVF or ICSI) nor the presence of areas of dense cytoplasmic granulation or larger vacuoles affected the zygote in terms of halo performance. Furthermore, it was demonstrated that the pronuclear pattern and halo formation are two distinct parameters (19). In contrast to the pronuclear pattern, no association between halo formation and genetic status of the fertilized egg has been observed (52).

CONCLUSION

During evaluation of zygote morphology, it has to be considered that both halo and pronuclear formation follow a fixed schedule. Since direct ooplasmic placement of a viable spermatozoon is performed in ICSI, thus bypassing most steps of fertilization (including acrosome reaction and zona binding), the further course of development will be somewhat accelerated as compared to conventional IVF. It is of interest that more physiological sperm selected on the basis of its potential to bind to hyaluronic acid did not influence the pronuclear score (53).

Pronuclear morphology and halo characteristics turned out to be unstable independent factors within the dynamic process of fertilization. The degree and morphology of the halo per se have no influence on further outcome. However, the presence of such a halo had positive predictive power. Consequently, halo formation in combination with optimal pronuclear patterns (e.g., those with alignment of fused nucleoli) will characterize a subgroup of oocytes showing a developmental advantage compared to zygotes lacking these positive predictors.

This is in line with recent findings indicating that during syngamy those zygotes with an accelerated breakdown of the pronuclear membranes at 22–25 hours post-insemination or post-injection implanted significantly more frequently than those with delayed dissolution (54). This is not to forget the reported positive correlation between the occurrence of the first mitotic division and the rates of implantation and clinical pregnancy (55–57).

Recently, promising strategies have been published combining the morphological information of zygote stage with other developmental stages (58–62). In detail, sequential assessment of cultured human embryos allowed for accurate prognosis in terms of good-quality blastocyst development (60,61). Others (58) found a relatively high outcome predictability after IVF using a combined score for zygote und embryo morphology and growth rate. Finally, day-3 embryo transfer with combined evaluation at the pronuclear and cleavage stage compared favorably with day-5 blastocyst transfer (59).

This suggests that zygote stage, although being an important developmental phase, should not be used solitarily as a prognostic parameter, but rather morphological information from day 1 should be pooled with that of earlier and/or later stages in order to maximize benefit and minimize the numbers of embryos transferred.

REFERENCES

1. Nagy ZP, Janssenswillen C, Janssens R et al. Timing of oocyte activation, pronucleus formation, and cleavage in humans after intracytoplasmic sperm injection (ICSI) with testicular spermatozoa and after ICSI or *in-vitro* fertilization on sibling oocytes with ejaculated spermatozoa. *Hum Reprod* 1998; 13: 1606–12.
2. van Wissen B, Wolf JP, Bomsel-Helmreich O et al. Timing of pronuclear development and first cleavages in human embryos after subzonal insemination: Influence of sperm phenotype. *Hum Reprod* 1995; 10: 642–8.
3. Montag M, Van der Ven H. Evaluation of pronuclear morphology as the only selection criterion for further embryo culture and transfer: Results of a prospective multicentre study. *Hum Reprod* 2001; 16: 2384–9.
4. Payne D, Flaherty SP, Barry MF et al. Preliminary observations on polar body extrusion and pronuclear formation in human oocytes using time-lapse video cinematography. *Hum Reprod* 1997; 12: 532–41.
5. Ciray HN, Campbell A, Agerholm IE et al. Proposed guidelines on the nomenclature and annotation of dynamic human embryo monitoring by a time-lapse user group. *Hum Reprod* 2014; 29: 2650–60.

6. Azzarello A, Hoest T, Mikkelsen AL. The impact of pronuclei morphology and dynamicity on live birth outcome after time-lapse culture. *Hum Reprod* 2012; 27: 2649–57.
7. Van Blerkom J, Davis P, Merriman J et al. Nuclear and cytoplasmic dynamics of sperm penetration, pronuclear formation and microtubule organization during fertilization and early preimplantation development in the human. *Hum Reprod Update* 1995; 1: 429–61.
8. Scott L. The biological basis of non-invasive strategies for selection of human oocytes and embryos. *Hum Reprod Update* 2003; 9: 137–249.
9. Tesarik J, Kopecny V. Development of human male pronucleus: Ultrastructure and timing. *Gamete Res* 1989; 24: 135–49.
10. Van Blerkom J. Occurrence and developmental consequences of aberrant cellular organization in meiotically mature oocytes after exogenous ovarian hyperstimulation. *J Electron Microsc Tech* 1990; 16: 324–46.
11. Scott LA, Smith S. The successful use of pronuclear embryo transfers the day following oocyte retrieval. *Hum Reprod* 1998; 13: 1003–13.
12. Tesarik J, Greco E. The probability of abnormal preimplantation development can be predicted by a single static observation on pronuclear stage morphology. *Hum Reprod* 1999; 14: 1318–23.
13. Tesarik J, Junca AM, Hazout A et al. Embryos with high implantation potential after intracytoplasmic sperm injection can be recognized by a simple, noninvasive examination of pronuclear morphology. *Hum Reprod* 2000; 15: 1396–99.
14. Scott LA, Alvero R, Leondires M. The morphology of human pronuclear embryos is positively related to blastocyst development and implantation. *Hum Reprod* 2000; 15: 2394–403.
15. Wright G, Wiker S, Elsner C et al. Observations on the morphology of pronuclei and nucleoli in human zygotes and implications for cryopreservation. *Hum Reprod* 1990; 5: 109–15.
16. Scott L. Pronuclear scoring as a predictor of embryo development. *Reprod Biomed Online* 2003; 6: 201–14.
17. Ludwig M, Schöpper B, Al-Hasani S, Diedrich K. Clinical use of a PN stage score following intracytoplasmic sperm injection: impact on pregnancy rates under the conditions of the German embryo protection law. *Hum Reprod* 2000; 15: 325–9.
18. Wittemer C, Bettahar-Lebugle K, Ohl J. Zygote evaluation: An efficient tool for embryo selection. *Hum Reprod* 2000; 15: 2591–7.
19. Ebner T, Moser M, Sommergruber M et al. Presence, but not type or degree of extension, of a cytoplasmic halo has a significant influence on preimplantation development and implantation behaviour. *Hum Reprod* 2003; 18: 2406–12.
20. Arroyo G, Veiga A, Santaló J et al. Developmental prognosis for zygotes based on pronuclear pattern: Usefulness of pronuclear scoring. *J Assist Reprod Genetics* 2007; 14: 173–81.
21. Salumets A, Hydén-Granskog C, Suikkari AM et al. The predictive value of pronuclear morphology of zygotes in the assessment of human embryo quality. *Hum Reprod* 2001; 16: 2177–81.
22. Balaban B, Urman B, Isiklar A et al. The effect of pronuclear morphology on embryo quality parameters and blastocyst transfer outcome. *Hum Reprod* 2001; 16: 2357–61.
23. Balaban B, Yakin K, Urman B et al. Pronuclear morphology predicts embryo development and chromosome constitution. *Reprod Biomed Online* 2004; 8: 695–700.
24. Chen CK, Shen GY, Horng SG et al. The relationship of pronuclear stage morphology and chromosome status at cleavage stage. *J Assist Reprod Genetics* 2003; 20: 413–20.
25. Kahraman S, Kumtepe Y, Sertyel S et al. Pronuclear morphology scoring and chromosomal status of embryos in severe male infertility. *Hum Reprod* 2002; 17; 3193–200.
26. Gianaroli L, Magli MC, Ferraretti AP et al. Pronuclear morphology and chromosomal abnormalities as scoring criteria for embryo selection. *Fertil Steril* 2003; 80: 341–9.
27. Arroyo G, Santaló J, Parriego M et al. Pronuclear morphology, embryo development and chromosome constitution. *Reprod Biomed Online* 2010; 20: 649–55.
28. Nicoli A, Palomba S, Capodanno F et al. Pronuclear morphology evaluation for fresh *in vitro* fertilization (IVF) and intracytoplasmic sperm injection (ICSI) cycles: A systematic review. *J Ovarian Res* 2013; 12: 64.
29. Alpha Scientists in Reproductive Medicine and ESHRE Special Interest Group of Embryology. The Istanbul consensus workshop on embryo assessment: Proceedings of an expert meeting. *Hum Reprod* 2011; 26: 1270–83.
30. Sakkas D, Shoukir Y, Chardonnens D et al. Early cleavage of human embryos to the two-cell stage after intracytoplasmic sperm injection as an indicator of embryo viability. *Hum Reprod* 1998; 13: 182–7.
31. Garello C, Baker H, Rai J et al. Pronuclear orientation, polar body placement, and embryo quality after intracytoplasmic sperm injection and *in-vitro* fertilization: Further evidence for polarity in human oocytes? *Hum Reprod* 1999; 14: 2588–94.
32. Kattera S, Chen C. Developmental potential of human pronuclear zygotes in relation to their pronuclear orientation. *Hum Reprod* 2004; 19: 294–9.
33. Edwards RG, Beard HK. Oocyte polarity and cell determination in early mammalian embryos. *Mol Hum Reprod* 1997; 3: 863–905.
34. Munné S, Cohen J. Chromosome abnormalities in human embryos. *Hum Reprod Update* 1997; 6: 842–55.

35. Plachot M. Chromosome analysis of oocytes and embryos. In: *Preimplantation Genetics*. Verlinsky Y, Kuliev (eds). Plenum Press, New York, NY, pp. 103–12.
36. Staessen C, Janssenwillen C, Devroey P et al. Cytogenetic and morphological observations of single pronucleated human oocytes after *in-vitro* fertilization. *Hum Reprod* 1993; 8: 221–3.
37. Sultan KM, Munné S, Palermo GD et al. Chromosomal status of uni-pronuclear human zygotes following *in-vitro* fertilization and intracytoplasmic sperm injection. *Hum Reprod* 1995; 10: 132–6.
38. Staessen C, Van Steirteghem AC. The chromosomal constitution of embryos developing from abnormally fertilized oocytes after intracytoplasmic sperm injection and conventional *in-vitro* fertilization. *Hum Reprod* 1997; 12: 321–7.
39. Levron J, Munné S, Willadsen S et al. Male and female genomes associated in a single pronucleus in human zygotes. *Biol Reprod* 1995; 52: 653–7.
40. Goud P, Goud A, Van Oostveldt P et al. Fertilization abnormalities und pronucleus size asynchrony after intracytoplasmic sperm injection are related to oocyte post maturity. *Fertil Steril* 1999; 72: 245–52.
41. Sadowy S, Tomkin G, Munné S et al. Impaired development of zygotes with uneven pronuclear size. *Zygote* 1998; 6: 137–41.
42. Manor D, Drugan A, Stein D et al. Unequal pronuclear size—A powerful predictor of embryonic chromosome anomalies. *J Assist Reprod Genetics* 1999; 16: 385–9.
43. Stalf T, Herrero J, Mehnert C et al. Influence of polarization effects and pronuclei on embryo quality and implantation in an IVF program. *J Assist Reprod Genetics* 2002; 19: 355–62.
44. Zollner U, Zollner KP, Hartl G et al. The use of a detailed zygote score after IVF/ICSI to obtain good quality blastocysts: The German experience. *Hum Reprod* 2002; 17: 1327–33.
45. Barnett DK, Kimura J, Bavister BD. Translocation of active mitochondria during hamster preimplantation embryo development studied by confocal laser scanning microscopy. *Dev Dyn* 1996; 205: 64–72.
46. Wu GJ, Simerly C, Zoran SS et al. Microtubule and chromatin dynamics during fertilization and early development in rhesus monkeys, and regulation by intracellular calcium ions. *Biol Reprod* 1996; 55: 260–70.
47. Bavister BD, Squirrell JM. Mitochondrial distribution and function in oocytes and early embryos. *Hum Reprod* 2000; 15(Suppl 2): 189–98.
48. Sousa M, Barros A, Silva J et al. Developmental changes in calcium content of ultrastructurally distinct subcellular compartments of pre-implantation human embryos. *Mol Hum Reprod* 1997; 3: 83–90.
49. Diaz G, Setzu M, Zucca A et al. Subcellular heterogeneity of mitochondrial membrane potential: Relationship with organelle distribution and intercellular contacts in normal, hypoxic and apoptotic cells. *J Cell Sci* 1999; 112: 1077–84.
50. Van Blerkom J, Davis P, Alexander S. Differential mitochondrial distribution in human pronuclear embryos leads to disproportionate inheritance between blastomeres: Relationship to microtubular organization, ATP content and competence. *Hum Reprod* 2000; 15: 2621–33.
51. Motta PM, Nottola SA, Makabe S et al. Mitochondrial morphology in human fetal and adult gene cells. *Hum Reprod* 2000; 15(Suppl): 129–47.
52. Coskun S, Hellani A, Jaroudi K et al. Nuclear precursor body distribution in pronuclei is correlated to chromosomal embryos. *Reprod Biomed Online* 2003; 7: 86–90.
53. Van den Bergh M, Fahy-Deshe M, Hohl MK. Pronuclear zygote score following intracytoplasmic injection of hyaluronan-bound spermatozoa: A prospective randomized study. *Reprod Biomed Online* 2009; 19: 796–801.
54. Fancsovits P, Toth L, Takacz ZF et al. Early pronuclear breakdown is a good indicator of embryo quality and viability. *Fertil Steril* 2005; 84: 881–7.
55. Shoukir Y, Campana A, Farley T et al. Early cleavage of *in-vitro* fertilized human embryos to the 2-cell stage: A novel indicator of embryo quality und viability. *Hum Reprod* 1997; 12: 1531–6.
56. Sakkas D, Percival G, D'Arcy Y et al. Assessment of early cleaving in *in vitro* fertilized human embryos at the 2-cell stage before transfer improves embryo selection. *Fertil Steril* 2001; 76: 1150–6.
57. Lundin K, Bergh C, Hardarson T. Early embryo cleavage is a strong indicator of embryo quality in human IVF. *Hum Reprod* 2001; 16: 2652–7.
58. De Placido G, Wilding M, Strina I et al. High outcome predictability after IVF using a combined score for zygote und embryo morphology und growth rate. *Hum Reprod* 2002; 17: 2402–9.
59. Rienzi L, Ubaldi F, Iacobelli M et al. Day 3 embryo transfer with combined evaluation at the pronuclear and cleavage stage compares favourably with day 5 blastocyst transfer. *Hum Reprod* 2002; 17: 1852–5.
60. Lan KC, Huang FJ, Lin YC et al. The predictive value of using a combined Z-score und day 3 embryo morphology score in the assessment of embryo survival on day 5. *Hum Reprod* 2003; 18: 1299–306.
61. Neuber E, Rinaudo P, Trimarchi JR et al. Sequential assessment of individually cultured human embryos as an indicator of subsequent good quality blastocyst development. *Hum Reprod* 2003; 18: 1307–12.
62. Alvarez C, Taronger R, Garcia-Garrido C et al. Zygote score and status 1 or 2 days after cleavage and assisted reproduction outcome. *Int J Gynaecol Obstet* 2008; 101: 16–20.

Culture systems for the human embryo 16

DAVID K. GARDNER and MICHELLE LANE

INTRODUCTION

Embryo culture is frequently mistaken for a relatively simple procedure. In reality, it is a complex task, requiring proactive quality control and quality assurance programs to ensure the optimum performance of the laboratory and equipment, together with a high level of training for embryologists. Furthermore, a sufficient number of suitable incubation chambers are required to maintain a stable environment for development *in vitro*. Hence, embryo culture is far more involved than simply using the appropriate culture media formulations. Consequently, in order to optimize embryo development *in vitro* and maintain viability to ensure the delivery of a healthy baby, it is essential to consider embryo culture as a system in its entirety. The embryo culture system consists of the media, macromolecules, gas phase, type of medium overlay, the culture vessel, the incubation chamber, ambient air quality, and even the embryologists themselves. The concept of an embryo culture system successfully highlights the interactions that exist not only between the embryo and its physical surroundings, but also between all parameters within the laboratory (Figure 16.1). Only by taking such a holistic approach can one optimize embryo development *in vitro* and maintain success rates.

Working *in vitro* (literally "in glass") means that stressors can be present in the culture system, which are not evident within the lumen of the female reproductive tract. Stressors identified in the embryology laboratory that can have a negative impact on gametes and embryos include: transient temperature shifts as gametes and embryos are manipulated; changes to the levels of carbon dioxide and hence changes in pH when embryos are taken in and out of an incubator; potential physical stress should pipetting be too vigorous; atmospheric oxygen; and the accumulation of ammonium from amino acids. Of concern is that these stressors have the capacity to interact with each other and create an even greater negative synergy (10).

Finally, it is also important to appreciate that it is not feasible to make a good embryo from poor-quality gametes (the current investigations on oocyte rejuvenation through mitochondrial transfer have yet to be validated). Rather, the role of the laboratory is to maintain the inherent viability of the oocyte and sperm from which the embryo is derived. Ultimately, the success of *in vitro* fertilization (IVF) is also dependent on the quality of the ovarian stimulation decided by the physician and the preparation/development of a receptive endometrium, as well as on patient factors including the impact of their lifestyle choices (especially diet), hence emphasizing the need for a broader perspective of patient management as well as laboratory management. In order to ensure consistent successful outcomes, it is paramount that appropriate communication pathways exist between physicians and scientists to ensure all variables are considered and discussed, and that action plans are in place so that changes can be rapidly implemented in response to any concerns.

THE HUMAN EMBRYO IN CULTURE

Serendipitously for the field of human IVF, the human embryo exhibits a considerable degree of plasticity, enabling it to develop under a wide variety of culture conditions. Indeed, it appears that the human preimplantation embryo is the most resilient of all mammalian species studied to date. However, this should be perceived as a reflection of the ability of the human embryo to adapt to its surroundings and not our ability to culture it. Undoubtedly, having to adapt to suboptimal collection and/or culture conditions comes at the cost of impaired viability and potentially compromised pregnancy outcomes (11,12). Therefore, it is important to focus on the generation of healthy embryos, as it is clear that embryo development in culture, even to the blastocyst stage, does not necessarily equate to the development of a viable embryo (13). Implantation rate (fetal heart rate, as opposed to fetal sac) is an important parameter to report, is extremely important in evaluating the performance of the IVF laboratory, and provides relatively quick information on cycle performance. However, the definition of viability is best described as the ability of the embryo to implant successfully and give rise to a normal, healthy term baby. Subsequently, live birth rates should always be reported and considered, as they reflect the true efficacy of a given IVF system.

Today, clinics are not only faced with a multitude of embryo culture media to choose from and whether to employ a reduced oxygen concentration, but also with the decision of whether to transfer at the cleavage or the blastocyst stage. However, with the publication of an evidence-based Cochrane review (14) and meta-analysis (15) demonstrating a clear increase in pregnancy and implantation rates and reduced pregnancy loss following blastocyst culture, and with a move to performing preimplantation genetic screening through trophectoderm biopsy, there is an increasing awareness and demand for laboratories to be able to support extended culture (13). It is the aim of this chapter to discuss the types of media and culture systems currently available and to describe how they can be implemented in a clinical setting irrespective of the day of transfer.

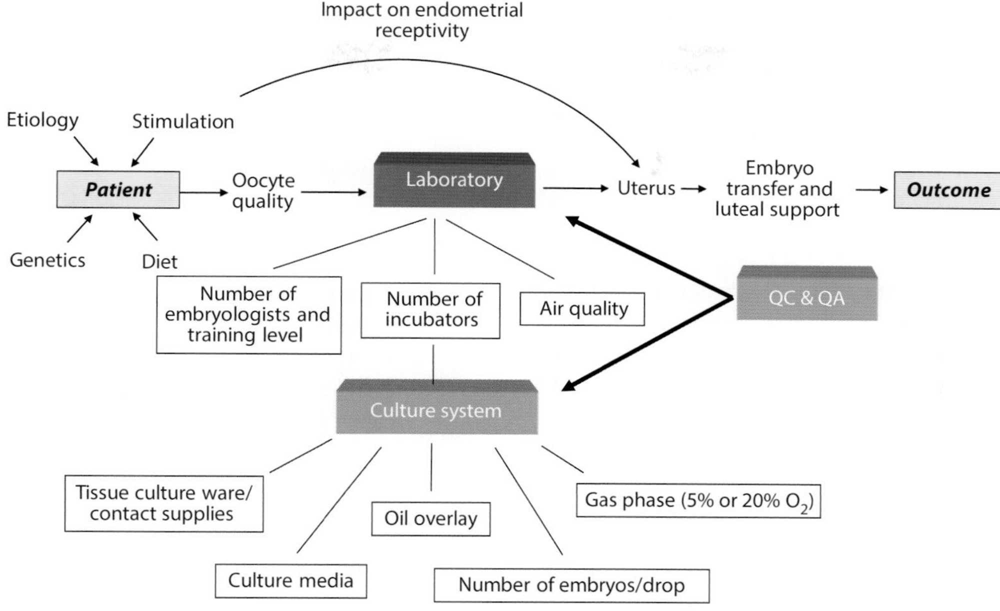

Figure 16.1 The relationship between patient stimulation, the laboratory, and transfer outcome in human *in vitro* fertilization (IVF). This figure serves to illustrate the complex and interdependent nature of human IVF treatment. For example, the stimulation regimen used not only impacts on oocyte quality (and hence embryo physiology and viability (1)), but can also affect subsequent endometrial receptivity (2–5). Furthermore, the health and dietary status of the patient can have a profound effect on the subsequent developmental capacity of the oocyte and embryo (6,7). The dietary status of patients attending the IVF clinic is typically not considered as a compounding variable, but growing data would indicate this should be otherwise. In the schematic, the laboratory has been broken down into its core components, only one of which is the culture system. The culture system has in turn been broken down into its components, only one of which is the culture media. Therefore, it would appear rather simplistic to assume that by changing only one part of the culture system (i.e., culture media) one is going to mimic the results of a given laboratory or clinic. One of the biggest impacts on the success of a laboratory and culture system is the level of QC and QA in place. For example, one should never assume that anything coming into the laboratory that has not been pretested with a relevant bioassay (e.g., mouse embryo assay [MEA]) is safe merely because a previous lot has performed satisfactorily. Only a small percentage of the contact supplies and tissue culture ware used in IVF comes suitably tested. Therefore, it is essential to assume that everything entering the IVF laboratory without a suitable pretest is embryotoxic until proven otherwise. In our programs, the one-cell MEA is employed to prescreen every lot of tissue culture ware that enters the program (i.e., plastics that are approved for tissue culture). Around 25% of all such material fails the one-cell MEA (in a simple medium lacking protein after the first 24 hours) (8). Therefore, if one does not perform QC to this level, one in four of all contact supplies used clinically will be embryotoxic. In reality, many programs cannot allocate the resources required for this level of QC and when embryo quality is compromised in the laboratory it is the media that are held responsible, when in fact the lab ware is often the culprit. *Abbreviations*: QA, quality assurance; QC, quality control. (Modified from Gardner DK, Lane M. *Reprod Biomed Online* 2003; 6: 470–81, with permission.) (9)

IMPACT OF SINGLE-EMBRYO TRANSFER ON THE LABORATORY

It is evident that with the development of enhanced culture systems and better methods for embryo selection (see Chapter 17) and cryopreservation (Chapters 22 and 23), the move to single-embryo transfer (SET) for most patients is now a practical reality. Indeed, in several countries this is mandated. Far from being exceptional, SET (or single-blastocyst transfer) is now considered best practice for the majority of patients that seek IVF treatment (16) (Chapter 58). One of the impacts of SET is the increased reliance on a successful cryopreservation program. Therefore, an important consideration in assessing the efficacy of any culture system is its ability to produce high-quality embryos that can survive cryopreservation by either freezing and thawing, or by vitrification followed by warming, as this has significant implications for cumulative pregnancy rates per retrieval. As we shall reveal, the culture conditions used to support embryo development have a profound effect on cryopreservation outcome.

DYNAMICS OF EMBRYO AND MATERNAL PHYSIOLOGY

Before attempting to culture any cell type, be it embryonic or somatic, it is important to consider the physiology of the cell in order to establish its nutrient requirements. The mammalian embryo represents an intriguing situation in that it undergoes significant changes in its physiology, molecular regulation, and metabolism during the preimplantation period. The preimplantation human embryo is a highly dynamic entity that changes its needs as development proceeds. Indeed, it goes from being one of the most quiescent tissues in the body (the oocyte) to being amongst the most metabolically active (the blastocyst) within just four days (11,17,18). Interestingly, the pronucleate oocyte, like the metaphase II oocyte from which it was derived, exhibits relatively low levels of oxygen consumption and has a preference for the carboxylic acid pyruvate as its primary energy source (19,20). Lactate can be utilized as the sole substrate from the two-cell stage, but glucose is only consumed and utilized in relatively small amounts by the early embryo (21). The balance of mitochondrial and cytoplasmic metabolism is critical at these early stages of development for maintaining adequate levels of ATP production (22). However, despite the low levels of biosynthetic activity at these early stages of development, there is an increasing awareness of a significant amount of remodeling of the nucleus. For example, there are major changes in methylation and acetylation levels, with many of the processes involved still to be elucidated (23–25). Nevertheless, what is critical is that many key developmental events, such as activation of the egg and regulation of methylation and acetylation, are regulated by proteins whose activities are dependent on metabolic regulation (26–29). Therefore, maintenance of metabolic homeostasis at these early stages is paramount for the maintenance of viability. Consequently, the environment of the early embryo provided by the culture media continues to be a major focus of the culture system in the laboratory (11).

As development proceeds and energy demands increase with cell multiplication, transcription following activation of the embryonic genome, and the subsequent increase in protein synthesis, there is a concomitant increase in glucose utilization. By the blastocyst stage, the embryo exhibits high oxygen utilization and an ability to readily utilize glucose, along with other energy sources. Table 16.1 highlights some of the differences between the pre- and post-compacted embryo (17). In many ways, the physiology of the cells of the embryo prior to compaction, and hence before the formation of a transporting epithelium, can be likened to unicellular organisms (30). This in part explains why those amino acids present at high levels in the oviduct and classified as "non-essential" for tissue culture purposes are beneficial to the cleavage-stage embryo, as they confer stability to several key cell functions, as described below.

Within the human female reproductive tract, the nutrients available mirror the changing nutrient preference of the embryo. At the time when the embryo resides in the oviduct, the fluid within is characterized by relatively high concentrations of pyruvate (0.32 mM) and lactate (10.5 mM), and a relatively low concentration of glucose (0.5 mM) (31). In contrast, uterine fluid is characterized by relatively low levels of pyruvate (0.1 mM) and lactate (5.87 mM), and a higher concentration of glucose (3.15 mM), consistent with the changes in embryo energy production. The significance of these nutrient gradients in regulating embryo development has been questioned (32). However, it remains the contention of the authors that these nutrient gradients provide not only appropriate stage-specific energy substrates, but also provide stage-specific signals not just for metabolism, but also for the control of molecular signaling (18,29,33,34).

Table 16.1 Differences in embryo physiology pre- and post-compaction

Pre-compaction	Post-compaction
Low biosynthetic activity	High biosynthetic activity
Low QO_2	High QO_2
Pyruvate preferred nutrient	Glucose preferred nutrient
Requirement for specific amino acids including alanine, aspartate, glutamate, glycine, proline, serine, and taurine	Requirement for a more comprehensive group of amino acids
Maternal genome	Embryonic genome
Individual cells	Transporting epithelium
One cell type	Two distinct cell types: inner cell mass and trophectoderm

SUSCEPTIBILITY OF THE PREIMPLANTATION EMBRYO TO STRESS

There is an increasing understanding in mammalian embryology that the early embryo is highly adaptive to its environment. The embryo appears to have the ability to continue development, even to the blastocyst stage, at the cost of normal cellular processes and checkpoints that may be essential for viability. Therefore, as a result many embryos can appear to be morphologically normal while at a cellular level are actually highly perturbed and unlikely to be viable (12,30). It is clear from animal models, where invasive assessments allow additional insight, that disruptions to molecular pathways, including stress response pathways, frequently occur in the absence of any changes to embryo morphology. Furthermore, frequently these perturbations are permissive of implantation, affecting subsequent fetal growth (35–37). Consequently, a key focus of the embryology laboratory should be to ensure its gamete collection and culture system are able to maintain normal cellular development. Although the human embryo has a plasticity to adapt to its environment, as already highlighted, this is at a cost of cellular regulation either through metabolic adaptations or adaptations at a molecular level (12,30). Therefore, the laboratory should seek to employ systems that reduce these adaptations, thereby maintaining viability (10).

Cleavage-stage versus post-compaction embryos and stress

As a result of its more "primitive" physiology, the pre-compaction-stage embryo is highly susceptible to stress compared to the post-compaction-stage embryo. A stress

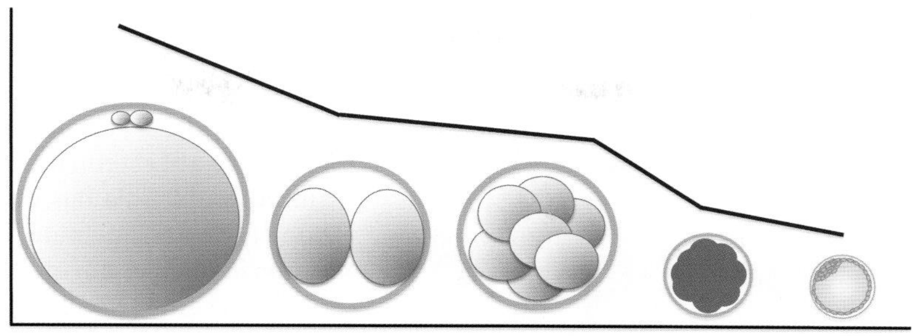

Figure 16.2 Relative impact of chemical and physical stress on the preimplantation embryo (from oocyte to blastocyst stage), representing the stage-specific differences in the embryo's response to stress. The fertilized oocyte is more sensitive than the cleavage-stage embryo, which in turn is more susceptible to stress than an embryo post-compaction. Of all stages, the blastocyst is least perturbed by such factors. (From Wale PL, Gardner DK. *Hum Reprod Update* 2016; 22: 2–22, with permission.)

applied *in vitro* at the pronucleate oocyte (2PN) to the eight-cell stage can have devastating effects on the normal cellular physiology and viability of the subsequent blastocyst and fetus (Figure 16.2) (30,38–40). At these early stages of development prior to activation of the embryonic genome, the embryo possesses only limited capacity at a molecular level to respond to a stress. In somatic cells, when a cell finds itself in a hostile environment it can activate a cascade of molecular signaling pathways to engage systems for maintaining normal cell function. However, the pre-compaction-stage embryo has a limited capacity for gene transcription (41) and therefore the human embryo prior to the eight-cell stage is highly vulnerable to any perturbed environment. At these early stages of embryo development prior to compaction, there is limited capacity to maintain normal cellular functions such as regulation of intracellular pH (pHi), alleviation of oxidative stress, and ionic homeostasis (12,30). Therefore, a stress applied prior to compaction can result in major disruptions to subsequent viability. In contrast, the application of the same stress post-compaction and post-embryonic genome activation typically has limited negative impact on subsequent developmental competence (30,39,40).

Further, it is apparent that effects of a stress can be masked at the level of morphological assessment and may only become evident downstream of the stress itself. For example, it has been shown that the detrimental effects of a stress applied at the early stage of development during handling and culture of the oocyte and 2PN may not be evident until the blastocyst stage. Even then, the effects may only be at a subcellular level with the embryo having reduced metabolic capacity, high levels of apoptosis, and an altered molecular profile, which ultimately result in a reduction in pregnancy rate (38–40). Therefore, the conditions employed for the collection and culture of the human cleavage-stage embryo directly affect the ability of the embryo to implant and form a viable pregnancy, independent of morphological assessments within the laboratory. The inability of morphology alone to distinguish viable and non-viable embryos highlights a major limitation in the field and reaffirms the need for the development of more diagnostic procedures to quantitate normal development (42) (see Chapter 17).

Composition of culture media

There are several extensive treatises on the composition of embryo culture media (20,43–50), and it is beyond the scope of this chapter to discuss in detail the role of individual medium components. However, two key components—amino acids and macromolecules—will be considered briefly due to their significant impact on cycle outcome. Understanding their effects on embryo physiology will greatly assist clinics to make a more informed decision regarding their choice of culture media.

Amino acids

It is certainly the case that the human embryo can grow in the absence of amino acids. The real question is: *how well* do they develop in their absence and how healthy are the resultant embryos? There are several reasons for the inclusion of amino acids in embryo culture media. Oviduct and uterine fluids contain significant levels of free amino acids (51–56), while both oocytes and embryos possess specific transport systems for amino acids (57) to maintain an endogenous pool (58). Amino acids are readily taken up and metabolized by the embryo (59,60). Table 16.2 lists the roles amino acids fulfill during the pre- and peri-implantation period of mammalian embryo development.

Oviduct and uterine fluids are characterized by high concentrations of the amino acids alanine, aspartate, glutamate, glycine, proline, serine, and taurine (51–56). With the exception of taurine, the amino acids at high concentrations in oviduct fluid bear striking homology to those amino acids present in Eagle's non-essential amino acids (71). Studies on the embryos of several mammalian species, such as mouse (72–75), hamster (76,77), sheep (78,79), cow (80,81), and human (82,83), have all demonstrated that the inclusion of amino acids in the culture medium enhances embryo development to the blastocyst stage.

Significantly, it has been demonstrated that the preimplantation embryo exhibits a switch in amino acid requirements as development proceeds. Up to the

Table 16.2 Functions of amino acids during preimplantation mammalian embryo development

Role	Reference
Biosynthetic precursors	(61)
Energy source	(62)
Regulators of energy metabolism	(11,22)
Osmolytes	(63)
Buffers of intracellular pH	(64)
Antioxidants	(65)
Chelators	(66)
Signaling	(67,68)
Regulation of differentiation	(69,70)

eight-cell stage, non-essential amino acids and glutamine increase cleavage rates (i.e., those amino acids present at the highest levels in oviduct fluid stimulate the cleavage-stage embryo) (69,81,84). However, after compaction, non-essential amino acids and glutamine increase blastocoel formation and hatching, while the essential amino acids stimulate cleavage rates and increase development of the inner cell mass (ICM) in the blastocyst (38,69). Recently, the essential amino acid threonine has been shown to be important in the maintenance of pluripotency in mouse embryonic stem cells (85). Importantly, amino acids have been reported to increase the viability of cultured embryos from several species after transfer to recipients (43,69,79), as well as increasing embryo development in culture. In the mouse, equivalent implantation rates to *in vivo*-developed blastocysts have been achieved when pronucleate oocytes were cultured with non-essential amino acids to the eight-cell stage followed by culture with all 20 amino acids from the eight-cell stage to the blastocyst (69).

The terms "non-essential" and "essential" have little meaning in terms of embryo development and differentiation; rather, they reflect the requirements of certain somatic cells *in vitro* (71). More appropriate terminology would reflect the ability of the non-essential group to stimulate early cleavage (cleavage amino acids [CAAs]), while the essential group stimulate the development of the ICM. The reasons for this switch undoubtedly stem from the nature of the CAAs: they act as strong intracellular buffers of pH due to their zwitterionic nature (76), and they are able to chelate toxins. As discussed, prior to compaction the blastomeres of the mammalian embryo appear to behave like unicellular organisms and therefore use exogenous amino acids to regulate their homeostasis. In contrast, the generation of a transporting epithelium postcompaction, enables, the embryo to regulate its internal environment and is not as dependent on the non-essential amino acids to regulate intracellular function (64).

It has been shown that even a transient exposure (of about five minutes) of mouse zygotes to medium lacking amino acids impairs subsequent developmental potential, providing further evidence of the significance of amino acids (86). During this five-minute period in a simple medium the zygote loses its entire endogenous pool of amino acids, which takes several hours of transport to replenish after returning the embryo to medium with amino acids. This has direct implications for the collection of oocytes, and more importantly the manipulation of denuded oocytes during intracytoplasmic sperm injection (ICSI), where the inclusion of amino acids in the holding medium will decrease or prevent intracellular stress (see below).

Similarly, the work of Ho et al. (87) on gene expression in mouse embryos goes some way to confirming this hypothesis, in that gene expression in mouse embryos cultured in the presence of amino acids was comparable to that of embryos developed *in vivo*. In contrast, mouse embryos cultured in the absence of amino acids (i.e., in a medium based on a simple salt solution) exhibited aberrant gene expression and altered imprinting of the H19 gene (88). Hence, the clinical use of any medium lacking amino acids, whether it be for gametes or embryos, should no longer be considered appropriate.

Cautionary tale

Even though the formulations of embryo culture media have improved significantly over the years, and for the most part have become more physiological in their basis, there is nothing physiological about a polystyrene culture dish. Therefore, one has to be careful about *in vitro* artifacts induced by a static environment. A good example of this is the production of ammonium by both embryo metabolism of amino acids (89) and by the spontaneous breakdown of amino acids in the culture medium once incubated at 37°C (Figure 16.3a) (72). Ammonium build-up in culture medium not only has negative effects on embryo development and differentiation in culture (72,78,90), but can also affect subsequent fetal growth rates and normality at a concentration of around 300 μM (38,91). Furthermore, it has been shown that ammonium affects embryo metabolism, pHi regulation, and gene expression in both the mouse and human (92–94), and that perturbations induced by ammonium are further compromised by its interaction with atmospheric oxygen (discussed in more detail later) (95).

As amino acids are such important regulators of embryo development, it is essential to alleviate this *in vitro* problem. The immediate answer is to renew the culture medium, thereby bringing the ammonium concentration under control. A second and complementary solution is to replace the most labile amino acid, glutamine, with a dipeptide form such as alanyl-glutamine. This dipeptide has the advantage of not breaking down at 37°C. Therefore, media containing this stable form of glutamine produce significantly lower levels of ammonium.

Although there is some debate as to the level of concern one should place on ammonium toxicity in culture medium (96,97), there are growing data to support the appearance of ammonium in the culture medium

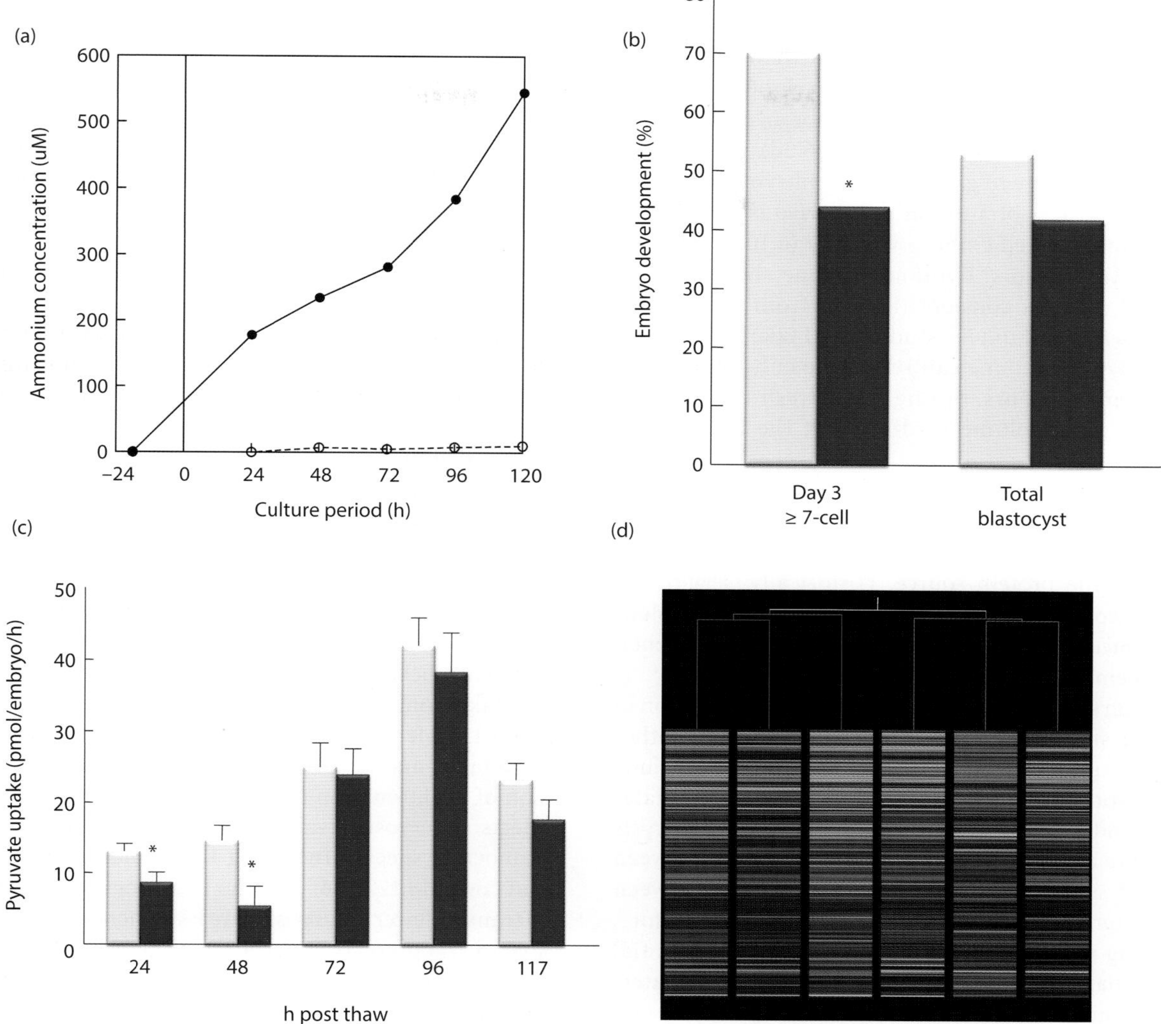

Figure 16.3 (a) Production of ammonium in the culture medium (lacking embryos) by the spontaneous breakdown of amino acids in culture media. Solid circles, $KSOM^{AA}$; open circles, G1/G2. The media were placed in the incubator at 4 p.m. the day before culture for equilibration purposes. The line at time zero represents when embryos would be placed into culture (although these measurements were taken in the absence of embryos). Medium $KSOM^{AA}$ contains 1 mM glutamine and therefore releases significant levels of ammonium into the culture medium. Media G1/G2 do not contain glutamine, but rather the stable dipeptide form, alanyl-glutamine, and therefore these media do not release significant levels of ammonium. At a concentration of just 75 μmol/L, ammonium can induce a 24 hour developmental delay in mouse fetal development by day 15 and induces the neural tube defect exencephaly in 20% of all fetuses. (b) Ammonium significantly reduces the development of the cleavage-stage human embryo. Pronucleate oocytes were exposed to an increasing ammonium gradient (93). Control media (open bars), presence of ammonium (red bars); significantly different from no ammonium, $p < 0.05$. (c) Ammonium significantly compromises human embryo metabolism. Pyruvate uptake was significantly reduced by ammonium at 24 and 48 hours of culture. Control media (open bars), presence of ammonium (red bars); significantly different from no ammonium, $p < 0.05$. (d) Ammonium significantly impairs human blastocyst gene expression. Heat map representation with hierarchical clustering of altered genes in human blastocysts following ammonium exposure and separation of control (green lines) and three ammonium (red lines) samples into distinct branches. Gene expression is related to color, with red representing the highest levels of gene up-regulation and blue representing down-regulation. ([b,c,d] From Gardner DK et al. *Reproduction* 2013; 146: 49–61, with permission.)

over time (72,90,98,99) (Figure 16.3a) and its toxicity to embryos, including those of humans (90,93). Indeed, an analysis of the impact of culture media composition on live birth rates and the subsequent development of the children conceived has been reported by Dumoulin and colleagues (100,101). In their studies, the effects of two commercial media were analyzed in a day-2 transfer program, and it was determined that differences existed in embryo growth kinetics and subsequent birth weight, which persisted through the first two years of life. Only one of the two culture media used contained free glutamine, and it was culture in this medium that resulted in delays in development and reduced birth weight, likely because the embryos were exposed to levels of ammonium known to adversely effect human embryo development and physiology (Figure 16.3b through 16.3d).

Notably, exposure of gametes and embryos to increasing concentrations of ammonium *in vivo* is not consistent with maintained embryo viability (6,102,103). It is, therefore, the authors' opinion that one should err on the side of caution, consider the data from animal and human *in vitro* and *in vivo* studies, and take appropriate action; for example, one can renew the culture medium at least every 48 hours, or one can refresh the medium by adding more volume to dilute out the ammonium present.

Macromolecules

Most culture media for the human embryo contain serum albumin as the protein source. Historically, serum was employed worldwide; however, the use of serum is no longer condoned due its extensive documented detrimental effects on embryos (79,104–107).

Although serum albumin is a relatively pure fraction of blood, it is still contaminated with fatty acids and other small molecules. The latter have been shown to include an embryotrophic factor, citrate, which stimulates cleavage and growth in rabbit morulae and blastocysts (108). There are significant differences not only between sources of serum albumin (109,110), but also between batches from the same source (109,111,112). Therefore, when using serum albumin preparations, it is essential that each batch is screened for its ability to adequately support mouse embryo development and human sperm survival prior to clinical use. Furthermore, new concerns with regards to the use of human serum albumin have been raised since it has been revealed that serum albumin, added as the protein supplement, is the source of detectable levels of di(2-ethylhexyl)phthalate and mono(2-ethylhexyl)phthalate, as well as polybrominated diphenyl ethers in human embryo culture media (113,114). In addition to these compounds, serum albumin preparations also contain variable levels of contaminants that include carbohydrates, amino acids, transition metals, growth factors and miRNAs. These contaminants will modify the compositions of the base media in a way that is variable between batches and is uncontrolled (115). Such data imply that the use of serum albumin in clinical IVF warrants renewed consideration.

To this end, recombinant human albumin is available, which eliminates the problems inherent with using blood-derived products and can lead to the standardization of media formulations. Recombinant human albumin has now been shown to be as effective as blood-derived albumin in supporting fertilization (116) and embryo development, and its efficacy has been proven in a prospective randomized trial (117). Significantly, embryos cultured in the presence of recombinant albumin exhibit an increased tolerance to cryopreservation (118). Historically, its clinical use has been restricted by price; however, with costs of such recombinant products falling, it makes this an appropriate time to re-evaluate its clinical use.

A further macromolecule present in the female reproductive tract is hyaluronan, which in the mouse uterus increases at the time of implantation (119). Hyaluronan is a high-molecular-mass polysaccharide that can be obtained endotoxin- and prion-free from a yeast fermentation procedure. Not only can hyaluronan improve mouse and bovine embryo culture systems (120,121), but its use for embryo transfer results in a significant increase in embryo implantation (120,122,123). In the largest prospective trial to date, which enrolled 1282 cycles of IVF, it was determined that the use of hyaluronan-enriched medium was associated with significant increases in clinical pregnancy rates and implantation rates, both for day-3 and day-5 embryo transfers. The beneficial effect was most evident in women who were >35 years of age, women who had only poor-quality embryos available for transfer, and women who had previous implantation failures (123,124). A recent Cochrane report confirmed improved pregnancy and take-home baby rates when hyaluronan was included in the transfer medium (125).

Notably, another highly significant effect of the inclusion of hyaluronan in the culture medium is its beneficial effects on cryosurvivability of cultured embryos from a number of species, including the human, mouse, sheep, and cow (118,122,126–128). As IVF programs are moving to transfer fewer embryos, there is an increasing need to be able to cryopreserve supernumerary embryos. The ability of culture systems to increase cryosurvival and therefore increase cumulative pregnancy outcomes is an important factor in deciding which culture system to use in the laboratory. In Figure 16.4, the effects of culture medium composition on the cryosurvival and subsequent implantation of human embryos is shown. Embryos were cultured in media with or without hyaluronan prior to slow freezing at the cleavage stage. Both survival and viability were higher if the embryos had been cultured in the presence of hyaluronan.

Monoculture or sequential media: one size fits all or a tailored approach?

It was established in the 1960s that it was feasible to culture the one-cell mouse embryo to the blastocyst stage in medium lacking amino acids. In the intervening decades, it has become apparent that amino acids have a significant role to play during embryo development (discussed above), and that medium should ideally be renewed/replenished at least every 48 hours to ensure minimal accumulation of embryotoxic ammonium (129). From a practical point of view, therefore, the amount of work and embryo manipulations required are the same whether one is working with sequential media or a monophasic system (i.e., one medium formulation for the entire preimplantation period).

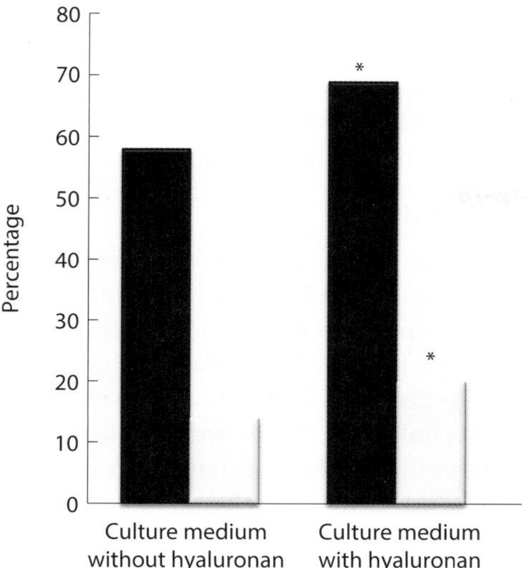

Figure 16.4 Effect of culture medium on the subsequent cryosurvival of cleavage-stage human embryos. Embryos were cultured either in medium without (n = 1235) or with elevated hyaluronan (n = 1351). Solid bars represent survival rate assessed as greater than or equal to 50% of blastomeres being intact. Open bars represent implantation rates as assessed by fetal heart beat at the eight-week scan. * Significantly different, $p < 0.05$.

However, the two approaches to embryo culture do have some fundamental differences. Specifically, monoculture is based on the principle of letting the embryo choose what it wants during development. In contrast, sequential media were developed to accommodate the dynamics of embryo nutrition and to mirror the environment of the female reproductive tract (in which the embryo is exposed to a gradient of nutrients as it passes along the oviduct into the uterus) (31,55,56). The significance of these nutrient gradients to the embryo in culture warrants further research as existing data on the mouse indicate that such gradients *in vitro* do impact embryo viability following transfer. For example, when the mouse zygote is cultured to the eight-cell stage and then transferred, embryo viability is highest after exposure of the embryo to a high lactate concentration (>20 mM D/L-lactate), while when the embryo is cultured post-compaction to the blastocyst stage, viability is highest after exposure to lower levels of lactate (<5 mM D/L-lactate) (130). These data support the hypothesis that the physiology of the developing conceptus is regulated by the concentrations of nutrients available at specific stages of development (33).

With the advent of time-lapse microscopy, we have seen the emergence of media designed specifically for the purpose of uninterrupted embryo culture, with the aim of minimizing the build-up of ammonium (131). These media have been shown to be effective, but further work is warranted in this area, such as the development of sequential media *in situ*, upon which existing media drops are not renewed but supplemented with a second formulation to give rise to a modified culture environment.

How far behind embryo development *in vivo* is development *in vitro*?

Historically, embryos cultured *in vitro* lag behind their *in vivo*-developed counterparts (132,133). However, with the development of sequential media based on the premise of meeting the changing requirements of the embryo and minimizing trauma, coupled with the use of reduced oxygen concentrations in the gas phase, *in vivo* rates of embryo development can now be attained *in vitro* in the mouse (11,134). The one proviso is that each laboratory must have sufficient-quality systems in place to ensure the optimum operation of a given culture system. Such advances in culture systems represent a significant development for the laboratory, for now there exists a means of producing blastocysts at the same time and with the same cell number and allocation to the ICM as embryos developed in the female tract (9,50). Using culture media in a highly controlled environment, as detailed throughout this book, it is possible to attain high rates of human embryo development to the blastocyst stage. Using an oocyte donor model to evaluate the efficacy of culture approaches, where the age of the oocyte is typically under 30 years, it is possible not only to obtain a blastocyst formation rate of 65%, but the resultant viability (as determined by fetal heart beat following transfer) is >65% (Table 16.3) (129). As such, oocyte donors represent as close to a human "gold standard" as one can have in an infertility clinic. With this in mind, ensuring one can attain blastocyst development of greater than 50% and implantation rates of over 50% when using donated oocytes is a good potential starting point for introducing blastocyst culture clinically, or for patients under 35 years of age.

Culture systems

Several key components of the culture system are reviewed here, none of which should be considered in isolation as all directly impact upon media performance.

Incubation chamber

Whatever incubation chamber is chosen, a key to successful embryo culture is to minimize perturbations in the atmosphere around the embryo. The two key perturbations to avoid are pH and temperature changes. This means that ideally the environment in which the embryo is placed is not disturbed during the culture period. Practically, this is

Table 16.3 Viability of human embryos conceived *in vitro* using an oocyte donor model

Mean blastocyst development (%)	65.1
Mean number of blastocysts transferred	2.05
Mean age of recipient (years)	40.3
Fetal heart beat (per blastocyst transferred) (%)	68.0
Clinical pregnancy rate (per retrieval) (%)	85.2
Twins (%)	59.9

difficult to achieve in a busy clinical laboratory. The use of an individual incubation chamber, such as a modular incubator chamber or glass desiccator (such as that used to grow Louise Brown), which can be purged with the appropriate gas mix, can alleviate such concerns. Using such incubator chambers, each patient's embryos can be completely isolated within an incubator, with the gas phase and, for the most part, temperature being unaffected when the incubator door is opened. We like to consider such chambers as "a womb with a view." However, a downside of this approach is that only three modular chambers can be placed in one incubator, thereby necessitating the acquisition of sufficient incubators. An alternative to the use of modular chambers is the use of inner doors within an incubator to significantly reduce fluctuations in the gaseous environment upon opening the incubator door. Several incubator manufacturers make incubators with inner doors. A more recent move has been the production of incubators with a greatly reduced working volume, such that rather than two double stacks of conventional incubators (giving four working chambers), one can now have three rows of smaller incubators, stacked three high, giving a total of nine chambers. This approach allows the successful allocation of one chamber to just one or two patients, thereby stabilizing the culture environment.

Incubators with infrared (IR) as opposed to thermocouple CO_2 sensors are quicker at regulating the internal environment of the chamber and are less sensitive to environmental factors and subsequently are better able to maintain a constant CO_2 level in the incubator. Therefore, incubators equipped with IR sensors will provide a more stable environment for embryo development. With regards to temperature changes, incubators with an air jacket are less susceptible to large temperature fluctuations than those with a water jacket. Again, the use of inner doors will aid in minimizing environmental fluctuations within the chamber.

Alternatives to classic tissue culture incubators are bench top mini-incubators with constant flow chambers, which allow for direct heat transfer between the chamber and culture vessel. Such chambers also allow for a direct flow of premixed gas, therefore minimizing changes in pH. More recently, such chambers have seen the inclusion of time-lapse capability, facilitating the constant monitoring of embryos without the need to remove them from their culture environment. Consequently, this approach has been shown to have inherent advantages for embryo development by minimizing handling and variations in temperature and pH (10,135).

What is evident is that it is imperative to have sufficient numbers of incubator chambers to match the caseload. This is especially true when performing extended culture. It is important to consider the number of times an incubator will be opened in a day and to keep this to a minimum. It is advisable to have separate incubators for media equilibration and for embryo culture, thereby minimizing the amount of access to incubators containing embryos. It can also be useful to have a mixture of incubator chambers for overnight or longer-term cultures, as well as benchtop models that recover quickly for manipulations such as denuding and ICSI. Consistent high rates of implantation are achieved if an incubation chamber is used for just two to three patients per week. Space can be optimized through the use of smaller incubation chambers.

pH and carbon dioxide

When discussing pH, it is worth considering that the pHi of the embryo is around 7.2 (136–138), while the pH of the media routinely range from 7.25 to 7.4. Specific media components, such as lactic and amino acids, directly affect and buffer pHi, respectively. Of the two isomers of lactate, D- and L-lactate, only the L-lactate form is biologically active. However, both the D- and L-lactate forms decrease pHi of the embryo (138). Therefore, it is advisable to use only the L-isomer of lactate and not a medium containing both the D- and L-lactate forms. While high concentrations of lactate in the culture medium can drive pHi down (138), amino acids increase the intracellular buffering capacity and help maintain the pHi at around 7.2 (64). As the embryo has to maintain pHi against a gradient when incubated at pH 7.4, it would seem prudent to culture embryos at a lower external pH. The pH of a CO_2/bicarbonate-buffered medium is not easy to quantitate. A pH electrode can be used, but one must be quick, and the same technician must take all readings to ensure consistency. A preferred and more accurate approach is to take samples of medium and measure the pH with a blood-gas analyzer. A final method necessitates the presence of phenol red in the culture medium and the use of Sorenson's phosphate buffer standards. This method allows visual inspection of a medium's pH with a tube in the incubator and is accurate to 0.2 pH units (20,46).

When using bicarbonate-buffered media, the concentration of CO_2 has a direct impact on the medium's pH (46). Although most media work over a wide range of pH (7.2–7.4), it is preferable to ensure that pH does not go over 7.4. Therefore, it is advisable to use a CO_2 concentration of between 6% and 7% to yield a medium pH of around 7.3. The amount of CO_2 in the incubation chamber can be calibrated with a Fyrite® (Bacharach, New Kensington, PA, USA), although such an approach is only accurate to $\pm1\%$. A more suitable method is to use a handheld IR metering system, such as that made by Vaisalla, which can be calibrated and are accurate to around 0.2%.

When using a CO_2/bicarbonate-buffered medium, it is essential to minimize the amount of time the culture dish is out of a CO_2 environment to prevent increases in pH. To facilitate this, modified pediatric isolettes designed to maintain temperature, humidity, and CO_2 concentration can be used. However, should it not be feasible to use an isolette, then the media used can be buffered with either 20–23 mM 4-(2-hydroxyet4hyl)-1-piperazineethane sulfonic acid (HEPES) (139) or 3-(*N*-morpholino)propanesulfonic acid (MOPS) (140) together with 5–2 mM bicarbonate (141). Such buffering systems do not require a CO_2 environment, and can be used for short term incubation of <10 mins. An oil overlay also reduces the speed of CO_2 loss and the associated increase in pH.

Oxygen

The concentration of oxygen in the lumen of the rabbit oviduct is reported to be 2%–6% (142,143), whereas the oxygen concentration in the oviduct of the hamster and rhesus monkey is ~8% (144). Interestingly, the oxygen concentration in the uterus is lower than in the oviduct, ranging from 5% in the hamster and rabbit to 1.5% in the rhesus monkey (144).

Importantly, it has been demonstrated that optimum embryo development of all non-human mammalian species occurs at an oxygen concentration below 10% (109,145,146). The fact that human embryos can grow at atmospheric oxygen concentration (~20%) and give rise to viable pregnancies has led to some confusion regarding the optimal concentration for embryo culture. Consequently, the validity of having to use a reduced oxygen concentration for human embryo culture is continually challenged. The continued use of 20% oxygen in a human IVF culture system is a good example of something that has been used for over three decades and does give results; however, the question remains: does 20% oxygen adversely affect the physiology of the developing embryo before implantation?

It was initially established in the mouse model that 20% oxygen impacts embryo development by as early as the first cleavage (Figure 16.5) (147). Interestingly, it was determined that 20% oxygen is detrimental to embryo development at all stages, but with the greatest detrimental effects being imparted at the cleavage stages (147). These findings have now been evaluated clinically, and it has been determined that 20% oxygen reduces developmental rates and delays completion of the third cell cycle (148), indicating a heightened sensitivity to oxidative stress during the cleavage stages. Furthermore, it has been established in animal models that embryos cultured to the blastocyst stage in the presence of 20% oxygen have altered gene expression and perturbed proteomes compared to embryos developed *in vivo* (30,149,150). In contrast, culture in 5% oxygen had significantly less effect on both embryonic gene expression and proteome. Similarly, 20% oxygen has been shown to adversely affect embryonic metabolism (12). Recent data have revealed that not only does 20% oxygen compromise the utilization of both carbohydrates and amino acids throughout the preimplantation period (94), but that atmospheric oxygen also impairs the ability of the embryo to regulate against an ammonium stress (95). Therefore, not only does oxygen induce its own trauma on the embryo, but it also increases the embryo's susceptibility to other stressors present in the culture system or laboratory (10). Furthermore, atmospheric oxygen has recently been linked to changes to the embryonic epigenome (for reviews, see [10,151]).

Clinical data, including a randomized controlled trial, support this move to more physiological conditions in showing that lower oxygen concentrations increase both implantation and live birth rates (152–155). However, in spite of the animal and clinical data describing the detrimental effects of atmospheric oxygen, it has been reported in a recent online survey in which 265 clinics from 54 different countries participated that <25% of IVF human embryo culture is performed exclusively under physiological (~5%) oxygen (156). Although this survey represents only a small fraction of the world's IVF clinics, what is notable from an extensive literature review of the past 10 years is a clear geographic difference with regard to the use of 5% oxygen. The authors of this chapter presented a case for the clinical introduction of physiological oxygen in human IVF over 25 years ago (46). In the intervening two decades, the rationale for the discontinuation of atmospheric oxygen has become compelling. Here, we therefore make a further plea for the cessation of embryonic stress through the exposure of human embryos to 20% oxygen.

Incubation vessel and the embryo:volume ratio

Culture of embryos in drops of culture medium under an oil overlay is the preferred and effective method of culturing embryos. Within the lumen of the female reproductive tract the developing embryo is exposed to microliter volumes of fluid (157). In contrast, the embryo grown *in vitro* is subject to relatively large volumes of medium of up to 1 mL. Consequently, any autocrine factor(s) produced by the developing embryo will be diluted and may therefore become ineffectual. It has been demonstrated in the mouse that cleavage rate and blastocyst formation increase when embryos are grown in groups (of up to 10) or reduced volumes (around 20 μL) (158–160). Of greatest significance is the observation that decreasing the incubation volume significantly increases embryo viability (160) due to an increase in ICM development. Similar results have been obtained with sheep (78) and cow embryos (161). It is therefore apparent that the preimplantation mammalian embryo produces a factor(s) capable of stimulating development of both itself and surrounding embryos. Furthermore, embryos of one species can be used to promote the development and differentiation of another (162).

In order to culture in such reduced volumes (of 20–50 μL), an oil overlay is required. Although the use of an oil overlay is time-consuming, it prevents the evaporation of media, thereby reducing the harmful effects of increases in osmolality, and reduces changes in pH caused by a loss of CO_2 from the medium when culture dishes are taken out of the incubator for embryo examination. An embryo-tested paraffin oil is highly recommended. Such an overlay also serves another purpose in being able to trap a number of volatile organic compounds.

The benefits of using drops of medium under oil would obviously be negated should the oil be embryotoxic. Therefore, care must be taken in selecting and storing oil, which if done incorrectly will lead to it becoming toxic. Oil should be stored in the dark and in glass. It should not be stored for extended periods in the incubator. Oil should never be aliquoted into tissue culture flasks as these are styrene based and oils are able to leach styrene from such containers at high rates over time. Always use a batch of oil prescreened with an appropriate mouse embryo bioassay

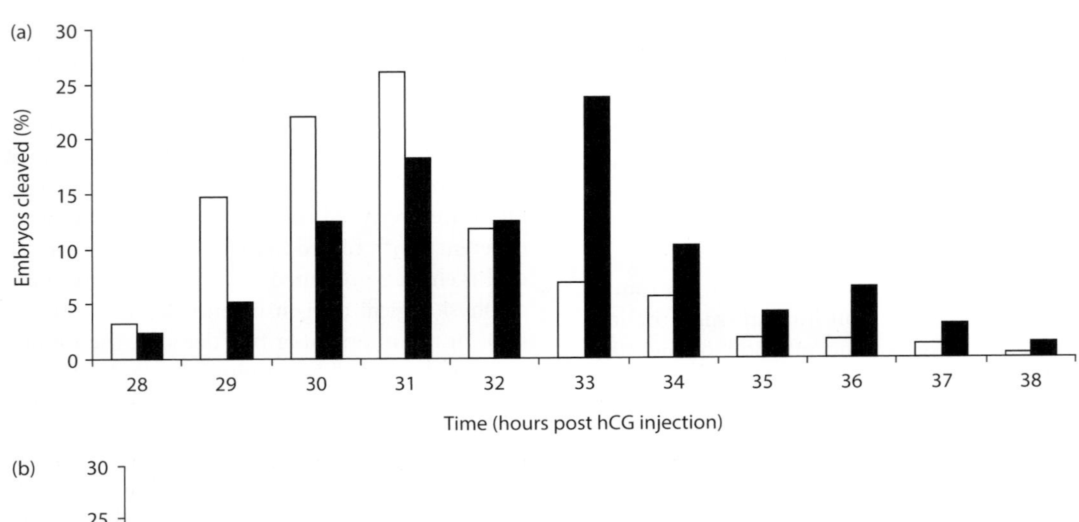

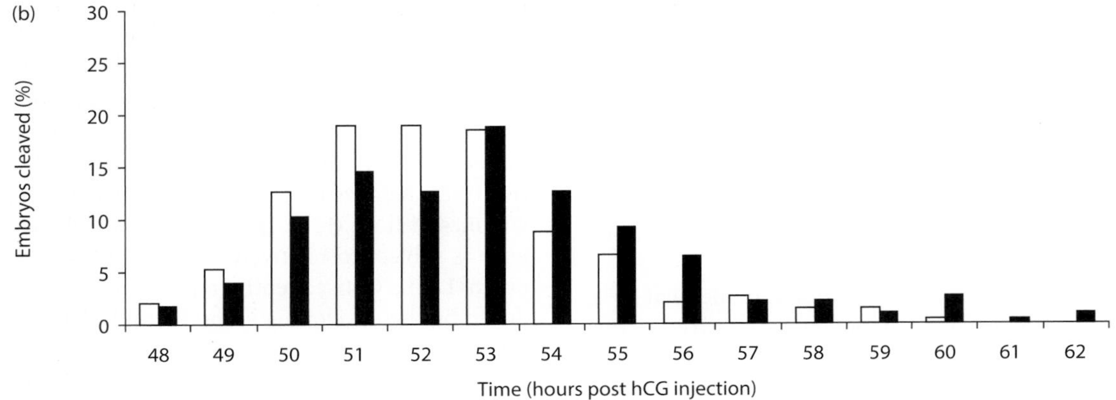

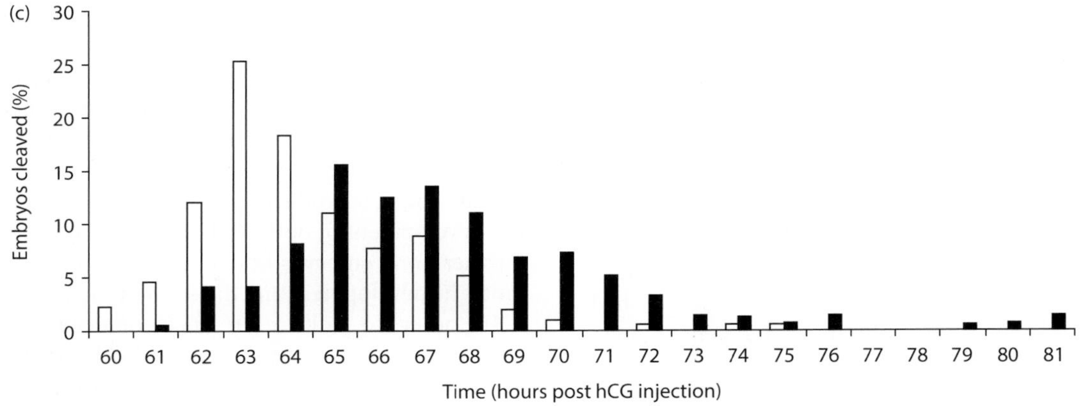

Figure 16.5 Distribution of cleavage timing for the (a) first, (b) second, and (c) third cleavage divisions of mouse pronucleate oocytes cultured in either 5% or 20% oxygen. White bars represent 5% oxygen concentration and black bars represent 20% oxygen concentration. As development progresses, one can see a significant cumulative delay in embryo development induced by 20% oxygen. *Abbreviation*: hCG, human chorionic gonadotropin. (From Wale PL, Gardner DK. *Reprod Biomed Online* 2010; 21: 402–10, with permission.)

before clinical use. Oil toxicity may not necessarily show up by simply culturing mouse embryos to the blastocyst stage. Rather, one should also look for signs of necrosis, which is most evident at the blastocyst stage, and perform cell counts on the blastocysts developed.

Medium storage

Commercially available culture media have several labile components and it is therefore important to know how to handle and store such solutions. Two of the most labile components are amino acids and vitamins. Glutamine is the most labile amino acid and produces the highest levels of ammonium of any amino acid. Therefore, it is paramount when using culture media containing amino acids that they are placed in the incubator for the minimum time required for equilibration, and they should certainly never be stored in the incubator. Fortunately, glutamine can be replaced with alanyl-glutamine, a dipeptide that is stable at 37°C. Vitamins are light sensitive and therefore care should be taken to minimize exposure to light by storing the culture media in the dark.

Quality control

Establishing an appropriate quality control system for the IVF laboratory is a prerequisite in the establishment of a successful laboratory (Chapter 2). The types of bioassays conducted for this have been the focus of much discussion (8). In reality, there is no perfect model for the human, save for the very patients we treat. Consequently, it is important to understand the limitations of the assays performed and to use data obtained from bioassays in an appropriate fashion. Quality control should not be limited to the culture media used, but should include all contact supplies and gases used in an IVF procedure. The bioassay we favor is the culture of pronucleate mouse oocytes in protein-free media. There has been a lot of conflicting data regarding the use of the mouse embryo bioassay, but by adjusting conditions, one can not only increase the sensitivity of the assay, but also quantitate quality with it.

First of all, the stage at which the embryo is cultured has an impact on development. Mouse embryos collected at the pronucleate stage do not tend to fare as well in culture as those collected at the two-cell stage. Second, the strain of mice is important. Embryos from hybrid parents have a decided advantage in culture and do not represent the diverse genetic background one is dealing with in an infertility clinic. Therefore, a random-bred strain of mice provides greater genetic diversity (163). Third, the embryo cultures should be performed in the absence of protein, as protein has the ability to mask the effects of any potential toxins present. Reports that mouse embryos can develop in culture in medium prepared using tap water (164,165) should be interpreted carefully after taking into account the strain of mouse, types of media used, and supplementation of medium with protein. Silverman et al. (164) used Ham's F-10. This medium contains amino acids, which can chelate any possible toxins present in the tap water (e.g., heavy metals). George et al. (165) included high levels of bovine serum albumin in their zygote cultures to the blastocyst. Albumin can chelate potential embryotoxins and thereby mask the effects of any present in the culture medium (166,167). Furthermore, all such studies used blastocyst development as the sole criterion for assessing embryo development. Blastocyst development is a poor indicator of embryo quality and does not accurately reflect developmental potential (69). Therefore, rates of development should be determined by scoring the embryos at specific times during culture. Key times to examine the embryos include the morning of day 3 to determine the extent of compaction, the afternoon of day 4 to determine the degree of blastocyst formation, and the morning of day 5 to assess the initiation of hatching. This latter approach can now be readily applied through the utilization of time-lapse microscopy (168).

Finally, the embryos that form blastocysts in a given time, typically on the morning of day 5, should have their cell numbers determined, as blastocyst cell number is a good indicator of subsequent developmental potential. When new components of certain culture media can affect the development of the ICM directly, such as essential amino acids, a differential nuclear stain should be performed in order to determine the extent of ICM development. By using such an approach, it is possible to identify potential problems in culture media before they are used clinically. In our experience, around 25% of all contact supplies fail such prescreening (8). Although some of the contact supplies that fail the bioassay are not outright lethal, they do compromise embryo development. If undetected, this would result in reduced clinical pregnancy rates. Consequently, this helps to explain periodic changes in clinical pregnancy rates and emphasizes the significance of an ongoing quality control program. There are an increasing number of products on the market that are prescreened for embryo toxicity. However, it is worth noting that not all testing is the same and that it is worth understanding the sensitivity of the assay used before introduction of an item into the laboratory. However, irrespective of the testing, all supplies should be tracked as they enter the laboratory to confirm efficacy for human embryos.

On what day should embryo transfer be performed?

For the past three decades, the majority of embryos conceived through IVF have been transferred between days 1 and 3 at either the pronucleate or cleavage stages. The reason for this stems primarily from the inability of past culture systems to support the development of viable blastocysts at acceptable rates. However, with the advent of sequential culture media (13), it became feasible to perform day-5 blastocyst transfers as a matter of routine in an IVF clinic (169,170). This now facilitates an answer to the question: on which day of embryo development should embryos be transferred? Before answering this question, the potential advantages and disadvantages of blastocyst culture and transfer are considered.

Blastocyst transfer: advantages and disadvantages

The potential advantages of blastocyst culture and transfer have been well documented (171–174). Advantages include:

1. Synchronizing embryonic stage with the female tract. This is important as the levels of nutrients within the fallopian tube and uterus do differ, and therefore the premature transfer of the cleavage-stage embryo to the uterus could result in metabolic stress (11). Furthermore, the uterine environment during a stimulated cycle cannot be considered normal. Certainly, it is known from animal studies that the hyperstimulated female tract is a less-than-optimal environment for the developing embryo, resulting in impaired embryo and fetal development (2,175,176). Therefore, it would seem prudent to shorten the length of time an embryo is exposed to such an environment before implantation.
2. When embryos are selected for transfer at the two- to eight-cell stage, the embryonic genome has only just

begun to be transcribed (41,177), and therefore it is not possible to identify from within a given cohort those embryos with the highest developmental potential. Only by culturing embryos past the maternal/embryonic genome transition and up to the blastocyst does it become realistic to identify those embryos with limited or no developmental potential. Assessment of pronucleate-stage oocytes in order to select embryos for transfer (178) has reportedly increased implantation rates, while others (179) have used a scoring system on day 3 to increase implantation rates. However, assessment of the embryos at either the pronucleate oocyte or cleavage stages can at best be considered as an assessment of the oocyte. The quality of the oocyte is important, as the quality of the developing embryo is ultimately dependent on the quality of gametes from which it is derived, but it provides limited information regarding true embryo developmental potential and eliminates the impact of the male gamete on development.

3. Not all fertilized oocytes are normal, and therefore a percentage always exists that is not destined to establish a pregnancy or go to term. Factors contributing to embryonic attrition include an insufficiency of stored oocyte-coded gene products and a failure to activate the embryonic genome (180). The culmination of this is that many abnormal embryos arrest during development *in vitro*. So by culturing embryos to the blastocyst stage, one has already selected against those embryos with little if any developmental potential. Sandalinas and colleagues (181) have confirmed that some chromosomally abnormal human embryos can reach the blastocyst stage *in vitro*. However, even though aneuploid embryos form blastocysts at lower rates than their euploid counterparts, this means blastocyst culture cannot be used as the sole means of identifying chromosomally abnormal embryos.
4. Uterine contractions have been negatively correlated with embryo transfer outcome, possibly by the expulsion of embryos from the uterine cavity (182). Uterine junctional zone contractions have been quantitated and found to be strongest on the day of oocyte retrieval (183). All patients exhibited such contractions on days 2 and 3 after retrieval, but contractility decreased and was barely evident on day 4. It is therefore feasible that the transfer of blastocysts on day 5 is, by default, associated with reduced uterine contractions and therefore there is less chance for embryonic expulsion and loss (184).
5. Cryopreservation of embryos at the blastocyst stage appears more successful than at earlier stages (185).
6. Trophectoderm biopsy and analysis enable the removal of more cells compared to cleavage-stage embryos, which facilitates the use of newer technologies such as next-generation sequencing (186,187). There is also some suggestion that trophectoderm biopsy is less invasive than using cleavage-stage embryos for preimplantation genetic screening (188).

The potential disadvantage of extended embryo culture in a program where only blastocyst culture and transfer is offered is the possibility that a patient will not have a morula or blastocyst for transfer. Certainly, there has been an increase in the percentage of patients who do not have an embryo transfer from 2.9% on day 3 to 6.7% on day 5 in one clinic (170), and from 1.3% on day 3 to 2.8% on day 5 in another (169). Interestingly, in spite of the increase in patients not having an embryo transfer, there was a significant increase in pregnancy rate per retrieval with blastocyst culture, due to a significant increase in implantation rates.

There is significant evidence to show that in many laboratories blastocyst transfer can be more successful than cleavage-stage transfer. However, this has not been universal and is likely due to the interactions of all of the components that we have described above from ovarian stimulation, culture media and system, oxygen levels, training levels, and numbers of embryologists, as well as quality control (Figure 16.1).

In a meta-analysis of prospective trials in which equal numbers of embryos were transferred, it was concluded that, "The best available evidence suggests that the probability of live birth after fresh IVF is significantly higher after blastocyst-stage embryo transfer as compared to cleavage-stage embryo transfer when equal number of embryos are transferred…" (15). Additionally, in the most recent Cochrane report on blastocyst transfer, there was a significant difference in live birth rate per couple favoring blastocyst transfer (14).

In support of such analyses, from a model previously developed to determine which patients should have SET, it was determined that pregnancy outcome was more favorable with day 5 than day 3 transfer (189). As well as the published prospective randomized trials, there are retrospective studies that have concluded that day 5 transfer exhibits significant benefits for human ART in both nonselected and specific patient populations (169,170,190).

For patients receiving oocyte donation, blastocyst culture and transfer is the most effective course of treatment. Oocytes from donors generally represent a more viable cohort of gametes, as they tend to come from young, fertile women. Embryos derived from oocyte donors tend to reach the blastocyst stage at a higher frequency than those from IVF patients, and tend to be of higher quality. It is possible to attain an implantation rate of >65% when transferring blastocysts to recipients whose mean age is over 40 (Table 16.3) (191). Such data not only reflect the competency of modern embryo culture systems, but also emphasize the need to move to SETs, especially when performing day 5 transfers (192).

Toward SET

Several reviews have discussed the development of scoring systems used in clinical IVF and their significance in identifying the most viable embryo(s) for transfer (193–195) (see also Chapter 17). Certainly with newer types of embryo culture media, implantation rates are increasing whether embryos are transferred at the cleavage stage or blastocyst. It is envisaged that for most patients, blastocyst culture and transfer will be the most effective means of

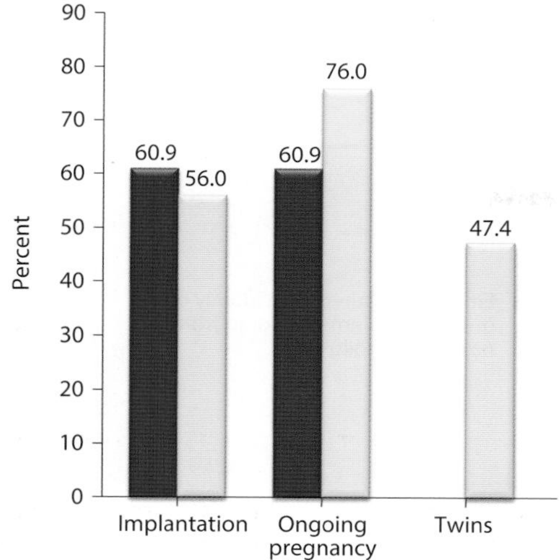

Figure 16.6 *In vitro* fertilization outcomes following the transfer of either one or two blastocysts. Blue bars represent the transfer of a single blastocyst (group I); yellow bars represent the transfer of two blastocysts (group II). Implantation and pregnancy rates were not statistically different between the two groups of patients. There were no twins in group I in contrast to 47.4% twins in group II. (From Gardner DK et al. *Fertil Steril* 2004; 81: 551–5, with permission.)

being able to transfer a single embryo while maintaining high pregnancy rates, as it is evident that blastocyst score is highly predictive of implantation potential. A prospective randomized trial of one versus two blastocysts transferred in patients with 10 or more follicles has been performed. The data in Figure 16.6 indicate that it is possible to transfer a single blastocyst and obtain an ongoing pregnancy rate of 60% (192). Subsequent trials of single-blastocyst transfer versus cleavage-stage embryo transfer have confirmed the higher implantation rate of the later-stage embryo. It has also been established that fetal loss is significantly less following blastocyst transfer (196).

Cumulative pregnancy rates per retrieval: The significance of cryopreservation

The introduction of blastocyst culture was met with much speculation as not all laboratories were able to cryopreserve blastocysts that were not transferred. However, with the development of more suitable slow-freezing procedures, it is now possible to obtain implantation and ongoing pregnancy rates of greater than 30% and 60%, respectively, using frozen–thawed blastocysts (185). Furthermore, clinical data following blastocyst vitrification are even more encouraging. It has now been demonstrated that the move to blastocyst vitrification is associated with a significant increase in clinical pregnancy (50% increase) and live birth rates (40% increase) compared with those obtained with slow freezing (197). Consequently, cumulative pregnancy data for cleavage- and blastocyst-stage embryos must be re-examined and be based upon cycles where vitrified blastocysts were utilized. The latter has been reported to result in pregnancy rates and outcomes equivalent to, or even greater than, fresh transferred blastocysts (197–199). Furthermore, the ability of a given culture system to support embryo cryosurvival is of utmost significance, with media containing hyaluronan conferring great advantage in this regard (50,126).

FUTURE DEVELOPMENTS IN EMBRYO CULTURE SYSTEMS

A subject already touched upon in this chapter is the toxicity of oxygen, plausibly through the induction of reactive oxygen species. As a result of the growing data on the pathologies induced by atmospheric oxygen, there has been a resurgence of interest in the role of antioxidants in facilitating embryo development (200,201). When present as a group, specific antioxidants have been shown to improve transfer outcome in the mouse model (201). An area not discussed in this text has been the role of growth factors in regulating embryo development in culture and subsequent fetal development. Although such factors are abundant in the fluids of the human female reproductive tract (202) and have effects on animal embryo viability (203), they are conspicuously absent from clinical embryo culture media. An exception to this is a study on the effects of granulocyte-macrophage colony-stimulating factor (GM-CSF) (204). However, it was reported that GM-CSF only had a beneficial effect when the levels of human serum albumin were reduced in the medium, an observation also previously reported in the mouse model (205). Therefore, further research on the effects of such factors at the physiological, genomic, and proteomic levels is required in order to lead to a better understanding of their roles in human IVF media (206–208).

As discussed previously, there is nothing physiological about the physical conditions in which embryos are cultured. Rather than a static drop of medium, the future may engage perfusion culture systems, enabling the embryo to be exposed to a flux of nutrients and factors (Figure 16.7) (43,209,210) (see Chapter 31). This latter approach has the advantage of being able to expose embryos to numerous gradients and fresh media throughout development. Furthermore, samples of medium can be taken and analyzed for carbohydrates (211), amino acids (212), and other factors related to implantation potential post-transfer (213) (see Chapter 17). Research in this area is growing, and the application of novel elastomers together with soft lithography is starting to produce new generations of chips capable of moving sub-microliter volumes accurately for both culture and analysis (209,210,214).

CONCLUSIONS

The culture system in the clinical laboratory is one part of the overall treatment cycle. Good oocytes, derived from appropriate stimulation regimes, are able to give rise to good embryos. However, it is not feasible to obtain good embryos from poor oocytes. After culture, the embryo transfer technique and subsequent luteal support administered have an impact on cycle outcome.

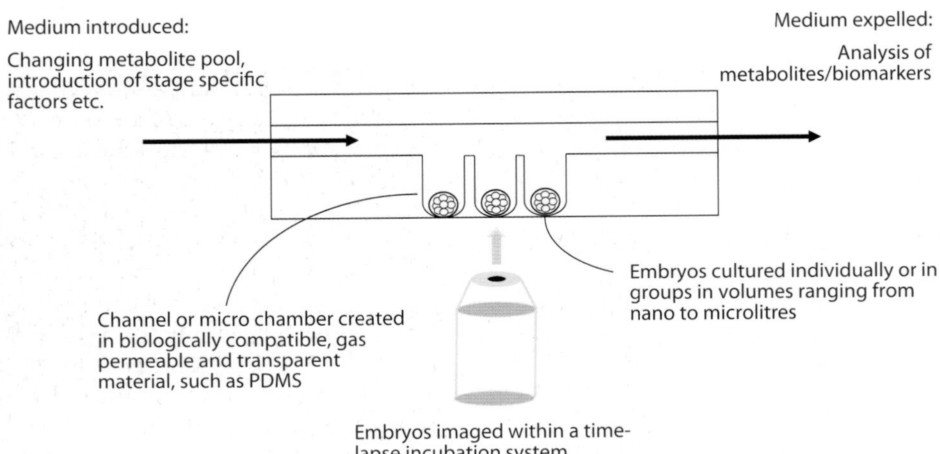

Figure 16.7 Schematic of an embryo perfusion culture system. Culture media are continuously passed over the embryo(s). The composition of the culture media can be changed according to the specific requirements of each stage of embryonic development. Toxins such as ammonium are not able to build up and impair embryo development, while more labile components of the culture system are not denatured. Further, media can be sampled in real time to quantitate embryo physiology. (Modified from Gardner DK. *Cell Biol Int* 1994; 18: 1163–79.)

Significant improvements in culture media formulations and embryo culture systems have conclusively provided better conditions for the human embryo to develop in the laboratory. The ability to culture embryos to the blastocyst stage has facilitated the introduction of the safer practice of SETs for an increasing number of patients, including those undergoing oocyte donation or who are <38 years of age and in their first cycle, and increasingly in conjunction with preimplantation genetic screening.

It is evident that culture conditions affect the ability of embryos to survive cryopreservation. As we move closer to the day when single-embryo/blastocyst transfer is considered the standard of care, it becomes more important than ever to ensure embryos are given the best chance of being cryopreserved for transfer at a later date, thereby increasing the efficiency of each oocyte retrieval procedure.

In this chapter, we have outlined how human embryos can be successfully cultured. Ongoing investment in quality management and quality control ensures that an IVF laboratory will run at its highest level of performance and that results will remain consistent over time.

Embryo culture

In order to perform oocyte isolation, preparation for ICSI, or embryo manipulation outside a CO_2 incubator, there are two distinct approaches: one can use media that have a second buffer system in them, such as MOPS or HEPES (both of which will keep the pH of the medium relatively constant in air); or one can employ a pediatric isolette-type system. The latter maintains both temperature and CO_2 and negates the use of buffer systems other than bicarbonate. Both approaches can be made to work effectively.

Embryo culture should be performed in a reduced O_2 environment (typically 5%, but the optimum value below 10% is yet to be determined) and 5%–7% CO_2 depending on the media system chosen and altitude. It is advisable to minimize the number of observations made outside the incubator during embryo development and to minimize the number of cases per incubator. It is also essential that all contact supplies, media, oil, and so on are prescreened with a suitable test (8).

Pronucleate oocytes to day-3 culture

Embryo manipulation (following fertilization assessment)

Once the cumulus is removed, then all manipulations should be performed using a glass capillary-style pipette or a displacement pipette. Fine control can be attained with both approaches. It is important to use a pipette with the appropriate-sized tip (days 1–3; around 200 μM). Using the appropriate-sized tip minimizes the volumes of culture medium moved with each embryo, which typically should be less than 1 μL. Such volume manipulation is a prerequisite for successful culture.

Setting up culture dishes (day 1 to day 3)

At around 4 p.m. on the day of oocyte retrieval, label pretested 60 mm dishes with the patient's name. Using a single-wrapped tip, rinse the tip once first, then place 6 × 25 μL drops of phase 1 medium onto the plate. Four drops should be at the 3, 6, 9, and 12 o'clock positions (for embryo culture), and the fifth and sixth drops should be in the middle of the dish (wash drops). Immediately cover drops with 9 mL of prescreened paraffin oil. Prepare no more than two plates at one time. Using a new tip for each drop, first rinse the tip and then add a further 25 μL of medium to each original drop. Immediately place the dish in the incubator.

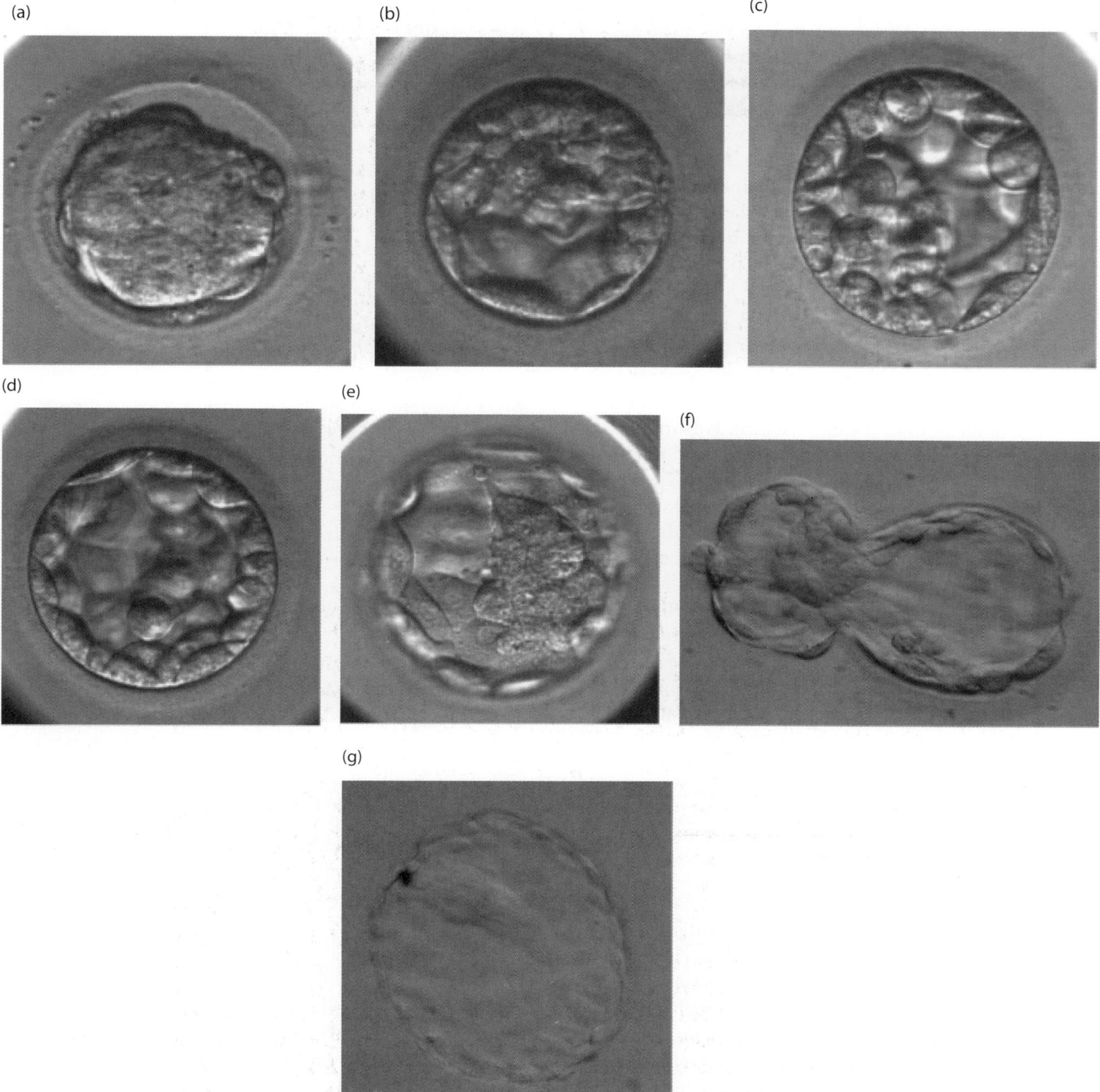

Figure 16.8 Human embryos on the morning of day 5 (four days of culture from the pronucleate oocyte stage). Embryos were cultured from the pronucleate oocyte until midday on day 3 in medium G1.3. Cleavage-stage embryos were then washed in medium G2.3 and culture in G2.3 for a further 48 hours. (a) 0—morula or lesser stage (no blastocoel cavity seen); (b) 1—early blastocyst (blastocoel less than half the volume of the embryo); (c) 2—blastocyst (blastocoel greater than or equal to half of the volume of the embryo); (d) 3—full blastocyst (blastocoel completely fills the embryo); (e) 4—expanded blastocyst (zona thinning and overall increase in size); (f) 5—hatching blastocyst (trophectoderm has started to herniate through the zona); (g) 6—hatched blastocyst (blastocyst has completely escaped from the zona).

Gently remove the lid of the dish and set at an angle on the side of the plate. Dishes must gas in the incubator for a minimum of four hours (this is the minimal measured time for the media to reach correct pH under oil).

For each patient, set up a wash dish at the same time as the culture dishes. Place 1 mL of phase 1 medium into the center of an organ well dish. Place 2 mL of medium into the outer well. Place immediately into the incubator. If working outside an isolette, use HEPES/MOPS-buffered medium with amino acids. This should not be placed in a CO_2 incubator, but rather warmed on a heated stage.

Morning of day 1

Culture in phase 1 medium

Following removal of the cumulus cells, embryos are transferred to the organ well dish and washed in the center well drop of medium in the culture dish. Washing entails picking up the embryo two to three times and moving it around within the well. Embryos should then be washed in the two center drops in the culture dish and up to four embryos placed in each drop of the culture medium. Four is the maximum number of embryos that can be cultured in each drop due to their nutrient requirements. More than four embryos may result in a significant depletion of the nutrient pool by the embryos. This will result in no more than 16 embryos per dish. Return the dish to the incubator immediately. It is advisable to culture embryos in at least groups of two. Therefore, for example, for a patient with six embryos it is best to culture in two groups of three and not four and two or five and one. On day 3, embryos can be transferred to the uterus in an appropriate hyaluronan-enriched transfer medium.

Day-3 embryos to the blastocyst

Setting up culture dishes (day 3 to day 5)

On day 3 before 8:30 a.m., label a 60 mm dish with the patient's name. Using a single-wrapped tip, rinse the tip once first, then place 6×25 μL drops of phase 2 medium onto the plate as described for Phase I. Immediately cover with 9 mL of oil. Never prepare more than two plates at one time. Using a new tip for each drop, rinse the tip and then add a further 25 μL of medium to each original drop. Immediately place the dish in the incubator. Gently remove the lid and set on the side of the plate.

For each patient, set up one wash dish per 10 embryos. Place 1 mL of phase 2 medium into the center of an organ well dish. Place 2 mL of medium into the outer well. Place immediately into the incubator. Dishes must gas in the incubator for a minimum of four hours. If working outside an isolette, use HEPES/MOPS-buffered medium with amino acids. This should not be placed in a CO_2 incubator, but rather warmed on a heated stage.

For each patient, set up one sorting dish before 8:30 a.m. Place 1 mL of phase 2 medium into the center of an organ well dish. Place 2 mL of medium into the outer well. Place immediately into the incubator. If working outside an isolette, use HEPES/MOPS-buffered medium with amino acids. This should not be placed in a CO_2 incubator, but rather warmed on a heated stage.

Culture in phase 2 medium

Moving embryos from phase 1 to phase 2 media should occur between 9 a.m. and midday. Wash embryos in the organ well thoroughly. Washing entails picking up the embryo two to three times and moving it around within the well.

Transfer embryos to the sorting dish and group like embryos together. Rinse through the wash drops of medium and again place up to four embryos in each drop of phase 2 medium. This will result in no more than 16 embryos per dish. Return the dish to the low-O_2 incubator immediately. If working outside an isolette, use HEPES/MOPS-buffered medium with amino acids in the sorting dish. This should not be placed in a CO_2 incubator, but rather warmed on a heated stage.

An alternative strategy for sequential culture is to supplement the phase 1 medium directly with the phase 2 medium, making this sequential media *in situ*. The phase 2 medium can be formulated to give the desired concentration of nutrients upon direct addition to the phase 1 medium, while concomitantly facilitating the dilution of end products of metabolism, such as ammonium.

On the morning of day 5, embryos should be scored (Figure 16.8) (215) (see Chapter 17) and the two top scoring embryos selected for transfer. Transfers should be performed in a medium enriched with hyaluronan. Any blastocysts not transferred can be cryopreserved. Should an embryo not have formed a blastocyst by day 5, then it should be cultured in a fresh drop of the phase 2 medium for 24 hours and assessed on day 6. Embryos at different stages of development are shown in Figure 16.8. For more details on blastocyst grading, see Chapter 17 and References 216, 217.

REFERENCES

1. Hardy K, Robinson FM, Paraschos T, Wicks R, Franks S, Winston RM. Normal development and metabolic activity of preimplantation embryos *in vitro* from patients with polycystic ovaries. *Hum Reprod* 1995; 10: 2125–35.
2. Van der Auwera I, Pijnenborg R, Koninckx PR. The influence of *in-vitro* culture versus stimulated and untreated oviductal environment on mouse embryo development and implantation. *Hum Reprod* 1999; 14: 2570–4.
3. Simon C, Garcia Velasco JJ, Valbuena D et al. Increasing uterine receptivity by decreasing estradiol levels during the preimplantation period in high responders with the use of a follicle-stimulating hormone step-down regimen. *Fertil Steril* 1998; 70: 234–9.
4. Ertzeid G, Storeng R. The impact of ovarian stimulation on implantation and fetal development in mice. *Hum Reprod* 2001; 16: 221–5.

5. Kelley RL, Kind KL, Lane M, Robker RL, Thompson JG, Edwards LJ. Recombinant human follicle-stimulating hormone alters maternal ovarian hormone concentrations and the uterus and perturbs fetal development in mice. *Am J Physiol Endocrinol Metab* 2006; 291: E761–70.
6. Gardner DK, Stilley K, Lane M. High protein diet inhibits inner cell mass formation and increases apoptosis in mouse blastocysts developed *in vivo* by increasing the levels of ammonium in the reproductive tract. *Reprod Fertil Dev* 2004; 16: 190.
7. Kwong WY, Wild AE, Roberts P, Willis AC, Fleming TP. Maternal undernutrition during the preimplantation period of rat development causes blastocyst abnormalities and programming of postnatal hypertension. *Development* 2000; 127: 4195–202.
8. Gardner DK, Reed L, Linck D, Sheehan C, Lane M. Quality control in human *in vitro* fertilization. *Semin Reprod Med* 2005; 23: 319–24.
9. Gardner D, Lane M. Towards a single embryo transfer. *Reprod Biomed Online* 2003; 6: 470–81.
10. Wale PL, Gardner DK. The effects of chemical and physical factors on mammalian embryo culture and their importance for the practice of assisted human reproduction. *Hum Reprod Update* 2016; 22: 2–22.
11. Gardner DK. Changes in requirements and utilization of nutrients during mammalian preimplantation embryo development and their significance in embryo culture. *Theriogenology* 1998; 49: 83–102.
12. Lane M, Gardner DK. Understanding cellular disruptions during early embryo development that perturb viability and fetal development. *Reprod Fertil Dev* 2005; 17: 371–8.
13. Gardner DK Lane M. Culture and selection of viable blastocysts: A feasible proposition for human IVF? *Hum Reprod Update* 1997; 3: 367–82.
14. Glujovsky D, Farquhar C, Quinteiro Retamar AM, Alvarez Sedo CR, Blake D. Cleavage stage versus blastocyst stage embryo transfer in assisted reproductive technology. *Cochrane Database Syst Rev* 2016; 6: CD002118.
15. Papanikolaou EG, Kolibianakis EM, Tournaye H et al. Live birth rates after transfer of equal number of blastocysts or cleavage-stage embryos in IVF. A systematic review and meta-analysis. *Hum Reprod* 2008; 23: 91–9.
16. Adashi EY, Barri PN, Berkowitz R et al. Infertility therapy-associated multiple pregnancies (births): An ongoing epidemic. *Reprod Biomed Online* 2003; 7: 515–42.
17. Gardner DK, Wale PL. Analysis of metabolism to select viable human embryos for transfer. *Fertil Steril* 2013; 99: 1062–72.
18. Gardner DK, Harvey AJ. Blastocyst metabolism. *Reprod Fertil Dev* 2015; 27: 638–54.
19. Leese HJ. Metabolism of the preimplantation mammalian embryo. *Oxf Rev Reprod Biol* 1991; 13: 35–72.
20. Gardner DK, Lane M. Embryo culture systems. In: *In Vitro Fertilization: A Practical Approach*. Gardner DK (ed.). New York, NY: Informa Healthcare, 2007, pp. 221–82.
21. Hardy K, Hooper MA, Handyside AH, Rutherford AJ, Winston RM, Leese HJ. Non-invasive measurement of glucose and pyruvate uptake by individual human oocytes and preimplantation embryos. *Hum Reprod* 1989; 4: 188–91.
22. Lane M, Gardner DK. Mitochondrial malate-aspartate shuttle regulates mouse embryo nutrient consumption. *J Biol Chem* 2005; 280: 18361–7.
23. Ratnam S, Mertineit C, Ding F et al. Dynamics of Dnmt1 methyltransferase expression and intracellular localization during oogenesis and preimplantation development. *Dev Biol* 2002; 245: 304–14.
24. Huang JC, Lei ZL, Shi LH et al. Comparison of histone modifications in *in vivo* and *in vitro* fertilization mouse embryos. *Biochem Biophys Res Commun* 2007; 354: 77–83.
25. Lucifero D, La Salle S, Bourc'his D, Martel J, Bestor TH, Trasler JM. Coordinate regulation of DNA methyltransferase expression during oogenesis. *BMC Dev Biol* 2007; 7: 36.
26. Dumollard R, Marangos P, Fitzharris G, Swann K, Duchen M, Carroll J. Sperm-triggered [Ca^{2+}] oscillations and Ca^{2+} homeostasis in the mouse egg have an absolute requirement for mitochondrial ATP production. *Development* 2004; 131: 3057–67.
27. Gangaraju VK, Bartholomew B. Mechanisms of ATP dependent chromatin remodeling. *Mutat Res* 2007; 618: 3–17.
28. Pepin D, Vanderhyden BC, Picketts DJ, Murphy BD. ISWI chromatin remodeling in ovarian somatic and germ cells: Revenge of the NURFs. *Trends Endocrinol Metab* 2007; 18: 215–24.
29. Harvey AJ, Rathjen J, Gardner DK. Metaboloepigenetic regulation of pluripotent stem cells. *Stem Cells Int* 2016; 2016: 1816525.
30. Gardner DK, Lane M. *Ex vivo* early embryo development and effects on gene expression and imprinting. *Reprod Fertil Dev* 2005; 17: 361–70.
31. Gardner DK, Lane M, Calderon I, Leeton J. Environment of the preimplantation human embryo *in vivo*: Metabolite analysis of oviduct and uterine fluids and metabolism of cumulus cells. *Fertil Steril* 1996; 65: 349–53.
32. Summers MC. A brief history of the development of the KSOM family of media. *Hum Fertil (Camb)* 2014; 17(Suppl 1): 12–6.
33. Lane M, Gardner DK. Lactate regulates pyruvate uptake and metabolism in the preimplantation mouse embryo. *Biol Reprod* 2000; 62: 16–22.
34. Gardner DK. Lactate production by the mammalian blastocyst: Manipulating the microenvironment for uterine implantation and invasion? *Bioessays* 2015; 37: 364–71.

35. Feuer SK, Camarano L, Rinaudo PF. ART and health: Clinical outcomes and insights on molecular mechanisms from rodent studies. *Mol Hum Reprod* 2013; 19: 189–204.
36. Bloise E, Feuer SK, Rinaudo PF. Comparative intrauterine development and placental function of ART concepti: Implications for human reproductive medicine and animal breeding. *Hum Reprod Update* 2014; 20: 822–39.
37. Calle A, Fernandez-Gonzalez R, Ramos-Ibeas P et al. Long-term and transgenerational effects of *in vitro* culture on mouse embryos. *Theriogenology* 2012; 77: 785–93.
38. Lane M, Gardner DK. Increase in postimplantation development of cultured mouse embryos by amino acids and induction of fetal retardation and exencephaly by ammonium ions. *J Reprod Fertil* 1994; 102: 305–12.
39. Zander DL, Thompson JG, Lane M. Perturbations in mouse embryo development and viability caused by ammonium are more severe after exposure at the cleavage stages. *Biol Reprod* 2006; 74: 288–94.
40. Rooke JA, McEvoy TG, Ashworth CJ et al. Ovine fetal development is more sensitive to perturbation by the presence of serum in embryo culture before rather than after compaction. *Theriogenology* 2007; 67: 639–47.
41. Braude P, Bolton V, Moore S. Human gene expression first occurs between the four- and eight-cell stages of preimplantation development. *Nature* 1988; 332: 459–61.
42. Gardner DK, Meseguer M, Rubio C, Treff NR. Diagnosis of human preimplantation embryo viability. *Hum Reprod Update* 2015; 21: 727–47.
43. Gardner DK. Mammalian embryo culture in the absence of serum or somatic cell support. *Cell Biol Int* 1994; 18: 1163–79.
44. Bavister BD. Culture of preimplantation embryos: Facts and artifacts. *Hum Reprod Update* 1995; 1: 91–148.
45. Leese HJ. Metabolic control during preimplantation mammalian development. *Hum Reprod Update* 1995; 1: 63–72.
46. Gardner DK, Lane M. Embryo culture systems. In: *Handbook of In vitro Fertilization*, 2nd edition. Trounson A, Gardner DK (eds). Boca Raton, FL: CRC Press, 1999, pp. 205–64.
47. Pool TB. Recent advances in the production of viable human embryos *in vitro. Reprod Biomed Online* 2002; 4: 294–302.
48. Summers MC, Biggers JD. Chemically defined media and the culture of mammalian preimplantation embryos: Historical perspective and current issues. *Hum Reprod Update* 2003; 9: 557–82.
49. Lane M, Gardner DK. Embryo culture medium: Which is the best? *Best Pract Res Clin Obstet Gynaecol* 2007; 21: 83–100.
50. Gardner DK. Dissection of culture media for embryos: The most important and less important components and characteristics. *Reprod Fertil Dev* 2008; 20: 9–18.
51. Perkins JL, Goode L. Free amino acids in the oviduct fluid of the ewe. *J Reprod Fertil* 1967; 14: 309–11.
52. Casslen BG. Free amino acids in human uterine fluid. Possible role of high taurine concentration. *J Reprod Med* 1987; 32: 181–4.
53. Miller JG, Schultz GA. Amino acid content of preimplantation rabbit embryos and fluids of the reproductive tract. *Biol Reprod* 1987; 36: 125–9.
54. Gardner DK, Leese HJ. Concentrations of nutrients in mouse oviduct fluid and their effects on embryo development and metabolism *in vitro. J Reprod Fertil* 1990; 88: 361–8.
55. Harris SE, Gopichandran N, Picton HM, Leese HJ, Orsi NM. Nutrient concentrations in murine follicular fluid and the female reproductive tract. *Theriogenology* 2005; 64: 992–1006.
56. Hugentobler SA, Diskin MG, Leese HJ et al. Amino acids in oviduct and uterine fluid and blood plasma during the estrous cycle in the bovine. *Mol Reprod Dev* 2007; 74: 445–54.
57. Van Winkle LJ. Amino acid transport regulation and early embryo development. *Biol Reprod* 2001; 64: 1–12.
58. Schultz GA, Kaye PL, McKay DJ, Johnson MH. Endogenous amino acid pool sizes in mouse eggs and preimplantation embryos. *J Reprod Fertil* 1981; 61: 387–93.
59. Gardner DK, Clarke RN, Lechene CP, Biggers JD. Development of a noninvasive ultramicrofluorometric method for measuring net uptake of glutamine by single preimplantation mouse embryos. *Gamete Res* 1989; 24: 427–38.
60. Rieger D, Loskutoff NM, Betteridge KJ. Developmentally related changes in the metabolism of glucose and glutamine by cattle embryos produced and co-cultured *in vitro. J Reprod Fertil* 1992; 95: 585–95.
61. Crosby IM, Gandolfi F, Moor RM. Control of protein synthesis during early cleavage of sheep embryos. *J Reprod Fertil* 1988; 82: 769–75.
62. Rieger D, Loskutoff NM, Betteridge KJ. Developmentally related changes in the uptake and metabolism of glucose, glutamine and pyruvate by cattle embryos produced *in vitro. Reprod Fertil Dev* 1992; 4: 547–57.
63. Van Winkle LJ, Haghighat N, Campione AL. Glycine protects preimplantation mouse conceptuses from a detrimental effect on development of the inorganic ions in oviductal fluid. *J Exp Zool* 1990; 253: 215–9.
64. Edwards LJ, Williams DA, Gardner DK. Intracellular pH of the mouse preimplantation embryo: Amino acids act as buffers of intracellular pH. *Hum Reprod* 1998; 13: 3441–8.

65. Liu Z, Foote RH. Development of bovine embryos in KSOM with added superoxide dismutase and taurine and with five and twenty percent O_2. *Biol Reprod* 1995; 53: 786–90.
66. Lindenbaum A. A survey of naturally occurring chelating ligands. *Adv Exp Med Biol* 1973; 40: 67–77.
67. Wu G, Morris SM, Jr. Arginine metabolism: Nitric oxide and beyond. *Biochem J* 1998; 336(Pt 1): 1–17.
68. Martin PM, Sutherland AE, Van Winkle LJ. Amino acid transport regulates blastocyst implantation. *Biol Reprod* 2003; 69: 1101–8.
69. Lane M, Gardner DK. Differential regulation of mouse embryo development and viability by amino acids. *J Reprod Fertil* 1997; 109: 153–64.
70. Martin PM, Sutherland AE. Exogenous amino acids regulate trophectoderm differentiation in the mouse blastocyst through an mTOR-dependent pathway. *Dev Biol* 2001; 240: 182–93.
71. Eagle H. Amino acid metabolism in mammalian cell cultures. *Science* 1959; 130: 432–7.
72. Gardner DK, Lane M. Amino acids and ammonium regulate mouse embryo development in culture. *Biol Reprod* 1993; 48: 377–85.
73. Dumoulin JC, Evers JL, Bakker JA, Bras M, Pieters MH, Geraedts JP. Temporal effects of taurine on mouse preimplantation development *in vitro. Hum Reprod* 1992; 7: 403–7.
74. Dumoulin JC, Evers JL, Bras M, Pieters MH, Geraedts JP. Positive effect of taurine on preimplantation development of mouse embryos *in vitro. J Reprod Fertil* 1992; 94: 373–80.
75. Gardner DK, Lane M. The 2-cell block in CF1 mouse embryos is associated with an increase in glycolysis and a decrease in tricarboxylic acid (TCA) cycle activity: Alleviation of the 2-cell block is associated with the restoration of *in vivo* metabolic pathway activities. *Biol Reprod* 1993; 49(Suppl 1): 152 (Abstract).
76. Bavister BD, McKiernan SH. Regulation of hamster embryo development *in vitro* by amino acids. In: *Preimplantation Embryo Development.* Bavister BD (ed.). New York, NY: Springer-Verlag, 1992, pp. 57–72.
77. McKiernan SH, Clayton MK, Bavister BD. Analysis of stimulatory and inhibitory amino acids for development of hamster one-cell embryos *in vitro. Mol Reprod Dev* 1995; 42: 188–99.
78. Gardner DK, Lane M, Spitzer A, Batt PA. Enhanced rates of cleavage and development for sheep zygotes cultured to the blastocyst stage *in vitro* in the absence of serum and somatic cells: Amino acids, vitamins, and culturing embryos in groups stimulate development. *Biol Reprod* 1994; 50: 390–400.
79. Thompson JG, Gardner DK, Pugh PA, McMillan WH, Tervit HR. Lamb birth weight is affected by culture system utilized during *in vitro* pre-elongation development of ovine embryos. *Biol Reprod* 1995; 53: 1385–91.
80. Takahashi Y, First NL. *In vitro* development of bovine one-cell embryos influence of glucose, lactate, amino acids and vitamins. *Theriogenology* 1992; 37: 963–78.
81. Steeves TE, Gardner DK. Temporal and differential effects of amino acids on bovine embryo development in culture. *Biol Reprod* 1999; 61: 731–40.
82. Devreker F, Winston RM, Hardy K. Glutamine improves human preimplantation development *in vitro. Fertil Steril* 1998; 69: 293–9.
83. Devreker F, Van den Bergh M, Biramane J, Winston RL, Englert Y, Hardy K. Effects of taurine on human embryo development *in vitro. Hum Reprod* 1999; 14: 2350–6.
84. Lane M, Gardner DK. Nonessential amino acids and glutamine decrease the time of the first three cleavage divisions and increase compaction of mouse zygotes *in vitro. J Assist Reprod Genet* 1997; 14: 398–403.
85. Wang J, Alexander P, Wu L, Hammer R, Cleaver O, McKnight SL. Dependence of mouse embryonic stem cells on threonine catabolism. *Science* 2009; 325: 435–9.
86. Gardner DK, Lane M. Alleviation of the '2-cell block' and development to the blastocyst of CF1 mouse embryos: Role of amino acids, EDTA and physical parameters. *Hum Reprod* 1996; 11: 2703–12.
87. Ho Y, Wigglesworth K, Eppig JJ, Schultz RM. Preimplantation development of mouse embryos in KSOM: Augmentation by amino acids and analysis of gene expression. *Mol Reprod Dev* 1995; 41: 232–8.
88. Doherty AS, Mann MR, Tremblay KD, Bartolomei MS, Schultz RM. Differential effects of culture on imprinted H19 expression in the preimplantation mouse embryo. *Biol Reprod* 2000; 62: 1526–35.
89. Gardner DK, Lane M, Stevens J, Schoolcraft WB. Noninvasive assessment of human embryo nutrient consumption as a measure of developmental potential. *Fertil Steril* 2001; 76: 1175–80.
90. Virant-Klun I, Tomazevic T, Vrtacnik-Bokal E, Vogler AK M., Meden-Vrtovec H. Increased ammonium in culture medium reduces the development of human embryos to the blastocyst stage. *Fertil Steril* 2006; 85: 526–8.
91. Sinawat S, Hsaio WC, Flockhart JH, Kaufman MH, Keith J, West JD. Fetal abnormalities produced after preimplantation exposure of mouse embryos to ammonium chloride. *Hum Reprod* 2003; 18: 2157–65.
92. Lane M, Gardner DK. Ammonium induces aberrant blastocyst differentiation, metabolism, pH regulation, gene expression and subsequently alters fetal development in the mouse. *Biol Reprod* 2003; 69: 1109–17.
93. Gardner DK, Hamilton R, McCallie B, Schoolcraft WB, Katz-Jaffe MG. Human and mouse embryonic development, metabolism and gene expression are altered by an ammonium gradient *in vitro. Reproduction* 2013; 146: 49–61.

94. Wale PL, Gardner DK. Oxygen regulates amino acid turnover and carbohydrate uptake during the preimplantation period of mouse embryo development. *Biol Reprod* 2012; 87: 24.
95. Wale PL, Gardner DK. Oxygen affects the ability of mouse blastocysts to regulate ammonium. *Biol Reprod* 2013; 89: 75.
96. Biggers JD, McGinnis LK, Summers MC. Discrepancies between the effects of glutamine in cultures of preimplantation mouse embryos. *Reprod Biomed Online* 2004; 9: 70–3.
97. Menezo YR, Guerin P. Preimplantation embryo metabolism and embryo interaction with the *in vitro* environment. In: *Human Preimplantation Embryo Selection*. Elder K, Cohen J (ed.). London, U.K.: Informa healthcare, 2007, pp. 191–200.
98. Nakazawa T, Ohashi K, Yamada M et al. Effect of different concentrations of amino acids in human serum and follicular fluid on the development of one-cell mouse embryos *in vitro*. *J Reprod Fertil* 1997; 111: 327–32.
99. Lane M, Gardner DK. Removal of embryo-toxic ammonium from the culture medium by *in situ* enzymatic conversion to glutamate. *J Exp Zool* 1995; 271: 356–63.
100. Dumoulin JC, Land JA, Van Montfoort AP et al. Effect of *in vitro* culture of human embryos on birthweight of newborns. *Hum Reprod* 2010; 25: 605–12.
101. Kleijkers SH, van Montfoort AP, Smits LJ et al. IVF culture medium affects post-natal weight in humans during the first 2 years of life. *Hum Reprod* 2014; 29: 661–9.
102. He Y, Hakvoort TB, Vermeulen JL, Lamers WH, Van Roon MA. Glutamine synthetase is essential in early mouse embryogenesis. *Dev Dyn* 2007; 236: 1865–75.
103. McEvoy TG, Robinson JJ, Aitken RP, Findlay PA, Robertson IS. Dietary excesses of urea influence the viability and metabolism of preimplantation sheep embryos and may affect fetal growth among survivors. *Anim Reprod Sci* 1997; 47: 71–90.
104. Dorland M, Gardner DK, Trounson A. Serum in synthetic oviduct fluid causes mitochondrial degeneration in ovine embryos. *Reprod Fertil (Abstr Ser)* 1994; 13: 70.
105. Khosla S, Dean W, Brown D, Reik W, Feil R. Culture of preimplantation mouse embryos affects fetal development and the expression of imprinted genes. *Biol Reprod* 2001; 64: 918–26.
106. Wrenzycki C, Herrmann D, Keskintepe L et al. Effects of culture system and protein supplementation on mRNA expression in pre-implantation bovine embryos. *Hum Reprod* 2001; 16: 893–901.
107. Young LE, Fernandes K, McEvoy TG et al. Epigenetic change in IGF2R is associated with fetal overgrowth after sheep embryo culture. *Nat Genet* 2001; 27: 153–4.
108. Gray CW, Morgan PM, Kane MT. Purification of an embryotrophic factor from commercial bovine serum albumin and its identification as citrate. *J Reprod Fertil* 1992; 94: 471–80.
109. Batt PA, Gardner DK, Cameron AW. Oxygen concentration and protein source affect the development of preimplantation goat embryos *in vitro*. *Reprod Fertil Dev* 1991; 3: 601–7.
110. McKiernan SH, Bavister BD. Different lots of bovine serum albumin inhibit or stimulate *in vitro* development of hamster embryos. *In Vitro Cell Dev Biol* 1992; 28: 154–6.
111. Kane MT. Variability in different lots of commercial bovine serum albumin affects cell multiplication and hatching of rabbit blastocysts in culture. *J Reprod Fertil* 1983; 69: 555–8.
112. Bar-Or D, Bar-Or R, Rael LT, Gardner DK, Slone DS, Craun ML. Heterogeneity and oxidation status of commercial human albumin preparations in clinical use. *Crit Care Med* 2005; 33: 1638–41.
113. Takatori S, Akutsu K, Kondo F, Ishii R, Nakazawa H, Makino T. Di(2-ethylhexyl)phthalate and mono(2-ethylhexyl)phthalate in media for *in vitro* fertilization. *Chemosphere* 2012; 86: 454–9.
114. Akutsu K, Takatori S, Nakazawa H, Makino T. Detection of polybrominated diphenyl ethers in culture media and protein sources used for human *in vitro* fertilization. *Chemosphere* 2013; 92: 864–9.
115. Morbeck DE, Paczkowski M, Fredrickson JR et al. Composition of protein supplements used for human embryo culture. *J Assist Reprod Genet* 2014; 31: 1703–11.
116. Bavister BD, Kinsey DL, Lane M, Gardner DK. Recombinant human albumin supports hamster *in-vitro* fertilization. *Hum Reprod* 2003; 18: 113–6.
117. Bungum M, Humaidan P, Bungum L. Recombinant human albumin as protein source in culture media used for IVF: A prospective randomized study. *Reprod Biomed Online* 2002; 4: 233–6.
118. Lane M, Maybach JM, Hooper K, Hasler JF, Gardner DK. Cryo-survival and development of bovine blastocysts are enhanced by culture with recombinant albumin and hyaluronan. *Mol Reprod Dev* 2003; 64: 70–8.
119. Zorn TM, Pinhal MA, Nader HB, Carvalho JJ, Abrahamsohn PA, Dietrich CP. Biosynthesis of glycosaminoglycans in the endometrium during the initial stages of pregnancy of the mouse. *Cell Mol Biol (Noisy-le-grand)* 1995; 41: 97–106.
120. Gardner DK, Rodriegez-Martinez H, Lane M. Fetal development after transfer is increased by replacing protein with the glycosaminoglycan hyaluronan for mouse embryo culture and transfer. *Hum Reprod* 1999; 14: 2575–80.
121. Palasz AT, Rodriguez-Martinez H, Beltran-Brena P et al. Effects of hyaluronan, BSA, and serum on bovine embryo *in vitro* development, ultrastructure, and gene expression patterns. *Mol Reprod Dev* 2006; 73: 1503–11.
122. Dattena M, Mara L, Bin TA, Cappai P. Lambing rate using vitrified blastocysts is improved by culture with BSA and hyaluronan. *Mol Reprod Dev* 2007; 74: 42–7.

123. Urman B, Yakin K, Ata B, Isiklar A, Balaban B. Effect of hyaluronan-enriched transfer medium on implantation and pregnancy rates after day 3 and day 5 embryo transfers: A prospective randomized study. *Fertil Steril* 2007; 90: 604–12.
124. Bontekoe S, Blake D, Heineman MJ, Williams EC, Johnson N. Adherence compounds in embryo transfer media for assisted reproductive technologies. *Cochrane Database Syst Rev* 2010; 7: CD007421.
125. Bontekoe S, Heineman MJ, Johnson N, Blake D. Adherence compounds in embryo transfer media for assisted reproductive technologies. *Cochrane Database Syst Rev* 2014; 2: CD007421.
126. Balaban B, Urman B. Comparison of two sequential media for culturing cleavage-stage embryos and blastocysts: Embryo characteristics and clinical outcome. *Reprod Biomed Online* 2005; 10: 485–91.
127. Stojkovic M, Kolle S, Peinl S et al. Effects of high concentrations of hyaluronan in culture medium on development and survival rates of fresh and frozen–thawed bovine embryos produced *in vitro*. *Reproduction* 2002; 124: 141–53.
128. Palasz AT, Brena PB, Martinez MF et al. Development, molecular composition and freeze tolerance of bovine embryos cultured in TCM-199 supplemented with hyaluronan. *Zygote* 2008; 16: 39–47.
129. Gardner DK, Lane. Embryo culture systems. In: *Handbook of In Vitro Fertilization*. Fourth Edition. Gardner DK, Simon C (eds). CRC Press, Boca Raton, 2017; pp. 205–244.
130. Gardner DK, Sakkas D. Mouse embryo cleavage, metabolism and viability: Role of medium composition. *Hum Reprod* 1993; 8: 288–95.
131. Hardarson T, Bungum M, Conaghan J et al. Noninferiority, randomized, controlled trial comparing embryo development using media developed for sequential or undisturbed culture in a time-lapse setup. *Fertil Steril* 2015; 104: 1452–59.e1-4.
132. Bowman P, McLaren A. Cleavage rate of mouse embryos *in vivo* and *in vitro*. *J Embryol Exp Morphol* 1970; 24: 203–7.
133. Harlow GM, Quinn P. Development of preimplantation mouse embryos *in vivo* and *in vitro*. *Aust J Biol Sci* 1982; 35: 187–93.
134. Gardner DK, Lane M. Culture of viable mammalian embroys. In: *Principles of Cloning*. Second Edition, Cibelli J, Lanza R, Campbell K, West MD (eds). Academic Press, San Diego, 2014; pp. 63–84.
135. Meseguer M, Rubio I, Cruz M, Basile N, Marcos J, Requena A. Embryo incubation and selection in a time-lapse monitoring system improves pregnancy outcome compared with a standard incubator: A retrospective cohort study. *Fertil Steril* 2012; 98: 1481–9.e10.
136. Phillips KP, Leveille MC, Claman P, Baltz JM. Intracellular pH regulation in human preimplantation embryos. *Hum Reprod* 2000; 15: 896–904.
137. Lane M, Baltz JM, Bavister BD. Regulation of intracellular pH in hamster preimplantation embryos by the sodium hydrogen (Na^+/H^+) antiporter. *Biol Reprod* 1998; 59: 1483–90.
138. Edwards LJ, Williams DA, Gardner DK. Intracellular pH of the preimplantation mouse embryo: Effects of extracellular pH and weak acids. *Mol Reprod Dev* 1998; 50: 434–42.
139. Quinn P, Barros C, Whittingham DG. Preservation of hamster oocytes to assay the fertilizing capacity of human spermatozoa. *J Reprod Fertil* 1982; 66: 161–8.
140. Lane M, Gardner DK. Preparation of gametes, *in vitro* maturation, *in vitro* fertilization, embryo recovery and transfer. In: *A Laboratory Guide to the Mammalian Embryo*. Gardner DK, Lane M, Watson AJ (eds). New York, NY: Oxford Press, 2004: pp. 24–40.
141. Gardner DK, Lane M. Mammalian preimplantation embryo culture. *Methods Mol Biol* 2014; 1092: 167–82.
142. Mastroianni L, Jr., Jones R. Oxygen tension within the rabbit fallopian tube. *J Reprod Fertil* 1965; 147: 99–102.
143. Ross RN, Graves CN. O_2 levels in female rabbit reproductive tract. *J Anim Sci* 1974; 39: 994.
144. Fischer B, Bavister BD. Oxygen tension in the oviduct and uterus of rhesus monkeys, hamsters and rabbits. *J Reprod Fertil* 1993; 99: 673–9.
145. Quinn P, Harlow GM. The effect of oxygen on the development of preimplantation mouse embryos *in vitro*. *J Exp Zool* 1978; 206: 73–80.
146. Thompson JG, Simpson AC, Pugh PA, Donnelly PE, Tervit HR. Effect of oxygen concentration on *in-vitro* development of preimplantation sheep and cattle embryos. *J Reprod Fertil* 1990; 89: 573–8.
147. Wale PL, Gardner DK. Time-lapse analysis of mouse embryo development in oxygen gradients. *Reprod Biomed Online* 2010; 21: 402–10.
148. Kirkegaard K, Hindkjaer JJ, Ingerslev HJ. Effect of oxygen concentration on human embryo development evaluated by time-lapse monitoring. *Fertil Steril* 2013; 99: 738–44 e4.
149. Katz-Jaffe MG, Linck DW, Schoolcraft WB, Gardner DK. A proteomic analysis of mammalian preimplantation embryonic development. *Reproduction* 2005; 130: 899–905.
150. Rinaudo PF, Giritharan G, Talbi S, Dobson AT, Schultz RM. Effects of oxygen tension on gene expression in preimplantation mouse embryos. *Fertil Steril* 2006; 86: 1252–65, 1265.e1–36.
151. Gardner DK. The impact of physiological oxygen during culture, and vitrification for cryopreservation, on the outcome of extended culture in human IVF. *Reprod Biomed Online* 2016; 32: 137–41.
152. Meintjes M, Chantilis SJ, Douglas JD et al. A controlled randomized trial evaluating the effect of lowered incubator oxygen tension on live births in a predominantly blastocyst transfer program. *Hum Reprod* 2009; 24: 300–7.

153. Nanassy L, Peterson CA, Wilcox AL, Peterson CM, Hammoud A, Carrell DT. Comparison of 5% and ambient oxygen during days 3–5 of *in vitro* culture of human embryos. *Fertil Steril* 2010; 93: 579–85.
154. Waldenstrom U, Engstrom AB, Hellberg D, Nilsson S. Low-oxygen compared with high-oxygen atmosphere in blastocyst culture, a prospective randomized study. *Fertil Steril* 2009; 91: 2461–65.
155. Bontekoe S, Mantikou E, van Wely M, Seshadri S, Repping S, Mastenbroek S. Low oxygen concentrations for embryo culture in assisted reproductive technologies. *Cochrane Database Syst Rev* 2012; 7: CD008950.
156. Christianson MS, Zhao Y, Shoham G et al. Embryo catheter loading and embryo culture techniques: Results of a worldwide web-based survey. *J Assist Reprod Genet* 2014; 31: 1029–36.
157. Leese HJ. The formation and function of oviduct fluid. *J Reprod Fertil* 1988; 82: 843–56.
158. Wiley LM, Yamami S, Van Muyden D. Effect of potassium concentration, type of protein supplement, and embryo density on mouse preimplantation development *in vitro*. *Fertil Steril* 1986; 45: 111–9.
159. Paria BC, Dey SK. Preimplantation embryo development *in vitro*: Cooperative interactions among embryos and role of growth factors. *Proc Natl Acad Sci USA* 1990; 87: 4756–60.
160. Lane M, Gardner DK. Effect of incubation volume and embryo density on the development and viability of mouse embryos *in vitro*. *Hum Reprod* 1992; 7: 558–62.
161. Ahern TJ, Gardner DK. Culturing bovine embryos in groups stimulates blastocyst development and cell allocation to the inner cell mass. *Theriogenology* 1998; 49: 194.
162. Spindler RE, Crichton EG, Agca Y et al. Improved felid embryo development by group culture is maintained with heterospecific companions. *Theriogenology* 2006; 66: 82–92.
163. Khan Z, Wolff HS, Fredrickson JR, Walker DL, Daftary GS, Morbeck DE. Mouse strain and quality control testing: Improved sensitivity of the mouse embryo assay with embryos from outbred mice. *Fertil Steril* 2013; 99: 847–54.e2.
164. Silverman IH, Cook CL, Sanfilippo JS, Yussman MA, Schultz GS, Hilton FH. Ham's F-10 constituted with tap water supports mouse conceptus development *in vitro*. *J In Vitro Fert Embryo Transf* 1987; 4: 185–7.
165. George MA, Braude PR, Johnson MH, Sweetnam DG. Quality control in the IVF laboratory: *In-vitro* and *in-vivo* development of mouse embryos is unaffected by the quality of water used in culture media. *Hum Reprod* 1989; 4: 826–31.
166. Fissore RA, Jackson KV, Kiessling AA. Mouse zygote development in culture medium without protein in the presence of ethylenediaminetetraacetic acid. *Biol Reprod* 1989; 41: 835–41.
167. Flood LP, Shirley B. Reduction of embryotoxicity by protein in embryo culture media. *Mol Reprod Dev* 1991; 30: 226–31.
168. Wolff HS, Fredrickson JR, Walker DL, Morbeck DE. Advances in quality control: Mouse embryo morphokinetics are sensitive markers of *in vitro* stress. *Hum Reprod* 2013; 28: 1776–82.
169. Wilson M, Hartke K, Kiehl M, Rodgers J, Brabec C, Lyles R. Integration of blastocyst transfer for all patients. *Fertil Steril* 2002; 77: 693–6.
170. Marek D, Langley M, Gardner DK, Confer N, Doody KM, Doody KJ. Introduction of blastocyst culture and transfer for all patients in an *in vitro* fertilization program. *Fertil Steril* 1999; 72: 1035–40.
171. Menezo YJ, Guerin JF, Czyba JC. Improvement of human early embryo development *in vitro* by coculture on monolayers of Vero cells. *Biol Reprod* 1990; 42: 301–6.
172. Lopata A. The neglected human blastocyst. *J Assist Reprod Genet* 1992; 9: 508–12.
173. Olivennes F, Hazout A, Lelaidier C et al. Four indications for embryo transfer at the blastocyst stage. *Hum Reprod* 1994; 9: 2367–73.
174. Scholtes MC, Zeilmaker GH. A prospective, randomized study of embryo transfer results after 3 or 5 days of embryo culture in *in vitro* fertilization. *Fertil Steril* 1996; 65: 1245–8.
175. Ertzeid G, Storeng R. Adverse effects of gonadotrophin treatment on pre- and postimplantation development in mice. *J Reprod Fertil* 1992; 96: 649–55.
176. Ertzeid G, Storeng R, Lyberg T. Treatment with gonadotropins impaired implantation and fetal development in mice. *J Assist Reprod Genet* 1993; 10: 286–91.
177. Taylor DM, Ray PF, Ao A, Winston RM, Handyside AH. Paternal transcripts for glucose-6-phosphate dehydrogenase and adenosine deaminase are first in the human preimplantation embryo at the three- to four-cell stage. *Mol Reprod Dev* 1997; 48: 442–8.
178. Scott LA, Smith S. The successful use of pronuclear embryo transfers the day following oocyte retrieval. *Hum Reprod* 1998; 13: 1003–13.
179. Gerris J, De Neubourg D, Mangelschots K, Van Royen E, Van de Meerssche M, Valkenburg M. Prevention of twin pregnancy after *in-vitro* fertilization or intracytoplasmic sperm injection based on strict embryo criteria: A prospective randomized clinical trial. *Hum Reprod* 1999; 14: 2581–7.
180. Tesarik J. Developmental failure during the preimplanation period of human embryogenesis. In: *The Biological Basis of Early Human Reproductive Failure*. Van Blerkom J (ed.). New York, NY: Oxford University Press, 1994, pp. 327–44.
181. Sandalinas M, Sadowy S, Alikani M, Calderon G, Cohen J, Munne S. Developmental ability of chromosomally abnormal human embryos to develop to the blastocyst stage. *Hum Reprod* 2001; 16: 1954–8.

182. Fanchin R, Righini C, Olivennes F, Taylor S, de Ziegler D, Frydman R. Uterine contractions at the time of embryo transfer alter pregnancy rates after *in-vitro* fertilization. *Hum Reprod* 1998; 13: 1968–74.
183. Lesny P, Killick SR, Tetlow RL, Robinson J, Maguiness SD. Uterine junctional zone contractions during assisted reproduction cycles. *Hum Reprod Update* 1998; 4: 440–5.
184. Fanchin R, Ayoubi JM, Righini C, Olivennes F, Schonauer LM, Frydman R. Uterine contractility decreases at the time of blastocyst transfers. *Hum Reprod* 2001; 16: 1115–9.
185. Veeck LL. Does the developmental stage at freeze impact on clinical results post-thaw? *Reprod Biomed Online* 2003; 6: 367–74.
186. Fragouli E, Lenzi M, Ross R, Katz-Jaffe M, Schoolcraft WB, Wells D. Comprehensive molecular cytogenetic analysis of the human blastocyst stage. *Hum Reprod* 2008; 23: 2596–608.
187. Schoolcraft WB, Fragouli E, Stevens J, Munne S, Katz-Jaffe MG, Wells D. Clinical application of comprehensive chromosomal screening at the blastocyst stage. *Fertil Steril* 2010; 94: 1700–6.
188. Scott RT, Jr., Upham KM, Forman EJ, Zhao T, Treff NR. Cleavage-stage biopsy significantly impairs human embryonic implantation potential while blastocyst biopsy does not: A randomized and paired clinical trial. *Fertil Steril* 2013; 100: 624–30.
189. Hunault CC, Eijkemans MJ, Pieters MH et al. A prediction model for selecting patients undergoing *in vitro* fertilization for elective single embryo transfer. *Fertil Steril* 2002; 77: 725–32.
190. Balaban B, Urman B, Alatas C, Mercan R, Aksoy S, Isiklar A. Blastocyst-stage transfer of poor-quality cleavage-stage embryos results in higher implantation rates. *Fertil Steril* 2001; 75: 514–8.
191. Schoolcraft WB, Gardner DK. Blastocyst culture and transfer increases the efficiency of oocyte donation. *Fertil Steril* 2000; 74: 482–6.
192. Gardner DK, Surrey E, Minjarez D, Leitz A, Stevens J, Schoolcraft WB. Single blastocyst transfer: A prospective randomized trial. *Fertil Steril* 2004; 81: 551–5.
193. Cummins JM, Breen TM, Harrison KL, Shaw JM, Wilson LM, Hennessey JF. A formula for scoring human embryo growth rates in *in vitro* fertilization: Its value in predicting pregnancy and in comparison with visual estimates of embryo quality. *J In Vitro Fert Embryo Transf* 1986; 3: 284–95.
194. Steer CV, Mills CL, Tan SL, Campbell S, Edwards RG. The cumulative embryo score: A predictive embryo scoring technique to select the optimal number of embryos to transfer in an *in-vitro* fertilization and embryo transfer programme. *Hum Reprod* 1992; 7: 117–9.
195. Scott L. The biological basis of non-invasive strategies for selection of human oocytes and embryos. *Hum Reprod Update* 2003; 9: 237–49.
196. Papanikolaou V. Early pregnancy loss is significantly higher after day 3 single embryo transfer that after day 5 single blastocyst transfer in GnRH antagonist stimulated IVF cycles. *Reprod Biomed Online* 2006; 12: 60–5.
197. Li Z, Wang YA, Ledger W, Edgar DH, Sullivan EA. Clinical outcomes following cryopreservation of blastocysts by vitrification or slow freezing: A population-based cohort study. *Hum Reprod* 2014; 29: 2794–801.
198. Takahashi K, Mukaida T, Goto T, Oka C. Perinatal outcome of blastocyst transfer with vitrification using cryoloop: A 4-year follow-up study. *Fertil Steril* 2005; 84: 88–92.
199. Roy TK, Bradley CK, Bowman MC, McArthur SJ. Single-embryo transfer of vitrified–warmed blastocysts yields equivalent live-birth rates and improved neonatal outcomes compared with fresh transfers. *Fertil Steril* 2014; 101: 1294–301.
200. Silva E, Greene AF, Strauss K, Herrick JR, Schoolcraft WB, Krisher RL. Antioxidant supplementation during *in vitro* culture improves mitochondrial function and development of embryos from aged female mice. *Reprod Fertil Dev* 2015; 27: 975–83.
201. Truong TT, Soh YM, Gardner DK. Antioxidants improve mouse preimplantation embryo development and viability. *Hum Reprod* 2016; 31: 1445–54.
202. Hannan NJ, Paiva P, Meehan KL, Rombauts LJ, Gardner DK, Salamonsen LA. Analysis of fertility-related soluble mediators in human uterine fluid identifies VEGF as a key regulator of embryo implantation. *Endocrinology* 2011; 152: 4948–56.
203. Binder NK, Evans J, Gardner DK, Salamonsen LA, Hannan NJ. Endometrial signals improve embryo outcome: Functional role of vascular endothelial growth factor isoforms on embryo development and implantation in mice. *Hum Reprod* 2014; 29: 2278–86.
204. Ziebe S, Loft A, Povlsen BB et al. A randomized clinical trial to evaluate the effect of granulocyte-macrophage colony-stimulating factor (GM-CSF) in embryo culture medium for *in vitro* fertilization. *Fertil Steril* 2013; 99: 1600–9.
205. Karagenc L, Lane M, Gardner DK. Granulocyte-macrophage colony-stimulating factor stimulates mouse blastocyst inner cell mass development only when media lack human serum albumin. *Reprod Biomed Online* 2005; 10: 511–8.
206. Kawamura K, Chen Y, Shu Y et al. Promotion of human early embryonic development and blastocyst outgrowth *in vitro* using autocrine/paracrine growth factors. *PLoS One* 2012; 7: e49328.
207. Thouas GA, Dominguez F, Green MP, Vilella F, Simon C, Gardner DK. Soluble ligands and their receptors in human embryo development and implantation. *Endocr Rev* 2015; 36: 92–130.
208. Thouas GA, Potter DL, Gardner DK. Microfluidic devices for the analysis of gamete and embryo

physiology. In: *Human Gametes and Preimplantation Embryos: Assessment and Diagnosis*. Gardner DK, Sakkas D, Seli E, Wells D (eds). New York, NY: Springer, 2013, pp. 281–99.

209. Suh RS, Phadke N, Ohl DA, Takayama S, Smith GD. Rethinking gamete/embryo isolation and culture with microfluidics. *Hum Reprod Update* 2003; 9: 451–61.
210. Wheeler MB, Walters EM, Beebe DJ. Toward culture of single gametes: The development of microfluidic platforms for assisted reproduction. *Theriogenology* 2007; 68(Suppl 1): S178–89.
211. Lane M, Gardner DK. Selection of viable mouse blastocysts prior to transfer using a metabolic criterion. *Hum Reprod* 1996; 11: 1975–78.
212. Brison DR, Houghton FD, Falconer D et al. Identification of viable embryos in IVF by non-invasive measurement of amino acid turnover. *Hum Reprod* 2004; 19: 2319–24.
213. Gardner DK, Sakkas D. Assessment of embryo viability: The ability to select a single embryo for transfer—A review. *Placenta* 2003; 24(Suppl B): S5–12.
214. Urbanski JP, Thies W, Rhodes C, Amarasinghe S, Thorsen T. Digital microfluidics using soft lithography. *Lab Chip* 2006; 6: 96–104.
215. Gardner DK, Schoolcraft WB. *In vitro* culture of human blastocyst. In: *Towards Reproductive Certainty: Fertility and Genetics Beyond 1999*. Jansen R, Mortimer D (eds). Carnforth, U.K.: Parthenon Publishing, 1999, pp. 378–88.
216. Gardner DK, Stevens, J., Sheehan, CB, Schoolcraft, WB. Analysis of blastocyst morphology. In: *Human Preimplantation Embryo Selection*. Elder KCJ (ed.). London, U.K.: Informa Healthcare, 2007, pp. 79–87.
217. Gardner DK, Balaban B. Assessment of human embryo development using morphological criteria in an era of time-lapse, algorithms and "OMICS": Is looking good still important? *Mol Hum Rep* 2016; 22: 704–18.

Evaluation of embryo quality

Analysis of morphology and physiology

17

DENNY SAKKAS and DAVID K. GARDNER

INTRODUCTION

Worldwide, the utilization of assisted reproduction technologies (ARTs) continues to increase annually. In 2006, over 1 million cycles were registered in the international report on ART monitoring (1). Subsequently, by 2011, it was reported that 1.5 million ART cycles were being performed each year, with an estimated 350,000 babies born worldwide (2). Well over half a million treatment cycles are initiated annually in the U.S.A., Europe, Australia, and New Zealand alone (3–5). This increasing trend of ART utilization has been driven by the steady improvement in delivery rates, improved access to care in many areas, and the relative ineffectiveness of other treatment options. The proportion of infants born after ART in Europe now ranges from 0.1% to 3.9% of all live-born children (6,7).

Historically, acceptable success rates through *in vitro* fertilization (IVF) were attained, in many cases, only through the simultaneous transfer of multiple embryos. However, over the past decade, this trend has changed dramatically. In the U.S.A., an average of 2.8 embryos were transferred in women <38 years of age in 2003 compared to 1.9 embryos per patient in 2013 (8). A further trend has been a shift to transferring embryos after cryostorage into a more receptive uterine environment, which has also led to lower numbers of embryos transferred (8).

The risks to both mother and baby related to multiple gestations are well documented and include maternal hypertension, preterm delivery, low birth weight, and a dramatic increase in the relative risk for cerebral palsy (reviewed in [9–12]). These complications lead to a higher incidence of medical, perinatal, and neonatal complications and a 10-fold increase in healthcare costs compared to a singleton delivery (13). Decreasing the prevalence of multiple gestations in IVF can only be achieved by the transfer of a single embryo.

In many countries including Norway, Sweden, Denmark, Belgium, England, Italy, and Germany, legal restrictions have been implemented governing the number of embryos that can be transferred in a given IVF cycle. For example, in most Scandinavian countries and Belgium, governments have set a legal limit of single-embryo transfer (i.e., only one embryo to be transferred per cycle) for specific patient groups, while many other European countries have restricted the number of transferred embryos to a maximum of two. In other parts of the world, where no legal restrictions exist, the onus is on the individual clinic (as well as the patient) to decrease the number of embryos transferred so that an acceptable balance can be achieved between the risks associated with multiple gestations and "acceptable" pregnancy rates. In Australia and New Zealand, this was achieved by clinicians and patients willingly shifting to single-embryo transfer, with the proportion increasing from 69.7% in 2009 to 79.2% in 2013 (14). A similar achievement was obtained in Quebec, Canada (15). Notably, in the U.S.A., the Practice Committee of the American Society for Reproductive Medicine and the Practice Committee of the Society for Assisted Reproductive Technology have now stipulated under what circumstances single-embryo transfer should take place (16). The current indications are that in the future all countries currently lacking legislation will be compelled via legal, financial, and/or moral obligation to restrict the number of embryos transferred in order to minimize the risk of multiple gestations.

A major issue in limiting the number of embryos transferred remains the apparent inability to accurately estimate the reproductive potential of individual embryos within a cohort of embryos using the existing selection techniques, which largely depend upon morphological evaluation. Faced with the scenario that we, the worldwide IVF community, will in the future have to select only one or at most two embryos for transfer, we will be forced to make certain choices. The first may be to rely on milder stimulation protocols, hence generating a lower number of eggs at collection. Paradoxically, the generation of a smaller number of oocytes could lead to a greater percentage of viable embryos within a given cohort (17,18) and a more receptive endometrium (19–23). The second choice (which is not exclusive from the first) is to improve the selection process for defining the quality of individual embryos so that the ones we choose for transfer are more likely to implant, thereby significantly decreasing the time to pregnancy. This chapter will discuss several strategies in selection criteria that will help us with this second choice.

MORPHOLOGY AS AN ASSESSMENT TOOL

For over 30 years, morphological assessment has been the primary means of the embryologist for selecting which embryo(s) to replace. From the early years of IVF, it was noted that embryos cleaving faster and those of better morphological appearance were more likely to lead to a pregnancy (24,25). Morphological assessment systems have subsequently evolved over the past three decades and, in addition to the classical parameters of cell number and fragmentation, numerous other characteristics have been examined, including: pronucleate oocyte morphology;

early cleavage to the two-cell stage; top-quality embryos on successive days; and various forms of sequential assessment of embryos (see reviews in [26–28]). Further, the ability to culture and assess blastocyst-stage embryos has significantly improved embryo selection on the basis of morphology (29). Concomitantly, in the past few years, we have seen the advent of commercially available video imaging technologies that shed new light on how we interpret and use the morphological features of the embryo (see Chapter 18 and [30]). Here, we briefly describe some of the historical papers that examined key morphogenic events and the key times at which they should take place in the laboratory.

THE PRONUCLEATE OOCYTE

The many transformations that take place during the fertilization process make this a highly dynamic stage to assess. The oocyte contains the majority of the developmental materials and maternal mRNA, for ensuring that the embryo reaches the four- to eight-cell stage. In human embryos, embryonic genome activation has been shown to occur between the four- to eight-cell stages (31). The quality of the oocyte therefore plays the lead role in determining embryo development and subsequent viability.

A number of studies postulated that embryo quality can be predicted at the pronucleate oocyte stage. Separate studies by Tesarik and Scott (32,33) concentrated on the predictive value of the nucleoli. Tesarik and Greco (32) proposed that the normal and abnormal morphology of the pronuclei were related to the developmental fate of human embryos. They retrospectively assessed the number and distribution of nucleolar precursor bodies (NPBs) in each pronucleus of fertilized oocytes that led to embryos that implanted. The characteristics of these pronucleate oocytes were then compared to those that led to failures in implantation. The features that were shared by pronucleate oocytes that had 100% implantation success were: (i) the number of NPBs in both pronuclei never differed by more than three; and (ii) the NPBs were always polarized or not polarized in both pronuclei, but never polarized in one pronucleus and not in the other. Pronucleate oocytes not showing the above criteria were more likely to develop into preimplantation embryos that had poor morphology and/or experienced cleavage arrest. The presence of at least one embryo which had shown the above criteria at the pronuclear stage in those transferred, led to a pregnancy rate of 22/44 (50%) compared to only 2/23 (9%) when none were present.

A further criterion of pronucleate oocytes that may affect embryo morphology is the orientation of pronuclei relative to the polar bodies. Oocyte polarity is clearly evident in non-mammalian species. In mammals, the animal pole of the oocyte may be estimated by the location of the first polar body, whereas after fertilization, the second polar body marks the embryonic pole (34). In human oocytes, a differential distribution of various factors within the oocyte has been described and anomalies in the distribution of these factors, in particular the side of the oocyte believed to contain the animal pole, are thought to affect embryo development and possibly fetal growth (35,36). Following from this hypothesis, Garello et al. (37) examined pronuclear orientation, polar body placement, and embryo quality to ascertain if a link existed between a plausible polarity of oocytes at the pronuclear stage and further development. The most interesting observation involved the calculation of angle β (Figure 17.1), which represented the angle between a line drawn through the axis of the pronuclei and the position of the furthest polar body. It was determined that as the angle β increased there was a concurrent decrease in the morphological quality of preimplantation-stage human embryos. Hence it was

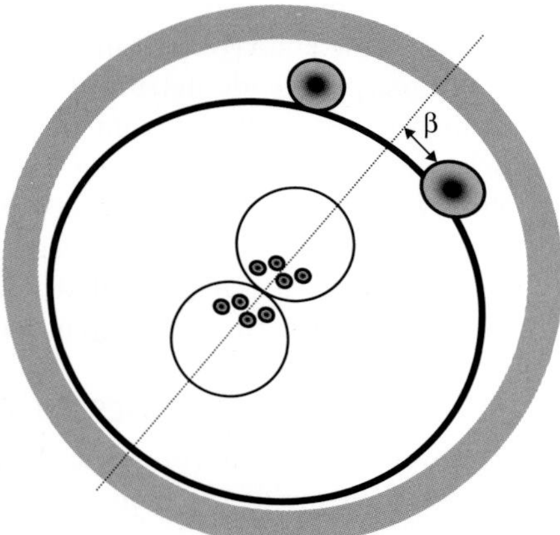

18–19 hrs post insemination/injection

Ideal features shared by pronucleate oocytes that have high viability:

(i) the number of nucleolar precursor bodies (NPBs) in both pronuclei never differed by more than three

(ii) the NPBs are always polarized or nonpolarized in both pronuclei but never polarized in one pronucleus and not in the other

(iii) the angle β from the axis of the pronuclei and the furthest polar body is less than 50°

Figure 17.1 Ideal features shared by pronucleate oocytes that have high viability as described by Tesarik and Greco (32), Garello et al. (37), and Scott and Smith (39). At 18-19 hours post-insemination/injection: (i) the number of NPBs in both pronuclei never differed by more than three; (ii) the NPBs are always polarized or not polarized in both pronuclei, but never polarized in one pronucleus and not in the other; and (iii) the angle from the axis of the pronuclei and the furthest polar body is less than 50°. *Abbreviation*: NPB, nucleolar precursor body.

postulated that the misalignment of the polar body might be linked to cytoplasmic turbulence, thereby disturbing the delicate polarity of the zygote. To this day, the question about polarity in the oocyte and its importance in influencing embryo viability is still not well understood (38).

In a further study, Scott and Smith (39) devised an embryo score on day 1 on the basis of alignment of pronuclei and nucleoli, the appearance of the cytoplasm, nuclear membrane breakdown, and cleavage to the two-cell stage. Patients who had an overall high embryo score (>15) had pregnancy and implantation rates of 34/48 (71%) and 49/175 (28%), respectively, compared to only 4/49 (8%) and 4/178 (2%) in the low-embryo score group. The use of pronuclear scoring has been reviewed by Scott (40). A report by Wong et al. (41) has also shown that success in progression to the blastocyst stage can be predicted with >93% sensitivity and specificity by measuring three dynamic, noninvasive imaging parameters to the four-cell stage. Furthermore, the timing of pronuclear events has been confirmed to be correlative to implantation potential by video imaging. Aguilar et al. (42) showed that the timings at which second polar body extrusion (3.3–10.6 hours), pronuclear fading (22.2–25.9 hours), and length of S-phase (5.7–13.8 hours) occurred were all linked successfully to embryo implantation. The same group also confirmed that the method of fertilization—intracytoplasmic sperm injection (ICSI) or routine IVF—was also important in determining how these parameters should be evaluated (43).

CLEAVAGE STAGE EMBRYOS

Historically, the most widely used criteria for selecting the best embryos for transfer have been based on cell number and morphology (24). A vast number of variations on this theme have been published. Some of the key studies have been presented by Gerris et al. (44) and Van Royen et al. (45), who employed strict embryo criteria to select single embryos for transfer. These did not, however, differ greatly from a paper published in the 1980s by Cummins et al. (24), who also described key cleavage events linked with viability. What constitutes a "top-quality" embryo? These "top-quality" embryos had the following characteristics: four or five blastomeres on day 2 and at least seven blastomeres on day 3 after fertilization, absence of multinucleated blastomeres, and <20% of fragments on day 2 and day 3 after fertilization. When these criteria were utilized in a prospective randomized clinical trial comparing single- and double-embryo transfers, it was found that in 26 single-embryo transfers where a top-quality embryo was available, an implantation rate of 42.3% and an ongoing pregnancy rate of 38.5% were obtained. In 27 double-embryo transfers, an implantation rate of 48.1% and an ongoing pregnancy rate of 74% were obtained. A larger study analyzing the outcomes of 370 consecutive single top-quality embryo transfers in patients younger than 38 years showed that the pregnancy rate after single top-quality embryo transfer was 51.9% (46). The same group of authors also provided evidence of the importance of multinucleation as part of the equation in selecting top-quality embryos (47).

The majority of studies that have used and reported embryo selection criteria on the basis of cell number and morphology do so by stating that embryos were selected on day 2 or day 3. As discussed by Bavister (48), one of the most critical factors in determining selection criteria was to ascertain strict time points to compare the embryos. Sakkas and colleagues therefore used cleavage to the 2-cell stage at 25 hours post-insemination or microinjection as the critical time point for selecting embryos (49–51). In a larger series of patients, it was found that 45% of patients undergoing IVF or ICSI have early-cleaving 2-cell embryos. Patients who have early-cleaving 2-cell embryos allocated for transfer on days 2 or 3 have significantly higher implantation and pregnancy rates (51). Furthermore, nearly 50% of the patients who have two early-cleaving 2-cell embryos transferred achieve a clinical pregnancy (Figure 17.2). The most convincing data supporting the usefulness of early-cleaving 2-cell embryos is that provided by single-embryo transfer (52,53). In one study, Salumets et al. (52) showed that when transferring single embryos, a significantly higher clinical pregnancy rate was observed after transfer of early-cleaving (50%) rather than non early cleaving (26.4%) embryos. The embryos that cleave early to the 2-cell stage have also been reported to have a significantly higher blastocyst formation rate (54,55). Another study by Guerif et al. (55) reported the sequential growth of 4042 embryos individually cultured from day 1 to days 5–6. Pronuclear morphology on day 1 and early cleavage, cell number, and fragmentation rate on day 2 were evaluated for each zygote. Interestingly, early cleavage and cell number on day 2 were the most powerful parameters to predict the development of a good-morphology blastocyst on day 5. Video imaging has aided in refining these timing events and now numerous algorithms exist (41,56) that help incorporate both cleavage and timing in predicting both blastocyst

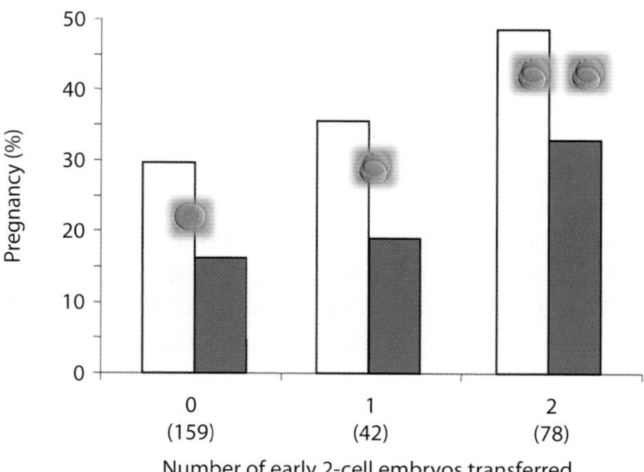

Figure 17.2 The percentages of clinical pregnancies (light columns) and implantation rates (dark columns) in relation to whether patients had zero, one, or two early-cleavage embryos transferred. The numbers in parentheses indicate the numbers of cycles per group.

development and implantation potential (57,58). Although some of these selection methodologies have shown promise (59–61), the jury is still out on how they may improve the move to single-embryo transfer. One well-conducted randomized trial has indicated that the addition of time-lapse morphokinetic data may not significantly improve clinical reproductive outcomes in all patients and in those with blastocyst transfers (62). Interestingly, this study and another by Ergin et al. (63) found that the time-lapse systems may provide extra information about multinucleation in embryos that could improve embryo selection.

MORULA STAGE EMBRYOS

One somewhat overlooked stage has been the morula stage. Why this has not been used as an assessment tool is interesting, but mostly stems from a need to not over-observe embryos and a lack of definitive historical morphological assessment during this stage. With the introduction of time-lapse analysis, we can now readily visualize and analyze key morphogenic events around the time at which the first epithelium of the conceptus is formed. Studies now indicate that a day 4 scoring system could be successfully adopted and implemented (64) and provide single-embryo transfer rates similar to day 5 single-embryo transfers (65). The adoption of such a strategy has, however, not been broadly accepted.

BLASTOCYST STAGE EMBRYOS

Blastocyst transfer is increasing in utilization due to: the increased efficacy of culture systems (see Chapter 16); the commercial availability of sequential, one-step, and time-lapse culture media; improvements in blastocyst cryopreservation made possible through vitrification (66–68); the continued reports of increased success rates after blastocyst transfer compared to cleavage stage (69–71); and the move to the biopsy of the trophectoderm for preimplantation genetic screening (30,72–75).

The type of blastocyst obtained is, however, of critical importance. As with the scoring of embryos during the cleavage stages, time and morphology are key in selecting the best blastocyst. The scoring assessment for blastocysts devised by Gardner and Schoolcraft (76) is one of the most widely adopted. In effect, even the Alpha Scoring System is a numerical interpretation of the Gardner scale (77,78). The Gardner scoring system is based on the expansion state of the blastocyst and on the consistency of the inner cell mass (ICM) and trophectoderm cells (Figure 17.3). Examples of high-quality blastocysts and an explanation of the alphanumeric grading system are shown in Figure 17.4. Using such a grading system, it was determined that when two high-scoring blastocysts (>3AA; i.e., expanded blastocoel with compacted ICM and cohesive trophectoderm epithelium) are transferred, a clinical pregnancy and implantation rate of >80% and 69%, respectively, can be attained (79). When two blastocysts not achieving these scores (<3AA) are transferred, the clinical pregnancy and implantation rate are significantly lower: 50% and 33%, respectively (80). Although reduced from the values obtained with top-scoring blastocysts, it is evident that early blastocysts on day 5 still have high developmental potential.

Recently, a more detailed analysis of whether the ICM or trophectoderm provides greater predictive weight for embryo selection concluded that the predictive strength of the trophectoderm grade was greater compared to the ICM for selecting the best blastocyst for embryo replacement (81). It has been suggested that even though ICM is important, a competent trophectoderm is essential at this stage of embryo development, allowing successful hatching and implantation. This has subsequently been validated by a number of studies (82–86) that all highlighted the need for high trophectoderm grading in relation to pregnancy. Interestingly, one study found that a poor ICM grading was also related to higher miscarriage rates (87).

The time of blastocyst formation is also crucial. When cases where only day 5 and day 6 frozen blastocysts were compared to those frozen on or after day 7 and transferred, the pregnancy rates were 7/18 (38.9%) and 1/16 (6.2%), respectively (88). In these cases, expanded blastocysts with a definable ICM and trophectoderm were frozen. These results show that even though blastocysts can be obtained, a crucial factor is when they form blastocysts. When taking this into account, the best blastocysts would be those that develop by day 5. Selecting the fastest blastocysts has historically caused concerns about creating a bias in sex selection, as Menezo et al. (89) reported that blastocysts transferred after development in co-culture gave rise to the birth of more male offspring. Milki et al. (90) also reported that combined data from the literature show a male-to-female ratio of 57.3%:42.7% in blastocyst transfer compared to 51.2%:48.8% in day 3 embryo transfer ($p = 0.001$). Recently, the Australian and New Zealand registry was used to show that blastocyst culture may skew the male outcome to 54.1% (91). Other evidence also now indicates that faster-growing blastocysts could be preferentially male (92). Ebner et al. (93) presented a correlation between trophectoderm quality and not only live birth outcome, but also that male blastocysts had a 2.53-times higher chance of exhibiting better trophectoderm quality. Significantly, Meintjes and colleagues (94) observed skewing in the sex ratio of babies following embryo culture at atmospheric oxygen and blastocyst transfer, with significantly more males (58.5%) being born. However, when human embryos were cultured in the presence of 5% oxygen, the sex ratio at birth was restored to 51.9% males. Consequently, any differences in sex ratio during culture may be attributed to the presence of one or more stressors in the culture system, such as atmospheric oxygen.

Some groups have attempted to correlate blastocyst rates not only with gender, but also the overall ploidy status of the embryo. This has been a particular goal of time-lapse systems, but has not been conclusive. In one study, Campbell and colleagues reported that the timing of formation of the blastocoel was delayed in aneuploid embryos (95). Time to the start of blastulation of <100 hours after insemination and the morphokinetic scoring system used in the time lapse morphokinetics group were independently associated with implantation. The association

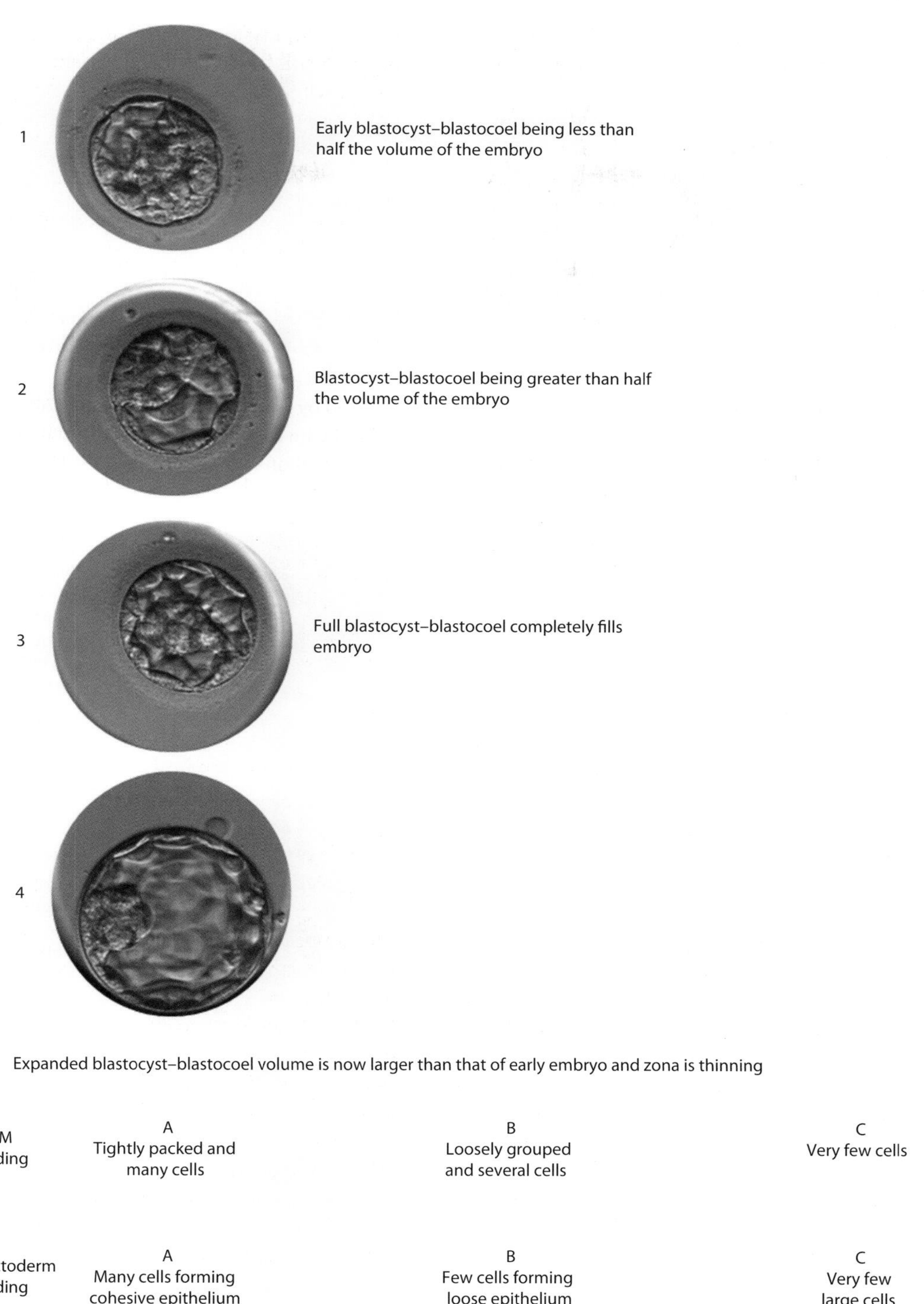

Figure 17.3 The blastocyst grading system. *Abbreviation*: ICM, inner cell mass. (Modified from Gardner DK, Schoolcraft WB. *In vitro* culture of human blastocysts. In: *Towards Reproductive Certainty: Infertility and Genetics Beyond.* Jansen R, Mortimer D (eds). Carnforth, U.K.: Parthenon Press, 1999, p. 378.)

between cleavage parameters and prediction of aneuploidy, however, remains controversial (96). Recently, one study has shed more light on this relationship, indicating that aneuploidy correlates with significant differences in the duration of the first mitotic phase when compared with euploid embryos (97). This, however, was on a small set of embryos and needs subsequent validation.

A STRATEGY FOR SELECTING THE BEST EMBRYO BY MORPHOLOGY

The above selection criteria have all shown that they generate some benefit in identifying individual embryos that have high viability. Curiously, one thing that video imaging seems to be teaching us is to not only investigate the things that go right, but also the

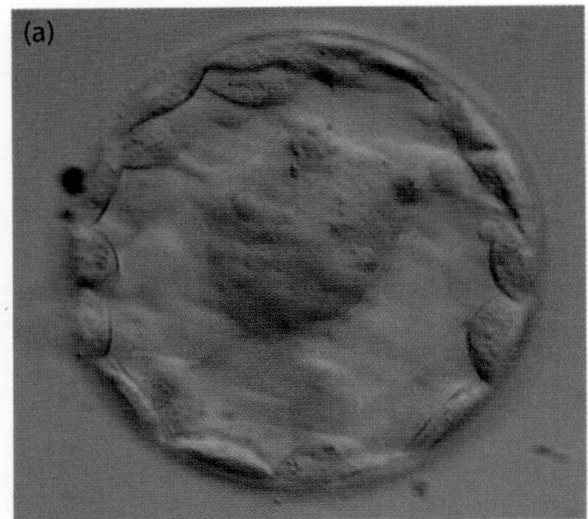

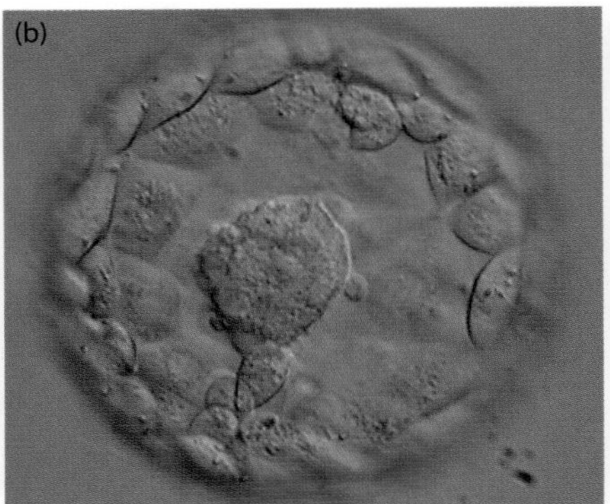

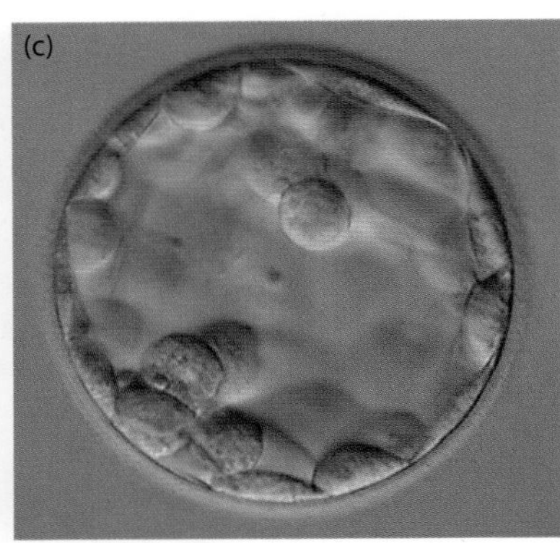

Figure 17.4 Day 5 human blastocysts using the grading system reported by Gardner and Schoolcraft (76). Blastocysts in (a) and (b) would both score 4AA, but the embryo in (c) would only score 4CA due to the apparent absence of an inner cell mass, in spite of the development of an excellent trophectoderm. See Figure 17.3 for an explanation of the embryo score.

things that go wrong. Although video imaging has aimed to develop selection algorithms looking for positive selection features related to embryo implantation potential, it has also shown us that numerous events can be used to deselect embryos from the transfer pool. One of the most evident deselection events seems to be direct cleavage to the three-cell stage (59).

How do we implement a strategy for selecting a single embryo when we have many embryos to choose from? A few schools of thought are now being adopted for embryo selection. The first is a multiple-step scoring system that encompasses all the above criteria. The use of sequential scoring systems has been shown to be beneficial by a number of authors (45,54,98). However, one analysis by Racowsky et al. (99) reported that multiple analysis for day 3 embryos was not beneficial. Here, we propose scenarios for sequential embryo assessment. A modification of the options available to perform sequential embryo assessment is considered below using the following criteria:

18–19 hours post-insemination/ICSI (Figure 17.1):

Identification of pronucleate oocytes

The pronuclei are examined for:

a. Symmetry
b. The presence of even numbers of NPBs
c. The positioning of the polar bodies

25–26 hours post-insemination/ICSI (Figure 17.5):

a. Embryos that have already cleaved to the two-cell stage
b. Zygotes that have progressed to nuclear membrane breakdown

42–44 hours post-insemination/ICSI (Figure 17.5):

a. Number of blastomeres should be greater than or equal to four
b. Fragmentation of less than 20%
c. No multinucleated blastomeres

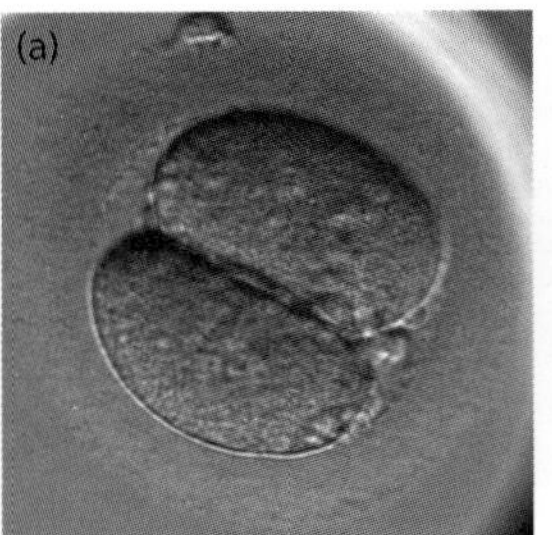

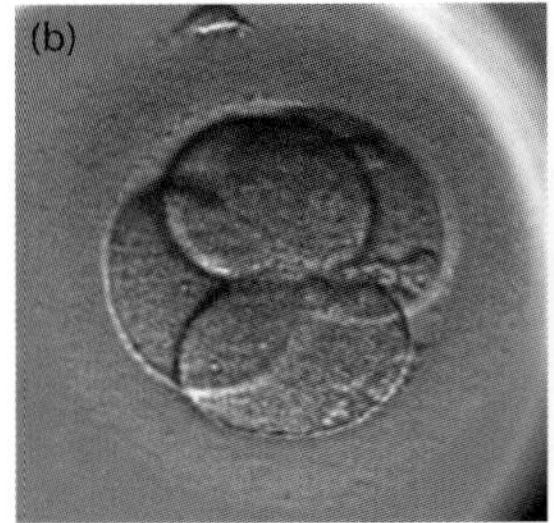

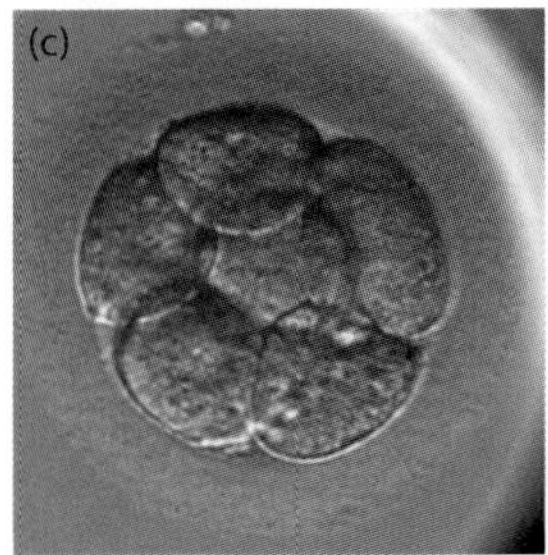

Figure 17.5 Ideal features of embryos scored at 25–26 hours, 42–44 hours, and 66–68 hours post-insemination/intracytoplasmic sperm injection. For more detail on the scoring criteria, see Sakkas et al. (27), Shoukir et al. (49), and Van Royen et al. (45). (a) 25–26 hours post-insemination/injection—embryo should be at the two-cell stage with equal blastomeres and no fragmentation. (b) 42–44 hours post-insemination/injection—embryo should have four or more blastomeres and less than 20% fragmentation. (c) 66–68 hours post-insemination/injection—embryo should have eight or more blastomeres and less than 20% fragmentation.

66–68 hours post-insemination/ICSI (Figure 17.5):

a. Number of blastomeres should be greater than or equal to eight
b. Fragmentation of less than 20%
c. No multinucleated blastomeres

106–108 hours post-insemination/ICSI (Figures 17.3 and 17.4):

a. The blastocoel cavity should be full
b. ICM should be numerous and tightly packed
c. Trophectoderm cells should be numerous and cohesive

Which of the above criteria would be the most important? If sequential embryo assessment is used to select the best embryos, we could envisage a fluid selection process that would mark embryos as they develop. The above criteria would therefore be seen as ideal hurdles of development. At every step an embryo would be given a positive mark when it reached the ideal criteria of a certain stage. It would, however, be possible that an embryo may not pass one step, but would pass the hurdle at a following step. The embryo or embryos attaining the best criteria at each step would therefore be the ones that would be selected for transfer. For example, if we are attempting to transfer a single embryo to a patient, the following scenario could be envisaged: an embryo may not pass any of the earlier hurdles, but still form a high-grade blastocyst on day 5. If this were the most successful of the cohort of embryos, then this would be the one selected. If, however, six blastocysts were observed on day 5, all of equally high grade, then the blastocyst that had achieved the most positive scores at each of the previous hurdles could be transferred. If the shortened protocol was used and only day 2 was the previous score, then the best-looking day 2 embryos would be ranked as better. Furthermore, patients who have low numbers of embryos and have transfer on days 2 or 3 could be assessed using the initial criteria, and the embryo that passed the initial hurdles would be selected. Proposed schedules of embryo selection are given in Figure 17.6, taking into account different strategies or assessment criteria. It is important to note that to date the strongest criteria of selection appear to be the selection of a high-quality blastocyst on day 5 of development (55,79). Since we first developed and advocated this approach to embryo selection (27) and then developed it further to include a weighted score for each stage (100), such data have been incorporated into many algorithms for use with time-lapse microscopy to facilitate both embryo deselection and selection.

So as well as the choice of cleavage versus blastocyst transfer, we are now also confronted with the choice of assessing multiple stages by either repeated manual or time-lapse assessments. Interestingly, many groups have looked at minimizing their assessment of embryos and culturing all embryos to the blastocyst stage, where the blastocyst morphology can potentially provide stronger evidence of viability (81). This would possibly involve scoring fertilization on day 1, assessment of embryos on day 2, and then leaving embryos in culture until days 5 and 6 when they are assessed for transfer or cryopreservation at the blastocyst stage. Observing embryos on day 2 may allow some patients to be transferred earlier if the clinic chooses. For example, the clinic may want to set a limit on how many four-cell embryos they need to continue blastocyst culture (Table 17.1). Data from Boston IVF indicate that a patient of any age with at least three good four-cell embryos on day 2 has over an 80% chance of having a blastocyst for transfer or cryopreservation.

A practical issue for performing such a selection process is that embryos need to be cultured in individual drops. This may remove any necessary benefits of culturing embryos in groups (101–103). A further practical issue when working without a time-lapse system is that embryos will need to be observed more often. However, using a drop culture system under oil with adequate heating control of all microscope stages will greatly reduce pH and temperature fluctuations (104). In prolonged culture, pronuclear assessment, changeover into new media on day 3, and assessment of the blastocyst are already performed. The extra assessment periods would be the checking of early-cleaving two-cell embryos and assessment of embryos on day 2. An optional observation could also include that of the polar body placement, as described by Garello et al. (37). A further observation would be to determine the degree of blastulation on the afternoon of day 4, with this reflecting the speed at which a given embryo is developing. Fortuitously, the move to commercialize real-time imaging of embryos has now placed the above sequential assessment procedure closer to a practical reality, removing any concerns related to constant visualization of the embryos away from the incubator (41,56,104). The further development of this type of imaging system is covered in Chapter 18. However, the scoring regimens described in detail in this chapter will serve all those clinical laboratories that do not have access to time-lapse analysis.

So it is evident that with improved culture conditions, together with suitable grading systems, it is possible to dramatically increase implantation rates, decrease the number of embryos transferred, and increase the live birth rate. However, this approach raises two issues: firstly, if the laboratory in question is not performing blastocyst transfer, then it cannot rely on advanced grading systems; and secondly, morphology will only tell us a limited amount about the physiological status of the embryo. The rest of this chapter is therefore devoted to the application of novel tests of embryonic function. It is assumed that such tests must be noninvasive for adoption into clinical use. Therefore, methods that can be considered as semi-invasive (i.e., those that involve embryo biopsy prior to cell analysis) are not considered here and are discussed in other chapters within this book.

BEYOND EMBRYO MORPHOLOGY: THE NONINVASIVE QUANTIFICATION OF EMBRYO PHYSIOLOGY

The inherent ease for the laboratory to assess various morphological markers makes it the preferred assessment technique to transfer embryos. However, its overall

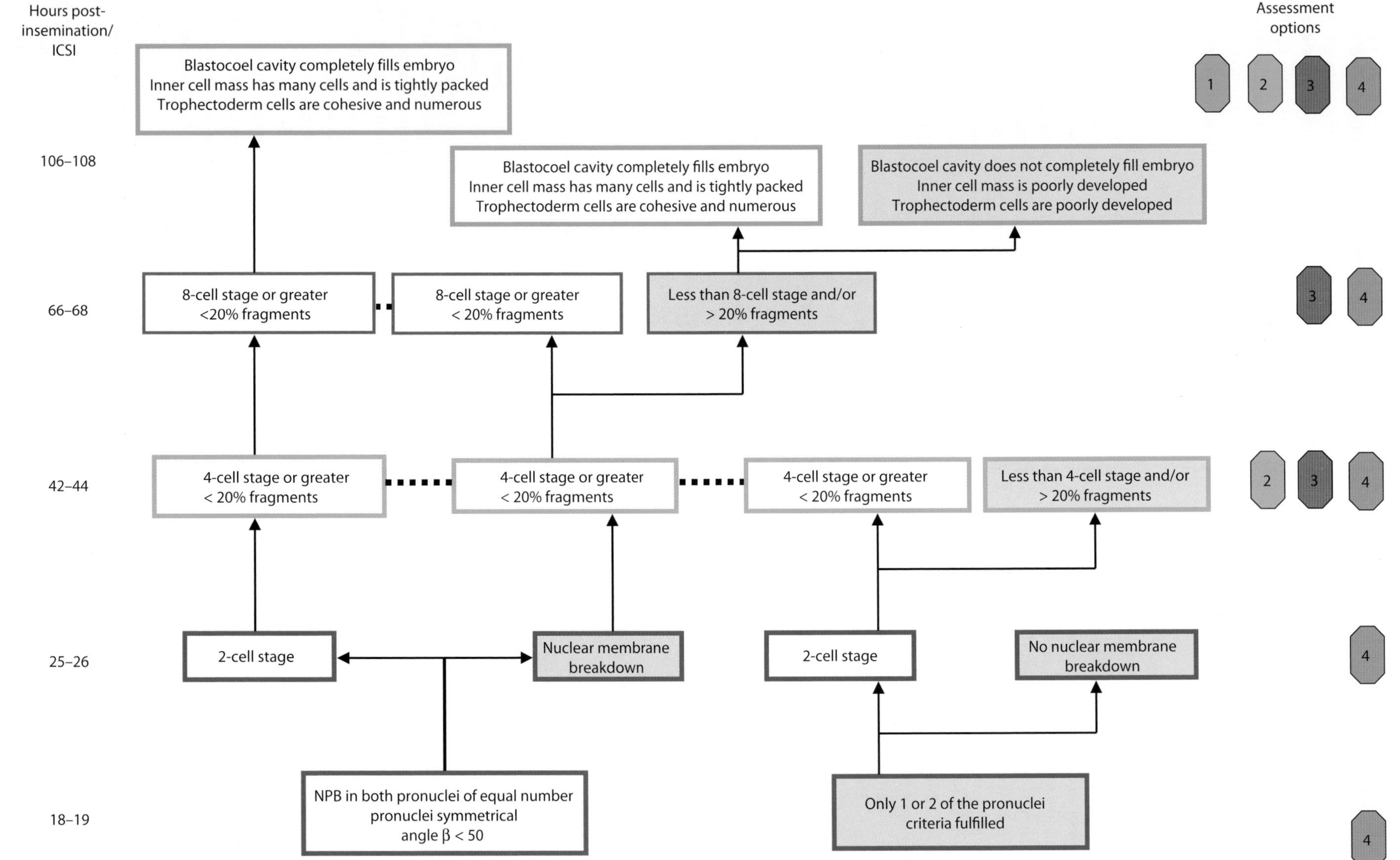

Figure 17.6 A strategy for selecting a single embryo for transfer using different morphological assessment options. Number 1 would entail a single assessment only at the blastocyst stage (green); number 2 (light blue) would allow triaging of patients on day 2 followed by assessment at the blastocyst stage; number 3 (red) would allow triaging of patients on days 2 and 3 followed by assessment at the blastocyst stage; number 4 (dark blue) would allow triaging of patients on each days 1, 2, and 3 followed by assessment at the blastocyst stage. *Abbreviations*: ICSI, intracytoplasmic sperm injection; NPB, nucleolar precursor body.

Table 17.1 The probability of obtaining at least 1–6 blastocysts for transfer or cryopreservation in relation to having three, four, five, or six good four-cell embryos on day 2.

Age (years)	Number of four-cell embryos on day 2	At least One blastocyst	Two blastocysts	Three blastocysts	Four blastocysts	Five blastocysts	Six blastocysts
<35	6	99.8%	97.8%	88.6%	65.4%	32.6%	7.8%
	5	99.4%	94.7%	77.0%	43.5%	11.9%	
	4	98.6%	87.7%	57.0%	18.3%		
	3	95.8%	72.3%	27.9%			
35–37	6	99.6%	95.8%	81.8%	54.0%	23.0%	4.6%
	5	98.9%	91.1%	67.9%	33.3%	7.6%	
	4	97.4%	81.9%	47.2%	12.8%		
	3	93.5%	64.5%	21.4%			
38–40	6	99.3%	94.8%	79.1%	50.2%	20.3%	3.8%
	5	98.7%	89.7%	64.8%	30.4%	6.6%	
	4	96.9%	79.7%	44.1%	11.3%		
	3	92.6%	61.9%	19.5%			

The data are from an analysis of over 15,000 fertilized embryos left for culture to the blastocyst stage. The darker shade shows when the chance is >80% and lighter shade shows when the chance is between 70% and 80%.

effectiveness has been questioned, and there are numerous reports of irregular morphological and morphokinetic parameters at early stages of *in vitro* development leading to live births (105). The fact remains that even with the adoption of more complex forms of assessment, morphology will remain a very practical means of embryo assessment. A number of quantitative techniques have been trialed that attempt to monitor the uptake of specific nutrients by the embryo from the surrounding medium, and to detect the secretion of specific metabolites and factors into the medium (Figure 17.7). Such approaches have strived to measure such changes in culture media and to fulfill three key criteria below so that they can be applicable in IVF clinics:

1. They must have the ability to measure the change without damaging the embryo.
2. They must have the ability to measure the change quickly (this requirement may, however, be lower, as the success of vitrification and possible move away from fresh transfers [106] may circumvent the need for a rapid test).
3. They must have the ability to measure the change consistently and accurately.

The analysis of metabolite levels within spent embryo culture media fulfills the above criteria, and has been one method examined to augment the analysis of embryo morphology as a means of embryo selection. Three approaches have been evaluated: analysis of carbohydrate utilization; the turnover of amino acids; and the analysis of the embryonic metabolome. The first two approaches could be considered analyses of the activity of specific metabolic pathways, whereas analysis of the metabolome should be considered as the systematic analysis of the inventory of metabolites that represent the functional phenotype at the cellular level. Depending upon the technology employed to analyze the metabolome, one does not necessarily obtain identification of specific metabolites, but rather one is able to create an algorithm that relates to cell function and hence to potential viability.

Analysis of carbohydrate utilization

A relationship between metabolic activity and embryo development and viability has been established over several decades (107). As early as 1970, Menke and McLaren revealed that mouse blastocysts, developed in basic culture conditions, lost their ability to oxidize glucose (108). This initial observation was followed by several studies that elucidated changes in embryo metabolism associated with loss of developmental capacity *in vitro* (reviewed in [109]). In 1980, Renard et al. (110) observed that day 10 cattle blastocysts that had an elevated glucose uptake developed better, both in culture and *in vivo* after transfer than those blastocysts with a low glucose uptake. In 1987, using the then relatively new technique of noninvasive microfluorescence, Gardner and Leese (111) measured glucose uptake by individual day 4 mouse blastocysts prior to transfer to recipient females. Those embryos that went to term had a significantly higher glucose uptake in culture than those embryos that failed to develop after transfer. This work was then built on by Lane and Gardner (112), who showed that the glycolytic rate of mouse blastocysts could be used to select embryos for transfer prospectively. Morphologically identical mouse blastocysts with equivalent diameters were identified using metabolic criteria as "viable" prior to transfer and had a fetal development of 80%. In contrast, those embryos that exhibited an abnormal metabolic profile (compared to *in vivo*-developed controls) developed at

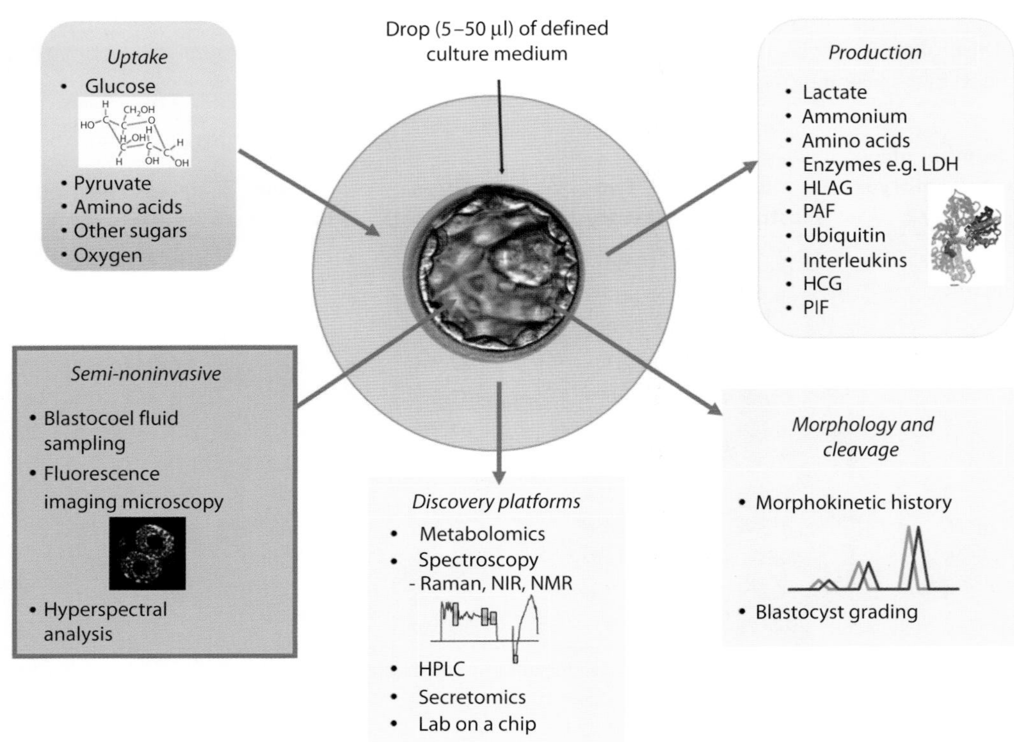

Figure 17.7 Options for the noninvasive analysis of human embryo nutrient consumption and metabolite/factor production. Individual blastocysts are incubated in 5.0–50.0 μL volumes of defined medium. Serial or end point samples of medium can then be removed for analysis and an indirect measurement of metabolic pathways can be ascertained by measuring uptake or production of various factors or using discovery platforms. Noninvasive platforms can also include current morphology and cleavage criteria using static or time-lapse measurements. Semi-noninvasive platforms are also in development using novel microscopy platforms or examining the blastocoelic fluid. *Abbreviations*: HPLC, high-performance liquid chromatography; NMR, nuclear magnetic resonance; PAF, platelet-activating factor; PIF, preimplantation factor; HLAG, human leukocyte antigen G; LDH, Lactate dehydrogenase; HCG, human chorionic gonadotropin.

a rate of only 6%. Clearly, such data provide dramatic evidence that metabolic function is linked to embryo viability (Figures 17.8 and 17.9), and that perturbations in the relative activity of metabolic pathways is associated with loss of cell function, leading to compromised development post-transfer (113).

Analysis of the relationship between human embryo nutrition and subsequent development *in vitro* (114,115) has been undertaken. Gardner et al. (114), determined that glucose consumption on day 4 by human embryos was twice as high in those embryos that went on to form blastocysts. Subsequently, Gardner and colleagues (116) went on to confirm a positive relationship between glucose uptake and human embryo viability on day 4 and day 5 of development (Figure 17.10). Furthermore, the data generated indicate that nutrient utilization differs between male and female embryos, a phenomenon previously documented in other mammalian species (117,118). Currently, performing an accurate analysis of nutrient uptake by individual embryos is achieved using non-commercial fluorescence assays, which are limited to just a few laboratories worldwide. The widespread implementation and subsequent validation of this approach should be made possible through the development of chip-based devices capable of accurately quantitating sub-microliter volumes of medium (119–121).

Analysis of amino acid utilization

In studies on amino acid turnover by human embryos, Houghton et al. (115) determined that alanine release into the surrounding medium on day 2 and day 3 was highest in those embryos that did not form blastocysts. Subsequently, Brison et al. (122) reported changes in concentration of amino acids in the spent medium of human zygotes cultured for 24 hours in an embryo culture medium containing a mixture of amino acids using high-performance liquid chromatography. It was found that asparagine, glycine, and leucine utilized in the 24 hours following fertilization were significantly associated with clinical pregnancy and live birth following day 2 embryo transfer. Further analysis also revealed an association of aneuploidy and embryonic sex with amino acid turnover (123). Ongoing studies in this area have been slow, but could still help to identify the group of amino acids at each stage of development whose usage is linked with subsequent viability. Recent animal studies have revealed how dynamic the use of amino acids is and how uptake can be affected by other aspects of the culture

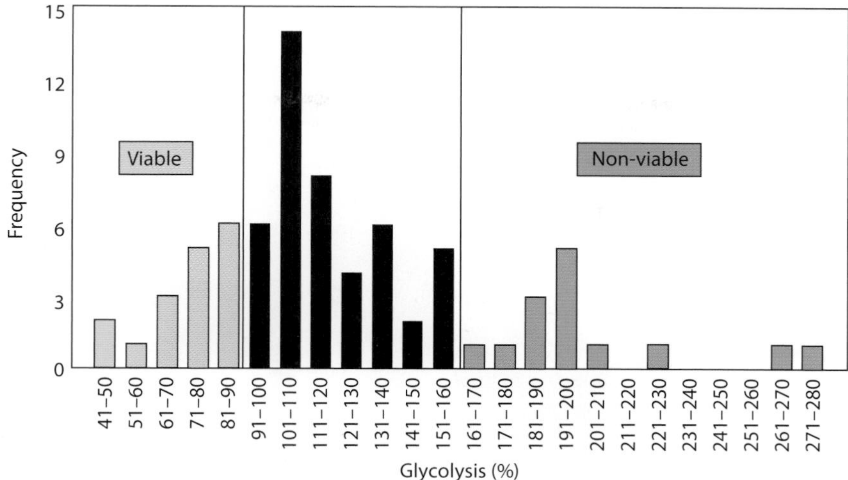

Figure 17.8 Distribution of glycolytic activity in a population of 79 morphologically similar mouse blastocysts cultured in medium DM1. The lowest 15% of glycolytic activity (<88%) were considered viable, while the highest 15% of the range (>160%) were deemed non-viable. (Adapted from Lane M, Gardner DK. *Hum Reprod* 1996; 11(9): 1975–8.)

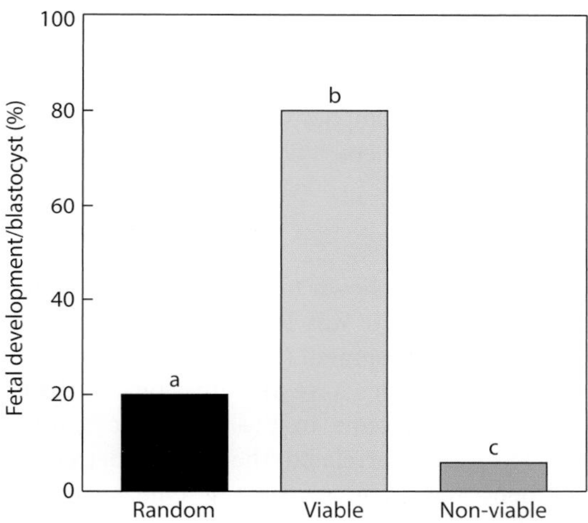

Figure 17.9 Fetal development of mouse blastocysts selected for transfer using glycolytic activity as a biochemical marker. "Viable" blastocysts were classified as those with a glycolytic rate close to *in vivo*-developed blastocysts (<88%), while "non-viable" blastocysts had a glycolytic rate in the highest 15% of the distribution (<160%). On each day of the experiment, a selection of blastocysts were transferred at random, along with those selected as either viable or non-viable. "a," "b," and "c" indicate significantly different populations ($p < 0.01$). (Adapted from Lane M, Gardner DK. *Hum Reprod* 1996; 11(9): 1975–8.)

system, such as oxygen and the accumulation of ammonium through the spontaneous breakdown and metabolism of amino acids (124,125). Consequently, data on the use of nutrients need to be carefully interpreted with regard to the conditions under which the embryos were developed.

Metabolomics

Evolving metabolomics technologies may allow us in the future to measure multiple factors in embryo culture media. Initial and encouraging metabolic studies indicated that embryos that result in pregnancy are different in their metabolomic profile compared to embryos that do not lead to pregnancies (126). Investigation of the metabolome of embryos, as detected in the culture media they grow in using targeted spectroscopic analysis and bioinformatics, revealed differences in some initial proof-of-principle studies (126).

Although a series of preliminary studies (127–131) showed a benefit of metabolomics-related techniques, they were largely based on retrospective studies and performed in a single research laboratory as distinct from a real clinical setting. The subsequent randomized clinical trials failed to show compelling benefits when comparing standard morphological techniques for embryo selection versus using the near-infrared (NIR) system to rank embryos within a cohort that had good morphology and were being selected for either transfer or cryopreservation (92,96–98). Similarly, although Katz-Jaffe et al. (132,133) revealed that the proteome of individual human blastocysts of the same grade differed between embryos, and also identified a number of secreted protein markers that could be used to identify the best embryo (133–135), a relationship between such biomarkers and subsequent viability has yet to be validated prospectively.

Although the use of metabolomic and proteomic platforms has yet to be proven and employed clinically, analysis of embryo function for its own sake can greatly enhance our understanding of development, and hence such approaches could ultimately assist in defining parameters that can be used in embryo selection. To this end, an analysis of the relationship between the morphokinetic development of embryos and their metabolic activity has been undertaken.

When morphometrics and metabolic analysis collide

By using a mouse model to analyze the relationship between key morphometric and metabolic data from individual IVF-derived embryos, Lee and colleagues determined

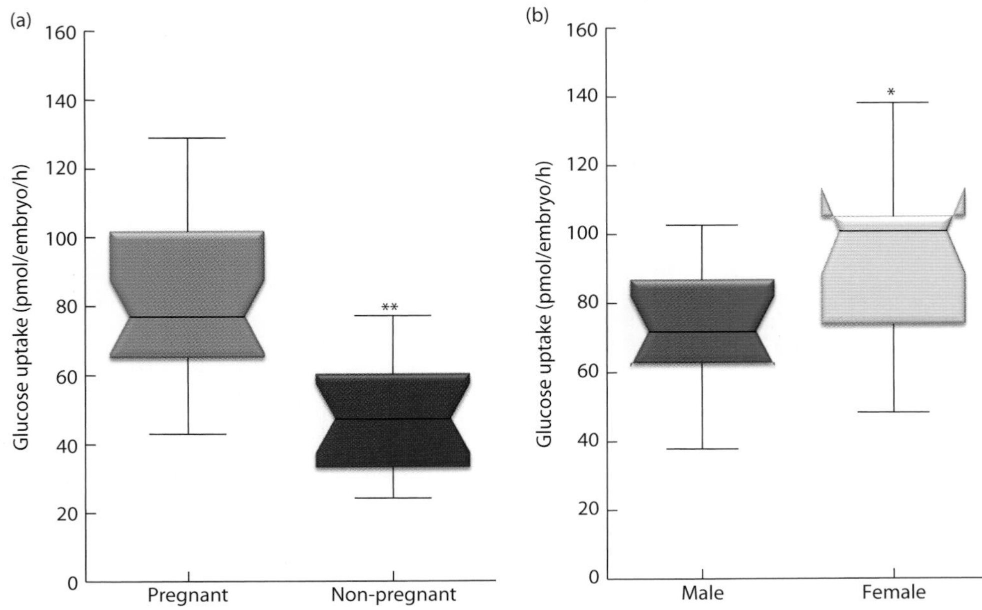

Figure 17.10 Relationship between glucose consumption on day 4 of development and human embryo viability and embryo sex. (a) Glucose uptake on day 4 of embryonic development and pregnancy outcome (positive fetal heart beat). Notches represent the confidence intervals of the medians, the depths of the boxes represent the interquartile ranges (50% of the data), and whiskers represent the 5% and 95% quartiles. The lines across the boxes are the median glucose consumptions. **, significantly different from pregnant ($p < 0.01$). (b) Glucose uptake by male and female embryos on day 4 of development. *, significantly different from male embryos ($p < 0.05$). (Adapted from Gardner DK et al. *Hum Reprod* 2011; 26(8): 1981–6.)

that blastocysts developing from those embryos exhibiting early cleavage (and hence presumed to have a higher viability) possessed a metabolic profile of increased glucose uptake and reduced rates of glycolysis (and hence exhibiting metabolic characteristics of enhanced viability) (136). Furthermore, it was observed that blastocysts developed from embryos with early cleavage also consumed more aspartate, potentially reflecting a more active malate–aspartate shuttle, which has been implicated in the regulation of blastocyst metabolism and viability (137,138). Together, such data generate renewed excitement regarding the potential for noninvasive quantification of embryo physiology to assist in the selection of the most viable embryo for transfer, and the potential for combining two independent means of assessing the preimplantation embryo in order to improve the accuracy of selection.

Other specific factors

Other techniques have also been reported to measure metabolic parameters in culture media; however, they have yet to be tested in a clinical IVF setting. These include the self-referencing electrophysiological technique, which is a noninvasive measurement of the physiology of individual cells and monitors the movement of ions and molecules between the cell and the surrounding media (139,140). Another technique using a probe was initially developed by Unisense to noninvasively measure the oxygen consumption of developing embryos. Interestingly, although this technology was shown to correlate with bovine blastocyst development, it was less successful at predicting mouse embryo development (141,142).

A number of studies have also investigated the assessment of secreted factors in the embryo culture media (Figure 17.7) and correlated them with better embryo development and pregnancy rates. One such factor is soluble HLA-G (143,144), which is believed to protect the developing embryo from destruction by the maternal immune response. Soluble HLA-G has been found in media surrounding the early embryo and a number of papers have also reported that its presence correlates with the improved pregnancy potential of an embryo (145–147). However, some studies have raised some serious concerns regarding the use of HLA-G production as a marker of further developmental potential (148–150), and prospective clinical trials are needed to further evaluate this parameter. Included in the studies examining the secretion of factors in the media by embryos are numerous papers examining the secretion of platelet-activating factor (PAF). The clinical utility of PAF in an IVF setting has also yet to be stringently examined (see review in [151]). Other factors are currently under investigation, including one called the preimplantation factor, which has been reported to provide some indication of embryo viability when measured and to possibly improve embryo quality when placed in embryo culture media (152). Numerous other candidates have also been postulated and tested, including human chorionic gonadotropin (153,154) and interleukin-6 (155).

It is beyond question that markers do exist in the spent embryo culture media that are indicative of viability. The major benefits of a noninvasive type of technology is the fact that the technology can be used on spent media and the time taken to assess the samples is very short, making it possible to perform the analysis just prior to embryo transfer. Many research groups around the world are still attempting to make this a reality for the IVF clinic. Advances in microscopy may further increase our understanding regarding metabolic function through technologies such as hyperspectral analysis (156).

SUMMARY

Analysis of embryo morphology and the development of suitable grading systems have greatly assisted in the selection of human embryos for transfer. However, it is proposed that in the near future embryo selection will also be significantly aided by the noninvasive analysis of embryo physiology and function by using approaches that better quantify embryo metabolism. The addition of such technologies will be of immense value in helping both clinicians and embryologists to select more confidently the most viable embryos within a cohort, facilitating the move to single-embryo transfer.

REFERENCES

1. Mansour R, Ishihara O, Adamson GD et al. International committee for monitoring assisted reproductive technologies world report: Assisted reproductive technology 2006. *Hum Reprod* 2014; 29(7): 1536–51.
2. European Society of Human Reproduction and Embryology, 2011 World IVF Report. 2016. Available from https://www.eshre.eu/guidelines-and-legal/art-fact-sheet.aspx
3. De Mouzon MJ, Goossens V, Bhattacharya S et al. Assisted reproductive technology in Europe, 2006: Results generated from European registers by ESHRE. *Hum Reprod* 2010; 25(8): 1851–62.
4. National Summary and Fertility Clinic Reports, 2006. Center for Disease Control and Prevention. 2006. Available from https://www.cdc.gov/art/pdf/archived/2006art.pdf
5. Australian & New Zealand Assisted Reproduction Database (ANZARD) 2006 data. 2006. Available from https://npesu.unsw.edu.au/sites/default/files/npesu/data_collection/Assisted%20reproductive%20technology%20in%20Australia%20and%20New%20Zealand%202006.pdf
6. Nyboe AA, Goossens V, Bhattacharya S et al. Assisted reproductive technology and intrauterine inseminations in Europe, 2005: Results generated from European registers by ESHRE: ESHRE. The European IVF Monitoring Programme (EIM), for the European Society of Human Reproduction and Embryology (ESHRE). *Hum Reprod* 2009; 24(6): 1267–87.
7. National Summary and Fertility Clinic Reports, 2009. Center for Disease Control and Prevention. 2009. Available from https://www.cdc.gov/art/pdf/archived/art_2009_full.pdf
8. National Summary and Fertility Clinic Reports, 2013. Center for Disease Control and Prevention. 2013. Available from https://www.cdc.gov/art/pdf/2013-report/art-2013-fertility-clinic-report.pdf
9. Adashi EY, Barri PN, Berkowitz R et al. Infertility therapy-associated multiple pregnancies (births): An ongoing epidemic. *Reprod Biomed Online* 2003; 7(5): 515–42.
10. Collins J. Cost efficiency of reducing multiple births. *Reprod Biomed Online* 2007; 15(Suppl 3): 35–9.
11. Gerris J, De Sutter P, De Neubourg D et al. A real-life prospective health economic study of elective single embryo transfer versus two-embryo transfer in first IVF/ICSI cycles. *Hum Reprod* 2004; 19(4): 917–23.
12. Bromer JG, Ata B, Seli M, Lockwood CJ, Seli E. Preterm deliveries that result from multiple pregnancies associated with assisted reproductive technologies in the USA: A cost analysis. *Curr Opin Obstet Gynecol* 2011; 23(3): 168–73.
13. Ledger WL, Anumba D, Marlow N, Thomas CM, Wilson EC. The costs to the NHS of multiple births after IVF treatment in the UK. *BJOG* 2006; 113(1): 21–5.
14. Australian & New Zealand Assisted Reproduction Database (ANZARD) 2016 data. 2016. Available from https://npesu.unsw.edu.au/sites/default/files/npesu/data_collection/Assisted%20reproductive%20technology%20in%20Australia%20and%20New%20Zealand%202013.pdf
15. Bissonnette F, Phillips SJ, Gunby J et al. Working to eliminate multiple pregnancies: A success story in Quebec. *Reprod Biomed Online* 2011; 23(4): 500–4.
16. Practice Committee of American Society for Reproductive Medicine; Practice Committee of Society for Assisted Reproductive Technology. Criteria for number of embryos to transfer: A committee opinion. *Fertil Steril* 2013; 99(1): 44–6.
17. Inge GB, Brinsden PR, Elder KT. Oocyte number per live birth in IVF: Were Steptoe and Edwards less wasteful? *Hum Reprod* 2005; 20(3): 588–92.
18. Patrizio P, Sakkas D. From oocyte to baby: A clinical evaluation of the biological efficiency of *in vitro* fertilization. *Fertil Steril* 2009; 91(4): 1061–6.
19. Edgell TA, Rombauts LJ, Salamonsen LA. Assessing receptivity in the endometrium: The need for a rapid, non-invasive test. *Reprod Biomed Online* 2013; 27(5): 486–96.
20. Evans J, Hannan NJ, Hincks C, Rombauts LJ, Salamonsen LA. Defective soil for a fertile seed? Altered endometrial development is detrimental to pregnancy success. *PLoS One* 2012; 7(12): e53098.

21. Salamonsen LA, Evans J, Nguyen HP, Edgell TA. The microenvironment of human implantation: Determinant of reproductive success. *Am J Reprod Immunol* 2015; 75(3): 218–25.
22. Blesa D, Ruiz-Alonso M, Simon C. Clinical management of endometrial receptivity. *Semin Reprod Med* 2014; 32(5): 410–3.
23. Miravet-Valenciano JA, Rincon-Bertolin A, Vilella F, Simon C. Understanding and improving endometrial receptivity. *Curr Opin Obstet Gynecol* 2015; 27(3): 187–92.
24. Cummins J, Breen T, Harrison K, Shaw J, Wilson L, Hennessey J. A formula for scoring human embryo growth rates in *in vitro* fertilization: Its value in predicting pregnancy and in comparison with visual estimates of embryo quality. *J In Vitro Fert Embryo Transf* 1986; 3: 284–95.
25. Edwards R, Fishel S, Cohen J. Factors influencing the success of *in vitro* fertilization for alleviating human infertility. *J In Vitro Fert Embryo Transf* 1984; 1: 3–23.
26. De Neubourg D, Gerris J. Single embryo transfer—State of the art. *Reprod Biomed Online* 2003; 7(6): 615–22.
27. Sakkas D. *Evaluation of Embryo Quality: A Strategy for Sequential Analysis of Embryo Development with the Aim of Single Embryo Transfer.* London, U.K.: Martin Dunitz Press, 2001.
28. Sakkas D, Gardner DK. Noninvasive methods to assess embryo quality. *Curr Opin Obstet Gynecol* 2005; 17(3): 283–8.
29. Gardner DK, Surrey E, Minjarez D, Leitz A, Stevens J, Schoolcraft WB. Single blastocyst transfer: A prospective randomized trial. *Fertil Steril* 2004; 81(3): 551–5.
30. Gardner DK, Meseguer M, Rubio C, Treff NR. Diagnosis of human preimplantation embryo viability. *Hum Reprod Update* 2015; 21(6): 727–47.
31. Braude P, Bolton V, Moore S. Human gene expression first occurs between the four- and eight-cell stages of preimplantation development. *Nature* 1988; 332: 459–61.
32. Tesarik J, Greco E. The probability of abnormal preimplantation development can be predicted by a single static observation on pronuclear stage morphology. *Hum Reprod* 1999; 14: 318–23.
33. Scott L, Alvero R, Leondires M, Miller B. The morphology of human pronuclear embryos is positively related to blastocyst development and implantation. *Hum Reprod* 2000; 15(11): 2394–403.
34. Gardner R. The early blastocyst is bilaterally symmetrical and its axis of symmetry is aligned with the animal–vegetal axis of the zygote in mouse. *Development* 1997; 124: 289–301.
35. Antczak M, Van Blerkom J. Oocyte influences on early development: The regulatory proteins leptin and STAT3 are polarized in mouse and human oocytes and differentially distributed within the cells of the preimplantation stage embryo. *Mol Hum Reprod* 1997; 3(12): 1067–86.
36. Antczak M, Van Blerkom J. Temporal and spatial aspects of fragmentation in early human embryos: Possible effects on developmental competence and association with the differential elimination of regulatory proteins from polarized domains. *Hum Reprod* 1999; 14(2): 429–47.
37. Garello C, Baker H, Rai J et al. Pronuclear orientation, polar body placement, and embryo quality after intracytoplasmic sperm injection and *in-vitro* fertilization: Further evidence for polarity in human oocytes? *Hum Reprod* 1999; 14(10): 2588–95.
38. Coticchio G, Guglielmo MC, Albertini DF et al. Contributions of the actin cytoskeleton to the emergence of polarity during maturation in human oocytes. *Mol Hum Reprod* 2014; 20(3): 200–7.
39. Scott LA, Smith S. The successful use of pronuclear embryo transfers the day following oocyte retrieval. *Hum Reprod* 1998; 13(4): 1003–13.
40. Scott L. Pronuclear scoring as a predictor of embryo development. *Reprod Biomed Online* 2003; 6(2): 201–14.
41. Wong CC, Loewke KE, Bossert NL et al. Non-invasive imaging of human embryos before embryonic genome activation predicts development to the blastocyst stage. *Nat Biotechnol* 2010; 28(10): 1115–21.
42. Aguilar J, Motato Y, Escriba MJ, Ojeda M, Munoz E, Meseguer M. The human first cell cycle: Impact on implantation. *Reprod Biomed Online* 2014; 28(4): 475–84.
43. Cruz M, Garrido N, Gadea B, Munoz M, Perez-Cano I, Meseguer M. Oocyte insemination techniques are related to alterations of embryo developmental timing in an oocyte donation model. *Reprod Biomed Online* 2013; 27(4): 367–75.
44. Gerris J, De Neubourg D, Mangelschots K, Van Royen E, Van de Meerssche M, Valkenburg M. Prevention of twin pregnancy after *in-vitro* fertilization or intracytoplasmic sperm injection based on strict embryo criteria: A prospective randomized clinical trial. *Hum Reprod* 1999; 14(10): 2581–7.
45. Van Royen E, Mangelschots K, De Neubourg D et al. Characterization of a top quality embryo, a step towards single-embryo transfer. *Hum Reprod* 1999; 14(9): 2345–9.
46. De Neubourg D, Gerris J, Mangelschots K, Van Royen E, Vercruyssen M, Elseviers M. Single top quality embryo transfer as a model for prediction of early pregnancy outcome. *Hum Reprod* 2004; 19(6): 1476–9.
47. Van Royen E, Mangelschots K, Vercruyssen M et al. Multinucleation in cleavage stage embryos. *Hum Reprod* 2003; 18(5): 1062–9.
48. Bavister B. Culture of preimplantation embryos: Facts and artefacts. *Hum Reprod Update* 1995; 1: 91–148.
49. Shoukir Y, Campana A, Farley T, Sakkas D. Early cleavage of *in-vitro* fertilized human embryos to the 2-cell stage: A novel indicator of embryo quality and viability. *Hum Reprod* 1997; 12(7): 1531–6.

50. Sakkas D, Shoukir Y, Chardonnens D, Bianchi PG, Campana A. Early cleavage of human embryos to the two-cell stage after intracytoplasmic sperm injection as an indicator of embryo viability. *Hum Reprod* 1998; 13(1): 182–7.
51. Sakkas D, Percival G, D'Arcy Y, Sharif K, Afnan M. Assessment of early cleaving *in vitro* fertilized human embryos at the 2-cell stage before transfer improves embryo selection. *Fertil Steril* 2001; 76(6): 1150–6.
52. Salumets A, Hyden-Granskog C, Makinen S, Suikkari AM, Tiitinen A, Tuuri T. Early cleavage predicts the viability of human embryos in elective single embryo transfer procedures. *Hum Reprod* 2003; 18(4): 821–5.
53. Van Montfoort AP, Dumoulin JC, Kester AD, Evers JL. Early cleavage is a valuable addition to existing embryo selection parameters: A study using single embryo transfers. *Hum Reprod* 2004; 19(9): 2103–8.
54. Neuber E, Rinaudo P, Trimarchi JR, Sakkas D. Sequential assessment of individually cultured human embryos as an indicator of subsequent good quality blastocyst development. *Hum Reprod* 2003; 18(6): 1307–12.
55. Guerif F, Le Gouge A, Giraudeau B et al. Limited value of morphological assessment at days 1 and 2 to predict blastocyst development potential: A prospective study based on 4042 embryos. *Hum Reprod* 2007; 22(7): 1973–81.
56. Meseguer M, Herrero J, Tejera A, Hilligsoe KM, Ramsing NB, Remohi J. The use of morphokinetics as a predictor of embryo implantation. *Hum Reprod* 2011; 26(10): 2658–71.
57. Herrero J, Meseguer M. Selection of high potential embryos using time-lapse imaging: The era of morphokinetics. *Fertil Steril* 2013; 99(4): 1030–4.
58. Conaghan J, Chen AA, Willman SP et al. Improving embryo selection using a computer-automated time-lapse image analysis test plus day 3 morphology: Results from a prospective multicenter trial. *Fertil Steril* 2013; 100(2): 412–9.
59. Basile N, Vime P, Florensa M et al. The use of morphokinetics as a predictor of implantation: A multicentric study to define and validate an algorithm for embryo selection. *Hum Reprod* 2015; 30(2): 276–83.
60. Meseguer M, Rubio I, Cruz M, Basile N, Marcos J, Requena A. Embryo incubation and selection in a time-lapse monitoring system improves pregnancy outcome compared with a standard incubator: A retrospective cohort study. *Fertil Steril* 2012; 98(6): 1481–9.
61. Rubio I, Galan A, Larreategui Z et al. Clinical validation of embryo culture and selection by morphokinetic analysis: A randomized, controlled trial of the EmbryoScope. *Fertil Steril* 2014; 102(5): 1287–94.
62. Goodman LR, Goldberg J, Falcone T, Austin C, Desai N. Does the addition of time-lapse morphokinetics in the selection of embryos for transfer improve pregnancy rates? A randomized controlled trial. *Fertil Steril* 2016; 105(2): 275–85.e10.
63. Ergin EG, Caliskan E, Yalcinkaya E et al. Frequency of embryo multinucleation detected by time-lapse system and its impact on pregnancy outcome. *Fertil Steril* 2014; 102(4): 1029–33.
64. Ebner T, Moser M, Shebl O, Sommergruber M, Gaiswinkler U, Tews G. Morphological analysis at compacting stage is a valuable prognostic tool for ICSI patients. *Reprod Biomed Online* 2009; 18(1): 61–6.
65. Feil D, Henshaw RC, Lane M. Day 4 embryo selection is equal to day 5 using a new embryo scoring system validated in single embryo transfers. *Hum Reprod* 2008; 23(7): 1505–10.
66. Sparks AE. Human embryo cryopreservation-methods, timing, and other considerations for optimizing an embryo cryopreservation program. *Semin Reprod Med* 2015; 33(2): 128–44.
67. Cobo A, de los Santos MJ, Castello D, Gamiz P, Campos P, Remohi J. Outcomes of vitrified early cleavage-stage and blastocyst-stage embryos in a cryopreservation program: Evaluation of 3,150 warming cycles. *Fertil Steril* 2012; 98(5): 1138–46.
68. Alpha Scientists In Reproductive Medicine. The Alpha consensus meeting on cryopreservation key performance indicators and benchmarks: Proceedings of an expert meeting. *Reprod Biomed Online* 2012; 25(2): 146–67.
69. Zander-Fox DL, Tremellen K, Lane M. Single blastocyst embryo transfer maintains comparable pregnancy rates to double cleavage-stage embryo transfer but results in healthier pregnancy outcomes. *Aust N Z J Obstet Gynaecol* 2011; 51(5): 406–10.
70. Gardner DK. The impact of physiological oxygen during culture, and vitrification for cryopreservation, on the outcome of extended culture in human IVF. *Reprod Biomed Online* 2016; 32(2): 137–41.
71. Blake DA, Proctor M, Johnson NP. The merits of blastocyst versus cleavage stage embryo transfer: A Cochrane review. *Hum Reprod* 2004; 19(4): 795–807.
72. Scott RT Jr., Upham KM, Forman EJ et al. Blastocyst biopsy with comprehensive chromosome screening and fresh embryo transfer significantly increases *in vitro* fertilization implantation and delivery rates: A randomized controlled trial. *Fertil Steril* 2013; 100(3): 697–703.
73. Treff NR, Forman EJ, Scott RT, Jr. Next-generation sequencing for preimplantation genetic diagnosis. *Fertil Steril* 2013; 99(6): e17–8.
74. Forman EJ, Hong KH, Treff NR, Scott RT. Comprehensive chromosome screening and embryo selection: Moving toward single euploid blastocyst transfer. *Semin Reprod Med* 2012; 30(3): 236–42.
75. Schoolcraft WB, Treff NR, Stevens JM, Ferry K, Katz-Jaffe M, Scott RT, Jr. Live birth outcome with trophectoderm biopsy, blastocyst vitrification, and single-nucleotide polymorphism microarray-based comprehensive chromosome screening in infertile patients. *Fertil Steril* 2011; 96(3): 638–40.

76. Gardner DK, Schoolcraft WB. *In vitro* culture of human blastocysts. In: *Towards Reproductive Certainty: Infertility and Genetics Beyond*. Jansen R, Mortimer D (eds). Carnforth, U.K.: Parthenon Press, 1999, pp. 378–88.
77. Alpha Scientists in Reproductive Medicine and ESHRE Special Interest Group of Embryology. The Istanbul consensus workshop on embryo assessment: Proceedings of an expert meeting. *Hum Reprod* 2011; 26(6): 1270–83.
78. Alpha Scientists in Reproductive Medicine: ESHRE Special Interest Group of Embryology. Istanbul consensus workshop on embryo assessment: Proceedings of an expert meeting. *Reprod Biomed Online* 2011; 22(6): 632–46.
79. Gardner DK, Lane M, Stevens J, Schlenker T, Schoolcraft WB. Blastocyst score affects implantation and pregnancy outcome: Towards a single blastocyst transfer. *Fertil Steril* 2000; 73(6): 1155–8.
80. Gardner DK, Stevens J, Sheehan CB, Schoolcraft WB. Morphological assessment of the human blastocyst. In: *Analysis of the Human Embryo*. Elder KT, Cohen J (eds). Taylor & Francis, London, England: 2007, pp. 79–87.
81. Ahlstrom A, Westin C, Reismer E, Wikland M, Hardarson T. Trophectoderm morphology: An important parameter for predicting live birth after single blastocyst transfer. *Hum Reprod* 2011; 26(12): 3289–96.
82. Hill MJ, Richter KS, Heitmann RJ et al. Trophectoderm grade predicts outcomes of single-blastocyst transfers. *Fertil Steril* 2013; 99(5): 1283–9.
83. Chen X, Zhang J, Wu X et al. Trophectoderm morphology predicts outcomes of pregnancy in vitrified–warmed single-blastocyst transfer cycle in a Chinese population. *J Assist Reprod Genet* 2014; 31(11): 1475–81.
84. Thompson SM, Onwubalili N, Brown K, Jindal SK, McGovern PG. Blastocyst expansion score and trophectoderm morphology strongly predict successful clinical pregnancy and live birth following elective single embryo blastocyst transfer (eSET): A national study. *J Assist Reprod Genet* 2013; 30(12): 1577–81.
85. van der Weiden RM. Trophectoderm morphology grading reflects interactions between embryo and endometrium. *Fertil Steril* 2013; 100(4): e23.
86. Honnma H, Baba T, Sasaki M et al. Trophectoderm morphology significantly affects the rates of ongoing pregnancy and miscarriage in frozen–thawed single-blastocyst transfer cycle *in vitro* fertilization. *Fertil Steril* 2012; 98(2): 361–7.
87. Van den Abbeel E, Balaban B, Ziebe S et al. Association between blastocyst morphology and outcome of single-blastocyst transfer. *Reprod Biomed Online* 2013; 27(4): 353–61.
88. Shoukir Y, Chardonnens D, Campana A, Bischof P, Sakkas D. The rate of development and time of transfer play different roles in influencing the viability of human blastocysts. *Hum Reprod* 1998; 13(3): 676–81.
89. Menezo YJ, Chouteau J, Torello J, Girard A, Veiga A. Birth weight and sex ratio after transfer at the blastocyst stage in humans. *Fertil Steril* 1999; 72(2): 221–4.
90. Milki AA, Jun SH, Hinckley MD, Westphal LW, Giudice LC, Behr B. Comparison of the sex ratio with blastocyst transfer and cleavage stage transfer. *J Assist Reprod Genet* 2003; 20(8): 323–6.
91. Dean JH, Chapman MG, Sullivan EA. The effect on human sex ratio at birth by assisted reproductive technology (ART) procedures—An assessment of babies born following single embryo transfers, Australia and New Zealand, 2002–2006. *BJOG* 2010; 117(13): 1628–34.
92. Alfarawati S, Fragouli E, Colls P et al. The relationship between blastocyst morphology, chromosomal abnormality, and embryo gender. *Fertil Steril* 2011; 95(2): 520–4.
93. Ebner T, Tritscher K, Mayer RB et al. Quantitative and qualitative trophectoderm grading allows for prediction of live birth and gender. *J Assist Reprod Genet* 2016; 33(1): 49–57.
94. Meintjes M, Chantilis SJ, Douglas JD et al. A controlled randomized trial evaluating the effect of lowered incubator oxygen tension on live births in a predominantly blastocyst transfer program. *Hum Reprod* 2009; 24(2): 300–7.
95. Campbell A, Fishel S, Bowman N, Duffy S, Sedler M, Thornton S. Retrospective analysis of outcomes after IVF using an aneuploidy risk model derived from time-lapse imaging without PGS. *Reprod Biomed Online* 2013; 27(2): 140–6.
96. Rienzi L, Capalbo A, Stoppa M et al. No evidence of association between blastocyst aneuploidy and morphokinetic assessment in a selected population of poor-prognosis patients: A longitudinal cohort study. *Reprod Biomed Online* 2015; 30(1): 57–66.
97. Vera-Rodriguez M, Chavez SL, Rubio C, Reijo Pera RA, Simon C. Prediction model for aneuploidy in early human embryo development revealed by single-cell analysis. *Nat Commun* 2015; 6: 7601.
98. Fisch JD, Rodriguez H, Ross R, Overby G, Sher G. The Graduated Embryo Score (GES) predicts blastocyst formation and pregnancy rate from cleavage-stage embryos. *Hum Reprod* 2001; 16(9): 1970–5.
99. Racowsky C, Ohno-Machado L, Kim J, Biggers JD. Is there an advantage in scoring early embryos on more than one day? *Hum Reprod* 2009; 24(9): 2104–13.
100. Gardner DK, Sakkas D. Assessment of embryo viability: The ability to select a single embryo for transfer—A review. *Placenta* 2003; 24(Suppl B): S5–12.
101. Wiley LM, Yamami S, Van Muyden D. Effect of potassium concentration, type of protein supplement, and embryo density on mouse preimplantation development *in vitro*. *Fertil Steril* 1986; 45(1): 111–9.
102. Lane M, Gardner DK. Effect of incubation volume and embryo density on the development and viability of mouse embryos *in vitro*. *Hum Reprod* 1992; 7(4): 558–62.

103. Gardner DK, Lane M, Spitzer A, Batt PA. Enhanced rates of cleavage and development for sheep zygotes cultured to the blastocyst stage *in vitro* in the absence of serum and somatic cells: Amino acids, vitamins, and culturing embryos in groups stimulate development. *Biol Reprod* 1994; 50(2): 390–400.
104. Wale PL, Gardner DK. The effects of chemical and physical factors on mammalian embryo culture and their importance for the practice of assisted human reproduction. *Hum Reprod Update* 2016; 22(1): 2–22.
105. Stecher A, Vanderzwalmen P, Zintz M et al. Transfer of blastocysts with deviant morphological and morphokinetic parameters at early stages of *in-vitro* development: A case series. *Reprod Biomed Online* 2014; 28(4): 424–35.
106. Shapiro BS, Daneshmand ST, Garner FC, Aguirre M, Hudson C. Freeze-all can be a superior therapy to another fresh cycle in patients with prior fresh blastocyst implantation failure. *Reprod Biomed Online* 2014; 29(3): 286–90.
107. Rieger D. The measurement of metabolic activity as an approach to evaluating viability and diagnosing sex in early embryos. *Theriogenology* 1984; 21: 138–49.
108. Menke TM, McLaren A. Mouse blastocysts grown *in vivo* and *in vitro*: Carbon dioxide production and trophoblast outgrowth. *J Reprod Fertil* 1970; 23(1): 117–27.
109. Gardner DK. Changes in requirements and utilization of nutrients during mammalian preimplantation embryo development and their significance in embryo culture. *Theriogenology* 1998; 49(1): 83–102.
110. Renard JP, Philippon A, Menezo Y. *In-vitro* uptake of glucose by bovine blastocysts. *J Reprod Fertil* 1980; 58(1): 161–4.
111. Gardner DK, Leese HJ. Assessment of embryo viability prior to transfer by the noninvasive measurement of glucose uptake. *J Exp Zool* 1987; 242(1): 103–5.
112. Lane M, Gardner DK. Selection of viable mouse blastocysts prior to transfer using a metabolic criterion. *Hum Reprod* 1996; 11(9): 1975–8.
113. Gardner DK, Wale PL. Analysis of metabolism to select viable human embryos for transfer. *Fertil Steril* 2013; 99(4): 1062–72.
114. Gardner DK, Lane M, Stevens J, Schoolcraft WB. Noninvasive assessment of human embryo nutrient consumption as a measure of developmental potential. *Fertil Steril* 2001; 76(6): 1175–80.
115. Houghton FD, Hawkhead JA, Humpherson PG et al. Non-invasive amino acid turnover predicts human embryo developmental capacity. *Hum Reprod* 2002; 17(4): 999–1005.
116. Gardner DK, Wale PL, Collins R, Lane M. Glucose consumption of single post-compaction human embryos is predictive of embryo sex and live birth outcome. *Hum Reprod* 2011; 26(8): 1981–6.
117. Gardner DK, Larman MG, Thouas GA. Sex-related physiology of the preimplantation embryo. *Mol Hum Reprod* 2010; 16(8): 539–47.
118. Sturmey RG, Bermejo-Alvarez P, Gutierrez-Adan A, Rizos D, Leese HJ, Lonergan P. Amino acid metabolism of bovine blastocysts: A biomarker of sex and viability. *Mol Reprod Dev* 2010; 77(3): 285–96.
119. Urbanski JP, Johnson MT, Craig DD, Potter DL, Gardner DK, Thorsen T. Noninvasive metabolic profiling using microfluidics for analysis of single preimplantation embryos. *Anal Chem* 2008; 80(17): 6500–7.
120. Thouas GA, Potter DL, Gardner DK. Microfluidic device for the analysis of gamete and embryo physiology. In: *Human Gametes and Preimplantation Embryos: Assessment and Diagnosis*. Gardner DK, Seli E, Wells D, Sakkas D (eds). New York, NY: Springer, 2013, pp. 281–99.
121. Swain JE, Lai D, Takayama S, Smith GD. Thinking big by thinking small: Application of microfluidic technology to improve ART. *Lab Chip* 2013; 13(7): 1213–24.
122. Brison DR, Houghton FD, Falconer D et al. Identification of viable embryos in IVF by non-invasive measurement of amino acid turnover. *Hum Reprod* 2004; 19(10): 2319–24.
123. Picton HM, Elder K, Houghton FD et al. Association between amino acid turnover and chromosome aneuploidy during human preimplantation embryo development *in vitro*. *Mol Hum Reprod* 2010; 16(8): 557–69.
124. Wale PL, Gardner DK. Oxygen affects the ability of mouse blastocysts to regulate ammonium. *Biol Reprod* 2013; 89(3): 75.
125. Wale PL, Gardner DK. Oxygen regulates amino acid turnover and carbohydrate uptake during the preimplantation period of mouse embryo development. *Biol Reprod* 2012; 87(1): 24, 1–8.
126. Seli E, Sakkas D, Scott R, Kwok SC, Rosendahl SM, Burns DH. Noninvasive metabolomic profiling of embryo culture media using Raman and near-infrared spectroscopy correlates with reproductive potential of embryos in women undergoing *in vitro* fertilization. *Fertil Steril* 2007; 88(5): 1350–7.
127. Seli E, Vergouw CG, Morita H et al. Noninvasive metabolomic profiling as an adjunct to morphology for noninvasive embryo assessment in women undergoing single embryo transfer. *Fertil Steril* 2010; 94(2): 535–42.
128. Vergouw CG, Botros LL, Roos P et al. Metabolomic profiling by near-infrared spectroscopy as a tool to assess embryo viability: A novel, non-invasive method for embryo selection. *Hum Reprod* 2008; 23(7): 1499–504.
129. Scott R, Seli E, Miller K, Sakkas D, Scott K, Burns DH. Noninvasive metabolomic profiling of human embryo culture media using Raman spectroscopy predicts embryonic reproductive potential: A prospective blinded pilot study. *Fertil Steril* 2008; 90(1): 77–83.
130. Seli E, Bruce C, Botros L, Henson M et al. Receiver operating characteristic (ROC) analysis of day 5 morphology grading and metabolomic viability

score on predicting implantation outcome. *J Assist Reprod Genet* 2011; 28(2): 137–44.
131. Ahlstrom A, Wikland M, Rogberg L, Barnett JS, Tucker M, Hardarson T. Cross-validation and predictive value of near-infrared spectroscopy algorithms for day-5 blastocyst transfer. *Reprod Biomed Online* 2011; 22(5): 477–84.
132. Katz-Jaffe MG, Schoolcraft WB, Gardner DK. Analysis of protein expression (secretome) by human and mouse preimplantation embryos. *Fertil Steril* 2006; 86(3): 678–85.
133. Katz-Jaffe MG, Gardner DK, Schoolcraft WB. Proteomic analysis of individual human embryos to identify novel biomarkers of development and viability. *Fertil Steril* 2006; 85(1): 101–7.
134. Katz-Jaffe MG, McReynolds S, Gardner DK, Schoolcraft WB. The role of proteomics in defining the human embryonic secretome. *Mol Hum Reprod* 2009; 15(5): 271–7.
135. Krisher RL, Schoolcraft WB, Katz-Jaffe MG. Omics as a window to view embryo viability. *Fertil Steril* 2015; 103(2): 333–41.
136. Lee YS, Thouas GA, Gardner DK. Developmental kinetics of cleavage stage mouse embryos are related to their subsequent carbohydrate and amino acid utilization at the blastocyst stage. *Hum Reprod* 2015; 30(3): 543–52.
137. Mitchell M, Cashman KS, Gardner DK, Thompson JG, Lane M. Disruption of mitochondrial malate–aspartate shuttle activity in mouse blastocysts impairs viability and fetal growth. *Biol Reprod* 2009; 80(2): 295–301.
138. Gardner DK, Harvey AJ. Blastocyst metabolism. *Reprod Fertil Dev* 2015; 27(4): 638–54.
139. Trimarchi JR, Liu L, Porterfield DM, Smith PJ, Keefe DL. A non-invasive method for measuring preimplantation embryo physiology. *Zygote* 2000; 8(1): 15–24.
140. Trimarchi JR, Liu L, Smith PJ, Keefe DL. Noninvasive measurement of potassium efflux as an early indicator of cell death in mouse embryos. *Biol Reprod* 2000; 63(3): 851–7.
141. Ottosen LD, Hindkjaer J, Lindenberg S, Ingerslev HJ. Murine pre-embryo oxygen consumption and developmental competence. *J Assist Reprod Genet* 2007; 24(8): 359–65.
142. Lopes AS, Larsen LH, Ramsing N et al. Respiration rates of individual bovine *in vitro*-produced embryos measured with a novel, non-invasive and highly sensitive microsensor system. *Reproduction* 2005; 130(5): 669–79.
143. Kovats S, Main EK, Librach C, Stubblebine M, Fisher SJ, DeMars R. A class I antigen, HLA-G, expressed in human trophoblasts. *Science* 1990; 248(4952): 220–3.
144. Jurisicova A, Casper RF, MacLusky NJ, Mills GB, Librach CL. HLA-G expression during preimplantation human embryo development. *Proc Natl Acad Sci USA* 1996; 93(1): 161–5.
145. Noci I, Fuzzi B, Rizzo R et al. Embryonic soluble HLA-G as a marker of developmental potential in embryos. *Hum Reprod* 2005; 20(1): 138–46.
146. Sher G, Keskintepe L, Nouriani M, Roussev R, Batzofin J. Expression of sHLA-G in supernatants of individually cultured 46-h embryos: A potentially valuable indicator of "embryo competency" and IVF outcome. *Reprod Biomed Online* 2004; 9(1): 74–8.
147. Yie SM, Balakier H, Motamedi G, Librach CL. Secretion of human leukocyte antigen-G by human embryos is associated with a higher *in vitro* fertilization pregnancy rate. *Fertil Steril* 2005; 83(1): 30–6.
148. Menezo Y, Elder K, Viville S. Soluble HLA-G release by the human embryo: An interesting artefact? *Reprod Biomed Online* 2006; 13(6): 763–4.
149. Sageshima N, Shobu T, Awai K et al. Soluble HLA-G is absent from human embryo cultures: A reassessment of sHLA-G detection methods. *J Reprod Immunol* 2007; 75(1): 11–22.
150. Sargent I, Swales A, Ledee N, Kozma N, Tabiasco J, Le Bouteiller P. sHLA-G production by human IVF embryos: Can it be measured reliably? *J Reprod Immunol* 2007; 75(2): 128–32.
151. O'Neill C. The role of PAF in embryo physiology. *Hum Reprod Update* 2005; 11(3): 215–28.
152. Stamatkin CW, Roussev RG, Stout M et al. Preimplantation factor (PIF) correlates with early mammalian embryo development-bovine and murine models. *Reprod Biol Endocrinol* 2011; 9: 63.
153. Xiao-Yan C, Jie L, Dang J, Tao L, Xin-Ru L, Guang-Lun Z. A highly sensitive electrochemiluminescence immunoassay for detecting human embryonic human chorionic gonadotropin in spent embryo culture media during IVF–ET cycle. *J Assist Reprod Genet* 2013; 30(3): 377–82.
154. Strom CM, Bonilla-Guererro R, Zhang K et al. The sensitivity and specificity of hyperglycosylated hCG (hhCG) levels to reliably diagnose clinical IVF pregnancies at 6 days following embryo transfer. *J Assist Reprod Genet* 2012; 29(7): 609–14.
155. Dominguez F, Meseguer M, Aparicio-Ruiz B, Piqueras P, Quinonero A, Simon C. New strategy for diagnosing embryo implantation potential by combining proteomics and time-lapse technologies. *Fertil Steril* 2015; 104(4): 908–14.
156. Sutton-McDowall ML, Purdey M, Brown HM et al. Redox and anti-oxidant state within cattle oocytes following *in vitro* maturation with bone morphogenetic protein 15 and follicle stimulating hormone. *Mol Reprod Dev* 2015; 82(4): 281–94.

Evaluation of embryo quality

18

Time-lapse imaging to assess embryo morphokinesis

NATALIA BASILE, ANDREA RODRIGO CARBAJOSA, and MARCOS MESEGUER

INTRODUCTION

In vitro fertilization (IVF) programs are coming closer every day to the goal of reducing multiple pregnancies while maintaining good clinical results. The transfer of a single embryo is progressively becoming a reality, and this is the result of major improvements in different areas. From a clinical point of view, two major achievements are worth mentioning: first, physicians have learned to handle the stimulation drugs that are more pure, more powerful, and more comfortable for the patient; and second, an increased knowledge of the pathophysiology of ovarian hyperstimulation syndrome has made the frequency of this syndrome almost anecdotal. On the other hand, concerns about the "epidemic" of multiple gestations have raised awareness of the risks not only to the mother (gestational diabetes, hypertension, and anemia), but also to the babies—extreme prematurity, low birth weight, children with neurological damage, and so on—not to mention the psychological burden and suffering of the parents and the tremendous health costs that it entails. From the laboratory point of view, several achievements are worth mentioning as well: studies on embryo metabolism have led to the formulation of suitable culture media. In the early 1990s, the introduction of intracytoplasmic sperm injection (ICSI) revolutionized the treatment of male infertility and genetic screening became the gold standard for the selection of aneuploid embryos. Vitrification came along, and preservation of fertility was no longer a utopia for modern women; the wave of the "omics" initiated an era of noninvasiveness for studying human embryos in the laboratory, and most recently, the introduction of imaging systems allowed us to assess embryos in a different way: through their morphokinetics.

TIME-LAPSE TECHNOLOGY

Traditional embryo assessment is based on time-point evaluations. Through this approach, embryo categories are normally based on the number of blastomeres and nuclei, the percentage of fragments, cell symmetry, and the quality of the inner cell mass (ICM) and trophectoderm (TE). Even though great knowledge has been achieved through this approach, it has been demonstrated that embryo status can markedly change within a few hours (1–4). In addition, inter- and intra-observer variability are commonly described problems (5), probably due to the subjective nature surrounding traditional morphological assessment (3,6–10). In theory, increasing the number of observations could provide better information on the development of the embryo and therefore improve its assessment (3,11,12). However, increased handling and higher evaluation frequencies will expose the embryo to undesirable changes in temperature, humidity, and gas composition (11–13).

Time-lapse systems (TMS) represent a solution to this problem. In 1997, Payne et al. (14) developed time-lapse cinematography to manage intermittent observation of the process of oocyte fertilization. Later on, the observation period was augmented while maintaining optimal culture conditions (2) and nowadays TMS allow the complete observation of the entire process of embryo development in the IVF laboratory. The two main advantages of these systems are: (1) improved and stable culture conditions; and (2) the determination of objective and accurate markers, both quantitative and qualitative (3). In addition, we should mention that there is: reduced handling and human risk; minimization of culture media, gas, and oil; detection of abnormal events that would normally occur between observations; reduced inter- and intra-observer variability; and reduced numbers of hours needed by the embryologist in the laboratory (15).

Morphokinetics, defined as the combination of the embryo appearance (morphology) and the timing in which cellular events occur, has been introduced as a new concept to improve embryo selection. The use of this strategy could allow single-embryo transfers (SETs) without jeopardizing the overall IVF success (16), becoming very attractive especially in European countries in which legislation is stricter about the number of embryos transferred (15).

Models on the market

There are different options of TMS available on the market. Some of them present all the items integrated into one single piece of equipment (e.g., EmbryoScope® [Vitrolife], Geri® [Genea Biomedx], and Miri® TL [Esco Medical]). Others offer the option of introducing a microscope inside an available incubator (e.g., Primo Vision® [Vitrolife] and The Eeva™ Test [Merck-Serono]). Tables 18.1 and 18.2 describe the clinical and technical features of all the TMS available on the market.

Table 18.1 Technical features compared between the time-lapse systems available on the market

Technical feature	EmbryoScope®	Primovision™	Eeva™ test	Geri®	Miri® TL
Microscopy	Phase contrast	Phase contrast	Dark field	Phase contrast	Phase contrast
Image capture frequency	Every 10 minutes	Every 10 minutes	Every 5 minutes	Every 5 minutes	Every 5 minutes
Focusing levels	7	Several	1	Several	Several
Patients per system	6	1	1	6	6
Embryos per dish	12	16	12	16	14
Integrated incubator	Yes	No	No	Yes	Yes
Data analysis	Manual	Manual	Real time	Manual	Manual

Table 18.2 Clinical features compared between the time-lapse systems available on the market

Clinical feature	EmbryoScope®	Primovision™	Eeva™ test	Geri®	Miri® TL
Automatic assessment	No	No	Yes	No	No
Worker dependent	Yes	Yes	No	Yes	Yes
Time consuming	Yes	Yes	No/automatic	Yes	Yes
Selection algorithm	Set by the user	Set by the user	Preset	Set by the user	Set by the user
Blastocyst formation prediction by day 3	No	No	Yes	No	No
Implantation prediction by day 3	Yes	Yes	Yes	No	No
Prospective validated	Yes	No	Yes	No	No

Kinetic parameters (individual plus calculated)

As described in the proposed guidelines on the nomenclature and annotation of dynamic human embryo monitoring by a time-lapse user group, we can define the following morphokinetic "individual" variables (17):

t0	Time of IVF or mid-time of microinjection (ICSI/intracytoplasmic morphologically selected sperm injection)
tPB2	The second polar body completely detached from the oolemma
tPN	Fertilization is confirmed
tPNa	Appearance of individual pronuclei; tPN1a, tPN2a; tPN3a, etc.
tPNf	Time of pronuclei disappearance; tPN1f; tPN2f, etc.
tZ	Time of PN scoring
t2 to t9	Time to two to nine discrete cells
tSC	First evidence of compaction
tMf/p	End of compaction "f" corresponds to full compaction; "p" corresponds to partial compaction
tSB	Initiation of blastulation
tByz	Full blastocyst "y" corresponds to morphology of ICM "z" corresponds to morphology of TE cells
tEyz	Initiation of expansion; first frame of zona thinning
tHNyz	Herniation; end of expansion phase and initiation of hatching
tHDyz	Fully hatched blastocyst

Additionally, we can define "calculated" variables that represent a certain cell stage or cycle duration (Figure 18.1):

VP	tPNf – tPNa	Pronucleous (PN) duration
ECC1	t2 – tPB2	Duration of first cell cycle
ECC2	t4 – t2	Duration of second cell cycle Duration of single blastomere cycle: cc2a = t3 – t2; cc2b = t4 – t2
ECC3	t8–t4	Duration of third cell cycle Duration of single blastomere cell cycle: cc3a = t5 – t4; cc3b = t6 – t4; cc3c = t7 – t4; cc3d = t8 – t4
s2	t4 – t3	Synchronization of cell divisions
s3	t8 – t5	Synchronization of cleavage pattern
dcom		Duration of compaction tMf – tSC (full compaction); tMp – tSC (partial compaction)

(*Continued*)

dB	tB – tSB	Duration of blastulation
dexp	tHN – tE	Duration of blastocyst expansion
dcol	tBCend(n) – tBCi(n)	Duration of blastocyst collapse "n" is number of episodes of collapse and re-expansion
dre – exp tre – exp end(n) – tre – expi(n)		Duration of re-expansion
dHN	tHN – tHD	Duration of herniation

BLASTOCYST DEVELOPMENT STUDIES

Kinetic markers have been associated with good-quality embryos and the prediction of blastocyst formation (Table 18.3).

In 2010, Wong et al. analyzed kinetic parameters of 100 embryos that were cultured up to days 5 or 6 of development (18). Three parameters were founded to be predictors of blastocyst formation: P1—duration of the first cytokinesis (14.3 ± 6.0 minutes); P2—interval between the end of the first mitosis and the initiation of the second mitosis (11.1 ± 2.2 hours); and P3—the synchrony between the second and third mitosis (1.0 ± 1.6 hours). The authors concluded that embryo development to the blastocyst stage could be predicted with 94% sensitivity and 93% specificity after using those parameters. Embryos with one or more values outside these ranges were expected to arrest. The time of completion of the second and third mitosis was also analyzed by Hashimoto et al., who observed that high-scoring blastocysts took significantly shorter times for these divisions (19).

Hlinka et al. (20) analyzed 180 embryos that resulted in 28 pregnancies. After calculating the average duration of the interphases and cleavages of a subset of implanting embryos, the authors established a uniform time-patterning of cleavage clusters (c) and interphases (i); more specifically: i2 = 11 ± 1, i3 = 15 ± 1, i4 = 23 ± 1 hours; c2 = 15 ± 5, c3 = 40 ± 10, c4 = 55 ± 15 hours. Embryos falling within these values showed a higher rate of blastocyst development than those falling outside this range (88.2% vs. 13.3%). In addition, higher morphological abnormality rates were observed in embryos falling outside the optimal ranges.

In a retrospective cohort study, Cruz et al. (21) monitored 834 embryos. Mean timings for the variables t2, t3, t4, t5, tM, cc2, and s2 were calculated for embryos that developed to blastocyst and for those that did not. Quartiles were defined for each parameter in association with the proportions of good- and poor-morphology blastocysts. Finally, optimal ranges were proposed as follows: t2, 24.3–27.9 hours; t3, 35.4–40.3 hours; t5, 48.8–56.6 hours; s2, <0.76 hours; cc2, <11.9 hours. The following deselection criteria were also recorded: uneven blastomere size at the two-cell stage and abrupt division from zygote to a three-blastomere embryo. In general, it was observed that embryos performing earlier cleavages had significantly higher developmental potential to day 5. Therefore, the capability of reaching the blastocyst stage seemed to be related to early embryo division kinetics.

In 2013, Chamayou et al. (22) reported time intervals of morphokinetic parameters identified as predictors of embryo competence. In this retrospective study, embryos were divided into three groups: implanted (n = 72), non-implanted (n = 106), and arrested (n = 66). Each kinetic parameter for every single embryo was compared and significant differences were found. The authors concluded that day-3 embryos develop into viable blastocysts when their kinetic parameters met the following ranges: t1 (18.4–30.9 hpi [hours post insemination]), t2 (21.4–34.8 hpi), t4 (33.1–57.2 hpi), t7 (46.1–82.5 hpi), t8 (46.4–97.8 hpi), tC – tF (7.7–22.9 hpi), and s3 (0.7–30.8 hpi).

A couple of prospective studies were performed in 2013. Kirkegaard et al. (23) analyzed 571 embryos from good-prognosis patients and reported three markers linked to high-quality blastocysts: duration of the first cytokinesis; duration of the three-cell stage; and direct cleavage to the

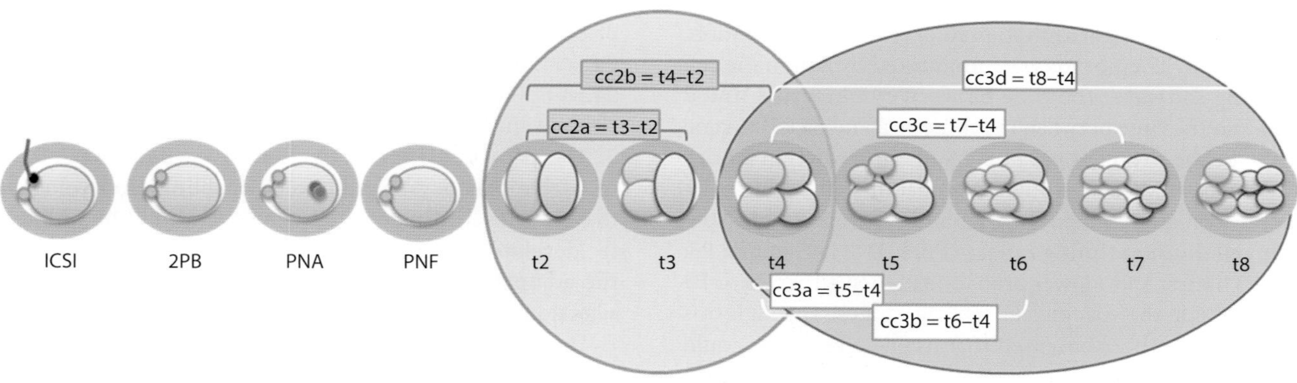

Figure 18.1 Graphical representation of kinetic variables up to the eight-cell stage. *Abbreviations*: ICSI, intracytoplasmic sperm injection; 2PB, 2 polar bodies; PNa, pronucleaous appereance; PNF, pronuecleous fading.

Table 18.3 Studies associating blastocyst formation with kinetic markers

Author	Study design	Embryos (n)	Embryo origin	Time-lapse system	Predictive marker identified
Wong et al. (18)	Retrospective study	100	Supernumerary frozen2PN	Modified Olympus IX-70/71; CKX-40/41	First cytokinesis, P2 and P3
Hashimoto et al. (19)	Experimental study	80	Donated human embryos for research	Biostation CT	Durations of second (t4 – t3) and third mitotic divisions (t8 – t5)
Hlinka et al. (20)	Retrospective study	180	Clinical IVF routine	Primovision	c2, c3, and c4; i2, i3, and i4
Cruz et al. (21)	Retrospective cohort study	834	Oocyte donation cycles	EmbryoScope	t4, s2, DC3 cells, and tM; UN2 cells
Chamayou et al. (22)	Retrospective study	224	Fresh oocyte ICSI treatments	EmbryoScope	t1, t2, t4, t7, t8, tC–tF, and s3
Kirkegaard et al. (23)	Prospective cohort study	571	Fresh oocyte ICSI treatments	EmbryoScope	First cytokinesis, t3, and DC3 cells
Conaghan et al. (24)	Prospective multicenter cohort study	233	Fresh oocyte ICSI treatments	Eeva	P2 and P3
Kirkegaard et al. (25)	Retrospective multicenter study	1519	Fresh oocyte ICSI treatments	EmbryoScope	P2 and P3
Cetinkaya et al. (26)	Retrospective observational cohort study	3354	Clinical IVF routine	EmbryoScope	CS2
Yang et al. (27)	Prospective observational study	345	Metaphase I donated for research	Primovision	Cleavage patterns
Milewski et al. (28)	Retrospective observational study	432	Fresh oocyte ICSI treatments	EmbryoScope	t2, t5, cc2, and SC
Storr et al. (29)	Prospective cohort study	380	Fresh oocyte ICSI treatments	EmbryoScope	s3, t8, and tEB
Motato et al. (30)	Retrospective study	7483	Clinical IVF routine	EmbryoScope	tM; t8 – t5

Abbreviations: ICSI, intracytoplasmic sperm injection; IVF, *in vitro* fertilization.

three-cell, all of which had comparable predictive values but no connection to implantation results. Conaghan et al. (24) conducted a two-phase multicenter study to develop and validate an algorithm to predict blastocyst formation. A total of 1727 embryos were monitored by automatic cell tracking software. The time between cytokinesis 1 and 2 (P2) and the time between cytokinesis 2 and 3 (P3) turned out to be the strongest parameters in the prediction model. The results indicated a higher probability of usable blastocyst formation when both P2 and P3 were within specific cell division timing ranges (P2, 9.33–11.45 hours; P3, 0–1.73 hours) and a lower probability when either P2 or P3 were outside the specific cell timing ranges. Through this model, the authors observed that usable blastocysts could be predicted with a specificity of 84.2% (95% CI = 78.7%–88.5%), a sensitivity of 58.8% (95% CI = 47.0%–69.7%), a positive predictive value (PPV) of 54.1% (95% CI = 42.8%–64.9%), and a negative predictive value (NPV) of 86.6% (95% CI = 81.3%–90.6%). By comparison, the same prediction based on morphology alone was achieved with a specificity of 52.1% (95% CI = 39.7%–64.6%), a sensitivity of 81.8% (95% CI = 70.6%–92.9%), a PPV of 34.5% (95% CI = 31.5%–37.5%), and a NPV of 90.9% (95% CI = 87.3%–94.5%). The authors concluded that the use of this algorithm significantly improved the specificity (84.2% vs. 52.1%; $p < 0.0001$) and PPV (54.1% vs. 34.5%; $p < 0.01$) of usable blastocyst predictions, enabling embryologists to better discriminate which embryos would be unlikely to develop to blastocyst. Therefore, they recommend the adjunctive use of this algorithm to improve embryo selection.

The Conaghan model was tested retrospectively by a different group using a set of 1519 transferred embryos with known clinical outcome (25). According to the algorithm, embryos were classified as usable or non-usable. The difference in implantation rate between the usable group and the whole cohort was 30%, indicating that implantation rates could increase using this model. In addition, the percentage of non-usable embryos that resulted in implantation was 50.6%, raising concerns regarding the discarding of viable embryos. Even though the Conaghan model was developed for blastocyst formation and the end point of this study was clinical outcome, the authors expressed that implanted embryos should derive from the usable embryo group and not from the non-usable group (or at least not in such high proportions). The possible explanation for these findings, according to the authors, could be that the model is based on narrow time intervals.

In 2015, Cetinkaya et al. (26) studied 17 kinetic markers in 3354 embryos cultured up to day 5. The parameters t8 – t5, cleavage synchronicity from four to eight cells (CS4–8), and cleavage synchronicity from two to eight cells (CS2–8) were found to be good indicators. In particular, CS2–8, defined as ([t3 – t2] + [t5 – t4])/(t8 – t2), was selected as the best predictor on day 3 for blastocyst formation and quality (area under the curve [AUC] = 0.786). The authors concluded that relative timings (time intervals and relative ratios) were better indicators of development than absolute time points that cannot be standardized for general applicability in different laboratories.

Yang et al. (27) took a different approach and developed a study to describe different types of abnormal divisions and how they may affect the developmental potential of the embryo. Seven types of divisions within two categories were defined according to the impact caused on blastocyst development. Category 1 consisted of divisions with low impact on the development potential: normal division, uneven blastomere formation, and appearance of big fragments. Category 2 consisted of divisions with high impact on embryo development: direct cleavage, fragmentation, developmental arrest, and disordered division. By taking this into consideration, a hierarchical classification model was developed based on the division patterns during the three initial embryo cleavages rather than on morphokinetic parameters as in previous studies. Day-3 embryos were then classified into six categories of A–F according to the number and category of the abnormal cleavages they had presented. More specifically: (A) embryos that had normal cleavage in the initial three cleavages; (B) embryos that had category 1 behaviors in all three cleavages; (C) embryos undergoing category 1 behaviors in the initial two cleavages and category 2 behaviors in the third cleavage; (D) embryos that showed category 1 behaviors in the first cleavage and one of the two blastomeres (partial) showed category 2 behaviors in the second cleavage; (E) embryos that showed category 1 behaviors in the first cleavage and two blastomeres (all) showed category 2 behaviors in the second cleavage; and (F) embryos that showed category 2 behaviors in the first cleavage. The model was validated in a prospective observational study in which images from 345 embryos were acquired. The study revealed that 72.2% of the embryos presented at least one abnormal division. According to the model, the blastocyst formation rate decreases from 94.8% to 21.2%, the good-quality blastocyst formation rate decreases from 70.8% to 3.8%, and the implantation rate (for those that were transferred) decreases from 67% to 0% as we proceed from A to F.

In a study by Milewski et al., the parameters t2, t3, t4, t5, cc2, and s2 were measured and differences were observed between embryos that reached the blastocyst stage and embryos that arrested. A total of 432 embryos were analyzed. The resultant data for each parameter were divided into four intervals (C1–C4) and score values were assigned in order to find out which parameter values corresponded to the highest blastocyst development rate. The highest ones generally belonged to compartments C3 and C2. The extreme compartments—C1 and C4—had the lowest rates. A univariate logistic regression analysis concluded that all the studied parameters were significantly associated with blastocyst development. However, after multivariate logistic regression, only the t2, t5, and cc2 parameters were taken into account and combined into a new parameter (SC), defined as the predictor of development to blastocyst (28).

Storr et al. recorded the timings of 380 blastocysts and found eight significant prediction markers of top-quality blastocysts: s3, t6, t7, t8, tM, tSB, tB, and tEB. Out of these potential predictors, s3 was identified as the one with the best individual discriminatory capacity before compaction (AUC = 0.585, 95% CI = 0.534–0.635), and tEB was identified as the best predictor regardless of embryo stage (AUC = 0.727, 95% CI = 0.675–0.775). By combining ts3, tEB, and t8, a model with higher discriminatory capacity for predicting top-quality embryos was proposed (29).

Finally, the most recent study on blastocyst prediction was published by Motato et al. in 2016 (30). This was a three-phase observational, retrospective, single-center clinical study in which the authors describe the events associated with blastocyst formation and implantation based on the largest sample size ever described with time-lapse monitoring.

Phase 1 consisted of embryo scoring based on a classification tree to select embryos with higher blastocyst formation probabilities. The observed correlations between morphokinetic parameters and blastocyst formation were the basis for a proposed hierarchical classification procedure to select viable embryos with a high blastocyst formation potential. A detailed retrospective analysis of cleavage times was made for 7483 zygotes. A total of 17 parameters were studied and several were significantly correlated with blastocyst formation and implantation. The most predictive parameters for blastocyst formation were time of morula formation, tM (81.28–96.0 hours after ICSI), and t8 – t5 (≤8.78 hours) or time of transition of five-blastomere embryos to eight-blastomere embryos with a receiver operating characteristic curve (ROC) value = 0.849 (95% CI = 0.835–0.854). These parameters were less predictive of implantation, with a ROC value of 0.546 (95% CI = 0.507–0.585).

Phase 2 focused on the blastocysts transferred and implantation rate. Owing to a lack of a relationship between the previously described variables and implantation potential, the authors identified new variables by comparing transferred blastocysts (n = 383) that implanted with those that did not implant (n = 449). Once again they analyzed 17 morphokinetic parameters and identified the variables time for expansion blastocyst, tEB (107.9–112.9 hours after ICSI), and t8 – t5 (5.67 hours after ICSI) as predicting blastocyst implantation, with a ROC value of 0.591 (95% CI = 0.552–0.630). Using these data, a hierarchical model representing a classification tree was proposed. The model subdivided blastocysts into four categories from A to D with higher or lower implantation rates (i.e., from 72.2% in category A to 39.7% in category D).

Phase 3 consisted of validation of the implantation model. After the conclusion of phase 2, the created model was validated on an independent data set composed of 257 embryos and 123 blastocysts with known implantation rates (known implantation data [KID] embryos), giving a ROC of 0.596 (95% CI = 0.526–0.666; $p = 0.008$).

The authors concluded that the inclusion of kinetic parameters into score evaluations could improve blastocyst selection criteria as well as predict blastocyst formation with high accuracy. In addition, the proposed models classify embryos according to their probabilities of blastocyst stage and implantation.

IMPLANTATION STUDIES

In addition to blastocyst formation, the scientific community has also correlated kinetic markers to embryo implantation as an end point (Table 18.4).

Starting in 2008, Lemmen et al. (31) retrospectively compared time-lapse recordings of a small group of embryos transferred at the four-cell stage that resulted in eight pregnancies. In this case, the authors observed that nuclei appearance in the first blastomere following the first cleavage was faster in embryos that implanted versus those that did not, and that nuclei appearance in the first two blastomeres was significantly more synchronous ($p < 0.05$).

Three years later, Meseguer et al. (1) published a study where several parameters were correlated with embryo implantation. The study was based on 247 KID embryos and it developed a hierarchical model that subdivided embryos into six categories from A to F. Four of these categories (A–D) were further subdivided into two sub-categories: (+) or (–). The hierarchical classification procedure starts with a morphological screening of all embryos in a cohort to eliminate those embryos that are clearly not viable (i.e., highly abnormal, atresia, or clearly arrested embryos). Those embryos that are clearly not viable are discarded and not considered for transfer (category F). The next step in the model is to exclude embryos that fulfill any of the three exclusion criteria: (i) uneven blastomere size at the two-cell stage; (ii) abrupt division from one to three or more cells; or (iii) multi-nucleation at the four-cell stage (category E). The subsequent levels in the model follow a strict hierarchy based on the binary timing variables t5, s2, and cc2. First, if the value of t5 falls inside the optimal range (48.8–56.6 hours), the embryo is categorized as A or B. If the value of t5 falls outside the optimal range (or if t5 has not yet been observed at 64 hours), the embryo is categorized as C or D. If the value of s2 falls inside the optimal range (≤0.76 hours), the embryo is categorized as A or C depending on t5; similarly, if the value of s2 falls outside the optimal range, the embryo is categorized as B or D depending on t5. Finally, the embryo is categorized with the extra plus (+) if the value for cc2 is inside the optimal range (≤11.9 hours; A+, B+, C+, or D+) and is categorized with a minus (–) as A–, B–, C–, or D– if the value for cc2 is outside the optimal range (Figure 18.2).

In 2012, Azzarello et al. (32) performed a prospective study transferring 159 embryos and proposed the variable "time of pronuclear breakdown" as a predictor of pregnancy. In this study, the pronuclear breakdown of embryos resulting in live births occurred significantly later than those that did not. In fact, the authors proposed the limit of 20 hours and 45 minutes and recommended to avoid transferring embryos presenting pronuclear breakdowns at earlier times.

In the same year, Hlinka et al. (20) proposed a novel method to predict implantation. The model relied on cleavage ratings of the embryos; more specifically, time-patterning of cleavage clusters and interphases were used to select the highest-quality embryos. The diagnostic relation between blastocyst implantation and cleavage success was 100% specific for all the embryos analyzed (n = 180) and all the pregnancies resulted from timely cleaved embryos.

Direct cleavage is another parameter that has been correlated with implantation. Meseguer et al. (1) initially observed this phenomenon based on 247 KID embryos. Later on, these findings were confirmed by a multicenter retrospective study performed by Rubio et al. (33). In this case, the number of embryos analyzed was much higher (n = 5225) and embryo implantation for embryos presenting direct cleavage from two to three cells (DC2–3 <5 hours) was statistically lower than for those with a normal cleavage pattern. Only 1 out of 109 embryos with DC2–3 resulted in clinical pregnancy.

The impact of extrinsic factors on embryo kinetics and their relation with implantation has been studied as well. In 2013, Freour et al. (34) focused on women who smoked, and the authors observed that embryo divisions occurred later in smokers than in non-smokers, resulting in worse outcomes for the first group. The authors analyzed 191 embryos and indicated t4 and s3 as the most relevant kinetic parameters with respect to implantation. According to the distributions of these two variables, implantation was significantly higher in the first two quartiles. Embryos were graded as A or B depending on the optimal range defined for t4 (A = inside the range and B = outside the range). In addition, embryos were given a "+" or "–" value according to the optimal range of s3 ("+" = inside the range and "–" = outside the range). The

Table 18.4 Implantation studies

	Study design	Total number of embryos	Embryo origin	Time-lapse system	Predictive marker identified/ utilized
Lemen et al. (2008)	Retrospective study	19	IVF/ICSI cycles	Nikon Diaphot 300 microscope with camera in a closed system	Nuclei appearance in the first blastomere
Meseguer et al. (2011)	Retrospective study	247	ICSI cycles	EmbryoScope	t5, s2, cc2, UN 2 cell, MN 4 cell, DC 1–3 cells
Arazello et al. (2012)	Prospective study	159	ICSI cycles	EmbryoScope	PN breakdown
Hlinka et al. (2012)	Retrospective study	114	ICSI cycles	Primovision	c2, c3 and c4; i2, i3 and i4
Rubio et al. (2012)	Multicenter retrospective study	5225 (1659 transferred)	IVF cycles from donated and autologous oocytes	EmbryoScope	DC 2–3 cells
Freour et al. (2013)	Retrospective analysis and prospectivelly collected database	191	ICSI cycles	EmbryoScope	t4 and s3
Chamayou et al. (2013)	Retrospective study	178	ICSI cycles	EmbryoScope	cc3
Kirkgaard et al. (2013a)	Prospective cohort study	84	ICSI cycles	EmbryoScope	None
Rubio et al. (2014)	Prospective randomized control trial	2638	ICSI cycles from donated oocytes	EmbryoScope	T5; s2; cc2; UN 2 cell; MN 4 cell; DC 1–3 cells
Aguilar et al. (2012)	Retrospective cohort study	1448	ICSI cycles from donated oocytes	EmbryoScope	Time to 2PB; PF; length of S-phase
Basile et al. (2014)	Retrospective multicentric study	1122	ICSI cycles from donated and autologous oocytes	EmbryoScope	Cc2, t3, t5, UN 2 cell, MN 4 cell, DC 1–3 cells
Vermilea et al. (2014)	Retrospective multicentric study	331	IVF/ICSI cycles	Eeva	P2 and P3
Freour et al. (2015)	Retrospective study	528	ICSI cycles	EmbryoScope	t5, s2, cc2, UN 2 cell, MN 4 cell, DC 1–3 cells
Dominguez et al. (2015)	Retrospective cohort study	28	ICSI cycles from donated oocytes	EmbryoScope	Cc2
Adamson et al. (2016)	Prospective concurrent cohort studyl		ICSI and IVF cycles from autologous oocytes	Eeva	P2 and P3
Goodman et al. (2016)	Prospective randomized control trial	2092	ICSI and IVF cycles from autologous oocytes	Embryoscope	Cc2, s2, t5, s3, tSB, MN, irregular division

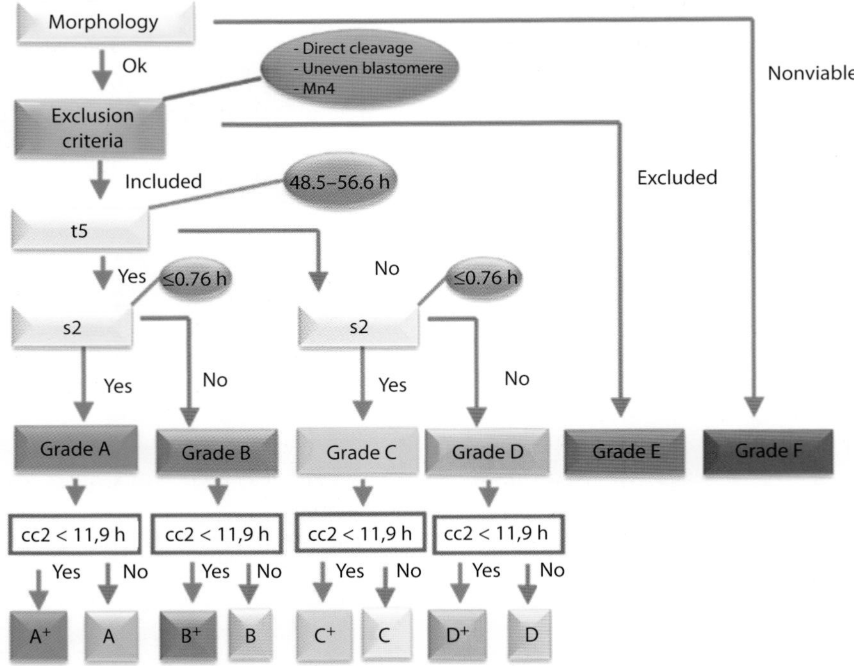

Figure 18.2 Original embryo categorization algorithm. (From Meseguer M et al. *Hum Reprod* 2011; 26: 2658–71, reproduced with permission.)

authors validated this classification model in a database including all transferred embryos, observing implantation rates of 38.7%, 33.3%, 30.7%, and 15.3% for A+, A–, B+, and B– categories, respectively. The proportions of A+ and A– embryos were higher in non-smoker patients.

Chamayou et al. (22) retrospectively compared morphokinetic parameters of 72 implanted and 106 non-implanted embryos. No differences were found for PN appearance, PN disappearance, t1, t2, t4, t7, t8, tC–tF, and s3 parameters. The authors concluded that these markers were not predictors of implantation, but that they could predict embryo development to the blastocyst stage. In this study, the only predictor marker of implantation and production of a viable pregnancy was cc3. Embryos with cc3 between 9.7 and 21 hours seemed to have the highest probability of implantation and clinical pregnancy.

As opposed to many authors, Kirkegaard et al. (23) showed no differences in the timings of cellular division or embryonic stage between implanted and non-implanted embryos. The study was based on the observation of 84 SETs. The author identified the duration of first cytokinesis, duration of the three-cell stage, and direct cleavage to three cells as predictors of high-quality embryo development but not of implantation or pregnancy. Therefore, this group concluded that a universal algorithm for optimal timing might not be feasible.

Validation of Meseguer et al.'s algorithm from 2001 (1) came along with a triple-blind randomized prospective controlled trial published by Rubio et al. (35). In this study, 405 patients were included in the control group in which embryos were selected based purely on morphology and 438 patients were included in the study group in which embryos were selected based on the algorithm. Implantation rates were significantly higher in the study group (44.9%; 95% CI = 41.4%–48.4%) versus the control group (37.1%; 95% CI = 33.6%–40.7%). In addition, the ongoing pregnancy rate was also higher in the study group versus the control group (54.5%; 95% CI = 49.6%–59.2% vs. 45.3%; 95% CI = 40.3%–50.4%). The authors concluded that morphokinetic variables allow us to reject embryos with lower implantation probabilities while distinguishing those with higher implantation probabilities. Selecting embryos through kinetic markers may therefore improve reproductive outcomes (35).

A second randomized control trial published by a different group reached similar results, although they were not able to achieve statistical significance (36). As opposed to Rubio et al.'s study (35), in which both study groups had different culture conditions (standard incubator vs. EmbryoScope), one of the strengths of this study was that it was the first one to evaluate all embryos cultured within identical culture conditions and to demonstrate whether the addition of continuously monitored morphokinetic parameters improved clinical outcomes compared with conventional once-daily morphologic assessment. The study anticipated a 10% increase and although it did not reach statistical significance, there were increased clinical pregnancy and implantation rates with the use of the additional parameters. In addition, the time of the start of blastulation, the absence of multinucleation, and the use of a score based on morphology and kinetics were significant predictors of implantation. The authors concluded that in this dynamic and evolving field, larger studies were needed to confirm their findings.

In 2014, Aguilar et al. (37) studied the human's first cell cycle and its impact on implantation based on morphokinetics. To this aim, the authors conducted a retrospective analysis of 1448 transferred embryos and compared the timings of second polar extrusion, first and second pronuclear appearance, pronuclear abuttal, pronuclear fading, and length of S-phase between implanted and non-implanted embryos. The time ranges successfully linked to implantation were 3.3–10.6 hours for second polar body extrusion, 22.2–25.9 hours for pronuclear fading, and 5.7–13.8 hours for the length of S-phase.

In 2015, Basile et al. (38) continued the study by Meseguer et al. (1) and published an improved version of the algorithm by studying a larger data set of embryos from four different IVF clinics. To that aim, a sequential approach was adopted by the authors. During phase 1 of the study, an algorithm was developed taking into consideration morphokinetic data of 754 KID embryos that were selected for transfer based only on conventional morphological criteria. The new algorithm included the variables t3, cc2, and t5 in combination with morphology and exclusion criteria (direct cleavage [DC], uneven blastomere [UBS], and multinucleation at day 4 [MN]) and classified embryos from A to E according to their implantation potential (Figure 18.3). Subsequently, during phase 2 of the study, the predictive ability of this new algorithm was tested by applying it to embryo classification in a different group of IVF patients (885 cycles). Considering only cycles with known implantation (100% or 0% implantation, n = 1137), a significant decrease in implantation rate (IR) was observed as embryo categories decreased from A to E. More specifically: A = 32%, B = 28%, C = 26.25%, D = 20.19%, and E = 17% ($p < 0.001$).

Another study by VerMilyea et al. (39) established the relationship between implantation and three embryo categories derived from a computer-automated TMS. The system classified embryos into the categories high, medium, or low based on the variables P2 and P3. According to this multicenter study (205 patients), implantation rates were significantly linked to the three categories; more specifically: 37%, 35%, and 15% for high, medium, and low, respectively. In addition, the clinical pregnancy rate for patients that had one or more "high" transferred embryos was significantly higher (51% vs. 34%; $p = 0.02$).

A most recent study published by Adamson et al. in 2016 (40) tested the same technology in a prospective way. The aim of the study was to prove if an automatic time-lapse test (TL-test) combined with traditional morphology improves day-3 implantation rates compared with morphology alone. Two concurrently collected groups of patients were compared: those who received a day-3 transfer with the use of the TL-test together with morphology (test group); and those who received a day-3 transfer with the use of morphology alone (control group). To further assess the impact of the automated TL-test score, the authors evaluated the implantation potential of embryos assigned by the TL-test as categories TL-high versus TL-low among all transferred embryos (TL-high: duration of two-cell stage within 9.33–11.45 hours and duration of three-cell stage within 0–1.73 hours; TL-low: outside the TL-high ranges) and among those with only good morphology. Analysis of the study's primary end point—implantation rate—showed a significantly higher implantation rate for day-3 transfer among the test group (30.2%, 58/192) than the control group (19.0%, 84/442;

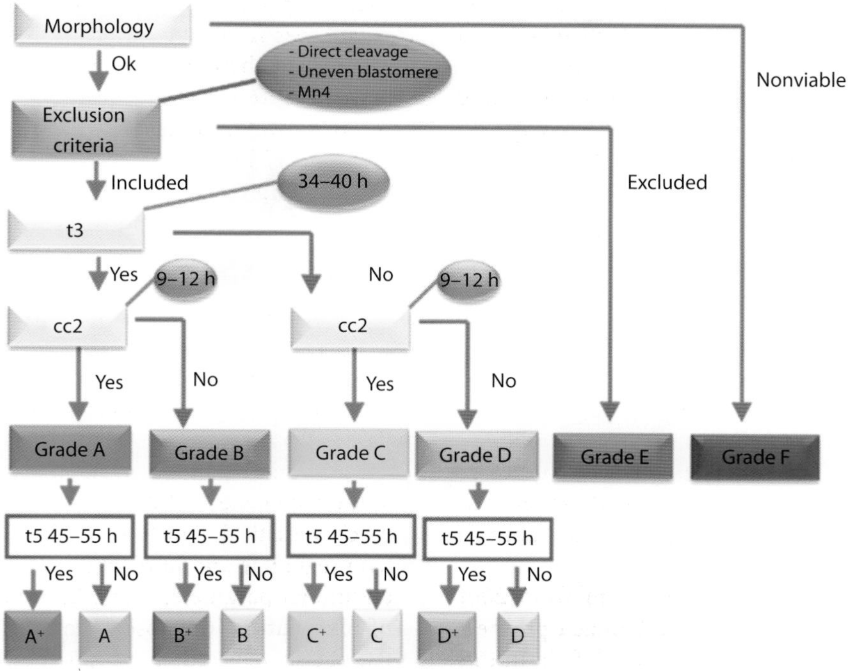

Figure 18.3 Revised embryo categorization algorithm. (From Basile N, Caiazzo M, Meseguer M. *Curr Opin Obstet Gynecol* 2015; 27: 193–200, reproduced with permission.)

p = 0.003). The clinical pregnancy rate was also significantly higher among the test group (46.0%, 45/98) than the control group (32.1%, 71/ 221; p = 0.02). Within the test group, patients receiving at least one TL-high embryo had significantly higher implantation rates than patients receiving only TL-low embryos (36.8% vs. 20.6%). TL-high compared with TL-low embryos had significantly higher implantation rates (44.7% vs. 20.5%). Among morphologically good embryos, TL-high embryos were more likely to implant than TL-low embryos (44.1% vs. 20.6%). The authors concluded that the noninvasive TL-test adds valuable information to traditional morphologic grading and that it should be used to increase clinicians' confidence in recommending elective SET with day-3 transfer, and that we would expect higher implantation rates and higher clinical pregnancy rates, as well as reduced multiple pregnancy rates, compared with patients with embryos not assessed by the TL-test.

Limitations on the external performance and the universal use of published algorithms have been addressed (41). In a study published by Freour et al. (34), an external validation of Meseguer et al.'s algorithm (1) was performed in an unselected patient population. The model was applied showing a heterogeneous distribution of implantation rates in the resultant categories. In addition, correlation coefficients were significantly lower than the ones in the originally study. However, a simplified version of the model (in which only the two main morphokinetic variables—t5 and s2—were consider and not cc2) performed acceptably. The authors explained that the differences could be the result of variations in oxygen culture conditions, oocyte source (donor cycles vs. autologous cycles), restrictions in the studied population, and/or the stimulation protocols used. The conclusion was that a hierarchical prediction model should not be used universally in an unselected population; it should be center specific.

The combination of technologies may be the key to improving results in the future. Dominguez et al. (42) combined proteomics and time-lapse analysis of implanted (n = 16) and non-implanted (n = 12) embryos. After logistic regression analysis, the model identified the presence or absence of protein interleukin-6 and the duration of cc2 as the most relevant embryo features. Based on these results, the authors developed a hierarchical model (Figure 18.4) based on these two variables, classifying embryos into four categories of A–D. Implantation rates are expected to decrease as we move on from A to D as observed in this study (A = 88.8%, B = 66.6%, C = 57%, and D = 33%) (40).

ANEUPLOIDY STUDIES

The correlation between euploidy and embryo kinetics has been studied as well (Table 18.5).

In 2010, Wong et al. (18) collected single embryos for gene expression analysis and revealed that embryos with P1, P2, and P3 outside of the optimal ranges exhibited abnormal RNA patterns for embryo cytokinesis, microRNA biogenesis, and maternal mRNA reserve, suggesting that embryo fate may be predetermined and inherited very early in development (by the four-cell stage).

Chavez et al. (43) subsequently observed that euploid embryos clustered tightly in the P1, P2, or P3 window, which was predictive of blastocyst formation according to Wong et al.'s study (18). Performing further molecular analysis, the authors discovered that fragmentation dynamics, together with P1, P2, and P3, could potentially distinguish euploid from aneuploid embryos at the four-cell stage, considering that the fragments contained

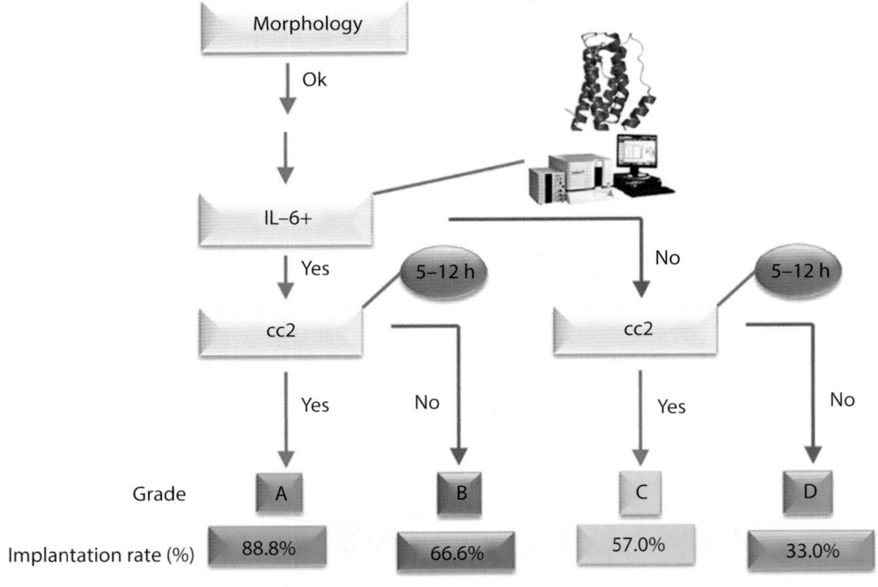

Figure 18.4 Combined embryo categorization algorithm. (From Dominguez F et al. *Fertil Steril* 2015; 104: 908–14, reproduced with permission.)

Table 18.5 Studies correlating euploidy and embryo kinetics

Author	Study design	N	TL system	Biopsy day	PDG technology	Parameters with significantly differences founded
Chavez (2012)	Prospective observational	75	Custom-built microscope	D3	aCGH	P1, P2, P3 and fragmentation
Campbell (2013a)	Retrospective cohort	98	Embryoscope	D5	aCGh/SNP array	tSB and tB
Basile (2014)	Retrospective cohort	504	Embryoscope	D3	aCGH	t5 – t2 and cc3
Rienzi (2015)	Longitudinal cohort	455	Embryoscope	D5	CCS	None
Chawla (2015)	Retrospective cohort	460	Embryoscope	D3	aCGH	tPNf, t2, t5, cc2, cc3, t5 – t2
Vera-Rodriguez (2015)	Prospective observational	85	Eeva	D3	aCGH	Time between PN disappearance and the start of 1st cytokinesis; 3 to 4 cell

nuclear DNA, kinetochore proteins, and whole chromosomes as detected by fluorescence *in situ* hybridization.

In 2013, Campbell et al. (44) elaborated an aneuploidy risk model based on the differences of tSB and tB between euploid and aneuploid embryos that had undergone TE biopsy. The model included three categories: low risk, tB <122.9 hpi and tSB <96.2 hpi; medium risk, tB <122.9 hpi and tSB 96.2 hpi; and high risk, tB 122.9 hpi (34). The same group in a different study (45) applied this model to evaluate its effectiveness and potential clinical impact for unselected IVF patients without undergoing preimplantation genetic screening after analyzing KID embryos. The study revealed significant differences in fetal heart rate (72.7, 25.5, and 0 beats per minute) and live birth rate (61.1%, 19.2%, and 0%) between the three categories low, medium, and high, respectively. This demonstrates that time-lapse imaging using defined morphokinetic data classify human preimplantation embryos according to their risk of aneuploidy without performing biopsy and preimplantation genetic screening, and that this correlates well with clinical outcomes.

In the following year, Basile et al. (46) also correlated morphokinetics with embryo aneuploidy based on 77 patients undergoing genetic screening due to recurrent miscarriage or implantation failure. In this case, embryo biopsy was performed on day 3 of development and the total number of embryos analyzed was 504. A logistic regression analysis was used to select and organize which observed timing events (expressed as binary variables inside or outside the optimal range) were most relevant to selecting embryos with higher probabilities of being chromosomally normal. The model identified t5 – t2 (odds ratio [OR] = 2.853, 95% CI = 1.763–4.616) followed by cc3 (OR = 2.095, 95% CI = 1.356–3.238) as the most relevant variables related to normal chromosomal content. An algorithm for embryo selection based on these two variables classified embryos from A to D (Figure 18.5)

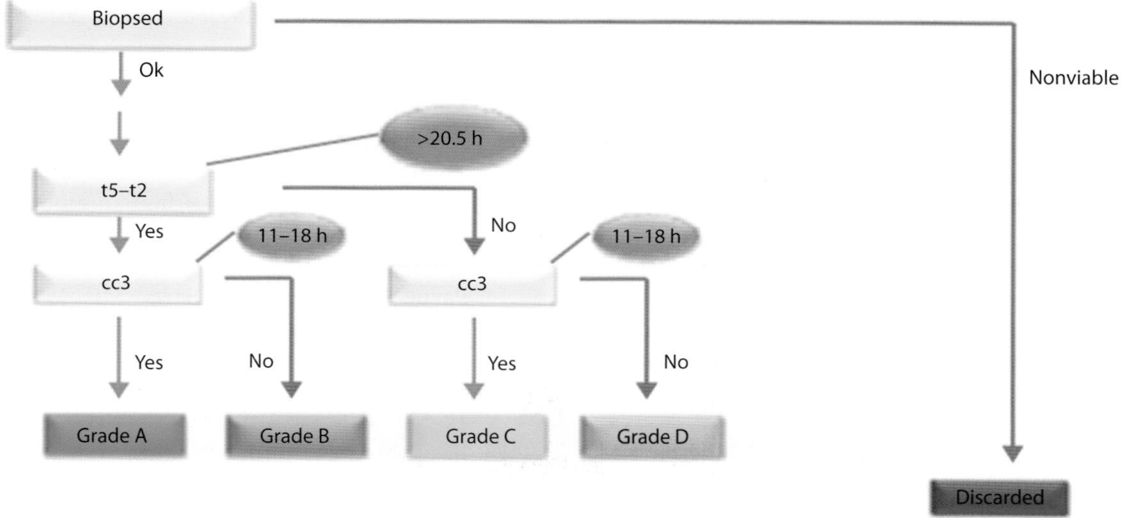

Figure 18.5 Embryo selection algorithm. (From Basile N et al. *Fertil Steril* 2014; 101: 699–704, reproduced with permission.)

with significant differences in the percentages of normal embryos as we move on from A to D. More specifically, A = 35.9%, B = 26.4%, C = 12.1%, and D = 9.8% ($p < 0.001$).

As opposed to the previous studies, Rienzi et al. (47) reported no correlation at all between 16 commonly detected morphokinetic parameters and embryo ploidy. This was a longitudinal cohort study conducted using 455 blastocysts from 138 patients at increased risk of aneuploidy because of advance maternal age, history of unsuccessful IVF treatments, or both. The analyzed parameters included t2, t3, t4, t5, t8, ccl, cc2, s2, s3, cc3, cc3/cc2, t5-t2, syngamy, tSB, tSC, and tB.

Finally, in 2015, two studies observed correlations between embryo kinetics and euploidy. The first one, reported by Chawla et al. (48), identified tPNf, t2, t5, cc2, cc3, and t5 – t2 as parameters that significantly differed between chromosomally normal and abnormal embryos. The second one by Vera-Rodriguez et al. (49) combined chromosomal assessment and single-cell quantitative reverse transcription polymerase chain reaction (RT-qPCR) to simultaneously obtain information from all the blastomeres of human embryos until approximately the eight-cell stage ($n = 85$). According to their results, the chromosomal status of aneuploid embryos ($n = 26$) correlates with significant differences in the duration of the first mitotic phase when compared with euploid embryos ($n = 28$). Moreover, gene expression profiling in this study suggested that a subset of genes is differentially expressed in aneuploid embryos during the first 30 hours of development.

CONCLUSION

Static observations obtained from standard microscopes have contributed significantly to our knowledge of embryo development; however, it is becoming more challenging to identify embryos with the highest implantation potential due to the static and notoriously subjective character of this type of morphological evaluation. The study of embryo kinetics through time-lapse technology has given rise to new markers for embryo selection, representing a new and excitingly powerful tool for viewing cellular activity and embryogenesis in a coherent and uninterrupted manner that is otherwise not available through standard microscopy. The current chapter presents an overview of the most recent studies that describe the use of this new technology in the IVF laboratory. It is our opinion that standard morphological assessment should remain the gold standard when initiating embryo evaluation; however, if possible, it should be complemented with the detection of kinetic markers known to improve clinical results. This new approach will allow the embryologist to perform a more accurate and objective embryo selection, and therefore the goal of SET slowly becomes more tangible.

REFERENCES

1. Meseguer M, Herrero J, Tejera A, Hilligsoe KM, Ramsing NB, Remohi J. The use of morphokinetics as a predictor of embryo implantation. *Hum Reprod* 2011; 26: 2658–71.
2. Mio Y, Maeda K. Time-lapse cinematography of dynamic changes occurring during *in vitro* development of human embryos. *Am J Obstet Gynecol* 2008; 199: 660.e1–5.
3. Gardner DK, Meseguer M, Rubio C, Treff NR. Diagnosis of human preimplantation embryo viability. *Hum Reprod Update* 2015; 21: 727–47.
4. Alpha Scientists in Reproductive Medicine and ESHRE Special Interest Group of Embryology. The Istanbul consensus workshop on embryo assessment: Proceedings of an expert meeting. *Hum Reprod* 2011; 26: 1270–83.
5. Baxter B, Allison E. Interobserver and intraobserver variation in day 3 embryo grading. *Fertil Steril* 2006; 86: 1608–15.
6. Kaser DJ, Racowsky C. Clinical outcomes following selection of human preimplantation embryos with time-lapse monitoring: A systematic review. *Hum Reprod Update* 2014; 20: 617–31.
7. Paternot G, Wetzels A, Thonon F et al. Intra- and interobserver analysis in the morphological assessment of early stage embryos during an IVF procedure: A multicentre study. *Reprod Biol Endocrinol* 2011; 9: 127.
8. Sundvall L, Ingerslev HJ, Breth Knudsen U, Kirkegaard K. Inter- and intra-observer variability of time-lapse annotations. *Hum Reprod* 2013; 28: 3215–21.
9. Arce JC, Ziebe S, Lundin K, Janssens R, Helmgaard L, Sorensen P. Interobserver agreement and intraobserver reproducibility of embryo quality assessments. *Hum Reprod* 2006; 21: 2141–8.
10. Scott L. The biological basis of non-invasive strategies for selection of human oocytes and embryos. *Hum Reprod Update* 2003; 9: 237–49.
11. Meseguer M, Rubio I, Cruz M, Basile N, Marcos J, Requena A. Embryo incubation and selection in a time-lapse monitoring system improves pregnancy outcome compared with a standard incubator: A retrospective cohort study. *Fertil Steril* 2012; 98: 1481–9. e10.
12. Kirkegaard K, Ahlstrom A, Ingerslev HJ, Hardarson T. Choosing the best embryo by time lapse versus standard morphology. *Fertil Steril* 2015; 103: 323–32.
13. Zhang JQ, Li XL, Peng Y, Guo X, Heng BC, Tong GQ. Reduction in exposure of human embryos outside the incubator enhances embryo quality and blastulation rate. *Reprod Biomed Online* 2010; 20: 510–15.
14. Payne D, Flaherty SP, Barry MF, Matthews CD. Preliminary observations on polar body extrusion and pronuclear formation in human oocytes using time-lapse video cinematography. *Hum Reprod* 1997; 12: 532–41.
15. Basile N, Caiazzo M, Meseguer M. What does morphokinetics add to embryo selection and *in-vitro* fertilization outcomes? *Curr Opin Obstet Gynecol* 2015; 27(3): 193–200.

16. Herrero J, Meseguer M. Selection of high potential embryos using time-lapse imaging: The era of morphokinetics. *Fertil Steril* 2013; 99: 1030–34.
17. Ciray HN, Campbell A, Agerholm IE et al. Proposed guidelines on the nomenclature and annotation of dynamic human embryo monitoring by a time-lapse user group. *Hum Reprod* 2014; 29: 2650–60.
18. Wong CC, Loewke KE, Bossert NL et al. Non-invasive imaging of human embryos before embryonic genome activation predicts development to the blastocyst stage. *Nat Biotechnol* 2010; 28: 1115–21.
19. Hashimoto S, Kato N, Saeki K, Morimoto Y. Selection of high-potential embryos by culture in poly(dimethylsiloxane) microwells and time-lapse imaging. *Fertil Steril* 2012; 97: 332–7.
20. Hlinka D, Kalatova B, Uhrinova I et al. Time-lapse cleavage rating predicts human embryo viability. *Physiol Res* 2012; 61: 513–25.
21. Cruz M, Garrido N, Herrero J, Perez-Cano I, Munoz M, Meseguer M. Timing of cell division in human cleavage-stage embryos is linked with blastocyst formation and quality. *Reprod Biomed Online* 2012; 25: 371–81.
22. Chamayou S, Patrizio P, Storaci G et al. The use of morphokinetic parameters to select all embryos with full capacity to implant. *J Assist Reprod Genet* 2013; 30: 703–10.
23. Kirkegaard K, Kesmodel US, Hindkjaer JJ, Ingerslev HJ. Time-lapse parameters as predictors of blastocyst development and pregnancy outcome in embryos from good prognosis patients: A prospective cohort study. *Hum Reprod* 2013; 28: 2643–51.
24. Conaghan J, Chen AA, William SP et al. Improving embryo selection using a computer-automated time-lapse image analysis test plus day 3 morphology: Results from a prospective multicenter trial. *Fertil Steril* 2013; 100: 412–9.e5.
25. Kirkegaard K, Campbell A, Agerholm I et al. Limitations of a time-lapse blastocyst prediction model: A large multicentre outcome analysis. *Reprod Biomed Online* 2014; 29: 156–8.
26. Cetinkaya M, Pirkevi C, Yelke H, Colakoglu YK, Atayurt Z, Kahraman S. Relative kinetic expressions defining cleavage synchronicity are better predictors of blastocyst formation and quality than absolute time points. *J Assist Reprod Genet* 2015; 32: 27–35.
27. Yang S, Shi J, Gong J et al. Cleavage pattern predicts developmental potential of day 3 human embryos produced by IVF. *Reprod Biomed Online* 2015; 30: 625–34.
28. Milewski R, Kuc P, Kuczynska A, Stankiewicz B, Lukaszuk K, Kuczynski W. A predictive model for blastocyst formation based on morphokinetic parameters in time-lapse monitoring of embryo development. *J Assist Reprod Genet* 2015; 32: 571–79.
29. Storr A, Venetis CA, Cooke S, Susetio D, Kilani S, Ledger W. Morphokinetic parameters using time-lapse technology and day 5 embryo quality: A prospective cohort study. *J Assist Reprod Genet* 2015; 32: 1151–60.
30. Motato Y, de Los Santos MJ, Escriba MJ, Ruiz BA, Remohí J, Meseguer M. Morphokinetic analysis and embryonic prediction for blastocyst formation through an integrated time-lapse system. *Fertil Steril* 2016 ; 105: 376–84.
31. Lemmen JG, Agerholm I, Ziebe S. Kinetic markers of human embryo quality using time-lapse recordings of IVF/ICSI-fertilized oocytes. *Reprod Biomed Online* 2008; 17: 385–91.
32. Azzarello A, Hoest T, Mikkelsen AL. The impact of pronuclei morphology and dynamicity on live birth outcome after time-lapse culture. *Hum Reprod* 2012; 27: 2649–57.
33. Rubio I, Kuhlmann R, Agerholm I et al. Limited implantation success of direct-cleaved human zygotes: A time-lapse study. *Fertil Steril* 2012; 98: 1458–63.
34. Freour T, Dessolle L, Lammers J, Lattes S, Barriere P. Comparison of embryo morphokinetics after *in vitro* fertilization–intracytoplasmic sperm injection in smoking and nonsmoking women. *Fertil Steril* 2013; 99: 1944–50.
35. Rubio I, Galan A, Larreategui Z et al. Clinical validation of embryo culture and selection by morphokinetic analysis: A randomized, controlled trial of the EmbryoScope. *Fertil Steril* 2014; 102: 1287–94.e5.
36. Goodman LR, Goldberg J, Falcone T, Austin C, Desai N. Does the addition of time-lapse morphokinetics in the selection of embryos for transfer improve pregnancy rates? A randomized controlled trial. *Fertil Steril* 2016; 105: 275–85.
37. Aguilar J, Motato Y, Escriba MJ, Ojeda M, Munoz E, Meseguer M. The human first cell cycle: Impact on implantation. *Reprod Biomed Online* 2014; 28: 475–84.
38. Basile N, Vime P, Florensa M et al. The use of morphokinetics as a predictor of implantation: A multicentric study to define and validate an algorithm for embryo selection. *Hum Reprod* 2015; 30: 276–83.
39. VerMilyea MD, Tan L, Anthony JT et al. Computer-automated time-lapse analysis results correlate with embryo implantation and clinical pregnancy: A blinded, multi-centre study. *Reprod Biomed Online* 2014; 29: 729–36.
40. Adamson GD, Abusief ME, Palao L, Witmer J, Palao LM, Gvakharia M. Improved implantation rates of day 3 embryo transfers with the use of an automated time-lapse-enabled test to aid in embryo selection. *Fertil Steril* 2016; 105: 369–75.
41. Kirkegaard K. Choosing the best embryo by time lapse versus standard morphology. *Fertil Steril* 2014; 103: 323–32.

42. Dominguez F, Meseguer M, Aparicio-Ruiz B, Piqueras P, Quinonero A, Simon C. New strategy for diagnosing embryo implantation potential by combining proteomics and time-lapse technologies. *Fertil Steril* 2015; 104: 908–14.
43. Chavez SL, Loewke KE, Han J et al. Dynamic blastomere behavior reflects human embryo ploidy by the four-cell stage. *Nat Commun* 2012; 3: 1251.
44. Campbell A, Fishel S, Bowman N, Duffy S, Sedler M, Hickman CF. Modelling a risk classification of aneuploidy in human embryos using non-invasive morphokinetics. *Reprod Biomed Online* 2013; 26: 477–85.
45. Campbell A, Fishel S, Bowman N, Duffy S, Sedler M, Thornton S. Retrospective analysis of outcomes after IVF using an aneuploidy risk model derived from time-lapse imaging without PGS. *Reprod Biomed Online* 2013; 27: 140–6.
46. Basile N, Nogales Mdel C, Bronet F et al. Increasing the probability of selecting chromosomally normal embryos by time-lapse morphokinetics analysis. *Fertil Steril* 2014; 101: 699–704.
47. Rienzi L, Capalbo A, Stoppa M et al. No evidence of association between blastocyst aneuploidy and morphokinetic assessment in a selected population of poor-prognosis patients: A longitudinal cohort study. *Reprod Biomed Online* 2015; 30: 57–66.
48. Chawla M, Fakih M, Shunnar A et al. Morphokinetic analysis of cleavage stage embryos and its relationship to aneuploidy in a retrospective time-lapse imaging study. *J Assist Reprod Genet* 2015; 32: 69–75.
49. Vera-Rodriguez M, Chavez SL, Rubio C, Reijo Pera RA, Simon C. Prediction model for aneuploidy in early human embryo development revealed by single-cell analysis. *Nat Commun* 2015; 6: 7601.

Evaluation of embryo quality 19

Proteomic strategies

MANDY KATZ-JAFFE

INTRODUCTION

Unlike the human genome that is relatively fixed and steady throughout the human body, the human proteome (protein complement to the genome) is by several orders of magnitude more complex, diverse, and dynamic. Any single gene can produce a heterogeneous population of proteins that can be further modified by post-translational modifications such as phosphorylation. The result is a human proteome estimated at considerably over a million proteins to only ~25,000 human genes (1). Several studies have indicated that the genome's transcriptome (mRNA expression levels) does not necessarily predict the abundance or functional activity of proteins (2,3). Rather, it is the human proteome that significantly contributes to physiological homeostasis in any cell or tissue (4). Various biological conditions including age, gender, diet, lifestyle, medication, and disease, among others, directly impact the composition of the human proteome in any particular cell or tissue, generating a unique proteomic signature (5). The characterization of protein signatures during embryonic development has the potential to address a variety of unresolved topics, with the ultimate goal of expanding our knowledge of embryonic cellular processes and the evolution of viability assays.

Relatively little is known regarding the proteome of the human preimplantation embryo, particularly the protein production of the blastocyst just prior to implantation. The task begins with identifying the proteins expressed, including those proteins changing in response to internal and external stimuli. These individual proteins can then be quantified and characterized, at the same time examining their interactions during embryonic development. In order to elucidate embryonic cellular architecture and function, a detailed understanding of the complexity at the protein level is essential. Of particular interest is the cell surface proteome, as it may pinpoint key molecules associated with implantation including cell surface receptors as well as the protein–protein interactions occurring between the developing embryo and the surrounding maternal environment (6).

The preimplantation embryonic stage represents the most difficult challenge due to the combined effect of limited numbers of cells and minimal protein expression, resulting in extremely low levels of total protein available for analysis—only 27 ng of protein in a single mouse embryo (7).

THE EMBRYONIC PROTEOME

Two-dimensional polyacrylamide gel electrophoresis (2D-PAGE) is at present the standard technique for separation of total protein. This technology separates proteins in the horizontal dimension by isoelectric focusing (a pH gradient range of typically 3–10) and in the vertical dimension by molecular weight in a polyacrylamide gel gradient (8). 2D-PAGE is efficient at differential protein quantitation and detecting post-translational modifications with starting amounts of total protein isolated from typically 10^6 cells. Limitations to this technology include a long processing time, weak detection of low-concentration proteins, and the inability to capture or resolve very acidic or basic proteins, membrane proteins, as well as very small- or large-molecular-weight proteins (8).

Protein databases involving 2D-PAGE that represent the entire mouse preimplantation period from fertilization to the blastocyst stage have been constructed to provide a means of studying protein synthesis and characterizing protein changes (9,10). 2D-PAGE was performed through the analysis of radiolabeled proteins after embryos were exposed to one to three hours of incubation in a high concentration of radiolabeled amino acids. After protein resolution, spots were detected by fluorography and a software program assembled the images into protein databases (9). Comparison of the proteins between the eight-cell mouse embryo and the fully expanded mouse blastocyst database identified a total of 43 spots, approximately 3% of all total spots, which were only detected at the eight-cell stage, and 75 spots identified solely at the blastocyst stage (10).

2D-PAGE use in the field of embryology has been limited due to the requirement for larger amounts of starting template as well as the lack of robustness and degree of labor intensity. Consequently, protein-based studies have concentrated on identifying and localizing individual proteins by western blot analysis. Two insulin-responsive glucose transporter isoforms (GLUT4 and GLUT8) and the insulin receptor proteins were confirmed by western blot analysis as being present in rabbit blastocysts (11). Another study observed the expression of stress-activated protein kinase/Jun kinase (SAPK/JNK) phosphoproteins and p38 mitogen-activated protein kinases (MAPKs) by western blotting from groups of over 100 mouse embryos (12). A limitation of this approach is that proteins do not function individually, but within pathways, thus the analysis of the embryonic proteome as a whole is critical.

Mass spectrometry (MS) has rapidly become the key technology in proteomics, allowing for rapid identification and quantitation of proteins, including low-expression proteins. An array of templates can be applied, including tissues, cells, and biological fluids. MS involves an ion source for the production of charged species in the gas phase and the analyzer, which separates ions by their mass-to-charge (m/z) ratio. The commonly used ionization methods include electrospray ionization, matrix-assisted laser desorption/ionization (MALDI), and surface-enhanced laser desorption/ionization (SELDI) and are most commonly coupled to time-of-flight (TOF), ion trap, or quadrupole analyzers. Post-translational modifications are also identifiable since the modification will change the m/z ratio of a protein. Protein identification can then be performed by protease digestion to generate specific fragments from well-characterized cleavage products. These fragments are identifiable following tandem MS (MS/MS) analysis and protein database searching (13).

A comprehensive proteomics approach has been applied to study the mammalian oocyte; however, in these studies, the starting template is still considerable. In one study, approximately 200 porcine oocytes were used to separate and visualize proteins of interest by 2D-PAGE, with an even larger starting template used for peptide profiling by MALDI-TOF MS and peptide sequencing by liquid chromatography (LC)–MS/MS (14). More recently, Vitale et al. (15) used 2D-PAGE and MS to identify differentially expressed proteins during murine oocyte maturation. Five hundred germinal vesicle (GV) and metaphase II (MII) oocytes were extracted and resolved on 2D gels stained with silver. A total of 12 proteins were observed to be differentially expressed between the GV and MII stages. These proteins were then characterized by MS with the identification of nucleoplasmin 2 (Npm2), an oocyte-restricted protein (15). Another study investigated mature mouse cumulus–oocyte complexes, identifying 156 individual proteins following 2D-PAGE and MS. Several protein families were discovered that may play important roles in ovarian follicular development (16).

With further advances in proteomic technologies, the identification and quantitation of very small quantities of proteins has become more of a reality. SELDI-TOF MS involves the application of small sample volumes (in the microliter range) and enables detection of both the low- and higher-molecular-weight proteins, with the optimal range for the technology being at <20 kDa. The sensitivity is stated to be in the picomole to femtomole range, making proteomic profiling of diverse and limited biological samples possible. This technology is also capable of studying samples based on activated surfaces for pre-selection including hydrophobic interaction, anion or cation exchange, and metal affinity capture (17). Bound proteins are laser activated, thereby liberating gaseous ions by desorption/ionization. The TOF tube is under a vacuum, which causes smaller ions to travel faster towards the detector, thereby allowing for separation of these ions according to the mass-to-charge ratio (m/z). The technology has been applied to a variety of biological sources including serum (18) and cell lysates (19), with specific focus on oncoproteomics and the early detection, metastatic ability, and therapeutic outcome of an assortment of different cancers through associated biomarkers (20). Biomarkers can be defined as candidate proteins or peptides that are either down- or up-regulated in response to different physiological states. Pregnancy-related problems have also been the subject of SELDI-TOF MS studies searching for early detection of conditions including ectopic pregnancy (21) and neonatal sepsis (22). Some concerns regarding this technology involve the dynamic and sensitive nature of the proteome to variables during sample collection, handling, processing, and storage as well as peaks prejudiced by MS calibration and instrument drift (23).

The development of a zeptoproteomics approach using SELDI-TOF MS has led to the characterization of protein profiles representing individual murine and human embryos across all stages of preimplantation development (24,25). Due to the multifactorial nature of mammalian embryonic development, panels of proteins specific to each of the individual stages were successfully identified, allowing for the possibility of utilizing these panels to accurately gauge the level of perturbation of a biological system and effectively diagnose developmental competence (Figure 19.1) (24). The individual human embryonic proteome demonstrated that human blastocysts with similar morphologies do not typically have identical protein signatures (25). These data are consistent with the observations that human blastocysts from the same patient with similar morphologies vary greatly in their metabolic fingerprint (26). Furthermore, specific blastocyst developmental stages displayed differential protein expression profiles, as shown by the significant up- and down-regulation of biomarkers in expanded blastocysts compared to early blastocysts (25). Taken as a whole, human blastocyst morphology could be recognized according to specific individual protein signatures with significant differences in protein expression related to specific blastocyst developmental time points and/or degeneration (Figure 19.2) (25). A panel of upregulated biomarkers distinguished arrested embryos from developing blastocysts (Figure 19.3). Candidate identification implicated both apoptotic and growth-inhibiting pathways (25). It is also probable that some of these differential proteins or peptides are secreted by the embryo, reflecting a signature of developmental competence.

THE EMBRYONIC SECRETOME

With the knowledge that blastocyst morphology could be recognized according to specific protein expression (25), it is proposed that developmentally viable embryos will also possess a unique proteome profile, with some of these expressed proteins secreted into the surrounding environment (secretome). Analysis of the embryonic proteome, as described in the above section, represents a destructive approach. On the other hand, analysis of the embryonic secretome is a noninvasive method suitable for clinical application.

Currently, the selection of embryos for transfer is based on morphological indices (27). Though successful, the field of assisted reproduction technology would benefit from more quantitative and noninvasive methods of

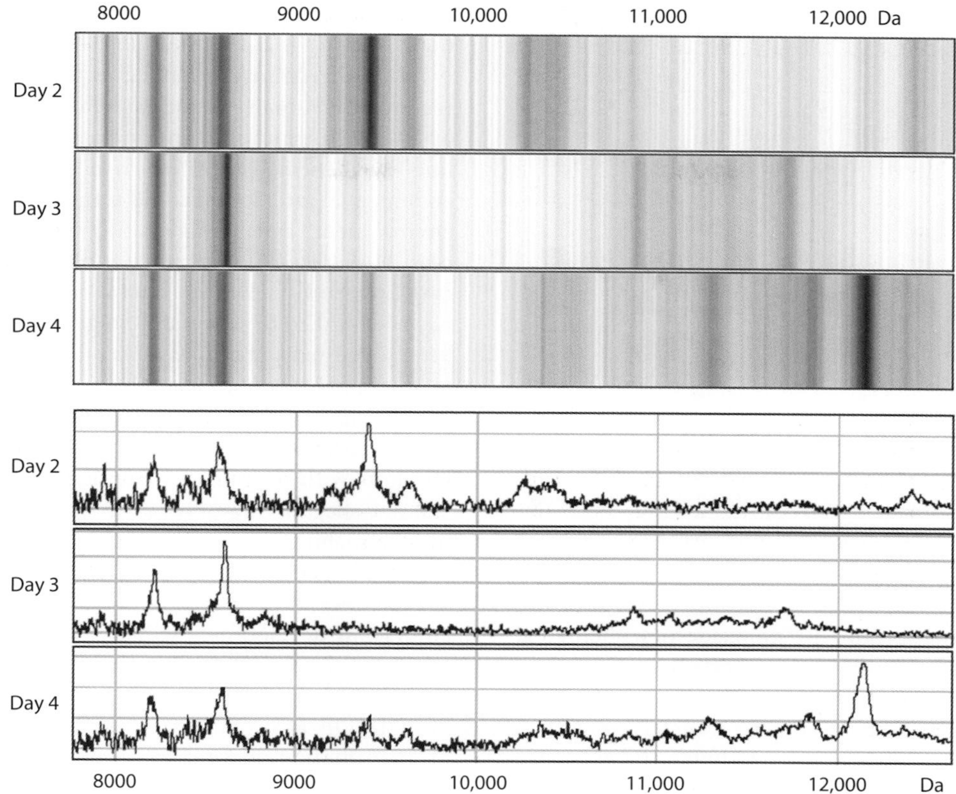

Figure 19.1 Protein profiling signatures across preimplantation embryonic development in the m/z range of 8000–12,000 Da. (Data are shown as the original spectra and gel view; Katz-Jaffe MG et al. *Reproduction* 2005; 130: 899–905.)

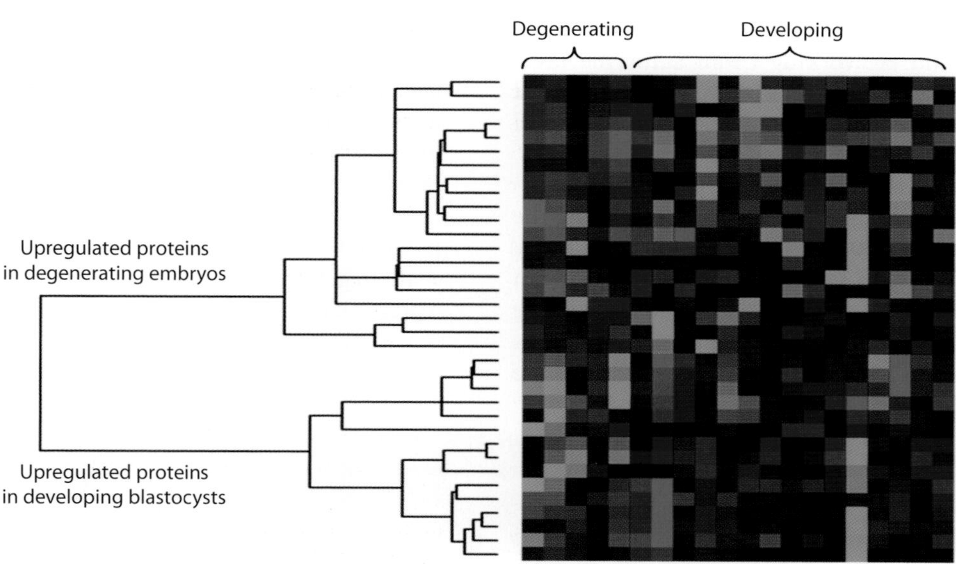

Figure 19.2 A heat map segregating developing human blastocysts and degenerate human embryos according to protein signatures. Each column of squares represents an individual human embryo, while each row of squares represents an individual protein profile. Clustering analysis facilitates the grouping of similar protein expression profiles. Two major clusters were classified as shown on the left of the heat map. The top cluster identifies proteins that are up-regulated (red) in degenerating embryos, while the bottom cluster identifies proteins that are up-regulated (red) in developing blastocysts. Red = up-regulated proteins; green = down-regulated proteins. (Adapted from Katz-Jaffe MG et al. *Fertil Steril* 2006; 85: 101–7.)

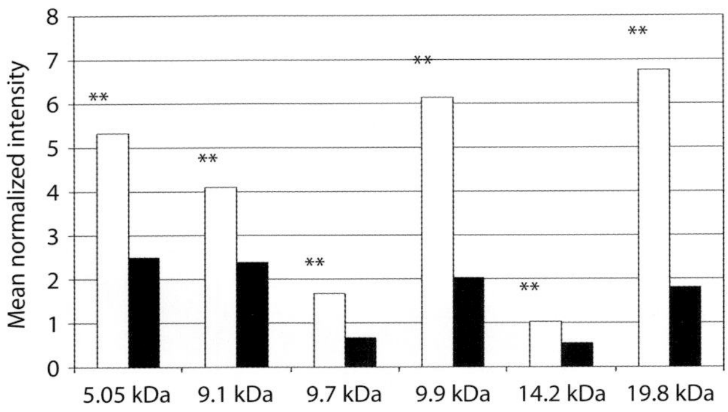

Figure 19.3 Negatively charged proteins showing significant differential expression related to blastocyst morphology. Open bars, degenerating embryos; solid bars, developing blastocysts. ** significantly different from developing blastocysts ($p < 0.01$). (Adapted from Katz-Jaffe MG et al. *Fertil Steril* 2006; 85: 101–7.)

viability determination to run alongside morphological assessment. These quantitative methods hold the promise of improving *in vitro* fertilization (IVF) success rates as well as optimizing single-embryo transfer (28). There have been several studies that have shown the existence of soluble factors secreted by human embryos that could impact either or both developmental competence and implantation. The initial studies of the human embryonic secretome involved targeted analysis of individual proteins and molecules. The soluble factor 1-o-alkyl-2-acetyl-sn-glycero-3-phosphocholine (PAF) has been identified as one of the first targeted molecules. PAF was shown to be produced and secreted by mammalian embryos during preimplantation development (29). Secreted PAF could be working in an autocrine fashion as a survival factor, as well as influencing maternal physiology alterations including platelet activation and immune function (29).

Leptin, a 16 kDa small pleotrophic peptide, was also observed to be secreted by human blastocysts during the interaction between the embryo and endometrial epithelial cells (EECs) (30). In this study, competent human blastocysts secreted higher leptin concentrations into the surrounding medium than arrested embryos. Leptin has been hypothesized to interact with leptin receptors in the maternal endometrium during the window of implantation (31).

In another study by Sakkas et al., a soluble molecule secreted by human blastocysts that modulates regulation of HOXA10 expression in an epithelial endometrial cell line was identified (32). This form of reciprocal embryo–endometrial interaction could transform the local uterine environment, directly impacting the implantation process. More recently, the presence of soluble human leukocyte antigen G (sHLA-G) in embryo spent culture media has been linked to successful pregnancy outcome and has been suggested as a noninvasive marker to predict embryo quality and implantation success, especially when used in conjunction with current morphological embryo assessment methods. These results, however, have not been absolute, with pregnancies having been established from sHLA-G-negative embryos (33,34), as well as data revealing the inability to measure sHLA-G production in some supernatants (35).

It is more than likely that the multifactorial nature of embryonic development will dictate a panel of molecules to assess developmental competence and/or implantation potential rather than just the single variable. The SELDI-TOF MS analysis of proteins in the secretome of mammalian embryos throughout preimplantation development highlighted distinctive protein signatures at each 24-hour developmental stage (Table 19.1) (36). These signatures uniquely identified an embryo, independent of morphology. Comparison of mouse and human secretomes across preimplantation development revealed similar patterns and few differences between species (36).

Subsequent analysis revealed protein expression only at specific 24-hour developmental time points, while other proteins were observed through several embryonic stages, particularly occurring either before or after the activation of the embryonic genome (36). Examples are shown in Figure 19.4; the light gray boxes highlight the profiles of several biomarkers only secreted during the first 24 hours from day 1 to day 2 of mouse embryonic development ($p < 0.05$). Other biomarkers were observed to be secreted at all stages of embryonic development with increasing expression towards the blastocyst stage, as shown in Figure 19.4 (dark gray box; $p < 0.05$). In addition, the expression of numerous biomarkers was only observed after the

Table 19.1 Each stage of mammalian embryonic development revealed a panel of significant biomarkers that were only detected in the drops of spent *in vitro* fertilization culture media at specific stages of development ($p < 0.05$)

Stage of embryonic development	No. of proteins/ biomarkers	Description of events
Day 1–2	~20 candidate peaks	Maternal control of early embryonic development
Day 2–3	~12 candidate peaks	Embryonic genome activated
Day 3–4	~20 candidate peaks	Embryonic proteins translated
Day 4–5	~20 candidate peaks	Initiation of blastocyst implantation

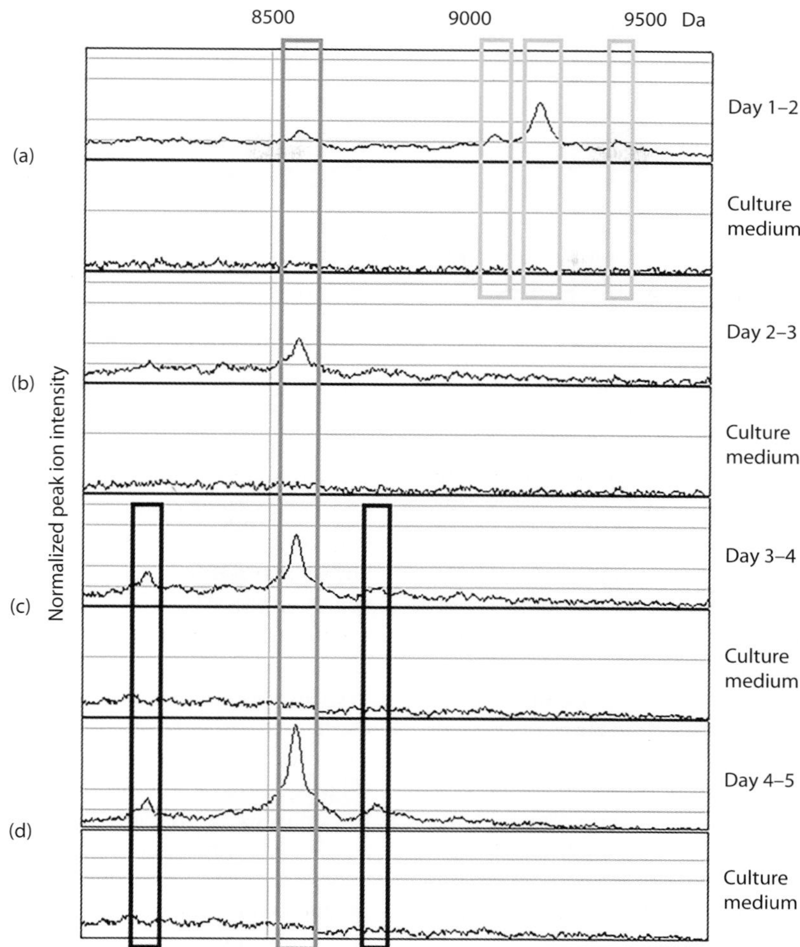

Figure 19.4 Protein profiles enhanced around the 7–10 kDa range for the secretome of each individual stage of mouse embryonic development. The bottom profiles for each 24 hours are from the control drops of media cultured under exact incubation conditions without embryos. (a) Days 1–2; (b) days 2–3 (c); days 3–4; and (d) days 4–5. Dark gray box displays protein expression across all developmental stages and light gray boxes highlight day 1–2 maternal protein expression, while black boxes indicate protein expression after the activation of the embryonic genome. (Adapted from Katz-Jaffe MG et al. *Fertil Steril* 2006; 86: 678–85.)

activation of the embryonic genome (Figure 19.4; black boxes). The transition from maternal inherited transcripts and proteins to the activation of the embryonic genome and the expression of key embryonic proteins must occur for continued embryonic development (37). Thus, embryos with a correctly activated embryonic genome, and hence a fully functional embryonic proteome, may have a higher potential of developmental competence.

Secretome analysis on day 5 was directly correlated with continuing blastocyst development, including the identification of differentially expressed biomarkers. The profile of an 8.5 kDa protein that was secreted every 24 hours from day 2 to day 5 of human embryonic development, with significantly increasing intensity towards the blastocyst stage, was also directly associated with ongoing development (Figure 19.5). The near lack of expression of this 8.5 kDa protein/biomarker from degenerating embryos, in conjunction with its high expression in developing blastocysts, potentially indicates an association between this biomarker and ongoing blastocyst development (Figure 19.5; $p < 0.05$) (36). Initial identification of this 8.5 kDa biomarker involving reverse-phase chromatography, sodium dodecylsulfate PAGE, trypsin digest, MS/MS, and database peptide sequence searching indicated that the best candidate was ubiquitin. Ubiquitin is a component of the ubiquitin-dependent proteasome system that is involved in a number of physiological processes including proliferation and apoptosis. Secreted ubiquitin has been shown to be up-regulated in body fluids in certain disease states, providing evidence for an increase in protein turnover (38,39). In addition, ubiquitin has been implicated in playing a crucial role during mammalian implantation by directing the activities and turnover of key signaling molecules (40).

Protein microarrays have also been utilized to generate human secretome protein profiles (41). In a retrospective study, 120 antibody targets were used to compare implanted versus non-implanted blastocyst-conditioned media. Due to the requirement of at least 10 pg/mL of

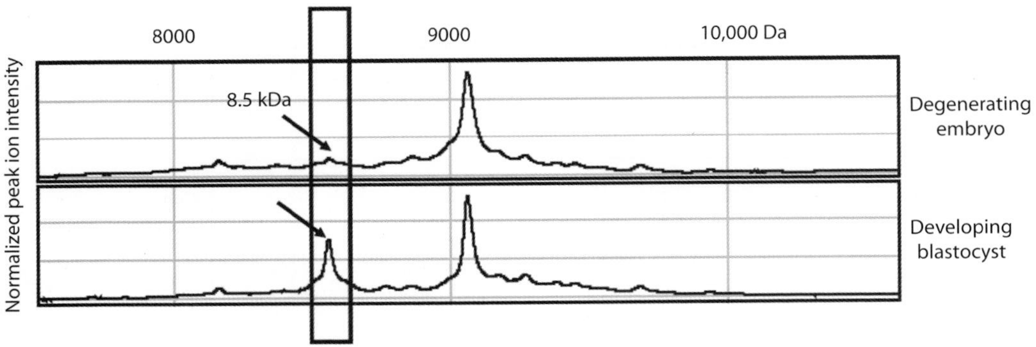

Figure 19.5 The expression of this 8.5 kDa protein/biomarker appears to be directly associated with ongoing blastocyst development. The black box highlights differences in protein expression across morphologically different day-5 embryos. (Adapted from Katz-Jaffe MG et al. *Fertil Steril* 2006; 86: 678–85.)

protein, samples were pooled following single-embryo transfer after classification of pregnancy outcome. An increased expression of the soluble TNF receptor 1 and interleukin-10 (IL-10) and a decreased expression of MSP-α, SCF, CXCL13, TRAILR3, and MIP-1β were observed in the conditioned media compared to the control media (41). In addition, the presence of two significantly decreased proteins, CXCL13 and granulocyte-macrophage colony-stimulating factor (GM-CSF), was observed in the pooled implanted blastocyst-conditioned media compared to non-implantation. These results reflect other studies showing that GM-CSF may promote embryo development and implantation when present in both human and mice blastocyst culture media (42).

In a follow-up study conducted by the same lab, the protein secretome profiles of an EEC co-culture system were compared with a sequential microdrop culture media system, revealing differential protein secretome profiles (43). Several molecules were increased in the EEC co-culture profile including IL-6, PLGF, and BCL (CXCL13), while other proteins were decreased (consumed), such as FGF-4, IL-12p40, VEGF, and uPAR. IL-6 was the most secreted protein by the EEC co-culture system and in subsequent experiments using an IL-6 enzyme-linked immunosorbent assay (ELISA) the sequential culture media secretome of viable blastocysts displayed an increased uptake compared to non-implanting blastocysts, suggesting a potential role for IL-6 in blastocyst development and implantation (43).

An essential requirement for healthy embryo and fetal development is the presence of all 23 pairs of human chromosomes (euploidy). Typically, embryos produced from aneuploid embryos (incorrect number of chromosomes) have little potential of forming a viable pregnancy. Indeed, over 60% of first trimester miscarriages are associated with chromosomal aneuploidy (44). To date, only invasive biopsy techniques that potentially could compromise outcome are able to screen for chromosomal aneuploidies in IVF embryos.

Using an LC–MS/MS platform, the protein secretome profile of pooled euploid blastocysts was notably different from the protein secretome profile of pooled aneuploid blastocysts (45). Nine potential candidate biomarkers characteristically classified chromosome aneuploidy with the most significant differentially expressed protein, lipocalin-1. Lipocalin-1 was shown to be increased in expression in the aneuploid protein secretome and was confirmed in individual samples with a commercially available lipocalin-1 ELISA kit (Uscn, Life Science, Inc.) (Figure 19.6). Further MS/MS experiments that included the analysis of the secretome from euploid blastocysts resulting in negative implantation showed the same expression profile of lipocalin-1 in spent IVF culture media from euploid blastocyst resulting in pregnancy (45). This suggests that the altered expression levels of

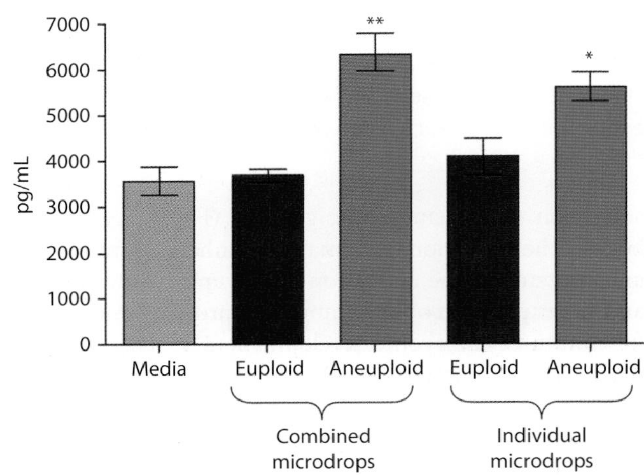

Figure 19.6 Lipocalin-1 concentration in the human embryonic protein secretome was measured by enzyme-linked immunosorbent assay and statistically analyzed by a Student t-test. Control media (n = 5); combined microdrops from euploid (n = 12) and aneuploid (n = 12) blastocysts (**$p < 0.01$); individual microdrops from euploid (n = 4) and aneuploid (n = 4) blastocysts (*$p < 0.05$). Control media = gray bar; euploid secretome = blue bars; aneuploid secretome = red bars. (Adapted from McReynolds S et al. *Fertil Steril* 2011; 95: 2631–3.)

lipocalin-1 are related to aneuploidy and not to failed implantation, revealing its potential as a biomarker for noninvasive aneuploidy screening. In these experiments, protein secretome analysis clearly discriminated between euploid and aneuploid blastocysts (45).

Human chorionic gonadotropin (hCG) is produced by trophoblast cells throughout pregnancy and is one of the most studied markers of embryonic development. Gene expression studies have revealed expression of hCG isoforms as early as the cleavage-stage embryo, leading Butler et al. to investigate the presence of hCG isoforms in preimplantation embryo culture media (46). A total of 118 embryos from 16 patients undergoing routine infertility treatment were analyzed using a highly sensitive and qualitative approach including commercial and "in-house" immunoassays, as well as a MALDI-TOF MS platform. Their results revealed hCG-β subunit expression in spent culture media from the pronuclear stage through to the blastocyst, with suggestion of potential correlation with quality in early preimplantation embryos (46).

Another strategy being investigated in the development of a diagnostic tool for embryo viability is combining protein secretome analysis with other embryo selection techniques, specifically time-lapse technology (47). Dominguez et al. examined embryonic morphokinetic data and analyzed seven proteins by multiplex immunoassay in the spent media of 16 embryos that implanted and 12 embryos that did not implant. Logistic regression analysis was performed revealing that the presence/absence of IL–6 and the duration of the second cycle (cc2) were the most relevant features for embryo selection (47). Combining these two parameters into a hierarchical model showed a relationship with the presence of IL-6 and 5–12-hour cc2 associated with significantly higher implantation rates (47). It is important to note that the sample size in this study was very small and therefore further clinical corroboration with a larger sample size is obligatory to confirm the validity of these results.

Protein identification and association of biomarkers with embryonic developmental competence, IVF outcome, and chromosome constitution is a promising area under investigation. An important variable that requires consideration when interpreting protein secretome data is the protein supplement either included or added into commercial embryo culture media. These non-declared proteins vary from batch to batch, with well over 100 having been identified, and can be problematic when attempting to identify potential biomarkers to distinguish normal and abnormal embryo development (48). Nevertheless, with appropriate controls and experimental design, protein secretome data provide insight into the unique molecular events occurring during embryonic development, including revealing some of the complex dialogs between the developing embryo and its maternal environment. This research could also translate into a cost-effective, high-throughput, and reliable assay for assessment of human embryonic viability. From a clinical perspective, noninvasive quantification of human embryonic viability, incorporating or in conjunction with comprehensive chromosome screening, will lead to routine implementation of single-embryo transfers, with higher implantation rates, reductions in pregnancy losses, and increased singleton deliveries.

CONCLUSIONS AND FUTURE PERSPECTIVES

Continuing advances in proteomic technologies have instigated novel studies to characterize the proteins expressed, as well as secreted, by the mammalian embryo during all stages of preimplantation development. This information has the potential to provide insight into the cellular function and biological processes during embryonic development and the implantation process. In addition, this technology could be of value in the development of noninvasive viability assays that, in conjunction with current morphologically based selection methods and perhaps other "omics" technologies, may increase IVF success rates whilst reducing the number of embryos transferred.

Looking towards the future, the emergence of nanotechnologies will be fundamental to the detection of low-abundance biomarkers in complex biological systems. Advances incorporating nanofluidics, nanoparticles, and nanostructures promise microscopic-volume liquid handling and the monitoring of concentration changes that have never before been detectable, as well as the potential for separation- and label-free protein analysis (49). The advent of the field of nanoproteomics will offer exciting opportunities to discover diagnostic biomarkers of preimplantation embryonic development and viability.

REFERENCES

1. Kenyon GL, DeMarini DM, Fuchs E et al. Defining the mandate of proteomics in the post-genomics era: Workshop report. *Mol Cell Proteomics* 2002; 1: 763–80.
2. Gygi SP, Rochon Y, Franza BR, Aebersold R. Correlation between protein and mRNA abundance in yeast. *Mol Cell Biol* 1999; 19: 1720–30.
3. Wulfkuhle JD, Liotta LA, Petricoin EF. Proteomic applications for the early detection of cancer. *Nat Rev Cancer* 2003; 3: 267–75.
4. Espina V, Dettloff KA, Cowherd S, Petricoin EF, Liotta LA. Use of proteomic analysis to monitor responses to biological therapies. *Expert Opin Biol Ther* 2004; 4: 83–93.
5. Petricoin EF, Liotta LA. Clinical applications of proteomics. *J Nutr* 2003; 133: 2476S–84S.
6. Hachey DL, Chaurand P. Proteomics in reproductive medicine: The technology for separation and identification of proteins. *J Reprod Immunol* 2004; 63: 61–73.
7. Brinster RL. Protein content of the mouse embryo during the first five days of development. *J Reprod Fertil* 1967; 13: 413–20.
8. Patton WF. Detection technologies in proteome analysis. *J Chromatogr B Analyt Technol Life Sci* 2002; 771: 3–31.

9. Latham KE, Garrels JI, Chang C, Solter D. Analysis of embryonic mouse development: Construction of a high-resolution, two-dimensional gel protein database. *Appl Theor Electroph* 1992; 2: 163–70.
10. Shi CZ, Collins HW, Garside WT, Buettger CW, Matschinsky FM, Heyner S. Protein databases for compacted eight-cell and blastocyst-stage mouse embryos. *Mol Reprod Develop* 1994; 37: 34–47.
11. Navarette Santos A, Tonack S, Kirstein M, Kietz S, Fischer B. Two insulin-responsive glucose transporter isoforms and the insulin receptor are developmentally expressed in rabbit preimplantation embryos. *Reproduction* 2004; 128: 503–16.
12. Wang HM, Zhang X, Qian D et al. Effect of ubiquitin–proteasome pathway on mouse blastocyst implantation and expression of matrix metalloproteinases-2 and -9. *BOR* 2004; 70: 481–7.
13. Liebler DC. *Introduction to Proteoemics, Tools for the New Biology*. Totowa, NJ: Humana Press, 2002.
14. Ellederova Z, Halada P, Man P, Kubelka M, Motlik J, Kovarova H. Protein patterns of pig oocytes during *in vitro* maturation. *BOR* 2004; 71: 1533–9.
15. Vitale AM, Calvert ME, Mallavarapu M et al. Proteomic profiling of murine oocyte maturation. *Mol Reprod Dev* 2006; 74: 608–16.
16. Meng Y, Liu XH, Ma X et al. The protein profile of mouse mature cumulus–oocyte complex. *Biochim Biophys Acta* 2007; 1774: 1477–90.
17. Seibert V, Wiesner A, Buschmann T, Meuer J. Surface-enhanced laser desorption ionization time-of-flight mass spectrometery (SELDI TOF-MS) and ProteinChip technology in proteomics research. *Pathol Res Pract* 2004; 200: 83–94.
18. Cazares LH, Diaz JI, Drake RR, Semmes OJ. MALDI/SELDI protein profiling of serum for the identification of cancer biomarkers. *Methods Mol Biol* 2007; 428: 125–40.
19. Jansen C, Hebeda KM, Linkels M et al. Protein profiling of B-cell lymphomas using tissue biopsies: A potential tool for small samples in pathology. *Cell Oncol* 2008; 30: 27–38.
20. Cho WC. Contribution of oncoproteomics to cancer biomarker discovery. *Mol Cancer* 2007; 6: 25.
21. Gerton GL, Fan XJ, Chittams J et al. A serum proteomics approach to the diagnosis of ectopic pregnancy. *Ann NY Acad Sci* 2004; 1022: 306–16.
22. Buhimschi CS, Bhandari V, Hamar BD et al. Proteomic profiling of the amniotic fluid to detect inflammation, infection and neonatal sepsis. *PLoS Med* 2007; 4: e18.
23. Poon TC. Opportunities and limitations of SELDI-TOF-MS in biomedical research: Practical advices. *Expert Rev Proteomics* 2007; 4: 51–65.
24. Katz-Jaffe MG, Linck DW, Schoolcraft WB, Gardner DK. A proteomic analysis of mammalian preimplantation embryonic development. *Reproduction* 2005; 130: 899–905.
25. Katz-Jaffe MG, Gardner DK, Schoolcraft WB. Proteomic analysis of individual human embryos to identify novel biomarkers of development and viability. *Fertil Steril* 2006; 85: 101–7.
26. Gardner DK, Lane M, Stevens J, Schoolcraft WB. Noninvasive assessment of human embryo nutrient consumption as a measure of developmental potential. *Fertil Steril* 2001; 76: 1175–80.
27. Ebner T, Moser M, Sommergruber M, Tews G. Selection based on morphological assessment of oocytes and embryos at different stages of preimplantation development: A review. *Hum Reprod Update* 2003; 9: 251–62.
28. Sakkas D, Gardner DK. Noninvasive methods to assess embryo quality. *Curr Opin Obstet Gynecol* 2005; 17: 283–8.
29. O'Neill C. The role of paf in embryo physiology. *Hum Reprod Update* 2005; 11: 215–28.
30. Gonzalez RR, Caballero-Campo P, Jasper M et al. Leptin and leptin receptor are expressed in the human endometrium and endometrial leptin secretion is regulated by the human blastocyst. *J Clin Endocrinol Metab* 2000; 85: 4883–8.
31. Cervero A, Horcajadas JA, Dominguez F, Pellicer A, Simon C. Leptin system in embryo development and implantation: A protein in search of a function. *Reprod Biomed Online* 2005; 10: 217–23.
32. Sakkas D, Lu C, Zulfikaroglu E, Neuber E, Taylor HS. A soluble molecule secreted by human blastocysts modulates regulation of HOXA10 expression in an epithelial endometrial cell line. *Fertil Steril* 2003; 80: 1169–74.
33. Noci I, Fuzzi B, Rizzo R, Melchiorri L et al. Embryonic soluble HLA-G as a marker of developmental potential in embryos. *Hum Reprod* 2005; 20: 138–46.
34. Fisch JD, Keskintepe L, Ginsburg M, Adamowicz M, Sher G. Graduated embryo score and soluble human leukocyte antigen-G expression improve assisted reproductive technology outcomes and suggest a basis for elective single-embryo transfer. *Fertil Steril* 2007; 87: 757–63.
35. Sargent I, Swales A, Ledee N, Kozman N, Tabiasco J, Le Bouteiller P. sHLA-G production by human IVF embryos: Can it be measured reliably? *J Reprod Immunol* 2007; 75: 128–32.
36. Katz-Jaffe MG, Schoolcraft WB, Gardner DK. Quantification of protein expression (secretome) by human and mouse preimplantation embryos. *Fertil Steril* 2006; 86: 678–85.
37. Telford NA, Watson AJ, Schultz GA. Transition from maternal to embryonic control in early mammalian development: A comparison of several species. *Mol Reprod Dev* 1990; 26: 90–100.
38. Delbosc S, Haloui M, Louedec L. Proteomic analysis permits the identification of new biomarkers of arterial wall remodeling in hypertension. *Mol Med* 2008; 14: 383–94.

39. Sandoval JA, Hoelz DJ, Woodruff HA et al. Novel peptides secreted from human neuroblastoma: Useful clinical tools? *J Pediatr Surg* 2006; 41: 245–51.
40. Wang Y, Puscheck EE, Lewis JJ, Trostinskaia AB, Wang F, Rappolee DA. Increases in phosphorylation of SAPK/JNK and p38MAPK correlate negatively with mouse embryo development after culture in different media. *Fertil Steril* 2005; 83: 1144–54.
41. Dominguez F, Gadea B, Esteban FJ, Horcajadas JA, Pellicer A, Simon C. Comparative protein-profile analysis of implanted versus non-implanted human blastocysts. *Hum Reprod* 2008; 23: 1993–2000.
42. Robertson SA. GM-CSF regulation of embryo development and pregnancy. *Cytokine Growth Factor Rev* 2007; 18: 287–98.
43. Dominguez F, Gadea B, Mercader A, Esteban FJ, Pellicer A, Simon C. Embryologic outcome and secretome profile of implanted blastocysts obtained after coculture in human endometrial epithelial cells versus the sequential system. *Fertil Steril* 2010; 93: 774–82.
44. Martinez MC, Mendez C, Ferro J, Nicolas M, Serra V, Landeras J. Cytogenetic analysis of early nonviable pregnancies after assisted reproduction treatment. *Fertil Steril* 2010; 93: 289–92.
45. McReynolds S, Vanderlinden L, Stevens J, Hansen K, Schoolcraft WB, Katz-Jaffe MG. Lipocalin-1 a potential marker for non-invasive aneuploidy screening. *Fertil Steril* 2011; 95: 2631–3.
46. Butler SA, Luttoo J, Freire MO, Abban TK, Borrelli PT, Iles RK. Human chorionic gonadotropin (hCG) in the secretome of cultured embryos: Hyperglycosylated hCG and hCG-free beta subunit are potential markers for infertility management and treatment. *Reprod Sci* 2013; 20: 1038–45.
47. Dominguez F, Meseguer M, Aparicio-Ruiz B, Piqueras P, Quinonero A, Simon C. New strategy for diagnosing embryo implantation potential by combining proteomics and time-lapse technologies. *Fertil Steril* 2015; 104: 908–14.
48. Dyrlund TF, Kirkegaard K, Toftgaard Poulsen E et al. Unconditional commercial embryo culture media contain a large variety of non-declared proteins: A comprehensive proteomics analysis. *Hum Reprod* 2014; 29: 2421–30.
49. Kobeissy FH, Gulbakan B, Alawieh A et al. Post-genomics nanotechnology is gaining momentum: Nanoproteomics and applications in life sciences. *OMICS* 2014; 18: 111–31.

The human oocyte
Controlled-rate cooling

CARLOTTA ZACÀ and ANDREA BORINI

20

INTRODUCTION

Thanks to the new protocols that have been developed, which have improved the application of oocyte cryopreservation, this procedure is today one of the techniques that can be used in clinical practice and is an important option for women planning to undergo *in vitro* fertilization (IVF) treatment (1–9).

This technique may be used to rescue cycles at high risk of ovarian hyperstimulation syndrome, for failure to obtain sperm, in oocyte donation programs, in the treatment of congenital infertility disorders or premature ovarian failure (POF), as an alternative to embryo freezing, or, for fertile women, as an alternative to electively delay in childbearing.

Supernumerary oocyte freezing is the best way to optimize stimulation cycles and cumulative results. Oocyte cryopreservation also represents an option for single women about to undergo gonadotoxic treatments that may compromise their chances to conceive (10–12).

The initial attempts to freeze oocytes were published about 40 years ago using mouse oocytes (13), but the first pregnancies obtained with the use of human frozen oocytes were reported in the 1980s by Chen (14) and Al-Hasani et al. (15). Cryopreservation of human oocytes, because of the characteristics of that kind of cell, has several technical difficulties associated with the unique properties of the human mature oocyte (size, sensitivity to low temperature, high water content, low surface-to-volume ratio, and suboptimal plasma membrane permeability).

As a consequence of these typical features, human oocytes risk retaining more water and are more likely to encounter ice formation. Over the years, there have been several changes to cryopreservation methods (2,16–18) to ensure adequate dehydration and to avoid damage to chromosomes and the meiotic spindle, the cytoskeleton, and cortical granules (19,20).

Egg freezing has been considered for a long period to be an experimental procedure, mainly due to the characteristics of this particular cell and because of considerable concerns about egg freezing itself, due to the lack of cryobiological data.

BIOPHYSICAL PRINCIPLES OF CONTROLLED-RATE COOLING AND METHODOLOGY

Cryobiology is the branch of biology that studies the effects of low temperatures on living systems. The basic principles of cryobiology must be well known in order to get good results. Cryopreservation requires the biological sample to be brought to cryogenic temperature (−196°C) at which biological, chemical, and physical activities come to a stop. The factors playing a fundamental role in cryopreservation are biophysical—such as cryoprotectant and speed—and morphological—such as dimensions and quality of sample. For these reasons, cryopreservation of human oocytes, because of their unique features of size and physiology, experiences several difficulties.

The high water content (75%–85%), related to the large cell size, can convert into ice crystals at low temperatures, generating significant and irreversible damage to the cellular ultrastructure. In addition to this, the cytoplasmic oocyte is also characterized by a high sensitivity of the cytoskeleton to low temperatures (21). These elements lead to relevant difficulties in the successful application of the technique.

Over the years, changes have been made to cryopreservation methods with the aim of reducing intracellular ice crystal formation and improving results in terms of biological and clinical outcomes. To obtain those results, reaching a sufficient dehydration is mandatory, and this can be done thanks to specific molecules called cryoprotectant agents (CPAs) that can be differently mixed in order to maximize the outcome. A common feature among these compounds is their ability to interact with water via hydrogen bonding; prior to slow cooling, they lower the freezing point of the solution and allow greater cell dehydration without excessive shrinkage (22).

Cryoprotectants can be divided into two groups according to their characteristics and their ability to pass through the cell membrane:

- *Permeating agents*: Substances chemically characterized as having a relatively low molecular weight and able to penetrate the lipid bilayer of the cell, but more slowly than water. This group of agents includes glycerol, ethylene glycol (EG), dimethyl sulfoxide (DMSO), and 1,2-propanediol (PROH). Permeating cryoprotectants are able to penetrate the cell membrane during cooling. They replace intracellular water through an osmotic process, decrease the formation of intracellular ice crystals, lower the freezing point of the solution, and support enhanced cellular dehydration during freezing.
- *Non-permeating agents*: These have a high molecular weight so they remain in the extracellular solution because of their size, and they include sugars and other macromolecules such as sucrose, raffinose, and trehalose. Non-permeating cryoprotectants, which are unable to cross the cell membrane because of their

molecular size, generate an osmotic gradient that causes cell dehydration and decreases the intracellular water content; consequently, there is a lower likelihood of intracellular ice crystal formation as the temperature drops. The most frequently used non-permeating agents are trehalose and sucrose.

Permeating and non-permeating agents are usually used in association; their capability to replace water, which is so important at low temperatures, also means that they are characterized by an innate toxicity if they are used on cells at physiological temperatures. Toxicity is proportional to exposure time and concentration. The basic task of the CPAs is to reduce possible damage due to ice crystal formation inside the cell, which is the principal cause of cryopreservation damage.

During the procedure, they are added and removed gradually in order to reduce excessive osmotic gradients that may arise during the process. It is also essential to balance the benefit of the slow addition of the cryoprotectants with the detrimental effects caused by the consequent increase in exposure time.

Ice formation is affected by the characteristics of the permeability of the cell, by the surface/volume relationship of the cell, and by the cooling rate, so for each type of cell, a specific curve of cooling must be identified to obtain an optimal survival.

An important aspect that plays a key role in biological and medical procedures is reproducibility: in this case, it is related to the temperature at which dehydration/rehydration solutions are used.

In controlled-rate cooling, thanks to automated machines, the decrease in temperature is finely regulated and recorded; indeed, it is achieved using a computerized freezing system consisting of a computer and freezing chamber connected by a pump to a cylinder from which liquid nitrogen is extracted in gaseous form. The temperature reduction curve to be achieved is saved on the computer; according to the temperature detected by the temperature sensor, the computer opens and closes the solenoid valve and regulates the introduction of gaseous nitrogen into the freezing chamber, thus permitting controlled temperature lowering.

An example of the reproducibility of this protocol is provided by the comparison of four studies that were carried out with large numbers of patients using the same slow-freezing method (Table 20.1). From these data, it is possible to observe that survival, fertilization, cleavage, and implantation rates were rather similar, despite the fact that the four studies were conducted in different centers.

In slow-freezing protocols, two-step dehydration is normally carried out before cooling the cell to subzero temperatures. In the first phase of dehydration, concentrations of permeating CPAs (1.0–1.5 mol/L) are utilized to remove water from the cell, preventing ice formation. The most widely used cryoprotectants in this phase are PROH, DMSO, or EG. The presence of permeating CPA in the extracellular media creates an osmotic gradient that draws water out of the cell. The oocyte, once dehydrated and shrunk, returns to near the original volume as the cryoprotectant enters the cell, replacing the water. This causes a double flux across the membrane (the water exits the cell while the CPA enters) that influences both the intracellular solute concentration and the cell volume (Figure 20.1). The extreme extent of shrinkage and swelling can cause damage or even cell death because of the osmotic stress acting on the oocyte membrane.

In the second phase, a non-permeating CPA is usually added to minimize the phenomenon of shrinkage. The most common agents successfully applied are sucrose and trehalose (22,29,30). This new agent creates a second-phase

Table 20.1 Oocyte cryopreservation outcomes generated in four different studies adopting the same freezing protocol

	Borini et al. (23)	Levi Setti et al. (24)	De Santis et al. (25)	Parmegiani et al. (26)
Patients	146	120	66	75
Thaws	201	159	68	93
Oocytes:				
Thawed	927	1087	396	437
Survived (%)	687 (74)	760 (69)	282 (71.2)	328 (75.1)
Microinjected	589	687	194	264
2PN	448 (76)	464 (67)	156 (80.4)	227 (86)
Embryos:				
Cleaved	404 (90)	413 (89)	142 (91)	198 (87.2)
Mean transferred	2.1 ± 0.8	–	–	–
Pregnancies (% per ET)	18 (9.7)	18 (12.4)	6 (9.5)	16 (19.3)
Implantations (%)	21 (5.2)	19 (5.7)	7 (5.7)	(9.6)
Implantation efficiency per thawed oocyte	2.6%	1.9%	2.6%	–

Abbreviations: 2PN, two pronuclei; ET, embryo transfer.

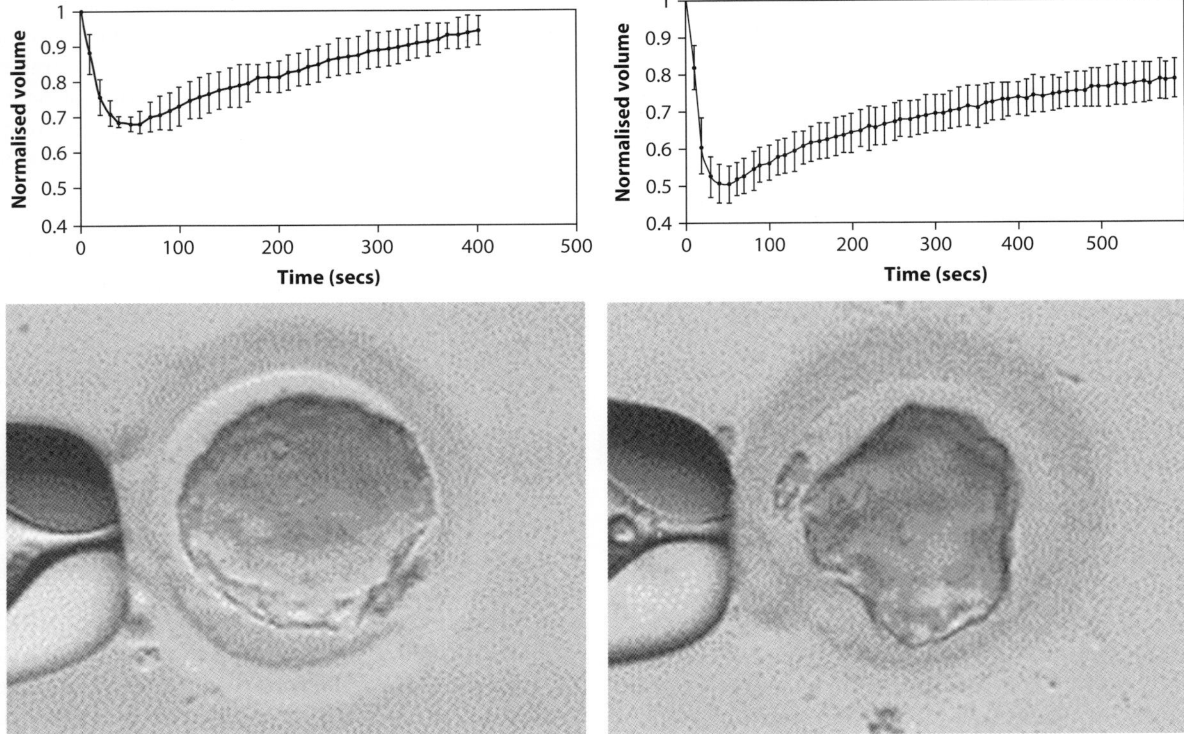

Figure 20.1 Mean ± SD normalized volumes of human oocytes during exposure to 1.5 mol/L 1,2-propanediol (27) (left) or ethylene glycol (28) (right) at 25°C. The magnitude and kinetics of volume changes are dictated by the relative oolemma permeability to water and cryoprotective agent (CPA). Low permeability to CPA and, consequently, more pronounced volume reduction may cause major transient perturbations of the original spherical shape (right).

dehydration in which the shrinkage rate is faster with a higher reduction of the cell volume before freezing (Video 20.1). This phenomenon decreases the later likelihood of intracellular ice crystal formation.

Afterwards, the sample is slowly cooled, and once the sample temperature has been lowered to −6 to −8°C, ice nucleation (seeding) is induced to provoke ice formation in extracellular water. Controlled ice formation during freezing is recognized as a key factor in determining oocyte viability as the ice crystals do not enter the cell because of the marginally higher osmolarity (lower freezing point) of the intracellular environment. Following the seeding, the concentration of the solutes in the non-frozen fraction gradually increases as water is incorporated into the extracellular ice crystals. The increasing concentration in the solutes generates an osmotic gradient across the cell membrane, which draws out more water, causing the dehydration of the cell. At this point, the samples can be plunged directly into liquid nitrogen.

During thawing, cell rehydration is usually obtained by its exposure to decreasing concentrations of the permeating cryoprotectant in order to return to a physiological condition; in this phase, rapid temperature transition is preferred to prevent the recrystallization of water, with the potential for ice crystal damage. Cell rehydration is usually performed by a stepwise dilution of the intracellular CPA present in the freezing media, together with a high concentration of the extracellular CPA, such as sugar, which acts as an osmotic buffer. As the permeating cryoprotectant gradually diffuses out of the oocyte, the concentration of the non-permeating cryoprotectant gradually decreases, until the oocyte goes back to standard culture medium (Video 20.2).

An optimal exposure should aim to minimize osmotic stress while avoiding chemical toxicity and allowing sufficient permeation and dehydration to achieve protection from freezing injury.

PREPARATION AND SELECTION OF FREEZABLE OOCYTES

Cryopreservation of human oocytes, contrary to sperm cryopreservation, has faced greater technical difficulties arising directly from the nature of this particular cell.

The cryopreservation of female gametes faces many difficulties due to morphological features such as their size and physiology: the human female gamete is the largest cell in the human body, with a low surface/volume ratio and with a high cytoplasmic water content (75%–85%). At the same time, it only has a small amount of water-permeable membrane itself; water tends to remain inside the cell during cooling procedures, leading to the formation of ice crystals that are lethal because they can cause mechanical damage to the cytoplasmic organelles and result in degeneration of the cell. The selection of freezable eggs is certainly a difficult choice for embryologists. Just after retrieval, the oocyte is surrounded by two types of somatic granulosa cells: cumulus oophorus cells, which are more dispersed, and corona radiata cells, which are in contact with the zona pellucida. The cumulus oophorus and corona radiata cells, together with the oocyte, constitute the cumulus–corona–oocyte complex. During the collection of the oocytes of a stimulated cycle, the embryologist, using a stereomicroscope, can observe and evaluate the complexes that have typical morphological characteristics related to the stage of maturation. The cumulus–corona–oocyte complex of a human mature oocyte (metaphase II) is characterized by expanded cells that form a characteristic radiating structure. The presence of the cumulus might influence the exchange of water and CPAs during dehydration and rehydration of the oocytes, and that ultimately has an effect on the cryopreservation procedure. Few studies are available in the literature about the influence of the cumulus on the freezing outcome. One of the first papers in this area was published by Gook et al. (31); it analyzed intact cumulus or totally decumulated oocytes frozen using the protocol initially described by Lassalle et al. for embryo cryopreservation (32). A higher survival rate was observed in the group without cumulus compared with the cumulus-enclosed complexes (69% vs. 48%, respectively).

When choosing suitable oocytes for cryopreservation it is important to assess oocyte maturity and quality, so the complete denudation of the cumulus–corona complex using hyaluronidase enzyme and mechanical pipetting before freezing is recommended, since the presence of cumulus cells does not allow us to effectively evaluate nuclear maturity and cytoplasm characteristics.

It is generally accepted that a "morphologically normal" human mature oocyte should have a round, clear zona pellucida, a reduced perivitelline space containing a single and non-fragmented first polar body, and a uniform or moderately granular cytoplasm, with no inclusions. There are several different cytoplasmic and extracytoplasmic abnormalities; in fact, after ovarian hyperstimulation, some of the retrieved oocytes exhibit one or more morphological cytoplasmic or extracytoplasmic abnormalities (33–35).

The cytoplasm can be dark, homogenously granulous, or located in the middle; it can also have vacuoles, various formations that are formed from endoplasmic reticulum. It is also possible to find oocytes with a larger diameter termed "giant" that are generally discarded because of their abnormal chromosomes (36). Also, the extracytoplasmic abnormalities seem to be associated with oocyte function and embryo development. Abnormalities of the zona pellucida, perivitelline space, and first polar body are part of this category. It is preferable to cryopreserve only "morphologically normal" oocytes since cytoplasmic and extracytoplasmic abnormalities seem to affect oocyte competence. Unfortunately, methods to assess the quality of the oocytes are usually invasive and thus non-conservative.

TIME OF CRYOPRESERVATION

During the routine procedure, eggs are cultured for several hours following retrieval before insemination. The interval time is about 40 hours after human chorionic gonadotropin (hCG) administration; this is the time required for the oocytes to undergo nuclear and cytoplasmic maturation.

With oocyte cryopreservation, one of the concerns is the risk of creating a discontinuity in life during the critical period between recovery and fertilization. The ideal interval time in which the oocyte should be frozen is still under discussion.

In our unpublished study of 213 cycles on the total culture time (pre-freezing and post-thawing), we found a total time of less than seven hours compared to seven to eight hours and up eight hours of total culture is associated with greater clinical results in terms of pregnancy rate (31.8%, 27.8%, and 16.1%, respectively) and implantation rate (21.3%, 15.7%, and 10.4%, respectively) (Table 20.2).

In a clinical retrospective study involving 75 patients and 93 oocyte thawings, Parmegiani et al. (26) achieved significantly improved embryo quality and clinical outcome when oocyte cryopreservation was performed within two hours from retrieval. Lappi et al. confirmed these results (37) in a retrospective study on 311 thawing cycles using a slow-freezing protocol with 1.5 M PROH and 0.3 M sucrose. Oocytes frozen within 40 hours of hCG administration showed significantly higher pregnancy and implantation rates compared with eggs cryopreserved more than 40 hours after hCG administration (22% vs. 12% pregnancy/transfer, $p < 0.05$; and 13% vs. 7% implantation, $p < 0.05$). No difference was found in the time between end of thawing and microinjection. These studies show that the timing of oocyte cryopreservation seems to play a key role in determining the clinical outcome after thawing. In particular, the time post-hCG administration at which freezing is carried out is very important to determine the potential development of oocytes from the frozen cycles.

METHODOLOGY

Slow-freezing procedure

The oocytes are decumulated mechanically and enzymatically two hours after transvaginal retrieval to detect the metaphase II oocytes suitable for the slow-freezing procedure.

1. The solutions are placed at room temperature (RT; 22°C–24°C) before use. Just before starting, the cryofreezer is turned on. It is necessary to print a label with the name, surname, freezing date, couple code, and numbers of the oocytes and put it on the straw. One to a maximum of three oocytes per straw are loaded. Then, an adapted syringe is connected to each straw, a weighted ID rod is prepared, and a 170 μm denuding pipette is set up.
2. For each oocyte or group of oocytes, 0.6 mL of the equilibration solution (ES; 1.5 M PROH) is dispensed in well 1 and 0.6 mL of loading solution (LS; 1.5 M PROH

Table 20.2 Unpublished data on the effects of total culture time (pre-freezing and post-thawing) on clinical results

	Pre-freeze + post-thaw culture time		
	<7 hours	7–8 hours	>8 hours
Mean age (years)	36.0	35.3	35.4
Cycles	22	54	137
Thawed oocytes	108	266	686
Survival rate (%)	88/108 (81.5)	210/266 (78.9)	539/686 (78.6)
Fertilization rate (%)	49/62 (79.0)	129/155 (83.2)	330/402 (82.1)
Cleavage rate (%)	47/49 (95.9)	127/129 (98.4)	310/330 (93.9)
ET	22	54	137
Pregnancy rate/cycle (%)	7/22 (31.8)	15/54 (27.8)	22/137 (16.1)
Pregnancy rate/ET (%)	7/22 (31.8)	15/54 (27.8)	22/137 (16.1)
Implantation rate (%)	10/47 (21.3)	20/127 (15.7)	32/309 (10.4)
Implantation rate/thawed oocytes (%)	10/108 (9.3)	20/266 (7.5)	32/686 (4.7)

Abbreviation: ET, embryo transfer.

+ 0.2 M sucrose) is dispensed in well 2 of a four-well plate labeled with the patient's surname, name, and couple code.

3. The denuded mature oocytes are transferred from their culture media to the ES and incubated for 10 minutes. After this time, the oocytes are moved to the LS beginning with the first incubated oocyte. The passage between one solution and the other is carried out by collecting the oocytes with a 170 μm denuding pipette in a small amount of solution. Within five minutes of the first oocytes having been incubated in the LS, it is necessary to proceed with loading the oocyte into the straw.
4. First, a small amount of LS and then an air bubble is loaded, and subsequently LS containing the oocyte is loaded into the middle of the liquid. Then, another air bubble and, at the end, another small amount of the same solution are loaded.
5. The straw is then separated from the adapted syringe. Each weighted ID rod is inserted into the straw and it is sealed on both sides. The straws are placed into the automated cryo-freezer when the temperature is around 20°C.
6. The sample is slowly cooled from +20°C to −7°C at a rate of −2°C/minute. Manual seeding is performed at −7°C (temperature maintained for 10 minutes). During this time, the straws are removed rapidly but not completely to induce ice crystals by touching the straw with very cold metal forceps in proximity to the first small amount of LS nearby the filter. Then, the temperature decreases to −30°C at a rate of −0.3°C/minute and then rapidly decreases to −150°C at a rate of −50°C/minute. An acoustic and visual signal indicates the end of the freezing program. Finally, the straws are directly plunged into a goblet of liquid nitrogen and finally stored into the dewar at −196°C.

Rapid-thawing procedure

1. Thawing solutions (TSs) are at room temperature (22°C–24°C). In this phase, it is necessary to prepare the sterile gauze, sterile scissors, adjustor syringe, 170 μm denuding pipette, timer, 30°C water bath, Petri dish, and a four-well plate for each straw to thaw labeled with patient's surname, name, and couple code.
2. The TSs are dispensed into individual wells of the four-well plate: 0.5 mL of TS1 (1 M PROH + 0.3 M sucrose) in well 1, 0.5 mL of TS2 (0.5 M PROH + 0.3 M sucrose) in well 2, 0.5 mL of TS3 (0.3 M sucrose) in well 3, and finally 0.5 mL of TS4 (phosphate-buffered saline) in well 4.
3. The samples are removed from the liquid nitrogen. The straw is taken out from the liquid nitrogen and kept in air for 30 seconds (at RT). Immediately after this, the straw is put for 40 seconds in a 30°C water bath. Subsequently, the straw is dried gently with surgical gauze and is cut at one end with the small sterile scissors and attached to the adapted syringe.
4. The other extremity is cut and the solution containing oocytes is emptied into a Petri dish under the stereo-zoom microscope to immediately visualize the oocytes. As soon as the oocytes are seen, they are moved into TS1 and incubated for five minutes. After this time, the oocytes are moved into TS2 and incubated for five minutes, then into TS3 and TS4 for 10 minutes each. At the end of the thawing procedure, oocyte integrity is evaluated with the inverted microscope. The thawed and surviving oocytes are cultured until insemination time.

All the steps of slow-freezing and rapid-thawing procedures are carried out by two people: the operator and a second person who assists the operator during the procedure.

CRYODAMAGE

The oocyte, in addition to surviving the cryopreservation, needs to develop into a viable embryo to be able to result in a pregnancy. Survival after thawing is certainly crucial, but does not necessarily coincide with cell integrity. It has been widely demonstrated that there are several structures that must be preserved in order to consider the oocyte functional and suitable to progress towards generation, because low temperatures may induce sublethal damage or alteration to different organelles and structures, such as the zona pellucida, cortical granules, mitochondria, and meiotic spindle.

The zona pellucida is a trilaminar structure consisting of glycoproteins that can be damaged by cryopreservation. This structure has the function of controlling fertilization in physiological conditions, binding the male gamete, and initiating the acrosome reaction of the sperm. If this structure is damaged during freezing, an abnormal or failed fertilization can be the outcome. There is evidence that cryopreservation, irrespective of the adopted method, causes hardening of the zona pellucida through premature cortical granule release, which then acts as a barrier to fertilization (38–40). If standard insemination techniques are used, a reduction of normal fertilization rates (41) would occur. Supplementation of the solutions of cryopreservation with a protein component has allowed us to reduce the phenomenon of zona hardening (40), despite equal premature release of the granules taking place. After the introduction in 1992 of the intracytoplasmic sperm injection (ICSI) by Palermo et al. (41), it was possible to bypass the hardened zona, leading to improved fertilization and live birth rates (8,42,43).

Another structure that can be damaged by cryopreservation is the meiotic spindle, which is composed of microtubules and is important for chromosome segregation. At the time of fertilization, upturn of meiosis takes place, separating the chromatids attached to the meiotic spindle, expelling one set into the second polar body and the other into the female pronucleus (44). The meiotic spindle apparatus is a dynamic structure and it has been demonstrated to depolymerize when exposed to low temperatures (45). Nevertheless, after a return to normal conditions, the spindle is able to significantly reassemble (21,46,47). This structure must work correctly to achieve accurate chromosome segregation; subsequent impaired repolymerization at warming may lead to misaggregation of chromatids and aneuploidy (48).

During the slow-freezing procedure, the oocyte experiences a drastic change in temperature that can be detrimental for the spindle; on the other hand, CPAs play an important role in protecting the spindle. Unfortunately, in order to have accurate information, cytogenetic or confocal analyses should be performed on oocytes after thawing, with a consequent loss of viability.

The introduction of the PolScope (orientation-independent polarized light microscope) has enabled the study of the dynamic behavior of the meiotic spindle, permitting repetitive observations *in vivo* (49). Microtubules are responsible for spindle birefringence and their density is measured by retardance. With this noninvasive alternative technique that allows us to preserve oocyte viability, it has been demonstrated that microtubule depolymerization starts at about 32°C and that a complete breakdown is reached within a few minutes of the start of cooling (50), confirming results previously achieved by invasive techniques that focused on the relationship between temperature and spindle behavior. In addition to this, further studies showed that the meiotic spindles of thawed oocytes derive from "*de novo*" reconstruction (51).

Several authors attempted to visualize the reappearance of the spindle after rewarming by applying different slow-freezing protocols. Rienzi et al. (51) used a 1.5 M PROH plus 0.1 M sucrose mixture and showed recovery in 37% of the oocytes immediately after thawing; after a transient disappearance, the spindle was present in all the eggs that survived within three hours of incubation at 37°C. Similar data were published by our group (52) using a comparable freezing protocol with a higher sucrose concentration (0.3 M). Immediately after thawing, only 22.9% of oocytes showed a weak birefringence signal, while only 1.2% of oocytes displayed a high signal. After three hours of culture, 49.4% of the oocytes showed a weak birefringence while 18.1% showed a high-intensity signal. There was a statistically significant increase in signal restoration after three hours of culture ($p < 0.001$). We (53) studied a larger cohort of eggs and demonstrated a 90% signal restoration after one hour of culture. The authors stated that post-thaw culture could be considerably shortened to one hour. Furthermore, they speculated that a short culture time could be beneficial to the whole cryopreservation procedure, making the risk of aging *in vitro* less likely, which may occur after thawing if the oocytes are incubated for longer periods in preparation for insemination.

A further demonstration was obtained by confocal microscopy (54), where fresh control oocytes were compared with frozen eggs fixed at different times after thawing (zero, one, two, or three hours). All the control oocytes displayed normal bipolar spindles. Directly after thawing at $T = 0$, a significant reduction of oocytes with bipolar spindles (59.1%) was observed, while after one hour of culture (T1), 85.7% regained bipolar spindles. Oocytes cultured for a longer period (two or three hours) displayed 73.7% and 72.7% bipolar spindles, respectively.

Unfortunately, Coticchio et al. (55) demonstrated that while the PolScope is useful for showing the presence and the dynamics of the spindle, the morphometric evaluation of the spindle through the PolScope is not consistent with confocal analysis.

Another set of structures that are sensitive to freezing are the mitochondria. It was displayed (with transmission electron microscopy [TEM]) long since a damage of these structures in response to a lowering of the temperature to 0°C in the presence or absence of DMSO (56). Nottola et al. revealed the presence of mitochondrial damage by comparing fresh with frozen oocytes using PROH and different concentrations of sucrose (0.1 and 0.3 M), while areas of microvacuolation have been described in the presence of high concentrations of sucrose (0.3 M). These areas may be correlated with a reduced potential of embryonic development after thawing (57).

In 2009, Gualtieri et al. (58) confirmed these data by TEM, detecting a decrease in cortical granules and microvacuolation in oocytes cryopreserved with PROH and 0.3 M sucrose.

In fresh samples, mitochondria had a regular shape with few short cristae, whereas in the frozen–thawed group, a high percentage of oocytes (72%) showed a variable and, in some cases, very high fraction of mitochondria with decreased electron density of the matrix or ruptures of the outer and inner membranes. Moreover, in those oocytes, the mitochondrial damage was associated with smooth endoplasmic reticulum swelling.

It is possible to speculate that the damage caused by the freezing of mitochondria and endoplasmic reticulum may be reflected in the altered regulation of calcium homeostasis. This might partially explain the low implantation rates obtained with this protocol (5,23).

Our recent study by transmission electron microscopy (59) has shown that vacuolation appears as a form of cell damage during slow freezing and, to a lesser extent, during vitrification. The data published in 2011 by Gualtieri et al. (60) demonstrate and confirm that cryopreservation may generally induce a number of such damages: intracytoplasmic microvacuolation, exocytosis of cortical granules, and degeneration of mitochondria.

SURVIVED OOCYTES AND INSEMINATION

The survival rate is important, especially when a limited number of cells are available for cryopreservation. Intracellular water is essential, and equally relevant is its shift across the cell membrane to equalize the vapor pressure gradient as a result of ice formation in the external solute with reduced temperature (61).

The importance of the rate of outward flow of water and the surface area/volume ratio of the cell was clearly demonstrated by the different survival rates observed in oocytes cryopreserved in the same conditions at different developmental stages. Movement of water out of the oocyte is achieved by use of a cryoprotectant (61), providing an osmotic gradient and, in the case of permeating cryoprotectants, limiting shrinkage by replacing the lost water. The rate at which a permeating cryoprotectant diffuses into the oocyte differs between cryoprotectants and is temperature dependent (27).

A relevant indicator of the efficiency of the oocyte cryopreservation process is the survival rate. The most evident cryodamage is the lysis of the cell membrane as a result of intracellular ice. Over the years, improvements of protocols for human oocyte cryopreservation have led to an increase in the survival rate. Initial oocyte cryopreservation with DMSO was associated with survival rates that ranged between 20% and 30% (62–65). Substituting the permeating cryoprotectant with PROH and adding 0.1 M sucrose have doubled the survival rate. The evolution of the protocols has also led to increasing the sucrose concentration from 0.1 to 0.2 or 0.3 M during dehydration, increasing the survival rate up to 60%–80% (5,23,25,66–68). These changes have led survival rates of around 70% when performing the protocol with 0.2 M sucrose (18,69–71) and slightly higher (74%) when using 0.3 M sucrose (23,66,67,72).

Morphologically, a mature human egg surviving after cryopreservation should look like a fresh human egg; however, survival does not mean capacity for fertilization. In order to identify the right time for the microinjection after thawing, it is important to balance carefully the recovery time that oocytes need in order to restore the meiotic spindle with oocyte aging, which must be avoided.

In our study (73) on 375 thawing cycles, evidence has shown that the time before freezing does not compromise the final outcome. Instead, a more important role is played by the post-thawing culture time. This result can probably be associated with the protective effect that cumulus cells exert on the oocyte, limiting its aging; thus, denuded oocytes might be more sensitive to damage.

The insemination of surviving oocytes takes place not earlier than one hour or at maximum two hours after the end of the thawing procedure in order to avoid exceeding the total culture time and to recover the meiotic spindle after thawing.

DEVELOPMENTAL PERFORMANCE OF FROZEN–THAWED OOCYTES

Much information is available in the literature about the relationship between different freezing conditions and the embryo's ability to resume the mitotic cycle. This factor can help predict the implantation potential of frozen–thawed embryos (74). By contrast, little is known about the early developmental competence of embryos coming from frozen eggs.

Development rate, which is correlated with implantation potential, seems to be compromised after cryopreservation with high sucrose concentrations (0.3 M). A study published by Konc et al. in 2008 (68) showed a significant delay in development on day 2 (four-cell stage) in embryos derived by oocytes cryopreserved using the 0.3 M sucrose procedure when compared to embryos from fresh oocytes (17% vs. 66%).

Additional evidence of this trend is reported in a study conducted by our group (75) where we compared the frequency of early cleavage, cell number, and degree of fragmentation in embryos derived from sibling fresh and frozen–thawed oocytes of patients undergoing IVF treatment in order to determine potential differences. We observed that very few embryos (7%) had undergone early cleavage at 25 hours post-insemination compared with most of the embryos resulting from fresh oocytes (59%).

These data are consistent with the hypothesis that, to some extent, the implantation potential of embryos developed from frozen oocytes may be affected by freezing with high sucrose concentrations.

This trend has been confirmed by a study (76) that analyzed the impact of high sucrose concentrations on embryo development. The data show different oocyte development and growth after cryopreservation in comparison with the corresponding sibling fresh oocytes. This gives an estimation of the effects caused by freezing and thawing and, indirectly, of the expectations related to oocyte cryobanking. The differences were independent of age, suggesting that the mechanisms regulating oocyte activation and the first cleavage divisions are especially sensitive to low temperatures.

By contrast oocytes cryopreserved in 0.2 M sucrose generated 50% of embryos with at least four cells on day 2 (18), indicating no impact on embryo development with this protocol.

In any case, it has been remarked by different authors that high cleavage rates are not necessarily related to high implantation potential (23,24,68). In these publications, high rates of cleavage (90%–93%) resulted in scarce implantation rates (5%–6%).

Conversely, when our group (77) compared the developmental ability of embryos derived from sibling fresh and frozen–thawed oocytes using a protocol with differential sucrose concentrations (0.2 M freezing stage and 0.3 M thawing stage), the outcomes were different. Embryos from fresh and frozen oocytes were assessed by comparing fertilization rate, cleavage rate, and the number of blastomeres at 42–44 hours after microinjection. In 85 fresh cycles, 244 oocytes were inseminated, while in 104 frozen cycles, 357 out of 525 oocytes survived after thawing (68%) and 248 were microinjected. Normal fertilization rates were comparable and high in both fresh and frozen groups (81.9% and 81.4%, respectively). Cleavage rates were 96.5% and 93.1% and the rates of four-cell embryos were 47.0% and 47.2% in fresh and frozen groups, respectively. The overall implantation rate of embryos developed from frozen oocytes was 15.7%, while this frequency increased to 26.9% in cases in which at least two four-cell embryos were transferred.

Following cryopreservation, the early developmental ability of frozen–thawed oocytes does not appear to be affected in comparison to that of sibling non-frozen oocytes. Moreover, from these preliminary studies, it is possible to affirm that the timing of the first cleavage gives some understanding of the implantation potential of embryos coming from cryopreserved eggs.

CLINICAL RESULTS OF OOCYTE CRYOPRESERVATION

The first pregnancy achieved with cryopreserved human oocytes was obtained by Chen in 1986 (14). The author, on the basis of the high survival rates obtained with cryopreserved mouse oocytes, adopted the same technique to cryopreserve human eggs, mechanically reducing the cumulus oophorus and using DMSO as the cryoprotectant.

From this event onwards, several steps forward have been taken, leading to numerous studies validating the technique (3,31,78). The first approach applied to oocytes was the same as for the freezing of embryos developed by Lassalle et al. (32), based on the use of solutions 1.5 M PROH plus 0.1 M sucrose (loading) for freezing and progressive dilutions of PROH (1.0 and 0.5 M) with an unchanged concentration of sucrose (0.2 M) for thawing. Unfortunately, the results were not comparable with the embryo outcomes.

The first preliminary results regarding survival, fertilization, and embryonic development using human eggs were provided by Gook and colleagues (31,79), but the first pregnancy and subsequent live birth with this protocol combined with ICSI as a method of insemination dates back to 1997 (8).

In 2004, our group (4) provided the first data on a significant number of patients (68 pairs), showing an implantation rate of 16.4% and a good percentage of pregnancies per transfer (25.4%), despite the low survival and fertilization rates (37% and 45.4%, respectively). Over the years, with the aim of improving biological and clinical results, the freezing protocol has therefore undergone several changes.

The turning point arrived in 2001 when Fabbri et al. (2) increased the concentration of sucrose to 0.1 M (34%), 0.2 M (60%), and 0.3 M (82%) in the solutions of both freezing and thawing, reported higher percentages of recovery after thawing. The exposure times were maintained unchanged, and so was the lowering temperature curve. Consequently, the increase in survival could be directly correlated with greater dehydration of the oocyte. The reduced amount of water inside the cell avoided ice crystal formation, improving post-thaw recovery.

The increase of non-permeating cryoprotectants led to greater dehydration of the oocyte and, consequently, a higher survival rate. Several authors (80–82) subsequently confirmed the improvement provided by these variations; Chen (82) obtained survival (75%) and fertilization rates (67%) comparable to those described by Fabbri et al. (2) and satisfactory pregnancy and implantation rates (33% and 11%, respectively).

Later, due to a change in Italian law (40/2004), oocyte cryopreservation became an important tool in the IVF routine. Since just three eggs could be inseminated and embryo freezing was not allowed, oocyte cryopreservation was the only option available to avoid repeated stimulation cycles. As a consequence, several reports have been published since then. In 2006, Chamayou et al. (72) compared results arising from fresh cycles and cycles of freezing (0.3 M sucrose) within the same cohort of oocytes. There were no significant differences in terms of fertilization between the two groups, while embryos derived from frozen oocytes showed a reduced rate of cleavage and significantly reduced embryo quality.

In 2006, by applying the same protocol to 146 patients and 201 cycles of freezing oocytes, our group (23) obtained satisfactory data in terms of survival and fertilization rates (74% and 76%, respectively), but low pregnancy and implantation rates per patient (12.3% and 5.2%, respectively). Further confirmation of these data came from other groups (5,83).

In 2007, in a retrospective study, De Santis et al. (25) compared the first protocol (0.1 M sucrose) with the one introduced by Fabbri et al. in 2001 (0.3 M sucrose) (2); the results showed significant improvements in survival and fertilization rates in the presence of high concentrations of sucrose, but higher pregnancy and implantation rates with 0.1 M sucrose. This study has allowed us to speculate that excessive dehydration of the oocyte could, to some extent, affect embryonic development.

Following this observation and the review of the initial protocol, in 2007, our group (18) introduced a fundamental change that has resulted in the maintenance of good survival (75.9%) and fertilization rates (76.2%) and, simultaneously, an improvement in pregnancy (21.8%) and implantation rates per patient (13.5%). The results obtained by this protocol have been confirmed in a further study published in 2012 (84). Bianchi et al. (18) tried to modulate sucrose concentrations during freezing–thawing in order to optimize the dehydration–rehydration conditions and to avoid excess shrinkage. In previous osmotic response experiments (85), it emerged that after around three minutes of exposure to 1.5 M PROH in the presence of 0.3 M sucrose, oocyte volume decreases rapidly, reaching values below the 30% threshold excursion, which may be detrimental to cell viability. With a reduced sucrose concentration (0.2 M), the 30% volume change is not reached until after 10 minutes of exposure. Therefore, dehydration may be achieved more slowly and less traumatically.

The employed procedure resumes in general the original idea of Lassalle et al. (32) while maintaining a difference in sucrose concentration between the freezing solution (0.2 M) and the thawing solution (0.3 M) (Table 20.3). On the one hand, this allows us to avoid excessive dehydration of the egg cell at the time of freezing and, on the other hand, to foster a more controlled rehydration during thawing.

In 2010, Borini et al. (86) published a final and homogeneous analysis of data that were derived from the comparison between fresh and oocyte freezing–thawing cycles offered by a multicenter observational study relating to eight IVF centers with a high number of patients. The protocol used a two-step PROH–sucrose-based solution and, out of 2046 patients, the overall survival rate was 55.8%. An overall pregnancy rate above 14% was achieved with a good degree of reproducibility in all the clinics. Regardless of the variability of the different clinics analyzed, the

Table 20.3 Schematic description of a slow cooling rate protocol involving the use of 0.2 and 0.3 mol/L sucrose for dehydration and rehydration, respectively

Dehydration		
Solution	**Time**	**Temperature**
1.5 mol/L PROH	10 minutes	24°C
1.5 mol/L PROH, 0.2 mol/L sucrose	5 minutes	24°C
Controlled-rate cooling		
Ramp	**Thermal interval**	
1	−20 to −8°C, −2.0°C/minute	
2	−8°C, hold for 10 minutes; seed at about 30% of ramp	
3	−8°C to −30°C, −0.3°C/minute	
4	−30°C to −150°C, −50.0°C/minute	
5	−150°C, hold for 10 minute, then plunge into LN_2	
Thawing		
Time	**Temperature**	
30 seconds	24°C	
40 seconds	30°C, water bath	
Rehydration		
Solution	**Time**	**Temperature**
1.0 mol/L PROH, 0.3 mol/L sucrose	5 minutes	24°C
0.5 mol/l PROH, 0.3 mol/L sucrose	5 minutes	24°C
0.3 mol/L sucrose	10 minutes	24°C
Buffer	10 minutes	24°C

Note: Solutions are prepared in phosphate-buffered saline media and supplemented with 10 mg/mL of human serum albumin.

Abbreviations: LN_2, liquid nitrogen; PROH, 1,2-propanediol.

percentage of success is greater in fresh cycles, but it is equally clear the additional result that oocyte cryopreservation brings to cumulative result for stimulating cycle. Considered the additional results obtained by thawing of cryopreserved oocytes, the probability per patients to get a live birth in a single ovarian stimulation cycle is increased compared to the probability given only by a fresh cycle.

In fact, if embryo cryopreservation is not possible or the risk of hyperstimulation syndrome is present, oocyte freezing should be offered to patients.

In 2014, Parmegiani et al. (87) evaluated and proposed the application of rapid warming in oocytes cryopreserved by the slow-freezing technique protocol (0.3 M sucrose). Following the warming, a group of oocytes were parthenogenetically activated and the other group was assigned for evaluation of the configuration of the meiotic spindle. Warmed oocytes show increased survival (90.2% vs. 74.6%; $p = 0.005$) and a greater number of blastomeres ($p = 0.042$) than those on which standard thawing had been applied.

It is possible to argue that, to date, oocyte cryopreservation has been one of the biggest steps forward in the optimization of clinical practice; indeed, improving the results arising from freezing gave us the chance to obtain a more satisfactory cumulative pregnancy rate.

SAFETY OF OOCYTE CRYOPRESERVATION

Another important aspect, besides the outcome, is the safety of oocyte cryopreservation. The first report that analyzed this issue was published by Porcu et al. in 2000 (88). The paper shows the results of obstetric complications, perinatal outcomes, and children's follow-up regarding 17 pregnancies from cryopreserved oocytes. These initial observations reported reassuring data about the children: no malformations have been reported and the follow-up showed normal physical and cognitive development in all of newborns.

These reassuring observations were confirmed in subsequent studies carried out on 70 children (88) and 105 babies (89). In the latter, a mean gestational age at birth of 38.9 weeks and a mean birth weight of 3353 g in singletons (73 babies) and 2599 g in twins (32 babies) were reported.

In 2009, Noyes et al. (90) published a report with more data on 963 babies born from cryopreserved oocytes using slow-freezing or vitrification techniques between 1986 and 2008. The number of babies born was almost the same using slow freezing and vitrification (308 from slow freezing, 289 from vitrification, and 12 from a combination of both protocols). The rate of single pregnancies was 81% compared to 19% for multiples. The rate of birth anomalies (1.3%) was found to be comparable with that of spontaneous pregnancy. The birth anomalies observed were three ventricular septal cardiac defects, one choanal atresia, one biliary atresia, one Rubinstein–Taybi syndrome, one club-foot, and one skin hemangioma.

Another review published in 2009 by Wennerholm et al. (91) reported data concerning children born from oocyte cryopreservation (148 from slow freezing and 221 from vitrification). Even though the data were limited, the weight at birth of newborns was within the normal range. These studies confirm that babies born from frozen oocytes have no significant differences in abnormalities compared with naturally conceived children.

In addition to this, information on the duration of storage (92) shows that there are no differences between oocytes cryopreserved with slow freezing and thawed after up to 48 months compared to earlier thaws in terms of survival, fertilization, cleavage, embryo quality, implantation, and live birth rates (Table 20.4).

A recent study published in 2015 (93) demonstrate that embryos that survived to cultures to the blastocyst stages after long-term oocyte cryopreservation display equivalent rates of aneuploidy, implantation, and live birth compared with blastocysts derived from fresh oocytes. The duration of oocyte cryostorage (3.5 years) suggests that long-term storage has no detrimental effect on chromosomal

Table 20.4 Recently reported rates of survival, fertilization, cleavage, and implantation following oocyte cryopreservation

Reference	Method	No. of thawed oocytes	Survival (%)	2PN (%)	Cleavage (%)	Implantation (%)
Borini et al. (23)	PROH/0.3–0.3 mmol/L sucrose	927	74.1	76.1	90.2	5.2
Boldt et al. (6)	PROH/Na-depleted	190	59.5	67.9	n.r.	15.9
Chamayou et al. (72)	PROH/0.3–0.3 mmol/L sucrose	337	78.0	67.9	77.3	5.6
Levi Setti et al. (24)	PROH/0.3–0.3 mmol/L sucrose	1087	69.0	67.5	89.1	5.7
Bianchi et al. (18)	PROH/0.2–0.3 mmol/L sucrose	325	75.1	77.3	93.0	16.7
De Santis et al. (25)	PROH/0.3–0.3 mmol/L sucrose	396	71.2	80.4	91.0	5.7
Parmegiani et al. (26)	PROH/0.3–0.3 mmol/L sucrose	437	75.1	86.0	87.2	9.6
Konc et al. (68)	PROH/0.3–0.3 mmol/L sucrose	110	76.0	76.0	86.0	15.4
Magli et al. (76)	PROH/0.3–0.3 mmol/L sucrose	997	72.8	73.0	88.0	n.r.
Borini et al. (86)	PROH/0.2–0.3 mmol/L sucrose	5093	55.8	73.8	n.r.	10.1
Gook et al. (12)	PROH/0.2–0.2 mmol/L sucrose	289	75.8	67.6	90.5	18.2
Bianchi et al. (84)	PROH/0.2–0.3 mmol/L sucrose	2458	71.8	77.9	94.5	13.5

Abbreviations: 2PN, two pronuclei; PROH, 1,2-propanediol; n.r., not recorded.

competence or live birth outcomes, further supporting the safety and efficacy of this rapidly growing technology. Consequently, oocyte cryopreservation techniques should no longer be considered experimental (94).

SUMMARY

Cryopreservation of human oocytes is an important tool used in the IVF routine, as it deals successfully with legal, ethical, and moral issues related to embryo cryopreservation.

This technique may be used in different situations: to rescue cycles complicated by ovarian hyperstimulation syndrome; when there is failure to obtain sperm; in oocyte donation programs; in the treatment of congenital infertility disorders or POF; as an alternative to embryo freezing; or, for fertile women, as an alternative to electively delays of childbearing. Freezing of supernumerary oocytes is the best way to optimize stimulation cycles and cumulative results. Oocyte cryopreservation also provides an option for single women to undergo gonadotoxic treatments that may compromise their chances to conceive. The structural features of mature human oocytes mean that their cryopreservation is fraught with complex difficulties; indeed, after the initial disappointment due to the low survival rate, several changes have been made over the years to cryopreservation methods in order to improve results in terms of biological and clinical outcomes. The fertilization and cleavage performance levels of frozen–thawed oocytes are now not so different from those of fresh sibling oocytes. What now becomes clear is the fact that certain oocyte cryopreservation protocols may affect cell division and have thus been associated with low implantation rates. Other freezing methods instead seem not to affect the post-implantation development and are going to be used in laboratories as alternatives to embryo freezing.

Some studies that have also analyzed the safety of oocyte cryopreservation demonstrate that live birth rates from cryopreserved eggs do not significantly differ in terms of abnormalities compared with naturally conceived children.

VIDEOS

Video 20.1 Oocyte slow freezing. The video shows the first freezing step in which the oocytes are exposed to the equilibration solution and subsequently to the loading solution. In this last one is visible as, with the addition of non-permeating cryoprotectant (sucrose), greater shrinkage with a stronger reduction of the cell volume takes place. https://youtu.be/tTjI4KONANc

Video 20.2 Oocyte thawing. The video shows exposure to solutions with decreasing concentrations of cryoprotectants during thawing procedures, leading to gradual oocyte rehydration. https://youtu.be/O2v7_bapYIY

REFERENCES

1. Fabbri R, Porcu E, Marsella T et al. Oocyte cryopreservation. *Hum Reprod* 1998; 13(Suppl 4): 98–108.
2. Fabbri R, Porcu E, Marsella T, Rocchetta G, Venturoli S, Flamigni C. Human oocyte cryopreservation: New perspectives regarding oocyte survival. *Hum Reprod* 2001; 16: 411–6.
3. Porcu E, Fabbri R, Damiano G et al. Clinical experience and applications of oocyte cryopreservation. *Mol Cell Endocrinol* 2000; 169: 33–7.
4. Borini A, Bonu MA, Coticchio G, Bianchi V, Cattoli M, Flamigni C. Pregnancies and births after oocyte cryopreservation. *Fertil Steril* 2004; 82: 601–5.
5. Levi Setti PE, Albani E, Novara PV, Cesana A, Morreale G. Cryopreservation of supernumerary oocytes in IVF/ICSI cycles. *Hum Reprod* 2006; 21: 370–5.
6. Boldt J, Tidswell N, Sayers A, Kilani R, Cline D. Human oocyte cryopreservation: 5-year experience with a sodium-depleted slow freezing method. *Reprod Biomed Online* 2006; 13: 96–100.
7. Ubaldi F, Anniballo R, Romano S et al. Cumulative ongoing pregnancy rate achieved with oocyte vitrification and cleavage stage transfer without embryo selection in a standard infertility program. *Hum Reprod* 2010; 25: 1199–205.
8. Porcu E, Fabbri R, Seracchioli R, Ciotti PM, Magrini O, Flamigni C. Birth of a healthy female after intracytoplasmic sperm injection of cryopreserved human oocytes. *Fertil Steril* 1997; 68: 724–6.
9. Levi Setti PE, Porcu E, Patrizio P, Vigiliano V, de Luca R, d'Aloja P, Spoletini R, Scaravelli G. Human oocyte cryopreservation with slow freezing versus vitrification. Results from the National Italian Registry data, 2007–2011. *Fertil Steril* 2014; 102(1): 90–95.
10. Yang D, Brown SE, Nguyen K et al. Live birth after the transfer of human embryos developed from cryopreserved oocytes harvested before cancer treatment. *Fertil Steril* 2007; 87(6): 1469.e1–1469.e4.
11. Porcu E, Venturoli S, Damiano G et al. Healthy twins delivered after oocyte cryopreservation and bilateral ovariectomy for ovarian cancer. *Reprod Biomed Online* 2008; 17(2): 265–7.
12. Gook DA, Edgar DH. Implantation rates of embryos generated from slow cooled human oocytes from young women are comparable to those of fresh and frozen embryos from the same age group. *J Assist Reprod Genet* 2011; 28(12): 1171–6.
13. Whittingham DG. Fertilization *in vitro* and development to term of unfertilized mouse oocytes previously stored at −196°C. *J Reprod Fertil* 1977; 49: 89–94.
14. Chen C. Pregnancy after human oocyte cryopreservation. *Lancet* 1986; 1(8486): 884–6.
15. Al-Hasani S, Diedrich K, van der Ven H, Krebs D. Initial results of the cryopreservation of human oocytes. *Geburtshilfe Frauenheilkd* 1986; 46(9): 643–4.
16. Stacheki JJ, Willadsen SM. Cryopreservation of mouse oocytes using a medium with low sodium content: Effect of plunge temperature. *Cryobiology* 2000; 40: 4–12.

17. Boldt J, Tidswell N, Sayers A, Kilani R, Cline D. Human oocytes cryopreservation: 5-year experience with a sodium-depleted slow freezing method. *Reprod Biomed Online* 2006; 13: 96–100.
18. Bianchi V, Coticchio G, Distratis V et al. Differential sucrose concentration during dehydration (0.2 mol/L) and rehydration (0.3 mol/L) increases the implantation rate of frozen human oocytes. *Reprod Biomed Online* 2007; 14: 64–71.
19. Elliot K, Whelan J (eds). *CIBA Foundation Symposium 52—The Freezing of Mammalian Embryos.* Amsterdam, The Netherlands: Elsevier, 1977.
20. Ashwood-Smith MJ, Farrant J. (eds). *Low Temperature Preservation in Medicine and Biology.* Bath, U.K.: Pitman Press, 1980.
21. Pickering SJ, Johnson MH. The influence of cooling on the organization of the meiotic spindle of the mouse oocyte. *Hum Reprod* 1987; 2: 207–16.
22. Ashwood-Smith MJ. Mechanisms of cryoprotectant action. *Symp Soc Exp Biol* 1987; 41: 395–406.
23. Borini A, Sciajno R, Bianchi V, Sereni E, Flamigni C, Coticchio G. Clinical outcome of oocyte cryopreservation after slow cooling with a protocol utilizing a high sucrose concentration. *Hum Reprod* 2006; 21(2): 512–7.
24. Levi Setti PE, Albani E, Novara PB et al. Cryopreservation of supernumerary oocytes in IVF/ICSI cycles. *Hum Reprod* 2006; 21: 370–5.
25. De Santis L, Cino I, Rabellotti E, Papaleo E, Calzi F, Fusi FM, Brigante C, Ferrari A. Oocyte cryopreservation: Clinical outcome of slow-cooling protocols differing in sucrose concentration. *Reprod Biomed Online* 2007; 14(1): 57–63.
26. Parmegiani L, Cognigni GE, Bernardi S et al. Freezing within 2 h from oocytes retrieval increases the efficiency of human oocyte cryopreservation when using slow freezing/rapid protocol with high sucrose concentration. *Hum Reprod* 2008; 23: 1771–7.
27. Paynter SJ, O'Neil L, Fuller BJ, Shaw RW. Membrane permeability of human oocytes in the presence of the cryoprotectant propane-1,2-diol. *Fertil Steril* 2001; 75: 532–8.
28. De Santis L, Coticchio G, Paynter S, Albertini D, Hutt K, Cino I, Iaccarino M, Gambardella A, Flamigni C, Borini A. Permeability of human oocytes to ethylene glycol and their survival and spindle configurations after slow cooling cryopreservation. *Hum Reprod* 2007; 22: 2776–83.
29. Eroglu A, Toner M, Toth T. Beneficial effect of micro-injected trehalose on the cryosurvival of human oocytes. *Fertil Steril* 2002; 77: 152–8.
30. Wright D, Eroglu A, Toner M, Toth T. Use of sugar in cryopreservation of human oocytes. *Reprod Biomed Online* 2004; 9: 179–86.
31. Gook DA, Osborn SM, Johnston WI. Cryopreservation of mouse and human oocytes using 1,2-propanediol and the configuration of the meiotic spindle. *Hum Reprod* 1993; 8: 1101–9.
32. Lassalle B, Testart J, Renard JP. Human embryo features that influence the success of cryopreservation with the use of 1,2 propanediol. *Fertil Steril* 1985; 44: 645–51.
33. Ebner T, Moser M, Tews G. Is oocyte morphology prognostic of embryo developmental potential after ICSI? *Reprod Biomed Online* 2006; 12: 507–12.
34. Balaban B, Urman B, Sertac A, Alatas C, Aksoy S, Mercan R. Oocyte morphology does not affect fertilization rate, embryo quality and implantation rate after intracytoplasmic sperm injection. *Hum Reprod* 1998; 13: 3431–3.
35. Balaban B, Urman B. Effect of oocyte morphology on embryo development and implantation. *Reprod Biomed Online* 2006; 12: 608–15.
36. Balakier H, Bouman D, Sojecki A, Librach C, Squire JA. Morphological and cytogenetic analysis of human giant oocytes and giant embryos. *Hum Reprod* 2002; 17: 2394–401.
37. Lappi M, Magli MC, Muzzonigro F et al. Early time of freezing affects the clinical outcome of oocyte cryopreservation. *Hum Reprod* 2009; 24(Suppl 1): 90.
38. Ghetler Y, Skutelsky E, Ben Nun I, Ben Dor L, Amihai D, Shalgi R. Human oocyte cryopreservation and the fate of cortical granules. *Fertil Steril* 2006; 86: 210–6.
39. Carroll J, Depypere H, Matthews CD. Freeze–thaw-induced changes of the zona pellucida explains decreased rates of fertilization in frozen–thawed mouse oocytes. *J Reprod Fert* 1990; 90: 547–53.
40. Carroll J, Wood MJ, Whittingham DG. Normal fertilization and development of frozen thawed mouse oocytes: Protective action of certain macromolecules. *Biol Reprod* 1993; 48: 606–12.
41. Palermo G, Joris H, Devroey P, Van Steirteghem AC. Pregnancies after intracytoplasmic injection of single spermatozoon into an oocyte. *Lancet* 1992; 340: 17–8.
42. Gook DA, Schiewe MC, Osborn SM, Asch RH, Jansen RP, Johnston WI. Intracytoplasmic sperm injection and embryo development of human oocytes cryopreserved using 1,2-propanediol. *Hum Reprod* 1995; 10: 2637–41.
43. Kazem R, Thompson LA, Srikantharajah A, Laing MA, Hamilton MPR, Templeton A. Cryopreservation of human oocytes and fertilization by two techniques: *In-vitro* fertilization and intracytoplasmic sperm injection. *Hum Reprod* 1995; 10: 2650–4.
44. Gook DA, Edgar DH. Human oocyte cryopreservation. *Hum Reprod Update* 2007; 13: 591–605.
45. Sathananthan AH, Kirby C, Trounson A, Philipatos D, Shaw J. The effects of cooling mouse oocytes. *J Assist Reprod Genet* 1992; 9: 139–48.
46. Zenzes MT, Bielecki R, Casper RF, Leibo SP. Effects of chilling to 0 degrees C on the morphology of meiotic spindles in human metaphase II oocytes. *Fertil Steril* 2001; 75: 769–77.
47. Kopeika J, Thornhill A, Khalaf Y. The effect of cryopreservation on the genome of gametes and embryos: Principles of cryobiology and critical appraisal of the evidence. *Hum Reprod Update* 2015; 21: 209–27.

48. Stachecki JJ, Munne S, Cohen J. Spindle organization after cryopreservation of mouse, human, and bovine oocytes. *Reprod Biomed Online* 2004; 8: 664–77.
49. Oldenbourg R. A new view on polarization microscopy. *Nature* 1996; 381: 811–2.
50. Wang WH, Meng L, Hackett RJ, Oldenbourg R, Keefe DL. Limited recovery of meiotic spindles in living human oocytes after cooling–rewarming observed using polarized light microscopy. *Hum Reprod* 2001; 16: 2374–8.
51. Rienzi L, Martinez F, Ubaldi F et al. PolScope analysis of meiotic spindle changes in living metaphase II human oocytes during the freezing and thawing procedures. *Hum Reprod* 2004; 19: 655–9.
52. Bianchi V, Coticchio G, Fava L et al. Meiotic spindle imaging in human oocytes frozen with a slow freezing procedure involving high sucrose concentration. *Hum Reprod* 2005; 20: 1078–83.
53. Sereni E, Sciajno R, Fava L et al. A PolScope evaluation of meiotic spindle dynamics in frozen–thaw oocytes. *Reprod Biomed Online* 2009; 19: 191–7.
54. Bromfield JJ, Coticchio G, Hutt K et al. Meiotic spindle dynamics in human oocytes following slow-cooling cryopreservation. *Hum Reprod* 2009; 24: 2114–23.
55. Coticchio G, Sciajno R, Hutt K et al. Comparative analysis of the metaphase II spindle of human oocytes through polarized light and high-performance confocal microscopy. *Fertil Steril* 2010; 93: 2056–64.
56. Sathananthan AH, Trounson A, Freeman L, Brady T. The effects of cooling human oocytes. *Hum Reprod* 1988; 3: 968–77.
57. Nottola SA, Coticchio G, De Santis L et al. Ultrastructural of human mature oocytes after slow cooling cryopreservation using different sucrose concentrations. *Hum Reprod* 2007; 22: 1123–33.
58. Gualtieri R, Iaccarino M, Mollo V, Prisco M, Iaccarino S, Talevi R. Slow cooling of human oocytes: Ultrastructural injuries and apoptotic status. *Fert Steril* 2009; 91: 1023–34.
59. Bianchi V, Macchiarelli G, Borini A, Lappi M, Cecconi S, Miglietta S, Familiari G, Nottola SA. Fine morphological assessment of quality of human mature oocytes after slow freezing or vitrification with a closed device: A comparative analysis. *Reprod Biol Endocrinol* 2014; 12: 110.
60. Gualtieri R, Mollo V, Barbato V, Fiorentino I, Iaccarino M, Talevi R. Ultrastructure and intracellular calcium response during activation in vitrified and slow-frozen human oocytes. *Hum Reprod* 2011; 26: 2452–60.
61. Mazur P, Rall WF, Leibo SP. Kinetics of water loss and the likelihood of intracellular freezing in mouse ova. Influence of the method of calculating the temperature dependence of water permeability. *Cell Biophys* 1984; 6: 197–213.
62. Al-Hasani S, Diedrich K, van der Ven H, Reinecke A, Hartje M, Krebs D. Cryopreservation of human oocytes. *Hum Reprod* 1987; 2: 695–700.
63. van Uem JF, Siebzehnrübl ER, Schuh B, Koch R, Trotnow S, Lang N. Birth after cryopreservation of unfertilized oocytes. *Lancet* 1987 1: 752–3.
64. Mandelbaum J, Junca AM, Plachot M, Alnot MO, Salat-Baroux J, Alvarez S, Tibi C, Cohen J, Debache C, Tesquier L. Cryopreservation of human embryos and oocytes. *Hum Reprod* 1988; 3(1): 117–9.
65. Siebzehnruebl ER, Todorow S, van Uem J, Koch R, Wildt L, Lang N. Cryopreservation of human and rabbit oocytes and one-cell embryos: A comparison of DMSO and propanediol. *Hum Reprod* 1989; 4(3): 312–7.
66. Chen SU, Lien YR, Tsai YY, Chang LJ, Ho HN, Yang YS. Successful pregnancy occurred from slowly freezing human oocytes using the regime of 1.5 mol/L 1,2-propanediol with 0.3 mol/L sucrose. *Hum Reprod* 2002; 17: 1412.
67. La Sala GB, Nicoli A, Villani MT, Pescarini M, Gallinelli A, Blickstein I. Outcome of 518 salvage oocyte-cryopreservation cycles performed as a routine procedure in an *in vitro* fertilization program. *Fertil Steril* 2006; 86(5): 1423–7.
68. Konc J, Kanyo K, Varga E, Kriston R, Cseh S. Births resulting from oocyte cryopreservation using a slow freezing protocol with propanediol and sucrose. *Syst Biol Reprod Med* 2008; 54: 205–10.
69. Yang D, Blohm P, Winslow K, Cramer L. A twin pregnancy after microinjection of human cryopreserved oocyte with a specially developed oocyte cryopreservation regime. *Fertil Steril* 1998; 70(Suppl 1): S239.
70. Winslow K, Yang D, Blohm P, Brown S, Jossim P, Nguyen K. Oocyte cryopreservation/a three year follow up of sixteen births. *Fertil Steril* 2001; 76(Suppl 1): S120–1.
71. Gook DA, Hale L, Edgar DH. Live birth following transfer of a cryopreserved embryo generated from a cryopreserved oocyte and a cryopreserved sperm: Case report. *J Assist Reprod Genet* 2007; 24: 43–5.
72. Chamayou S, Alecci C, Ragolia C, Storaci G, Maglia E, Russo E, Guglielmino A. Comparison of *in-vitro* outcomes from cryopreserved oocytes and sibling fresh oocytes. *Reprod Biomed Online* 2006; 12: 730–6.
73. Bianchi V, Lappi M, Bonu MA, Borini A. Elapsing time: A variable to consider in oocyte cryopreservation. *Hum Reprod* 2011; 26(Suppl 1): 197.
74. Edgar DH, Archer J, Bourne H. The application and impact of cryopreservation of early cleavage stage embryos in assisted reproduction. *Hum Fertil (Camb)* 2005; 8: 225–30.
75. Bianchi V, Coticchio G, Distratis V, Di Giusto N, Borini A. Early cleavage delay in cryopreserved human oocytes. *Hum Reprod* 2005; 20(Suppl 1): i54.
76. Magli MC, Lappi M, Ferraretti AP, Capoti A, Ruberti A, Gianaroli L. Impact of oocyte cryopreservation on embryo development. *Fertil Steril* 2010; 93: 510–6.

77. Coticchio G, Distratis V, Bianchi V et al. Fertilization and early developmental ability of cryopreserved human oocytes is not affected compared to sibling fresh oocytes. *Fertil Steril* 2007; 88(Suppl 1): 340.
78. Gook DA, Osborn SM, Bourne H, Johnston WI. Fertilization of human oocytes following cryopreservation; normal karyotypes and absence of stray chromosomes. *Hum Reprod* 1994; 9: 684–91.
79. Gook DA, Edgar DH. Cryopreservation of the human female gamete: Current and future issues. *Hum Reprod* 1999; 14: 2938–40.
80. Li XH, Chen SU, Zhang X, Tang M, Kui YR, Wu X, Wang S, Guo YL. Cryopreserved oocytes of infertile couples undergoing assisted reproductive technology could be an important source of oocyte donation: A clinical report of successful pregnancies. *Hum Reprod* 2005; 20: 3390–94.
81. Fosas N, Marina F, Torres PJ, Jové I, Martin P. Péerez N, Arnedo N, Marina S. The births of five Spanish babies from cryopreserved donated oocytes. *Hum Reprod* 2003; 18: 1417–21.
82. Chen SU, Lien YR, Chen HF, Chang LJ, Tsai YY, Yang YS. Observational clinical follow-up of oocyte cryopreservation using a slow-freezing method with 1,2-propanediol Plus sucrose followed by ICSI. *Hum Reprod* 2005; 20: 1975–80.
83. La Sala GB, Nicoli A, Villani MT, Pescarini M, Gallinelli A, Blickstein I. Outcome of 518 salvage oocyte cryopreservation cycles performed as routine procedure in an *in vitro* fertilization program. *Fertil Steril* 2006; 86: 1423–7.
84. Bianchi V, Lappi M, Bonu MA, Borini A. Oocyte slow freezing using a 0.2–0.3 M sucrose concentration protocol: Is it really the time to trash the cryopreservation machine? *Fertil Steril* 2012; 97(5): 1101–7.
85. Paynter SJ, Borini A, Bianchi V et al. Volume changes of mature human oocytes on exposure to cryoprotectant solutions used in slow cooling procedures. *Hum Reprod* 2005; 20: 1194–8.
86. Borini A, Levi Setti P.E, Anserini P, De Luca R, De Santis L, Porcu E, La Sala GB, Ferraretti A, Bartolotti T, Coticchio G, Scaravelli G. Multicentric observational study on slow-cooling oocyte cryopreservation: Clinical outcome. *Fertil Steril* 2010; 94: 1662–8.
87. Parmegiani L, Tatone C, Cognigni GE, Bernardi S, Troilo E, Arnone A, Maccarini AM, Di Emidio G, Vitti M, Filicori M. Rapid warming increases survival of slow-frozen sibling oocytes: A step towards a single warming procedure irrespective of the freezing protocol? *Reprod Biomed Online* 2014; 33: 614–23.
88. Porcu E, Fabbri R, Damiano G, Giunchi S, Fratto R, Ciotti PM, Venturoli S, Flamigni C. Clinical experience and applications of oocyte cryopreservation. *Mol Cell Endocrinol* 2000; 169: 33–7.
89. Borini A, Bianchi V, Bonu MA, Sciajno R, Sereni E, Cattoli M, Mazzone S, Trevisi MR, Iadarola I, Distratis V, Nalon M, Coticchio G. Evidence-based clinical outcome of oocyte slow cooling. *Reprod Biomed Online* 2007; 15: 175–81.
90. Noyes N, Porcu E, Borini A. Over 900 oocyte cryopreservation babies born with no apparent increase in congenital anomalies. *Reprod Biomed Online* 2009; 18: 769–76.
91. Wennerholm UB, Söderström-Anttila V, Bergh C, Aittomäki K, Hazekamp J, Nygren KG, Selbing A, Loft A. Children born after cryopreservation of embryos or oocytes: A systematic review of outcome data. *Hum Reprod* 2009; 24: 2158–72.
92. Parmegiani L, Garello C, Granella F, Guidetti D, Bernardi S, Cognigni GE, Revelli A, Filicori M. Long-term cryostorage does not adversely affect the outcome of oocyte thawing cycles. *Reprod Biomed Online* 2009; 19: 374–9.
93. Goldman KN, Kramer Y, Hodes-Wertz B, Noyes N, McCaffrey C, Grifo JA. Long-term cryopreservation of human oocytes does not increase embryonic aneuploidy. *Fertil Steril* 2015; 103: 662–8.
94. Practice Committees of American Society for Reproductive Medicine; Society for Assisted Reproductive Technology. Mature oocyte cryopreservation: A guideline. *Fertil Steril* 2013; 99: 37–43.

21 The human oocyte

Vitrification

MASASHIGE KUWAYAMA

INTRODUCTION

The past 50 years have yielded impressive breakthroughs in cryopreservation as applied to the discipline of reproductive biology. Techniques were usually derived in experimental and domestic animals and subsequently applied to humans. The first success in freezing cells was achieved in spermatozoa (1), followed by successful cryopreservation of preimplantation embryos at different stages of development (2–4). Since the first report in 1972 of the cryopreservation of mammalian embryos resulting in the birth of live mice offspring (2), attempts to cryopreserve human oocytes, similar to the results with oocytes of domestic animals, mostly failed for many years. However, the development of an ultra-rapid vitrification method now means that oocytes can be cryopreserved without loss of their viability, and such oocytes may be used clinically (5).

The reasons to cryopreserve human oocytes are widely known and were summarized recently (6,7). Common indications for this procedure include diseases and their treatments (i.e., to preserve the reproductive competence of young cancer patients who need irradiation of the pelvic region or chemotherapy, or who require surgical intervention before or during their reproductive age that may involve removal of ovaries). Another reason for cryopreservation is when patients have problems resulting from ovarian malfunction, including premature menopause, ovarian hyperstimulation syndrome, or poor response to ovarian stimulation. There are also legal, ethical, social, and practical problems that may require oocyte cryopreservation: some countries restrict or prohibit embryo cryopreservation, which only leaves the option to preserve oocytes; women may wish to delay motherhood for various reasons, such as career priorities; and there may be cases where there is no semen available after a successful oocyte retrieval, to mention a few examples.

However, as discussed in detail recently (6–9), in broader terms, oocyte cryopreservation is also needed to compensate for the unique situation of women in regards to reproduction. As in most mammalian species, women suffer more and sacrifice more for their offspring both physically and emotionally. Yet a woman's reproductive capability is restricted in terms of quantity and duration. Males produce millions of sperm in a single ejaculation, while females ovulate only one or two mature oocytes every 28 days. From the time that he reaches puberty, a man's reproductive capability is almost unlimited, while that of a woman (without considering special treatments) is limited to a period of just 15–20 years. Assisted reproductive techniques did not eliminate this difference. In fact, with the introduction of the procedure of intracytoplasmic sperm injection (ICSI) and successful cryopreservation of sperm, the gap has widened considerably. Apart from the practical goals, our moral duty is to help develop an efficient and safe oocyte cryopreservation method to enhance the reproductive capability of women.

Unfortunately, the task is rather demanding. Although the first pregnancy from a cryopreserved oocyte was achieved about 30 years ago (10), advances until recently were very slow. Generally, inefficiency and lack of consistency were the two main problems (11). Oocytes are unique cells; their large size, spherical shape, single cell number, and general fragility explain many of the difficulties that occur during cryopreservation.

Oocytes are often described as the largest cells of the mammalian body, and this represents a real challenge in cryopreservation. Cell volume is known to be a crucial parameter that determines the likelihood of success when a cell is cryopreserved. Viruses and bacteria, which have a very tiny volume, may survive deep freezing without any special treatment, such as use of cryoprotectants or controlled-rate cooling. Freezing of fibroblasts or epidermal cells is usually an easy and efficient routine task in tissue culture laboratories, and does not need any special instruments. Sperm cryopreservation can be efficiently performed with the use of a controlled-rate freezer. Early cleavage-stage embryos with individual blastomeres having 50% to as little as 10% of the original size of oocytes survive traditional slow-rate freezing very well, and their developmental competence is usually well preserved. Preantral and primary follicles can also be frozen successfully, in contrast to the large, fully developed, metaphase II (MII)-stage oocytes.

The near-spherical shape of the oocyte does not confer an advantage from the point of view of cryopreservation. During equilibration and dilution before and after cooling and warming, permeable cryoprotectants must be distributed rapidly and uniformly throughout the ooplasm. A large spherical object, such as an oocyte, has the lowest surface area/volume ratio of any geometric shape. An irregular object, such as a fibroblast or lymphocyte, has a much larger surface area/volume ratio and will equilibrate osmotically much faster than an oocyte.

The one-cell stage of an oocyte also severely limits options, as there is no margin for error. The single cell survives or it does not. Multicellular embryos may survive and develop even if more than 50% of their cells are damaged.

(This fact is clearly demonstrated by successful births resulting from bisected embryos of domestic animals.)

However, apart from the size, shape, and cell number, other factors may also play important roles in limiting successful oocyte cryopreservation. Germinal vesicle (GV)-stage oocytes and fertilized zygotes have almost exactly the same characteristics. However, zygotes are considerably more resistant to cryoinjuries, while GV-stage oocytes are even more sensitive than MII-stage oocytes. Factors that are known to influence their sensitivity include chilling injury, serious deformation of shape during exposure to and/or removal of cryoprotectants, and hardening of the zona pellucida.

Chilling injury is probably one of the least understood types of injuries during cryopreservation, involving damage to lipid droplets, lipid-rich membranes, and microtubules. The temperature zone at which such injury occurs is rather high, between +15°C (in some biological objects +20°C) and −5°C (12). The damage to lipids is irreversible and causes death of the oocytes. Compared to other species, the lipid content of human oocytes is relatively low. Yet, their sensitivity to chilling is still considerable, probably caused by membrane damage and depolymerization of microtubules, with all of the subsequent consequences, including misalignment of chromosomes and aneuploidy (13–17); however, the latter effect may be less detrimental than previously supposed (18). Chilling damage of membranes in human mature oocytes seems to be much more serious than at later developmental stages (e.g., zygotes), a possible cause for the well-known stage-dependent sensitivity (19).

As a result of osmotic effects, serious deformation of their shape may occur when oocytes are exposed to cryoprotectant solutions. However, in spite of the somewhat peculiar morphology that oocytes may exhibit during exposure to cryoprotectants, they do seem to tolerate these deformations rather well. Careful addition of cryoprotectants may minimize the deleterious effects of such morphological alterations. An alternative strategy, such as addition of cytoskeleton relaxants used with porcine embryos (20), may not be required in the human. On the other hand, during removal of the cryoprotectant, the spherical shape of the oocyte may allow only a minimal expansion; accordingly, the inrushing water may disrupt the cell membrane.

VITRIFICATION VERSUS TRADITIONAL FREEZING

During the past four decades, two major strategies for the cryopreservation of oocytes and embryos in mammalian species have been developed (21). Traditional slow-rate freezing establishes a delicate balance between various sources of injuries, while the principal goal of vitrification is to eliminate ice crystal formation entirely in the whole solution containing the embryos and oocytes. To achieve this ice-free, glass-like solidification of solutions, which may also be defined as an extremely increased viscosity, high cryoprotectant concentrations and/or very high cooling rates are required. To decrease the potential osmotic and toxic damage caused by cryoprotectants, recent vitrification methods have focused on increasing the cooling and warming rates (22–25). Most successful vitrification methods are based on use of extremely small volumes of solution containing the specimens and direct contact between this solution and liquid nitrogen.

One of these approaches—the minimum drop size method—was first applied by Arav (26), and further modified by Hamawaki et al. (27). Based on these earlier results, a novel method, called the Cryotop vitrification technique, was developed for the cryopreservation of oocytes and embryos (28). The Cryotop method has been used successfully to cryopreserve embryos from a wide variety of mammalian species, and has resulted in a considerable increase in the overall efficiency of the cryopreservation of human oocytes and embryos (29–32). More recently, based on these huge results and experiences using the Cryotop method for over 2 million clinical cases for 12 years in 65 countries, a noninvasive, 100% survival vitrification method called the Cryotec method was established by Dr. Kuwayama, again for the standard clinical protocol for human oocytes and embryos (7,33).

USE OF THE CRYOTEC VITRIFICATION METHOD TO CRYOPRESERVE HUMAN MII-PHASE OOCYTES

The following is a description of the steps that should be followed carefully to utilize the Cryotec method to its full capability.

Timing

Oocytes can be vitrified between one and six hours after ovum pick-up, and immediately after denudation (cumulus cell removal). ICSI can be performed within two to four hours after the oocytes have been warmed. This short time of culture is required to allow the oocytes to recover the plasticity of their membranes during the puncture by the ICSI needle.

Device

The Cryotec consists of a 1.0-mm wide, 20-mm long, 0.075-mm thick flexible filmstrip attached to a rigid plastic handle (Figure 21.1a). To protect the filmstrip and the sample cryopreserved on it, a 30-mm long transparent plastic cap is also provided to cover this part during storage in liquid nitrogen (Figure 21.1b). The device is sterilized, and should be handled under aseptic conditions and only for one cycle of vitrification.

Solutions

Media for all phases of vitrification are listed in Table 21.1. All solutions are serum and protein free.

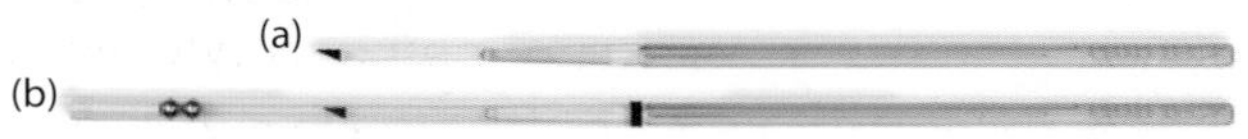

Figure 21.1 Cryotec vitrification container (a) without and (b) with cover cap.

Table 21.1 Solutions used for Cryotec vitrification

Name	Basic medium	Permeable cryoprotectants	Non-permeable cryoprotectants
Washing solution	m-MEM + HPC	–	–
Equlibration solution	m-MEM + HPC	7% EG, 7% DMSO	–
Vitrification solution	m-MEM + HPC	14.5% EG, 14.5% DMSO	0.5 M trehalose (endotoxin free)
Thawing solution	m-MEM + HPC	–	1.0 M trehalose (endotoxin free)
Dilution solution	m-MEM + HPC	–	0.5 M trehalose (endotoxin free)

Note: All chemicals except for those otherwise indicated are derived from Sigma Chemical Co. (St. Louis, MO).
Abbreviations: m-MEM, HEPES-buffered minimal essential medium; +HPC, maximum concentration of hydroxypropyl cellulose; EG, ethylene glycol; DMSO, dimethyl sulfoxide.

Working environment and preparation steps

The vitrification procedure has to be performed in a well-ventilated laboratory at room temperature of 25°C–27°C. Because all equilibration and dilution parameters described below were adjusted for this temperature, it is very important to warm media that have been stored in the refrigerator to 25°C–27°C. This is easily achieved by placing all the solutions and vials on a clean bench for more than one hour, preferably inside a laminar-flow hood. The only exception is the thawing solution (TS), which should be warmed to 37°C to obtain the highest warming rate of the vitrified oocytes. Note that the basic solution contains HEPES buffer as well as bicarbonate buffer, and has been adjusted to maintain the appropriate pH even when exposed to air. Therefore, a carbon dioxide incubator is not required for warming of solutions in closed vials.

Additional tools

Vitrification has to be performed in 300-μL volume three-well plates (Vitri-Plate, REPROLIFE, Tokyo, Japan; Figure 21.2). To obtain the optimum gradual change of osmolality of the extracellular solutions for the best post-thaw survival of the oocytes, it is very important that precise proportions of the volume of each solution and transferred solution be used. For practical reasons, a relatively small, thick-walled Styrofoam box (approximately 250 × 150 × 200 cm for length, width, and height) with a minimum of 3-cm thick walls and bottom is suggested, preferably with an appropriate Styrofoam cover. The box should be placed on a stable surface within easy reach but with little risk of accidentally spilling it or pouring off the liquid nitrogen. All safety instructions related to work with liquid nitrogen should be strictly followed. Points for selection of optimal sources and possible pre-treatment of liquid nitrogen will be discussed later. The Styrofoam box should also contain plastic racks for temporary storage of the device.

Cryotec vitrification requires adept handling of oocytes and embryos. For vitrification and warming, a relatively simple stereomicroscope equipped with a zoom lens and capable of providing sharp contrast images is appropriate. Except for special purposes, there is no need for an upright or inverted compound microscope or for fluorescent equipment. There is no need to restrict illumination if light sources are filtered for UV lights. Use microscope lights only when required.

Equilibration and cooling

Gently mix vials of pre-warmed equilibration solution (ES) and vitrification solution (VS) (one vial of each). Pour 300 μL of ES into well 1 and 300 μL of VS into wells 2 and 3 in the proper Vitri-Plate (Figure 21.2).

Before starting a vitrification procedure, check the quality and perivitelline space of the oocytes, compare it to the thickness of the zona pellucida, and record any characteristics that might affect oocyte survival. The equilibration and vitrification procedure consists of the following steps.

1. Place the oocytes in the center of the surface of the ES. The oocytes will begin to contract osmotically and they will sink by their own density to the bottom of the well (Figure 21.3).
2. Contraction of the oocytes should occur at the latest within 90 seconds after placing them into the ES. Wait for 12 minutes and observe the recovery of the oocytes. If full re-expansion of oocytes occurs (the perivitelline space should be the same as before equilibration), oocytes should be picked up for the next step. If the volumetric recovery of the oocytes is incomplete, continue the equilibration until 15 minutes all together. The recovery period can be used to prepare the liquid nitrogen container and to label the Cryotecs.

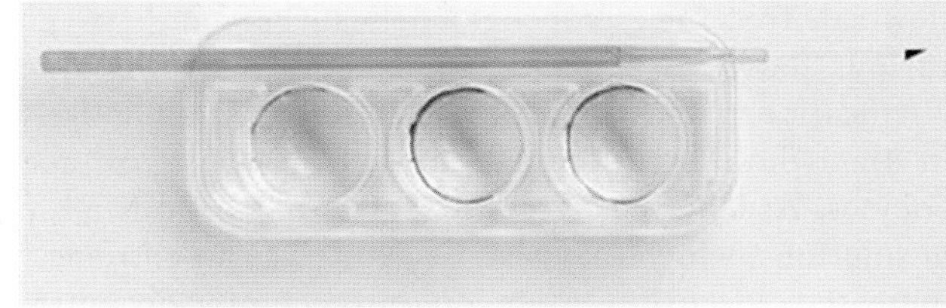

Figure 21.2 Vitrification plate.

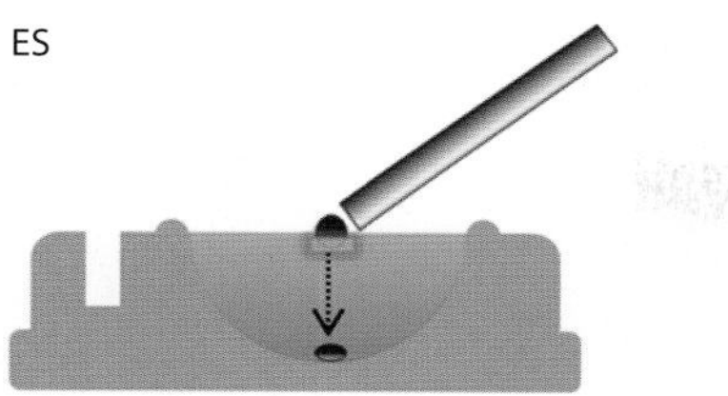

Figure 21.3 Equilibration of oocytes in ES. *Abbreviation*: ES, equilibration solution.

3. Pick up oocytes with the pipette and expel the oocytes at the middle depth of VS1 with ES. The oocytes will immediately float to the surface of VS1. Expel and wash the inside of the pipette with fresh VS, and pick up the oocytes and expel them again at the bottom of the VS. The oocytes will then very slowly float to the middle and stop. When the oocytes stop, it is the end of the equilibration step as the weight will have become the same inside and outside of the oocytes. Aspirate the oocytes at the tip of pipette to move to VS2 (Figure 21.4).
4. Expel the oocytes into the middle depth of VS2. Expel and aspirate fresh VS from the edge of the surface, and expel it outside of the well. Aspirate fresh VS2 again from the surface and mix the solution around the oocyte to confirm the oocytes to be shrunk in 3D (Figure 21.5). Expel and wash the inside of the pipette with fresh VS, and aspirate the oocytes at the tip of the pipette to put the oocytes onto the Cryotec set on the slit of the Vitri-Plate.
5. Pick up the oocytes with the pipette in the smallest possible amount of VS and place them on the strip of the Cryotec on the Vitri-Plate near the black triangle mark (Figure 21.6).
6. Immerse the Cryotec directly in the liquid nitrogen in the Styrofoam box and rapidly stir the Cryotec in the liquid nitrogen to obtain the maximum cooling rate (23,000°C/minute). While keeping the Cryotec submerged in liquid nitrogen, cover the strip of the Cryotec with the plastic cap using tweezers and then the fingers to ensure it is tightly closed (Figure 21.7).

Warming and dilution

An unopened vial of TS and a warming plate (Figure 21.8) should be pre-warmed to 37°C in an incubator for at least one hour. All other solutions should be kept at room temperature (i.e., 25°C–27°C).

Gently mix pre-warmed diluent solution (DS) and TS vials with an up-and-down movement. Pour 300 μL of DS into well 2 and 1.8 mL of 37°C TS into square well 1 of the warming plate.

The warming and dilution procedures consist of the following steps (dilution is also shown in Figure 21.8):

1. Using tweezers, remove the plastic cap of the Cryotec while it is still submerged in liquid nitrogen. This manipulation can be performed easily if the Styrofoam box is filled almost entirely with liquid nitrogen. The container should be positioned close to the microscope to avoid delay when transferring the Cryotec. The microscope should be focused at the center of the TS of the warming plate with low magnification.
2. Hold the Cryotec and look for the black mark while maintaining the tip submerged in liquid nitrogen. Remove the

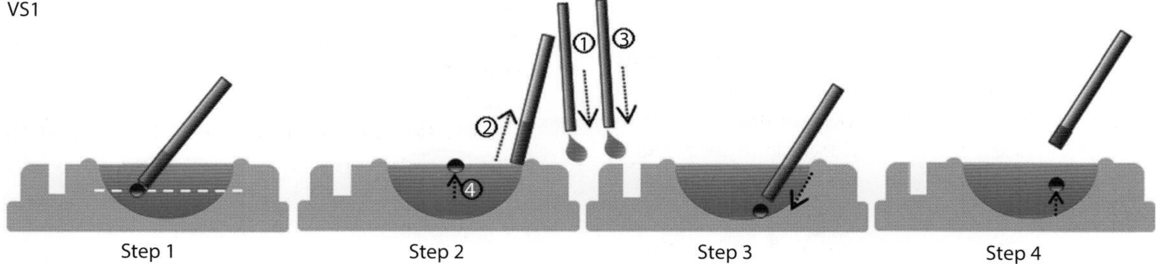

Figure 21.4 Equilibration of oocytes in VS1. *Abbreviation*: VS1, vitrification solution 1.

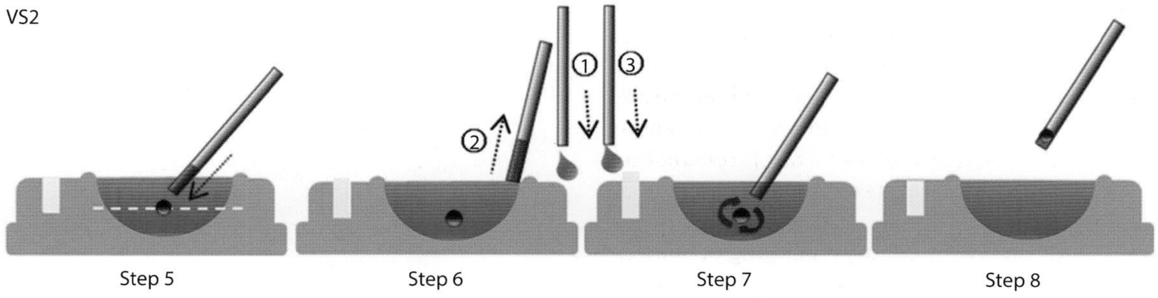

Figure 21.5 Confirmation of oocyte shrinkage in VS2. *Abbreviation*: VS2, vitrification solution 2.

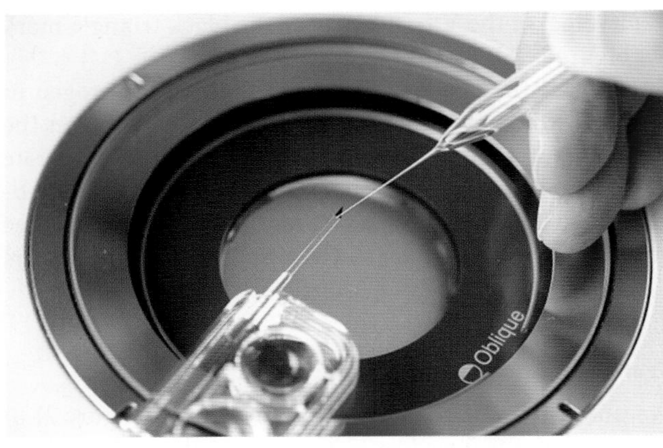

Figure 21.6 Easy loading of oocytes using Vitri-Plate.

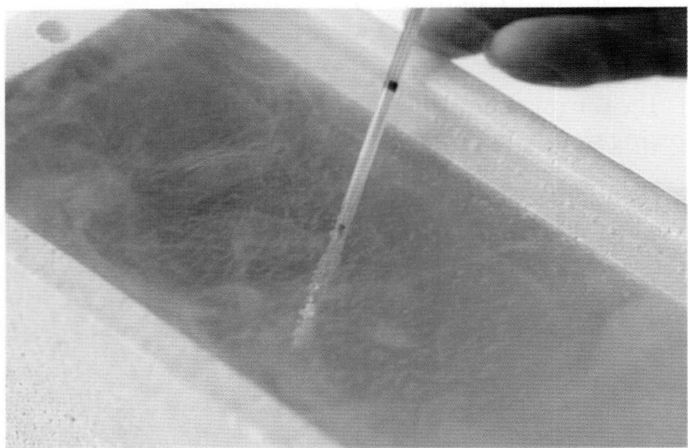

Figure 21.7 Vitrified oocytes on Cryotec in liquid nitrogen with tightly closed cover cap.

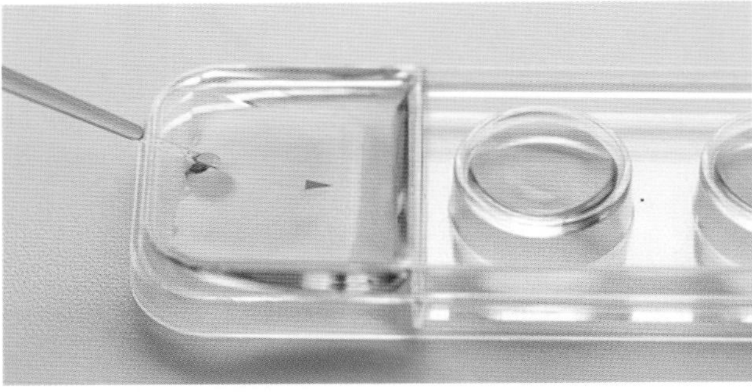

Figure 21.9 Warming: oocyte on Cryotec sheet in thawing solution in the warming plate.

Cryotec with a rapid movement from the liquid nitrogen and place the tip immediately into the middle of the square TS well of the warming plate (Figure 21.9).

3. Find the oocytes by adjusting the focus on the Cryotec sheet. One minute after immersing into TS, while keeping the Cryotec sheet in the middle of the TS, oocytes will separate themselves from the Cryotec sheet and will begin to float. Follow all movements of the oocytes continuously, as they will become transparent at this phase of the procedure and it is easy to lose them. Later, they will regain their normal appearance.
4. Gently pick up the oocytes in the pipette and aspirate an additional 3-mm long TS column to the tip of the pipette. Transfer the pipette to the bottom of the DS well and expel the contents gently to the center of the bottom (deepest place): first the TS media, allowing it to form a small "mountain" of fluid, then the oocytes at the bottom of this mountain. Then do nothing and wait for 3 minutes (Figure 21.10).

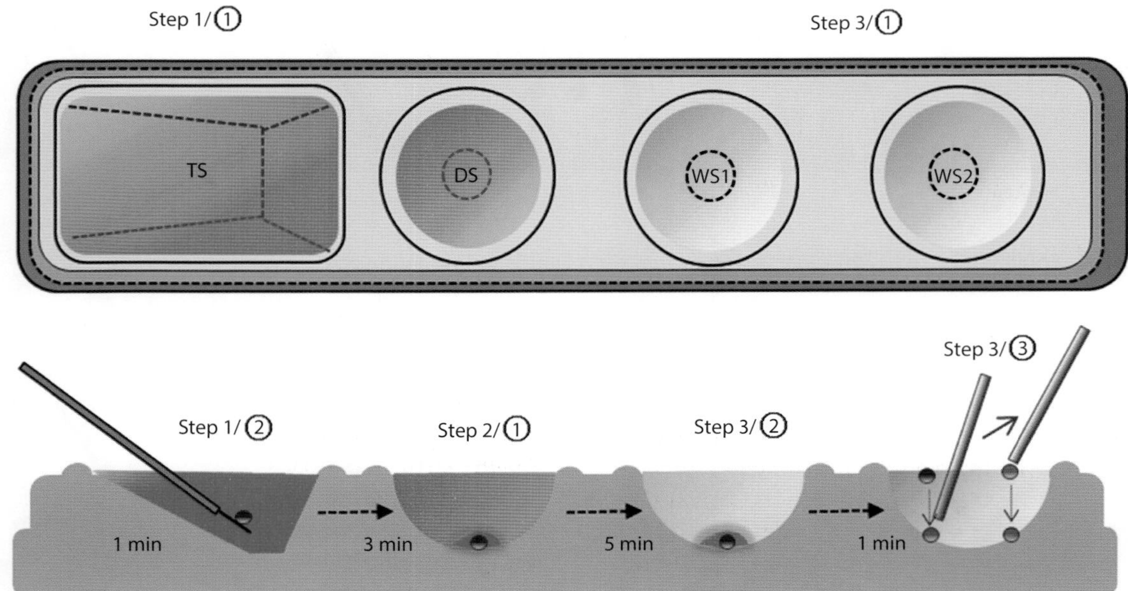

Figure 21.8 Warming plate and warming procedure of the Cryotec method. *Abbreviations*: DS, dilution solution; TS, thawing solution; WS1, washing solution 1; WS2, washing solution 2.

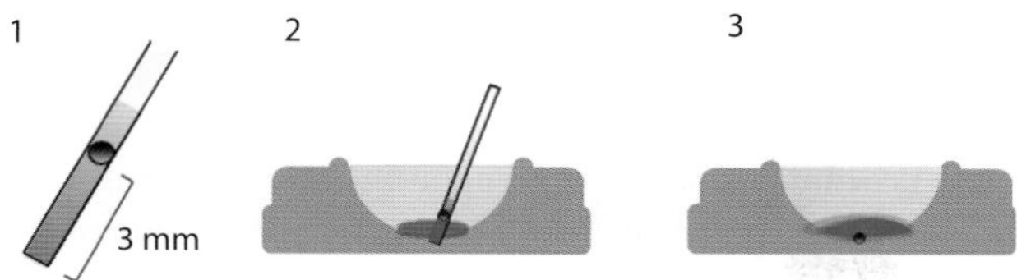

Figure 21.10 Gradual replacement of the solutions (thawing solution to dilution solution/dilution solution to washing solution).

5. Subsequently, the same method of transfer should be applied but with different solutions: oocytes will be placed at the bottom of the mountain formed from DS medium in the WS1 dish for 5 minutes, without any stirring or mixing of the media.
6. Place the oocytes onto the surface of WS2 and wait for 1 minute.
7. Finally, transfer the oocytes into the culture dish and examine their morphology under the stereomicroscope. ICSI can be performed after a recovery period of at least one hour.

The danger of liquid nitrogen-mediated disease transmission

Safety issues regarding open methods of vitrification have been discussed recently in detail (5,21,34). Liquid nitrogen may become contaminated with pathogenic agents and can transmit these agents to other samples stored in the same tank of liquid nitrogen. Under experimental conditions, transmission has also been demonstrated between embryological samples (35,36). Although no disease transmission related to liquid nitrogen-mediated contamination and embryo transfer has been reported for humans or for animals during the past 40 years, a theoretical danger exists and should be minimized with rational measures. According to most observations, hermetical isolation of samples from liquid nitrogen or medium during cooling and thawing considerably decreases cooling and warming rates and, as a consequence, also reduces survival of oocytes. One reasonable solution to this problem is to separate cooling and thawing of oocytes from their storage. Cooling can be performed in liquid nitrogen that is directly provided from the factory, has not been in contact with any other biological samples, and has been filtered before use (37,38). For storage, samples may be sealed in a pre-cooled, hermetically isolated container (e.g., 1-mL diameter cryobiosystem [CBS] straw; IMV, L'Aigle, France). An analog of the system has been used for open pulled straw (OPS) vitrification (36) and the required instrument is commercially available (VitSet, Minitüb, Landshut, Germany). At warming, the end of the 1-mL straw may be cut with sterile scissors while the rest of the straw is still submerged in liquid nitrogen, and the Cryotec can be quickly removed with narrow forceps for immersion into the proper medium. However, high post-warm survival rates of oocytes have not been obtained in these partially closed or fully closed systems, possibly because of the lower cooling and warming rates than those in ultra-rapid vitrification. The fact is that no viral transmission problems have occurred after more than 2.5 million cases of clinical applications of the Cryotop and Cryotec method for 16 years in 65 countries. This provides the best practical evidence to indicate the safety of this method with respect to possible liquid nitrogen-mediated disease transmission.

RESULTS ACHIEVED WITH CRYOTOP AND CRYOTEC VITRIFICATION OF HUMAN OOCYTES

The first baby born after human oocyte vitrification was achieved with the OPS technique (39). However, the survival rate was not very high and no replicate results have been reported. This is similar to the first success of human oocyte freezing in 1986 (10). The OPS method may briefly expose the VS to liquid nitrogen, and it contains more than 1 μL of VS, which may cause a lower cooling rate. Nevertheless, this technique does work very well for mammalian embryos, even if less efficiently for oocytes.

Before being cryopreserved, the potential development rate of oocytes is 100%. If some oocytes undergo serious damage during cryopreservation, those oocytes die, resulting in a lower overall survival rate. A lower survival rate is evidence of increasing damage caused by cryopreservation. Therefore, especially in clinical applications of vitrification, it is very important that the highest survival be attained not only for the efficiency of the treatment, but also to ensure the likelihood of producing normal, healthy babies. Such high post-warming survival of oocytes can be obtained using an ultra-rapid vitrification method.

In 2000, Kuwayama and Kato obtained the first pregnancy derived from vitrified oocytes using a minimal-volume cooling method (28). The protocol of this vitrification was improved and made easier for everyone's use, and named it the Cryotop method (28).

After the first successful report of oocyte vitrification with the Cryotop vitrification method in 2000 (28), the protocol has gradually become used around the world, being adapted for various clinical needs in each country.

In Japan, using this method, a 91% post-thaw survival rate, 90% fertilization rate, and 50% blastocyst formation rate after ICSI and *in vitro* culture were first reported (30). After embryo transfer, a pregnancy rate of 41% was achieved. The ultimate birth rate of those embryos that implanted was 83%. A total of 20 healthy babies were delivered in this clinical trial. This ultra-rapid vitrification method was used to establish the first oocyte bank for unmarried cancer patients in 2001. More than 600 oocytes from 112 patients have been cryopreserved for their future *in vitro* fertilization (IVF) treatment use.

In the U.S.A., Katayama et al. (29) repeatedly used the Cryotop method and achieved a post-thaw survival rate for oocytes of 97%, and they obtained the first live baby from a vitrified oocyte in the U.S.A. They also established an oocyte bank for unmarried cancer patients and for healthy women to preserve their fertility for social reasons in 2003.

In Spain, Cobo et al. (38) reported that the survival rate of 231 oocytes that were thawed after vitrification was 97%; the respective fertilization, cleavage, and blastocyst rates were 76%, 94%, and 49%. Embryo transfer performed on 23 patients resulted in a 65% pregnancy rate, although with a miscarriage rate of 20%. The Spanish team is the largest IVF unit in Europe and has used oocyte vitrification for an egg donation program (40). More than 1000 healthy babies have been born from oocytes that were vitrified by this team alone.

Recently, based on the wide-ranging experience of Cryotop vitrification, the reasons for lethal damage to the oocytes during the vitrification process became clear. These reasons are the lower viscosity of the solutions, the difficulty of judging completion of oocyte equilibration in VS, the difficulty of loading oocytes onto vitrification container sheets within a limited time, and the sticking of oocytes to the sheet at warming in TS, among others. These problems in the method were eliminated by using new finding additives: hydroxypropyl cellulose, improvement of equilibration using specific gravity difference, and improvements of vitrification and warming plates. For this purpose, Dr. Kuwayama, developer of the Cryotop method created and improved vitrification method named the Cryotec method (7).

As a result of personal communications with colleagues in over 40 countries, I estimate that more than 20,000 oocytes have been vitrified by the Cryotec method, and in most of the centers, the survival rates of vitrified oocytes after warming were 100%, and more than 2000 such healthy babies have been delivered thus far. The fact that such results have been reported by so many independent clinical groups in different countries with no direct or commercial connection for the past four years may indicate that a reliable clinical procedure to cryopreserve human oocytes has been obtained.

CONCLUSION

Cryopreservation of oocytes is regarded as one of the most demanding tasks of human assisted reproduction. With scrupulous attention to numerous details and proper application of the latest vitrification techniques, the efficiency of the procedure has been substantially improved. The Cryotec vitrification method has resulted in an almost 100% survival rate followed by excellent fertilization, blastocyst development, pregnancy, and births after embryo transfers (ETs), comparable to those achieved with non-vitrified control oocytes. The technique can be useful in diverse situations where oocyte storage is required or considered.

ACKNOWLEDGEMENTS

The author is very grateful to Prof. Stanley Leibo and Dr. Sofia Soto for their critical reading of the manuscript.

REFERENCES

1. Polge C, Smith AY, Parkes AS. Revival of spermatozoa after vitrification and dehydration at low temperatures. *Nature* 1949; 164: 666.
2. Whittingham DG, Leibo SP, Mazur P. Survival of mouse embryos frozen to −196°C and −269°C. *Science* 1972; 178: 411–4.
3. Wilmut I. The effect of cooling rate, warming rate, cryoprotective agent and stage of development on survival of mouse embryos during freezing and thawing. *Life Sci* 1972; 11: 1071–9.
4. Trounson A, Mohr L. Human pregnancy following cryopreservation, thawing, and transfer of an eight-cell embryo. *Nature* 1983; 305: 707–9.
5. Kuwayama M. Highly efficient vitrification for cryopreservation of human oocytes and embryos: The Cryotop method. *Theriogenology* 2007; 67: 73–80.
6. Kuwayama M, Cobo A, Vajta G. Vitrification of oocytes: General considerations and the use of the Cryotop method. In: *Vitrification in Assisted Reproduction*. Tucker MJ, Liebermann J (eds). London, U.K.: Informa Healthcare, 2008, pp. 119–28.
7. Gandhi G, Ramesh S, Khatoon A. Vitrification of oocytes: General considerations. In: *Vitrification in Assisted Reproduction*. U.K.: Springer, 2014, pp. 17–30.
8. Kuwayama M, Gandhi G, Kagalwala S. Ramani R. Vitrification: An overview. In: *Vitrification in Assisted Reproduction*. U.K.: Springer. 2014, pp. 1–7.
9. Kuwayama M, Gandhi G, Kagalwala S. Khatoon A. Oocyte banking: Current perspectives. In: *Vitrification in Assisted Reproduction*. U.K.: Springer, 2014, pp. 89–95.
10. Chen C. Pregnancy after human oocyte cryopreservation. *Lancet* 1986; 1(8486): 884–6.
11. Liebermann J, Tucker MJ. Comparison of vitrification and conventional cryopreservation of day 5 and day 6 blastocysts during clinical application. *Fertil Sterill* 2006; 86: 20–6.
12. Leibo SP, Martino A, Kobayashi S, Pollard JW. Stage-dependent sensitivity of oocytes and embryos to low temperatures. *Anim Reprod Sci* 1996; 42: 45–53.
13. Magistrini M, Szollosi D. Effects of cold and of isopropyl N-phenylcarbamate on the second meiotic spindle of mouse oocytes. *Eur J Cell Biol* 1980; 22: 699–707.
14. Sathananthan AH, Ng SC, Trounson AO, Bongso A, Ratnam SS, Ho J, Mok H, Lee MN. The effects of ultrarapid freezing on meiotic and mitotic spindles of oocytes and embryos. *Gamete Res* 1998; 21: 385–401.
15. Pickering SJ, Braude PR, Johnson MH, Cant A, Currie J. Transient cooling to room temperature can cause irreversible disruption of the meiotic spindle in the human oocyte. *Fertil Steril* 1990; 54: 102–8.
16. Fabbri R, Porcu E, Marsella T, Rocchetta G, Venturoli S, Flamigni C. Human oocyte cryopreservation: New perspectives regarding oocyte survival. *Hum Reprod* 2001; 16: 411–6.
17. Stachecki JJ, Munne S, Cohen J. Spindle organization after cryopreservation of mouse, human, and bovine oocytes. *Reprod Biomed Online* 2004; 8: 664–72.

18. Stachecki JJ, Munne S, Cohen J. Spindle organization after cryopreservation of mouse, human, and bovine oocytes. *Reprod Biomed Online* 2004; 8: 664–72.
19. Ghetler Y, Yavin S, Shalgi R, Arav A. The effect of chilling on membrane lipid phase transition in human oocytes and zygotes. *Hum Reprod* 2005; 20: 3385–9.
20. Dobrinsky JR, Pursel VG, Long CR, Johnson LA. Birth of piglets after transfer of embryos cryopreserved by cytoskeletal stabilization and vitrification. *Biol Reprod* 2000; 62: 564–70.
21. Vajta G, Nagy PZ. Are programmable freezers still needed in the embryo laboratory? Review on vitrification. *Reprod Biomed Online* 2006; 12: 779–96.
22. Martino A, Songsasen N, Leibo SP. Development into blastocysts of bovine oocytes cryopreserved by ultra-rapid cooling. *Biol Reprod* 1996; 54: 1059–69.
23. Vajta G, Holm P, Kuwayama M, Booth PJ, Jacobsen H, Greve T, Callesen H. Open pulled straw (OPS) vitrification: A new way to reduce cryoinjuries of bovine ova and embryos. *Mol Reprod Dev* 1998; 51: 53–8.
24. Lane M, Schoolcraft WB, Gardner DK. Vitrification of mouse and human blastocysts using a novel cryoloop container-less technique. *Fertil Steril* 1999; 72: 1073–8.
25. Lane M, Bavister BD, Lyons EA, Forest KT. Containerless vitrification of mammalian oocytes and embryos. *Nat Biotechnol* 2001; 17: 1234–6.
26. Arav A. Vitrification of oocytes and embryos. In: *New Trends in Embryo Transfer*. Lauria A, Gandolfi F (eds). Cambridge, U.K.: Portland Press, 1992, pp. 255–64.
27. Hamawaki A, Kuwayama M, Hamano S. Minimum volume cooling method for bovine blastocyst vitrification. *Theriogenology* 1999; 51: 165.
28. Kuwayama M, Kato O. All-round vitrification method for human oocytes and embryos. *J Assist Reprod Genet* 2000; 17: 477.
29. Katayama P, Stehlik J, Kuwayama M, Kato O, Stehlik E. High survival rate of vitrified human oocytes results in clinical pregnancy. *Fertil Steril* 2003; 80: 223–4.
30. Kuwayama M, Vajta G, Kato O, Leibo S. Highly efficient vitrification method for cryopreservation of human oocytes. *Reprod Biomed Online* 2005; 11: 300–8.
31. Kuwayama M, Vajta G, Ieda S, Kato O. Vitrification of human embryos using the CryoTip™ method. *Reprod Biomed Online* 2005; 11: 608–14.
32. Kuwayama M, Leibo S. Cryopreservation of human embryos and oocytes. *J Mamm Ova Res* 2010; 25: 79–86.
33. Dalvit G. Vitrification of day2–3 human embryos using various methods. In: *Vitrification in Assisted Reproduction*. U.K.: Springer, 2014, pp. 65–70.
34. Vajta G, Kuwayama M, Vanderzwalmen P. Disadvantages and benefits of vitrification. In: *Vitrification in Assisted Reproduction*. Tucker MJ, Liebermann J (eds). London, U.K.: Informa Healthcare, 2008, pp. 33–44.
35. Bielanski A, Nadin-Davis S, Sapp T, Lutze-Wallace C. Viral contamination of embryos cryopreserved in liquid nitrogen. *Cryobiology* 2000; 40: 110–6.
36. Bielanski A, Bergeron H, Lau PC, Devenish J. Microbial contamination of embryos and semen during long-term banking in liquid nitrogen. *Cryobiology* 2003; 46: 146–52.
37. Vajta G, Lewis IM, Kuwayama M, Greve T, Callesen H. Sterile application of the open pulled straw (OPS) vitrification method. *Cryo-Letters* 1998; 19: 389–92.
38. Cobo A, Kuwayama M, Pérez S, Ruiz A, Pellicer A, Remohi J. Comparison of concomitant outcome achieved with fresh and cryopreserved donor oocytes vitrified by the Cryotop method. *Fertil Steril* 2008; 89: 1657–64.
39. Kuleshova L, Gianaroli L, Magli C, Trounson A. Birth following vitrification of a small number of human oocytes. *Hum Reprod* 1999; 14: 3077–9.
40. Cobo A, Remohi J, Chang CC, Nagy ZP. Oocyte cryopreservation for donor egg banking. *Reprod Biomed Online* 2011; 11: 300–8.

The human embryo
Slow freezing

22

MARIUS MEINTJES

INTRODUCTION

Blastocyst culture and transfer are strongly desired, as they allow for increased embryo selection and consequently lead to significantly improved implantation and live birth rates (1). In contrast, cleavage-stage transfer programs are now more often finding themselves at a disadvantage. Transferring at the cleavage stage mostly necessitates the transfer of multiple embryos to be competitive and, as a result, is plagued with multiple implantations. Furthermore, the practice of transferring multiple cleavage-stage embryos does not easily lead to higher live birth rates anymore.

Even so, blastocyst culture for all patients has gained slow acceptance due to the intolerance of suboptimum culture systems and air quality, the increased utilization of low-O_2 culture, and, most importantly, the perceived inability to reliably cryopreserve supernumerary blastocysts for later use. Historically, the slow freezing of blastocysts was plagued with low survival rates, high rates of biochemical pregnancies, and frequent early miscarriages. Only a very few programs could consistently claim acceptable frozen–thawed blastocyst outcomes.

With the advent of blastocyst vitrification, consistently good cryopreservation outcomes became the norm for more clinics. Even the few programs with good slow-freezing results are now able to further improve their outcomes. Blastocyst vitrification contributed significantly to the movement towards not transferring during the fresh cycle and the liberal use of preimplantation genetic screening after trophoblast biopsy. For the first time, routine single-embryo transfers are becoming a reality, without losing a competitive advantage over day-2 and day-3 embryo transfer programs. Today, blastocyst culture and transfer is increasingly becoming the method of choice and, at least in some countries, has become the mainstream approach. For this reason, this chapter will focus on blastocysts, rather than on pronuclear or cleavage-stage embryos.

The question then is: why still talk about slow blastocyst freezing? Firstly, some lessons can be learned from slow freezing that may assist in optimizing current vitrification methods. Secondly, thousands of slow-frozen embryos will be presented for thawing in the foreseeable future, either as follow-up cycles or as donated embryos to infertile couples. It is proposed that the thawing rather than the freezing of slow-frozen blastocysts is the most critical step to ensuring a good outcome. Regardless of the slow-freezing technique applied in the past, careful attention to sound slow thawing will prove critical and allow good clinical outcomes years after these blastocysts were frozen.

THE ROLE OF PRE-FREEZE BLASTOCYST QUALITY

Regardless of the method of cryopreservation, the quality of the blastocyst before cryopreservation is paramount to a successful outcome. The quality of the pre-freeze blastocyst may be affected by the patient, culture conditions, and/or culture media. A small problem in the culture conditions or environment will be exacerbated with an additional two to four days of *in vitro* culture to the blastocyst stage. As an example, culture and cryopreservation of blastocysts should not be attempted without a reduced O_2 culture environment. It has been shown repeatedly that the implantation potential of blastocysts is disproportionately compromised by atmospheric O_2 culture when compared with cleavage-stage embryos (2). Similarly, the cryosurvivability of blastocysts is directly affected by the pre-freeze culture conditions such as the addition of hyaluronan to the culture medium (3).

POST-THAW INNER CELL MASS SURVIVAL

Timing of freezing and blastocyst selection before freezing

Unlike in the case of vitrification where the developmental stage or absolute quality of the blastocyst have little impact on warming outcomes, slow freezing appears to be temperamental regarding which blastocysts to freeze and, importantly, when to freeze them. With vitrification, an all-or-none rule seems to apply, where all of the blastocysts survive or, alternatively, there is no survival after warming. Frequently, post-thaw blastocysts after slow freezing may exhibit partial survival with preferential damage to the inner cell mass (ICM) cells. Therefore, best slow-freeze outcomes are observed if the biomass going into the freeze is optimized, meaning that one should freeze fully expanded blastocysts with compact ICMs (Figure 22.1). This allows for partial loss of cells after thawing with enough viable cells remaining to support implantation, hence the importance of paying attention to ICM quality (biomass), even before committing to slow freezing.

Earlier blastocysts, which are not fully expanded, or expanded blastocysts where individual ICM cells can still be counted tend to yield less than desired outcomes. Similarly, poor-quality blastocysts have a very low chance of surviving slow freezing and thawing (Figure 22.2). This is in stark contrast to current vitrification techniques where what goes in at the front end tends to come out after warming, regardless of quality. Furthermore, unlike in the case of vitrification, hatched blastocysts do not freeze well when slow-frozen. The resultant poor survival of partially hatched, slow-frozen blastocysts after biopsy is partly

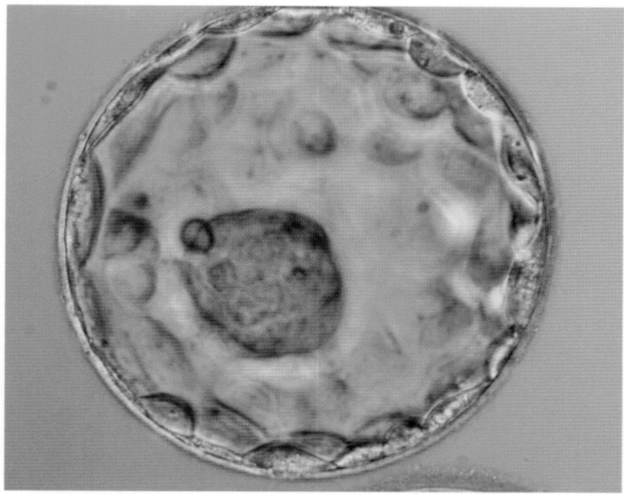

Figure 22.1 A fully expanded blastocyst with a compact inner cell mass containing many cells. This is an example of a blastocyst at the right stage for a slow freeze with an excellent chance of surviving the subsequent thaw. This blastocyst resulted in a live birth.

responsible for trophoblast biopsy not having been viable before the advent of reliable vitrification. Vitrification after trophoblast biopsy almost guarantees the survival of biopsied blastocysts.

ICM and trophoblast act different

Blastocysts consist of two distinct cell types: the ICM and trophoblast cells. These two cell types act differently during slow freezing and thawing, with ICM cells being the most sensitive. It is not uncommon for trophoblast cells to routinely survive thawing with compromised ICM cell survival or no ICM survival at all. In the human, unlike most other species, implantation is provisionally allowed in the absence of a viable ICM. This facilitation of implantation without a functional ICM and the preferential damage to ICM cells after thawing are frequently manifested as high biochemical pregnancy rates (a positive β-human chorionic gonadotropin [β-hCG] result failing to progress to a clinical pregnancy) and, commonly, first-trimester miscarriages. Several healthy post-thaw trophoblasts with no discernible ICMs were transferred, which resulted in clinical pregnancies, shortly followed by early miscarriages (Figure 22.3).

When considering the quality of the post-thaw ICM, patients with only poor-quality ICMs at the time of transfer had high rates of biochemical pregnancies or early miscarriages (4). However, ongoing pregnancies and live births are still possible, albeit at significantly lower rates. As illustrated in Figure 22.4, the observed clinical outcomes directly relate to ICM quality (4). Similarly, weak and/or damaged ICMs in the poor-quality ICM group may explain the high rate of biochemical pregnancies and the clinical pregnancy losses observed.

Efforts to optimize the recovery of slow-frozen blastocysts should focus, in part, on ICM survival. ICM survival may be improved by proper selection of blastocysts before cryopreservation (5), an optimal culture environment (low O_2 and proper macromolecule supplementation), and, specifically, the optimization of thaw solutions (6).

Modification of the thaw process to optimize ICM survival

Even though IVF programs today would likely not slow-freeze blastocysts anymore, thawing some of the thousands of blastocysts in the worldwide frozen inventory is still a reality. Therefore, paying attention to- and adapting

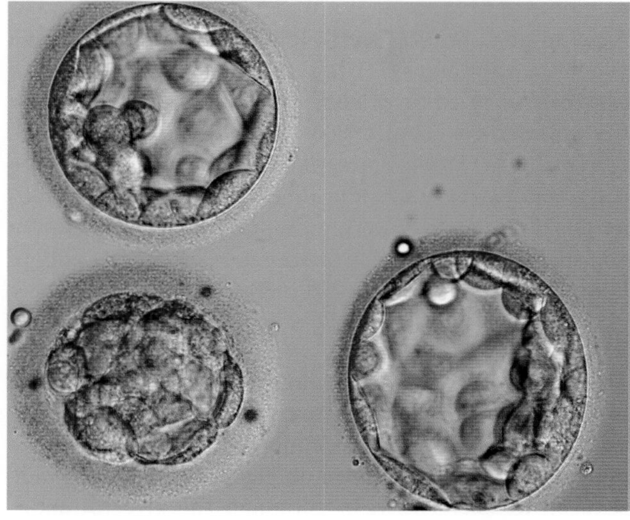

Figure 22.2 Examples of early blastocysts that are not yet fully expanded and, in addition, do not have a coherent inner cell mass. Slow-freezing blastocysts at this stage and with these quality inner cell masses seldom result in a good clinical outcome.

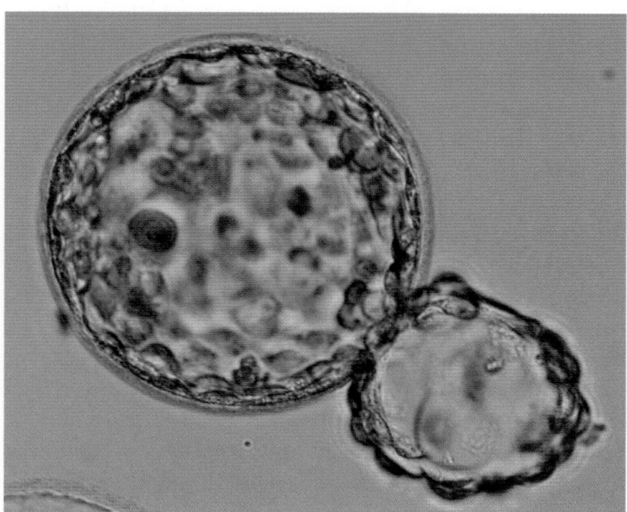

Figure 22.3 A hatching blastocyst 14 hours post-thaw with no discernable inner cell mass (ICM) and a healthy trophoblast. This blastocyst was frozen with a quality ICM. It is not uncommon for trophoblast cells to routinely survive thawing alongside compromised ICM cell survival or no ICM survival at all. After transfer, this blastocyst resulted in a biochemical pregnancy.

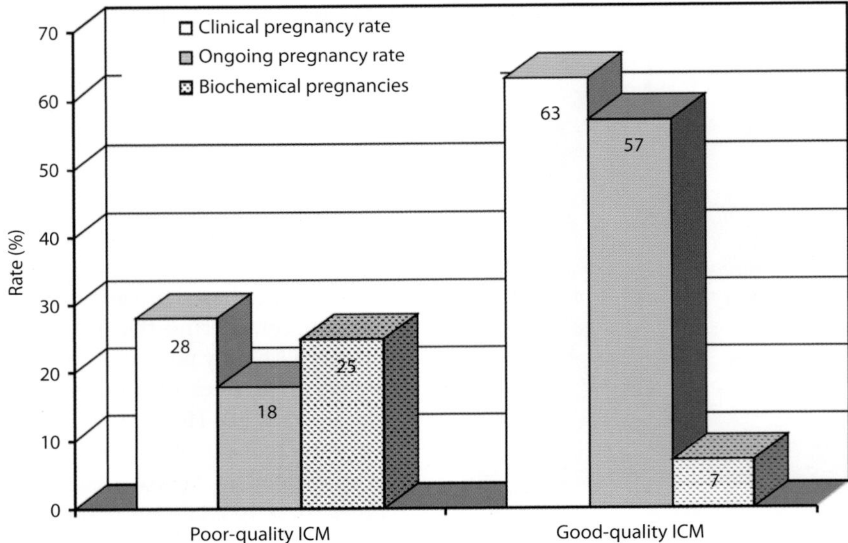

Figure 22.4 Clinical, ongoing, and biochemical (not resulting in a clinical pregnancy) pregnancies observed for slow-frozen, thawed blastocysts with poor- and good-quality ICMs. *Abbreviation*: ICM, inner cell mass.

to known cryobiological principles can ensure the best possible outcome when thawing slow-frozen blastocysts. When slow-freezing and thawing human blastocysts, cryoinjury can be incurred in at least three different ways (7). These may include organelle damage due to intracellular hyperosmosis during freezing, cell lysis during thawing, and physical ice crystal-induced damage to membranes and organelles during freezing and/or thawing.

During the freezing process, the blastomeres are dehydrated to reduce the chance of intracellular ice formation. The risk during freezing then pertains to extended intracellular hyperosmosis, resulting in organelle damage (Figure 22.5). This type of damage during freezing, therefore, may vary due to the extent and duration of the intracellular hyperosmotic state.

Damage during thawing relates to the rehydration of the thawing blastomeres. Water rushes into the cell faster than the permeable cryoprotectant (usually glycerol) can get out. The result is a temporary swelling and overextension of the blastomere (Figure 22.6). It appears that trophoblast cells can tolerate swelling better than ICM cells. Overextension of the blastomere will lead to cell lysis, which is by nature irreversible. In contrast, for slow freezing, there exists a possible spectrum of hyperosmotic freeze damage; damage incurred during thawing will either be absent (full recovery after temporary swelling) or result in lysis and complete blastomere death. However, in a given blastocyst, some cells may survive (more robust cells such as trophoblast cells) and others may undergo lysis (e.g., some ICM cells), hence the importance of designing the thaw protocol towards ICM survival and the importance of maximizing the ICM biomass before freezing. The presence of numerous cells in the ICM will increase the chance of a viable implantation even after losing some of the ICM cells during the thaw process. Lastly, intracellular ice crystal formation can damage the cell organelles during freezing and/or thawing when the rate of freezing is too fast (not allowing for timely dehydration) or the rate of thawing is too slow (refreezing of water that enters the hyperosmotic thawing cells).

Blastocyst freezing

Human blastocysts were first frozen using glycerol-based protocols developed for domestic animal blastocysts, without much use of non-permeable cryoprotectants such as sucrose. These protocols originally proved to be successful in the sheep (8) and the cow (9). When thawing these blastocysts, they were placed in a series of decreasing glycerol solutions with a total exposure to glycerol for as long as 110 minutes at room temperature (10). Later on, the survival rates were somewhat improved with pre-freeze co-culture and the addition of sucrose to the freezing and thawing steps, but still with a total glycerol exposure time of at least 31 minutes (11). Interestingly, cow embryos that were neither co-cultured nor exposed to hyaluronan before freezing did not survive slow-freeze protocols very well, confirming what we know today that pre-freeze culture conditions can have a significant impact on cryosurvivability (3). However, by lowering the freeze start temperature and slightly increasing the freeze rate, cryosurvivability of human blastocysts was further increased (12).

Blastocyst thawing

From this followed a perception that this long exposure to glycerol at room temperature was toxic to the embryos, as well as cumbersome and impractical. To resolve this perceived problem, the seven to eight thawing steps were reduced to only two (13). Although the glycerol exposure time and lengthiness of the thaw procedure were addressed, this approach created another unforeseen complication: ICM cells now frequently did not survive in adequate numbers, giving rise to reasonably positive β-hCG rates, but unacceptably high rates of biochemical

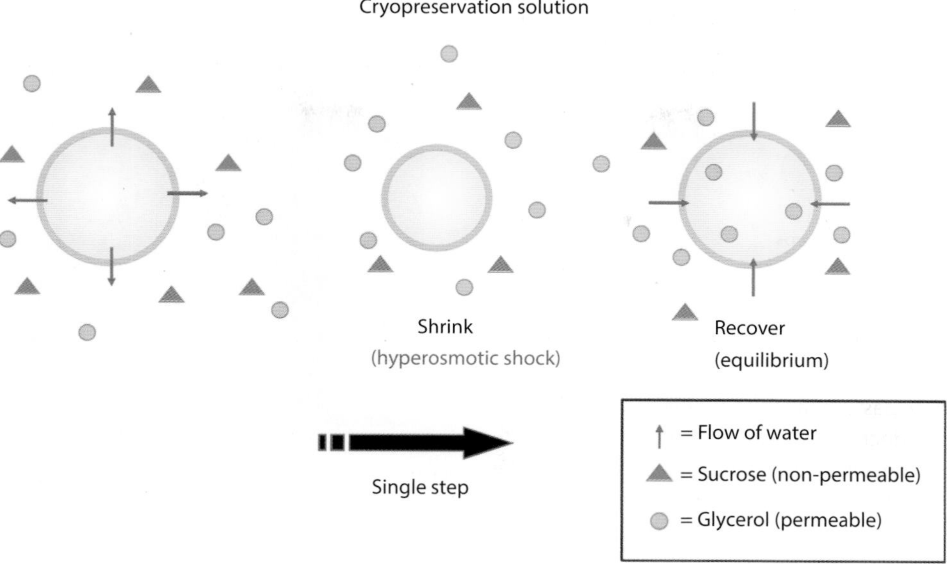

Figure 22.5 Illustration of the osmotic response of a single blastomere during a single freeze-dilution step. In general, water moves across the blastomere membrane faster than the permeable (glycerol) cryoprotectant. When the blastocyst is immersed in the first cryopreservation solution, water will rush out of the blastomere from a relatively high concentration to a lower concentration of water outside to attempt to achieve osmotic equilibrium. Water moving out will cause an initial shrinkage, resulting in a temporary hyperosmotic state inside the blastomere. During this hyperosmotic state, the blastomere is vulnerable to organelle damage. Next, glycerol will start to move into the blastomere from a high concentration outside to a low concentration inside to work towards glycerol equilibrium. Finally, water will follow the glycerol back into the blastomere to reach a final state of equilibrium. The blastomere now will be the same size as what it was before being immersed into the cryoprotectant solution. This sequence of events is repeated for each freeze step through increasing concentrations of cryoprotectants.

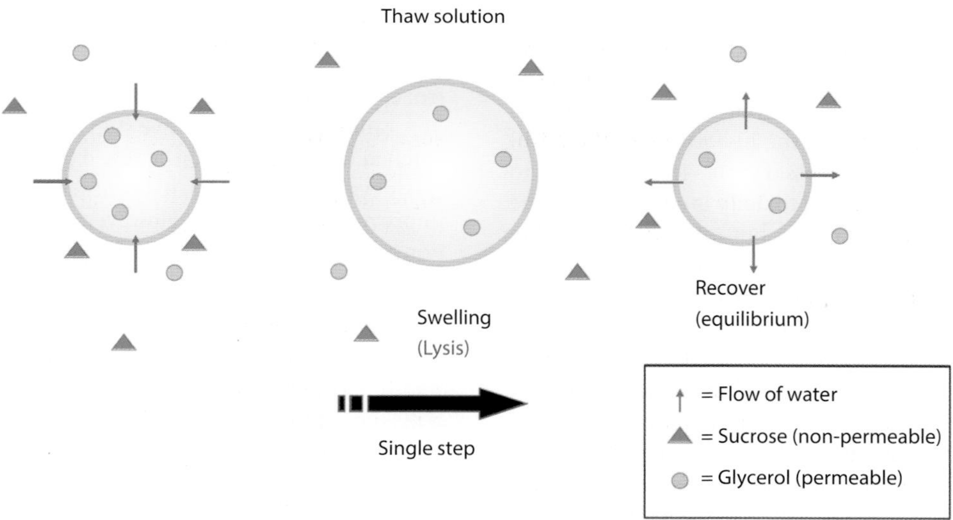

Figure 22.6 Illustration of the osmotic response of a single blastomere during a single thaw-dilution step. In general, water moves across the blastomere membrane faster than the permeable (glycerol) cryoprotectant. When the blastocyst is immersed in the first thaw solution, water will rush into the blastomere from a relatively high concentration outside to a lower concentration inside to attempt to achieve osmotic equilibrium. Water moving in will cause an initial swelling of the blastomere. If overextended at this stage, the blastomere will lyse, with irreversible damage leading to cell death. Next, glycerol will start to move out of the blastomere from a high concentration inside to a low concentration outside to work towards glycerol equilibrium. Finally, water will follow the glycerol back out of the blastomere to reach a final state of equilibrium. The blastomere now will be the same size as what it was before being immersed into the thaw solution. This sequence of events is repeated for each thaw step through decreasing concentrations of cryoprotectants.

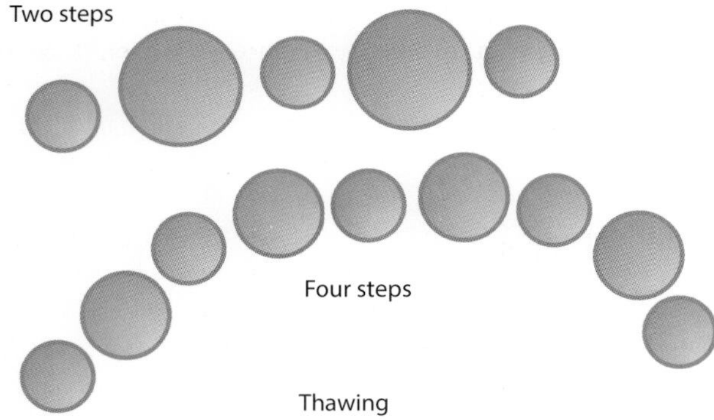

Figure 22.7 When passing the thawing blastocyst through four or more steps of decreasing glycerol solutions, the initial swelling of the blastomere is mild. In contrast, when using only two steps in the thawing procedure, swelling of the blastomere is more extreme, frequently leading to lysis.

pregnancies and miscarriages. When passing the thawing blastocyst through five or more steps of decreasing glycerol solutions, the initial swelling of the blastomere, when water rushes into the cell in response to the high intracellular concentration of glycerol, is mild (Figure 22.7). More thawing dilution steps follow the sound cryobiological principle of low rates of change in concentration (7). In contrast, when using only two steps in the thawing procedure, the amount of water rushing into the blastomere can overextend the blastomere plasma membrane, leading to lysis. The presence of impermeable solutes (such as sucrose) in the extracellular environment has proven to be critical to slowing down the initial rush of water into the blastomere, acting as an osmotic buffer (7). Knowing that at 37°C glycerol crosses the blastomere membrane and reaches transmembrane equilibrium in less than 60 seconds, it becomes clear that the historical long glycerol exposure times were unnecessary (14–16). The way to reduce the potential of glycerol toxicity is not to reduce the number of steps during thawing, but rather to reduce the time in each step, honoring the cryobiological principle of low rates of change in the glycerol concentration.

Applying these discussed principles, high ICM survival rates can be obtained as manifested by good clinical pregnancy rates, but importantly, without high miscarriage rates (Figure 22.8). Provided that embryos were properly cultured before cryopreservation (low O_2 concentration and optimum macromolecular supplementation), a live birth rate for day-5 frozen blastocysts of 54.6% was achieved (17). The optimized thawing protocols used to consistently achieve live birth rates over 50% are summarized in Table 22.1. Importantly, all solutions throughout the thawing protocol were supplemented with 12 mg/mL human serum albumin (HSA) or 20% serum substitute supplement (SSS) (v/v) and buffered with HEPES or MOPS. Thawing was conducted at 37°C and blastocysts were allowed to recover in the post-thaw recovery medium (regular culture medium supplemented with 12 mg/mL HSA or 20% SSS) for a minimum of four hours before transfer.

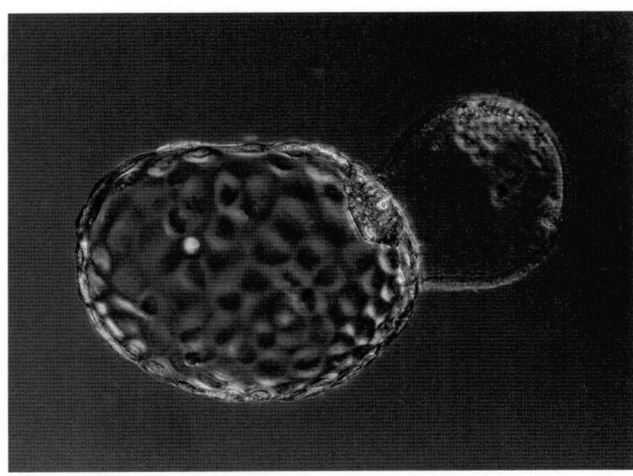

Figure 22.8 A fully hatched blastocyst after thawing and overnight culture. The inner cell mass can be clearly discerned with a healthy trophoblast, containing many cells. This transfer resulted in a live birth.

A PLACE FOR ASSISTED HATCHING OF FROZEN–THAWED BLASTOCYSTS?

In the 1980s and early 1990s, assisted hatching was proposed as a tool to assist implantation in embryos with a thick or tough zona pellucida (18). It later became clear that some of these observations might have resulted from inadequate media composition, specifically as a result of prolonged high glucose/phosphate exposure and/or a lack of specific amino acids, vitamins, or ethylenediaminetetraacetic acid (19). Regardless, it was also verified that the composition and function of the zona pellucida may change due to freezing and thawing (20,21). Therefore, it is tempting to speculate that assisted hatching may improve frozen–thawed blastocyst transfer outcomes.

A randomized prospective study (22) compared assisted-hatched (n = 76) and non-hatched (n = 76) frozen–thawed blastocyst transfer cycles. It was observed that implantations improved with hatching. However, these assisted implantations did not last, with no continued improvement in the ongoing pregnancy/live birth rate (Figure 22.9). It appears, then, that in this case assisted hatching allowed blastocysts to implant that should not otherwise have implanted and,

Table 22.1 Optimized thawing protocol for slow-frozen blastocysts

Step	Glycerol concentration	Sucrose concentration	Time in solution
1	5%	0.4 M	90 seconds
2	4%	0.2 M	90 seconds
3	3%	0.2 M	90 seconds
4	2%	0.2 M	90 seconds
5	1%	0.2 M	90 seconds
6	–	0.2 M	90 seconds
7	–	0.1 M	90 seconds
8	–	–	5 minutes

consequently, did not have the ability to result in a live birth. These results further suggest that assisted hatching may not contribute to increased live birth rates for slow-frozen blastocysts, but rather allow for miscarriages in patients that otherwise would have had a negative pregnancy.

DAY-5 AND DAY-6 CRYOPRESERVED BLASTOCYSTS

The exact timing and the blastocyst developmental stage at the time of slow-freezing may be imperative to optimizing frozen–thawed blastocyst pregnancy outcomes. Embryologists frequently face decisions in freezing expanding blastocysts with reduced cell numbers on day 5 or freezing them early the next day with increased cell numbers. However, when freezing too late, one risks ICM degeneration or *in vitro* hatching, which is not optimal for slow freezing.

It was observed that blastocysts frozen late on day 5 (n = 270) resulted in higher implantation and ongoing pregnancy/live birth rates than blastocysts frozen early on day 6 (n = 261) (Figure 22.10) (17). This same trend seems to hold true also for vitrified blastocysts, with a day-5 vitrified implantation rate of 62.3% (n = 73) and a day-6 vitrified implantation rate of 47.4% (n = 59). Interestingly, the euploidy rate was not different between day-5 (48%) and day-6 (53%) vitrified blastocysts (23). It is not possible to say if this observed difference was due to the day of freeze per se, or rather was a consequence of slower-developing embryos resulting in lower post-thaw pregnancy rates. The practical application of this information is to preferentially thaw day-5 embryos if given the opportunity to choose between day-5 frozen or day-6 frozen blastocysts.

DAY OF FREEZE AND SEX RATIO

It has been observed repeatedly that fresh blastocyst transfers may result in an increased male:female sex ratio in certain laboratories (24), especially under suboptimum culture conditions (25). Freezing the slower blastocysts (not selected for fresh transfer) may theoretically result in a normalization of the sex ratio in frozen–thawed blastocyst pregnancies. Indeed, the male:female sex ratio (57:43) of babies born from blastocysts frozen on day 5 (n = 150) was significantly skewed and similar to that reported for fresh blastocyst transfers (17). Interestingly, the male:female sex ratio (54:46) was not different and less pronounced for blastocysts frozen on day 6 (n = 151), similar to that seen after cleavage-stage transfer. All efforts should be made to optimize the pre-freeze culture conditions with appropriate macromolecule supplementation (such as hyaluronic acid) (3) and low-O_2 culture (2).

EXPECTATIONS FROM AN OPTIMIZED BLASTOCYST CRYOPRESERVATION PROGRAM

Even with the limitations of slow-rate blastocyst freezing, live birth rates close to those of fresh blastocyst transfers can be achieved. The optimization of a blastocyst cryopreservation program mandates a comprehensive approach. On the front end, a sound embryo culture system with special attention to the protein supplement and a low-O_2 environment has been shown to increase the number of blastocysts available for cryopreservation, improve the ICM quality, and increase blastocyst cryosurvivability. Critical timing of cryopreservation seems essential, as the success of slow-rate blastocyst cryopreservation appears to be developmental-stage specific. Freezing and thawing protocols/solutions are crucial; however, they are only a part of the overall cryopreservation program.

Table 22.2 summarizes age-specific results from our program that can be expected with slow-rate cryopreservation and thawing of blastocysts when attention is given to the factors mentioned. It is important to note that as patients are getting older, a smaller percentage of fertilized oocytes are frozen and fewer patients have any blastocysts to freeze. Not only the patient age, but also the number of oocytes

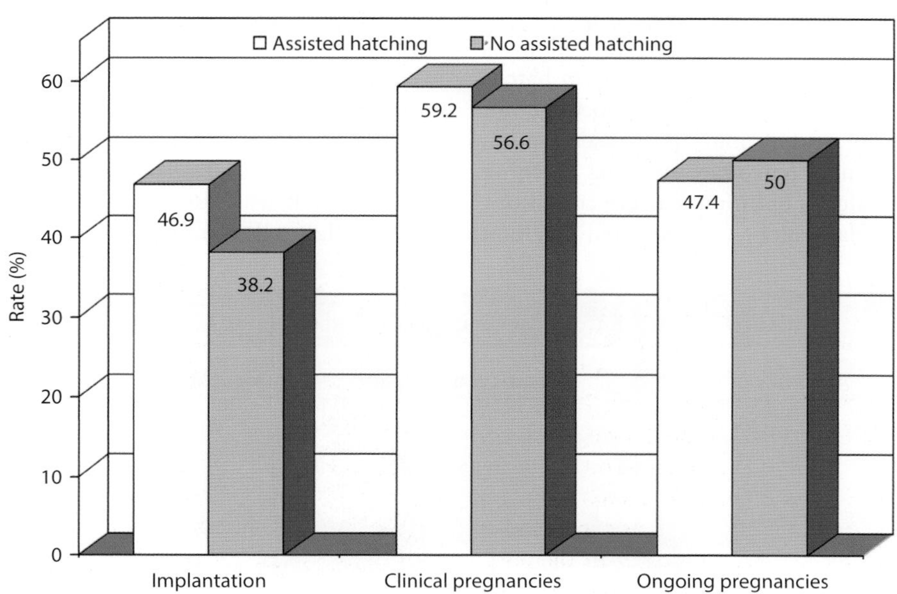

Figure 22.9 Implantation and pregnancy outcomes for frozen–thawed blastocyst transfers after assisted hatching.

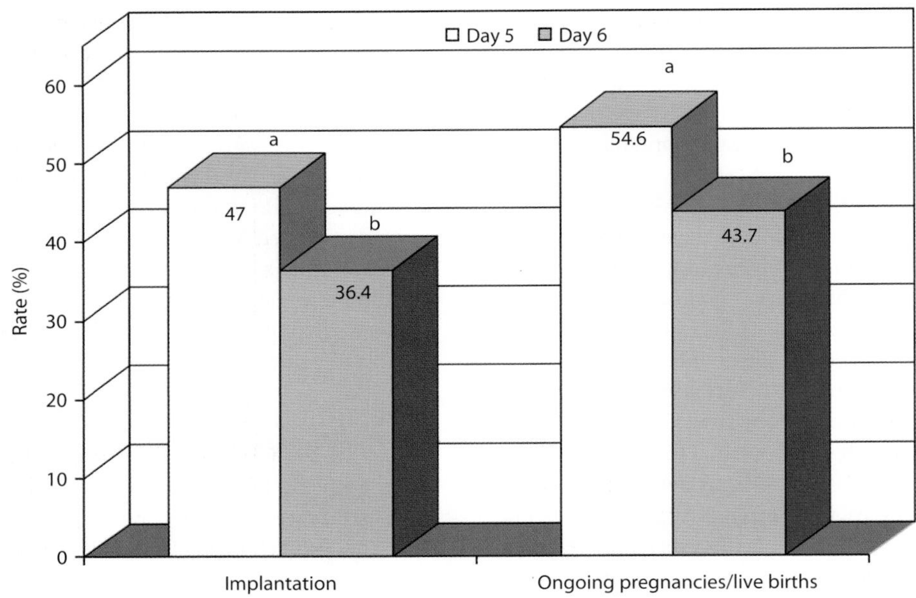

Figure 22.10 Day-5 and day-6 implantation and pregnancy outcomes for frozen–thawed blastocyst transfers.

retrieved per patient have direct effects on the number of blastocysts frozen for each patient. Significantly more blastocysts were frozen if more than 10 oocytes were recovered, regardless of the age group (26). However, as long as the same morphological-quality blastocysts are consistently frozen for all patient ages, fewer transfers for older patients may result, but ongoing pregnancy rates per transfer will not be significantly affected by the age of the patient.

CONCLUSIONS

It appears that the success of blastocyst cryopreservation and thawing depends on the ability to protect and recover a viable ICM. At the front end, the culture system should be optimized to produce a cryopreservation-resilient ICM. For slow freezing, the timing of the freeze is important in order to strike a balance between an optimum biomass to freeze and later ICM degeneration or *in vitro* hatching. In our experience, freezing of fully expanded but not hatched blastocysts before 118 hours post-insemination results in the best clinical outcomes. Assisted hatching seems to be of little value if optimum culture conditions are established in the laboratory (22). Assisted hatching may even be detrimental in that blastocysts may implant that are not capable of producing a live baby. In general, as patients are getting older, a smaller percentage of fertilized oocytes are frozen and fewer patients have any blastocysts to freeze. However, as long as the same morphological-quality blastocysts are consistently frozen, pregnancy rates per transfer will not be significantly affected by the age of the patient (26).

Regardless of the method of slow freezing, respectable live birth rates can be obtained with an optimized thaw protocol. The thawing protocol should protect the ICM, which is most sensitive to thawing. When concerned about long glycerol exposure times, one should not reduce the number of steps during thawing, but rather reduce the time in each step, honoring the principle of low rates of change of permeable and non-permeable cryoprotectants. When laboratories today are presented with the thaw of a slow-frozen blastocyst, they should refrain from using two-step protocols. When using only a two-step thawing protocol (with or without glycerol), a post-thaw injury may commonly result, with lysis of some or all of the ICM cells. Since trophoblast cells commonly survive even when using these

Table 22.2 Ongoing pregnancy/live birth outcomes for age-specific frozen–thawed blastocyst transfers

Patient age (years)	Number of transfers	Blastocysts/transfer	Implantations (%)	Ongoing/live births (%)
≤34	94	1.7	45.1	54
35–37	41	1.7	39.4	42
38–40	25	1.7	53.5	60
>40	6	1.7	50	67
Donor oocytes	47	1.9	40.9	60
Total	213	1.8	44.2	54

Source: Ward D et al. *Fertil Steril* 2005; 84(Suppl 1): S184 (abstr.).

suboptimum thawing protocols, implantation is still possible. Implantation of these compromised blastocysts frequently results in biochemical pregnancies or miscarriages.

When laboratories are presented with a blastocyst for slow thawing, the pre-freeze culture conditions, timing of cryopreservation, developmental stage, and other selection criteria for cryopreservation are not always known. However, even with the limitations of slow-rate blastocyst freezing, live birth rates close to those of fresh blastocyst transfers can still be achieved if attention is given to proper thawing.

REFERENCES

1. Alper MM, Brinsden P, Fischer R, Wikland M. To blastocyst or not to blastocyst? That is the question. *Hum Reprod* 2001; 16: 617–19.
2. Meintjes M, Chantilis SJ, Douglas SD, Rodriguez AJ, Guerami AR, Bookout DM, Barnett BD, Madden JD. A controlled randomized trial evaluating the effect of lowered incubator oxygen tension on live births in a predominantly blastocyst transfer program. *Hum Reprod* 2009; 24: 300–7.
3. Lane M, Maybach JM, Hooper K, Hasler JF, Gardner DK. Cryo-survival and development of bovine blastocysts are enhanced by culture with recombinant albumin and hyaluronan. *Mol Reprod Dev* 2003; 64: 70–8.
4. Rodriguez J, Douglas J, Bookout D, Guerami A, Madden J, Meintjes M. The effect of post-thaw blastocyst quality and the day of freeze on clinical outcome of a blastocyst cryopreservation programme. *Hum Reprod* 2002; 17(Suppl 1): 21 (abstr.).
5. Massip A. Cryopreservation of embryos from farm animals. *Reprod Domest Anim* 2001; 36: 49–55.
6. Emiliani S, Van den Bergh M, Vannin AS, Biramane J, Englert Y. Comparison of ethylene glycol, 1,2,-propanediol and glycerol for cryopreservation of slow-cooled mouse zygotes, 4-cell embryos and blastocysts. *Hum Reprod* 2000; 15: 905–10.
7. Pegg DE. The history and principles of cryopreservation. *Semin Reprod Med* 2002; 20(1): 5–14.
8. Willadsen SM. Factors affecting the survival of sheep embryos during deep-freezing and thawing. In: *The Freezing of Mammalian Embryos*. Elliot K, Whelan J (eds). Amsterdam, The Netherlands: Elsevier/North Holland, 1977, pp. 75–189.
9. Seidel GE, Elsden RP, Takeda T, Farrand GD. Field trials with cryopreserved bovine embryos. In: *Fertilization of the Human Egg In Vitro*. Beier HM, Lindner HR (eds). New York, NY: Springer-Verlag, 1983, pp. 343–52.
10. Cohen J, Simons RF, Edwards RG, Fehilly CB, Fishel SB. Pregnancies following the frozen storage of expanding human blastocysts. *J Assist Reprod Gen* 1985; 2: 59–64.
11. Ménézo Y, Nicollet B, Herbaut N, André D. Freezing co-cultured human blastocysts. *Fertil Steril* 1992; 58: 977–80.
12. Gardner DK, Lane M, Stevens J, Schoolcraft WB. Changing the start temperature and cooling rate in a slow freezing protocol increases human blastocyst viability. *Fertil Steril* 2003; 79: 401–10.
13. Ménézo Y, Veiga A. Cryopreservation of blastocysts. *Proceedings of the 10th World Congress on In Vitro Fertilization and Assisted Reproduction*. Vancouver, Canada, 1997; 49–53.
14. Kleinhans FW. Membrane permeability modelling: Kedem–Katchalsky vs a two-parameter formalism. *Cryobiology* 1998; 37: 271–89.
15. Leibo SP. Cryopreservation of oocytes and embryos: Optimization by theoretical versus empirical analysis. *Theriogenology* 2008; 69: 37–47.
16. Pfaff RT, Agca Y, Liu J, Woods EJ, Peter AT, Critser JK. Cryobiology of rat embryos 1: Determination of zygote membrane permeability coefficients for water and cryoprotectants, their activation energies and the development of improved cryopreservation methods. *Biol Reprod* 2000; 63: 1294–302.
17. De Kock A, Rodriguez A, Chantilis S, Guerami A, Madden J, Meintjes M. Clinical outcome and sex ratio for frozen blastocyst transfers as related to timing of blastocyst cryopreservation. *Fertil Steril* 2005; 84(Suppl 1): S176 (abstr.).
18. Cohen J, Alikani M, Trowbridge J, Rozenwaks Z. Implantation enhancement by selective assisted hatching using zona drilling of human embryos with poor prognosis. *Hum Reprod* 1990; 7: 686–91.
19. Lane M, Gardner D. Embryo culture medium: Which is the best? *Best Pract Res Clin Obstet Gyn* 2007; 21: 83–100.
20. Carroll J, Depypere H, Matthews CD. Freeze–thaw-induced changes in the zona pellucida explains decreased rates of fertilization in frozen–thawed mouse oocytes. *J Reprod Fertil* 1990; 90: 547–53.
21. Yi-Fan G, Chang-Fu L, Ge L, Guang-Xiu L. A comparative analysis of the zona pellucida birefringence of fresh and frozen–thawed human embryos. *Reproduction* 2010; 139: 121–7.
22. Adriaanse H, Perez O, Barnett BD, Madden JD, Chantilis SJ, Meintjes M. Assisted hatching of frozen–thawed blastocysts. Does it makes a difference? *Fertil Steril* 2004; 82(Suppl 2): S117 (abstr.).
23. Purcell S, Tilley B, Chantilis SJ, Lee K, Thomas M, Gada R, Meintjes M. The effect of the day of cryopreservation on FET success rates in PGS and non-PGS blastocysts. *Fertil Steril* 2015; 104: e194 (abstr.).
24. Tarín JJ, García-Pérez MA, Hermenegildo C, Cano A. Changes in sex ratio from fertilization to birth in assisted-reproductive-treatment cycles. *Reprod Biol Endocrinol* 2014; 12: 56.
25. Meintjes M, Chantilis S, Guerami A, Douglas J, Rodriguez A, Madden J. Normalization of the live-birth sex ratio after human blastocyst transfer from optimized culture conditions. *Fertil Steril* 2009; 92: S229–30 (abstr.).
26. Ward D, Chantilis S, Madden J, Bookout D, Guerami A, Meintjes M. Expectations for blastocyst cryopreservation and frozen–thawed blastocyst transfer outcomes. *Fertil Steril* 2005; 84(Suppl 1): S184 (abstr.).

The human embryo
Vitrification

23

ZSOLT PETER NAGY, CHING-CHIEN CHANG, and GÁBOR VAJTA

INTRODUCTION

Decades ago, most assisted reproductive technologies including *in vitro* fertilization (IVF) and cryopreservation of embryos by traditional freezing were applied to humans almost immediately after the first successes in some experimental or domestic species. However, there are some techniques where efforts to adopt a new approach were insufficient and sporadic, and consequently the practical application has been considerably delayed. Vitrification belongs to the latter group. Reasons for this delay may include the fact that cryopreservation of zygote-, cleavage-, and blastocyst-stage human embryos was more or less resolved by traditional freezing; vitrification has and still uses a seemingly very "undeveloped" manual technology compared to automatic traditional freezers and standardized, ready-to-use media. The high concentrations of cryoprotectants required for vitrification discouraged some potential users initially. Finally, none of the major suppliers were eager to replace their expensive freezing machines with the much simpler system required for vitrification (though very recently there have been some efforts to develop an instrument that would allow a "semi-automated" vitrification process [1]).

A decade ago, certain scientists moving to the human field from domestic animal embryology started to apply the technique, leading to the mass production of results regarding the applicability of vitrification in human fields. However, additional years were still required to get the approach acknowledged, to develop commercially available tools and kits, and to teach both distributors and consumers about the benefits of vitrification. Eventually, the overwhelming comparative evidence made clear to almost everybody that in all developmental stages, vitrification produces better survival and more competent oocytes/embryos than traditional freezing. Today, the rapidly increasing interest regarding vitrification creates novel problems such as diversity of tools and media, lack of information regarding ingredients, and inconsistency in teaching and application. Legal concerns on biosafety issues have also emerged, although no scientific proof exists about the magnitude or existence of any risks.

In this chapter, we summarize and compare the basic features of traditional freezing and vitrification, explain some special features of vitrification, and provide data about the efficiency of vitrification for the cryopreservation of human preimplantation-stage embryos at different developmental stages. We will also discuss how the highly efficient vitrification (of both embryo and oocyte) method has contributed to a paradigm shift in how assisted reproduction treatment is practiced today.

For terms and definitions, we accept and use the excellent review and suggestions of Shaw and Jones (2). For the basic principles of cryobiology, we refer to earlier reviews (3–6).

MAIN CRYOPRESERVATION APPROACHES

Within approximately the decade of the first successes with cryopreservation of mammalian embryos (7–11), the first human pregnancies were achieved (12,13). All these works have been performed with traditional slow freezing. Vitrification was first applied for the cryopreservation of mammalian embryos in 1985 (14), but was regarded as a curiosity and experimental procedure for almost a decade, when practical application was begun in domestic animal embryology and there were sporadic approaches in humans. Competitive vitrification strategies for human embryo and oocyte cryopreservation have only been developed 10–12 years ago.

The strategies of the two approaches are basically different. By far the most important source of damage at cryopreservation is ice crystal formation. To minimize this injury, application of various chemicals (cryoprotectants) is required, which, unfortunately, may also induce various injuries including toxic and osmotic damage.

Traditional slow-rate freezing creates a delicate balance between these factors. Embryos are typically exposed to 1–2-mol/L solutions of permeable and (less concentrated, if any) non-permeable cryoprotectants, then loaded into a 0.25-mL straw, sealed, and cooled to −6°C relatively rapidly, by placing the straws into a controlled-rate freezer. With the given cryoprotectant concentration, no spontaneous ice formation occurs at this temperature; however, ice nucleation can be induced by "seeding" (i.e., touching the straw with forceps that have been previously immersed into liquid nitrogen). This seeding is performed far from the embryo, and during the subsequent steps, this ice grows stepwise towards the embryo. The controlled-rate freezer is adjusted to allow very slow cooling (usually 0.3°C/minute, to around −30°C), then the straws are immersed in liquid nitrogen for final cooling and storage. In slow freezing, the toxic and osmotic damage caused by the relatively low concentrations of cryoprotectant solutions may not be too serious. However, this concentration is insufficient to avoid ice crystal formation; therefore, an additional manipulation is required to minimize the damage. It is the slow cooling and seeding that result in controlled growth of ice in the extracellular solution; consequently, considerable increases in the concentrations of ions, macromolecules, and other components, including cryoprotectants, occur in the remaining fluid. The slow rate of the procedure allows solution exchange between the extracellular and intracellular fluids without serious osmotic effects and deformation of the cells (this fact is reflected in the other name of the procedure: equilibrium freezing) (15).

The strategy of vitrification is much more radical. The main purpose (according to the cryobiological definition) is the complete elimination of ice formation in the whole solution the sample is cooled in.

Evidently, this can only be performed with the use of high cryoprotectant concentrations, which may theoretically induce serious toxic and osmotic damages. A huge variety of cryoprotectants have been tested so far, and although no consensus has yet been achieved regarding the best components, combinations, and concentrations, some principles have already been obtained (see later in the text). Cell shrinkage caused by non-permeable cryoprotectants and the incomplete penetration of permeable components may cause a relative increase in the intracellular concentration of macromolecules that is enough to hamper intracellular ice formation. Accordingly, vitrification belongs to the group of non-equilibrium cryopreservation methods.

Another possibility for minimizing the chance of ice formation during vitrification is to increase the cooling and warming rates. The higher the cooling rate, the lower the required cryoprotectant concentration is, and vice versa. Eventually, even the radical approach of vitrification has to establish a delicate balance, as it requires: (i) establishment of a safe system for maximal and reliable cooling (and warming) rates while avoiding consequent damage including fracture of the zona pellucida or the cells; and (ii) elimination or minimization of the toxic and osmotic effects of the high cryoprotectant concentrations needed to obtain and maintain the glass-like solidification.

There is, however, a small, poorly defined group of cryopreservation techniques that shares some features with both vitrification and slow-rate freezing. In this method, cryoprotectant concentrations are insufficient to establish vitrification (8,16–18). This approach has been established entirely empirically and does not meet any supposed requirements of cryopreservation in embryology. Although ice is formed in the solution, under certain (and sometimes unpredictable) conditions, embryos survive and develop further (19,20). However, the lack of control may result in inconsistent survival and developmental rates. On the other hand, some of the early experiments characterized as rapid freezing were in fact vitrifications (21,22).

INJURY AND PREVENTION DURING CRYOPRESERVATION

Exposition to deep subzero temperatures is a situation mammalian cells never meet under physiological circumstances. Injury may occur at all phases of the procedure.

During cooling, different types of damage may occur when embryos pass through three overlapping temperature zones.

Firstly, at relatively high temperatures between +15 and −5°C, chilling injury is the major factor, predominantly damaging the cytoplasmic lipid droplets and microtubules including the meiotic spindle (23–25). While the latter damage may be reversible, the former is always irreversible and contributes to the death of cryopreserved lipid-rich oocytes and embryos of some species.

Secondly, between −5 and −80°C, extracellular or predominantly intracellular ice crystal formation is the main source of injury.

Thirdly, temperatures between −50 and −150°C are postulated to cause fracture damage to the zona pellucida or the cytoplasm (although the mechanism and the actual temperature of occurrence is not entirely defined) (26). However, it is unlikely that zona fracture could occur as a simple consequence of osmotic stress, as suggested by Smith and Silva (5).

Storage below −150°C (typically in liquid nitrogen at −196°C) is probably the least dangerous phase of the cryopreservation procedure.

Importantly, accidental warming is probably the most frequent form of injury, putting vitrified samples at risk if not handled appropriately (27). The effect of background irradiation seems to be less harmful than supposed, and is not a significant source of DNA injury in a realistic time interval (i.e., years, decades, or even centuries) (28). There is increasing concern regarding possible disease transmission between the stored samples mediated by the liquid nitrogen, even though that there are no reported cases in the literature involving embryos.

At warming, the same types of injuries may occur as at cooling, though obviously in reverse order. One of the most likely reasons for injury is recrystallization during warming, which nearly always occurs. To avoid or minimize its potential damage, addition of certain components to the cryosolution has been investigated, as well adjusting the speed of warming (relative to the speed of cooling) (29,30).

Apart from these processes, there are some only partially understood injuries including damage to intracellular organelles, the cytoskeleton, and cell-to-cell contacts (31,32).

All embryos subject to cryopreservation may suffer considerable damage during cooling and warming. Fortunately, they also have a remarkable, sometimes surprising ability to fully or partially repair this damage, and in the best case to continue normal development. All cryopreservation methods try to decrease the damage and facilitate the regeneration process.

Cryoprotectants are a diverse group of simple or complex, permeable or non-permeable, organic or inorganic compounds with two common features: they are water soluble and they protect the cells from cryoinjuries. The range is wide, expanding from well-known, simple organic solvents such as ethanol to complex, partially known substances such as serum or egg yolk. Permeable cryoprotectants enter the cells and minimize ice formation by various mechanisms depending on their structure and chemical activity, while non-permeable cryoprotectants remain outside the cells and minimize ice formation by removing water from the cells by the osmotic effect. However, there are certain overlaps between the two groups, especially in vitrification methods, where the usually applied short exposure to the concentrated, theoretically permeable components do not allow full equilibrium; therefore, part of the effect of permeable cryoprotectants is dehydration as well. Additionally, both permeable and non-permeable components may have some other specific cryoprotectant effects, such as stabilization of cell membranes, the meiotic spindle, or other cellular structures (33). Unfortunately, most cryoprotectants have some negative effects including toxicity and, obviously, osmotic effects. Toxicity is usually in direct correlation with the concentration of the substance, temperature, and time of exposure, while the osmotic effect is mostly proportional to the concentration. In case of permeable or partially permeable cryoprotectants, the osmotic effect can be minimized by slow, stepwise addition and removal during equilibration and dilution, respectively. The mechanism and reasons for damage during cryopreservation as well as the precise protective mechanisms of cryoprotectants are poorly understood at present. Morphological observations of the intracellular structures during the actual phase of cooling (especially at subzero temperatures) are difficult; functional analysis of specific processes at a given moment is almost impossible. The most frequently applied approaches are to investigate the effects of cryoprotectants without cooling and warming, or to draw retrospective conclusions based on the damage that can be observed after warming. However, the effects of a given cryoprotectant may substantially differ at physiological and at low temperatures; thus, the retrospective analysis of damage may result in faulty conclusions. Considering these uncertainties, it is not surprising that the vast majority of existing cryopreservation techniques were established empirically, based on rough morphological changes observed under a stereomicroscope, and have been justified by the outcome (i.e., *in vitro* and *in vivo* survival). This is valid for the development and perfection of the vitrification technique, but also stands for the slow-freezing technology. Recent developments in sensitive diagnostic testing, related to quantification of oocyte's metabolome and proteome can help to further improve cryopreservation protocols (34).

VITRIFICATION

Cryoprotectants

No cryoprotectants exclusively designed or used for vitrification have been developed yet. However, some components and combinations (e.g., ethylene glycol, dimethyl sulfoxide [DMSO], and sucrose) are typically used for vitrification purposes, and the concentration of specific components is significantly higher at vitrification than in traditional or rapid freezing.

The most common permeable components are ethylene glycol, propylene glycol, acetamide, glycerol, raffinose, and DMSO, and these have been tested in various combinations (4,35). Due to its low toxicity, high permeability, and excellent ice-blocking ability, ethylene glycol is an almost indispensable component of all cryoprotectant solutions. However, a common strategy to decrease the specific toxicity of any one cryoprotectant is to use a mixture of two permeable cryoprotectants (i.e., a mixture of ethylene glycol and either DMSO, propylene glycol, or, less typically, other components). The mixture of ethylene glycol and DMSO now appears to be used frequently (36,37). According to some studies, the permeability of this mixture is higher than that of the individual components (38). It should be noted that the earlier concerns regarding the genotoxicity and cytotoxicity of DMSO have been dismissed (39,40).

Commonly used non-permeable cryoprotectants include monosaccharides and disaccharides, sucrose, trehalose, glucose, and galactose (41–43). Recently, sucrose has become almost a standard component of vitrification mixtures. This is true even though nearly all comparative investigations proved the superiority of trehalose. Sucrose as well as other sugars may not have any toxic effects at low temperatures, but may compromise embryo survival when applied extensively to counterbalance embryo swelling after warming (44–46), although this effect was not always demonstrated (47). Several polymers were also suggested for the purpose, including polyvinylpyrrolidine, polyethylene glycol, Ficoll, dextran and polyvinyl alcohol (48–53). However, from this group, the only widely used compound is Ficoll, predominantly in combination with ethylene glycol and sucrose (54). Various forms of protein supplementation have also been used, including egg yolk, but its optically dense appearance made microscopic manipulation rather difficult. High concentrations of sera of different origins as well as serum albumin preparations (55) are common additives. In the bovine model, recombinant albumin and hyaluronan were also effective (56). On the other hand, the use of antifreeze proteins isolated from arctic animals (57–59) has largely been abandoned. More recently, hydroxypropyl cellulose was investigated as a replacement for serum-derived protein for use in cryoprotectant solutions, and results from its use have been promising (60,61).

Another practical feature is the stepwise addition of increasing concentrations of cryoprotectants (55,62–64). After several early attempts, the two-step equilibration has become the most commonly used approach, with the first solution containing approximately 50% of the final cryoprotectant concentration. Embryos and oocytes are equilibrated for a relatively long period (5–15 minutes, or sometimes up to 21 minutes) in the first solution, then for a short period (~1 minute) in the second one (65–67). This approach may increase the toxic effect slightly, but provides much better protection for the whole cell, and may be especially beneficial in the case of large substances with a low surface/volume ratios, including oocytes or early-stage embryos. On the other hand, earlier attempts to cool the concentrated solution to 4°C in order to decrease toxicity have later been found to be unnecessary. Because of the much higher concentrations of cryoprotectant agents used in vitrification, it was initially assumed that intracellular concentrations of cryoprotectant agents are higher after vitrification than after slow freezing, raising concerns about the toxicity of these cryoprotectant agents. However, in a recent elegant study, it was demonstrated that intracellular concentrations of cryoprotectants are actually lower after vitrification than after slow freezing, despite exposure to higher concentrations of cryoprotectant solutions (68).

TOOLS OF CRYOPRESERVATION USED FOR VITRIFICATION

Plastic insemination straws or cryovials were used initially for vitrification experiments. These tools were not designed for the special purpose of vitrification, had a thick wall, and required a relatively large amount of solution for safe loading. Accordingly, the cooling and warming rates were quite limited (approximately 2500°C/minute for straws [69], and even less for cryovials). This relatively low rate was still hazardous to perform, as direct immersion into liquid nitrogen at cooling and transfer to a water bath at warming induced extreme pressure changes in the closed system and frequently led to the collapse or explosion of the straws and loss of the sample. Other consequences of these manipulations were the decreased and inconsistent rates: the temperature of the vapor of liquid nitrogen is variable, depending on many factors, and the definition of "room temperature" laboratory air may mean 5°C–7°C differences, even at the same place on the same day. Consequently, a minimum 5—7-mol/L cryoprotectant concentration was required, and chilling injury could not be lowered to the level occurring at slow freezing.

Some scientists have investigated the use of an instrument, called the VitMaster, to achieve higher cooling rates. (VitMaster is able to lower the temperature of liquid nitrogen from its boiling point of -196°C to around -208°C—applying vacuum—thus the nitrogen then changes from its liquid state to a slush, which prevents an insulating pocket of gas forming around the sample, resulting in faster cooling.) Although outcomes of vitrification using VitMaster tended to be somewhat better than "traditional" vitrification (70,71), its use has not become part of the daily routine (possibly because it is hard to vitrify a larger number of samples in a timely manner with this instrument). More recently, efforts were made to develop an instrument that can offer some level of automation for vitrifying samples (1). This "Gavi" system can automatically perform equilibration steps before closed vitrification is performed for embryos. The warming, however, has to be performed manually, and currently the system is not proven to perform equivalently for oocyte cryopreservation.

INCREASING COOLING RATES WITH NEW CARRIER TOOLS

Although the increased cooling and warming rates are well-known approaches to keeping the concentrations of cryoprotectants as low as possible and to minimizing the related toxic and osmotic injuries, this option has remained unexploited for a relatively long period of time. The first purpose-made tools were only produced approximately 20 years ago. Today, however, the opposite is the problem: a huge variety of tools, methods, and approaches are available, and without authentic comparative studies, the selection of the best choice is a serious problem for embryologists working in a routine human IVF laboratory.

The most logical way to increase cooling and warming rates is to decrease the volume of the solution that surrounds the sample and to establish direct contact between the sample and the liquid nitrogen.

Seemingly the simplest way to accomplish this task is direct dropping into liquid nitrogen (65,72–74). Unfortunately, to form a drop from a water-based solution requires a relatively large amount of solution (4–6 μL), and the drop does not sink immediately into the liquid nitrogen, because for the initial seconds the drop is surrounded by the vapor that is induced by the warm solution, and does not allow the sample to sink.

Accordingly, some carrier tools have been used to push the sample immediately below the level of the liquid nitrogen, to serve as a storage device after cooling, and to facilitate quick warming. Electron microscopic grids used for this completely different purpose proved the practical value of the idea first (72–76). In this system, the size of the drop surrounding the sample was extremely small, as after loading, most of it was removed by placing the grid on a filter membrane. The thermoconductive metal grid also contributed to improving the cooling and warming rates. Surprisingly, the solidified cryoprotectant solution fixed the sample safely to the grid during cooling and storage and released it easily after warming (77). However, the storage and handling of the tiny grid is a demanding task.

The first purpose-made tool for vitrification was the open pulled straw (OPS), a modification of a standard 0.25-mL plastic straw with decreased diameter and wall thickness. This modification enabled loading with the capillary effect, and the minimum volume decreased to approximately 0.5–1 μL (i.e., 5–10-times smaller than that of the original straw), resulting in an approximately 10-fold increase in the achievable cooling and warming rates and a 30% decrease of the cryoprotectant concentration required for vitrification. An additional benefit was related to the open system: no explosions of the straws occurred, and the fracture damage (with some precautions) could be entirely eliminated. The OPS has become the most widely used approach for ultra-rapid vitrification (78–86). According to preliminary experiments, by using recent equilibration and dilution parameters, results achieved with OPS vitrification of human oocytes and embryos are at least as good as with other commonly used vitrification tools.

The cryoloop is another approach using the small volume–direct contact principle (Figure 23.1). It consists of a small nylon loop attached to a holder and equipped with a container. It has been used for cryopreservation

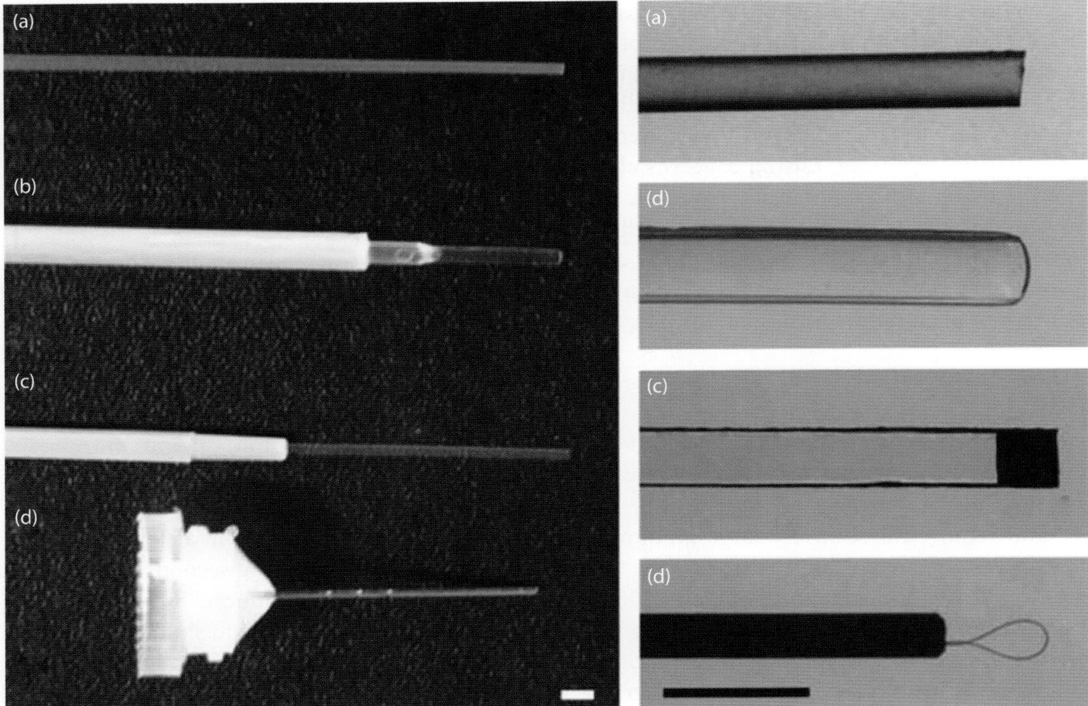

Figure 23.1 Examples for commercially available tools used as carriers for high-speed vitrification. (a) Open pulled straw (Minitüb, Landshut, Germany); (b) McGill Cryoleaf (MediCult, Jyllinge, Denmark); (c) Cryotop (Kitazato, Tokyo, Japan); (d) Cryoloop (Hampton Research, Aliso Viejo, CA). Bars represent 2 mm.

in crystallography and is now used widely for oocyte and embryo cryopreservation (87–90). The solution film bridging the hole of the loop is strong enough to hold the oocyte or the embryo, and with this minimal solution volume, the achievable cooling rate may be extremely high, up to an estimated 700,000°C/minute (91). Using this tool, safe cryopreservation can be achieved even in the vapor of liquid nitrogen (92,93).

The minimum drop size method of Arav et al. (94) consists of a small droplet of vitrification solution containing the oocyte or embryo placed on a solid surface that is immersed into liquid nitrogen. The approach was used later with some modifications called minimum volume cooling (95) or in the hemi-straw system (96), where the carrier tool was a cut-open straw.

Currently, the most commonly used tool for the vitrification of human oocytes and embryos is the Cryotop, an advanced version of the minimum volume cooling technology (67,95). It consists of a flexible transparent plastic film attached to a handle, and is also equipped with a protective tube to avoid damage to the film during storage in liquid nitrogen. The sample is loaded onto the film, the excess solution is removed, and the film is immersed in the liquid nitrogen. At warming, the Cryotop is quickly removed from the liquid nitrogen, and the film is immersed in the warming medium. This simple system, with appropriate solutions and equilibration parameters, triggered an exponential increase of the use of vitrification in human embryology. Since its introduction, a good number of studies have confirmed its value (97–99). Yet other carriers, such as the Cryolock and Cryotec, which are similar in their design to the Cryotop, are gaining more popularity and being used efficiently (100,101).

Cryopette is probably the first carrier that has been designed by aiming to combine the benefit of very-low-volume solutions with the benefit of a closed system. There are other closed carriers that have been investigated and tried for the use of embryo vitrification, including the Rapid-I (102,103) and the CBS-VIT High Security straw, demonstrating satisfactory outcomes (104,105). Based on published studies, it appears that closed systems are also able to provide adequate outcomes for embryo vitrification; however, open systems are more likely to provide superior results when oocytes are vitrified and to preserve the original physiological cell conditions (106,107).

The flowchart of a typical high-speed vitrification procedure is shown in Figure 23.2.

DECREASED VAPOR FORMATION FOR INCREASED COOLING RATES

One major limitation of the achievable cooling rates around the sample is the vapor that is formed around it at immersion. At −196°C, liquid nitrogen is at boiling point; accordingly, a submerged, warmer item will induce extensive evaporation around the sample, producing a thermoinsulating coat around the sample and decreasing the achievable cooling rate, especially at the initial moments when chilling injury may develop.

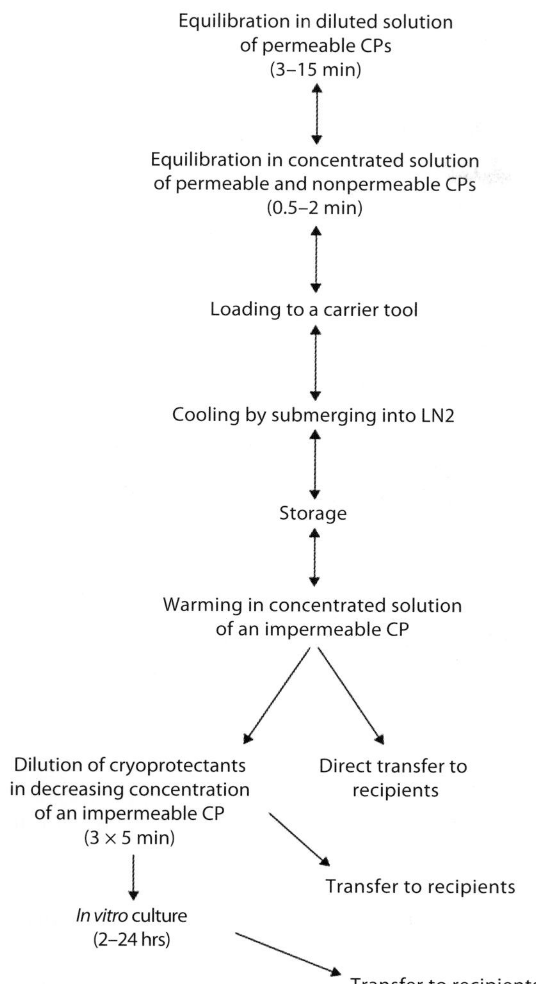

Figure 23.2 Flowchart of a typical high-speed vitrification procedure. *Abbreviations*: CP, cryoprotectant; LN2, liquid nitrogen.

One possible approach to avoiding this phenomenon is to expose liquid nitrogen to a vacuum for several minutes. Part of the liquid nitrogen will evaporate, and the rest will cool down to −203 to −207°C, at which point it starts to solidify (i.e., slush is formed). As the nitrogen escapes from the fragile boiling zone, the immersed sample creates minimal evaporation; consequently, the cooling rate becomes considerably higher (81,82,108).

The other way to eliminate the vapor is the use of precooled metal surfaces instead of the liquid nitrogen for cooling. This can be performed by immersing a metal block into liquid nitrogen (109), or by using a more sophisticated, commercially available version (CMV; Cryologic, Australia).

The freely available comparative data do not provide entirely convincing evidence regarding the superiority of these vapor-minimizing or vapor-free approaches compared to other vitrification procedures.

TRANSMISSION OF INFECTIOUS AGENTS

One of the concerns regarding the use of vitrification in human embryology is the potential risk of liquid nitrogen-mediated disease transmission. To understand this better, we need to consider the following:

1. Semen and oocyte collection, processing/handling, and cryopreservation protocols are not sterile procedures (110); consequently, the contents of virtually all stored straws and cryovials may be sources of infection.
2. In human embryology, liquid nitrogen may also be contaminated by the surfaces of straws, cryovials, racks, and other tools that are usually not handled fully aseptically. Accordingly, the presence of infective agents is not strictly related to leaky or open containers.
3. Seemingly sterile containers may not be as safe as supposed. Infection may occur in common straws in slow freezing (through the holes of incomplete sealing or pores of the plastic walls), and most cryovials do not have secure caps. A possible source of infection may also be the inappropriate decontamination of the outer walls of straws before loading and expelling.
4. Liquid nitrogen in storage tanks likely contains a number of commensal and potentially pathogenic environmental microorganisms (110).
5. Cases of liquid nitrogen-mediated transmission of pathogens (111–113) have been documented, but never in relation to cryopreserved oocytes or embryos. Disease transfer has occurred only on one occasion, where two leaky bags containing blood samples were stored in the same dewar (111).
6. According to the experiments of Bielanski et al. (114), cross-contamination may also occur during open embryo storage if one of samples is artificially infected. However, the volume of the microbes in this case was extremely high, a concentration that may never arise in clinical situations.
7. Not a single case of any disease transmission in assisted reproduction technology has been found to be related to liquid nitrogen-mediated cross-contamination, in spite of the enormous number of human sperm samples, embryos, and oocytes stored worldwide, neither related to traditional, supposedly closed (but very often leaky or inappropriately handled) systems, nor to open vitrification systems, in spite of the enormous focus on the latter. A study published in 2012 provided evidence from a real case scenario of the lack of risk of cross-contamination among seropositive patients, even when using an open device for vitrification (115).

There is no doubt that closed and properly handled systems should always be preferred, provided the outcome is comparable with that of open systems. Results achieved by using closed systems for cleavage-stage human embryos and blastocysts are promising (104,116,117). However, the fact that open systems are superior to closed ones for human oocyte vitrification proves the superiority of the former systems (67,118). A possible solution is to conduct cooling in sterilized liquid nitrogen (119,120) and store the samples in precooled, hermetically sealed containers afterwards (79,121). Alternatively, open carriers can also be stored in cryotanks where, instead of liquid, the vapor of nitrogen maintains the low storage temperature (122). A number of studies have demonstrated the efficiency of the vapor storage system for vitrified oocytes/embryos using open carriers in both animal and human systems (122–124). Concerns may also be raised regarding the applicability of closed systems for other chilling-sensitive objects, including cattle oocytes and early-stage embryos, porcine blastocysts, or human oocytes (125), regarding not just *in vitro* survival rates, but also *in vitro* development, pregnancies, and birth of healthy offspring.

WARMING

Previously, Rall (55) found that the high rate of survival of vitrified embryos can be achieved with rather slow warming rates. However, most vitrification methods use rapid warming procedures, and recently it has been demonstrated that warming rates may be even more important than cooling rates (126).

Closed systems are usually immersed into water baths, while open systems can be directly submerged into the medium; in this way, the warming and the first dilution are performed in a single step. This seemingly negligible difference may contribute considerably to the inferior results achieved with some closed systems consisting of a simple plastic or glass tube. After warming in the water bath, the surface has to be decontaminated quickly with a nontoxic but perfectly safe disinfectant, then the tube is cut and the sample is expelled into the appropriate medium. This means a significant delay between the warming and dilution; accordingly, the samples in this critical, very fragile phase are exposed for a relatively long period of time (5–10 seconds) to the concentrated cryoprotectants. Although a slight devitrification (occurrence of ice crystals) may occur, especially when the cryoprotectant level is kept at a minimum, this transitional change is usually restricted to a part of the embryo-containing medium and most probably does not involve intracellular crystal formation, and consequently does not cause significant harm in the embryos or oocytes (127), especially if the volume of the droplet is minimized (at the time of placing the embryo on the carrier).

In routine warming protocols of vitrified embryos, the dilution is a multistep procedure with decreasing concentrations of osmotic buffers (usually sucrose) to counterbalance the swelling caused by the permeable cryoprotectant that leaves the cells relatively slowly. This delicate, multistep dilution procedure seems to be indispensable for human embryos or oocytes, although one-step dilution without a significant decrease of *in vitro* survival was reported in some animal species including cattle (46,63,128) and pigs (129). Based on this approach, direct transfer methods after ultra-rapid vitrification of embryos resulted in offspring after transfer in cattle (130) and sheep (131). Interestingly, the commonly used warming protocol (for vitrified samples) may also be used very efficiently for slow-frozen oocytes/embryos, thus providing a simplified and standard warming protocol for all samples, irrespective of how they were frozen/vitrified (132).

FACTORS INFLUENCING THE OUTCOME

Species and genotype

There are well-demonstrated but poorly understood differences in sensitivity to cryoinjuries between different species in mammals. It appears that transparent oocytes and embryos are usually more resistant, while dense, dark ones are more fragile due to the increased lipid content. Accordingly, cryopreservation of light mouse embryos is a relatively easy task, cryopreservation of darker bovine embryos is a more difficult task, and cryopreservation of dense pig embryos is truly a challenge in cryobiology. In parallel with the lighter appearance of the cytoplasm, considerably increased survival rates were detected after both slow freezing (133) and vitrification (134–137). This approach also improves the *in vitro* survival of vitrified porcine blastocysts produced by somatic cell nuclear transfer (137,138).

It should also be noted that apart from the differences between species, in mice, differences between genotypes in the ability to develop after vitrification were also observed (139).

Developmental stage

The change in the size and shape of the cells is unprecedented in the first five to six days of mammalian development. A relatively simple spherical shape protected by an acellular outer layer develops into a complicated multicellular structure without external protection. Predictably, the extreme differences in morphology also correlate considerably with differences in sensitivity to cryoinjuries.

Generally, the earlier the development stage (starting from the germinal vesicle stage), the more sensitive oocytes and embryos are. However, although there is only a minimal difference between the size and shape, immature oocytes are usually more sensitive to cryopreservation than mature (metaphase II [MII]) oocytes (24,125,140). Membrane permeability related to the type and expression levels of aquaporin at different stages may also explain differences in cryoprotectant protection efficiency and thus differences in survival (141,142). Additionally, a very remarkable difference exists between the chilling sensitivities of unfertilized and fertilized human oocytes. A possible explanation for this phenomenon is the increased chilling sensitivity of membranes: the lipid phase transition at room temperature storage in human germinal vesicle- and MII-stage oocytes is 10–times higher than that of human pronuclear embryos (125).

In the human, the survival rates after slow freezing are not significantly different between zygotes, cleavage-stage embryos, and blastocysts (between 75% and 80% for each) (143–145). Similarly, in the human, survival rates after vitrification are not different for zygote-, cleavage-, or blastocyst-stage embryos (though at each stage vitrification provides a significantly higher survival rate) (146–148). The complex structure of blastocysts may give rise to additional problems. In humans, mechanical reduction of the blastocoel by puncturing or repeated pipetting improved survival and pregnancy rates (149–153). The

Table 23.1 Various vitrification techniques in embryology

System	Reference
Direct dropping into liquid nitrogen	Landa and Tepla (72)
Electron microscopic grids	Martino et al. (24)
Open pulled straw	Vajta et al. (79)
Glass micropipettes	Kong et al. (166)
Super-finely pulled open pulled straw	Isachenko et al. (167)
Gel-loading tips	Tominaga and Hamada (168)
Sterile stripper tip	Kuleshova and Lopata (121)
Flexipet denuding pipette	Liebermann et al. (169)
Fine-diameter plastic micropipette	Cremades et al. (170)
100-μL pipetting tip	Hredzak et al. (171)
Closed pulled straw	Chen et al. (172)
Sealed open pulled straws	Lopez-Bejar and Lopez-Gatius (173)
Cryotip	Kuwayama et al. (67)
Cryoloop	Lane et al. (87)
Nylon mesh	Matsumoto et al. (93)
Minimum drop size	Arav (174)
Minimum volume cooling	Hamawaki et al. (95)
Hemi-straw system	Vanderzwalmen et al. (96)
Cryotop	Kuwayama et al. (66)
VitMaster	Arav et al. (81)
Solid surface vitrification	Dinnyes et al. (109)

Source: Reprinted from Vajta G, Nagy ZP. Are programmable freezers still needed in the embryo laboratory? Review on vitrification. *Reprod Biomed Online* 2006; 12(6): 779–96 (175), with permission from Reproductive Healthcare Ltd.

usual explanation for this is that the large blastocoel may not be protected appropriately from ice crystal formation (149). Survival rates of blastocyst-stage embryos using vitrification are extremely high (usually above 95%), even without any additional "manipulation" (145). However, some studies demonstrated that blastocyst survival (and intactness) may be further increased after vitrification if the blastocoel is punctured, resulting in shrinkage—especially when the blastocyst is expanded—in human and in other species (153–156).

In vivo- versus *in vitro*-produced embryos

Due to the lack of *in vivo*-derived human embryos, such differences can only be evaluated in domestic and experimental animals (157). In these species, *in vivo*-produced embryos are more resistant to injuries—including cryoinjuries—than their *in vitro*-fertilized or cloned counterparts. Again, there might be some correlation between this and the increased lipid content of embryos produced in some *in vitro* systems. In general, the less that the morphological difference from the *in vivo* counterpart is detectable in the *in vivo*-produced embryos, the smaller the expected difference in survival after cryopreservation (158). Although total elimination of these differences is still impossible, according to the joint conclusion of many publications, vitrification seems to be especially appropriate to counterbalancing this handicap (159).

OUTCOMES AFTER EMBRYO VITRIFICATION

Domestic, experimental, and wild animals

There is an extensive literature of comparative experiments between slow freezing versus vitrification (some examples include [87,88,139,160–165]). The overwhelming majority of these papers prove the superiority of vitrification for the given purpose. Probably less than 10% of the studies did not find significant differences that were conducted at an early stage; however, the overwhelming majority of more recent studies clearly demonstrated the superiority of vitrification (Table 23.1). Moreover, there are situations where vitrification is uniquely or predominantly suitable to achieving the goal: most of these areas are summarized in Table 23.2.

Human embryos

In humans, the clinical pregnancy rate from embryo transfer after slow freezing is approximately two-thirds that from the fresh transfer of embryos (192), although new techniques have recently been introduced to restore (cleavage-stage) embryo viability (193,194). The theoretical possibility for improvement is supported by the results obtained in cattle, where the difference is no more than 10%–15%.

Initial studies have demonstrated the feasibility and potential superiority of vitrification for embryo cryopreservation (4,21,22,75,76,84,85,89,90,96,149,150,162,195–207).

Table 23.2 Examples in mammalian embryology where first success in cryopreservation was achieved by vitrification

Species, stage, system	References
Bovine immature oocytes for IVF	Vieria et al. (176)
Bovine *in vitro*-matured oocytes for IVF	Martino et al. (177); Vajta et al. (79)
Bovine *in vitro*-matured oocytes for somatic cell nuclear transfer	Hou et al. (178)
Bovine cytoplasts for embryonic cell nuclear transfer	Booth et al. (179)
Bovine early-stage IVF embryos	Vajta et al. (80); *in vitro* study
Bovine zona-included blastocysts generated by somatic cell nuclear transfer	French et al. (180)
Bovine zona-free blastocysts generated by somatic cell nuclear transfer	Tecirlioglu et al. (130)
Bovine transgenic blastocysts generated by somatic cell nuclear transfer	French et al. (181)
Ovine zona-included embryos generated by nuclear transfer	Peura et al. (182)
Porcine immature oocytes for ICSI	Fujihira et al. (183); *in vitro* study
Porcine *in vitro*-matured oocytes for ICSI	Fujihira et al. (184); *in vitro* study
Porcine *in vivo*–derived blastocysts	Kobayashi et al. (185)
Porcine *in vivo*–derived morulae	Berthelot et al. (186)
Porcine *in vitro*-produced blastocysts	Men et al. (187); *in vitro* study
Equine *in vivo*-matured oocytes	Maclellan et al. (188)
European polecat *in vivo*-derived morulae and blastocysts	Piltti et al. (189)
Siberian tiger *in vivo*–derived embryos	Crichton et al. (190); *in vitro* study
Minke whale immature oocytes for maturation	Iwayama et al. (191); *in vitro* study

Source: Reprinted from Vajta G, Nagy ZP. Are programmable freezers still needed in the embryo laboratory? Review on vitrification. *Reprod Biomed Online* 2006; 12(6): 779–96 (175), with permission from Reproductive Healthcare Ltd.

Note: Embryos and oocytes were not treated mechanically or chemically to prepare them for the vitrification. Full-term developments were reported except where otherwise indicated.

Abbreviations: ICSI, intracytoplasmic sperm injection; IVF, *in vitro* fertilization.

In 2005, however, three comparative investigations were published, and all three concluded that vitrification was a more efficient way to cryopreserve human embryos than slow-rate freezing (67,208,209). More recent comparative studies published in the literature have confirmed that vitrification is clearly more efficient than slow freezing used at different embryonic developmental stages (210–215). Accordingly, these representative comparisons have proved that vitrification is more efficient than slow-rate freezing for the cryopreservation of human embryos at all stages (216). In addition to these comparative studies, other non-comparative studies on the efficiency of vitrification have been published, applying the technique at different stages of pre-implantation embryo development, including zygote, cleavage, and blastocyst stages (117,147,152,215,217–221), as well as showing successful day-7 vitrification (222). Based on these reported improved outcomes, a consensus meeting was organized by Alpha Scientists, to set minimum standards and inspirational outcome parameters following cryopreservation that today set the standards worldwide (145).

Although several tools (carriers) and kits (vitrification solution kits) are currently available today for vitrification, two technologies related to the type of carriers have obtained more attention initially: the OPS, predominantly in the animal field; and the Cryotop for human areas. It should be emphasized, however, that the differences do not necessarily mean an unbreakable frontier. The OPS is more robust and is easy to perform even under compromised conditions, while the more delicate Cryotop method may be the best choice where an extremely high cooling rate is the primary objective. However, if properly applied, both OPS and Cryotop methods seem to be suitable for the given purposes. A good example to support this statement is that very healthy piglets were born after OPS vitrification and transfer of the extremely sensitive somatic cell-cloned blastocyst derived from delipated oocytes (138). As written earlier, there are now several new cryotools/carriers available on the market that are likely to be tested and used more widely for both embryo and oocyte vitrification. Storage time, as expected, had no impact on the outcomes of vitrified embryos (or vitrified oocytes), as different studies have established (223,224), if samples are stored and handled adequately, avoiding accidental warming.

Updated results obtained from the Reproductive Biology Associates, an IVF clinic, which was the first in the U.S.A. to apply embryo (and oocyte) vitrification in routine patient care using the Cryotop or Cryolock approaches, demonstrate equal or better outcomes with vitrification compared to slow freezing in comparable patient populations (see Table 23.3).

Vitrification and assisted reproduction technology services

Routine application of vitrification has spread out all over the world in recent years (215,225,226), resulting in a paradigm shift in how assisted reproduction treatment is performed.

Table 23.3 Outcomes of embryo cryopreservation–embryo transfer cycles comparing vitrification/warming with slow freezing/thawing (including 2PN/day-3 and blastocyst-stage cryopreserved embryos)

	Slow freeze	Vitrification	p-value
All thaws (two-pronuclear zygote [2PN]/day 3/blastocyst)			
Thaw–warm cycles	132	468	
Average age (years)	36.1	35.9	Non-significant
Embryos thawed/warmed	662	1307	
Embryos thawed/warmed per cycle	5.0	2.8	<0.001
Survived	529	1246	
Survival rate	79.9%	95.3%	<0.001
Clinical pregnancy rate	48.5%	59.6%	<0.05
Implantation rate	32.6%	39.0%	<0.01

The extremely high efficiency of vitrification applied on oocytes and embryos provides possibilities for novel patient services. Oocyte and embryo vitrification can now provide the base for fertility preservation for both medical and social reasons (227–231) and for donor egg banking (97,99), or for various other clinical conditions, such as hyperstimulation, failure to obtain sperm on the day of oocyte collection, or due to moral/ethical reasons for preferring egg preservation instead of embryo preservation (232–235), cryopreserving excess oocytes aspirated from intrauterine insemination patients with excess follicles (236).

This highly efficient embryo vitrification has opened up several new possibilities. One of the most important benefits relates to embryo biopsy and preimplantation genetic screening/diagnosis. In the past, survival of embryos after slow freeze/thaw following embryo biopsy was more than disappointing, strongly limiting the use of biopsy and genetic testing—mainly to be performed on day-3 cleavage-stage embryos or for polar body biopsy (237,238). Applying vitrification instead of slow freezing on biopsied embryos has significantly improved survival rates (208,239), and therefore this procedure has become routine when embryos are to be tested genetically (213,240). Additionally, biopsy timing can now be shifted from day 3 (or day 0/day 1) to day 5/day 6, when embryos develop to the blastocyst stage, as there is no more need to use these embryos for fresh transfer, as they will survive cryopreservation much better, usually perfectly. Biopsying embryos at the blastocyst stage has several advantages compared to earlier stages, especially compared to day-3-stage biopsy, as embryos are more resistant to the biopsy procedure, more cells can be removed (genetic testing can be more reliable), one is less likely to encounter mosaicism, and embryos will be transferred into a (possibly) more receptive uterine environment; all of these factors in combination result in very high pregnancy rates (240–243). Pregnancies and live births were also reported when vitrification was repeated on the same embryo at the same (or different) stage or after oocyte vitrification, or even after involving a trophectoderm biopsy, demonstrating the robustness of the technique (100,243–246). Because of the extremely high success rates obtained with vitrified embryos after biopsy, it seems a logical extension to think that other patients with different clinical conditions may also benefit from the "cryopreserve all" embryos approach and from performing transfer in a "cryo-cycle" (247). Rationally, patients at risk for ovarian hyperstimulation can clearly benefit from vitrifying all embryos (221); other study recommend "cryo embryos" for women with endometriosis (248), while some may consider applying this idea to all IVF patients, aiming for the benefit of a more receptive endometrium in a cryo-cycle for patients who have undergone ovarian stimulation (247,249). Additionally, patients with diminished ovarian reserve (irrespective of reproductive age) may also benefit, for the same reasons as the "cryopreserve all" strategy. Instead of performing a fresh transfer, all embryos or oocytes (typically vitrified at an early stage due to the low oocyte/zygote number) are cryopreserved and then transferred later into a "frozen embryo transfer cycle"/"frozen embryo replacement (FER) cycle" (either a natural or supplemented cycle) (250,251). In fact, there are fewer and fewer reasons to perform fresh embryo transfers, and one can expect that in the near future all/most IVF cycles will be "cryopreserve all" and embryo transfer will be performed in "FER cycles" only (247). Moreover, the high efficiency of embryo vitrification also strongly promotes single-embryo transfer. In the past, when slow-freezing was used, embryos frequently did not survive cryopreservation, thus prompting both clinicians and patients to use more embryos for fresh transfer, instead of freezing them. Today, using vitrification, the viability of the embryo post-warming is virtually equivalent to the viability prior to cryopreservation, which in combination with a more "natural" endometrium can benefit patients and offspring (252). Society for Assisted Reproductive Technology (SART) data show that the number of "FER cycles" has exponentially increased: in 2003 there were about 13,000 FER cycles, while 10 years later, in 2013, there were about 38,000 FER cycles, and at the same time the number of "fresh cycles" has remained about the same (Table 23.4). The fact that in this 10-year period the number of "FER cycles" has tripled is the direct

Table 23.4 Society for Assisted Reproductive Technology data from 2003 and 2013 showing the number of fresh and frozen cycles (from non-donor oocytes) and the outcomes after "FER"

	Thawed embryos from non-donor oocytes			
	<35	35–37	38–40	41–42
2003				
Number of transfers	7456	3302	2244	670
Percentage of transfers resulting in live births	29.5	28.3	22.6	16.9
Average number of embryos transferred	2.7	2.7	2.8	3.0
Number of fresh cycles	36,178	18,508	17,396	7635
2013				
Number of transfers	18,801	9602	7116	2731
Percentage of transfers resulting in live births	44.4	40.6	36.1	31.6
Average number of embryos transferred	1.7	1.6	1.7	1.8
Number of fresh cycles	36,958	18,508	16,853	9026

consequence of: improved embryo culture and the trend to cryopreserve embryos at the most potent stage, when developed to the blastocyst; increasing use of preimplantation genetic screening to deselect chromosomally abnormal embryos; and the effectiveness of vitrification, as well as taking advantage of a more receptive endometrium.

Safety of vitrification

In order for a new technique or technology to be fully accepted and applied worldwide, there are two critical points that need to be met: efficiency and safety. Vitrification of embryos/oocytes has been clearly demonstrated to provide extremely high efficiency, providing outcomes similar to those achieved by using fresh oocytes/embryos. However, safety is a point that is yet to be proven beyond any doubt. Initial studies presenting outcomes on live birth data (mainly gathered after oocyte vitrification) do not indicate any alarming or unexpected results or trends (217,243,245,253–257). More recent data on babies born after embryo vitrification continue to demonstrate the safety of the technique, not showing increased risks for birth defects or other live birth parameters (258–261). It would be most prudent for national or international IVF societies to organize the needed data collection through registries. Only a multicenter effort where most IVF clinics participate would be able to provide a sufficient amount of data in a reasonable period of time.

CONCLUSIONS

Vitrification as an approach to cryopreserving human embryos or oocytes has achieved remarkable success. With very few publications on clinical results and applications, today there are several dozens of papers demonstrating the efficient use of embryo/oocyte vitrification in human assisted reproduction, and most likely all (or virtually all) IVF clinics have switched from slow freezing to vitrification. This extraordinary achievement would not have been possible without the constant dedication and hard work of the few early pioneers, mainly coming from the field of veterinary medicine. On the safety of vitrification, any currently available data do not indicate a higher incidence of malformation, which is reassuring, but obviously needs to be confirmed on a much larger scale.

The overwhelming majority of the studies/publications support the application of vitrification by emphasizing its advantages: the simple, inexpensive, and rapid procedure leading to higher survival and developmental rates than those achievable with alternative methods. Concerns regarding disease transmission are theoretically justified, but safer methods are now available to mitigate this risk. Outstanding results like the breakthrough in human oocyte vitrification and the excellent (and improved) results on embryo cryopreservation have changed the way we practice routine IVF, providing more efficient and safer options for patients.

APPENDIX: EMBRYO/BLASTOCYST VITRIFICATION PROTOCOL

Vitrification

Materials

Equilibration solution (ES) is a 4-(2-hydroxyet4hyl)-1-piperazineethane sulfonic acid (HEPES)-buffered medium, 7.5% (v/v) each of dimethyl sulfoxide (DMSO) and ethylene glycol and 20% (v/v) serum protein substitute.

Vitrification solution (VS) is a HEPES-buffered medium, 15% (v/v) each of DMSO and ethylene glycol, 20% (v/v) serum protein substitute, and 0.5 M sucrose.

Cryolock® (Biodesign, Colombia).

Procedures

1. Bring one vial each of ES and VS to room temperature (20°C–27°C) for at least 30 minutes prior to freezing embryos.
2. Fill the liquid nitrogen reservoir with liquid nitrogen.
3. Determine the number of embryos to be vitrified.
4. Label each Cryolock with necessary information.
5. Prepare a four-well dish with 1.0 mL ES and 1.0 mL VS in each well.

6. Transfer the embryos to ES for 15 minutes.
7. Transfer the embryos to VS for 1 minute.
8. Load the embryos onto the Cryolock with a minimal volume.
9. Plunge the Cryolock into liquid nitrogen (cooling at a rate of −12,000°C/minute).
10. Move the plunged Cryolock to the liquid nitrogen freezer for long-term storage.

Warming

Materials

Thawing Solution (TS) is a HEPES-buffered medium, 1.0 M sucrose and 20% (v/v) serum protein substitute.

Dilution Solution (DS) is a HEPES-buffered medium, 0.5 M sucrose and 20% (v/v) serum protein substitute.

Washing Solution (WS) is a HEPES-buffered medium and 20% (v/v) serum protein substitute.

Procedures

1. Bring one vial each of TS, DS, and WS to room temperature (20°C–27°C) for at least 30 minutes prior to thawing embryos.
2. Fill the liquid nitrogen reservoir with liquid nitrogen.
3. Determine the number of embryos to be thawed.
4. Take the Cryolock out of the liquid nitrogen and quickly transfer embryos into TS (3 mL at 37°C), where embryos should stay for 1 minute.
5. Transfer the embryos into 1.0 mL DS for 3 minutes at room temperature.
6. Transfer the embryos into 1.0 mL WS for 10 minutes at room temperature.
7. Transfer the embryos into pre-equilibrated culture medium.

REFERENCES

1. Roy TK et al. Embryo vitrification using a novel semi-automated closed system yields *in vitro* outcomes equivalent to the manual Cryotop method. *Hum Reprod* 2014; 29(11): 2431–8.
2. Shaw JM, Jones GM. Terminology associated with vitrification and other cryopreservation procedures for oocytes and embryos. *Hum Reprod Update* 2003; 9(6): 583–605.
3. Fuller B. and Paynter S. Fundamentals of cryobiology in reproductive medicine. *Reprod Biomed Online* 2004; 9(6): 680–91.
4. Kasai M, Mukaida T. Cryopreservation of animal and human embryos by vitrification. *Reprod Biomed Online* 2004; 9(2): 164–70.
5. Smith GD, Silva ESCA. Developmental consequences of cryopreservation of mammalian oocytes and embryos. *Reprod Biomed Online* 2004; 9(2): 171–8.
6. Stachecki JJ, Cohen J. An overview of oocyte cryopreservation. *Reprod Biomed Online* 2004; 9(2): 152–63.
7. Whittingham DG, Leibo SP, Mazur P. Survival of mouse embryos frozen to −196 degrees and −269 degrees C. *Science* 1972; 178(59): 411–4.
8. Wilmut I, The effect of cooling rate, warming rate, cryoprotective agent and stage of development on survival of mouse embryos during freezing and thawing. *Life Sci II* 1972; 11(22): 1071–9.
9. Wilmut I, Rowson LE. Experiments on the low-temperature preservation of cow embryos. *Vet Rec* 1973; 92(26): 686–90.
10. Bank H, Maurer RR. Survival of frozen rabbit embryos. *Exp Cell Res* 1974; 89(1): 188–96.
11. Willadsen SM et al. Deep freezing of sheep embryos. *J Reprod Fertil* 1976; 46(1): 151–4.
12. Trounson A, Mohr L. Human pregnancy following cryopreservation, thawing and transfer of an eight-cell embryo. *Nature* 1983; 305(5936): 707–9.
13. Zeilmaker GH et al. Two pregnancies following transfer of intact frozen–thawed embryos. *Fertil Steril* 1984; 42(2): 293–6.
14. Rall WF, Fahy GM. Ice-free cryopreservation of mouse embryos at −196 degrees C by vitrification. *Nature* 1985; 313(6003): 573–5.
15. Mazur P. Equilibrium, quasi-equilibrium, and non-equilibrium freezing of mammalian embryos. *Cell Biophys* 1990; 17(1): 53–92.
16. Leibo SP, McGrath JJ, Cravalho EG. Microscopic observation of intracellular ice formation in unfertilized mouse ova as a function of cooling rate. *Cryobiology* 1978; 15(3): 257–71.
17. Kasai M, Niwa K, Iritani A. Survival of mouse embryos frozen and thawed rapidly. *J Reprod Fertil* 1980; 59(1): 51–6.
18. Wood MJ, Farrant J. Preservation of mouse embryos by two-step freezing. *Cryobiology* 1980; 17(2): 178–80.
19. Trounson A, Peura A, Kirby C. Ultrarapid freezing: A new low-cost and effective method of embryo cryopreservation. *Fertil Steril* 1987; 48(5): 843–50.
20. Shaw JM, Diotallevi L, Trounson A. Ultrarapid embryo freezing: Effect of dissolved gas and pH of the freezing solutions and straw irradiation. *Hum Reprod* 1988; 3(7): 905–8.
21. Barg PE, Barad DH, Feichtinger W. Ultrarapid freezing (URF) of mouse and human preembryos: A modified approach. *J In Vitro Fert Embryo Transf* 1990; 7(6): 355–7.
22. Feichtinger W, Hochfellner C, Ferstl U. Clinical experience with ultra-rapid freezing of embryos. *Hum Reprod* 1991; 6(5): 735–6.
23. Aman RR, Parks JE. Effects of cooling and rewarming on the meiotic spindle and chromosomes of *in vitro*-matured bovine oocytes. *Biol Reprod* 1994; 50(1): 103–10.
24. Martino A, Pollard JW, Leibo SP. Effect of chilling bovine oocytes on their developmental competence. *Mol Reprod Dev* 1996; 45(4): 503–12.
25. Zenzes MT et al. Effects of chilling to 0 degrees C on the morphology of meiotic spindles in human metaphase II oocytes. *Fertil Steril* 2001; 75(4): 769–77.

26. Rall WF, Meyer TK. Zona fracture damage and its avoidance during the cryopreservation of mammalian embryos. *Theriogenology* 1989; 31(3): 683–92.
27. Sansinena M et al. Implications of storage and handling conditions on glass transition and potential devitrification of oocytes and embryos. *Theriogenology* 2014; 82(3): 373–8.
28. Rall WF. Cryopreservation of mammalian embryos, gametes and ovarian tissues. Current issues and progress. In: *Assisted Fertilization and Nuclear Transfer in Mammals*. Wolf DP, Zelinski-Wooten M (eds). Totowa, NJ: Humana Press. 2001, pp. 173–87.
29. Chaytor JL et al. Inhibiting ice recrystallization and optimization of cell viability after cryopreservation. *Glycobiology* 2012; 22(1): 123–33.
30. Cha SK et al. Effects of various combinations of cryoprotectants and cooling speed on the survival and further development of mouse oocytes after vitrification. *Clin Exp Reprod Med* 2011; 38(1): 24–30.
31. Vincent C, Johnson MH. Cooling, cryoprotectants, and the cytoskeleton of the mammalian oocyte. *Oxf Rev Reprod Biol* 1992; 14: 73–100.
32. Massip A, Mermillod P, Dinnyes A. Morphology and biochemistry of *in-vitro* produced bovine embryos: Implications for their cryopreservation. *Hum Reprod* 1995; 10(11): 3004–11.
33. Chang CC et al. The oocyte spindle is preserved by 1,2-propanediol during slow freezing. *Fertil Steril* 2010; 93(5): 1430–9.
34. Gardner DK et al. Analysis of oocyte physiology to improve cryopreservation procedures. *Theriogenology* 2007; 67(1): 64–72.
35. dela Pena EC et al. Vitrification of mouse oocytes in ethylene glycol-raffinose solution: Effects of preexposure to ethylene glycol or raffinose on oocyte viability. *Cryobiology* 2001; 42(2): 103–11.
36. Ishimori H, Takahashi Y, Kanagawa H. Factors affecting survival of mouse blastocysts vitrified by a mixture of ethylene glycol and dimethyl sulfoxide. *Theriogenology* 1992; 38(6): 1175–85.
37. Ishimori H et al. Vitrification of bovine embryos in a mixture of ethylene glycol and dimethyl sulfoxide. *Theriogenology* 1993; 40(2): 427–33.
38. Vicente JS, Garcia-Ximenez F. Osmotic and cryoprotective effects of a mixture of DMSO and ethylene glycol on rabbit morulae. *Theriogenology* 1994; 42(7): 1205–15.
39. Aye M et al. Assessment of the genotoxicity of three cryoprotectants used for human oocyte vitrification: Dimethyl sulfoxide, ethylene glycol and propylene glycol. *Food Chem Toxicol* 2010; 48(7): 1905–12.
40. Lawson A, Ahmad H, Sambanis A. Cytotoxicity effects of cryoprotectants as single-component and cocktail vitrification solutions. *Cryobiology* 2011; 62(2): 115–22.
41. Ali, J, Shelton JN. Design of vitrification solutions for the cryopreservation of embryos. *J Reprod Fertil* 1993; 99(2): 471–7.
42. Kasai M. Cryopreservation of mammalian embryos. *Mol Biotechnol* 1997; 7(2): 173–9.
43. Wright DL et al. Use of sugars in cryopreserving human oocytes. *Reprod Biomed Online* 2004; 9(2): 179–86.
44. Kasai M. Nonfreezing technique for short-term storage of mouse embryos. *J In Vitro Fert Embryo Transf* 1986; 3(1): 10–4.
45. Kasai M et al. Survival of mouse morulae vitrified in an ethylene glycol-based solution after exposure to the solution at various temperatures. *Biol Reprod* 1992; 47(6): 1134–9.
46. Vajta G et al. Survival and development of bovine blastocysts produced *in vitro* after assisted hatching, vitrification and in-straw direct rehydration. *J Reprod Fertil* 1997; 111(1): 65–70.
47. Kuleshova LL et al. Sugars exert a major influence on the vitrification properties of ethylene glycol-based solutions and have low toxicity to embryos and oocytes. *Cryobiology* 1999; 38(2): 119–30.
48. Oda K, Gibbons WE, Leibo SP. Osmotic shock of fertilized mouse ova. *J Reprod Fertil* 1992; 95(3): 737–47.
49. Ohboshi S et al. Usefulness of polyethylene glycol for cryopreservation by vitrification of *in vitro*-derived bovine blastocysts. *Anim Reprod Sci* 1997; 48(1): 27–36.
50. Shaw JM et al. Vitrification properties of solutions of ethylene glycol in saline containing PVP, Ficoll, or dextran. *Cryobiology* 1997; 35(3): 219–29.
51. Naitana S et al. Polyvinyl alcohol as a defined substitute for serum in vitrification and warming solutions to cryopreserve ovine embryos at different stages of development. *Anim Reprod Sci* 1997; 48(2–4): 247–56.
52. Kuleshova LL, Shaw JM, Trounson AO. Studies on replacing most of the penetrating cryoprotectant by polymers for embryo cryopreservation. *Cryobiology* 2001; 43(1): 21–31.
53. Asada M et al. Effect of polyvinyl alcohol (PVA) concentration during vitrification of *in vitro* matured bovine oocytes. *Theriogenology* 2002; 58(6): 1199–208.
54. Kasai M et al. A simple method for mouse embryo cryopreservation in a low toxicity vitrification solution, without appreciable loss of viability. *J Reprod Fertil* 1990; 89(1): 91–7.
55. Rall WF. Factors affecting the survival of mouse embryos cryopreserved by vitrification. *Cryobiology* 1987; 24(5): 387–402.
56. Lane M et al. Cryo-survival and development of bovine blastocysts are enhanced by culture with recombinant albumin and hyaluronan. *Mol Reprod Dev* 2003; 64(1): 70–8.
57. Rubinsky B, Arav A, Devries AL. The cryoprotective effect of antifreeze glycopeptides from antarctic fishes. *Cryobiology* 1992; 29(1): 69–79.
58. Eto TK, Rubinsky B. Antifreeze glycoproteins increase solution viscosity. *Biochem Biophys Res Commun* 1993; 197(2): 927–31.

59. Wowk B et al. Vitrification enhancement by synthetic ice blocking agents. *Cryobiology* 2000; 40(3): 228–36.
60. Mori C et al. Hydroxypropyl cellulose as an option for supplementation of cryoprotectant solutions for embryo vitrification in human assisted reproductive technologies. *Reprod Biomed Online* 2015; 30(6): 613–21.
61. Coello, A. et al. A combination of hydroxypropyl cellulose and trehalose as supplementation for vitrification of human oocytes: a retrospective cohort study. *J Assist Reprod Genet* 2016; 33(3): 413–21.
62. Vanderzwalmen P et al. Vitrification of bovine blastocysts. *Theriogenology* 1998; 31: 270.
63. Saha S et al. Direct rehydration of *in vitro* fertilised bovine embryos after vitrification. *Vet Rec* 1994; 134(11): 276–7.
64. Szell AZ, Windsor DP. Survival of vitrified sheep embryos *in vitro* and *in vivo*. *Theriogenology* 1994; 42(5): 881–9.
65. Papis K, Shimizu M, Izaike Y. Factors affecting the survivability of bovine oocytes vitrified in droplets. *Theriogenology* 2000; 54(5): 651–8.
66. Kuwayama M et al. Highly efficient vitrification method for cryopreservation of human oocytes. *Reprod Biomed Online* 2005; 11(3): 300–8.
67. Kuwayama M et al. Comparison of open and closed methods for vitrification of human embryos and the elimination of potential contamination. *Reprod Biomed Online* 2005; 11(5): 608–14.
68. Vanderzwalmen P et al. Lower intracellular concentration of cryoprotectants after vitrification than after slow freezing despite exposure to higher concentration of cryoprotectant solutions. *Hum Reprod* 2013; 28(8): 2101–10.
69. Palasz AT, Mapletoft RJ. Cryopreservation of mammalian embryos and oocytes: recent advances. *Biotechnol Adv* 1996; 14(2): 127–49.
70. Cuello C et al. Vitrification of porcine embryos at various developmental stages using different ultrarapid cooling procedures. *Theriogenology* 2004; 62(1-2): 353–61.
71. Liu WX et al. Effects of different cryoprotectants and cryopreservation protocols on the development of 2–4 cell mouse embryos. *Cryo Letters* 2011; 32(3): 240–7.
72. Landa V, Tepla O. Cryopreservation of mouse 8-cell embryos in microdrops. *Folia Biol (Praha)* 1990; 36(3–4): 153–8.
73. Riha J et al. Vitrification of cattle embryos by direct dropping into liquid nitrogen and embryo survival after nonsurgical transfer. *Zivoc Viroba* 1994; 36: 113–20.
74. Yang BC, Leibo SP. Viability of *in vitro*-derived bovine zygotes cryopreserved in microdrops. *Theriogenology* 1999; 51: 178.
75. Choi DH et al. Pregnancy and delivery of healthy infants developed from vitrified blastocysts in an IVF-ET program. *Fertil Steril* 2000; 74(4): 838–9.
76. Cho HJ et al. An improved protocol for dilution of cryoprotectants from vitrified human blastocysts. *Hum Reprod* 2002; 17(9): 2419–22.
77. Son WY et al. Pregnancy resulting from transfer of repeat vitrified blastocysts produced by *in-vitro* matured oocytes in patient with polycystic ovary syndrome. *Reprod Biomed Online* 2005; 10(3): 398–401.
78. Vajta G et al. Vitrification of porcine embryos using the open pulled straw (OPS) method. *Acta Vet Scand* 1997; 38(4): 349–52.
79. Vajta G et al. Open pulled straw (OPS) vitrification: A new way to reduce cryoinjuries of bovine ova and embryos. *Mol Reprod Dev* 1998; 51(1): 53–8.
80. Vajta G et al. Sterile application of the open pulled straw (OPS) vitrification method. *Cryo Letters* 1998; 19: 389–92.
81. Arav A, Zeron Y, Ocheretny A. A new device and method for vitrification increases the cooling rate and allows successful cryopreservation of bovine oocytes. *Theriogenology* 2000; 53: 248.
82. Arav A et al. New trends in gamete's cryopreservation. *Mol Cell Endocrinol* 2002; 187(1-2): 77–81.
83. Chen SU et al. Open pulled straws for vitrification of mature mouse oocytes preserve patterns of meiotic spindles and chromosomes better than conventional straws. *Hum Reprod* 2000; 15(12): 2598–603.
84. El-Danasouri I, Selman H. Successful pregnancies and deliveries after a simple vitrification protocol for day 3 human embryos. *Fertil Steril* 2001; 76(2): 400–2.
85. Selman HA, El-Danasouri I. Pregnancies derived from vitrified human zygotes. *Fertil Steril* 2002; 77(2): 422–3.
86. Isachenko V et al. Modified vitrification of human pronuclear oocytes: efficacy and effect on ultrastructure. *Reprod Biomed Online* 2003; 7(2): 211–6.
87. Lane M et al. Containerless vitrification of mammalian oocytes and embryos. *Nat Biotechnol* 1999; 17(12): 1234–6.
88. Lane M, Schoolcraft WB, Gardner DK. Vitrification of mouse and human blastocysts using a novel cryoloop container-less technique. *Fertil Steril* 1999; 72(6): 1073–8.
89. Mukaida T et al. Successful birth after transfer of vitrified human blastocysts with use of a cryoloop containerless technique. *Fertil Steril* 2001; 76(3): 618–20.
90. Mukaida T, Takahashi K, Kasai M. Blastocyst cryopreservation: Ultrarapid vitrification using cryoloop technique. *Reprod Biomed Online* 2003; 6(2): 221–5.
91. Isachenko E et al. Vitrification of mammalian spermatozoa in the absence of cryoprotectants: From past practical difficulties to present success. *Reprod Biomed Online* 2003; 6(2): 191–200.
92. Larman MG, Sheehan CB, Gardner DK. Vitrification of mouse pronuclear oocytes with no direct liquid nitrogen contact. *Reprod Biomed Online* 2006; 12(1): 66–9.

93. Matsumoto H et al. Vitrification of large quantities of immature bovine oocytes using nylon mesh. *Cryobiology* 2001; 42(2): 139–44.
94. Arav A, Shehu D, Mattioli M. Osmotic and cytotoxic study of vitrification of immature bovine oocytes. *J Reprod Fertil* 1993; 99(2): 353–8.
95. Hamawaki AKM, Hamano S Minimum volume cooling method for bovine blastocyst vitrification. *Theriogenology* 1999; 51: 165.
96. Vanderzwalmen P et al. *In vitro* survival of metaphase II oocytes (MII) and blastocysts after vitrification in a hemi-straw (HS) system. *Fertil Steril* 2000; 74: S215–6.
97. Nagy ZP et al. Clinical evaluation of the efficiency of an oocyte donation program using egg cryo-banking. *Fertil Steril* 2009; 92(2): 520–6.
98. Chang CC et al. Human oocyte vitrification: *in-vivo* and *in-vitro* maturation outcomes. *Reprod Biomed Online* 2008; 17(5): 684–8.
99. Cobo A et al. Comparison of concomitant outcome achieved with fresh and cryopreserved donor oocytes vitrified by the Cryotop method. *Fertil Steril* 2008; 89(6): 1657–64.
100. Chang CC et al. Two successful pregnancies obtained following oocyte vitrification and embryo re-vitrification. *Reprod Biomed Online* 2008; 16(3): 346–9.
101. Gutnisky C et al. Evaluation of the Cryotech Vitrification Kit for bovine embryos. *Cryobiology* 2013; 67(3): 391–3.
102. Larman MG, Gardner DK. Vitrification of mouse embryos with super-cooled air. *Fertil Steril* 2011; 95(4): 1462–6.
103. Hashimoto S et al. A closed system supports the developmental competence of human embryos after vitrification: Closed vitrification of human embryos. *J Assist Reprod Genet* 2013; 30(3): 371–6.
104. Van Landuyt L et al. Outcome of closed blastocyst vitrification in relation to blastocyst quality: Evaluation of 759 warming cycles in a single-embryo transfer policy. *Hum Reprod* 2011; 26(3): 527–34.
105. Schiewe MC et al. Validation of microSecure vitrification (muS-VTF) for the effective cryopreservation of human embryos and oocytes. *Cryobiology* 2015; 71(2): 264–72.
106. Bonetti A et al. Ultrastructural evaluation of human metaphase II oocytes after vitrification: Closed versus open devices. *Fertil Steril* 2011; 95(3): 928–35.
107. Papatheodorou A et al. Open versus closed oocyte vitrification system: A prospective randomized sibling-oocyte study. *Reprod Biomed Online* 2013; 26(6): 595–602.
108. Huang CC et al. Successful pregnancy following blastocyst cryopreservation using super-cooling ultra-rapid vitrification. *Hum Reprod* 2005; 20(1): 122–8.
109. Dinnyes A et al. High developmental rates of vitrified bovine oocytes following parthenogenetic activation, *in vitro* fertilization, and somatic cell nuclear transfer. *Biol Reprod* 2000; 63(2): 513–8.
110. Bielanski, A et al. Microbial contamination of embryos and semen during long term banking in liquid nitrogen. *Cryobiology* 2003; 46(2): 146–52.
111. Tedder RS et al. Hepatitis B transmission from contaminated cryopreservation tank. *Lancet* 1995; 346(8968): 137–40.
112. Fountain D et al. Liquid nitrogen freezers: A potential source of microbial contamination of hematopoietic stem cell components. *Transfusion* 1997; 37(6): 585–91.
113. Berry ED et al. Bacterial cross-contamination of meat during liquid nitrogen immersion freezing. *J Food Prot* 1998; 61(9): 1103–8.
114. Bielanski A et al. Viral contamination of embryos cryopreserved in liquid nitrogen. *Cryobiology* 2000; 40(2): 110–6.
115. Cobo A et al. Viral screening of spent culture media and liquid nitrogen samples of oocytes and embryos from hepatitis B, hepatitis C, and human immunodeficiency virus chronically infected women undergoing *in vitro* fertilization cycles. *Fertil Steril* 2012; 97(1): 74–8.
116. Liebermann, J., Vitrification of human blastocysts: an update. *Reprod Biomed Online* 2009; 19(Suppl 4): 4328.
117. Vanderzwalmen P et al. Aseptic vitrification of blastocysts from infertile patients, egg donors and after IVM. *Reprod Biomed Online* 2009; 19(5): 700–7.
118. Vajta G, Rienzi L, Ubaldi FM. Open versus closed systems for vitrification of human oocytes and embryos. *Reprod Biomed Online* 2015; 30(4): 325–33.
119. Parmegiani, L et al. Sterilization of liquid nitrogen with ultraviolet irradiation for safe vitrification of human oocytes or embryos. *Fertil Steril* 2010; 94(4): 1525–8.
120. Parmegiani L et al. Efficiency of aseptic open vitrification and hermetical cryostorage of human oocytes. *Reprod Biomed Online* 2011; 23(4): 505–12.
121. Kuleshova LL, Lopata A. Vitrification can be more favorable than slow cooling. *Fertil Steril* 2002; 78(3): 449–54.
122. Cobo A et al. Storage of human oocytes in the vapor phase of nitrogen. *Fertil Steril* 2010; 94(5): 1903–7.
123. Eum JH et al. Long-term liquid nitrogen vapor storage of mouse embryos cryopreserved using vitrification or slow cooling. *Fertil Steril* 2009; 91(5): 1928–32.
124. Abdelhafez F et al. Vitrification in open and closed carriers at different cell stages: Assessment of embryo survival, development, DNA integrity and stability during vapor phase storage for transport. *BMC Biotechnol* 2011; 11: 29.
125. Ghetler Y et al. The effect of chilling on membrane lipid phase transition in human oocytes and zygotes. *Hum Reprod* 2005; 20(12): 3385–9.
126. Mazur, P, Seki S. Survival of mouse oocytes after being cooled in a vitrification solution to −196 degrees C at 95 degrees to 70,000 degrees C/min and warmed at 610 degrees to 118,000 degrees C/min: A new paradigm for cryopreservation by vitrification. *Cryobiology* 2011; 62(1): 1–7.

127. Shaw, J.M. et al. An association between chromosomal abnormalities in rapidly frozen 2-cell mouse embryos and the ice-forming properties of the cryoprotective solution. *J Reprod Fertil* 1991; 91(1): 9–18.
128. Vajta G et al. In-straw dilution of bovine blastocysts after vitrification with the open-pulled straw method. *Vet Rec* 1999; 144(7): 180–1.
129. Cuello C et al. *In vitro* development following one-step dilution of OPS-vitrified porcine blastocysts. *Theriogenology* 2004; 62(6): 1144–52.
130. Tecirlioglu RT et al. Birth of a cloned calf derived from a vitrified hand-made cloned embryo. *Reprod Fertil Dev* 2003; 15(7-8): 361–6.
131. Isachenko V et al. New technology for vitrification and field (microscope-free) warming and transfer of small ruminant embryos. *Theriogenology* 2003; 59(5-6): 1209–18.
132. Parmegiani L et al. Rapid warming increases survival of slow-frozen sibling oocytes: A step towards a single warming procedure irrespective of the freezing protocol? *Reprod Biomed Online* 2014; 28(5): 614–23.
133. Nagashima H et al. Removal of cytoplasmic lipid enhances the tolerance of porcine embryos to chilling. *Biol Reprod* 1994; 51(4): 618–22.
134. Dobrinsky JRNH, Pursel VG et al. Cryopreservation of swine embryos with reduced lipid content. *Theriogenology* 1999; 51: 164.
135. Beeb LF et al. Piglets born from centrifuged and vitrified early and peri-hatching blastocysts. *Theriogenology* 2002; 57(9): 2155–65.
136. Esaki R et al. Cryopreservation of porcine embryos derived from *in vitro*-matured oocytes. *Biol Reprod* 2004; 71(2): 432–7.
137. Du YKP, Zhang X et al. Successful vitrification of parthenogenetic porcine blastocysts produced from delipated *in vitro* matured oocytes. *Reprod Fert Dev* 2006; 18: 153.
138. Li R et al. Cloned transgenic swine via *in vitro* production and cryopreservation. *Biol Reprod* 2006; 75(2): 226–30.
139. Dinnyes, A, Wallace GA, Rall WF. Effect of genotype on the efficiency of mouse embryo cryopreservation by vitrification or slow freezing methods. *Mol Reprod Dev* 1995; 40(4): 429–35.
140. Men H, Monson RL, Rutledge JJ. Effect of meiotic stages and maturation protocols on bovine oocyte's resistance to cryopreservation. *Theriogenology* 2002; 57(3): 1095–103.
141. Edashige K et al. Artificial expression of aquaporin-3 improves the survival of mouse oocytes after cryopreservation. *Biol Reprod* 2003; 68(1): 87–94.
142. Edashige K, Sakamoto M, Kasai M. Expression of mRNAs of the aquaporin family in mouse oocytes and embryos. *Cryobiology* 2000; 40(2): 171–5.
143. Veeck LL. Does the developmental stage at freeze impact on clinical results post-thaw? *Reprod Biomed Online* 2003; 6(3): 367–74.
144. Pool TB, Leibo SP. Cryopreservation and assisted human conception. Introduction. *Reprod Biomed Online* 2004; 9(2): 132–3.
145. Alpha Scientists In Reproductive Medicine. The Alpha consensus meeting on cryopreservation key performance indicators and benchmarks: proceedings of an expert meeting. *Reprod Biomed Online* 2012; 25(2): 46–67.
146. Edgar DH, Gook DA. A critical appraisal of cryopreservation (slow cooling versus vitrification) of human oocytes and embryos. *Hum Reprod Update* 2012; 18(5): 536–54.
147. Wang XL et al. Outcomes of day 3 embryo transfer with vitrification using Cryoleaf: A 3-year follow-up study. *J Assist Reprod Genet* 2012; 29(9): 883–9.
148. Fernandez-Shaw S et al. Ongoing and cumulative pregnancy rate after cleavage-stage versus blastocyst-stage embryo transfer using vitrification for cryopreservation: Impact of age on the results. *J Assist Reprod Genet* 2015; 32(2): 177–84.
149. Vanderzwalmen P et al. Births after vitrification at morula and blastocyst stages: Effect of artificial reduction of the blastocoelic cavity before vitrification. *Hum Reprod* 2002; 17(3): 744–51.
150. Son WY et al. Pregnancy outcome following transfer of human blastocysts vitrified on electron microscopy grids after induced collapse of the blastocoele. *Hum Reprod* 2003; 18(1): 137–9.
151. Hiraoka K, Kinutani M, Kinutani K. Blastocoele collapse by micropipetting prior to vitrification gives excellent survival and pregnancy outcomes for human day 5 and 6 expanded blastocysts. *Hum Reprod* 2004; 19(12): 2884–8.
152. Raju GA et al. Vitrification of human early cavitating and deflated expanded blastocysts: Clinical outcome of 474 cycles. *J Assist Reprod Genet* 2009; 26(9–10): 523–9.
153. Iwayama H, Hochi S, Yamashita M. *In vitro* and *in vivo* viability of human blastocysts collapsed by laser pulse or osmotic shock prior to vitrification. *J Assist Reprod Genet* 2011; 28(4): 355–61.
154. Cao S et al. Retrospective clinical analysis of two artificial shrinkage methods applied prior to blastocyst vitrification on the outcome of frozen embryo transfer. *J Assist Reprod Genet* 2014; 31(5): 577–81.
155. Van Landuyt L et al. A prospective randomized controlled trial investigating the effect of artificial shrinkage (collapse) on the implantation potential of vitrified blastocysts. *Hum Reprod* 2015; 30(11): 2509–18.
156. Min SH et al. Forced collapse of the blastocoel enhances survival of Cryotop vitrified bovine hatching/hatched blastocysts derived from *in vitro* fertilization and somatic cell nuclear transfer. *Cryobiology* 2013; 66(2): 195–9.
157. Roth TL, Swanson WF, Wildt DE. Developmental competence of domestic cat embryos fertilized *in vivo* versus *in vitro*. *Biol Reprod* 1994; 51(3): 441–51.

158. Enright BP et al. Culture of *in vitro* produced bovine zygotes *in vitro* vs *in vivo*: Implications for early embryo development and quality. *Theriogenology* 2000; 54(5): 659–73.
159. Rizos D et al. Consequences of bovine oocyte maturation, fertilization or early embryo development *in vitro* versus *in vivo*: Implications for blastocyst yield and blastocyst quality. *Mol Reprod Dev* 2002; 61(2): 234–48.
160. Mahmoudzadeh AR et al. Optimization of a simple vitrification procedure for bovine embryos produced *in vitro*: Effect of developmental stage, two-step addition of cryoprotectant and sucrose dilution on embryonic survival. *J Reprod Fertil* 1995; 103(1): 33–9.
161. Wurth YA et al. Developmental potential of *in vitro* produced bovine embryos following cryopreservation and single-embryo transfer. *Theriogenology* 1994; 42: 1275–84.
162. Reinders JMC. From embryo to a calf after embryo transfer, a comparison of *in vivo* and *in vitro* produced embryos. *Theriogenology* 1995; 43: 306.
163. Agca Y et al. Transfer of fresh and cryopreserved IVP bovine embryos: Normal calving, birth weight and gestation lengths. *Theriogenology* 1998; 50(1): 147–62.
164. Sirisha K et al. Cryopreservation of zona-free cloned buffalo (*Bubalus bubalis*) embryos: Slow freezing vs open-pulled straw vitrification. *Reprod Domest Anim* 2013; 48(4): 538–44.
165. Zander-Fox D, Lane M, Hamilton H. Slow freezing and vitrification of mouse morula and early blastocysts. *J Assist Reprod Genet* 2013; 30(8): 1091–8.
166. Kong IK et al. Comparison of open pulled straw (OPS) vs glass micropipette (GMP) vitrification in mouse blastocysts. *Theriogenology* 2000; 53(9): 1817–26.
167. Isachenko VA, Vajta G. Double cryopreservtion of rat embryos at different developmental stages with identical vitrification protocol: The not properly understood phenomenon. *J Reprod Fertil* 2000; 26 Abstract series: 10.
168. Tominaga K, Hamada Y. Gel-loading tips as container for vitrification of *in vitro*-produced bovine embryos. *J Reprod Dev* 2001; 47: 259–65.
169. Liebermann J et al. Blastocyst development after vitrification of multipronuclear zygotes using the Flexipet denuding pipette. *Reprod Biomed Online* 2002; 4(2): 146–50.
170. Cremades N et al. Experimental vitrification of human compacted morulae and early blastocysts using fine diameter plastic micropipettes. *Hum Reprod* 2004; 19(2): 300–5.
171. Hredzak R et al. [Clinical experience with a modified method of human embryo vitrification]. *Ceska Gynekol* 2005; 70(2): 99–103.
172. Chen SU et al. Vitrification of mouse oocytes using closed pulled straws (CPS) achieves a high survival and preserves good patterns of meiotic spindles, compared with conventional straws, open pulled straws (OPS) and grids. *Hum Reprod* 2001; 16(11): 2350–6.
173. Lopez-Bejar M, Lopez-Gatius F. Nonequilibrium cryopreservation of rabbit embryos using a modified (sealed) open pulled straw procedure. *Theriogenology* 2002; 58(8): 1541–52.
174. Arav A. Vitrification of oocytes and embryos. In: *New Trends in Embryo Transfer.* Lauria AGF (ed.). Cambridge, U.K.: Portland Press, 1992, pp. 255–64.
175. Vajta G, Nagy ZP. Are programmable freezers still needed in the embryo laboratory? Review on vitrification. *Reprod Biomed Online* 2006; 12(6): 779–96.
176. Vieira AD et al. Calves born after open pulled straw vitrification of immature bovine oocytes. *Cryobiology* 2002; 45(1): 91–4.
177. Martino A, Songsasen N, Leibo SP. Development into blastocysts of bovine oocytes cryopreserved by ultra-rapid cooling. *Biol Reprod* 1996; 54(5): 1059–69.
178. Hou YP et al. Bovine oocytes vitrified by the open pulled straw method and used for somatic cell cloning supported development to term. *Theriogenology* 2005; 64(6): 1381–91.
179. Booth PJ et al. Full-term development of nuclear transfer calves produced from open-pulled straw (OPS) vitrified cytoplasts: Work in progress. *Theriogenology* 1999; 51(5): 999–1006.
180. French AJHV, Korfiatis NT et al. Viability of cloned bovine embryos following OPS vitrification. *Theriogenology* 2002; 57: 413.
181. French AJ, Lewis IM, Ruddock NT et al. Generation of aS1 casein gene transgenic calves by nuclear transfer. *Biol Reprod* 2003; 68: 240.
182. Peura TT et al. No differences in sheep somatic cell nuclear transfer outcomes using serum-starved or actively growing donor granulosa cells. *Reprod Fertil Dev* 2003; 15(3): 157–65.
183. Fujihira T, Kishida R, Fukui Y. Developmental capacity of vitrified immature porcine oocytes following ICSI: Effects of cytochalasin B and cryoprotectants. *Cryobiology* 2004; 49(3): 286–90.
184. Fujuhira T, Nagai H, Fukui Y. Relationship between equilibration times and the presence of cumulus cells, and effect of taxol treatment for vitrification of *in vitro* matured porcine oocytes. *Cryobiology* 2005; 51: 339–43.
185. Kobayashi S et al. Piglets produced by transfer of vitrified porcine embryos after stepwise dilution of cryoprotectants. *Cryobiology* 1998; 36(1): 20–31.
186. Berthelot F et al. Birth of piglets after OPS vitrification and transfer of compacted morula stage embryos with intact zona pellucida. *Reprod Nutr Dev* 2001; 41(3): 267–72.
187. Men H et al. Beneficial effects of serum supplementation during *in vitro* production of porcine embryos on their ability to survive cryopreservation by open pulled straw vitrification. *Theriogenology* 2005; 64(6): 1340–9.

188. Maclellan LJ et al. Pregnancies from vitrified equine oocytes collected from super-stimulated and non-stimulated mares. *Theriogenology* 2002; 58(5): 911–9.
189. Piltti K et al. Live cubs born after transfer of OPS vitrified–warmed embryos in the farmed European polecat (*Mustela putorius*). *Theriogenology* 2004; 61(5): 811–20.
190. Crichton EG et al. Efficacy of porcine gonadotropins for repeated stimulation of ovarian activity for oocyte retrieval and *in vitro* embryo production and cryopreservation in Siberian tigers (*Panthera tigris altaica*). *Biol Reprod* 2003; 68(1): 105–13.
191. Iwayama H et al. Effects of cryodevice type and donors' sexual maturity on vitrification of minke whale (*Balaenoptera bonaerensis*) oocytes at germinal vesicle stage. *Zygote* 2004; 12(4): 333–8.
192. Check JH et al. Fresh embryo transfer is more effective than frozen for donor oocyte recipients but not for donors. *Hum Reprod* 2001; 16(7): 1403–8.
193. Nagy ZP et al. Removal of lysed blastomeres from frozen–thawed embryos improves implantation and pregnancy rates in frozen embryo transfer cycles. *Fertil Steril* 2005; 84(6): 1606–12.
194. Elliott TA et al. Lysed cell removal promotes frozen–thawed embryo development. *Fertil Steril* 2007; 87(6): 1444–9.
195. Jelinkova L et al. Twin pregnancy after vitrification of 2-pronuclei human embryos. *Fertil Steril* 2002; 77(2): 412–4.
196. Vanderzwalmen P et al. Vitrification of human blastocysts with the Hemi-Straw carrier: Application of assisted hatching after thawing. *Hum Reprod* 2003; 18(7): 1504–11.
197. Vanderzwalmen P et al. Pregnancies after vitrification of human day 5 embryos. *Hum Reprod* 1997; 12(Suppl): 98.
198. Mukaida T et al. Vitrification of human embryos based on the assessment of suitable conditions for 8-cell mouse embryos. *Hum Reprod* 1998; 13(1O): 2874–9.
199. Park SP et al. Ultra-rapid freezing of human multipronuclear zygotes using electron microscope grids. *Hum Reprod* 2000; 15(8): 1787–90.
200. Saito H et al. Application of vitrification to human embryo freezing. *Gynecol Obstet Invest* 2000; 49(3): 145–9.
201. Yokota Y et al. Successful pregnancy following blastocyst vitrification: Case report. *Hum Reprod* 2000; 15(8): 1802–3.
202. Yokota Y et al. Birth of a healthy baby following vitrification of human blastocysts. *Fertil Steril* 2001; 75(5): 1027–9.
203. Liebermann J, Tucker MJ. Effect of carrier system on the yield of human oocytes and embryos as assessed by survival and developmental potential after vitrification. *Reproduction* 2002; 124(4): 483–9.
204. Reed ML et al. Vitrification of human blastocysts using the cryoloop method: Successful clinical application and birth of offspring. *J Assist Reprod Genet* 2002; 19(6): 304–6.
205. Son WY et al. Ongoing twin pregnancy after vitrification of blastocysts produced by *in-vitro* matured oocytes retrieved from a woman with polycystic ovary syndrome: Case report. *Hum Reprod* 2002; 17(11): 2963–6.
206. Isachenko V et al. Aseptic technology of vitrification of human pronuclear oocytes using open-pulled straws. *Hum Reprod* 2005; 20(2): 492–6.
207. Liebermann J, Tucker MJ. Vitrifying and warming of human oocytes, embryos, and blastocysts: Vitrification procedures as an alternative to conventional cryopreservation. *Methods Mol Biol* 2004; 254: 345–64.
208. Zheng WT et al. Comparison of the survival of human biopsied embryos after cryopreservation with four different methods using non-transferable embryos. *Hum Reprod* 2005; 20(6): 1615–8.
209. Stehlik E et al. Vitrification demonstrates significant improvement versus slow freezing of human blastocysts. *Reprod Biomed Online* 2005; 11(1): 53–7.
210. Balaban B et al. A randomized controlled study of human day 3 embryo cryopreservation by slow freezing or vitrification: Vitrification is associated with higher survival, metabolism and blastocyst formation. *Hum Reprod* 2008; 23(9): 1976–82.
211. Rezazadeh Valojerdi M et al. Vitrification versus slow freezing gives excellent survival, post warming embryo morphology and pregnancy outcomes for human cleaved embryos. *J Assist Reprod Genet* 2009; 26(6): 347–54.
212. Son WY et al. Comparison of survival rate of cleavage stage embryos produced from *in vitro* maturation cycles after slow freezing and after vitrification. *Fertil Steril* 2009; 92(3): 956–8.
213. Keskintepe L et al. Vitrification of human embryos subjected to blastomere biopsy for pre-implantation genetic screening produces higher survival and pregnancy rates than slow freezing. *J Assist Reprod Genet* 2009; 26(11–12): 629–35.
214. Wilding MG et al. Human cleavage-stage embryo vitrification is comparable to slow-rate cryopreservation in cycles of assisted reproduction. *J Assist Reprod Genet* 2010; 27(9-10): 549–54.
215. Sifer C et al. [Outcome of embryo vitrification compared to slow freezing process at early cleavage stages. Report of the first French birth]. *Gynecol Obstet Fertil* 2012; 40(3): 158–61.
216. AbdelHafez FF et al. Slow freezing, vitrification and ultra-rapid freezing of human embryos: A systematic review and meta-analysis. *Reprod Biomed Online* 2010; 20(2): 209–22.
217. Desai N et al. Cryoloop vitrification of human day 3 cleavage-stage embryos: post-vitrification development, pregnancy outcomes and live births. *Reprod Biomed Online* 2007; 14(2): 208–13.

218. Hong SW et al. Cryopreserved human blastocysts after vitrification result in excellent implantation and clinical pregnancy rates. *Fertil Steril* 2009; 92(6): 2062–4.
219. Hiraoka K, Kinutani M, Kinutani K. Vitrification of human hatched blastocysts: A report of 4 cases. *J Reprod Med* 2007; 52(5): 413–5.
220. Stachecki JJ et al. A new safe, simple and successful vitrification method for bovine and human blastocysts. *Reprod Biomed Online* 2008; 17(3): 360–7.
221. Selman H et al. Vitrification is a highly efficient method to cryopreserve human embryos in *in vitro* fertilization patients at high risk of developing ovarian hyperstimulation syndrome. *Fertil Steril* 2009; 91(4 Suppl): 1611–3.
222. Hiraoka K et al. Vitrified human day-7 blastocyst transfer: 11 cases. *Reprod Biomed Online* 2008; 17(5): 689–94.
223. Wirleitner B et al. The time aspect in storing vitrified blastocysts: Its impact on survival rate, implantation potential and babies born. *Hum Reprod* 2013; 28(11): 2950–7.
224. Cobo A et al. Six years' experience in ovum donation using vitrified oocytes: report of cumulative outcomes, impact of storage time, and development of a predictive model for oocyte survival rate. *Fertil Steril* 2015; 104(6): 1426–34.e8.
225. Achour R et al. [Embryo vitrification: First Tunisian live birth following embryo vitrification and literature review]. *Tunis Med* 2015; 93(3): 181–3.
226. Sparks AE. Human embryo cryopreservation-methods, timing, and other considerations for optimizing an embryo cryopreservation program. *Semin Reprod Med* 2015; 33(2): 128–44.
227. Knopman JM et al. Women with cancer undergoing ART for fertility preservation: a cohort study of their response to exogenous gonadotropins. *Fertil Steril* 2009; 91(4 Suppl): 1476–8.
228. Grifo JA, Noyes N. Delivery rate using cryopreserved oocytes is comparable to conventional *in vitro* fertilization using fresh oocytes: Potential fertility preservation for female cancer patients. *Fertil Steril* 2010; 93(2): 391–6.
229. Noyes N et al. Oocyte cryopreservation as a fertility preservation measure for cancer patients. *Reprod Biomed Online* 2010.
230. Lockwood G. Politics, ethics and economics: oocyte cryopreservation in the UK. *Reprod Biomed Online* 2003; 6(2): 151–3.
231. Bedoschi G, Oktay K. Current approach to fertility preservation by embryo cryopreservation. *Fertil Steril* 2013; 99(6): 1496–502.
232. Cobo A et al. New options in assisted reproduction technology: The Cryotop method of oocyte vitrification. *Reprod Biomed Online* 2008; 17(1): 68–72.
233. Nagy ZP et al. The efficacy and safety of human oocyte vitrification. *Semin Reprod Med* 2009; 27(6): 450–5.
234. Lin YH et al. Combination of cabergoline and embryo cryopreservation after GnRH agonist triggering prevents OHSS in patients with extremely high estradiol levels—A retrospective study. *J Assist Reprod Genet* 2013; 30(6): 753–9.
235. Imudia AN et al. Elective cryopreservation of all embryos with subsequent cryothaw embryo transfer in patients at risk for ovarian hyperstimulation syndrome reduces the risk of adverse obstetric outcomes: A preliminary study. *Fertil Steril* 2013; 99(1): 168–73.
236. Stoop D et al. Offering excess oocyte aspiration and vitrification to patients undergoing stimulated artificial insemination cycles can reduce the multiple pregnancy risk and accumulate oocytes for later use. *Hum Reprod* 2010; 25(5): 1213–8.
237. Joris H et al. Reduced survival after human embryo biopsy and subsequent cryopreservation. *Hum Reprod* 1999; 14(11): 2833–7.
238. Jericho H et al. A modified cryopreservation method increases the survival of human biopsied cleavage stage embryos. *Hum Reprod* 2003; 18(3): 568–71.
239. Schoolcraft WB, Katz-Jaffe MG. Comprehensive chromosome screening of trophectoderm with vitrification facilitates elective single-embryo transfer for infertile women with advanced maternal age. *Fertil Steril* 2013; 100(3): 615–9.
240. Grifo JA et al. Single thawed euploid embryo transfer improves IVF pregnancy, miscarriage, and multiple gestation outcomes and has similar implantation rates as egg donation. *J Assist Reprod Genet* 2013; 30(2): 259–64.
241. Schoolcraft WB et al. Clinical application of comprehensive chromosomal screening at the blastocyst stage. *Fertil Steril* 2010; 94(5): 1700–6.
242. Fragouli E et al. Comprehensive chromosome screening of polar bodies and blastocysts from couples experiencing repeated implantation failure. *Fertil Steril* 2010; 94(3): 875–87.
243. Schoolcraft WB et al. Live birth outcome with trophectoderm biopsy, blastocyst vitrification, and single-nucleotide polymorphism microarray-based comprehensive chromosome screening in infertile patients. *Fertil Steril* 2011; 96(3): 638–40.
244. Oakes MB et al. A case of oocyte and embryo vitrification resulting in clinical pregnancy. *Fertil Steril* 2008; 90(5): 2013.e5–8.
245. Peng W, Zhang J, Shu Y. Live birth after transfer of a twice-vitrified warmed blastocyst that had undergone trophectoderm biopsy. *Reprod Biomed Online* 2011; 22(3): 299–302.
246. Greco E et al. Successful implantation and live birth of a healthy boy after triple biopsy and double vitrification of oocyte–embryo–blastocyst. *Springerplus* 2015; 4: 22.
247. Shapiro BS et al. Clinical rationale for cryopreservation of entire embryo cohorts in lieu of fresh transfer. *Fertil Steril* 2014; 102(1): 3–9.
248. Mohamed AM et al. Live birth rate in fresh and frozen embryo transfer cycles in women with endometriosis. *Eur J Obstet Gynecol Reprod Biol* 2011; 156(2): 177–80.

249. Shapiro BS et al. Evidence of impaired endometrial receptivity after ovarian stimulation for *in vitro* fertilization: A prospective randomized trial comparing fresh and frozen–thawed embryo transfer in normal responders. *Fertil Steril* 2011; 96(2): 344–8.
250. Cobo A et al. Accumulation of oocytes: A new strategy for managing low-responder patients. *Reprod Biomed Online* 2012; 24(4): 424–32.
251. Vanderzwalmen P et al. Blastocyst transfer after aseptic vitrification of zygotes: An approach to overcome an impaired uterine environment. *Reprod Biomed Online* 2012; 25(6): 591–9.
252. Roy TK et al. Single-embryo transfer of vitrified–warmed blastocysts yields equivalent live-birth rates and improved neonatal outcomes compared with fresh transfers. *Fertil Steril* 2014; 101(5): 1294–301.
253. Chian RC et al. Obstetric outcomes following vitrification of *in vitro* and *in vivo* matured oocytes. *Fertil Steril* 2009; 91(6): 2391–8.
254. Noyes N, Porcu E, Borini A. Over 900 oocyte cryopreservation babies born with no apparent increase in congenital anomalies. *Reprod Biomed Online* 2009; 18(6): 769–76.
255. Rama Raju GA et al. Neonatal outcome after vitrified day 3 embryo transfers: A preliminary study. *Fertil Steril* 2009; 92(1): 143–8.
256. Shu Y, Peng W, Zhang J. Pregnancy and live birth following the transfer of vitrified–warmed blastocysts derived from zona- and corona-cell-free oocytes. *Reprod Biomed Online* 2010; 21(4): 527–32.
257. Wikland M et al. Obstetric outcomes after transfer of vitrified blastocysts. *Hum Reprod* 2010; 25(7): 1699–707.
258. Shi W et al. Perinatal and neonatal outcomes of 494 babies delivered from 972 vitrified embryo transfers. *Fertil Steril* 2012; 97(6): 1338–42.
259. Chen Y et al. Neonatal outcomes after the transfer of vitrified blastocysts: Closed versus open vitrification system. *Reprod Biol Endocrinol* 2013; 11: 107.
260. Li Z et al. Clinical outcomes following cryopreservation of blastocysts by vitrification or slow freezing: A population-based cohort study. *Hum Reprod* 2014; 29(12): 2794–801.
261. Devine K et al. Single vitrified blastocyst transfer maximizes liveborn children per embryo while minimizing preterm birth. *Fertil Steril* 2015; 103(6): 1454–60.e1.

Managing an oocyte bank

24

ANA COBO, PILAR ALAMÁ, JOSÉ MARÍA DE LOS SANTOS,
MARÍA JOSÉ DE LOS SANTOS, and JOSÉ REMOHÍ

INTRODUCTION

Nowadays, the challenge of the cryopreservation, long-term storage, and successful implantation of the female gamete is feasible thanks to vitrification. There is a large population that is currently benefiting from oocyte banks, such as cancer patients who need an option for fertility preservation before undergoing potentially sterilizing treatment (1) or women who wish to delay their motherhood due to a variety of reasons (2,3). Oocyte cryostorage brings additional advantages to assisted reproduction technology (ART) programs, being helpful in solving different clinical situations such as low-response patients (4), unpredictable availability of semen sample collection from the male partner, risk of suffering from ovarian hyperstimulation syndrome (5), or some other cases in which embryo transfer is not advisable (6). Undoubtedly, ovum donation programs have also been major beneficiaries of egg banking. Oocyte cryostorage is very useful for overcoming the most common drawbacks involved in ovum donation as currently applied, such as synchronization between donors and recipients, long waiting lists subject to the availability of a suitable donor, and, most important, the absence of a quarantine period.

In spite of its great value, oocyte cryostorage has not been a valid option until relatively recently, due to the lack of successful methodologies. The reasons behind the long period of failures in attempts to cryopreserve oocytes are well identified. Among them, the size and shape of the female gamete are two significant reasons. The female gamete is the largest cell of the human body, with a large content of water, leading to a higher probability of ice formation during the cryopreservation process. Chilling injury, defined as irreversible damage to the cytoskeleton (7) and cell membranes (8), following exposure of cells to low temperatures from +15 to –5°C before the nucleation of ice is another major factor responsible for cell death during cryopreservation (9). Ice crystal formation within the cytoplasm must be avoided at all costs in order to guarantee the survival and integrity of the cells when they are later thawed. Vitrification efficiently avoids chilling injury by direct passage from room temperatures to –196°C and so avoids ice formation (10). Vitrification employs both high cooling rates and high cryoprotectant concentrations (11). However, due to the potential toxicity of these compounds, the vitrification protocols have been modified in order to reduce damage. Additionally, efforts have also focused on increasing both the cooling and the warming rates in order to guarantee the viability of the cells (12,13). As a result, these days we count on several efficient approaches that are able to provide successful outcomes comparable to those achieved with fresh oocytes, thus making oocyte banking a reliable approach.

In this chapter, we will briefly review the clinical outcomes achieved with the use of vitrified oocytes in ovum donation, but we will primarily focus on the essential issues related to the management of the oocyte bank, including a description of the facilities, the equipment for storage, and liquid nitrogen (LN) supply. We will also evaluate the most relevant clinical aspects involved in the management of the oocyte bank, such as donor selection, preparation of recipients, and the matching process.

CLINICAL OUTCOME USING AN OOCYTE BANK FOR OVUM DONATION

Similar embryo development has been previously shown in embryos that originated from fresh versus vitrified oocytes in a sibling cohort study (14), whereas the clinical validation of using vitrified oocytes for egg donation was later demonstrated in a large randomized controlled clinical trial (15). Comparable obstetric and perinatal outcomes of the babies conceived using vitrified versus fresh oocytes have been recently demonstrated in a large study involving more than 2000 infants, suggesting the harmlessness of the technology (16).

The use of cryostored oocytes in a large ovum donation program has been evaluated recently (17). The overall survival rate analyzed in this large series including over 40,000 vitrified oocytes was 92.6%. The possible effects of storage time on the survival rate and clinical outcome was calculated in different time categories from less than six months until over five years, showing no impact on either survival rate or clinical outcome (17). We believe that this is very reassuring information since success after long-term storage guarantees the sustainability of the approach. The clinical, ongoing pregnancy, and delivery rates were 55.0%, 45.3%, and 37.6%, respectively, thus confirming the consistency of the results as compared to our previous findings (15,18). The likelihood of having surplus embryos available for additional cryotransfers was very high in this series due to the mean number of oocytes donated. The possibility of further cryotransfers increased cumulative outcomes, and thus maximized the yield of a single-donation cycle, which is precisely what we show herein. The cumulative delivery rate per donation cycle increased to over 70% after three cryotransfers and rose to nearly 80% after five cryotransfers. These results render the donation cycle highly efficient. This finding supports the previous observations we made about the absence of harmful effects of double vitrification (i.e., vitrified embryos developed from vitrified oocytes)

(19). The probability increases exponentially according to the number of oocytes consumed, and the patient can achieve a baby at any number of consumed oocytes with a probability of almost 100% when around three to four donation cycles are completed (17).

To date, we have notification of nearly 6000 babies born (n = 5989) after over 15,000 ovum donation cycles with vitrified oocytes (16,404), involving nearly 200,000 vitrified oocytes (n = 187,647) in the Instituto Valenciano de Infertilidad (IVI) group (unpublished data), revealing the great scope of this approach. At present, nearly 12,000 *in vitro* fertilization (IVF) cycles (n = 11,785) involving the use of own vitrified oocytes (~73,000 oocytes) have been performed at our centers (2787 babies born from whom we have notification), accounting for ~8000 children born from vitrified oocytes in our group.

LOGISTICS AND TECHNICAL ASPECTS RELATED TO THE OOCYTE BANK

Facilities

In accordance with European Directive 2004/23/EC, ART laboratories including centers or clinics, as well as banks of gametes, are considered tissue establishments and therefore are under the regulations and standards that were placed to prevent the transmission of infectious diseases of human tissues and cells.

Safety measures need to be implemented not only during procurement, testing, and processing, but also during preservation, distribution, use, and, of course, storage. Here, we will describe some of the technical features that an oocyte bank has to meet in order to fulfill the European regulations and so be qualified in the four following aspects: design, installation, operation, and performance.

Regarding the facilities, one of the aspects to be qualified in is related to location, air quality, and construction materials.

Location of the storage room

From the practical point of view, the storage room with the LN tanks should be located close to the IVF laboratory so the cryopreserved oocytes can be easily, rapidly, and successfully transferred to the storage room and into the LN tanks.

Concerning distribution purposes, having your own oocyte bank will be logistically easier for distribution and use. However, oocyte transport is also a feasible and safe option that will be revised in this chapter.

As far as dimensions are concerned, the storage room should be designed to allocate a sufficient number of tanks to the storage of the expected number of samples. Some experts suggest calculating the space based on a linear increment within a 10-year plan basis or to have an off-site storage room in case of urgent need for extra space (20,21).

Environmental variables

Although storage facilities might not need to strictly follow the same environmental criteria as procurement and processing facilities, it is recommended, at least for oocyte banking in vapor phase and semi-closed systems, to implement preventive measures in order to minimize bacterial and other airborne contaminations during storage. Such preventive measures can be implemented by installing high-efficiency particulate air filters within the air conditioning system to remove small particles (<0.3 mm); positive pressure could also be considered as an option.

Tissue establishments in Europe must achieve grade A-quality environmental air during procurement and processing, however, since fewer critical steps are performed in the storage areas, grade D-quality background air is acceptable.

The effects of volatile organic compounds (VOCs) on cryopreserved human oocytes and embryos have not yet been evaluated; therefore, it is difficult to assess the level of stringency in terms of VOC control in the storage room. Our recommendation would be to control and minimize VOCs by use of fixed or mobile versions of photo-catalytic oxidizing units or similar approaches.

With regards to temperature, ever though room temperature (22°C–23°C) should be adequate, setting up the room under a cold temperature might help to minimize the LN evaporation and water condensation that can facilitate microbial growth. Another approach can be undertaken by setting up a humidity controller.

Moreover, low-level oxygen sensors and alarm systems in case of LN leaks have to be put in place for safety reasons. As a part of the clinic's general emergency plan, the storage facility should also have generators or an uninterrupted power supply system in case of loss of electrical power.

Equipment

All our samples are cryopreserved by vitrification. This procedure, as currently performed, is entirely manually operated, making the use of any equipment to carry out the vitrification process itself unnecessary. The ease and efficiency of vitrification have brought about a turning point in the field of cryopreservation, making the whole process take no longer than 20 minutes (vitrification and warming) and involving very simple tools. However, the fact that the samples are vitrified and mostly contained in very low volumes represents a challenge for further handling, storage, and maintenance of the vitrified samples. Here, we describe the material and equipment needed for the proper storage of vitrified oocytes in our oocyte bank facilities.

Storage tank

The storage vessel can be traditional LN tanks or vapor tanks. In our oocyte bank facilities, we use vapor-phase storage tanks (CBS V1500; Custom Biogenic Systems, Bruce Township, MI), which contain an outer jacket with LN (Figure 24.1). This is responsible for cooling the storage area where the oocytes are maintained in a nitrogen gas atmosphere. The cold spreads from the vacuum-insulated jacket by convection and through vents in the storage compartment that expel the nitrogen vapor downwards to the bottom of the freezer, thus creating a flow of extremely cold air through the entire storage area (Figures 24.1 and 24.2).

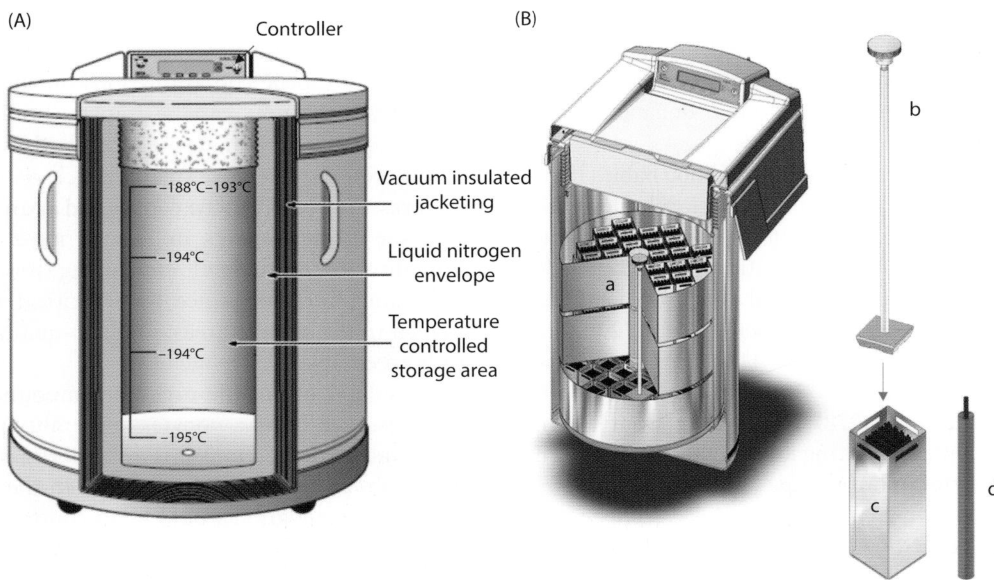

Figure 24.1 (A) Diagram to illustrate the inside of the tank, showing the jacket with liquid nitrogen and the vapor area for storage. (B) (a) Three storage levels assembled on a rotating carousel. (b) Retrieval tool to place and retrieve the canister (c). (d) Goblet containing the samples that are placed into the canisters.

The exceptional uniformity of temperature allows the whole storage tank to be used, achieving temperatures below –180°C at the upper level and –195°C at the bottom. Samples can be manipulated in safe temperature ranges (−180°C) thanks to the working area located on top of the storage area, thus avoiding any risk of accidental warming (Figure 24.2). Figure 24.3 shows the disposition of samples in the storage area. Nearly 11.000 Cryotops can be stored in each tank. An additional advantage of this storage system is that the supply of LN can be programmable, although it also can be performed manually. We have demonstrated the effectiveness of this storage vessel as a strategy for preventing the risk of cross-contamination due to direct contact with the LN, showing comparable results between vapor-stored oocytes versus those stored in conventional LN tanks (22).

For periodical cleaning and due to the more complex and sophisticated nature of these tanks, we recommend regular maintenance, which forces the emptying of the vessels and the temporary location of the samples in a backup tank intended for that purpose. The backup tank

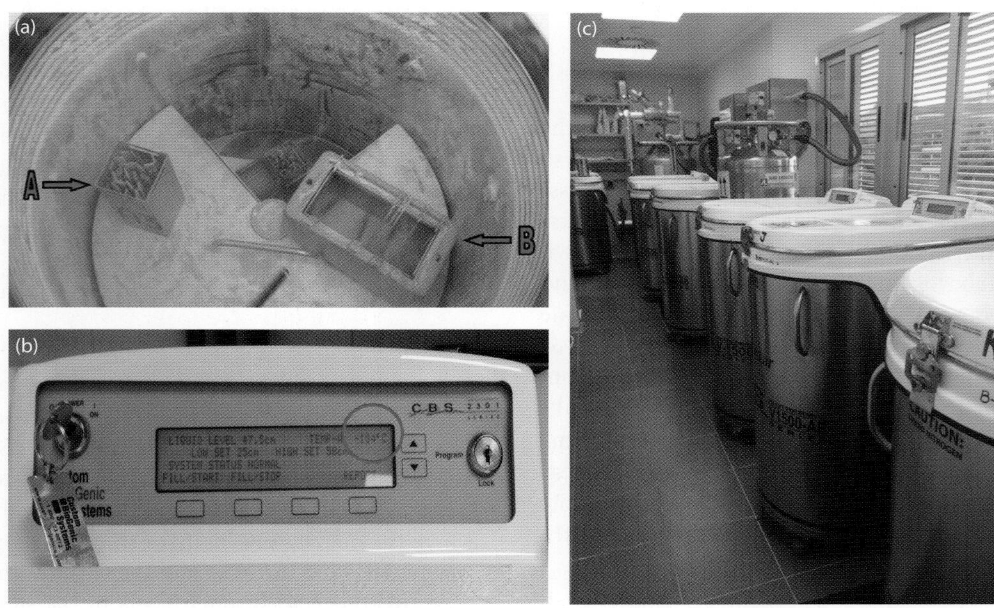

Figure 24.2 (a) Working area of the vapor tank showing a storage canister (A arrow) and the vitrification rack (B arrow) at the time of storing oocytes. (b) Display showing the temperature while manipulating the oocytes (−184°C). (c) Storage room.

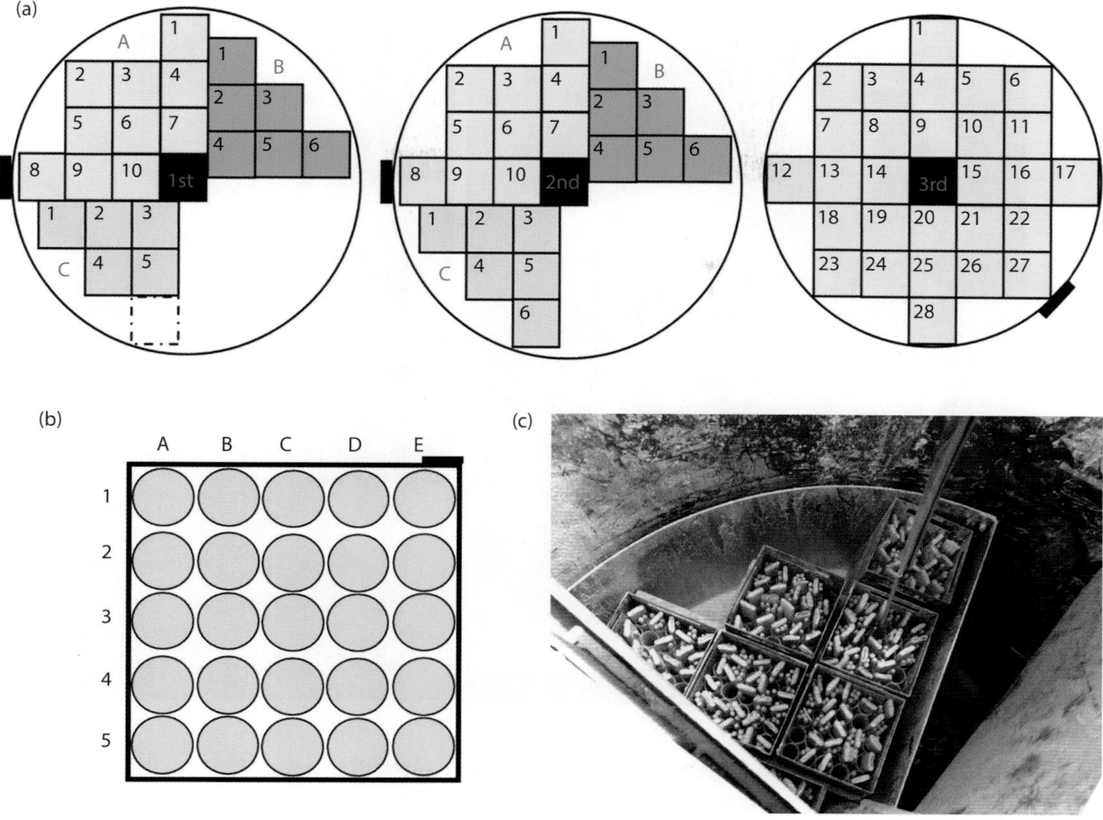

Figure 24.3 (a) Schematic drawing showing the arrangement and number of canisters for storage. Each canister is divided into 25 individual alphanumeric positions (b) for a total of 1800 positions in each tank. Each position can hold up to six Cryotops (10,800 Cryotops per bank). (c) Detail of some stored samples showing the canisters containing the goblets and Cryotops. Each goblet contains samples from individual donors. Placing samples from different patients in the same goblet is not allowed.

must provide the same safe conditions as the storage tank. The emptying for cleaning and maintenance should be scheduled in advance and needs to be performed following strict standard operating protocols.

Construction, nitrogen supply, and gas pipes

The types of construction materials should be similar to those used in procurement and processing facilities, consisting of smooth surfaces and being easy to clean. Perhaps one of the most particular considerations to be undertaken with regards to contraction materials are that the floor should be resistant to large changes of temperature so that it will not easily crack as a result of LN spills.

In our facilities, there are three essential elements for the nitrogen supply to the storage tanks: firstly, a large-scale reservoir of LN (cistern with 2400 L capacity able to supply LN to approximately 10 CBS V1500 vapor tanks) located outside the building (Figure 24.4); secondly, a pressurized tank fed by the reservoir; and thirdly, vapor storage tanks that receive supply from the pressurized tank. The circuit is controlled by an automated, programmable system (Simatic Siemens PLC HMI, Nürnberg, Germany). The system is able to control a number of adjustable parameters, such as minimum and maximum permissible levels, pressure of LN filling, and low-level and overfilling alarms.

The conduction system for LN should be completely insulated to avoid loss of temperature and excess condensation and to minimize the evaporation of LN during refilling maneuvers.

Additionally, individual valves allow the influx of LN into the jackets of the storage tanks. To prevent the impurities that LN may contain entering the storage tank, the use of a pre-filter is strongly recommended, as the presence of "debris" could cause serious problems to the valves of the storage tank (Figure 24.4c).

Nitrogen supply for the vitrification process

With the aim of purifying the LN used during the vitrification process, a specific ceramic filter is coupled to the pressurized tank (Figure 24.5). The Ceralin online filter (Air Liquide Medicinal, Paris, France) consists of a 0.1 µm ceramic membrane in accordance with U.S. Food and Drug Administration Guidelines on Aseptic Processing (1987) (23). The Ceralin online filter consists of two elements of liquid filtration connected in series and inserted into a section of the vacuum transfer line. The ceramic membrane is made from multiple layers formed into a multichannel element. It is housed in a vacuum-insulated pipe, itself installed close to the end-use point. During operation, LN flows through the filter and over the ceramic membrane. The result is

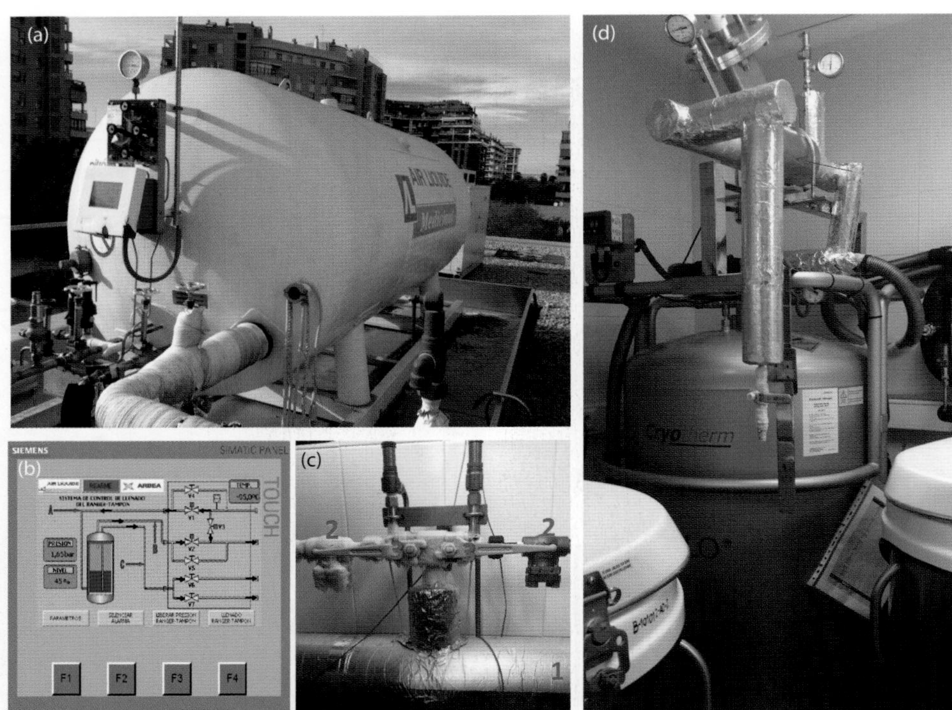

Figure 24.4 (a) Reservoir tank for liquid nitrogen (LN) storage (Air Liquide, Madrid, Spain). (b) Detail of the touchscreen controller of the system, showing the scheme for the filling of the pressurized tank. The filling of the pressurized tank (Apollo 350, Cryotherm, Kirchen (Sieg), Germany) begins at −130°C and is controlled by the system by actuating three solenoids (V1, V2, and V3). All the LN-phase gas coming from the reservoir tank via pipe A is disposed of in order to ensure that the pressurized tank is filled with liquid-phase nitrogen. The LN fills the pressurized tank (nurse tank) when the preset temperature is reached. The excess pressure generated during the filling phase is removed via pipe B. The valves automatically close when the filling is completed. LN is supplied to the vapor storage tanks via specific pipe C. In case of failure, the system can be handled manually by the action of the manual solenoids V4, V5, V6, and V7. (c) (1) Pipe with insulating coating for LN; (2) online wire mesh pre-filter; (3) entry valve for each tank. (d) Pressurized (nurse) tank. The arrow shows the ceramic filter Ceralin online.

high-purity LN with a bacteria count of less than 1 colony-forming unit (CFU)/L gas. Additionally, the large filtration area of the membrane and low level of contamination of LN means it is likely to be several decades before filter saturation. Periodic sampling for microbial assessment is needed.

Temperature monitoring system during storage

Vitrified samples, especially those loaded in minimum volume in the vitrification device, are extremely sensible to any change in temperature. For this reason, a temperature monitoring system is strongly advised as a part of the routine quality control (QC) of the cryolab. In our facilities, we use a system that allows continuous monitoring of the temperature of every storage tank in our unit (DataCare, ControlTemp, Barcelona, Spain). The system is able to provide numeric and graphic records (Figure 24.6) and to display alarms in real time with updates every second. A record of incidents occurring during the alarm can also be easily assessed, differentiating between active alarms or alarms that were active but are no longer in that state. In case of an alarm, the system sends alerts and warning messages to authorized personnel.

Safety during handling of LN

All safety measures for secure handling of LN must be observed. All laboratory personnel, especially embryologists/technicians in charge of the bank, vitrification, and all the related procedures, must be aware of the Material Safety Data Sheet for LN and should be informed of the potential hazards of its use. The banking area should be located in a well-ventilated room. The measurement of oxygen levels is highly advisable due to high concentrations of nitrogen potentially reducing the breathable oxygen in the air. Approved personal protective equipment for eyes, cryogenic gloves, lab coats, closed-toe shoes, and long pants are mandatory.

MANAGEMENT OF DONORS AND RECIPIENTS

Egg donor selection

Spanish Assisted Reproduction Law is based on legislation that was passed in November 1988 (Law 35/1988) (25). Although some countries already had regulations on or recommendations for ART at that time, Spain was the first country to create a specific law to cover this area of

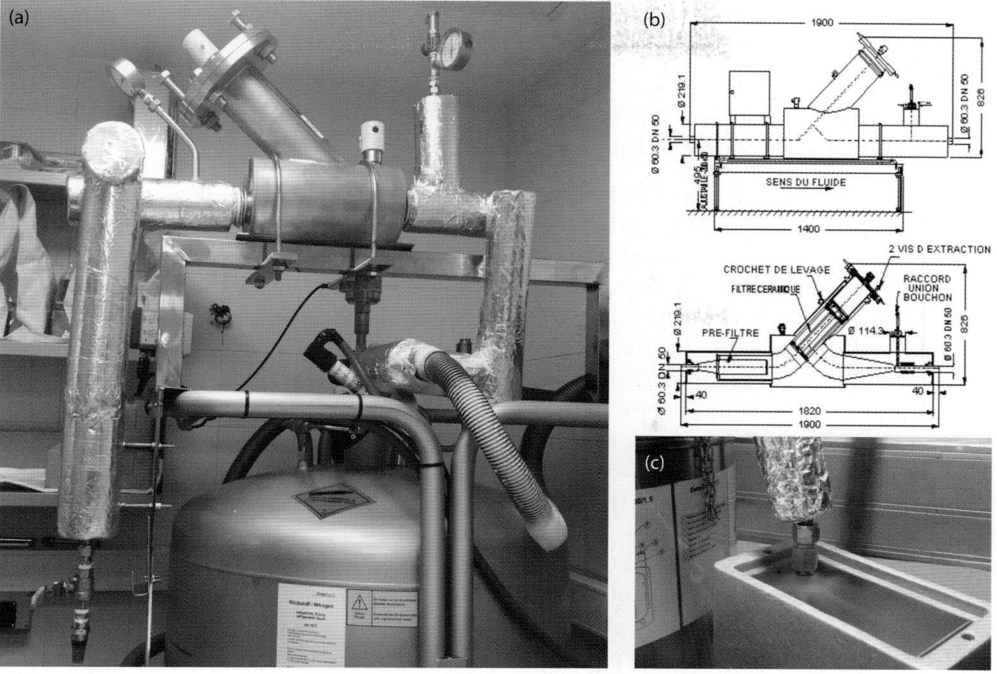

Figure 24.5 (a) Ceralin online filter (Air Liquide Medicinal, France). (b) Schematic illustration. (c) Collection of filtered liquid nitrogen in a sterile container used for vitrification.

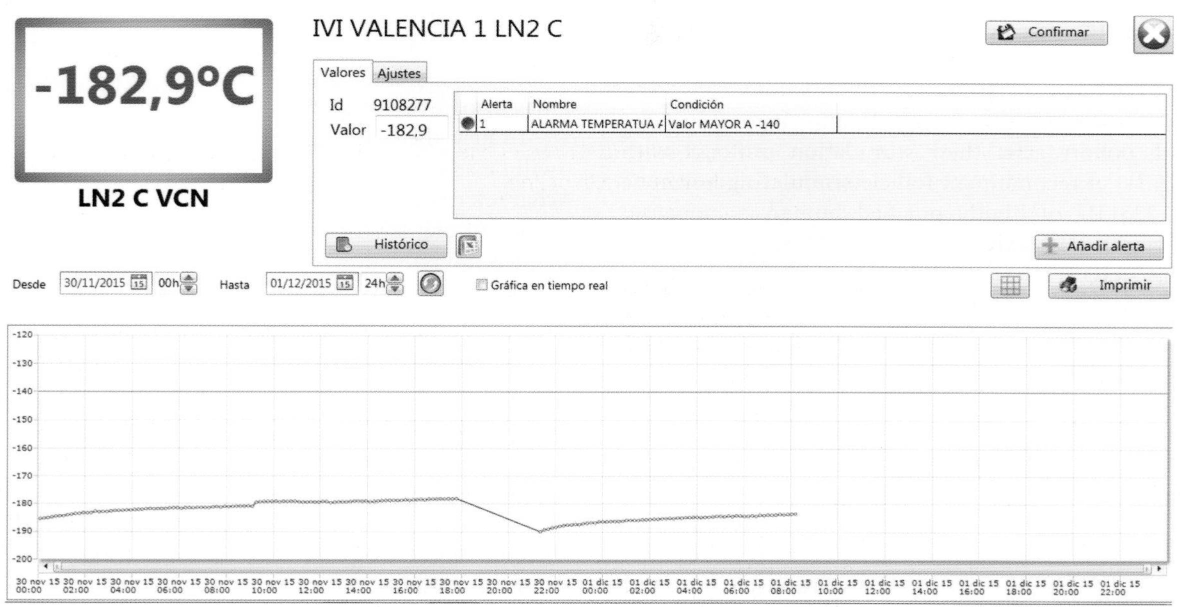

Figure 24.6 Data logger graphic representation of temperature measurement over a time period of one vapor storage tank.

medicine. Royal Decree 412/1996 and Ministerial Order of March 25, 1996, established donor requirements, as well as mandatory standard screening procedures, to rule out the transmission of genetic, hereditary, or infectious diseases (26). In 2006, a new Spanish Law on Assisted Reproduction was approved (Law 14/2006) (27), which determined requirements for gamete and embryo use and regulations on financial compensation.

The following are the most important topics included in Spanish Law on Egg Donation:

- Donation of human gametes is a formal, confidential contract between the donor and the reproductive medicine center. Identities of donors must remain anonymous.
- The donation cannot be revoked.

- The maximum number of children generated from a single donor's gametes should not exceed six.

To be accepted as an egg donor, women must be aged between 18 and 35 years and be healthy. The following steps are necessary to be admitted as an egg donor in our clinics:

- *Medical history*: During the first visit, an interview is conducted to complete the family and personal history.
- *Psychological screening*: Psychological evaluation and counseling by a qualified mental health professional. The donor will be asked to speak with a psychologist to ensure that she fully understands the benefits and risks of egg donation and is properly motivated to become a donor.
- *Gynecological examination*: Evaluation of the donor's menstrual cycles and a vaginal ultrasound are made to examine ovaries, to count antral follicles, and to ensure that there is no pathology in her ovaries. At the same time, body mass index is calculated.
- *Medical screening*: This involves testing for blood type, Rh factor, antibody screening, complete blood count, hemostasis, biochemistry, and infectious disease screening, such as for HIV, hepatitis C virus (HCV), and syphilis.
- *Genetic screening*: Blood tests for karyotype and carrier screening tests for severe recessive and X-linked childhood diseases based on next generation sequencing (NGS) are conducted (549 genes implicated in 623 disease phenotypes).

To begin the egg donation cycle, an oral contraceptive pill is taken for a maximum of 21 days, which starts on days 1 or 2 of the menses of the previous cycle (28). After a five-day washout period following taking the last pill, donors start their stimulation protocol with 150–225 IU of recombinant follicle-stimulating hormone (FSH), 225 IU of highly purified human menopausal gonadotropin (HP-hMG), or 150–225 IU of recombinant FSH plus 75 IU HP-hMG. Egg donors are monitored regularly during FSH injections to measure follicle growth and to ensure it is within an appropriate healthy range. Clinics use vaginal sonograms and blood tests to monitor follicle growth. Daily doses of 0.25 mg gonadotropin-releasing hormone (GnRH) antagonist (ganirelix or cetrorelix) start on day 5 of stimulation in both groups. Once follicles have matured enough for retrieval, a single dose of GnRH agonist is administered to trigger final oocyte maturation. Transvaginal oocyte retrieval takes place 36 hours after GnRH agonist administration. Donors receive light intravenous sedation for the egg retrieval procedure to ensure their comfort, and they rest for two hours at the clinic until they are discharged. In some cases, a post-retrieval vaginal scan is scheduled two to three days following egg retrieval (29).

OOCYTE RECIPIENTS

Oocyte recipients enter our egg donation program for one of the following main diagnoses: premature ovarian failure/menopause; failure to achieve pregnancy after at least three cycles of assisted reproduction techniques; genetic or chromosomal disorders; low response to controlled ovarian hyperstimulation; or recurrent miscarriages.

The vast majority of oocyte recipients undergo hormone-replacement therapy (HRT). In patients with ovarian function, depot GnRH agonist is administered in the mid-luteal phase of their cycle, or GnRH antagonist is administered daily with menstruation for five days. HRT is initiated on days 1–3 of the following cycle with oral estradiol valerate or an estradiol transdermal patch (30–32). Recipients without ovarian function are submitted to the same endometrial preparation protocol, but are not administered depot GnRH agonist. On days 15 or 16 of HRT, a transvaginal ultrasound is performed to measure endometrial thickness, and serum E2 and progesterone levels are tested. Most recipients are ready to receive embryos within two to three weeks of starting HRT, although administration of estradiol valerate can be maintained for a maximum of 50 days until a suitable donation becomes available. Micronized progesterone (800 mg/day vaginally) is initiated on the day after oocyte donation, and embryos are transferred in the blastocyst stage. The recipient continues taking estrogen and progesterone with a positive pregnancy test, and these hormonal supplements are then continued through 12 weeks of pregnancy.

Before treatment begins, the recipient undergoes preliminary testing. This assessment phase includes infectious disease screening (e.g., HIV, CHV, and syphilis) and blood type and Rh factor analysis for both parents. In women older than 45 years, a recent mammogram, full blood count, coagulation tests, and blood biochemistry may also be required.

To help the donor team select an egg donor, recipients will be asked to complete a form regarding their physical characteristics, such as hair color, weight, height, and eye color, among other traits.

It is advisable to collect a sperm sample if the partner lives far from the clinic.

Ovum donation synchronization

We consider many different factors during donor selection: we take into account race, reproductive history, and the physical characteristics that match those of the female partner, and we match blood type and genetic carrier screening. We call matching the time when we select a donor for a recipient after taking into account all the above-mentioned factors.

The timing for the matching procedure has been improved in the last years thanks to the establishment of egg-banking. However, it is important to note that in our current practice, we conduct donations both with fresh and vitrified oocytes, as long as fresh donations are still allowed in our country. Whether to conduct one strategy or another depends on different circumstances related to the availability of oocytes and the needs of the recipient.

Before introducing vitrification into our egg donation program, the numbers of donors and recipients in the clinic are determined at the time of matching: if there are many

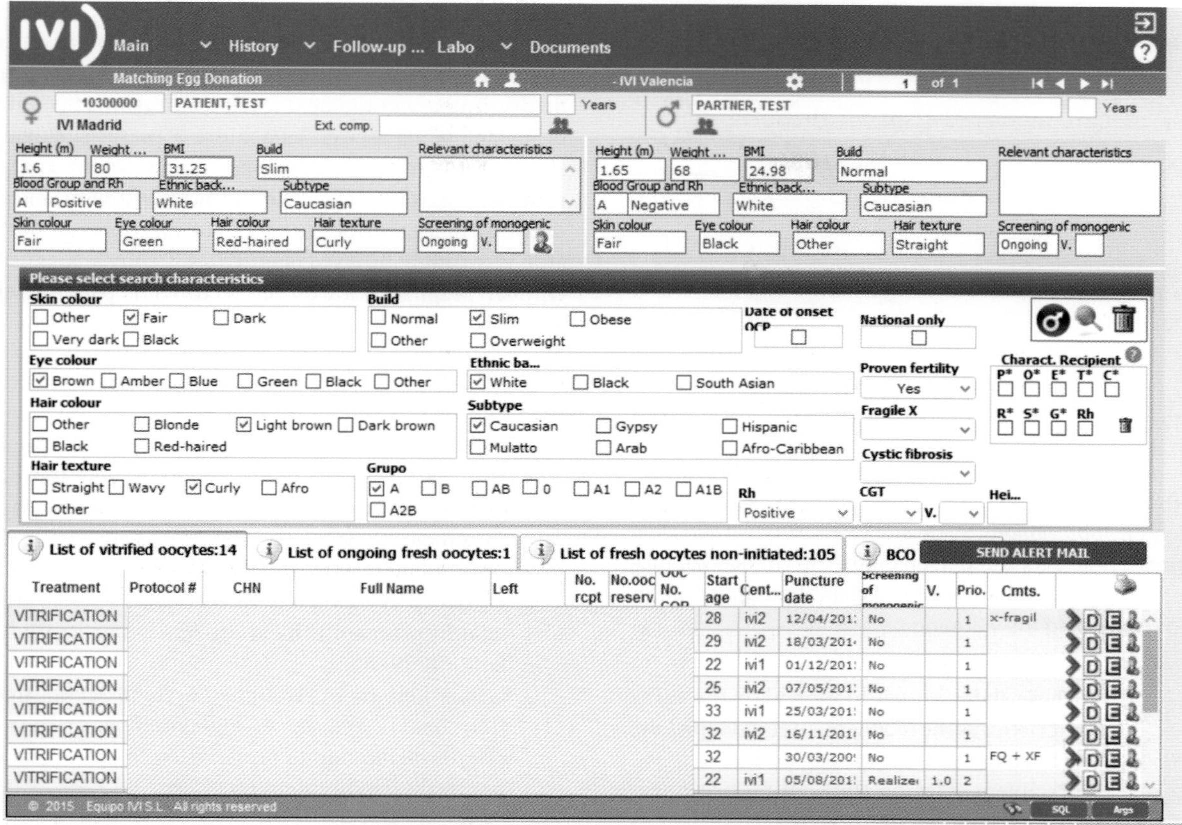

Figure 24.7 Matching sheet for donors and recipients (Equipo IVI S.L. ©).

donors, the matching between donors and recipients is done on the day of the donor's pickup. This means that sometimes recipients are on the waiting list for so many days that they may start bleeding. If, however, the clinic has very few donors needed for special considerations, then donors and recipients are synchronized. This means that recipients and donors start with ovarian stimulation (donors) and HRT (recipients) at the same time. The problem with this situation lies in there being an issue with the donor's stimulation (e.g., cancelations or fewer oocytes than expected). Then, the cycle has to be cancelled and the donation time is only indicative and cannot be officially scheduled (18). The likelihood of this happening underlines the importance of having a large egg donor bank with the availability of a large and varied number of stored oocytes that meet different characteristics.

In addition to the previous problems, about 65% of our recipients come from foreign countries. As such, we need to consider compatibility issues from a medical viewpoint and we must take into account the logistics of the process.

As our usual medical practice now has an egg bank, the time of matching the donor and the recipient depends on different aspects, such as if recipients need specific characteristics or have requested a specific date for embryo transfer.

- Recipients who need specific characteristics: Blood type (O negative, AB negative), specific race, screening for specific genetic diseases, or partners who would like to have another baby with the same donor as they had before:
  - First, we use our donor selection database and select one donor or two with the required characteristics. Sometimes there will be donors under stimulation with the required characteristics, and sometimes we call them to return to our clinic.
  - Second, all the oocytes obtained during pickup are vitrified for the recipient.
  - Finally, the recipient chooses the best time to schedule embryo transfer, and we provide them with instructions to begin HRT depending on embryo transfer.
- Recipients who do not need specific characteristics:
  - Recipients have a date for embryo transfer.
    - First, we reserve oocytes from our egg donor bank.
    - Second, the recipient begins HRT depending on embryo transfer.
    - Finally, we have two options:
      - We use fresh oocytes when we have a donor pickup scheduled on the same date as the donation (with the same characteristics as the partner). The reservation is cancelled in this case.
      - We use vitrified oocytes.
  - Recipients who do not have a date for embryo transfer:
    - The recipient begins HRT and remains on the waiting list.

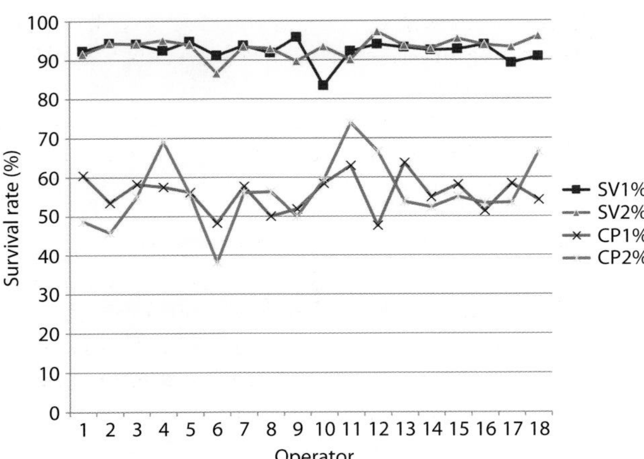

Figure 24.8 Survival and clinical outcomes according to the operator. *Abbreviations*: SV1% and CP1%, survival and clinical pregnancy rates for the person doing the vitrification procedure. SV2% and CP2%, survival and clinical pregnancy rates for the person doing the warming procedure.

- If on these dates an egg donor with the same characteristics as the recipient undergoes pickup, we use fresh oocytes for the egg donation.
- If the recipient stays on the waiting list longer than 20–25 days, we use oocytes from the egg donor bank.

We have created a software that allows us to manage the ovodonación program, which includes all the relevant information about the donors. This application includes donors under stimulation, donors with vitrified oocytes, and vitrified oocytes that are located at other IVI clinics. We have developed a matching application for our soft ward in which a list of best possible donors is supplied after the introduction of recipients' characteristics, including phenotype, blood type, and other especial features (Figure 24.7).

QC IN THE OOCYTE BANK

The cryolab, including the bank, is part of the IVF lab, and as such, it must be subjected to strict QC. In general, the same QC parameters for controlling the IVF lab are useful for the Cryolab as well (24). Accordingly, the cryolab needs to monitor and document the temperature, pH, osmolarity, and culture media, including vitrification solutions. The temperature of the storage tanks needs to be strictly controlled (Figure 24.6).

On the other hand, unlike other laboratory procedures, vitrification as currently performed is an entirely hand-operated procedure, for which outcomes are usually highly dependent on the embryologist/technician. Thus, in order to ensure efficiency, it should be performed only by highly skilled professionals who have undergone a long learning curve. Therefore, an adequate learning curve is also one of the most important requirements when performing vitrification that requires close attention. Our training program has produced satisfactory results since the introduction of vitrification in our clinical setting. It consists of different phases that gradually increase in difficulty. To pass to the next level, trainees must acquire the necessary skills as well as achieve a preset survival rate. Additionally, dynamic database management analysis is routinely performed in order to monitor the maintenance of competence. Periodic analysis of success rates per operator is strongly advised. Figure 24.8 shows survival and clinical pregnancy rates per technician performing the vitrification and warming procedures.

REFERENCES

1. Cobo A, Domingo J, Pérez S, Crespo J, Remohi J, Pellicer A. Vitrification, an effective new approach to oocyte banking in healthy women, could be applied in cancer patients to preserve their fertility. *Clin Transl Oncol* 2008; 10: 268–73.
2. Dondorp WJ, De Wert GM. Fertility preservation for healthy women: Ethical aspects. *Hum Reprod* 2009; 24(8): 1779–85.
3. Garcia-Velasco JA, Domingo J, Cobo A, Martinez M, Carmona L, Pellicer A. Five years' experience using oocyte vitrification to preserve fertility for medical and nonmedical indications. *Fertil Steril* 2013; 99(7): 1994–9.
4. Cobo A, Garrido N, Crespo J, Jose R, Pellicer A. Accumulation of oocytes: A new strategy for managing low-responder patients. *Reprod Biomed Online* 2012; 24(4): 424–32.
5. Herrero L, Pareja S, Losada C, Cobo AC, Pellicer A, Garcia-Velasco JA. Avoiding the use of human chorionic gonadotropin combined with oocyte vitrification and GnRH agonist triggering versus coasting: A new strategy to avoid ovarian hyperstimulation syndrome. *Fertil Steril* 2011; 95(3): 1137–40.
6. Herrero L, Pareja S, Aragones M, Cobo A, Bronet F, Garcia-Velasco JA. Oocyte versus embryo vitrification for delayed embryo transfer: An observational study. *Reprod Biomed Online* 2014; 29(5): 567–72.
7. Pickering SJ, Braude PR, Johnson MH, Cant A, Currie J. Transient cooling to room temperature can cause irreversible disruption of the meiotic spindle in the human oocyte. *Fertil Steril* 1990; 54(1): 102–8.
8. Ghetler Y, Yavin S, Shalgi R, Arav A. The effect of chilling on membrane lipid phase transition in human oocytes and zygotes. *Hum Reprod* 2005; 20(12): 3385–9.
9. Watson PF, Morris GJ. Cold shock injury in animal cells. *Symp Soc Exp Biol* 1987; 41: 311–40.
10. Liebermann J, Dietl J, Vanderzwalmen P, Tucker MJ. Recent developments in human oocyte, embryo and blastocyst vitrification: Where are we now? *Reprod Biomed Online* 2003; 7(6): 623–33.
11. Vajta G, Kuwayama M. Improving cryopreservation systems. *Theriogenology* 2006; 65(1): 236–44.
12. Kuwayama M, Vajta G, Ieda S, Kato O. Comparison of open and closed methods for vitrification of

human embryos and the elimination of potential contamination. *Reprod Biomed Online* 2005; 11(5): 608–14.

13. Seki S, Mazur P. Effect of warming rate on the survival of vitrified mouse oocytes and on the recrystallization of intracellular ice. *Biol Reprod* 2008; 79(4): 727–37.
14. Cobo A, Kuwayama M, Perez S, Ruiz A, Pellicer A, Remohi J. Comparison of concomitant outcome achieved with fresh and cryopreserved donor oocytes vitrified by the Cryotop method. *Fertil Steril* 2008; 89(6): 1657–64.
15. Cobo A, Meseguer M, Remohi J, Pellicer A. Use of cryo-banked oocytes in an ovum donation programme: A prospective, randomized, controlled, clinical trial. *Hum Reprod* 2010; 25(9): 2239–46.
16. Cobo A, Serra V, Garrido N, Olmo I, Pellicer A, Remohi J. Obstetric and perinatal outcome of babies born from vitrified oocytes. *Fertil Steril* 2014; 102(4): 1006–15.e4.
17. Cobo A, Garrido N, Pellicer A, Remohi J. Six years' experience in ovum donation using vitrified oocytes: Report of cumulative outcomes, impact of storage time, and development of a predictive model for oocyte survival rate. *Fertil Steril* 2015; 104(6): 1426–34.e1–8.
18. Cobo A, Remohi J, Chang CC, Nagy ZP. Oocyte cryopreservation for donor egg banking. *Reprod Biomed Online* 2011; 23(3): 341–6.
19. Cobo A, De Los Santos JM, Castellò D, Pellicer A, Remohi J. Effect of re-vitrification of embryos achieved following oocyte vitrification on the new born rate. *Fertil Steril* 2011; 96(3 Suppl): S73.
20. Vajta G, Reichart A. Designing and operating cryopreservation facilities. In: *A Practical Guide of Setting up an IVF Lab, Embryo, Culture Systems and Running the Unit.* Varghese AC, Sjöblom P, Jayaprakasan K (eds.). New Delhi, India: Jaypee Brothers Ltd, 2013, pp. 54–9.
21. Guide of the quality and safety of tissues and cells for human application, 2nd edition [database on the Internet]. EDQM, Council of Europe. 2015. Available from: https://www.edqm.eu/en/news/guide-quality-and-safety-tissues-and-cells-human-application-2nd-edition
22. Cobo A, Romero JL, Perez S, de los Santos MJ, Meseguer M, Remohi J. Storage of human oocytes in the vapor phase of nitrogen. *Fertil Steril* 2010; 94(5): 1903–7.
23. Cobo A, Castellò D, Weiss B, Vivier C, De la Macorra A, Kramp F. Highest liquid nitrogen quality for vitrification process: Micro bacteriological filtration of LN_2. *16th World Congress on In vitro Fertilization; 6th World Congress on In vitro Maturation*, Tokyo, Japan. Abstract book. 2011; 286.
24. Mortimer D, Pool TR, Cohen J. Introduction to quality management in assisted reproductive technology symposium. *Reprod Biomed Online* 2014; 28(5): 533–4.
25. Disposiciones generales Ley 35/1988, de 22 de Noviembre, sobre Técnicas de Reproducción Asistida. 1988; 33373–8.
26. Decreto R. Donación gametos. RD 412/1996: 11253–6.
27. LEY 14/2006, de 26 de mayo, sobre *Técnicas de Reproducción Humana Asistida*. 2006; 19947–56.
28. Remohi J, Vidal A, Pellicer A. Oocyte donation in low responders to conventional ovarian stimulation for *in vitro* fertilization. *Fertil Steril* 1993; 59(6): 1208–15.
29. Remohi J, Gartner B, Gallardo E, Yalil S, Simon C, Pellicer A. Pregnancy and birth rates after oocyte donation. *Fertil Steril* 1997; 67(4): 717–23.
30. Remohi J, Gutierrez A, Cano F, Ruiz A, Simon C, Pellicer A. Long oestradiol replacement in an oocyte donation programme. *Hum Reprod* 1995; 10(6): 1387–91.
31. Soares SR, Troncoso C, Bosch E et al. Age and uterine receptiveness: Predicting the outcome of oocyte donation cycles. *J Clin Endocrinol Metab* 2005; 90(7): 4399–404.
32. Soares SR, Velasco JA, Fernandez M, Bosch E, Remohi J, Pellicer A et al. Clinical factors affecting endometrial receptiveness in oocyte donation cycles. *Fertil Steril* 2008; 89(3): 491–501.

Severe male factor infertility

Genetic consequences and recommendations for genetic testing

25

KATRIEN STOUFFS, WILLY LISSENS, and SARA SENECA

OVERVIEW

Infertility associated with a severe male factor such as oligo-astheno-teratozoospermia (OAT) or azoospermia may be of genetic origin. This means that either the number or the structure of the chromosomes may be aberrant or a gene defect may be present. Two major reasons are indicated for genetic investigations in case of male infertility. One reason is to understand more about the possible causes of azoospermia or OAT. Another reason is to be able to offer genetic counseling to the patient, his partner, and his family whenever indicated. The role of genetic counseling in case of infertility has increased since the advent of assisted reproduction technology (ART) in general, and certainly since the introduction of intracytoplasmic sperm injection (ICSI), offering the possibility to have children to men with almost no spermatozoa (1–3). In the clinic, genetic investigations are usually performed when the azoospermia or oligozoospermia is part of a more complex disease or syndrome. Based on the available data, today a number of genetic tests should also be performed in case of infertility in an otherwise healthy male. In the majority of such cases it will be sufficient to start with the analysis of the karyotype in peripheral lymphocytes, a search for the presence of a Yq11 deletion on the long arm of the Y chromosome, and/or an analysis of the *CFTR* gene in couples in which the male partner has congenital bilateral absence of the vas deferens (CBAVD). More specific genetic investigations can be done if indicated.

GENETIC CAUSES OF MALE INFERTILITY

Chromosomal aberrations

It has been known for over 50 years that the presence of an extra X chromosome in males, resulting in a 47,XXY karyotype, causes Klinefelter syndrome, with testicular atrophy and non-obstructive azoospermia as main features (4,5). Since then, many chromosomal studies have been performed in series of infertile males, and the conclusions drawn from these studies are that constitutional chromosomal aberrations increase as sperm counts decrease.

From these studies it is also clear that the incidence of numerical sex chromosomal aberrations such as 47,XXY and 47,XYY is proportionally higher in males with azoospermia than in males with oligozoospermia, whereas structural chromosomal aberrations of autosomes such as Robertsonian (Figure 25.1a) and reciprocal (Figure 25.1b) translocations are proportionally more frequent in oligozoospermic males (Table 25.1) (6–8).

In azoospermic males it is also possible to find a 46,XX karyotype. In roughly 90% of these Klinefelter-like males the *SRY* gene, normally located close to the pseudoautosomal region of the short arm of the Y chromosome, is now, due to a crossing-over event during meiosis, present in that same region on one of the X chromosomes (9–11). The *SRY* gene, referring to the sex-determining region of the Y chromosome, has to be expressed to induce the sexual development of an embryo toward a male phenotype (12). In the remaining 10% of XX males, most probably other genes with functions in sexual development are involved. Spermatogenesis seems to be absent in these XX males, whereas in apparently non-mosaic Klinefelter patients a few spermatozoa can be found in testicular tissue. This can be explained by the absence of the long arm of the Y chromosome containing the azoospermia factor (AZF) regions in XX males. Spermatozoa obtained from Klinefelter patients have been used in ICSI procedures, and healthy as well as a few 47,XXY children have been born (reviewed in Fullerton et al. [13]).

Microdeletions on the long arm of the Y chromosome (Yq11)

The first azoospermic male patients in whom a deletion in the q11 region of the long arm of the Y chromosome (Yq11) was linked to their infertility were identified through conventional cytogenetic analysis (14). At that time the concept of the AZF region—the region lacking factors (genes) necessary for spermatogenesis due to a deletion—was introduced. Since that time, the structure of the Y chromosome, consisting of the gene-containing euchromatic parts (Yp and Yq11) and the polymorphic heterochromatic parts (Yq12), has been studied in much detail using more sensitive molecular techniques. These have also helped to define the AZF region better. In fact, the AZF region consists of three sub-regions: AZFa, AZFb, and AZFc. Deletions in these sub-regions are most of the time not readily detectable by cytogenetic analysis. Only the molecular results of a polymerase chain reaction investigation with in-house developed primer sets or a commercially available kit will reveal detailed information on the presence of deletions in this region. Almost 100 studies, including more than 13,000 infertile males with reduced sperm numbers from azoospermia to oligozoospermia, have since been conducted. A prevalence of around 7.4% of Yq microdeletions

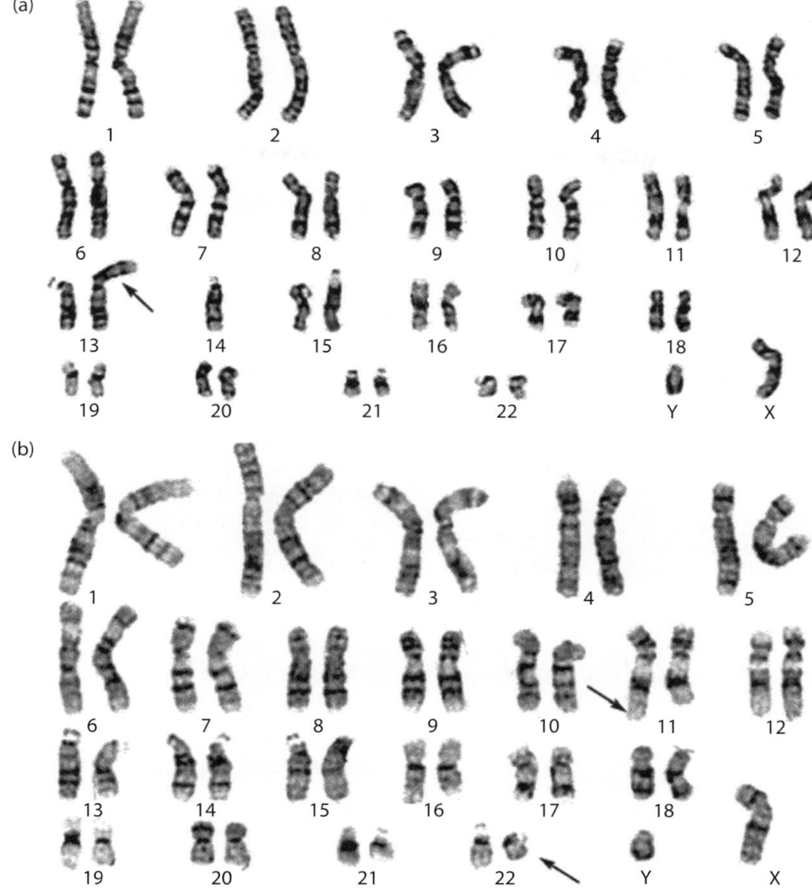

Figure 25.1 (a) 45,XY,der(13;14)(q10;q10) karyotype from a phenotypic normal male with a Robertsonian translocation of chromosomes 13 and 14 through centromeric fusion. (b) 46,XY,t(11;22)(q24.3;q12) karyotype from phenotypic normal male with a balanced reciprocal translocation of chromosome 11 and 22 with break points in 11q24.3 (↘) and 22q12 (↖).

can be deduced from these studies, and again the prevalence is higher in azoospermic (9.7%) than in oligozoospermic (6.0%) males (15). In most patients the deletions span the AZFb and/or AZFc regions, while in only a small number is the AZFa region deleted. Most deletions occur by intra-chromosomal homologous recombination between repeat sequences spread over the Yq11 region (16–18). These repeat sequences are either palindromes consisting of inverted repeat arms or intra-chromosomal repetitive sequences. Several genes have been identified in the AZF regions and they are being studied to clarify their role in spermatogenesis. It is of course evident that if these microdeletions cause the spermatogenic defect leading to a low to very low sperm count present in the ejaculate or to only a few sperm cells in the testes, these microdeletions will, through the use of ICSI, be transmitted to sons, who most probably will be infertile as well (19). However, ICSI children are currently still too young to evaluate their fertility or their sperm count. In a few exceptional cases, fertility has been described in AZFc-deleted fathers who transmitted the deletion to their now infertile sons (20–22). Age at investigation may play a role, as observed in one patient

Table 25.1 Incidence of chromosomal aberrations in infertile oligozoospermic and azoospermic males compared with newborns

Aberrations	Infertile males (n = 7876)	Oligozoospermia (n = 1701)	Azoospermia (n = 1151)	Newborns (n = 94,465)
Autosomes	1.3%	3.0%	1.1%	0.25%
Sex chromosomes	3.8%	1.6%	12.6%	0.14%
Total	5.1%	4.6%	13.7%	0.39%

Source: Summarized from Van Assche E, Bonduelle M, Tournaye H et al. Cytogenetics of infertile men. *Hum Reprod* 1996; 11: 1–26.

Table 25.2 Risk calculations for a child with cystic fibrosis (CF) or congenital bilateral absence of the vas deferens (CBAVD) in a case of CBAVD

	Male		Female			Risk
No testing	8/10	×	1/25	×	1/4	=1/125
Testing female						
Carrier	8/10	×	1	×	1/4	=1/5
No carrier	8/10	×	1/150	×	1/4	=1/750
Testing male + female						
Female carrier	CF/CF	×	1	×	1/2	=1/2
Female no carrier	CF/CF	×	1/150	×	1/2	=1/300
Female carrier	CF/5T	×	1	×	1/4	=1/4 (CF) =1/8 (CBAVD)

Note: If the CBAVD patient is not tested for CF mutations, his risk of having at least one CF mutation is 8/10; if his partner is not tested and Caucasian, her risk of being a carrier of one CF mutation is 1/25. A carrier has a risk of 1/2 to transmit the mutation. Two carriers have a risk of 1/4 to transmit their mutated gene at the same time. A CBAVD patient with two mutations will always transmit a mutated gene. Risks for CF can be calculated if none of the partners are tested, if only the female partner is tested, and if both partners are tested. In high-risk situations, pre-conceptional or preimplantation genetic diagnosis can be offered (91).

with an AZFc deletion being oligozoospermic and later on azoospermic (23).

CBAVD and cystic fibrosis

Men with CBAVD have obstructive azoospermia. Spermatogenesis is usually normal and sperm can be obtained through microsurgical epididymal sperm aspiration, testicular sperm extraction, percutaneous epididymal sperm aspiration, or epididymal or testicular fine-needle aspiration. This sperm can be used to fertilize oocytes *in vitro* through ICSI (2,24). CBAVD is known to be present in 97%–99% of male cystic fibrosis (CF) patients. CF is a frequent and by now well-known autosomal recessive disease in the Caucasian population with an incidence of approximately 1/2500. Many patients now surviving into their 30s and 40s suffer from severe lung disease and pancreatic insufficiency. Although, they are often too ill to reproduce, improved survival into adulthood generates interest in reproduction (25,26). The *CFTR* gene, encoding a protein involved in chloride transport across epithelial membranes, was shown to be responsible for CF due to malfunction of the protein when mutated (27–29).

CBAVD had also been observed in 1%–2% of apparently healthy infertile males, and in 6%–10% of men with obstructive azoospermia (30). When the *CFTR* gene was studied in these males, mutations or splice site variants in intron 8 (comprising the so-called 5T variant and the TG dinucleotide repeat upstream of it) interfering with gene expression were found in 80%–90% of them (31–36). In the remaining CBAVD patients no link could be found either with aberrant *CFTR* expression or with any other etiology. However, in these patients, CBAVD-associated urinary tract/renal malformations were observed (33,37,38). When performing ICSI with sperm from CBAVD males carrying *CFTR* mutations, their partners have to be tested for mutations in the same gene since the carrier frequency of CF mutations may be as high as 1/25 in Caucasians. If both partners carry *CFTR* mutations, the risk of having a child with CF is as high as 1/4 or 25%, or even 1/2 or 50% (Table 25.2). However, since the incidence and the type of *CFTR* mutations vary with ethnic origin as well as with geographical region, counseling and approaches to treatment will have to be adjusted. In high-risk situations, prenatal diagnosis or preimplantation genetic diagnosis (PGD) are indicated (see later).

Male infertility as part of a syndrome

These males all have a 46,XY normal karyotype. Most of the defects are monogenic and either the specific gene defect is known or a chromosomal locus is known or suggested (39). A number of these rather rare conditions that may be encountered in a fertility clinic have been summarized in Table 25.3. However, the (genetic) cause of male infertility remains unknown in many instances, and probably a large number of genes are involved.

Myotonic dystrophy is a rather common autosomal dominant syndrome causing muscular dystrophy with an incidence of 1/8000. The presence of an expanded CTG trinucleotide repeat in the *DMPK* gene interferes with its function (40–43). Symptoms can be very mild and restricted to cataract at an advanced age or, by contrast, very severe, as is the case in the congenital, often lethal form of the disease. Severity is related to the number of CTG repeats (44). In 60%–80% of male patients, testicular tubular atrophy will develop and cause OAT. When such spermatozoa are used to fertilize oocytes, the risk of transmitting the disease, often in a more severe form due to further expansion of the trinucleotide repeat (called anticipation), is 1/2 or 50%. Prenatal diagnosis or preferentially preimplantation diagnosis should be offered (45,46).

Kallmann syndrome is characterized by hypogonadotropic hypogonadism, due to impaired gonadotropin-releasing hormone secretion, and anosmia. X-linked as

Table 25.3 Some other known genetic causes of male infertility

Disease	Frequency	Clinic	Lab tests	Cause	Treatment	References
Myotonic dystrophy	1:8000	Male phenotype Myotonia	Normospermia/ oligospermia LH, FSH normal or ↗ T normal or ↘	AD "CTG" expansion in *DMPK* gene	ICSI PGD	(40–46)
Kallmann syndrome	1:10,000	Male phenotype Pubertal delay Anosmia	Azoospermia T, FSH, LH ↘ No response to GnRH test	X-linked Abnormal neuronal migration Point mutation in *KAL1* gene AR and AD forms exist as well	Hormonal substitution	(47–57)
Primary ciliary dyskinesia or immotile cilia syndrome	1:25,000	Male phenotype	Asthenozoospermia	AR Dynein deficiency Genetic heterogeneity (?)	ICSI	(58–60)
Kennedy disease or spinal bulbar muscular atrophy	1:50,000	Male (gynecomastia) Muscular atrophy	Oligozoospermia/ azoospermia T normal or ↘ LH, FSH ↗	X-linked "CAG" expansion in androgen receptor gene	ICSI or AID	(61,62)

Abbreviations: AD, autosomal dominant; AID, artificial insemination with donor sperm; AR, autosomal recessive; FSH, follicle-stimulating hormone; GnRH, gonadotropin-releasing hormone; ICSI, intracytoplasmic sperm injection; LH, luteinizing hormone; PGD, preimplantation genetic diagnosis; T, testosterone.

well as autosomal recessive and autosomal dominant inheritance forms exist. The X-linked form of Kallmann syndrome (*KAL1* gene) is the most frequent and the best known one (47). An autosomal dominant form of Kallmann syndrome is caused by mutations in the *FGFR1* gene (48). A possible interaction between the gene products of the *KAL1* and *FGFR1* genes has been suggested as an explanation for the higher prevalence of Kallmann syndrome in males than in females (49,50). In addition, mutations in four other genes have been implicated in Kallmann syndrome (51–53). Nevertheless, only about 30% of patients with a clinical diagnosis of Kallmann syndrome have mutations in one of the six genes identified so far (54). The presence of mutations in different genes of some individuals suggests that, at least in some patients, a possible digenic mode of inheritance of Kallmann syndrome exists (51,55,56). Hormonal treatment will stimulate spermatogenesis in patients with Kallmann syndrome (57). Genetic counseling is indicated.

Primary ciliary dyskinesia or immotile cilia syndrome is an autosomal recessive disease presenting with chronic respiratory tract disease, rhinitis, and sinusitis due to immotile cilia. Male patients are usually infertile because of asthenozoospermia (58). If the above symptoms are associated with situs inversus, the condition is called Kartagener syndrome (59,60). Men with this condition can reproduce with the help of ICSI. Genetic counseling is hampered because of the lack of knowledge of all genes involved in primary ciliary dyskinesia and Kartagener syndrome (60). However, if we accept the incidence of 1/25,000, the carrier frequency must be 1/80, which means that the risk of a man having an affected child is 1/160 ($1 \times 1/80 \times 1/2$).

Kennedy's disease or spinal and bulbar muscular atrophy is a neuromuscular disease causing muscular weakness that is associated with testicular atrophy and leads to oligozoospermia or azoospermia. It is an X-linked disease caused by an expanded (CAG) trinucleotide repeat in the transactivation domain of the androgen receptor gene (61,62). If treated with ICSI, genetic counseling is again indicated. However, point mutations in the androgen receptor gene might result in androgen insensitivity through impaired binding of dihydrotestosterone to the receptor, which will interfere with sexual development. The resulting syndrome is testicular feminization or androgen insensitivity syndrome, causing a (partial) female phenotype (63,64). The presenting problem here will not (only) be male infertility. Patients with an autosomal recessive 5α-reductase deficiency and therefore unable to synthesize dihydrotestosterone from testosterone may theoretically present at the clinic with azoospermia and pseudohermaphroditism (65,66).

Very rarely, patients with other mostly syndrome-associated genetic defects may consult at a male infertility clinic. Up to 80% of patients with Noonan syndrome present with oligozoospermia or azoospermia as a result of cryptorchidism (67). The diagnosis is so far based on other symptoms, including small stature, chest deformity, a rather typical facial dysmorphism, and congenital heart disease. Defects in a gene on chromosome 12q24.1, *PTPN11*, are responsible for approximately 40% of patients with Noonan syndrome (68). Another six genes involved in Noonan syndrome have been identified; all seven known genes account for around 60% of cases. Consequently, more (currently unknown) genes are involved in Noonan syndrome. The autosomal dominant inheritance asks for genetic counseling. Other possible patients may be affected by Aarskog–Scott syndrome with acrosomal sperm defects (69,70) or Beckwith–Wiedemann syndrome with cryptorchidism (71). Syndromes such as Bardet–Biedl syndrome and Prader–Willi syndrome, both presenting with hypogonadism, are associated with other major symptoms, including (severe) mental retardation, which limit procreation (72–74). Prader–Willi syndrome is an imprinting syndrome resulting from the absence of expression of the paternal alleles in the 15q11–q13 imprinted region (75–77). Other causes of male infertility include deficiencies in enzymes involved in the synthesis of testosterone (64,66), luteinizing hormone, and luteinizing hormone receptor (78,79).

Defects in energy production by the mitochondria have been implicated in male infertility. Mitochondria are the main sources of energy production for the cells through the process of oxidative phosphorylation. The synthesis of ATP occurs through the action of five enzyme complexes that are encoded by both nuclear genes and the small mitochondrial genome that is exclusively maternally inherited. Mitochondrial diseases usually evolve as multisystem disorders mainly affecting the central nervous system and muscles. In addition, these defects in respiratory function are believed to cause a decline in sperm motility because of depletion of ATP, which is necessary for flagellar propulsion of the spermatozoa. Reduced sperm motility and resulting male infertility have been well documented in several patients with mitochondrial encephalopathies caused by mitochondrial tRNA point mutations or (multiple) mtDNA deletions (80).

GLOBOZOOSPERMIA AND MACROZOOSPERMIA

Globozoospermia is a rare (<0.1%) cause of male infertility. A major characteristic of these round-headed spermatozoa is the malformation or absence of the acrosome (81). So far, at least three genes have been associated with this form of teratozoospermia in humans: *SPATA16*, *PICK1*, and *DPY19L2* (82–85). In all of these cases, the condition is inherited as an autosomal recessive disease. Variants in the *DPY19L2* gene are the most prevalent and can be detected in 60%–83.3% of patients with (type I) globozoospermia. Around 26.7%–73.3% of these patients are homozygous for a 200 kb deletion of the *DPY19L2* gene (86). Mutations in *PICK1* and *SPATA16* can be detected in patients with globozoospermia, although the prevalence is very low.

In another form of morphological abnormal spermatozoa (large-headed, multiflagellar, polyploid spermatozoa), a condition resulting in male infertility is caused by mutations in the *AURKC* gene, which is involved in chromosomal segregation and cytokinesis (87). The first mutation detected in this gene was a deletion of a single base pair (c.144delC). This mutation has been detected in patients of North African origin. Especially in a Magrebian population, it was estimated that ~1/50 are carriers of this mutation. A second recurrent mutation (p.Tyr248*) can be detected in European patients (88).

CONSEQUENCES AND RECOMMENDATIONS IN THE CLINIC

Genetic evaluation of infertile males before ART use

A personal history from the patient should be taken. In addition, a detailed pedigree should be drawn and completed for miscarriages or children (also deceased) with multiple congenital malformations in first- or second-degree relatives. It is also important to know about infertility in siblings or other family members. This information may suggest a possible chromosomal aberration such as a translocation (Figure 25.2a) or a monogenic disease like Kallmann syndrome (Figure 25.2b) or CF (Table 25.2). A thorough inquiry of the proband and his partner may pinpoint other hereditary diseases not necessarily causing infertility but causing morbidity or being lethal to offspring. A complete clinical examination of the proband and his partner is useful for establishing a clinical diagnosis of a disease or a syndrome associated with infertility such as Klinefelter syndrome or CF-linked CBAVD. This examination may also reveal other possible hereditary diseases not identified before. Since the couple is in such a case not aware of a genetic problem, they should be counselled before treatment starts. Complementary tests—mainly laboratory investigations—will help to confirm a clinical diagnosis. In case of male infertility, the personal history, the clinical examination, a semen analysis, and hormonal tests are sufficient to characterize most of the patients as being:

1. Infertile in association with other physical or mental problems.
2. Infertile but otherwise healthy. These patients can mostly be subdivided into oligozoospermic or eventually OAT males, and into males with obstructive or non-obstructive azoospermia. Rarely, patients with teratozoospermia are detected through semen analysis.

Genetic investigations will help to refine the diagnosis and to counsel the patient/couple accordingly. The above information will help to select the additional tests to be performed. In most cases of male infertility due to severe OAT or non-obstructive azoospermia, a peripheral karyotype should be performed, even if the family history is not suggestive of a chromosomal disorder (6–8). In the same cohort of patients, microdeletions of the AZF regions on Yq11 should be looked for in DNA from peripheral blood. The possibility of fertility treatment in couples in whom the male has an AZF deletion is strongly dependent on the type of deletion present (89). Deletions of AZFa or AZFb, or combinations including these regions, have a bad prognosis since no sperm cells will be produced and ICSI will not be possible. In contrast, spermatozoa can be found in about 70% of patients with a complete deletion of the AZFc region (89). For these patients ICSI will be possible.

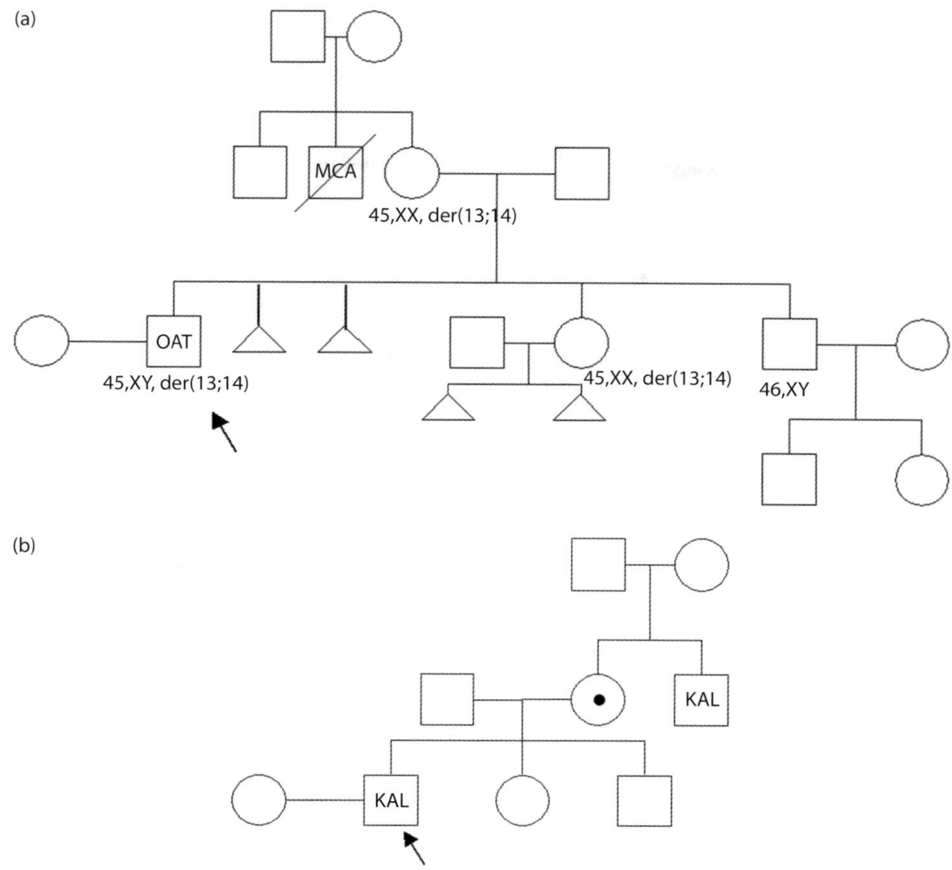

Figure 25.2 (a) Segregation of a Robertsonian translocation der(13;14) in a family: its consequences and recommendations. "OAT" (our proband ↖) presents with infertility due to Oligo-astheno-teratozoospermia. His sister had two miscarriages (Δ); his brother has two healthy children. His mother had two miscarriages (Δ), lost a brother born with multiple congenital anomalies (MCA), and has a healthy brother without children. This story is suggestive of a chromosomal translocation. The karyotype of "OAT" points to a Robertson translocation der(13;14) (Figure 25.1a). His mother and his sister have the same translocation explaining the recurrent miscarriages (Δ). These miscarriages are most probably resulting from a trisomy 14 or monosomy 13 or 14. The brother of "OAT" has a normal karyotype, which is perfectly possible. The MCA brother of the mother died and most probably had trisomy 13. "OAT" should be informed about all the above possible risks in case of pregnancy. In case of intracytoplasmic sperm injection, a preimplantation genetic diagnosis or a prenatal diagnosis should be offered. (b) X-linked Kallmann syndrome in a family: its consequences and recommendations. "KAL" (our proband ↖) has Kallmann syndrome. The family history fits with an X-linked transmission since the brother of the mother of "KAL" has the same disease. This means that the mother of "KAL" must be a carrier ⊙. Her daughter, the sister of our proband, therefore has a 50% risk of being a carrier and a 25% risk of having an affected son. Preimplantation or prenatal diagnosis should be discussed. If the wife of "KAL" becomes pregnant, boys will be healthy and fertile (because they inherit the Y chromosome of their father), while girls will always be carriers.

In men with non-obstructive azoospermia caused by CBAVD without anomalies of the urogenital tract, mutations in the *CFTR* gene should be looked for in the patient and, even more importantly, in his partner. At present it is possible to identify 85%–90% of carriers in the Caucasian population (90,91). Depending on whether *CFTR* mutations have been identified in the male patient and/or his female partner, the risk of conceiving a child with CF can be calculated (Table 25.2). These figures together with the type of mutations may be an indication for prenatal diagnosis or PGD (26,92,93). More specific tests should be performed if diseases such as Kennedy disease, Kallmann syndrome, myotonic dystrophy, immotile cilia syndrome, or other syndromes or diseases are suspected. In these cases it is again important not only to establish a correct diagnosis to treat appropriately, but also to counsel the proband and his family adequately concerning recurrence risks and prenatal or preimplantation diagnosis.

Genetic testing during ART use for severe male infertility

Genetic tests that can be performed during ART refer to PGD. They involve the genetic analysis (PGD) of one or two polar bodies before fertilization or the analysis of one or two blastomeres of the 8- to 10-cell embryo *in vitro* (94–99). The aim is to avoid the birth of a child with a genetic disease. PGD makes conventional prenatal diagnosis, eventually followed by termination of pregnancy, obsolete. PGD is a complex procedure because of the "single-cell" genetic diagnosis. It was developed and first applied in the clinic more than 20 years ago (100). At first, most of the PGDs performed were for CF, myotonic dystrophy, Huntington's disease, and Duchenne muscular dystrophy, but many others have since been performed for either infertile or fertile couples (96,98). For chromosomal aberrations, most PGDs have been done for reciprocal and Robertsonian translocations (101). In general, the take-home baby rate is of the same order of magnitude of 20%–25% as in ICSI cycles in general (2,3). A number of PGDs have been performed for Klinefelter patients in whom spermatozoa found in the testes were used to fertilize oocytes (13).

Genetic evaluation of pregnancies and children conceived through ICSI because of severe male infertility

Follow-up studies of pregnancies established and children born after the use of ICSI have been initiated as soon as this new procedure was applied in the clinic. From these still ongoing studies it became clear that the number of major malformations was comparable to the number of major malformations in *in vitro* fertilization (IVF) children, and possibly slightly higher than in naturally conceived children. Preliminary results on the psychomotor development of these children are also reassuring (102–109). The "*de novo*" chromosomal aberrations found at prenatal diagnosis indicate that numerical sex chromosomal anomalies are slightly increased when compared to a large newborn population. The incidence in the newborn after natural conception is 0.2%, but the incidence in ICSI children is 0.8%. This is a four-fold increase, but of course the overall incidence remains low (<1%). Apart from sex chromosome anomalies, *de novo*-balanced translocations have also been observed (107,109). These aberrations occurring in children of men with a normal peripheral karyotype could be related to chromosomal anomalies being present in their sperm but not in their lymphocytes (110–113).

CONTROVERSIES

To test or not to test

Some clinicians claim that now that ICSI is available to alleviate male infertility, it is sufficient to know whether these patients are oligozoospermic or azoospermic. Oligozoospermic and obstructive azoospermic males can be treated immediately and often successfully even if repetitive IVF cycles are necessary (114). Even in case of non-obstructive azoospermia, repeated testicular sperm extraction leads to a high sperm recovery rate that allows ICSI to be performed (115). It is probably true that in the majority of cases a healthy although maybe infertile child will be born. Nevertheless, in a number of cases (e.g., in the case of a chromosomal translocation) the treatment will fail and be repeated endlessly, or recurrent miscarriages will occur. Furthermore, a few CF children will be born and probably also a few other children with genetic disease that could have been avoided. Another option could be to not use ICSI further and so to leave decisions to nature.

Who to test?

Among those clinicians who are convinced that genetic tests are useful and among the geneticists performing the tests, the main ongoing discussion relates to which infertile male patients should karyotypes and Yq deletion tests be performed. With time, many do now agree on performing these genetic tests if the sperm count is below 1×10^6 or 5×10^6 spermatozoa/mL (116). However, chromosomal aberrations as well as Yq microdeletions have been found in patients with more than 5×10^6 spermatozoa/mL, although to a lesser extent (117). Based on a few reports, one can also wonder whether karyotype analysis of the female partners should be performed (118–120). Prenatal diagnosis through chorionic villus sampling or amniocentesis after ICSI should be discussed with the couple in view of the known increase in sex chromosomal aberrations in the offspring (107,109).

Genetic testing versus genetic screening

Genetic screening should not be confused with genetic testing. A screening test is offered to a "healthy" population. In that case, the persons who are tested have no particular problem, but they may be interested to know whether they are carriers of a particular gene mutation so as to take preventive measures. Examples are screening programs for CF, Tay–Sachs disease, and other diseases that are common in certain high-risk populations (121–124). Couples may want to know their carrier status before reproduction since, if both partners are carriers of such an autosomal recessive gene, the risk of having an affected child is 1/4. Such screening programs are not specific to infertile patients. However, a fertile couple with a 25% recurrence risk may choose to have prenatal diagnosis to prevent the birth of an affected child, while if the couple is infertile and can be helped with IVF/ICSI, they may prefer PGD (125).

PGD for aneuploidy screening

PGD for aneuploidy screening (preimplantation genetic screening [PGS]), an approach to select the "better" embryos for transfer after IVF/ICSI, is sometimes offered to selected groups of patients. The main indications suggested for PGS are advanced maternal age, repeated implantation failure, repeated miscarriage, and severe male factor infertility. Here, the embryos are biopsied and a variable number of chromosomes, usually 13, 16, 18, 21, 22, X, and Y, are enumerated using specific fluorescent *in situ* hybridization (FISH) probes. Embryos that are diploid for the chromosomes tested are then transferred without, of course, having information on the other chromosomes. The first observations reported that in women over 37 years of age, the IVF success rate increases (126), the rate of miscarriage decreases (127), and the implantation rate

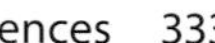

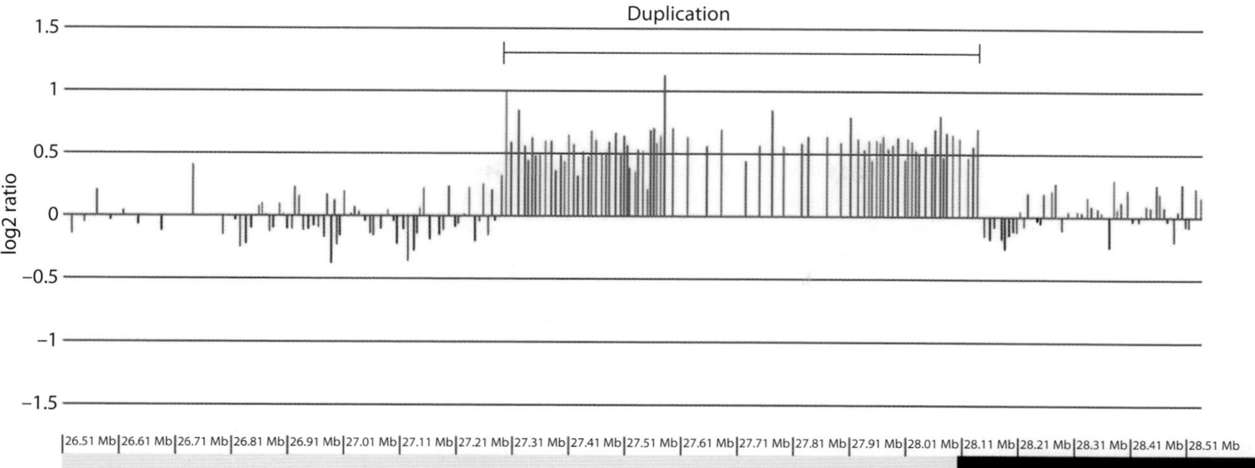

Figure 25.3 Example of a result obtained after array comparative genomic hybridization. The figure shows part of the genome where a duplication was detected in an infertile male patient.

per embryo increases (128–130). Since these early times, many studies have been performed, but little (or no) evidence was found that PGS increases live birth delivery rates. Recent studies focused on the use of polar bodies as the study material, in contrast to blastomeres that were used most of the time before, and other technologies (than FISH) were used, such as comparative genomic hybridization and single-nucleotide polymorphism arrays in PGS (131–135). Data are needed to evaluate the possible benefits of these new applications in aneuploidy screening for IVF embryos.

Is ICSI in case of severe male infertility safe?

Although the follow-up studies of pregnancies and children born after ICSI are reassuring, still a number of questions remain unanswered, one of them relating to concerns in terms of imprinting (106,136–142).

FUTURE FINDINGS

ICSI performed with ejaculated spermatozoa and later on with epididymal and testicular spermatozoa may be considered milestones in infertility treatment for the male patient. Today, very few men cannot be helped to have their own child. Research is ongoing to find other solutions for their fertility problems (143–147). However, some approaches are extremely controversial. ICSI has also triggered basic research in biology and genetics in order to gain more insight into gender development and spermatogenesis. Over recent years, many novel genes have been and are being identified. The development of whole-genome-scaled techniques (whole-exome sequencing and array comparative genomic hybridization) allow a better identification of disease-related abnormalities in known or novel genes (Figure 25.3). New findings will increase our knowledge and allow more accurate diagnosis and counseling, and probably new forms of treatment will become available.

CONCLUSION

In case of severe male infertility, good clinical practice requires genetic evaluation before, during, and after ART in order to properly treat and counsel the proband, the couple, and, eventually, the family. The aim is to inform the patients about possible risks, to improve the success rate of the ART treatment, and to avoid the birth of children affected with a severe genetic disease. Moreover, at present there are still many unknown causes of male infertility. More research in the field of genetics will provide us with a better understanding, as well as a better defining how great the risks are of transmitting infertility or possibly other genetic anomalies to the next generation.

REFERENCES

1. Palermo G, Joris H, Devroey P et al. Pregnancies after intracytoplasmic injection of single spermatozoon into an oocyte. *Lancet* 1992; 340: 17–8.
2. Devroey P, Van Steirteghem A. A review of ten years experience of ICSI. *Hum Reprod Update* 2004; 10: 19–28.
3. The ESHRE Capri Workshop Group. Intracytoplasmic sperm injection (ICSI) in 2006: Evidence and evolution. *Hum Reprod Update* 2007; 13: 515–26.
4. Jacobs PA, Strong JA. A case of human intersexuality having a possible XXY sex-determining mechanism. *Nature* 1959; 183: 302–3.
5. Forti G, Corona G, Vignozzi L et al. Klinefelter's syndrome: A clinical and therapeutical update. *Sex Dev* 2010; 4: 167–9.
6. Van Assche E, Bonduelle M, Tournaye H et al. Cytogenetics of infertile men. *Hum Reprod* 1996; 11: 1–26.
7. Yoshida A, Miura K, Shirai M et al. Cytogenetic survey of 1007 infertile males. *Urol Int* 1997; 58: 166–76.
8. Martin RH. Cytogenetic determinants of male fertility. *Hum Reprod Update* 2008; 14: 379–90.

9. Weil D, Wang I, Dietrich A et al. Highly homologous loci on the X and Y chromosomes are hot-spots for ectopic recombination resulting in XX maleness. *Nat Genet* 1994; 7: 414–9.
10. Schiebel K, Winkelmann M, Mertz A et al. Abnormal XY interchange between a novel isolated protein kinase gene, *PRKY*, and its homologue, PRKX, accounts for one third of all (Y+) XX males and (Y−) XY females. *Hum Mol Genet* 1997; 6: 1985–9.
11. Vorona E, Zitzmann M, Gromoll J et al. Clinical, endocrinological, and epigenetic features of the 46, XX male syndrome, compared with 47,XXY Klinefelter patients. *J Clin Endocrinol Metab* 2007; 92: 3458–65.
12. Sinclair AH, Berta P, Palmer MS et al. A gene from the human sex-determining region encodes a protein with homology to a conserved DNA-binding motif. *Nature* 1990; 346: 240–4.
13. Fullerton G, Hamilton M, Maheshwari A. Should non-mosaic Klinefelter syndrome men be labelled as infertile in 2009? *Hum Reprod* 2010; 25: 588–97.
14. Tiepolo L, Zuffardi O. Localization of factors controlling spermatogenesis in the nonfluorescent position of the human Y chromosome long arm. *Hum Genet* 1976; 34: 119–24.
15. Massart A, Lissens W, Tournaye H, Stouffs K. Genetic causes of spermatogenic failure. *Asian J Androl* 2012; 14: 40–8.
16. Skaletsky H, Kuroda-Kawaguchi T, Minx PJ et al. The male-specific region of the human Y chromosome is a mosaic of discrete sequence classes. *Nature* 2003; 423: 825–37.
17. Repping S, Skaletsky H, Lange J et al. Recombination between palindromes P5 and P1 on the human Y chromosome causes massive deletions and spermatogenic failure. *Am J Hum Genet* 2002; 71: 906–22.
18. Jobling MA. Copy number variation on the human Y chromosome. *Cytogenet Genome Res* 2008; 123: 253–62.
19. Silber SH. The Y chromosome in the era of intracytoplasmic sperm injection: A personal view. *Fertil Steril* 2011; 95: 2439–48.
20. Saut N, Terriou P, Navarro A et al. The human Y chromosome genes *BPY2*, *CDY1* and *DAZ* are not essential for sustained fertility. *Mol Hum Reprod* 2000; 6: 789–93.
21. Chang PL, Sauer MV, Brown S et al. Y chromosome microdeletion in a father and his four infertile sons. *Hum Reprod* 1999; 14: 2689–94.
22. Calogero AE, Garofalo MR, Barone N et al. Spontaneous transmission from a father to his son of a Y chromosome microdeletion involving the deleted in azoospermia (*DAZ*) gene. *J Endocrinol Invest* 2002; 25: 631–4.
23. Girardi SK, Mielnik A, Schlegel PN. Submicroscopic deletions in the Y chromosome of infertile men. *Hum Reprod* 1997; 12: 1635–41.
24. Sarkar NN. Intracytoplasmic sperm injection: An assisted reproductive technique and its outcome to overcome infertility. *J Obstet Gynaecol* 2007; 27: 347–53.
25. Sueblinvong V, Whittaker LA. Fertility and pregnancy: Common concerns of the aging cystic fibrosis population. *Clin Chest Med* 2007; 28: 433–43.
26. Keymolen K, Goossens V, De Rycke M et al. Clinical outcome of preimplantation genetic diagnosis for cystic fibrosis: The Brussels' experience. *Eur J Hum Genet* 2007; 15: 752–8.
27. Kerem B, Rommens JM, Buchanan JA et al. Identification of the cystic fibrosis gene: Genetic analysis. *Science* 1989; 245: 1073–80.
28. Riordan JR, Rommens JM, Kerem B et al. Identification of the cystic fibrosis gene: Cloning and characterization of complementary DNA. *Science* 1989; 245: 1066–73.
29. Rommens JM, Iannuzzi MC, Kerem B et al. Identification of the cystic fibrosis gene: Chromosome walking and jumping. *Science* 1989; 245: 1059–65.
30. Dubin L, Amelar RD. Etiologic factors in 1294 consecutive cases of male infertility. *Fertil Steril* 1971; 22: 469–74.
31. Anguiano A, Oates RD, Amos JA et al. Congenital bilateral absence of the vas deferens. A primarily genital form of cystic fibrosis. *JAMA* 1992; 267: 1794–7.
32. Chillon M, Casals T, Mercier B et al. Mutations in the cystic fibrosis gene in patients with congenital absence of the vas deferens. *N Engl J Med* 1995; 332: 1475–80.
33. Claustres M. Molecular pathology of the *CFTR* locus in male infertility. *Reprod Biomed Online* 2005; 10: 14–41.
34. Cuppens H, Cassiman JJ. *CFTR* mutations and polymorphisms in male infertility. *Int J Androl* 2004; 27: 251–6.
35. Lissens W, Mercier B, Tournaye H et al. Cystic fibrosis and infertility caused by congenital bilateral absence of the vas deferens and related clinical entities. *Hum Reprod* 1996; 11(Suppl 4): 55–80.
36. Groman JD, Hefferon TW, Casals T et al. Variation in a repeat sequence determines whether a common variant of the cystic fibrosis transmembrane conductance regulator gene is pathogenic or benign. *Am J Hum Genet* 2004; 74: 176–9.
37. Dumur V, Gervais R, Rigot JM et al. Congenital bilateral absence of the vas deferens in absence of cystic fibrosis. *Lancet* 1995; 345: 200–1.
38. Patrizio P, Zielenski J. Congenital absence of the vas deferens: A mild form of cystic fibrosis. *Mol Med Today* 1996; 1: 24–31.
39. Lissens W, Liebaers I, Van Steirteghem A. Male infertility. In: *Emery and Rimoin's Principles and Practice of Medical Genetics*. Rimoin DL, Connor JM, Pyeritz RE, Korf BC (eds). Philadelphia, PA: Elsevier, 2007, pp. 856–74.

40. Aslanidis C, Jansen G, Amemiya C et al. Cloning of the essential myotonic dystrophy region and mapping of the putative defect. *Nature* 1992; 355: 548–51.
41. Brook DJ, McCurrach ME, Harley HG et al. Molecular basis of myotonic dystrophy: Expansion of a trinucleotide (CTG) repeat at the 3′ end of a transcript encoding a protein kinase family member. *Cell* 1992; 68: 799–808.
42. Fu HY, Pizzuti A, Fenwick RG et al. An unstable triplet repeat in a gene related to myotonic muscular dystrophy. *Science* 1992; 255: 1256–8.
43. Mahadevan M, Tsilfidis C, Sabourin L et al. Myotonic dystrophy mutation: An unstable CTG repeat in the 3′ untranslated region of the gene. *Science* 1992; 255: 1253–5.
44. Hunter A, Tsilfidis C, Mettler G et al. The correlation of age of onset with CTG trinucleotide repeat amplification in myotonic dystrophy. *J Med Genet* 1992; 29: 774–9.
45. Sermon K, De Vos A, Van de Velde H et al. Fluorescent PCR and automated fragment analysis for the clinical application of preimplantation genetic diagnosis of myotonic dystrophy (Steinert's disease). *Mol Hum Reprod* 1998; 4: 791–6.
46. Sermon K, Seneca S, De Rycke M et al. PGD in the lab for triplet repeat diseases—Myotonic dystrophy, Huntington's disease and fragile-X syndrome. *Mol Cell Endocrinol* 2001; 183(Suppl 1): S77–85.
47. Rugarli EI, Ballabio A. Kallmann syndrome. From genetics to neurobiology. *JAMA* 1993; 270: 2713–16.
48. Dodé C, Levilliers J, Dupont JM et al. Loss-of-function mutations in *FGFR1* cause autosomal dominant Kallmann syndrome. *Nat Genet* 2003; 33: 463–5.
49. Ayari B, Soussi-Yanicostas N. *FGFR1* and anosmin-1 underlying genetically distinct forms of Kallmann syndrome are co-expressed and interact in olfactory bulbs. *Dev Genes Evol* 2007; 217: 169–75.
50. Cadman SM, Kim SH, Hu Y et al. Molecular pathogenesis of Kallmann's syndrome. *Horm Res* 2007; 67: 231–42.
51. Dodé C, Teixeira L, Levilliers J et al. Kallmann syndrome: Mutations in the genes encoding prokineticin-2 and prokineticin receptor-2. *PLoS Genet* 2006; 2: 1648–52.
52. Falardeau J, Chung WC, Beenken A et al. Decreased FGF8 signaling causes deficiency of gonadotropinreleasing hormone in humans and mice. *J Clin Invest* 2008; 118: 2822–31.
53. Kim HG, Kurth I, Lan F et al. Mutations in *CHD7*, encoding a chromatin-remodeling protein, cause idiopathic hypogonadotropic hypogonadism and Kallmann syndrome. *Am J Hum Genet* 2008; 83: 511–9.
54. Kaplan JD, Bernstein JA, Kwan A et al. Clues to an early diagnosis of Kallmann syndrome. *Am J Med Genet* 2010; 152: 2796–801.
55. Pitteloud N, Quinton R, Pearce S et al. Digenic mutations account for variable phenotypes in idiopathic hypogonadotropic hypogonadism. *J Clin Invest* 2007; 117: 457–63.
56. Sykiotis GP, Plummer L, Hughes VA et al. Oligogenic basis of isolated gonadotropin-releasing hormone deficiency. *Proc Natl Acad Sci USA* 2010; 107: 15140–4.
57. Büchter D, Behre HM, Kliesh S, Nieschlag E. Pulsatile GnRH or human chorionic gonadotropin/human menopausal gonadotropin as effective treatment for men with hypogonatropic hypogonadism: A review of 42 cases. *Eur J Endocrinol* 1998; 139: 298–303.
58. Cardenas-Rodriguez M, Badano JL. Ciliary biology: Understanding the cellular and genetic basis of human ciliopathies. *Am J Med Genet* 2009; 151: 263–80.
59. Afzelius BA. Immotile cilia syndrome: Past, present, and prospects for the future. *Thorax* 1998; 53: 894–7.
60. Sutherland MJ, Ware SM. Disorders of left–right asymmetry: Heterotaxy and situs inversus. *Am J Med Genet* 2009; 151: 307–17.
61. Igarashi S, Tanno Y, Onodera O et al. Strong correlation between the number of CAG repeats in androgen receptor genes and the clinical onset features of spinal and bulbar atrophy. *Neurology* 1992; 42: 2300–2.
62. Finsterer J. Perspectives of Kennedy's disease. *J Neurol Sci* 2010; 298: 1–10.
63. Quigley CA, De Bellis A, Marschke KB et al. Androgen receptor defects: Historical, clinical and molecular perspectives. *Endocr Rev* 1995; 16: 271–321.
64. Wisniewski AB, Mazur T. 46,XY DSD with female or ambiguous external genitalia at birth due to androgen insensitivity syndrome, 5α-reductase-2 deficiency, or 17-hydroxysteroid dehydrogenase deficiency: A review of quality of life outcomes. *Int J Pediatr Endocrinol* 2009; 2009: 567430.
65. Sinnecker GH, Hiort O, Dibbelt L et al. Phenotypic classification of male pseudo hermaphroditism due to steroid 5α-reductase 2 deficiency. *Am J Med Genet* 1996; 63: 223–30.
66. Chong CK. Practical approach to steroid 5alphareductase type 2 deficiency. *Eur J Pediatr* 2011; 170: 1–8.
67. Romano A, Allanson J, Dahlgren J et al. Noonan syndrome: Clinical features, diagnosis and management guidelines. *Pediatrics* 2010; 126: 746–59.
68. Tartaglia M, Mehler EL, Goldberg R et al. Mutations in *PTPN11*, encoding the protein tyrosine phosphatase SHP-2, cause Noonan syndrome. *Nat Genet* 2001; 29: 465–8.
69. Meschede D, Rolf C, Neugebauer DC et al. Sperm acrosome defects in a patient with Aarskog–Scott syndrome. *Am J Med Genet* 1996; 66: 340–2.

70. Orrico A, Galli L, Faivre L et al. Aarskog–Scott syndrome: Clinical update and report of nine novel mutations in the *FGD1* gene. *Am J Med Genet* 2010; 152: 313–18.
71. Choufani S, Shuman C, Weksberg R. Beckwith–Wiedemann syndrome. *Am J Med Genet* 2010; 154C: 343–54.
72. Beales PL, Elcioglu N, Woolf AS et al. New criteria for improved diagnosis of Bardet–Biedl syndrome: Results of a population survey. *J Med Genet* 1999; 36: 437–46.
73. Cassidy SB. Prader–Willi syndrome. *J Med Genet* 1997; 34: 917–23.
74. Baker K, Beales PL. Making sense of cilia in disease: The human ciliopathies. *Am J Med Genet* 2009; 151C: 281–95.
75. Horsthemke B, Dittrich B, Buiting K et al. Imprinting mutations on human chromosome 15. *Hum Mutat* 1997; 10: 329–37.
76. Feil R, Khosla S. Genomic imprinting in mammals. *Trends Genet* 1999; 15: 431–5.
77. Vogels A, Moerman P, Frijns JP, Bogaert GA. Testicular histology in boys with Prader–Willi syndrome: Fertile or infertile? *J Urol* 2008; 180: 1800–4.
78. Weiss J, Axelrod L, Whitcomb RW et al. Hypogonadism caused by a single amino acid substitution in the beta subunit of luteinizing hormone. *N Engl J Med* 1992; 326: 179–83.
79. Latronico AC, Segaloff DL. Naturally occurring mutations of the luteinizing-hormone receptor: Lessons learned about reproductive physiology and G protein-coupled receptors. *Am J Hum Genet* 1999; 65: 949–58.
80. Rajender S, Rahul P, Mahdi AA. Mitochondria, spermatogenesis and male infertility. *Mitochondrion* 2010; 10: 419–28.
81. Dam AH, Feenstra I, Westphal JR et al. Globozoospermia revisited. *Hum Reprod Update* 2007; 13: 63–75.
82. Dam AH, Koscinski I, Kremer JA et al. Homozygous mutation in *SPATA16* is associated with male infertility in human globozoospermia. *Am J Hum Genet* 2007: 813–20.
83. Liu G, Shi QW, Lu GX. A newly discovered mutation in *PICK1* in a human with globozoospermia. *Asian J Androl* 2010; 12: 556–60.
84. Harbuz R, Zouari R, Pierre V et al. Recurrent deletion of *DPY19L2* causes infertility in man by blocking sperm head elongation and acrosome formation. *Am J Hum Genet* 2011; 88: 351–61.
85. Koscinski I, Ellnati E, Fossard C et al. *DPY19L2* deletion as a major cause of globozoospermia. *Am J Hum Genet* 2011; 88: 344–50.
86. Coutton C, Escoffier J, Martinez G et al. Teratozoospermia: Spotlight on the main genetic actors in the human. *Hum Reprod Update* 2015; 21: 455–85.
87. Dieterich K, Soto Rifo R, Faure AK et al. Homozygous mutation of *AURKC* yields large-headed polyploid spermatozoa and causes male infertility. *Nat Genet* 2007; 39: 661–5.
88. Ben Khelifa M, Zouari R, Harbuz R et al. Identification of a new recurrent aurora kinase C mutation in both European and African men with macrozoospermia. *Mol Hum Reprod* 2011; 17: 762–8.
89. Stouffs K, Lissens W, Tournaye H et al. The choice and outcome of the fertility treatment of 38 couples in whom the male partner has a Yq microdeletion. *Hum Reprod* 2005; 20: 1887–96.
90. Dequeker E, Stuhrmann M, Morris MA et al. Best practice guidelines for molecular genetic diagnosis of cystic fibrosis and CFTR-related disorders—Updated European recommendations. *Eur J Hum Genet* 2009; 17: 51–65.
91. World Health Organisation. *The molecular genetic epidemiology of cystic fibrosis. Report of a joint meeting of WHO/ECFTN/ICF(M)A/ECFS*, 2004. Available from: www.who.int/genomics/publications/en/
92. Goossens V, Sermon K, Lissens W et al. Clinical application of preimplantation genetic diagnosis for cystic fibrosis. *Prenat Diagn* 2000; 20: 571–81.
93. Dreesen JC, Jacobs LJ, Bras M et al. Multiplex PCR of polymorphic markers flanking the *CFTR* gene; a general approach for preimplantation genetic diagnosis of cystic fibrosis. *Mol Hum Reprod* 2000; 6: 391–6.
94. Braude P, Pickering S, Flinter F, Ogilvie CM. Preimplantation genetic diagnosis. *Nat Rev Genet* 2002; 3: 941–53.
95. Sermon K, Van Steirteghem A, Liebaers I. Preimplantation genetic diagnosis. *Lancet* 2004; 363: 1633–41.
96. Geraedts JP, De Wert GM. Preimplantation genetic diagnosis. *Clin Genet* 2009; 76: 315–25.
97. Harper JC, Sengupta SB. Preimplantation genetic diagnosis: State of the ART 2011. *Hum Genet* 2011; 131: 175–86.
98. Simpson JL. Preimplantation genetic diagnosis at 20 years. *Prenat Diagn* 2010; 30: 682–95.
99. Handyside AH. Preimplantion genetic diagnosis after 20 years. *Reprod Biomed Online* 2010; 21: 280–2.
100. Handyside AH, Kontogianni EH, Hardy K et al. Pregnancies from biopsied human preimplantation embryos sexed by Y-specific DNA amplification. *Nature* 1990; 344: 768–70.
101. Harper JC, Coonen E, De Rycke M et al. ESHRE PGD Consortium data collection X: Cycles from January to December 2007 with pregnancy follow-up to October 2008. *Hum Reprod* 2010; 25: 2685–707.
102. Bonduelle M, Liebaers I, Deketelaere V et al. Neonatal data on a cohort of 2889 infants born after intracytoplasmic sperm injection (ICSI) (1991–1999) and of 2995 infants born after *in vitro* fertilization (IVF) (1983–1999). *Hum Reprod* 2002; 17: 671–94.

103. Bonduelle M, Van Assche E, Joris H et al. Prenatal testing in ICSI pregnancies: Incidence of chromosomal anomalies in 1586 karyotypes and relation to sperm parameters. *Hum Reprod* 2002; 17: 2600–14.
104. Bonduelle M, Ponjaert I, Van Steirteghem A et al. Developmental outcome of children born after ICSI compared to children born after IVF at the age of two years. *Hum Reprod* 2003; 19: 1–9.
105. Leunens L, Celestin-Westreich S, Bonduelle M, Liebaers I, Ponjaert-Kristoffersen I. Cognitive and motor development of 8-year-old children born after ICSI compared to spontaneously conceived children. *Hum Reprod* 2006; 21: 2922–9.
106. Sutcliffe AG, Ludwig M. Outcome of assisted reproduction. *Lancet* 2007; 370: 351–9.
107. Belva F, De Schrijver F, Tournaye H et al. Neonatal outcome of 724 children born after ICSI using non-ejaculated sperm. *Hum Reprod* 2011; 1752–8.
108. De Schepper J, Belva F, Schiettecatte J et al. Testicular growth and tubular function in prepubertal boys conceived by intracytoplasmic sperm injection. *Horm Res* 2009; 71: 359–63.
109. Woldringh GH, Besselink DE, Tillema AJ et al. Karyotyping, congenital anomalies and follow-up of children after intracytoplamic sperm injection with non-ejaculated sperm: A systemic review. *Hum Reprod Update* 2010; 16: 12–19.
110. Martin RH. Genetics of human sperm. *J Assist Reprod Genet* 1998; 15: 240–455.
111. Aran B, Blanco J, Vidal F et al. Screening for abnormalities of chromosomes X, Y, and 18 and for diploidy in spermatozoa from infertile men participating in an *in vitro* fertilization-intracytoplasmic sperm injection program. *Fertil Steril* 1999; 72: 696–701.
112. Vegetti W, Van Assche E, Frias A et al. Correlation between semen parameters and sperm aneuploidy rates investigated by fluorescence *in-situ* hybridization in infertile men. *Hum Reprod* 2000; 15: 351–65.
113. Egozcue S, Blanco J, Vendrell JM et al. Human male infertility: Chromosome anomalies, meiotic disorders, abnormal spermatozoa and recurrent abortion. *Hum Reprod Update* 2000; 6: 93–105.
114. Osmanagaoglu K, Tournaye H, Camus M et al. Cumulative delivery rates after intracytoplasmic sperm injection: 5 year follow-up of 498 patients. *Hum Reprod* 1999; 14: 2651–5.
115. Vernaeve V, Verheyen G, Goossens A et al. How successful is repeat testicular sperm extraction in patients with azoospermia? *Hum Reprod* 2006; 21: 1551–4.
116. Krausz C, Hoefsloot L, Simoni M et al. EAA/EMQN best practice guidelines form molecular diagnosis of Y-chromosomal microdeletions: State-of-the-art 2013. *Andrology* 2014; 2: 5–19.
117. Foresta C, Ferlin A, Gianaroli L, Dallapiccola B. Guidelines for the appropriate use of genetic tests in infertile couples. *Eur J Hum Genet* 2002: 303–12.
118. Meschede D, Lemcke B, Exeler JR et al. Chromosome abnormalities in 477 couples undergoing intracytoplasmic sperm injection-prevalence, types, sex distribution and reproductive relevance. *Hum Reprod* 1998; 13: 576–82.
119. van der Ven K, Peschka B, Montag M et al. Increased frequency of congenital chromosomal aberrations in female partners of couples undergoing intracytoplasmic sperm injection. *Hum Reprod* 1998; 13: 48–54.
120. Papanikolaou EG, Vernaeve V, Kolibianakis E et al. Is chromosome analysis mandatory in the initial investigation of normovulatory women seeking infertility treatment? *Hum Reprod* 2005; 20: 2899–903.
121. Riccaboni A, Lalatta F, Caliari I et al. Genetic screening in 2,710 infertile candidate couples for assisted reproductive techniques: Results of application of Italian guidelines for the appropriate use of genetic tests. *Fertil Steril* 2008; 89: 800–8.
122. Vallance H, Ford J. Carrier testing for autosomal recessive disorders. *Crit Rev Clin Lab Sci* 2003; 40: 473–97.
123. Kaback MM. Population-based genetic screening for reproductive counseling: The Tay–Sachs disease model. *Eur J Pediatr* 2000; 159(Suppl 3): 192–5.
124. Gason AA, Sheffield E, Bankier A et al. Evaluation of a Tay–Sachs disease screening program. *Clin Genet* 2003; 63: 386–92.
125. Liebaers I, Bonduelle M, Van Assche E et al. How far should we go with genetic screening in assisted reproduction? In: *Fertility and Reproductive Medicine. Proceedings of the XVI World Congress on Fertility and Sterility. San Francisco*. Kempers RD, Cohen J, Haney AF (eds). Amsterdam, The Netherlands: Elsevier Science BV, 1998; pp. 247–254.
126. Verlinsky Y, Cieslak J, Ivakhnenko V et al. Prevention of age-related aneuploidies by polar body testing of oocytes. *J Assist Reprod Genet* 1999; 16: 165–9.
127. Munné S, Magli C, Cohen J et al. Positive outcome after preimplantation diagnosis of aneuploidy in human embryos. *Hum Reprod* 1999; 14: 2191–9.
128. Gianaroli L, Magli MC, Ferraretti AP et al. Preimplantation diagnosis for aneuploidies in patients undergoing *in vitro* fertilization with a poor prognosis: Identification of the categories for what should be proposed. *Fertil Steril* 1999; 72: 837–44.
129. Staessen C, Platteau P, Van Assche E et al. Comparison of blastocyst transfer with or without preimplantation genetic diagnosis for aneuploidy screening in couples with advanced maternal age: A prospective randomized controlled trial. *Hum Reprod* 2004; 19: 2849–58.
130. Mastenbroek S, Twisk M, van Echten-Arends J et al. *In vitro* fertilization with preimplantation genetic screening. *N Engl J Med* 2007; 357: 9–17.
131. Geraedts J, Collins J, Gianarolli L et al. What next for preimplantation genetic screening? A polar body approach! *Hum Reprod* 2010; 25: 575–7.

132. Harper J, Coonen E, De Rycke M et al. What next for preimplantation genetic screening (PGS)? A position statement from the ESHRE PGD Consortium steering committee. *Hum Reprod* 2010; 25: 821–3.
133. Harper J, Harton G. The use of arrays in preimplantation genetic diagnosis and screening. *Fertil Steril* 2010; 94: 1173–7.
134. Geraedts J, Montag M, Magli MC et al. Polar body array CGH for prediction of the status of the corresponding oocyte. Part 1: Clinical results. *Hum Reprod* 2011; 26: 3173–80.
135. Magli MC, Montag M, Köster M et al. Polar body array CGH for prediction of the status of the corresponding oocyte. Part 2: Technical aspects. *Hum Reprod* 2011; 26: 3181–5.
136. De Rycke M, Liebaers I, Van Steirteghem A. Epigenetic risks related to assisted reproductive technologies. Risk analysis and epigenetic inheritance. *Hum Reprod* 2002; 17: 2487–94.
137. Cox GF, Burger J, Lip V et al. Intracytoplasmic sperm injection may increase the risk of imprinting defects. *Am J Hum Genet* 2002; 71: 162–4.
138. Debaun MR, Niemitz EL, Feinberg AP. Association of *in vitro* fertilization with Beckwith–Wiedemann syndrome and epigenetic alterations of *LIT1* and *H19*. *Am J Hum Genet* 2003; 72: 156–60.
139. Maher ER, Brueton LA, Bowdin SC et al. Beckwith–Wiedemann syndrome and assisted reproduction technology (ART). *J Med Genet* 2003; 40: 62–4.
140. Moll AC, Imhof SM, Cruysberg JRM et al. Incidence of retinoblastoma in children born after *in-vitro* fertilisation. *Lancet* 2003; 361: 309–10.
141. Diaz-Garcia C, Estella C, Perales-Puchalt A et al. Reproductive medicine and inheritance of infertility by offspring: The role of fetal programming. *Fertil Steril* 2011; 96: 536–45.
142. Weksberg R, Shuman C, Wilkins-Haug L et al. Workshop report: Evaluation of genetic and epigenetic risks associated with assisted reproductive technologies and infertility. *Fertil Steril* 2007; 88: 27–31.
143. Ko K, Schöler HR. Embryonic stem cells as a potential source of gametes. *Semin Reprod Med* 2006; 24: 322–9.
144. Ehmcke J, Wistuba J, Schlatt S. Spermatogonial stem cells: Questions, models and perspectives. *Hum Reprod Update* 2006; 12: 275–82.
145. Kubota H, Brinster RL. Technology insight: *In vitro* culture of spermatogonial stem cells and their potential therapeutic uses. *Nat Clin Pract Endocrinol Metab* 2006; 2: 99–108.
146. Nagy ZP, Chang CC. Artificial gametes. *Theriogenology* 2007; 67: 99–104.
147. Wyns C, Curaba M, Vanabelle B et al. Options for fertility preservation in prepubertal boys. *Hum Reprod Update* 2010; 16: 312–28.

Polar body biopsy and its clinical application

26

MARKUS MONTAG

INTRODUCTION

Polar body (PB) biopsy with subsequent analysis of chromosomal abnormalities was introduced in 1990 by Verlinsky et al. (1). This technique brought about the era of pre-conception genetic diagnosis as an alternative to preimplantation genetic diagnosis (PGD) of the embryo, which was proposed earlier by Handyside et al. (2). It is important to note that PB diagnosis gives direct information about the first and second PB and therefore only allows an indirect diagnosis of the maternal genetic or chromosomal constitution of the corresponding oocyte. In contrast, PGD of the embryo gives a direct diagnosis for the embryo and allows the detection of both maternally and paternally derived genetic or chromosomal contributions.

Consequently, embryo biopsy at the six- to eight-cell stage on day 3 was widely used, especially for preimplantation genetic screening (PGS) (3). However, since 2007, numerous randomized controlled trials reported that PGS by blastomere biopsy does not result in increased success rates (4–14), and several organizations published statements in which they no longer recommend using biopsy at the blastomere stage, at least for PGS (15,16). Since then, the overall trend goes in two different directions: PB biopsy and blastocyst biopsy (17). Obviously, PB biopsy does have limitations for the diagnosis of genetic diseases. But in view of aneuploidy screening to detect numerical chromosomal disorders that predominantly arise during meiosis in the oocyte (18,19), PB biopsy is a viable alternative, especially if combined with new diagnostic methods like array comparative genomic hybridization (aCGH), quantitative polymerase chain reaction (qPCR), or next-generation sequencing (NGS) for detecting all chromosomes (20–22). The present article gives an overview on the expectations and limitations of PB diagnosis and relevant technical details, with special emphasis on aneuploidy screening.

CLINICAL APPLICATION OF PB DIAGNOSIS

PB biopsy has been successfully used for the detection of numerical and structural chromosomal abnormalities in human oocytes (23,24) and for the diagnosis of monogenetic diseases (25).

PB biopsy and detection of numerical chromosomal abnormalities: PGS

Numerical chromosomal abnormalities are characterized by a wrong distribution of chromosomes or chromatids in the first or second PBs. These errors are strongly correlated to maternal age (19). Up to 70% of oocytes from women beyond 40 years of age can possess such a disorder (26). This explains why women with advanced maternal age have a lower chance for pregnancy and a higher risk to miscarry once they are pregnant. One possibility to reduce these risks and probably to increase the success rates is a screening for maternally derived chromosomal abnormalities of the oocyte. This can be achieved by PB diagnosis.

During the first meiotic division, the diploid chromosome content of an oocyte is reduced to two haploid chromosome sets, which both consist of paired chromatids. One paired chromatid set is extruded as part of the first PB. Sperm entry into an oocyte initiates the second meiotic division, whereby the set of paired chromatids is separated and a single chromatid set becomes part of the second PB. After the first meiotic division, the number of the chromosomes in the oocyte and the first PB should be identical and the same holds true for the number of chromatids following the second meiotic division. Numerical chromosomal abnormalities can be caused by non-disjunction, meaning that a whole chromosome is not directed to the proper compartment (either the oocyte or PB). Another mechanism is premature chromatid segregation into two single, separated chromatids, which has been suggested to occur frequently prior to the first meiotic division (27) and has been confirmed by clinical data (19). Premature chromatid segregation during meiosis I can either lead to a balanced situation, where both chromatids remain in the same compartment, or to an unbalanced situation, where the two chromatids are finally allocated to different compartments. Some of the unbalanced segregations that originate in meiosis I in the oocyte can be corrected in meiosis II during formation of the second PB (28), and can even give rise to a normal child (21).

PB biopsy and subsequent analysis of the first and second PBs by fluorescence *in situ* hybridization (FISH) or aCGH offers the possibility to detect numerical chromosome aberrations and to establish an indirect diagnosis for the corresponding oocyte (29). Alterations in the copy number in the first and second PBs indicate a trisomy for the resulting embryo if one copy is missing in the PBs or a monosomy if one signal is found in excess. Distinction of copy numbers is easily detected in FISH and in aCGH following the introduction of single-channel analysis (see below). aCGH has the advantage that all chromosomes can be investigated at once, whereas FISH has its limitations as only five to six chromosomes can be used in one hybridization round (30) and the efficacy of hybridization is reduced with each additional round (31).

Table 26.1 Success rates of polar body biopsy and aneuploidy screening in the international literature

Reference	Biopsied cells	No. of chromosomes	No. of cycles	No. of embryos per transfer	Clinical pregnancy rate
Biopsy using zona drilling by acidic Tyrode's solution					
Verlinsky et al. (32)	PB I/I + II	3	45	3.1	21.7%
Dyban et al. (33)	PB I/I + II	3	161	2.6	14.8%
Verlinsky et al. (34)	PB I/I + II	3	235	2.5	16.0%
Verlinsky et al. (35)	PB I/I + II	3	598	2.6	21.4%
Verlinsky et al. (36)	PB I/I + II	3	659	2.1	22.3%
Verlinsky et al. (25)	PB I/I + II	3/5	821	2.5	22.2%
Kuliev et al. (23)	PB I/I + II	3/5	1297	2.35	21.9%[a]
Biopsy using a 1.48-μm diode laser					
Montag et al. (61)	PB I	5	50	1.9	30.9%
Montag et al. (75)	PB I	5/6	110	1.8	26.6%
van der Ven et al. (37)	PB I/I + II	5/6	170	1.7	23.3%[b]

[a] Abortion rate: 23.7%.
[b] Abortion rate: 14.3%.
Abbreviation: PB, polar body.

PB biopsy and FISH for PGS have been clinically used since the early 1990s and the clinical outcomes have been described in numerous publications (Table 26.1). PB biopsy and aCGH are used clinically (19,20,38,39) and the results are considered to be controversial (see Delhanty [40] and section "Challenges in PB biopsy").

PB biopsy and detection of structural chromosomal aberrations

Structural chromosomal aberrations (e.g., balanced translocations) were found at a higher rate among infertile couples compared to the normal population (41–43). During meiosis, the pairing of homolog chromosomes is disturbed by a structurally aberrant chromosome and this may result in a partial aneuploidy in the oocyte. The risk for the extent of abnormal gametes is dependent on the size of the chromosome region involved in the translocation.

Usually only 10%–20% of all oocytes from a translocation carrier are either balanced or normal. Provided that the female is a carrier of a balanced translocation, PB biopsy allows selecting against abnormal oocytes using a reliable method for the genetic analysis. In the past, this has been achieved by FISH probes that were designed for each individual patient and covered the chromosomal breakpoints (44). Later, another technique was presented based on the combined use of centromeric and telomeric probes for FISH analysis of the chromosomes involved in the translocation (23). Recently, structural chromosomal disorders were successfully investigated by whole-genome amplification and aCGH (39). This approach offers the advantage of a combined screening test for structural as well as numerical aberrations, which seems to be especially beneficial for translocation patients (45).

PB biopsy and detection of monogenetic aberrations

The detection of monogenetic disorders by PB biopsy requires that the DNA of interest (e.g., the region containing the mutation) from the first and second PBs is accurately amplified by PCR. In addition to the general risk of contamination of PCR reagents and products with foreign DNA with a potential resulting misdiagnosis, specific problems need to be addressed in the case of PB biopsy. A major problem in single-cell PCR is the correct amplification of the region of interest, and it is known from numerous reports that in diploid cells, occasionally one allele will not amplify, also known as allele dropout (ADO) (46–50). Whereas this phenomenon will not lead to a misdiagnosis in homozygous mutant or homozygous wild-type single cells, the situation is different in heterozygous single cells and especially in PB diagnosis. Recombination and crossing-over of homologous chromatids frequently occurs during meiosis. As a result, the first PB may consist of one chromatid carrying the mutation of interest and one chromatid carrying the wild-type or normal sequence. In this case, ADO may directly lead to a misdiagnosis if crossing-over and ADO remain undetected. Only in the case that analysis of the second PB, which carries either a mutant or a normal chromatid, reveals a discrepant result from the first PB would the problem be recognized. Although ADO seems to be a frequent phenomenon in preimplantation diagnosis (PID) (between 1% and 25% and up to 40%) (51), the frequency of ADO in PB diagnosis is mainly unknown due to the low number of cases. Verlinsky (52) reported a frequency of ADO of 6% in 100 PBs that were analyzed.

Several strategies have been proposed to overcome this diagnostic problem, mainly co-amplification of polymorphic markers that are closely linked to the region of interest or the improvement of amplification efficiency through the use of nested primers (53). The use of PCR conditions that allow for continuous quantification of the PCR product (e.g., with fluorescent primers) will help to determine ADO or cases of preferential amplification of alleles. Although ADO has for a long time been recognized to be a substantial problem in PGD and especially PB diagnosis, a systematic evaluation of this phenomenon, which might eventually lead to strategies to decrease ADO rates, has only recently been begun (51).

Because in PB diagnosis only the maternal contribution to a potential genetic disease can be investigated, the isolated application of this technique is limited to selected genetic scenarios, such as autosomal dominant diseases with an affected mother or X-linked recessive and dominant diseases where the mother is the mutation carrier. In view of the increasing use of blastocyst biopsy, the majority of cases with a genetic disease will be offered this approach, which also has the advantage that several trophectoderm cells are usually biopsied and thus the amplification is much more robust for a reliable genetic diagnosis.

PB BIOPSY TECHNIQUES

For PB biopsy, timing is a crucial point. The first PB degenerates with time, and doing a biopsy later than 10 hours after ICSI may already result in lower hybridization efficiency. The second PB is formed around two to four hours after ICSI, but as it is firmly attached to the oolemma with a cytoplasmic strand and spindle remnants up to six hours after ICSI (54), the optimal time for biopsy is at 8–16 hours after ICSI. Recent data show that for testing of the second PB in aCGH, the amplification efficiency of the isolated DNA is lower if the biopsy is done before eight hours after ICSI (55). Based on this, one may conclude that the optimal timing for sequential biopsy is 4–10 hours after ICSI for the first PB and 8–16 hours after ICSI for the second PB. For simultaneous biopsy of the first and second PBs, an optimal time window is at 8–10 hours after ICSI.

Removal of PBs requires access to the perivitelline space through the zona pellucida (Video 26.1). For PB biopsy, acidic Tyrode's solution as a chemical means (56) cannot be used as it has a negative impact on further development if applied at the oocyte stage. Another method based on three-dimensional zona dissection was proposed by Cieslak et al. (57). Although this method can be performed with simple glass tools, multiple steps including dissection, release, and rotation of the oocyte are needed, and the procedure definitely requires skill and time.

The use of 1.48-μm diode laser drilling for PB biopsy was proposed in 1997 (58). Animal experimentation showed the potential of this method for PB biopsy and for assisted hatching (59) and allowed us to investigate its proper mode of application (60). For example, the size and position of laser-drilled openings can influence further embryonic development and, in particular, the mode of hatching at the blastocyst stage (61). Due to its ease, laser-assisted biopsy is now widely used for biopsy of blastomeres (62,63) and blastocyst cells (64), and its advantages compared to acidic Tyrode's solution have been reported (65), although a recent publication reported an effect of laser PB biopsy on embryo quality (66), which highlights that proper handling and application are crucial.

For laser-assisted PB biopsy, the size of the drilled opening is usually in the range of 20 μm, but it can be easily adjusted to the diameter of the aspiration capillary (Figure 26.1). As the capillary can be introduced through the laser-drilled opening, there is no need for a sharp aspiration needle. This allows the use of flame-polished, blunt-ended aspiration needles and greatly reduces the risk of damaging the PB, the blastomere, or the remaining oocyte or embryo. The procedure becomes safer, more accurate, and more reliable, thus allowing us to significantly reduce the number of cells that cannot be reliably diagnosed as a result of technical problems during the biopsy procedure (67). The performance of laser-assisted PB biopsy is shown in Table 26.2.

Another benefit is that laser drilling and subsequent biopsy can be performed without changing the culture dish or the capillaries in contrast to zona drilling using acidic Tyrode's solution. This may help to prevent contamination of samples to be diagnosed by sensitive techniques such as PCR.

The simultaneous removal of the first and second PBs is best accomplished if the oocyte is affixed to the holding capillary with the first PB at the 12 o'clock position and the second PB to the right of the first one but in the same focal plane. An opening is drilled at 2–3 o'clock and, by shoving the biopsy capillary into the perivitelline space, both PBs can be removed simultaneously, provided that the cytoplasmic bridge between the second PB and the oocyte is not too firm (Figure 26.1).

In all manipulation steps and zona opening techniques, it is important to drill only one opening, as two openings (e.g., to retrieve both PBs through separate openings) may cause problems at the time of hatching because the embryo could hatch through both openings simultaneously and therefore may get trapped within the zona (60). Another important point is to generate a sufficient opening, which allows consecutive hatching at the blastocyst stage, because smaller openings (<15 μm) may also cause trapping of the embryo followed by degeneration (60). Laser-drilled openings will stay permanently in the zona, and therefore gentle handling during subsequent transfer of oocytes to other media droplets and even during embryo transfer is recommend.

A position paper with relevant best practice guidelines for PB biopsy for PGD/PGS has been published by the European Society of Human Reproduction and Embryology (ESHRE) (68).

TRANSFER OF PBS FOR ANEUPLOIDY SCREENING BY FISH

Once both PBs are biopsied, the first and second PBs of an oocyte are placed together in a neighboring droplet of medium until all oocytes are biopsied. A special pretreatment of PBs like hypo-osmotic swelling or proteinase/pronase treatment is not necessary due to the small cytoplasmic content of PBs. For transfer onto the glass slide,

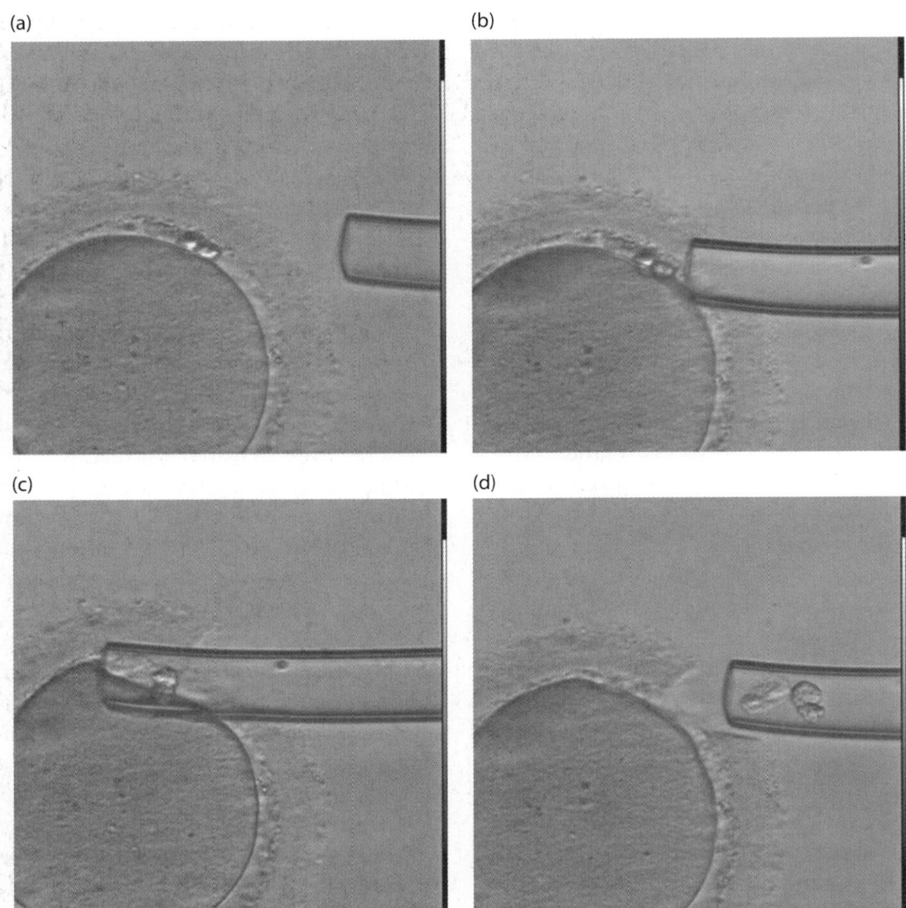

Figure 26.1 Simultaneous biopsy of the first and second polar bodies. For removal of the first and second polar bodies, the oocyte is held in a position where the polar bodies are located at 12 o'clock (a). An opening is drilled at 1–2 o'clock (b), which allows us to retrieve both polar bodies by sliding the capillary over them (c). If the second polar body is still firmly fixed to the oolemma, the capillary with the second polar body already inside is slowly forced towards the left in order to rupture the cytoplasmic bridge. Note the sharp border of the laser-drilled opening (d).

Table 26.2 Efficacy of laser-assisted polar body biopsy

Parameter	Value
Treatment cycles with polar body biopsy	174
No. of oocytes with biopsy	1245
No. of oocytes degenerated due to biopsy	5 (0.4%)
No. of polar bodies lost during biopsy/ transfer	20 (1.6%)
No. of polar bodies without hybridization signals	27 (2.2%)
No. of oocytes with fluorescence *in situ* hybridization results	1193 (95.8%)

the first and second PBs of one oocyte are removed from the medium drop and transferred with the biopsy capillary into a tiny drop (0.2 μL) of water placed on a clean glass slide (Figure 26.2). It is important to release the PBs at the bottom of the slide and to avoid floating in the droplet. The small volume guarantees that the PBs will attach to the slide within a small area and that the fluid will dry out very fast, which reduces the risk of a dislocation of the PBs on the slide. Nevertheless, the drying process must be observed under a stereomicroscope and the final location of the PBs after air-drying must be marked on top of the slide by encircling it with a suitable marker (diamond marker or tungsten pen). It is not absolutely required to distinguish the first and second PBs at that stage, as this becomes obvious during FISH analysis. With some experience, the first and second PBs from up to 12 oocytes can be placed within a round area of 10 mm, with each PB pair encircled using a marker. Fixation is performed with two to three drops of 10 μL methanol:acetic acid (3:1, ice-cold, –20°C) followed by a second fixation after air-drying using methanol at room temperature for 5 minutes. Once the slides are air-dried, 2.5 μL of hybridization solution is placed onto a 12-mm round cover slip, which is then inverted onto the area where the PBs are located. The cover slip should be sealed with rubber cement and additionally covered with a stretch of parafilm, which facilitates later removal of the cover slip after hybridization. The slide is then placed into a hybridization oven, where co-denaturation of the probe

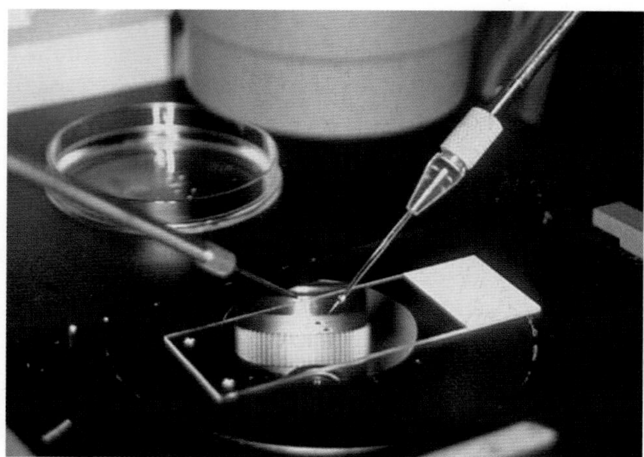

Figure 26.2 Transfer of isolated polar bodies onto a slide. The transfer of isolated polar bodies from the dish (seen in the background) into the droplet on the slide must be performed on the microscope stage. The setup shown here allows sliding of the dish used for biopsy backwards. Therefore, the aspiration capillary only needs to be lowered into the droplet for release of the polar body.

and the DNA of the PB occur at a temperature suitable for the probes used (usually around 68°C–73°C for up to 10 minutes). Hybridization is usually performed at 37°C. Centromeric probes require only 20–30 minutes of hybridization, whereas locus-specific probes require longer times. Commercially available multiprobe kits are usually hybridized for four to eight hours, followed by two rapid washing steps (73°C, 0.7 × sodium saline citrate [SSC] and 0.3% NP-40 for 7 minutes followed by 2 × SSC and 0.1% nonidet P-40 [NP-40] for 1 minute), which should be carried out exactly as described by the manufacturer. Following washing, a cover slip and antifade mounting media must be applied to the slide, which should then be stored immediately in the dark until FISH analysis.

FISH ANALYSIS AND INTERPRETATION OF RESULTS

Prior to analysis of the FISH results, the PBs located on the glass slide must be allocated under the microscope. This is rather easy if a circle is made around the area of PB deposition on top of the slide. The use of a 10× phase contrast objective usually allows for identification of the encircled area, and even the PBs can be identified in most cases (Figure 26.3). For FISH analysis, a 100× oil immersion objective with good transmission properties for the necessary wavelengths must be used. In the fluorescence-viewing mode, the right focal plane can be easily adjusted by focusing the diamond line followed by searching for the PBs within the encircled area. Once the PBs are allocated, it is recommended to view the different chromosome signals in the order that is proposed by the manufacturer of the kit, as certain fluorophores will fade more quickly compared to others.

Each chromosome should give two signals in the first PB and one signal in the second. An example of a first PB with a correct number of signals for chromosomes 13, 16, 18, 21, and 22 is shown (Figure 26.4), where chromosomes

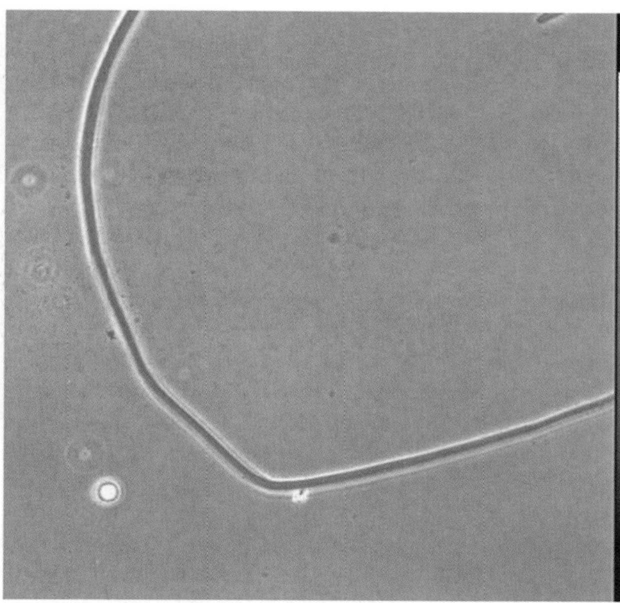

Figure 26.3 Identification of the polar body on the slide. This photograph is taken with a 10× phase contrast objective and the encircled area surrounding the polar body can be partially seen. The polar body appears gray-shaded and is marked by an arrow.

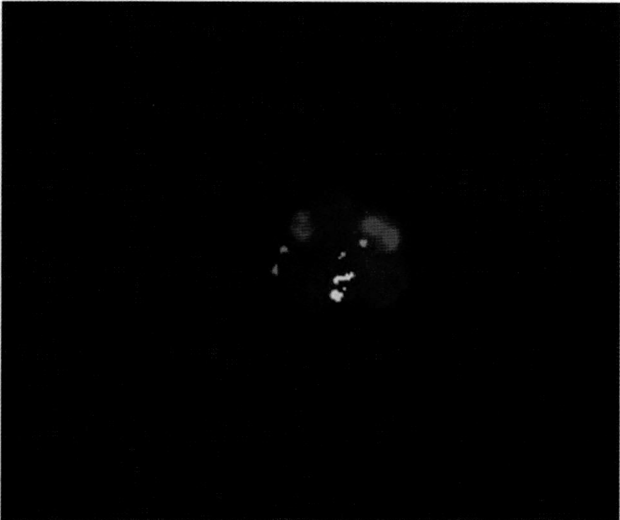

Figure 26.4 First polar body with correct signals for chromosomes 13, 16, 18, 21, and 22. This polar body shows two signals for each of the chromosomes under investigation. This picture is a composite overlay, where initially each chromosome probe was assembled as black and white using the appropriate filter set and, prior to overlay, signals were colored using a software program (chromosome 13: red, chromosomes 16 + 18: blue, chromosome 21: green, chromosome 22: yellow). The signals for chromosomes 16 and 18 are taken by a dual band pass filter set and therefore cannot be labeled with different colors. This mode of presentation also applies for the subsequent figures in terms of color.

16 and 18 are detected by centromere-specific probes and chromosomes 13, 21, and 22 are detected by locus-specific probes. It can be seen that the signals for chromosomes 16 and 18 can be clearly distinguished, despite the centromeric location of the probe. This is due to an early onset of chromatid separation within the first PB, which seems to start soon after oocyte retrieval, probably due to *in vitro* culture (69). In contrast, locus-specific probes will usually give good signals that are easy to evaluate, as the loci are located on the arms of the chromosome.

As mentioned earlier, most signals in the first PB are split signals due to premature chromatin segregation and, as demonstrated by several studies, unbalanced pre-division of chromatids is the most common origin of aneuploidy (27). The example in Figure 26.5 depicts a first PB where only the two signals for the two chromatids 18 are located side by side, whereas chromosomes 13, 16, 22, and X show a balanced pre-division and chromosome 21 shows an unbalanced pre-division with only one signal in the PB. The corresponding oocyte contains one additional chromatid 21 and therefore can develop trisomy 21.

A frequent problem in analysis of the first PB is the degeneration of chromatin, which may lead to speckled signals. This is most frequently observed for chromosomes 13 and 22. A diagnosis of aneuploidies or malsegregation is still possible, provided that the speckled regions are well separated from each other due to pre-division. Another problem is the high degree of fragmentation observed in first PBs (Figure 26.6). Obviously, all fragments can contain chromatin material and therefore it is obligatory to remove all fragments. In such a case, the drying process on the slide must be watched very carefully. If only one fragment is overlooked during FISH analysis, one may easily risk a misdiagnosis if one of the chromosomes under investigation is located in the missing fragment.

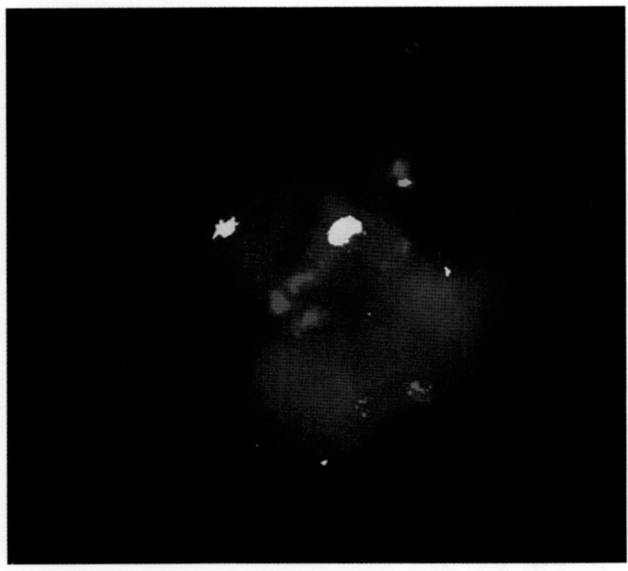

Figure 26.5 Chromosome segregation and trisomy 21. This polar body displays several common features, which can be observed during evaluation of fluorescence signals. Firstly, only signals for chromosome 18 are located side by side (blue dotted signals on the left), whereas all other chromosomes underwent pre-division of chromatids. Only one signal is present for chromosome 21 (green), which indicates that one additional chromatid 21 is present in the oocyte, and the embryo can develop trisomy 21 (chromosome 13: red, chromosome 16 + 18: blue, chromosome 21: green, chromosome 22: yellow—small dots, X chromosome: yellow—large dots).

Finally, PBs that are very advanced in the process of degeneration possess weak membranes that are likely to rupture during the fixation process. However, the chromatin will usually still affix to the glass slide after drying of the transfer droplet, although the signal will be spread and look like an elongated strand or bundle of DNA. Therefore, FISH analysis is still possible, but the signals will be scattered all over the encircled area, making interpretation of the results rather difficult.

TRANSFER OF PBS FOR ANEUPLOIDY SCREENING BY ACGH, QPCR, AND NGS

For aCGH, qPCR, and NGS, the first and second PBs must be transferred separately into individual PCR reaction tubes. This step should be performed in a laminar flow cabinet in order to avoid any contamination of the sample. Transfer can be easily accomplished by a 0.1–2.5-μL micropipette or by a stripping pipette used for oocyte denudation. Taking the PB into the pipette tip must be done under visual control using a stereomicroscope. Release of the PB in the PCR tube is best accomplished if the tube is prefilled with phosphate-buffered saline (PBS), the amount of which depends on the requirements of the subsequent amplification protocol. A usual protocol is 2.5 μL of PBS and, in this case, the tube should be pre-filled with 2.2 μL of PBS, and the transfer of a single PB is done in 0.3 μL of medium. After this, transfer tubes must be kept or stored in an upright position until amplification. Whole-genome amplification, labeling of amplified DNA, hybridization, and subsequent washing are usually performed according to the instructions provided by the manufacturer.

The standard procedure for aCGH is the labeling of the sample (PB) DNA by Cy3 and the labeling of male reference DNA with Cy5. Both labeled DNAs are then combined and co-hybridized on an array. For evaluation, the ratio of Cy3 versus Cy5 from that array is calculated by specific software. An example of such an analysis is shown in Figure 26.7a. Another recent approach uses a different strategy by which two samples (e.g., the first PB labeled with Cy3 and the second PB labeled with Cy5) are co-hybridized on one array and male and female reference DNAs labeled in Cy3/Cy5 and Cy5/Cy3 are co-hybridized as a dye-swap setup on two control arrays. The software hence calculates the Cy3 signal compared to both Cy5 from the male control array as well as to Cy5 from the female control array, which gives a much better resolution and supports a highly accurate analysis (Figure 26.7b and 26.7c).

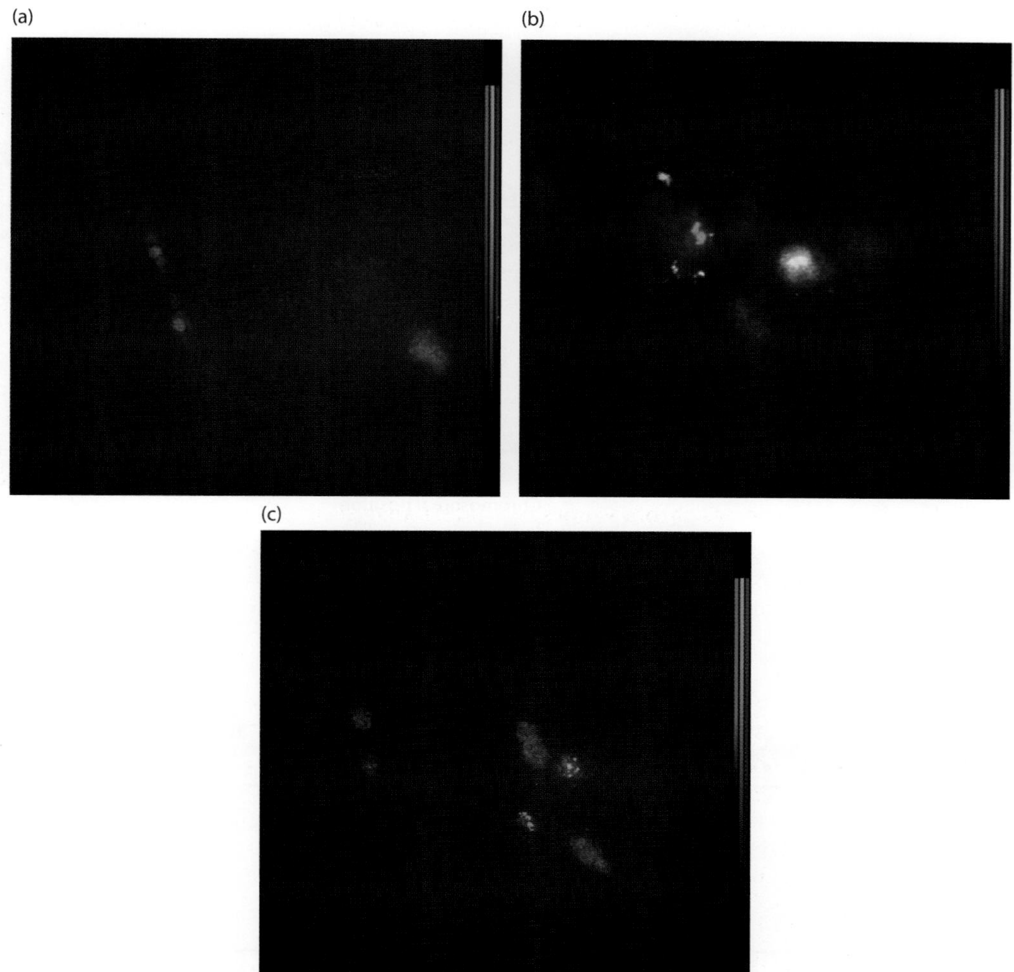

Figure 26.6 Fluorescence *in situ* hybridization analysis of a fragmented polar body. This example shows a highly fragmented polar body, where the fragments were located on the slide within a large area and consequently not all fragments could be viewed within one field. Following pre-division, both chromatids 18 (blue) are present in separated fragments (a). Two neighboring signals can be found for chromosomes 21 (green), 22 (yellow), and X (bright yellow—very close), but only one signal can be found for chromosome 16 (blue) (b). Chromosome 13 (red) is again located in two different fragments (c).

CHALLENGES OF PB BIOPSY AND DIAGNOSIS IN VIEW OF RECENT ADVANCEMENTS

There are certain pitfalls regarding PB biopsy and subsequent diagnosis of all chromosomes. As both PBs must be analyzed separately and as not all oocytes develop into a viable embryo, costs are more than double those of a day-5 diagnostic approach. Another challenge is the discussion of the correlation of aneuploidy results based on PB analysis. Some studies reported a high correlation for aneuploidy prediction based on PB analysis (49,70), whereas other studies question the accuracy of PB diagnosis due to the high incidence of post-zygotic errors (71,72). Reciprocal chromosome aneuploidies in the first and second PBs were considered to be problematic, but a recent study showed that this situation gives rise to normal euploid embryos (73), and the birth of a healthy child has been reported from an oocyte with reciprocal aneuploid PBs (21).

CONCLUSIONS

The pioneering work in PB diagnosis was performed by Yuri Verlinsky and Santiago Munné, and efficient biopsy techniques were elaborated by Cieslak et al. (57) and Montag et al. (58,59). This has led to a variety of (genetic and chromosomal) diagnostic applications following PB biopsy. Most cases of PB diagnosis have been performed for PGS using FISH analysis. More recently, PB biopsy followed by aCGH has been introduced for PGS (17,20,32,33,49), and the feasibility of this approach for a reliable diagnosis has been proven in a concordance analysis (20,49). Prospective randomized controlled trials to prove the benefits of PB diagnosis for aneuploidy screening in terms of higher pregnancy and birth rates are ongoing.

The cost-effectiveness of PB biopsy and analysis of all chromosomes for PGS is still a matter of debate. In addition, the controversial discussion on the relevance of aneuploidy results from PB analysis compared to those from trophectoderm

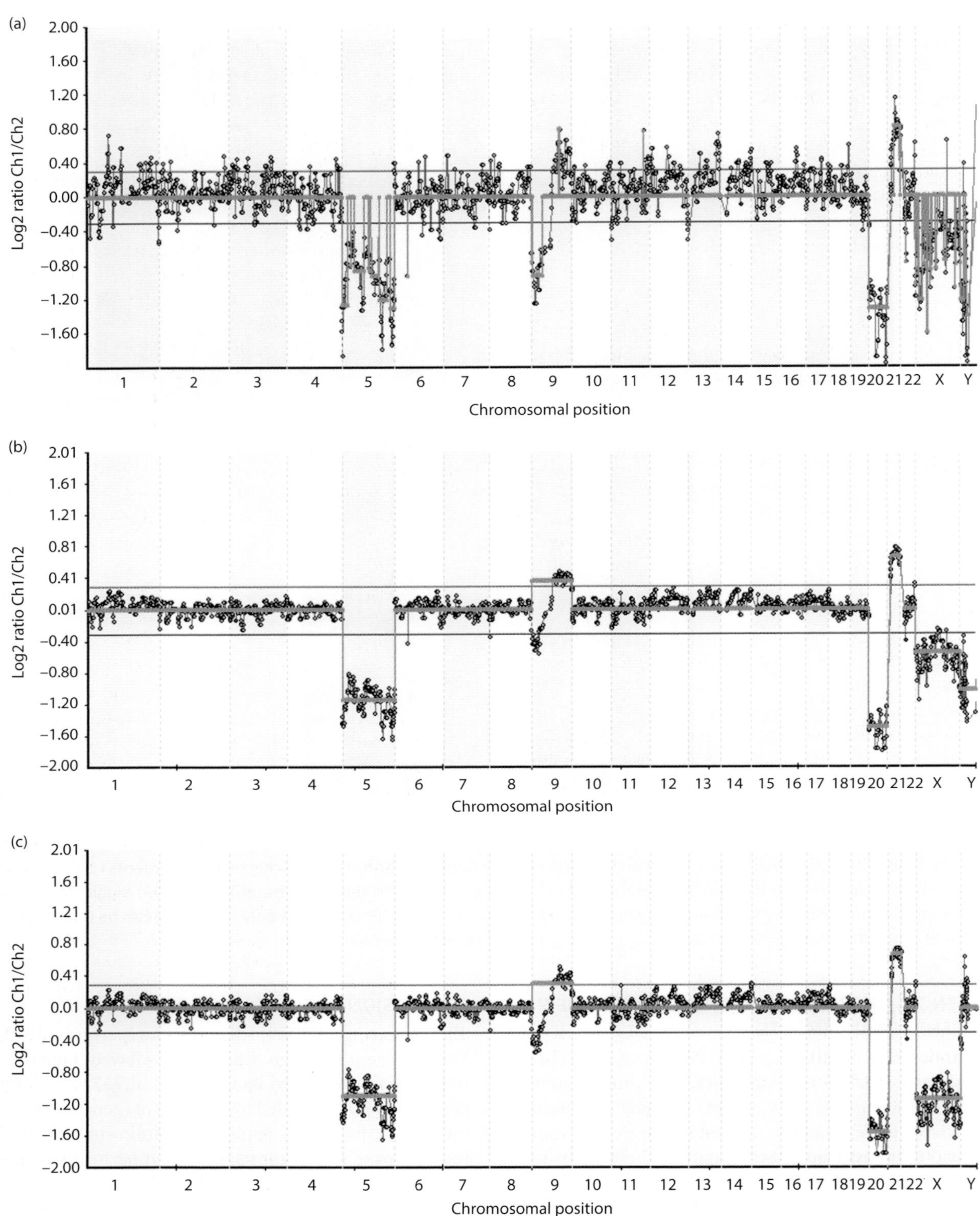

Figure 26.7 Array comparative genomic hybridization (aCGH) of polar bodies: conventional versus single-channel CGH. A standard evaluation of an aCGH experiment with first polar body DNA labeled with Cy3 and co-hybridized with male reference DNA labeled with Cy5. The ratio of Cy3 to Cy5 from the array is shown (a). Signals for chromosomes 5, 20, 21, 9p, and 9q are out of the mean ratio and indicate a loss or gain of chromosomes or chromatids. The same sample DNA was used in a single-channel experiment and the ratio of the first polar body DNA deviations were calculated with male (b) or female control DNA (c). The comparison shows that the single-channel experiment gives highly reduced background noise and that the quoting of the gonosomal aneuploidies becomes much easier.

biopsy reflects the limitations of this technology and underlines that the procedure itself must be continuously evaluated. Consequently, the use of PB diagnosis and aneuploidy screening should be primarily offered to patients at a high risk for maternal chromosomal aberrations and patients who are more likely to benefit from this therapy (74). The relevant data should be published continuously in order to enable an evaluation of this technique in view of evidence-based medicine. Finally, we may conclude that the use of a non-contact laser for PB biopsy is a safe and efficient approach (49,75).

VIDEOS

Video 26.1 Laser-assisted polar body biopsy: opening of the zona pellucida and removal of the first and second polar bodies. https://youtu.be/5sDc2XeEw6M

REFERENCES

1. Verlinsky Y, Ginsberg N, Lifchez A et al. Analysis of the first polar body: Preconception genetic diagnosis. *Hum Reprod* 1990; 5: 826–9.
2. Handyside AH, Kontogianni EH, Hardy K, Winston RML. Pregnancies from biopsied human preimplantation embryos sexed by Y-specific DNA amplification. *Nature* 1990; 244: 768–70.
3. Harper J. Introduction to preimplantation genetic diagnosis. In: *Preimplantation Genetic Diagnosis*, 2nd ed. Harper J (ed.). Cambridge, U.K.: Cambridge University Press, 2010, pp. 1–47.
4. Staessen C, Platteau P, Van Assche E et al. Comparison of blastocyst transfer with or without preimplantation genetic diagnosis for aneuploidy screening in couples with advanced maternal age: A prospective randomized controlled trial. *Hum Reprod* 2004; 19: 2849–58.
5. Stevens J, Wale P, Surrey ES, Schoolcraft WB. Is aneuploidy screening for patients aged 35 or over beneficial? A prospective randomized trial. *Fertil Steril* 2004; 82(Suppl 2): 249.
6. Mastenbroek S, Twisk M, Van Echten-Arends J et al. *In vitro* fertilization with preimplantation genetic screening. *N Engl J Med* 2007; 357: 9–17.
7. Blockeel C, Schutyser V, De Vos A et al. Prospectively randomized controlled trial of PGS in IVF/ICSI patients with poor implantation. *Reprod Biomed Online* 2008; 17: 848–54.
8. Hardarson T, Hanson C, Lundin K et al. Preimplantation genetic screening in women of advance maternal age decrease in clinical pregnancy rate: A randomized controlled trial. *Hum Reprod* 2008; 23: 2806–12.
9. Jansen RP, Bowman MC, de Boer KA et al. What next for preimplantation genetic screening (PGS)? Experience with blastocyst biopsy and testing for aneuploidy. *Hum Reprod* 2008; 23: 1476–78.
10. Mersereau JE, Pergament E, Zhang X, Milad MP. Preimplantation genetic screening to improve *in vitro* fertilization pregnancy rates: A prospective randomized controlled trial. *Fertil Steril* 2008; 90: 1287–9.
11. Staessen C, Verpoest W, Donoso P et al.. Preimplantation genetic screening does not improve delivery rate in women under the age of 36 following single-embryo transfer. *Hum Reprod* 2008; 23: 2818–25.
12. Meyer L, Klipstein S, Hazlett W et al. A prospective randomized controlled trial of preimplantation genetic screening in the "good prognosis" patient. *Fertil Steril* 2009; 91: 1731–8.
13. Schoolcraft WB, Katz-Jaffe MG, Stevens J et al. Preimplantation aneuploidy testing for infertile patients of advanced maternal age: A randomized prospective trial. *Fertil Steril* 2009; 92: 157–62.
14. Debrock S, Melotte C, Spiessens C et al. Preimplantation genetic screening for aneuploidy in embryos after *in vitro* fertilization (IVF) does not improve reproductive outcome in women over 35: A prospective controlled randomized trial. *Fertil Steril* 2010; 93: 364–73.
15. Anderson R, Pickering S. The current status of preimplantation genetic screening: British Fertility Society Policy and Practice Guidelines. *Hum Fertil* 2008; 11: 71–75.
16. Practice Committee of Society for Assisted Reproductive Technology, Practice Committee of American Society for Reproductive Medicine. Preimplantation genetic testing: A Practice Committee opinion. *Fertil Steril* 2008; 90(Suppl 1): S136–43.
17. Geraedts J, Collins J, Gianaroli L et al. What next for preimplantation genetic screening? A polar body approach! *Hum Reprod* 2010; 25: 575–7.
18. Nicolaidis P, Petersen MB. Origin and mechanisms of non-disjunction in human autosomal trisomies. *Hum Reprod* 1998; 13: 313–9.
19. Handyside AH, Montag M, Magli MC et al. Multiple meiotic errors caused by predivision of chromatids in woman of advanced maternal age undergoing *in vitro* fertilisation. *Eur J Hum Genet* 2012; 20: 742–7.
20. Geraedts J, Montag M, Magli MC et al. Polar body array CGH for prediction of the status of the corresponding oocyte. I. Clinical results. *Hum Reprod* 2011; 26: 3173–80.
21. Scott RT, Treff NR, Stevens J et al. Delivery of a chromosomal normal child from an oocyte with reciprocal aneuploid polar bodies. *J Assist Reprod Genet* 2012; 29: 533–7.
22. Wells D. Next-generation sequencing: The dawn of a new era for preimplantation genetic diagnostics. *Fertil Steril* 2014; 101: 1250–1.
23. Kuliev A, Cieslak J, Ilkevitch Y, Verlinsky Y. Chromosomal abnormalities in a series of 6733 human oocytes in preimplantation diagnosis for age-related aneuploidies. *Reprod Biomed Online* 2002; 6: 54–9.
24. Munné S, Sandalinas M, Escudero T et al. Outcome of preimplantation genetic diagnosis of translocations. *Fertil Steril* 2000; 73: 1209–18.
25. Verlinsky Y, Cieslak J, Ivakhenko V et al. Chromosomal abnormalities in the first and second polar body. *Mol Cell Endocrinol* 2001; 183S: 47–9.

26. Hassold T, Chiu D. Maternal age-specific rates of numerical chromosome abnormalities with special reference to trisomy. *Hum Genet* 1985; 70: 11–7.
27. Angell RR. Predivision in human oocytes at meiosis 1: A mechanism for trisomy formation in man. *Hum Genet* 1991; 86: 383–7.
28. Angell RR. Possible pitfalls in preimplantation diagnosis of chromosomal abnormailities based on polar body biopsy. *Hum Reprod* 1994; 9: 181–2.
29. Montag M, Köster M., Strowitzki T, Toth B. Polar body biopsy. *Fertil Steril* 2013; 100: 603–7.
30. Montag M, Limbach N, Sabarstinski M et al. Polar body biopsy and aneuploidy testing by simultaneous detection of six chromosomes. *Prenat Diagn* 2005; 25: 867–71.
31. Munné S. Preimplantation genetic diagnosis for infertility (preimplantation genetic screening). In: *Preimplantation Genetic Diagnosis*, 2nd ed. Harper J (ed.). Cambridge, U.K.: Cambridge University Press, 2010, pp. 203–9.
32. Verlinsky Y, Cieslak J, Freidin M et al. Pregnancies following pre-conception diagnosis of common aneuploidies by FISH. *Hum Reprod* 1995; 10: 1923–7.
33. Dyban A, Freidine M, Severova E et al. Detection of aneuploidy in human oocytes and corresponding first polar body by fluorescent *in situ* hybridisation. *J Assist Reprod Genet* 1996; 13: 73–8.
34. Verlinsky Y, Cieslak J, Ivakhenko V et al. Birth of healthy children after preimplantation diagnosis of common aneuploidies by polar body fluorescent *in situ* hybridization analysis. *Fertil Steril* 1996; 66: 126–9.
35. Verlinsky Y, Cieslak J, Ivakhenko V et al. Prepregnancy genetic testing for age-related aneuploidies by polar body analysis. *Genet Test* 1997/98; 4: 231–5.
36. Verlinsky Y, Cieslak J, Ivakhenko V et al. Prevention of age-related aneuploidies by polar body testing. *J Assist Reprod Genet* 1999; 16: 165–9.
37. van der Ven K, Montag M, van der Ven H. Polar body diagnosis—A step in the right direction? *Dtsch Arztebl Int* 2008; 105: 190–6.
38. Wells D, Escudero T, Levy B et al. First clinical application of comparative genomic hybridization and polar body testing for preimplantation genetic diagnosis of aneuploidy. *Fertil Steril* 2002; 78: 543–9.
39. Montag M, Köster K, van der Ven K, et al. Kombinierte Translokations- und Aneuploidieuntersuchungen nach Polkörperbiopsie und array-Comparative Genomic Hybridisation. *J Reproduktionsmed Endokrinol* 2010; 6: 498–502.
40. Delhanty JD. Is the polar body approach best for pre-implantation genetic screening? *Placenta* 2011; 32(Suppl 3): S268–70.
41. Stern C, Pertile M, Norris H et al. Chromosome translocations in couples with *in-vitro* fertilization implantation failure. *Hum Reprod* 1999; 14: 2097–101.
42. Van der Ven K, Peschka B, Montag M et al. Increased frequency of constitutional chromosomal aberrations in female partners of couples undergoing intracytoplasmic sperm injection (ICSI). *Hum Reprod* 1998; 13: 48–54.
43. Peschka B, Leygraaf J, van der Ven K et al. Type and frequency of chromosome aberrations in 551 couples undergoing intracytoplasmic sperm injection. *Hum Reprod* 1999; 14: 2257–63.
44. Munne S, Fung J, Cassel MJ et al. Preimplantation genetic analysis of translocations: Case-specific probes for interphase cell analysis. *Hum Genet* 1998; 102: 663–74.
45. Fiorentino F, Spizzichino L, Bono S et al. PGD for reciprocal and Robertsonian translocations using array comparative genomic hybridization. *Hum Reprod* 2011; 26: 1925–35.
46. Gitlin SA, Lanzendorf SE, Gibbons WE. Polymerase chain reaction amplification specifity: Incidence of allele-dropout using different DNA preparation methods for heterozygous single cells. *J Assist Reprod Genet* 1996; 13: 107–11.
47. Sermon K, Lissens W, Joris H et al. Clinical application of preimplantation diagosis for myotonic dystrophy. *Prenat Diagn* 1997; 17: 925–32.
48. Ray PF, Ao A, Taylor DM et al. Assessment of single blastomere analysis for preimplantation diagnosis of the delta F508 deletion causing cystic fibrosis in clinical practice. *Prenat Diagn* 1994; 18: 1402–12.
49. Rechitsky S, Strom C, Verlinsky O et al. Allele dropout in polar bodies and blastomeres. *J Assist Reprod Genet* 1998; 15: 253–7.
50. Hussey ND, Davis T, Hall JR et al. Preimplantation genetic diagnosis for b-thalassaemia using sequencing of single cell PCR products to detect mutations and polymorphic loci. *Mol Hum Reprod* 2002; 8: 1136–43.
51. Fiorentino F, Magli MC, Podini D et al. The minisequencing method: An alternative strategy for preimplantation genetic diagnosis of single gene disorders. *Reprod Biomed Online* 2003; 9: 399–410.
52. Verlinsky Y. Polar body-based preimplantation diagnosis for X-linked disorders. *Reprod Biomed Online* 2001; 4: 38–42.
53. Sermon K. Preimplantation genetic diagnosis for monogenic disorders: Multiplex PV three dimensional partial zona dissection for preimplantation genetic diagnosis and assisted hatching PCR and whole-genome amplification for gene analysis at the single cell level. In: *Preimplantation Genetic Diagnosis*, 2nd ed. Harper J (ed.). Cambridge, U.K.: Cambridge University Press, 2010, pp. 237–46.
54. Montag M, van der Ven K, van der Ven H. Polar body diagnosis. In: *Preimplantation Genetic Diagnosis*, 2nd ed. Harper J (ed.). Cambridge, U.K.: Cambridge University Press, 2010, pp. 166–74.

55. Magli C, Montag M, Köster M et al. Polar body array CGH for prediction of the status of the corresponding oocyte. I. Technical aspects. *Hum Reprod* 2011; 26: 3181–5.
56. Gordon JW, Talansky BE. Assisted fertilization by zona drilling: A mouse model for correction of oligospermia. *J Exp Zool* 1987; 239: 347–81.
57. Cieslak J, Ivakhenko V, Wolf G et al. Three-dimensional partial zona dissection for preimplantation genetic diagnosis and assisted hatching. *Fertil Steril* 1999; 71: 308–13.
58. Montag M, van der Ven K, Delacrétaz G et al. Efficient preimplantation genetic diagnosis using laser assisted microdissection of the zona pellucida for polar body biopsy followed by primed *in situ* labelling (PRINS). *J Assist Reprod Genet* 1997; 14: 455–6.
59. Montag M, van der Ven K, Delacrétaz G et al. Laser assisted microdissection of zona pellucida facilitates polar body biopsy. *Fertil Steril* 1998; 69: 539–42.
60. Montag M, van der Ven H. Laser-assisted hatching in assisted reproduction. *Croat Med J* 1999; 40: 398–403.
61. Montag M, Koll B, Holmes P, van der Ven H. Significance of the number of embryonic cells and the state of the zona pellucida for hatching of mouse blastocysts *in vitro* versu *in vivo*. *Biol Reprod* 2000; 62: 1738–44.
62. Licciardi F, Gonzalez A, Tang YX et al. Laser ablation of the mouse zona pellucida for blastomere biopsy. *J Assist Reprod Genet* 1995; 12: 462–6.
63. Boada M, Carrera M, De La Iglesia C et al. Successful use of a laser for human embryo biopsy in preimplantation genetic diagnosis: Report of two cases. *J Assist Reprod Genet* 1997; 15: 301–5.
64. Veiga A, Sandalinas M, Benkhalifa M et al. Laser blastocyst biopsy for preimplantation diagnosis in the human. *Zygote* 1997; 5: 351–4.
65. Joris H, de Vos A, Janssens R et al. Comparison of the results of human embryo biopsy and outcome of preimplantation genetic diagnosis (PGD) after zona drilling using acid Tyrode of a laser. *Hum Reprod* 2000; 15S: 53–54.
66. Levin I, Almog B, Shwartz T et al. Effects of laser polar-body biopsy on embryo quality. *Fertil Steril* 2012; 97: 1085–8.
67. Montag M, van der Ven K, van der Ven H. Erste klinische Erfahrungen mit der Polkörperdiagnostik in Deutschland. *J Fertil Reprod* 2002; 4: 7–12.
68. Harton GL, Magli MC, Lundin K et al. ESHRE PGD Consortium/Embryology Special Interest Group—Best practice guidelines for polar body and embryo biopsy for preimplantation genetic diagnosis/screening (PGD/PGS). *Hum Reprod* 2011; 26: 41–6.
69. Munne S, Dailey T, Sultan KM et al. The use of first polar bodies for preimplantation diagnosis of aneuploidy. *Mol Hum Reprod* 1995; 10: 1014–20.
70. Christopikou D, Tsorva E, Economou K, Shelley P, Davies S, Mastrominas M, Handyside A. Polar body analysis by array comparative genomic hybridization accurately predicts aneuploidies of maternal meiotic origin in cleavage stage embryos of women of advanced maternal age. *Hum Reprod* 2013; 28: 1426–34.
71. Treff NR, Scott RT, Jr., Su J, Campos J, Stevens J, Schoolcraft W, Katz-Jaffe M. Polar body morphology is not predictive of its cell division origin. *J Assist Reprod Genet* 2012; 29: 137–9.
72. Capalbo A, Bono S, Spizzichino L et al. Sequential comprehensive chromosome analysis on polar bodies, blastomeres and trophoblast: Insight into female meiotic errors and chromosomal segregation in the preimplantation window of embryo development. *Hum Reprod* 2013; 28: 509–18.
73. Forman EJ, Treff NR, Stevens JM, Garnsey HM, Katz-Jaffe MG, Scott RT, Jr., Schoolcraft WB. Embryos whose polar bodies contain isolated reciprocal chromosome aneuploidy are almost always euploid. *Hum Reprod* 2013; 28: 502–8.
74. Munne S, Sandalinas M, Escudero T et al. Improved implantation after preimplantation genetic diagnosis of aneuploidy. *Reprod Biomed Online* 2003; 7: 91–7.
75. Montag M, van der Ven K, Dorn C, van der Ven H. Outcome of laser-assisted polar body biopsy. *Reprod Biomed Online* 2004; 9: 425–9.

Preimplantation genetic diagnosis for infertility

27

JONATHAN LEWIN and DAGAN WELLS

INTRODUCTION

In vitro fertilization (IVF) treatment has revolutionized the treatment of infertility and is estimated to have led to more than 6 million births worldwide. However, despite the obvious benefits of IVF, it must be acknowledged that the process remains inefficient. Even after almost four decades of optimization, it is still the case that the majority of embryo transfers fail to produce a pregnancy. The problem worsens with advancing female age, with IVF success rates dropping with ever growing speed after the age of 35 years. The high failure rates are associated with significant financial and psychological costs to patients (1–3).

One explanation for why older women suffer low implantation and high miscarriage rates, both for natural and IVF pregnancies, is that they produce more aneuploid embryos (i.e., embryos containing cells with an incorrect number of chromosomes) (Figure 27.1). Long-standing evidence links spontaneous pregnancy losses with aneuploidy—karyotypes of tissue from miscarriages show aneuploid embryonic cells in over 50% of cases (4,5). Testing preimplantation embryos using a wide variety of methods consistently shows that aneuploidy is common in preimplantation embryos and increases markedly with female age (6–8).

There is good evidence from analysis of polar bodies that the great majority of aneuploidies detected in embryos are derived from the oocyte (9,10). This is especially true for reproductively older women and explains why the use of donor oocytes from young women results in higher IVF birth rates and lower miscarriage rates (11). Abnormalities of chromosome number, with the exception of trisomy 21 and sex chromosome aneuploidy, are essentially incompatible with life. The poor prognosis of older IVF patients can therefore likely be explained by the high rates of aneuploidy present in their oocytes (12,13).

One approach to improving the outcomes of IVF treatment for infertile patients is to test oocytes or embryos for the presence of aneuploidy, allowing euploid embryos to be identified and transferred to the uterus in preference to those that are aneuploid. This has given rise to a field of research and clinical practice termed preimplantation genetic screening (PGS). Traditionally, PGS has been offered to patients considered to be at elevated risk of producing aneuploid embryos, those of advanced reproductive age, couples experiencing recurrent implantation failure, and those with a history of multiple miscarriages. However, it is increasingly appreciated that younger women may also stand to gain from PGS, because they typically produce several embryos that can be selected between and, despite their age, still have appreciable levels of aneuploidy (14,15). By increasing the ability to identify embryos with a high likelihood of successful implantation, PGS may help to facilitate single-embryo transfer (SET), and therefore assist in the reduction of multiple pregnancy rates. As well as helping to avoid implantation failure and miscarriage associated with the transfer of aneuploid embryos, PGS is expected to avoid the vast majority of syndromes associated with aneuploidy (e.g., Down syndrome).

PGS BY FLUORESCENCE *IN SITU* HYBRIDIZATION

Initial attempts at PGS were focused on analysis of polar bodies removed from oocytes or cells (blastomeres) biopsied from cleavage-stage embryos. These methods had originally been developed in the late 1980s for preimplantation genetic diagnosis (PGD) of inherited conditions (16,17). Embryo biopsy was suggested to be safe, with the rate of blastocyst formation not significantly altered by the manipulation (18) and similar IVF pregnancy rates between biopsied and non-biopsied embryos (16). In the case of blastomere biopsy, a hole was typically made in the zona pellucida using acid Tyrode's solution. The cell (or on some occasions two cells) extracted was then fixed on a microscope slide and fluorescence *in situ* hybridization (FISH) was carried out using probes to detect specific chromosomes (19). Initially, only a handful of chromosomes could be examined, but over several years, technical innovations allowed the number of chromosomes tested to be expanded to cover about half of those in each cell (20).

Several non-randomized clinical trials provided evidence that PGS could be beneficial. The technique was first tested in couples with poor prognosis who were allowed to choose between assignment to PGS or the control group (21). The PGS group showed a significantly higher pregnancy rate (40% vs. 23%) and implantation rate (28% vs. 11.9%, $p \leq 0.05$). However, numbers in each group were small (11 and 17, respectively), and allowing the patients to choose which study group they would join could have introduced bias.

In a matched case-control study of 138 patients, the implantation rate was found to be significantly higher in PGS patients than age- and prognosis-matched controls (18% vs. 11%, $p < 0.05$) (22). This was particularly marked in patients who had no history of previously failed IVF cycles and who had a good fertilization rate, producing many embryos from which to choose morphologically and genetically.

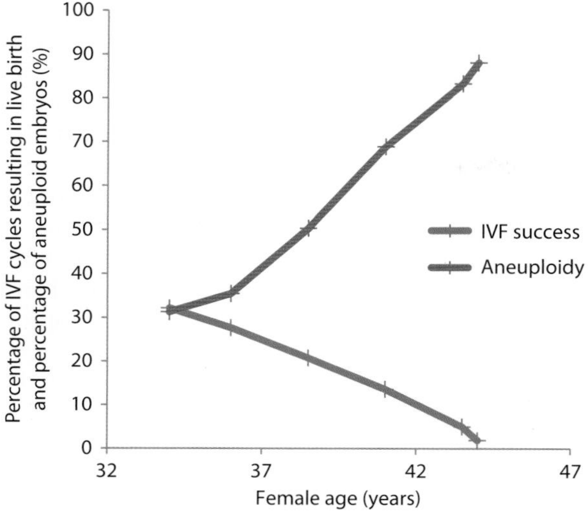

Figure 27.1 Aneuploid embryos (%) and live birth rate after IVF (%) with increasing maternal age. Beyond the age of 35 years, IVF success rates fall dramatically, while the percentage of embryos that are aneuploid increases. *Abbreviation*: IVF, *in vitro* fertilization. (Data derived from Franasiak JM et al. *J Assist Reprod Genet.* 2014; 31(11): 1501–9; Human Fertilisation and Embryology Association. IVF—Chance of success. Human Fertilisation and Embryology Authority 2014, Accessed February 17, 2016. Available from: http://www.hfea.gov.uk/ivf-success-rate.html.)

Despite these promising findings, the outcomes of subsequent randomized controlled trials (RCTs) were far less positive. A well-designed RCT of 400 prospectively randomized patients found no increase in viable pregnancy rate per embryo transfer or per IVF cycle, although it did produce a non-significant increase in implantation rate (17.1% vs. 11.5%) (23). Most alarmingly, in another RCT, the study had to be terminated before its completion due to the negative outcomes found in the PGS group (24).

The most worrisome piece of evidence against PGS came from a large, multicenter, double-blind RCT of patients with a mean age of approximately 38 years who underwent up to three cycles of IVF with either PGS or normal embryo selection, in which two embryos were consistently transferred (25). This found that controls had a significantly higher clinical pregnancy rate than the PGS group (44% vs. 30%, $p = 0.003$), as well as a higher live birth rate (35% vs. 24%, $p = 0.01$). However, this apparently well-constructed trial was highly criticized for its methodology (26). Firstly, PGS failed to produce a result in as many as 20% of embryos analyzed, and when these embryos were transferred, they resulted in only a 6% implantation rate, compared to 14% in the control group, implying severe damage to many of the embryos through poor biopsy technique. Furthermore, chromosomes 15 and 22, which are the second and third most common chromosomes to be aneuploid in miscarriages (27), were not analyzed in this study. By looking at success rates over three IVF cycles, this study also failed to recognize the benefits in first-cycle success and any decrease in time to pregnancy, which might be particularly important for older couples.

Nonetheless, further RCTs also failed to provide evidence of significant benefits to patients undergoing PGS using FISH (28), including in younger couples and those with a good prognosis (29,30). Although one small RCT showed a non-significant trend towards improved birth rates in the PGS group (31), a meta-analysis of prospective RCTs of cleavage-stage PGS by FISH showed a resounding lack of evidence to support its use (32).

WHY BLASTOMERE FISH IS NOT AN IDEAL TECHNIQUE

Although the theory behind PGS by FISH was reasonable, it is clear that technical issues inherent in the method limited its clinical potential. Researchers were interested in determining the number of chromosomes in individual cells, so the obvious choice of technique would have been metaphase karyotyping; yet this is not applicable in the context of PGS as the single cell biopsied is very rarely found to be in metaphase and cannot be cultured due to time constraints and technical difficulties. FISH had previously been used to sex embryos by checking for the presence of a single (Y) chromosome (33), and was extended for the purposes of PGS by simply adding new probes for other chromosomes. However, it was impossible to analyze all of the chromosomes in a cell using FISH because there were only five spectrally distinct fluorochromes available with which to label the probes, and because repeated rounds of FISH performed on the same fixed cell are associated with declining accuracy due to disintegration of the nucleus. The largest number of chromosomes that were reliably analyzed in a single study was 15, performed over three rounds, and this unsurprisingly revealed more aneuploidy and mosaicism than had been seen in previous studies (34). Inherent technical issues in FISH result in false-positive and false-negative results due to split signals, signal overlap, and loss of micronuclei (35), and as a result some laboratories experienced appreciable levels of test failures and errors, which were likely to impact on any improvement in IVF success that could be achieved (36).

Performing the analysis in cleavage-stage embryos rather than later stages is also likely to be suboptimal. Many cleavage-stage embryos arrest naturally, so performing analysis at a later stage has the advantage of requiring fewer embryos to be analyzed (36). Importantly, cleavage-stage embryos appear to be much more sensitive to biopsy than blastocysts, and there is a risk that the biopsy procedure itself may impair implantation rates (37). Also, mosaicism, the presence of one or more karyotypically distinct cell lines within the same embryo, which is common throughout preimplantation development, is at its most prevalent at the cleavage stage, posing significant problems for any diagnosis based upon a single cell. The failure to demonstrate clinical efficacy of protocols based upon blastomere FISH suggests that this strategy is not ideal, but does not necessarily invalidate the concept of PGS.

NEW TECHNOLOGIES AND ARRAY-BASED METHODS

While debate continued over the benefit of PGS using FISH, new genetic techniques were developed that could provide a comprehensive screening of all chromosomes with far greater accuracy. The first of these processes was metaphase comparative genomic hybridization (metaphase-CGH). In this method, DNA is extracted from the embryo biopsy and amplified using one of a number of techniques termed whole-genome amplification (WGA). This amplifies DNA from each chromosome in a way that reliably reflects the starting number of chromosomes. The amplified DNA is labeled with a fluorescent dye (usually green in color). The process is repeated for a sample known to be chromosomally normal, which is labeled with a different fluorochrome (usually red) and used as a reference. The test and reference DNA are mixed and added to chromosomes from a normal metaphase cell spread on a microscope slide. After washing, the color of fluorescence observed on individual chromosome indicates the relative amounts of test and control DNA derived from that chromosome, and thereby the ploidy of the embryo. Although this technique was shown to reliably detect aneuploidy in individual blastomeres (38,39), the process took at least three to four days, which was not ideal for clinical use as it did not allow time for transfer within the implantation window. However, it was possible to use this technique to screen for aneuploidy in the polar body of the oocyte with some success (40).

The process of chromosome analysis using CGH underwent increased automation and was greatly accelerated when metaphase chromosomes were replaced by microarrays. These consist of a solid support, such as a glass microscope slide, upon which a multitude of chromosome-specific DNA sequences are arrayed in individual spots. As with metaphase-CGH, differentially labeled test and control DNA samples are hybridized to these target sequences and the colors of the spots are indicative of the copy numbers of the chromosomes from which the sequences were derived (41). The analysis necessary for microarray-CGH (array-CGH [aCGH]) was much simplified compared with metaphase-CGH and, importantly, the time taken for the procedure was reduced to less than 24 hours, allowing the possibility of comprehensive chromosome screening in combination with a fresh embryo transfer (42). aCGH was not only highly accurate when compared with FISH, but it also detected 40% more aneuploidy, presumably due to the increased number of chromosomes analyzed (43).

Although accomplishing comprehensive chromosome screening in a reduced timeframe was a significant achievement, PGS at the blastocyst stage remained challenging due to the vary narrow window of time available for testing to be carried out. This often necessitated the cryopreservation of biopsied embryos to allow sufficient time for analysis before transfer. While for some clinics the introduction of vitrification had removed concerns about loss of embryo viability associated with cryopreservation, others continued to prefer a fresh transfer where possible. A rapid method of PGS, removing the necessity for cryopreservation of biopsied blastocysts, at least in theory, was soon developed and put into clinical practice (44). This technique applied quantitative polymerase chain reaction (qPCR) to amplify and measure the relative quantities of four specific loci per chromosome in just four hours and without the need for prior WGA. The only limitations of the method are issues with scalability (the number of samples that can be processed concurrently on one machine is relatively low) and an inability to reliably detect all forms of chromosome abnormality affecting fragments of chromosome rather than whole chromosomes.

Another method employed for the purpose of PGS has been analysis using single-nucleotide polymorphism (SNP) microarrays, of the type often used for genome-wide association studies (45). These arrays contain probes for tens of thousands of different SNPs that are distributed across all of the chromosomes. If DNA samples from the parents are examined alongside WGA products from the tested embryos, it is possible to trace the inheritance of individual alleles. Essentially, the large number of SNP probes provides a DNA fingerprint for each of the parental chromosomes and the presence/absence of these genetic signatures can be examined in the embryos. This not only reveals the presence of monosomies and trisomies of meiotic origin, but also reveals whether the affected chromosome was from the mother or the father. In addition to this qualitative approach to aneuploidy detection, quantitative analysis of the SNPs on the microarray is also possible, revealing whether or not the quantity of DNA from each chromosome is appropriate (46). Another benefit of analysis using SNP microarrays is that single-gene disorders can be diagnosed at the same time as aneuploidy. This is accomplished using linkage analysis, following the inheritance of polymorphisms surrounding/within a defective gene from parent(s) to embryos. This approach is sometimes referred to as karyomapping (47). The main drawback of SNP microarrays in the context of PGS is that they are more expensive than alternative methods and, although the protocol can be completed within 24 hours, it is longer and more time consuming than most others.

Most recently, next-generation sequencing (NGS) technology has been introduced for the purpose of PGS. Here, after embryo biopsy and WGA, the amplification products are fragmented, producing millions of short pieces of DNA, which are then simultaneously sequenced in parallel and aligned with reference to the known sequence of the human genome (48,49). The relative number of sequenced fragments derived from each chromosome provides an accurate indication of copy number in the sample. Although NGS is frequently used for whole-genome sequencing, in the context of PGS it is typical for less than 1% of the genome to be examined and thus the information obtained concerning the sequence of individual genes is negligible (50). Targeted NGS strategies (focusing on amplification and analysis of specified sequences) and methods involving deeper sequencing of the genome do have the potential to reveal information about individual genes if this is considered desirable. However, there are technical challenges and cost implications of applying such approaches to the PGD of single-gene disorders and so far NGS has seldom been used for this purpose.

In its current form, NGS has two advantages over other PGS methods. Firstly, the cost of comprehensive chromosome analysis using NGS is significantly less than those of other methods. Secondly, results obtained using NGS present a higher "dynamic range" (i.e., signal-to-noise ratio) than other methods, which allows subtle anomalies, especially chromosomal mosaicism in blastocyst biopsy samples, to be detected with greater certainty (51). Recent data suggest that embryos associated with mosaic trophectoderm biopsy specimens have diminished implantation potential, but could be considered for transfer in the absence of any euploid embryos and after appropriate patient counseling (52). The main drawbacks of NGS are a relatively complex workflow and the need to cryopreserve embryos after biopsy. The requirement for cryopreservation is not because of the time needed for NGS, although it is true that most protocols do not fit comfortably into the time available when carrying out a fresh transfer; rather, it is due to the need to run the sequencing equipment at full capacity. This is important for achieving the lowest possible costs of PGS, but usually means that samples (from several patients) must be accumulated over a few days, thus necessitating cryopreservation.

As well as advances in genetic testing, improvements to embryological practice have also contributed to the evolution of PGS. The development of blastocyst culture and trophectoderm biopsy have been particularly beneficial. Culturing the embryo to the blastocyst stage on day 5 selects out non-competent embryos, many of which arrest at earlier developmental stages (36). As a result, blastocyst culture is advantageous for IVF outcomes even without genetic testing (53). Blastocyst biopsy involves breach of the zona pellucida with a laser on day 3 or immediately prior to the procedure on days 5/6. Trophectoderm cells either herniate through the hole spontaneously or are actively drawn through it by suction. Three to ten of these cells (typically about five cells) can then be removed. The inner cell mass is not disturbed and therefore the technique does not affect cells that develop into the fetus. Trophectoderm biopsy is considered to pose significantly less risk to the embryo than cleavage-stage biopsy (37). Also, because several cells are taken, genetic tests tend to yield more robust data. Using some methods, especially NGS, mosaicism can be detected within the biopsy specimen. Blastocyst biopsy is increasingly becoming the first choice of biopsy method for PGS. Polar body biopsy is still currently used, but mostly in countries where genetic testing of the embryo itself is not permitted.

Blastocyst-stage PGS has also been facilitated by developments in cryopreservation, especially vitrification. This is of great importance because the time available for testing following biopsy at such a late stage of preimplantation development is very limited, in some cases necessitating cryopreservation. Vitrification of blastocysts after biopsy provides ample time for results to be generated and allows embryo transfer to be carried out at a time of optimal endometrial receptivity (54). The convergence of embryological and genetic advances is at the heart of the new generation of PGS strategies.

EVIDENCE FOR THE CLINICAL EFFICACY OF NEW PGS TECHNIQUES

Clinical trials involving the new generation of PGS techniques have produced encouraging results. The first indication that blastocyst biopsy combined with comprehensive chromosome screening might have overcome many of the limitations of earlier PGS methods came from a trial by Schoolcraft and colleagues. Although non-randomized, patients in PGS and control groups were well matched. Significantly improved ongoing pregnancy rates were observed for patients receiving PGS (68.9% vs. 44.8%, PGS vs. controls, $p < 0.0001$), despite fewer embryos being transferred (55). Another non-randomized study of 462 IVF cycles with PGS using aCGH demonstrated that the decrease in implantation rate typically seen with increasing maternal age was abolished by the transfer of euploid embryos (56), a similar effect to the use of donor oocytes from younger women (Figure 27.2) (11). This gives strength to the fundamental argument for the use of PGS—that aneuploidy (in this case increasing in frequency due to advancing age) is frequently responsible for the failure of IVF embryos to establish a pregnancy. The authors also compared the rate of pregnancy loss in these cycles to that

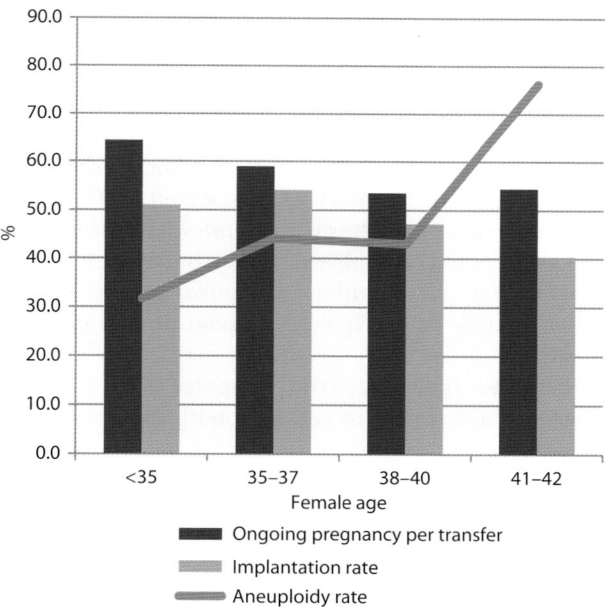

Figure 27.2 Pregnancy rate and implantation rate in different age categories after single-euploid embryo transfer. The usual dramatic decrease in *in vitro* fertilization success seen with age appears to be greatly reduced, while aneuploidy rates found in the biopsied blastocysts increase greatly over these age ranges. (Data derived from Harton GL et al. *Fertil Steril* 2013; 100: 1695–703.)

in patients undergoing IVF without PGS and found it to be significantly lower and unaltered by increasing age.

In a randomized trial assessing the use of PGS to assist in SET, patients were randomized to one of two groups: either SET after PGS or dual-embryo transfer with embryo selection based upon traditional morphological analysis and no PGS (57). The results showed similar pregnancy rates between the two groups, despite the PGS patients receiving half the number of embryos. However, in the control group, approximately half of all cycles resulted in a multiple pregnancy, compared with 0% in the study group. This demonstrates the selective power of PGS and indicates that it could support the use of SET, which is important for reducing multiple pregnancies and their associated risks (58). Although this trial demonstrates non-inferiority of SET after PGS compared to normal dual-embryo transfer, a third arm including patients undergoing SET without PGS would be required to give a clear indication of the effect of PGS itself.

A different study assessed how predictive a diagnosis of aneuploidy was for the outcome of an embryo transfer (59). Participants underwent dual-embryo transfer, and one of the two embryos transferred was analyzed by SNP array PGS, but the results were not revealed until the outcome of the embryo transfer was known. Depending on the outcome, either the baby or the products of conception could be tested to see whether it was from the tested embryo, thanks to the "fingerprinting" provided by the SNP array. The PGS results appeared highly predictive of the success of the cycle, with a negative predictive value of at least 96%.

Two RCTs have compared embryo selection using new PGS technologies with routine morphological analysis and again results have been positive. The first applied aCGH to blastocysts, with fresh transfer occurring on the following day, and reported a significantly higher ongoing pregnancy rate in the study group compared with the control group (69.1% vs. 41.7%, $p = 0.009$) (60). This was achieved in young patients with no prior failed IVF cycles, who produced many embryos, and all participants underwent SET only. As the authors recognize, these results cannot necessarily be extrapolated to poor-prognosis groups or patients.

The second randomized trial compared qPCR with morphological assessment in young, good-prognosis patients undergoing the transfer of one to two embryos (61). If patients produced two or more good-quality embryos by day 5, they were randomized to either undergo double-embryo transfer that day or PGS with embryo transfer on day 6. The PGS group showed a significantly improved implantation rate (79.8% vs. 63.2%, $p < 0.01$) and delivery rate (66.4% vs. 47.9%, $p < 0.01$), despite fewer embryos being transferred in the PGS group. However, the extra day of embryo culture required for PGS may have caused positive bias by adding a further round of embryo selection or increased endometrial receptivity, and blinding was lacking. Nevertheless, this study is one of the most rigorous that supports the use of PGS, and the improvement in delivery rates is promising.

RCTs investigating the clinical benefit of PGS show a significant benefit in young patients who produce many embryos. However, evidence for the benefit in older patients is still somewhat lacking. There are currently a number of ongoing, large, multicenter RCTs investigating the clinical benefits of using the new PGS techniques to help patients with infertility, which it is hoped will conclusively demonstrate whether PGS improves the clinical outcomes of IVF patients of poor prognosis (62).

THE CHALLENGE OF MOSAICISM

An emerging challenge facing embryo selection by PGS is the question of how to deal with mosaic embryos (i.e., those containing two or more cell lines with differing karyotypes). This usually occurs due to malsegregation of chromosomes during the early mitotic cleavage division, following fertilization. The result is a "mosaic" embryo, which may contain a mixture of normal diploid cells with aneuploid cells, or consist of a variety of different aneuploid cells. Early studies using FISH to analyze all the blastomeres within each embryo found that between 17% and 65% of cleavage-stage embryos were chromosomal mosaics, with the majority of these being diploid–aneuploid mosaics (34,63,64). A recent study using NGS has confirmed that approximately 30% of blastocysts are diploid–aneuploid mosaics (65).

There are two problems in the assessment of mosaic embryos. Firstly, the cells obtained from the biopsy may not be representative of the embryo as a whole. A "PGS-euploid" embryo that is used for transfer may contain mostly aneuploid cells and therefore fail to implant or miscarry. A "PGS-aneuploid" embryo may be mostly composed of euploid cells, resulting in the discarding of embryos with some reproductive potential. There is long-standing evidence that mosaicism is not always lethal to the embryo. Indeed, mosaic aneuploidy confined to placental tissues is seen in 1%–2% of pregnancies and in the vast majority of cases the corresponding fetus is chromosomally normal (66,67). Evidence from the early embryo is conflicting: while some have found discrepancies in the rates of aneuploidy between the inner cell mass and trophectoderm of blastocysts (68), other studies demonstrate that mosaicism shows no preference for a particular tissue at these early stages of development (69).

The other problem is that the clinical implications of mosaicism are not yet fully understood. Until recently, it has not been possible to observe mosaicism in an embryo before implantation, because cleavage-stage biopsy only produces one cell to test. Even most array-based methods only detect mosaicism if present in at least 30% of biopsied cells (70). There have been cases where known mosaic embryos have been used for IVF and produced chromosomally normal pregnancies (71), which has led some to believe that there may be corrective mechanisms within the embryo, such as blastomere exclusion, multi-polar divisions, endoreduplication of chromosomes, and fragment resorption (72). However, evidence suggests that mosaic embryos are far less likely to implant and produce pregnancies than those associated with an entirely euploid biopsy specimen, so normal embryos should be used preferentially, if available (73).

The newest NGS-based methods are far more sensitive at detecting the presence of mosaicism. While previously a mosaic embryo would have simply been classed as normal or abnormal in chromosome number, some can now be accurately placed in a third "mosaic" class, leading to improved estimation of their reproductive potential. It is hoped that this will be reflected in the results of future clinical trials using NGS.

CONCLUSION

The concept of PGS is founded on the reasonable hypothesis that screening for aneuploidy in preimplantation embryos, where it is common and associated with poor outcome, can assist in the identification of embryos of high potential. If prioritized for transfer, such embryos should deliver increased implantation rates and lower risks of miscarriage and chromosomal syndromes. The initial PGS method of blastomere biopsy and FISH showed promise, but ultimately failed to produce convincing results in RCTs. New techniques of trophectoderm biopsy and array-based methods are technically far superior, as they allow the testing of all chromosomes at a more appropriate developmental stage. Evidence that the new generation of PGS techniques succeed in improving IVF treatment outcomes is rapidly accumulating. Currently, most of the published data support the use of PGS for patients of good prognosis (younger women, those producing multiple blastocysts, etc.). Data from RCTs concerning the benefits of PGS for older patients and others of poor prognosis are still lacking, although some encouraging nonrandomized data have been presented. The coming years are likely to see further improvements in PGS technologies and reductions in the cost to patients of accessing this method of embryo selection. Additional clinical trials will shed light on the efficacy of PGS in distinct patient groups and it is hoped that after many years of debate and controversy a consensus view on the value of PGS will finally emerge.

REFERENCES

1. Piette C, De Mouzon J, Bachelot A, Spira A. *In-vitro* fertilization: Influence of women's age on pregnancy rates. *Hum Reprod* 1990; 5(1): 56–9.
2. Lintsen AME, Eijkemans MJC, Hunault CC et al. Predicting ongoing pregnancy chances after IVF and ICSI: A national prospective study. *Hum Reprod* 2007; 22(9): 2455–62.
3. Garrisi JG, Colls P, Ferry KM, Zheng X, Garrisi MG, Munné S. Effect of infertility, maternal age, and number of previous miscarriages on the outcome of preimplantation genetic diagnosis for idiopathic recurrent pregnancy loss. *Fertil Steril* 2009; 92(1): 288–95.
4. Daniely M, Aviram-Goldring A, Barkai G, Goldman B. Detection of chromosomal aberration in fetuses arising from recurrent spontaneous abortion by comparative genomic hybridization. *Hum Reprod* 1998; 13(4): 805–9.
5. Hassold TJ, Matsuyama A, Newlands IM et al. A cytogenetic study of spontaneous abortions in Hawaii. *Ann Hum Genet* 1978; 41(4): 443–54.
6. Delhanty JD, Griffin DK, Handyside AH et al. Detection of aneuploidy and chromosomal mosaicism in human embryos during preimplantation sex determination by fluorescent *in situ* hybridisation, (FISH). *Hum Mol Genet* 1993; 2(8): 1183–5.
7. Munné S, Alikani M, Tomkin G, Grifo J, Cohen J. Embryo morphology, developmental rates, and maternal age are correlated with chromosome abnormalities. *Fertil Steril* 1995; 64(2): 382–91.
8. Hassold T, Hunt P. To err (meiotically) is human: The genesis of human aneuploidy. *Nat Rev Genet* 2001; 2(4): 280–91.
9. Verlinsky Y, Cieslak J, Ivakhnenko V et al. Preimplantation diagnosis of common aneuploidies by the first- and second-polar body FISH analysis. *J Assist Reprod Genet* 1998; 15(5): 285–9.
10. Fragouli E, Alfarawati S, Goodall NN, Sánchez-García JF, Colls P, Wells D. The cytogenetics of polar bodies: Insights into female meiosis and the diagnosis of aneuploidy. *Mol Hum Reprod* 2011; 17(5): 286–95.
11. Wang YA, Farquhar C, Sullivan EA. Donor age is a major determinant of success of oocyte donation/recipient programme. *Hum Reprod* 2012; 27(1): 118–25.
12. Franasiak JM, Forman EJ, Hong KH et al. Aneuploidy across individual chromosomes at the embryonic level in trophectoderm biopsies: Changes with patient age and chromosome structure. *J Assist Reprod Genet* 2014; 31(11): 1501–9.
13. Human Fertilisation and Embryology Association. IVF—Chance of success. Human Fertilisation and Embryology Authority 2014, Accessed February 17, 2016. Available from: http://www.hfea.gov.uk/ivf-success-rate.html
14. Baart EB, Martini E, van den Berg I et al. Preimplantation genetic screening reveals a high incidence of aneuploidy and mosaicism in embryos from young women undergoing IVF. *Hum Reprod* 2006; 21(1): 223–33.
15. Goossens V, Harton G, Moutou C, Traeger-Synodinos J, Van Rij M, Harper JC. ESHRE PGD Consortium data collection IX: Cycles from January to December 2006 with pregnancy follow-up to October 2007. *Hum Reprod* 2009; 24(8): 1786–810.
16. Handyside A H, Kontogianni EH, Hardy K, Winston RM. Pregnancies from biopsied human preimplantation embryos sexed by Y-specific DNA amplification. *Nature* 1990; 344(6268): 768–70.
17. Verlinsky Y, Rechitsky S, Evsikov S et al. Preconception and preimplantation diagnosis for cystic fibrosis. *Prenat Diagn* 1992; 12: 103–10.
18. Hardy K, Martin KL, Leese HJ, Winston RM, Handyside AH. Human preimplantation development *in vitro* is not adversely affected by biopsy at the 8-cell stage. *Hum Reprod* 1990; 5(6): 708–14.

19. Munné S, Lee A, Rosenwaks Z, Grifo J, Cohen J. Diagnosis of major chromosome aneuploidies in human preimplantation embryos. *Hum Reprod* 1993; 8(12): 2185–91.
20. Abdelhadi I, Colls P, Sandalinas M, Escudero T, Munné S. Preimplantation genetic diagnosis of numerical abnormalities for 13 chromosomes. *Reprod Biomed Online* 2003; 6(2): 226–31.
21. Gianaroli L, Fiorentino A, Magli MC, Garrisi J, Ferraretti AP, Munné S. Preimplantation genetic diagnosis increases the implantation rate in human *in vitro* fertilization by avoiding the transfer of chromosomally abnormal embryos. *Fertil Steril* 1997; 68(6): 1128–31.
22. Munné S, Sandalinas M, Escudero T et al. Improved implantation after preimplantation genetic diagnosis of aneuploidy. *Reprod Biomed Online* 2003; 7(1): 91–7.
23. Staessen C, Platteau P, Van Assche E et al. Comparison of blastocyst transfer with or without preimplantation genetic diagnosis for aneuploidy screening in couples with advanced maternal age: A prospective randomized controlled trial. *Hum Reprod* 2004; 19(12): 2849–58.
24. Hardarson T, Hanson C, Lundin K et al. Preimplantation genetic screening in women of advanced maternal age caused a decrease in clinical pregnancy rate: A randomized controlled trial. *Hum Reprod* 2008; 23(12): 2806–12.
25. Mastenbroek S, Twisk M, van Echten-Arends J et al. *In vitro* fertilization with preimplantation genetic screening. *N Engl J Med* 2007; 357(1): 9–17.
26. Munné S, Cohen J, Simpson JL. *In vitro* fertilization with preimplantation genetic screening. *N Engl J Med* 2007; 357(17): 1769–70.
27. Lathi RB, Westphal LM, Milki AA. Aneuploidy in the miscarriages of infertile women and the potential benefit of preimplanation genetic diagnosis. *Fertil Steril* 2008; 89(2): 353–7.
28. Debrock S, Melotte C, Spiessens C et al. Preimplantation genetic screening for aneuploidy of embryos after *in vitro* fertilization in women aged at least 35 years: A prospective randomized trial. *Fertil Steril* 2010; 93(2): 364–73.
29. Meyer LR, Klipstein S, Hazlett WD, Nasta T, Mangan P, Karande VC. A prospective randomized controlled trial of preimplantation genetic screening in the "good prognosis" patient. *Fertil Steril* 2009; 91(5): 1731–8.
30. Stevens J, Wale P, Surrey ES, Schoolcraft WB, Gardner DK. Is aneuploidy screening for patients aged 35 or over beneficial? A prospective randomized trial. *Fertil Steril* 2004; 82: S249.
31. Schoolcraft WB, Katz-Jaffe MG, Stevens J, Rawlins M, Munne S. Preimplantation aneuploidy testing for infertile patients of advanced maternal age: A randomized prospective trial. *Fertil Steril* 2009; 92(1): 157–62.
32. Mastenbroek S, Twisk M, van der Veen F, Repping S. Preimplantation genetic screening: A systematic review and meta-analysis of RCTs. *Hum Reprod Update* 2011; 17(4): 454–66.
33. Penketh RJ, Delhanty JD, van den Berghe JA et al. Rapid sexing of human embryos by non-radioactive *in situ* hybridization: Potential for preimplantation diagnosis of X-linked disorders. *Prenat Diagn* 1989; 9(7): 489–99.
34. Baart EB, van den Berg I, Martini E, Eussen HJ, Fauser BCJM, Van Opstal D. FISH analysis of 15 chromosomes in human day 4 and 5 preimplantation embryos: The added value of extended aneuploidy detection. *Prenat Diagn* 2007; 27(1): 55–63.
35. Velilla E, Escudero T, Munné S. Blastomere fixation techniques and risk of misdiagnosis for preimplantation genetic diagnosis of aneuploidy. *Reprod Biomed Online* 2002; 4(3): 210–7.
36. Munné S, Grifo J, Cohen J, Weier HU. Chromosome abnormalities in human arrested preimplantation embryos: A multiple-probe FISH study. *Am J Hum Genet* 1994; 55(1): 150–9.
37. Scott RT, Upham KM, Forman EJ, Zhao T, Treff NR. Cleavage-stage biopsy significantly impairs human embryonic implantation potential while blastocyst biopsy does not: A randomized and paired clinical trial. *Fertil Steril* 2013; 100(3): 624–30.
38. Wells D, Sherlock JK, Handyside AH, Delhanty JD. Detailed chromosomal and molecular genetic analysis of single cells by whole genome amplification and comparative genomic hybridisation. *Nucleic Acids Res* 1999; 27(4): 1214–8.
39. Voullaire L, Wilton L, Slater H, Williamson R. Detection of aneuploidy in single cells using comparative genomic hybridization. *Prenatal Diagnosis.* 1999; 19(9): 846–51.
40. Sher G, Keskintepe L, Keskintepe M et al. Oocyte karyotyping by comparative genomic hybrydization provides a highly reliable method for selecting "competent" embryos, markedly improving *in vitro* fertilization outcome: A multiphase study. *Fertil Steril* 2007; 87(5): 1033–40.
41. Vermeesch JR, Melotte C, Froyen G et al. Molecular karyotyping: Array CGH quality criteria for constitutional genetic diagnosis. *J Histochem Cytochem* 2005; 53(3): 413–22.
42. Hellani A, Abu-Amero K, Azouri J, El-Akoum S. Successful pregnancies after application of array-comparative genomic hybridization in PGS-aneuploidy screening. *Reprod Biomed Online* 2008; 17(6): 841–7.
43. Gutiérrez-Mateo C, Colls P, Sánchez-García J et al. Validation of microarray comparative genomic hybridization for comprehensive chromosome analysis of embryos. *Fertil Steril* 2011; 95(3): 953–8.
44. Treff NR, Tao X, Ferry KM, Su J, Taylor D, Scott RT. Development and validation of an accurate quantitative real-time polymerase chain reaction-based

assay for human blastocyst comprehensive chromosomal aneuploidy screening. *Fertil Steril* 2012; 97(4): 819–24.

45. LaFramboise T. Single nucleotide polymorphism arrays: A decade of biological, computational and technological advances. *Nucleic Acids Res* 2009; 37(13): 4181–93.
46. Treff NR, Su J, Tao X, Levy B, Scott RT. Accurate single cell 24 chromosome aneuploidy screening using whole genome amplification and single nucleotide polymorphism microarrays. *Fertil Steril* 2010; 94(6): 2017–21.
47. Handyside AH, Grifo J, Prates R, Tormasi S, Fischer J, Munne S. Validation and first clinical application of karyomapping for preimplantation diagnosis (PGD) of Gaucher disease combined with 24 chromosome screening. *Fertil Steril* 2010; 94(4): S79–80.
48. Kung A, Munné S, Bankowski B, Coates A, Wells D. Validation of next-generation sequencing for comprehensive chromosome screening of embryos. *Reprod Biomed Online* 2015; 31(6): 760–9.
49. Fiorentino F, Biricik A, Bono S et al. Development and validation of a next-generation sequencing-based protocol for 24-chromosome aneuploidy screening of embryos. *Fertil Steril* 2014; 101(5): 1375–82.
50. Wells D, Kaur K, Grifo J et al. Clinical utilisation of a rapid low-pass whole genome sequencing technique for the diagnosis of aneuploidy in human embryos prior to implantation. *J Med Genet* 2014; 51(8): 553–62.
51. Zheng H, Jin H, Liu L, Liu J, Wang W-H. Application of next-generation sequencing for 24-chromosome aneuploidy screening of human preimplantation embryos. *Mol Cytogenet* 2015; 8(1): 38.
52. Munne S, Grifo J, Wells D. Mosaicism: "survival of the fittest" versus "no embryo left behind". *Fertil Steril* 2016; 105(5): 1146–9.
53. Gardner DK, Vella P, Lane M, Wagley L, Schlenker T, Schoolcraft WB. Culture and transfer of human blastocysts increases implantation rates and reduces the need for multiple embryo transfers. *Fertil Steril* 1998; 69(1): 84–8.
54. Cobo A, De Los Santos MJ, Castellò D, Gámiz P, Campos P, Remohí J. Outcomes of vitrified early cleavage-stage and blastocyst-stage embryos in a cryopreservation program: Evaluation of 3,150 warming cycles. *Fertil Steril* 2012; 98(5): 1138–46.
55. Schoolcraft WB, Fragouli E, Stevens J, Munne S, Katz-Jaffe MG, Wells D. Clinical application of comprehensive chromosomal screening at the blastocyst stage. *Fertil Steril* 2010; 94(5): 1700–6.
56. Harton GL, Munné S, Surrey M et al. Diminished effect of maternal age on implantation after preimplantation genetic diagnosis with array comparative genomic hybridization. *Fertil Steril* 2013; 100: 1695–703.
57. Forman EJ, Hong KH, Ferry KM et al. *In vitro* fertilization with single euploid blastocyst transfer: A randomized controlled trial. *Fertil Steril* 2013; 100(1): 100–7.e1.
58. Baruffi RLR, Mauri AL, Petersen CG et al. Single-embryo transfer reduces clinical pregnancy rates and live births in fresh IVF and Intracytoplasmic Sperm Injection (ICSI) cycles: A meta-analysis. *Reprod Biol Endocrinol* 2009; 7: 36.
59. Scott RT, Ferry K, Su J, Tao X, Scott K, Treff NR. Comprehensive chromosome screening is highly predictive of the reproductive potential of human embryos: A prospective, blinded, nonselection study. *Fertil Steril* 2012; 97(4): 870–5.
60. Yang Z, Liu J, Collins GS et al. Selection of single blastocysts for fresh transfer via standard morphology assessment alone and with array CGH for good prognosis IVF patients: Results from a randomized pilot study. *Mol Cytogenet* 2012; 5(1): 24.
61. Scott RT, Upham KM, Forman EJ et al. Blastocyst biopsy with comprehensive chromosome screening and fresh embryo transfer significantly increases *in vitro* fertilization implantation and delivery rates: A randomized controlled trial. *Fertil Steril* 2013; 100(3): 697–703.
62. Lee E, Illingworth P, Wilton L, Chambers GM. The clinical effectiveness of preimplantation genetic diagnosis for aneuploidy in all 24 chromosomes (PGD-A): Systematic review. *Hum Reprod* 2015; 30(2): 473–83.
63. Munné S, Weier HU, Grifo J, Cohen J. Chromosome mosaicism in human embryos. *Biol Reprod* 1994; 51(3): 373–9.
64. Harper JC, Coonen E, Handyside AH, Winston RM, Hopman AH, Delhanty JD. Mosaicism of autosomes and sex chromosomes in morphologically normal, monospermic preimplantation human embryos. *Prenat Diagn* 1995; 15(1): 41–9.
65. Grifo J, Colls P, Ribustello L, Escudero T, Liu E, Munne S. Why do array-CGH (aCGH) euploid embryos miscarry? Reanalysis by NGS reveals undetected abnormalities which would have prevented 56% of the miscarriages. *Fertil Steril* 2016; 104(3): e14.
66. Kalousek DK, Vekemans M. Confined placental mosaicism. *J Med Genet* 1996; 33(7): 529–33.
67. Kalousek DK, Dill FJ. Chromosomal mosaicism confined to the placenta in human conceptions. *Science* 1983; 221(4611): 665–7.
68. Liu J, Wang W, Sun X et al. DNA microarray reveals that high proportions of human blastocysts from women of advanced maternal age are aneuploid and mosaic. *Biol Reprod* 2012; 87(6): 148.
69. Johnson DS, Cinnioglu C, Ross R et al. Comprehensive analysis of karyotypic mosaicism between trophectoderm and inner cell mass. *Mol Hum Reprod* 2010; 16(12): 944–9.
70. Werner MD, Leondires MP, Schoolcraft WB et al. Clinically recognizable error rate after the transfer of comprehensive chromosomal screened euploid embryos is low. *Fertil Steril* 2014; 102(6): 1613–8.

71. Greco E, Minasi MG, Fiorentino F. Healthy babies after intrauterine transfer of mosaic aneuploid blastocysts. *N Engl J Med* 2015; 373(21): 2089–90.
72. Carbone L, Chavez SL. Mammalian pre-implantation chromosomal instability: Species comparison, evolutionary considerations, and pathological correlations. *Syst Biol Reprod Med* 2015; 61(6): 321–35.
73. Fragouli E, Alfarawati S, Spath K, Tarozzi N, Borini A, Wells D. The developmental potential of mosaic embryos. *Fertil Steril* 2016; 104(3): e96.

28 Genetic analysis of the embryo

YUVAL YARON, LIRAN HIERSCH, VERONICA GOLD,
SAGIT PELEG-SCHALKA, and MIRA MALCOV

INTRODUCTION

For couples at risk of transmitting a genetic disease, preimplantation genetic diagnosis (PGD) and transfer of disease-free embryos offer alternatives to prenatal diagnosis by chorionic villous sampling or amniocentesis, followed by therapeutic abortion of affected fetuses. Molecular PGD was initially employed for embryo sexing in couples at risk for X-linked diseases. The technique used polymerase chain reaction (PCR) to amplify Y chromosome-specific sequences, and only embryos diagnosed as females were transferred (1). During the last two decades, the range of genetic abnormalities that can be detected by PGD has increased exponentially and in fact it may be performed for virtually any genetic disorder for which the mutation has been detected. PGD can also be employed in carriers of cancer predisposition genes and other late-onset genetic conditions. This, however, raises many ethical and practical questions. For instance, familial adenomatous polyposis (FAP) is an autosomal dominant syndrome with almost 100% risk of colorectal cancer without prophylactic colectomy. In a study including 20 individuals with FAP, 95% would consider undergoing prenatal testing and 90% would consider PGD (2). In comparison, carriers of *BRCA1* or *BRCA2* mutations are at risk for breast and/or ovarian cancer, but at a comparatively lower risk of developing malignancy. A similar survey conducted among such carriers revealed that 75% felt it was acceptable to offer PGD for this indication, but only 14% of patients contemplating a future pregnancy would consider PGD themselves (3).

Moreover, it is possible to perform combined PGD and human leukocyte antigen (HLA) typing. This may prove beneficial in cases where the parents already have a child affected with a genetic disease amenable to bone marrow transplantation. In this approach, any future sibling produced by PGD may not only be free of the familial disease, but will also be a suitable bone marrow donor for the affected child. This approach has been successfully employed for Fanconi's anemia (4), and has been coined "savior sibling." However, the use of PGD for HLA typing, particularly in the absence of a genetic disease, and its use in screening embryos for susceptibility to cancer and late-onset diseases, as well as for gender selection, raise important ethical concerns.

Lastly, PGD for chromosomal imbalances, such as in balanced translocation carriers, has been traditionally performed using fluorescence *in situ* hybridization (FISH). It has recently been suggested that this can also be performed using PCR-based techniques (5). Recently, array comparative genomic hybridization (aCGH) has been introduced to PGD, particularly for aneuploidy screening. However, aCGH may also be used for the diagnosis of embryos with unbalanced reciprocal or Robertsonian translocations (6).

Despite its promise, PGD is still limited by technical difficulties due to the minute amount of genetic material and the inherent pitfalls of the PCR, such as amplification failure, allele dropout (ADO), and foreign DNA contamination. There is also a rather narrow window of opportunity for performing diagnosis (within hours) to enable embryo transfer without jeopardizing pregnancy rates. This chapter will review the various aspects of the genetic analysis of preimplantation embryos.

BASIC PRINCIPLES OF PGD

Polymerase chain reaction

Single-cell molecular analysis for PGD was made possible by PCR, which was first introduced in the mid-1980s. The technique enriches a DNA sample for one specific oligonucleotide fragment, the PCR product or amplicon. The technique uses a pair of short oligonucleotide fragments—primers—that are homologous to stretches of genomic DNA at a locus of interest. The PCR thermocycler is programmed to perform successive cycles consisting of denaturation at temperatures >90°C, during which the double-stranded template DNA melts into two separate single strands; annealing, in which the primers attach to their region of homology; and extension, during which new nucleotides (dNTPs) are added in succession to recreate a double-stranded DNA molecule by the enzymatic action of the thermostable Taq polymerase. The resulting new strands serve as templates for the subsequent cycles. After 30–40 such cycles, the initial minute quantity of DNA is amplified to the extent that it can actually be visualized by methods such as radioactive labeling, ethidium bromide, or silver staining. The PCR products may be further subjected to a variety of analytic techniques that determine the presence of point mutations, small deletions or insertions, or for analysis of linked polymorphic genetic markers. Finally, the precise composition of the amplified fragment may be studied by direct sequencing.

The number of cycles that may be performed in standard PCR is limited by a gradual decline in amplification efficiency with each subsequent cycle. This is partly due to the decrease in the activity of the Taq polymerase over time. Another reason is the "fraying" of the amplicon edges by the exonuclease activity of Taq polymerase. This causes the amplicons to become unsuitable templates for further amplification because their primer annealing sites become eroded.

Due to these limitations, when the number of initial DNA template molecules is limited, as in a single-cell PGD analysis, the quantity of amplified DNA may be insufficient for a complete molecular analysis. The two-step, nested primer PCR approach offers a solution to this problem by allowing sufficient amplification of even a single DNA copy. The method employs a first pair of outer primers, designed to amplify the region of interest in the primary PCR reaction. The PCR product of the primary PCR reaction is then further amplified using a second set of inner or nested primers. The use of nested primers that are proximal to the annealing site of the outer primers increases amplification efficiency since the nested primers anneal to sites that have not been eroded. This technique also decreases the rate of non-specific amplification.

Pitfalls of PCR in PGD

The precise diagnosis by PCR relies on several key elements: adequately functioning reagents such as primers, dNTPs, and Taq polymerase; the presence of an adequate tested DNA template; and the lack of any DNA contamination. Perturbations in any of these elements may lead to misdiagnosis. In particular, PCR for PGD has three potential pitfalls: amplification failure, ADO, and contamination.

Amplification failure

Amplification by PCR is unsuccessful in approximately 10% of isolated blastomeres, regardless of their genotype. The main reasons for amplification failure include biopsy technique, premature cell lysis, lysis protocol used, and PCR conditions (7,8). There appears to be an association between embryo or blastomere morphology and the success rate of PCR amplification. Cells that appear to be anucleate and those derived from arrested or fragmented embryos have low amplification efficiency (9,10). In such cells, the DNA may be degraded or entirely absent. Adequate positive and negative controls must be used to establish and fine-tune the PCR protocol and to ensure the integrity of the results. This is of particular importance in cases where the diagnosis is based on detection of deletions, such as in Duchenne muscular dystrophy (DMD). When in such cases an allele is not amplified, one must be certain that this is indeed due to a deletion and not secondary to amplification failure.

Allele dropout

ADO occurs when only one of the two alleles present in a cell is amplified to a detectable level. ADO is equally likely to affect either of the alleles in a heterozygous cell and thus it is not possible to predict which allele will be "dropped out" in a given reaction. The most significant implication of ADO is misdiagnosis of heterozygous embryos, particularly in PGD of dominant disorders. In such cases, the absence of the mutated allele due to ADO may result in misdiagnosis of an affected fetus as a normal one. Likewise, ADO may be responsible for misdiagnosis of recessive disorders in affected compound heterozygotes, where if only one of the mutations is detected, the embryo may be mistaken for a heterozygote (11). The reported frequency of ADO varies widely. In most experiments, the rate of ADO is reported to be 5%–20%, although in some cases ADO has been shown to affect over 30% of single-cell amplifications (10,12–16), or none of the cells (17).

The causes of ADO are still not fully understood. Current hypotheses include inaccessibility of the DNA template due to an imperfect denaturing temperature or incomplete cell lysis and DNA degradation prior to PCR. Ray and Handyside (13) demonstrated that an increase in denaturing temperature from 90 to 96°C during PCR may be associated with a four-fold reduction in ADO at the cystic fibrosis locus and an 11-fold reduction at the β-globin locus. The use of alkaline lysis buffer or lysis buffer containing proteinase K and detergent have also been suggested to reduce ADO (13,18). Degenerated and apoptotic cells show increased ADO, probably due to partial degradation of the DNA strands. It has been suggested that ADO is higher in blastomeres than in other cell types (15). This may be explained, at least partly, by the higher rate of haploidy of blastomeres (19).

In cases of diagnosis of dominant disorders or recessive diseases when both parents carry different mutations, measures should be taken to avoid or reduce the risk of ADO. A number of PGD protocols have been suggested that achieve this goal, most based on advanced techniques such as multiplex PCR in order to include flanking polymorphic markers, quantitative fluorescent (QF) PCR, reverse transcription (RT) PCR, and others, as will be described in the following sections. Other less sensitive detection methods may "overlook" the minimally amplified allele, resulting in ADO (12,16,20). The significant frequency of ADO resulting in misdiagnosis has led many PGD centers to use two cells from each embryo for genetic analysis. This problem may be overcome with the use of karyomapping, which is discussed later in this chapter.

Contamination

Contamination is one of the greatest obstacles to the analysis of specific genes in single cells (21). In the setting of PGD, there may be three main sources of possible contamination. First, paternal genome contamination may arise from the fact that many spermatozoa are still embedded in the zona pellucida after *in vitro* fertilization (IVF), and may thus be mistakenly sampled with the blastomere, second polar body, or trophoectoderm cells during embryo biopsy. Intracytoplasmic sperm injection (ICSI) using a single sperm that is injected into the oocyte completely abolishes this possibility. Accordingly, most PGD units routinely use ICSI for all PGD cases in which diagnosis relies on PCR. The second source of possible contamination may arise from maternal cumulus cells adherent to the oocytes. Stripping of the cumulus cells from the zona pellucida is performed mechanically and/or by enzymes to reduce this risk. Finally, external contamination either from laboratory technicians or from PCR products generated during previous experiments is yet another source of contamination. The risk of external contamination is influenced by the number of PCR cycles required for sufficient amplification of the DNA. Thus, with a starting template of only one genome, the risk of contamination with exogenous DNA sequences is a particularly concerning problem that must be avoided by the use of adequate safety measures, as will be described below.

Advanced molecular methods for PGD

Multiplex PCR

Multiplex PCR refers to the simultaneous amplification of more than one fragment in the same PCR reaction using more than one pair of unrelated primers (12,15,16,22). One or more primer pairs amplify the DNA fragment containing the locus to be tested, while the other(s) serve as a positive control within the same reaction. Amplification of multiple loci within the same multiplex PCR reaction is possible in single blastomeres. This requires careful primer design and reaction optimization to ensure that all primer sets amplify efficiently under the same conditions including annealing temperatures and concentrations of the different reagents in the PCR buffer, such as $MgCl_2$. Careful design of primers is mandated in order to avoid primer dimer formation, interaction between different PCR products, and interaction of primers with products. The primers should be designed such that the product of each PCR primer pair is of a different size so that it may be distinguished by gel electrophoresis. Alternatively, different fluorescent tags can be used for each primer pair.

Successful multiplex PCR reactions enable simultaneous assessment of numerous loci (22). Multiplex PCR reaction may include assays for specific gene defects, unique sequences of specific chromosomes, and linked-informative polymorphic markers. This allows both the analysis of the disease mutation, assessment of aneuploidy, and a reduction in the risk of contamination and ADO (14,15,23–26). This strategy is particularly useful for the PGD of dominant disorders, in which one primer set amplifies the region of mutation, while the other amplifies a polymorphic marker that is linked with the tested gene (24,27). The probability of ADO affecting both the mutation site and the linked polymorphic site is very low, and decreases as more polymorphic markers are tested. This decreases both false-positive and false-negative results.

Fluorescent PCR

The PCR products are commonly separated by gel electrophoresis, and their migration depends chiefly on their size. The standard visualization techniques include radioactive labeling, ethidium bromide, or silver staining. These techniques are rather insensitive, requiring a relatively large amount of DNA. Moreover, they cannot distinguish between products of a relatively similar size, nor provide an adequate estimate of quantity. Fluorescent PCR employs primers tagged with a fluorescent dye, which label the resulting amplicons, enabling detection by florescence-based DNA sequencers using a module such as GeneScan™ (Applied Biosystems-Thermo Fisher Scientific Inc., Waltham, MA, USA). A laser beam scans the acrylamide gel as the fluorescent products pass across the laser path by means of electrophoresis. The different fluorescent dyes absorb the light at a particular wavelength and emit fluorescence at a different wavelength. The emitted light passes through a filter, is digitally amplified, and is analyzed by a computer. With this technique, it is possible to separate, detect, and analyze the fluorescent-labeled PCR products with sensitivity that is 1000-times greater than that achieved using conventional methods (28). This method also has a higher fragment-size resolution and is able to distinguish between products having a size difference of even 1–2 bp. Thus, several primer sets can be multiplexed even if their product sizes only vary slightly.

This approach significantly reduces the likelihood of ADO resulting from preferential amplification, since even minimally amplified alleles are detected (12,16,20). In addition, since the detection efficiency is several magnitudes higher, fewer PCR cycles are required, thereby reducing the risk of contamination. Moreover, since fewer cycles are needed, less time is required for the complete analysis. Using this approach, Sermon et al. (20) have successfully reduced the rate of ADO by a factor of four in the diagnosis of myotonic dystrophy, and Findlay et al. (12) reported an accurate diagnosis in as many as 97% of cases.

Quantitative fluorescent PCR

QF-PCR provides information on the ploidy of the cell (29). It amplifies specific DNA sequences unique for each chromosome, such as short tandem repeat (STR) markers, which are composed of a varying number of nucleotide repeats (2–5 bp) and are highly polymorphic. Normal individuals are usually heterozygous for such polymorphic markers; that is, they have a different number of repeats, and therefore have different-sized alleles. During the initial exponential phase of PCR amplification, the amount of DNA product is proportional to the original number of repeats (30). Disomic individuals thus produce different-sized alleles with a ratio of 1:1, whereas trisomic DNA samples produce either three alleles of different lengths at a ratio of 1:1:1 (trisomic tri-allelic) or two alleles of the same size at a ratio of 2:1 (trisomic di-allelic) (29). This method has been successfully used in prenatal diagnosis of aneuploidy (31). In PGD, however, QF-PCR is only reliable in identifying tri-allelic trisomies, since the interpretation of di-allelic trisomies is problematic due to the possibility of preferential amplification (16).

Whole-genome amplification

The most significant limitation of single-cell analysis is the small amount of DNA. As mentioned previously, multiplex PCR is one way to overcome this problem. In addition, methods designed to achieve non-specific amplification of the entire genome—that is, whole-genome amplification (WGA)—have been developed (21,32). These techniques amplify a large proportion of the entire genome, thereby allowing further analyses by specific PCR reactions, enabling confirmation of diagnosis by alternative methods or the analysis of other genes.

There are several WGA techniques, which are outlined in the following sections.

Primer extension preamplification

Primer extension preamplification (PEP) is a WGA method designed mainly for use in single cells. Using random sequence primers of 15 bp, PEP has been claimed to amplify at least 70% of the genome in more than 30 copies (32). This, however, is likely to be a rather conservative estimate, since Paunio et al. (33) reported that PEP yields at least 1000 copies of the genome, and Wells and Sherlock (21) have suggested that more than of 90% of genomic sequences are represented in PEP amplification products. One of the drawbacks of PEP is the time required, which is usually more than 12 hours. Sermon et al. (34) have successfully adopted a modified protocol that requires less than six hours, and Tsai (35) has improved the efficiency through further technical modifications. Several autosomal recessive, dominant, and X-linked disorders have been successfully detected in single cells using PEP, including Tay–Sachs disease, cystic fibrosis, hemophilia A, DMD, and FAP (14,36,37).

Degenerate oligonucleotide-primed PCR

A second form of WGA called degenerate oligonucleotide-primed PCR (DOP-PCR) has been recently applied to PGD (21,38). DOP-PCR amplifies a similar proportion of the genome as does PEP, but to a greater extent, providing sufficient DNA for over 100 subsequent PCR amplifications (21), or for other analytical procedures such as comparative genomic hybridization (CGH). It has been shown that by using a combination of DOP-PCR, CGH, and QF-PCR, it is possible to determine the copy number of each chromosome and conduct various molecular studies on single cells and blastomeres (21,39).

Multiple displacement amplification

Multiple displacement amplification (MDA) is a recently developed non-PCR-based method that has been utilized for clinical samples with limited DNA content, providing high yields of relatively long fragments (>10 kb) with uniform and reliable representation across the genome (40). In MDA, annealing of exonuclease-resistant random hexamers to a DNA template is followed by strand-displacement DNA synthesis at a constant temperature of 30°C, without the need for cyclic DNA denaturation (40,41). The strand-displacing mechanism is accomplished by the Φ29 DNA polymerase (40) or the *Bacillus stearothermophilus* DNA polymerase large fragment (42). This mechanism allows increasing random priming events that form a network of hyper-branched DNA structures that generate thousands of copies of the original DNA in only a few hours (42,43). It appears that MDA is more advantageous due to decreased rates of unspecific amplification artifacts (44), incomplete coverage of loci (33), strong amplification bias (40), and the short length of the DNA products (45).

The Φ29 enzyme has been widely preferred over *B. stearothermophilus* DNA polymerase due to its superior sequence fidelity (41,46) and its higher processivity (number of nucleotides incorporated per single DNA polymerase/DNA-binding event), the highest to be described for a DNA polymerase (40,47,48). This attribute explains its low amplification bias (less than threefold) compared with DOP- and PEP-PCR methods (10^2- and 10^6-fold) (40).

Hellani et al. (49) and Handyside et al. (50) published the first successful reports of single-cell MDA from lymphocytes and blastomeres with further analysis of aCGH and nested PCR for 20 different loci, respectively. Despite these advantages, ADO is not completely eliminated (46), with observed ADO rates of 10%–31%.

In the setting of PGD, MDA has significant advantages: it obviates the need to set up unique single-cell protocols, such that following MDA, second round PCR may employ standard PCR protocols commonly used in molecular labs. In addition, the large quantity of DNA uniformly representing the entire genome allows subsequent analyses of a variety of other loci (46) for both diagnosis and research. Yet, the technique is not widely used in established PGD units. This may be due to higher rates of ADO, cost, and time required.

In 2006, Renwick et al. coined the term "preimplantation genetic haplotyping," which utilizes MDA with subsequent multiplex PCR of a fixed set of numerous disease-associated polymorphic markers. This allows the determination of the high-risk haplotype by linkage analysis using a single protocol for each disease, without the need to establish a specific protocol for each different mutation (51). Although the same test can be applied to several couples without considering or even identifying the mutation they carry, it has several limitations: it requires additional informative family members to determine phase (i.e., to determine which is the mutation-associated parental haplotype); it requires the use of various informative disease-linked markers; and the occurrence of recombination events could lead to misdiagnosis (46).

Polymorphic markers

Multiplex PCR and WGA allow the analysis of both the tested gene for mutation and polymorphic genetic markers such as STRs, also known as microsatellites, in a process referred to as "DNA fingerprinting." This technique is useful for ruling out contamination from various sources described earlier, and thus improves the reliability of the diagnosis. The amplification of one or more highly polymorphic STRs allows the determination of the source of amplified DNA (52). As mentioned previously, polymorphic STRs consist of a varying number of repeats of a 2–5 bp motif, present in introns throughout the genome. At each informative STR locus, each parent has two alleles of varying repeat numbers, resulting in two amplicons of different lengths in each individual. The resulting embryo will have inherited only one allele from each parent. Any deviation from the expected inheritance of one allele from each parent is indicative of contamination, be it maternal, paternal, or external (12,16,52).

Polymorphic STRs can also be used in the actual diagnosis when the exact mutation causing the disease is unknown. In such cases, polymorphic markers in close proximity or within the disease locus are used to evaluate whether the embryo has inherited the affected allele. Intragenic markers and tightly linked ones are preferred as they are unlikely to be separated from the mutation by recombination during meiosis. In order to perform such a linkage analysis, the parents and both healthy and affected siblings are analyzed to determine which polymorphic marker is inherited along with the disease. Such a strategy has been used for the diagnosis of Marfan syndrome, the first autosomal dominant disorder to be tested by PGD (53), and DMD. In the latter, only 60% of DMD patients exhibit detectable, large-scale deletions in the dystrophin gene. Since this is the largest known human gene, spanning more than 2 million base pairs, it is often impossible to detect small deletions or point mutations (54). Linkage analysis has also been suggested for the diagnosis of disease with large trinucleotide repeat expansions, such as fragile X and myotonic dystrophy (20,55). Single-cell analysis of the expanded portion of the expanded repeat region may lead to misdiagnosis due to difficulty in PCR amplification. Alternatively, it is possible to diagnose with certainty unaffected embryos by the detection of the normal maternal and paternal *FMR1* repeat region (56). In addition, polymorphic markers may be used in combination with direct mutation analysis to increase the precision and reliability of the diagnosis. Searching for suitable polymorphic markers is possible using available publications/National Center for Biotechnology Information–Sequence-Tagged Sites (NCBI-STS) databases, as well as online programs such as GeneLoc and HapMap, among others.

PCR-based PGD for translocation carriers

Traditionally, PGD for reciprocal and Robertsonian translocations was performed using FISH approaches. While generally successful, these techniques are subject to errors due to problems of signal and cell overlap, suboptimal hybridization, and interpretation difficulties due to the presence of mosaicism, among others. In contrast, molecular methods are usually associated with a lower error rate and are more reproducible. In addition, multiple polymorphic markers may be employed to increase precision and reliability and decrease the rate of ambiguous results. Furthermore, with Robertsonian translocation cases where there is the risk of uniparental disomy, the use of PCR-based methods with informative markers can ensure embryos demonstrating biparental inheritance are chosen (5).

MUTATION ANALYSIS

All the above-mentioned PCR techniques amplify the DNA of a single cell to a detectable level. In disorders caused by large-scale deletions, such as DMD or spinal muscular atrophy, the actual PCR amplification reaction is sufficient for making a diagnosis since it is based on the lack of amplification of the corresponding deleted portion of the gene. In other disorders caused by trinucleotide expansion, such as fragile X or myotonic dystrophy, the disease allele is significantly larger than the normal one, and amplicon size may also be diagnostic. More commonly, however, the amplified fragment harboring the mutation is indistinguishable from the normal one using standard visualization methods such as gel electrophoresis. In such cases, further analysis of the amplified fragment is required for mutation detection. Whenever the targeted mutation is precisely known, specific methods can be devised for the detection of the particular mutation. This is preferred to scanning methods that are used to search for mutations that have not been characterized. Scanning methods include heteroduplex analysis, single-strand conformational polymorphism, denaturant gradient gel electrophoresis, and others. These methods are based on the fact the normal DNA strands, mutant DNA strands, and various combinations thereof often have varying electrophoretic migratory properties under different conditions, allowing us to distinguish between them. These techniques often assist in scanning for a mutation in diseases that are caused by numerous different mutations. While PGD using these techniques has been reported in conditions such as β-thalassemia (57–59), it is preferred to limit their use to the initial mutation screen in the affected family members. Once the specific fragment of the gene harboring the mutation has been detected by these methods, further analysis is mandated using direct sequencing. The latter provides bona fide evidence of the mutation, and also facilitates the development of direct diagnostic techniques such as restriction endonuclease (RE) digestion of DNA or amplification refractory mutation system (ARMS).

RE DIGESTION

Alterations in the DNA sequence caused by mutations may often lead to the creation or abolition of specific RE recognition sites. These bacterially derived enzymes recognize specific DNA sequences and cleave the DNA strand at or near to the recognition site. When the precise mutation is known, a restriction enzyme may be selected that differentially cleaves the normal DNA strand but not the mutant one, or vice versa. Following electrophoresis, it is possible to distinguish the digested from the non-digested products and thereby detect the presence or absence of the mutation. Many mutations alter the recognition site of at least one of the many possible commercially available restriction enzymes.

As an example, the *ZFX* and *ZFY* genes located on the X and Y chromosomes, respectively, can be distinguished according to differences in the size of the fragments produced by the restriction enzyme HaeIII. This allows sex determination to be performed more accurately than that based on the presence or lack of amplification of the Y chromosome-specific *SRY* gene.

Amplification refractory mutation system

ARMS employs three primers in the PCR reaction: a common primer that anneals upstream of the mutation site and two other primers that differ slightly, each specific for either the normal or mutant alleles. The site-specific primers may be designed to vary in length, to contain a restriction site, or are tagged by different fluorescent markers (16). Any of these methods would facilitate the distinction of amplicons produced by either the normal or mutant allele. Since this test results in selective amplification of both the mutant and normal alleles, it is considered to be a safer method than the detection of the mutant allele alone. Using this technique in the multiplex PCR approach, it is possible to identify several different mutations, such as for cystic fibrosis, in a single-cell PCR reaction (60).

Mini-sequencing

Mini-sequencing (SnaPshot™) permits analysis of very small DNA fragments amplified by PCR, based on primer extension. It has been suggested that smaller amplicons have a lower rate of ADO. This would potentially improve the reliability of PGD without the need for extensive optimization for individual mutations. Bermudez et al. reported single-cell protocols for the diagnoses of cystic fibrosis, sickle cell anemia, and β-thalassemia using this technique (61).

DNA microarray technology

DNA microarrays or "chips" allow the simultaneous detection of up to thousands of different polymorphisms or mutations in defined genes. Numerous oligonucleotide probes (usually 20–25 bp) are arrayed in microscopic, predefined regions on a solid surface such as a thumbnail-sized glass slide. The probes are complementary to known mutations in defined genes or single-nucleotide polymorphisms (SNPs) throughout the genome. The microarray is hybridized with a fluorescent-labeled test DNA and the fluorescent signal is detected and digitally analyzed. Hybridization is indicative of a match between the test DNA and the specific oligonucleotide probe. For each possible mutation, several slightly varied probes may be used to increase sensitivity.

Array comparative genomic hybridization

Aneuploidy, or chromosome number imbalance, represents a major cause of spontaneous abortions (62–64). FISH for the detection of aneuploidy is discussed elsewhere in this textbook. The major drawback of FISH, however, lies in the fact that only a limited set of chromosomes can be analyzed in a single cell, usually 5–10. aCGH following WGA is an alternative to interphase FISH (65) that may be used to screen for *all* aneuploidies in single blastomeres (66–68) and polar bodies (69,70). In CGH, test and reference DNA samples are labeled with two different fluorochromes and co-hybridized to normal human metaphase spread on a microscope slide (71,72). A computerized imaging system calculates the fluorescence ratio for each fluorochrome at each chromosomal locus. Deviation from a 1:1 ratio indicates a change in DNA copy number (i.e., deletion, duplication, trisomy, etc.) (72).

aCGH is a simpler, more uniform technique that employs selected genomic regions printed onto a solid surface as hybridization probes. This eliminates the use of metaphase spreads that are non-uniform, and enables higher resolution, depending on the number, density, and size of the genomic probe printed on the array (71–73).

Le Caignec et al. (71) detected chromosomal imbalances from single lymphoblasts, fibroblasts, and blastomeres by aCGH following WGA by MDA. This approach may be preferable to aCGH following DOP-PCR that was reported Hu et al. (74).

aCGH has the potential to become an important method for aneuploidy diagnosis and screening in the setting of PGD, to a greater extent than standard FISH, allowing a larger number of abnormalities to be detected (71). It has been suggested that full-genome aneuploidy screening for embryo selection would enhance implantation rates (71).

Next-generation sequencing aneuploidy screening

Recent advances in next-generation sequencing (NGS) have now enabled an even more robust method for aneuploidy screening of human embryos. DNA amplified from single embryos and fragments is individually sequenced in parallel. The number of fragments from each chromosome is proportional to the chromosome copy number. Any deviation from the norm may be interpreted as aneuploid. This method provides a resolution of 800,000–1,000,000 fragment reads per embryo and may therefore detect not only trisomy or monosomy, but also sub-microscopic copy number variants. In addition, this test may be scaled by using the pooling of different samples in the same run by adding "barcoded" index primers. In this way, the cost of testing of each embryo may be reduced. Comparison to aCGH demonstrated full concordance but increased dynamic range, making interpretation much easier (75,76).

Karyomapping

Conventional PCR-based protocols for PGD have several limitations. Despite advances in DNA amplification technology, careful design and validation of the methods for reliable single-cell analysis remain challenging tasks. In particular, the individual design and validation of accurate multiplex PCR protocols for every new PGD case require time and resources. Thus, many couples requiring PGD may have to wait for several weeks or months before the laboratory is ready (77). In addition, although current PGD techniques for single-gene disorders are highly accurate and reliable for the detection of the specific disorder for which they were designed, many are not readily compatible with methods used for comprehensive chromosome screening (78,79).

In order to overcome these shortcomings, karyomapping, an alternative method to conventional PCR-based protocols, was introduced (80). Karyomapping uses an array platform that interrogates about 300,000 SNPs spread across the entire human genome. These SNPs are initially genotyped in both parents as well as affected and unaffected family members. Each chromosomal region has a unique SNP fingerprint, which is further used to identify the parental origin of each chromosome segment and is unique for every individual, as a result of independent segregation of parental chromosomes and the pattern of non-recombinant and recombinant chromosomes (80). Thus, by comparing SNP patterns obtained from parents and other family members, it is possible to reconstruct the haplotypes at each specific disease locus. In this way it is possible to deduce the combination of SNPs associated with the chromosome carrying the mutant gene. Since the SNPs are distributed throughout the genome, it obviates the need to design specific primers and conditions for each case. While the specific mutation in question is not analyzed, the multitude of gene-linked SNPs increases the reliability of this analysis. Furthermore, this approach becomes particularly attractive when multiple loci need to be interrogated, such as when testing for two genetic disease or when HLA matching is also required.

While karyomapping accurately identifies the inheritance of single-gene defects in preimplantation embryos (81,82), it can also be used for the diagnosis of *de novo* deletions, which are otherwise undetectable using conventional PGD technology (83). Although no large-scale studies comparing the rate of diagnosis of karyomapping to conventional PCR analysis exists, karyomapping was found to offer a more comprehensive assessment of the region of interest (99.6% vs. 96.8%) in 55 PGD cases involving 281 blastocysts (77).

Another key advantage of karyomapping is that it can be used for the diagnosis of potentially any familial single-gene disorder with no need for the development of a patient-specific test, greatly reducing the time required for work-up prior to PGD. Finally, the detection of individual parental chromosomes using SNPs allows trisomies of meiotic origin and monosomies to be ascertained.

Nonetheless, the ability of karyomapping to accurately diagnose single-gene disorders can be hampered by several factors. Challenging diagnoses via karyomapping can be expected when the number of SNPs around a gene of interest is relatively small, thereby reducing the number of informative SNPs. This is often the case with genes located in the sub-telomeric region (77). In addition, since karyomapping is based on the identification of the four different parental haplotypes, consanguineous couples may pose a challenge, as the number of informative SNPs in these cases may even be lower. Finally, cases in which couples with *de novo* mutations of a single-gene disorder are assessed with no other affected relatives available can also be challenging for karyomapping-based diagnosis. This can be overcome by using SNP analysis combined with direct mutation analysis in paternal sperm. Since haploid sperm contains only a single copy of each paternal chromosome, the combination of direct mutation analysis and SNP analysis can determine the two paternal haplotypes.

LABORATORY TECHNIQUES IN PGD

PGD at the single-cell level is a multistep, complex procedure. The various pitfalls outlined previously necessitate adequate calibration of the techniques employed to avoid misdiagnosis. Due to ethical limitations, single human blastomeres are difficult to obtain; therefore, different PGD centers have developed different protocols, and there is as yet no uniform method. Because of the numerous genetic disorders that are amenable to PGD, it is impossible to provide suitable protocols for all of them. Instead, some of the commonly used laboratory methods will be described in the following sections.

General safety measures

It is highly recommended that a physically separated site be used for template preparation, PCR assembly, and product analysis. The equipment and reagents used for single-cell PCR should be solely reserved for this purpose and should never be allowed to come into contact with previously amplified DNA samples. To avoid contamination, lab technicians should wear disposable outer clothing, caps, masks, shoe covers, and powder-free gloves that are kept in the room. In order to avoid external contamination from previously amplified DNA, some centers use a room kept under constant positive pressure. All equipment and required disposable supplies such as tubes, racks, and pipettes are to be kept in the room.

Glassware should be sterilized and aerosol-resistant pipette tips should be used. All reagents and solutions should be DNA free, sterilized by autoclaving, filtered through a 0.22 mM filter or by UV irradiation. All reagents should be prepared in a fume hood equipped with UV light. These safety measures, however, should not be considered as substitutes for efforts to avoid the possibility of external contamination occurring in the first place.

The PCR reagents should be rigorously tested prior to any clinical case to ensure that they have not become contaminated. It is recommended that all PCR reagents (minus Taq polymerase) be prepared in excess and aliquoted to reduce the amount of pipetting and sampling from the stock preparation. Sample aliquots may then be tested while the remainder is frozen until use.

To detect contamination in the analyzed sample, a negative control should be used consisting of all PCR reagents, substituting the template DNA or blastomere with an aliquot of the final blastomere wash buffer. To eliminate contamination by sperm, ICSI is employed.

The choice of positive controls

A variety of cells harboring the mutation of interest may be used as positive controls, such as buccal cells, cumulus cells, lymphocytes, or lymphoblasts. To reduce the chance of misdiagnosis due to ADO, it is possible to biopsy and analyze two blastomeres from the same embryo (12,14,84). The isolated single cells may also be used for calibration of the PGD techniques and for testing the precision, sensitivity, and reliability of the single-cell PCR strategy.

Buccal cells may be obtained from patients by mouthwashing with double-distilled water or by scraping the inside of the cheek with a sterile cotton swab and suspending the smear in phosphate-buffered saline (PBS). The suspension is centrifuged at 7.5 g for 5 minutes. The cell pellet is washed three times in PBS, and cells are resuspended and isolated using a pulled glass micropipette under an inverted microscope. Single cells are then washed several times in PBS microdrops to ensure that indeed only a single cell is aspirated and transferred to sterile PCR tubes for further use (85,86).

Cumulus cells may be obtained by incubating the retrieved oocyte in IVF culture medium supplemented with 80 IU hyaluronidase. Separated cumulus cells are then rinsed with IVF culture medium, washed in PBS, and transferred to sterile PCR tubes using a pulled glass micropipette under a stereomicroscope (33).

Lymphocytes may be isolated from peripheral blood by the Ficoll-Paque method, washed three times in PBS, resuspended, and diluted in culture medium on a glass slide. Individual cells are then selected using a pulled glass micropipette under an inverted microscope, washed three times in PCR buffer (50 mM KCl, 10 mM Tris-HCl, pH 8.3) supplemented with 0.01% polyvinylpyrrolidone (PVP), and transferred to sterile PCR tubes for further use. Lymphocytes may be used fresh or frozen–thawed. For freezing, lymphocytes are washed three times in PBS, resuspended in autologous plasma, and 20 μL of concentrated lymphocytes are added to 40 μL of fetal calf serum, 120 μL of RPMI 1640 Medium (Biological Industries Israel Beit-Haemek), and 20 μL of dimethyl sulfoxide (DMSO) and kept in liquid nitrogen until required. Cells can be stored for up to a year. Thawing is performed by several washes with culture medium (87).

A lymphoblast cell line carrying the known mutation is probably the best choice, since its establishment provides a perpetual source of cells with a known genetic composition. The cell line is achieved by transformation of peripheral blood lymphocytes with Epstein–Barr virus (88). Once the cell line is established, single cells may be aspirated and transferred to 1.5 mL Eppendorf tubes, washed three times with PBS, resuspended in 50 μL PBS, and kept at 4°C until use (89).

Embryonic cell isolation

Embryo biopsy is described in detail in Chapter 14. For the purpose of genetic analysis of the embryo, the single biopsied nucleated cells are washed several times in droplets of PCR buffer (50 mM KCl, 10 mM Tris-HCl, pH 8.3) supplemented with 0.01% PVP or 4 mg/mL bovine serum albumin (BSA) in a Petri dish using a pulled micropipette. PVP or BSA are used in order to prevent adherence of the cells to the pipette. The isolated cell is transferred in a minimal volume of washing buffer to a PCR tube containing lysis buffer or water, and can be frozen immediately at −80°C until use. Alternatively, the cells can be lysed immediately and then frozen (12,13,55,87,90,91).

Cell lysis

Lysis of the single embryonic cells and exposure of their genetic material to the PCR reagents is one of the most critical steps, and greatly affects ADO rates and the efficiency and reliability of PGD (18). Among several options, the three most commonly used lysis solutions are water, alkaline lysis buffer, and proteinase K/sodium dodecyl sulfate (SDS) buffer. There is as yet no consensus as to which is superior.

Water

Single blastomeres are washed three times in PBS transferred under visual control by pulled micropipettes to PCR tubes containing 60 μL biotechnology-grade water. An aliquot from the last washing droplet is added to a PCR tube containing 60 μL water, to serve as a negative control. Lysis is accomplished by two cycles of freezing in liquid nitrogen and thawing, and then boiling for 10 minutes. Lysates can be stored until use at −20°C (12).

Alkaline lysis buffer

Single cells are transferred as above to PCR tubes containing 5 μL alkaline lysis buffer (200 mM KOH and 50 mM dithiothreitol). For immediate use, samples are placed at −80°C for at least 30 minutes and undergo immediate lysis by incubation at 65°C for 10 minutes. Alternatively, samples may be immediately lysed, frozen, and stored (not longer than 1 week) at −80°C until further processing (87,92). After lysis, 5 μL neutralization buffer (300 mM/L KCl, 900 mM/L Tris-HCl, pH 8.3, 200 mM/L HCl) is added. Lysates are centrifuged briefly and placed on ice for immediate use or stored at −20°C until use (93).

Proteinase K/SDS buffer

Single blastomeres are washed three times in PBS or PCR buffers supplemented with 0.01% PVP or BSA and transferred individually to PCR tubes containing 5 μL proteinase K/SDS buffer (17 mM SDS and 400 ng/mL proteinase K) (85,94). Samples are incubated at 50°C for 1 hour followed by denaturation at 99°C for 15 minutes to inactivate the enzyme. Lysates can be stored at −80°C until use (57,86).

Primary and nested PCR conditions

For the primary PCR reaction, the following are mixed with the biopsied cell lysate to a final volume of 50 μL: PCR buffer (10 mM Tris-HCl, 50 mM KCl, and 2.5 mM $MgCl_2$, pH 8.3), 0.3 mM dNTP, 1–2 U Taq polymerase, and 0.5 mM outer primers. It is recommended to perform optimization of the reaction by using different $MgCl_2$ concentrations and different pH conditions. Amplification efficiency can be improved by addition of one or more of the following ingredients: glycerol, gelatin, betain, DMSO, $(NH_4)SO_4$, or detergent.

The PCR thermocycler program begins with a prolonged stage of initial denaturation at 95°C for 6 minutes. This has been shown to correlate with reductions in ADO rates (92). This is followed by 30 cycles of denaturation at 94°C for 1 minute, annealing at 52°C–65°C (according to the primer's melting temperature) for 1 minute, and extension at 72°C for 1 minute. Final extension at 72°C for 10 minutes is usually performed. The specificity of the reaction can be improved by using "hot start."

For secondary or nested PCR, 2–5 μL of the primary PCR product serves as the template to be used with the nested primers. In the nested PCR reaction, the duration and temperature of the initial denaturation step may be reduced and the $MgCl_2$ concentration can be lowered. DMSO is not required for this step. Other reagents and PCR conditions may be similar to those used in the primary PCR reaction (9,17).

Multiplex PCR

According to the standard protocol, each 50 μL reaction includes 1–1.5 U Taq polymerase, 0.3 mM for each dNTP, 0.5–2.5 mM $MgCl_2$, and 0.1–0.5 mM of each primer. The reaction's 10× PCR buffer is usually composed of 500 mM KCl and 100 mM Tris-HCl (pH 8.3), but at least one of the following ingredients is usually added: glycerol, gelatin, betain, DMSO, $(NH_4)SO_4$, or detergent. The PCR thermocycler program begins with initial denaturation at 96°C for 5 minutes (ensuring appropriate accessibility to the DNA strands). This is followed by 30 cycles at 94°C for 45 seconds, at 52°C–56°C for 60 seconds, and at 72°C for 60 seconds. Final extension of 5–15 minutes at 72°C is usually performed.

If ethidium bromide gel electrophoresis analysis is performed, nested PCR is usually required. After primary PCR is performed, a 2–5 μL aliquot of the product serves as the DNA template for the nested PCR reaction.

Primer extension preamplification

This method is based on multiple rounds of extensions using a random mixture of 15-base oligonucleotides as primers. Theoretically, the mixture contains up to 1×10^9 different primers. The PEP-PCR reaction in a final volume of 60 μL includes: 33 mM random primers, 10× PCR buffer (100 mM Tris-HCl, pH 8.3, 25 mM $MgCl_2$, 1 mg/mL gelatin, and 500 mM KCl), 0.1 mM dNTPs, and 5 U of Taq polymerase. The PCR buffer should be K^+-free if the cell was lysed by an alkaline lysis buffer. The reaction is carried out in 50 cycles of the following: denaturation at 92°C for 1 minute, annealing at 37°C for 2 minutes, a programmed ramping step of 10 seconds/°C until 55°C, and extension at 55°C for 4 minutes (32,33,37).

Improvement of amplification can be achieved by raising the denaturation temperature, elongating the denaturation period, raising the pH of the buffer from 8.3 to 8.8, modifying the $MgCl_2$ and gelatin concentrations, reducing the KCl concentration, and using a more thermostable DNA polymerase or one that has minimal exonuclease activity. Addition of glycerol, betain, BSA, detergents, spermidine, and $(NH_4)SO_4$ may also improve the product yield. Primers should be dissolved in Tris-HCl 5–10 mM (pH 8.3) and not in Tris-EDTA (TE) buffer to prevent the chelation of Mg^{2+} ions by ethylenediaminetetraacetic acid. The PEP-PCR product should produce an even smear on ethidium bromide gel electrophoresis. A 2–10 μL aliquot of the PEP product serves as the template for subsequent PCR reactions amplifying the mutation-containing fragment, linked polymorphic markers, and for sex determination.

Degenerated oligonucleotide-primed PCR

DOP-PCR is based on multiple rounds of extensions using a universal primer containing a 6 bp degenerate region representing all possible nucleotide combinations, flanked with GC-rich short sequences to improve hybridization to genomic DNA.

The DOP-PCR reaction mixture in a final volume of 100 μL contains 2.0 mM degenerated primers and 10× PCR buffer (100 mM Tris-HCl, pH 8.3, 25 mM $MgCl_2$, and 500 mM KCl [however, the buffer should be K^+-free if the cell was lysed by alkaline lysis buffer], 0.2 mM dNTPs, and 2.5 U Taq polymerase) (95). Thermal cycling conditions are as follows: prolonged initial denaturation step at 94°C for 9 minutes, then eight cycles of denaturation at 94°C for 1 minute, annealing at 30°C for 1.5 minutes, and extension at 72°C for 3 minutes, followed by 50 cycles of denaturation at 94°C for 1 minute, annealing at 62°C for 1 minute, and extension at 72°C for 1.5 minutes. Final extension is at 72°C for 8 minutes (21). As for PEP, amplification efficiency may be improved by adding and changing the reaction ingredients and by gradually increasing the extension time after the first 10 cycles.

Multiple displacement amplification

MDA is based on DNA amplification using a bacteriophage DNA polymerase and exonuclease-resistant, phosphorothioate-modified random hexamer oligonucleotide primers in an isothermal strand displacement reaction. It is achieved using bacteriophage Φ29 DNA polymerase, hexamer primers, and reaction buffer, according to the manufacturer's instructions (GenomiPhi v2 DNA Amplification Kit, GE Healthcare, Chicago, IL, USA or Repli-G Kit, Qiagen, Crawley, U.K.). The samples are incubated at 30°C for 2–6 hours, followed by a 3–10-minute incubation at 65°C to inactivate the enzyme. Amplified products can undergo subsequent diverse analyses, such as CGH.

Fluorescent PCR

Fluorescent PCR is performed in a final volume of 25 μL of 10× PCR buffer containing 15 mM $MgCl_2$ and 0.2 mM of each dNTP, as well as fluorescent-tagged primers at a final concentration of 0.05 mM. After a "hot-start," 0.6–1.5 U of Taq polymerase is added to the reaction mix. Initial denaturation is first performed at 95°C for 5 minutes, followed by 36 cycles of denaturation at 94°C for 60 seconds, annealing at 60°C for 60 seconds, and extension at 72°C for 60 seconds. The reaction is completed with a final extension at 70°C for 10 minutes. Due to its high sensitivity, nested PCR is usually not necessary (16,84,96).

Restriction enzyme digestion

For each different restriction enzyme, different conditions, such as buffer, temperature, and concentration, are specified in the commercially available kits. Some PCR reagents may interfere with the digestion reaction. To avoid this, PCR products can be purified by absorption of the DNA fragments onto glass fibers in the presence of chaotropic salts, then washed and eluted with a low-salt buffer or water. The isolated fragment may then be subjected to the restriction enzyme and buffer, incubated for 1–2 hours at 37°C, and resolved by electrophoresis on agarose or acrylamide gels.

Products detection

Ethidium bromide gel electrophoresis

An aliquot of the PCR products is applied onto an agarose or acrylamide gel containing 0.05% ethidium bromide and visualized under UV light. One lane is provided for a "DNA ladder" containing a mixture of DNA fragments of known sizes. This allows the determination of the size, presence, and a measure of quantity of the resulting fragments. This technique, however, is neither sensitive nor accurate because it does not detect PCR products if the amplification yield is low, nor does it allow for distinguishing between alleles differing in length by a few base pairs.

GeneScan

Following fluorescent PCR, size separation is performed on an acrylamide gel or using a capillary method, which is available in some sequencers. Fragment sizes are automatically determined for each PCR product. Each primer set is labeled with a different fluorescent marker; therefore, the products may be distinguished according to their specific emission wavelengths. The relative quantity of each PCR product may also be determined by the relative intensities of their fluorescence. Using a weight marker standard within each lane makes it possible to distinguish between products with a size difference of as little as 1–2 bp. The results are demonstrated as diagrams with colored peaks (12,16).

REFERENCES

1. Handyside AH, Kontogianni EH, Hardy K, Winston RM. Pregnancies from biopsied human preimplantation embryos sexed by Y-specific DNA amplification. *Nature* 1990; 344: 768–70.
2. Kastrinos F, Stoffel EM, Balmaña J, Syngal S. Attitudes toward prenatal genetic testing in patients with familial adenomatous polyposis. *Am J Gastroenterol* 2007; 102: 1284–90.
3. Menon U, Harper J, Sharma A, Fraser L, Burnell M, El Masry K, Rodeck C, Jacobs I. Views of BRCA gene mutation carriers on preimplantation genetic diagnosis as a reproductive option for hereditary breast and ovarian cancer. *Hum Reprod* 2007; 22: 1573–7.
4. Verlinsky Y, Rechitsky S, Schoolcraft W, Strom C, Kuliev A. Preimplantation diagnosis for Fanconi anemia combined with HLA matching. *JAMA* 2001; 285: 3130–3.
5. Traversa MV, Carey L, Leigh D. A molecular strategy for routine preimplantation genetic diagnosis in both reciprocal and Robertsonian translocation carriers. *Molecular Human Reproduction* 2010; 16: 329–337.
6. Alfarawati S, Fragouli E, Colls P, Wells D. First births after preimplantation genetic diagnosis of structural chromosome abnormalities using comparative genomic hybridization and microarray analysis. *Hum Reprod* 2011; 26: 1560–74.
7. Sermon K, Lissens W, Nagy ZP, Van Steirteghem A, Liebaers I. Simultaneous amplification of the two most frequent mutations of infantile Tay-Sachs disease in single blastomeres. *Hum Reprod* 1995; 10: 2214–7.
8. Kontogianni EH, Griffin DK, Handyside AH. Identifying the sex of human preimplantation embryos in X-linked disease: amplification efficiency of a Y-specific alphoid repeat from single blastomeres with two lysis protocols. *J Assist Reprod Genet* 1996; 13: 125–32.
9. Cui KH, Matthews CD. Nuclear structural conditions and PCR amplification in human preimplantation diagnosis. *Mol Hum Reprod* 1996; 2: 63–71.
10. Ray PF, Ao A, Taylor DM, Winston RM, Handyside AH. Assessment of the reliability of single blastomere analysis for preimplantation diagnosis of the delta F508 deletion causing cystic fibrosis in clinical practice. *Prenat Diagn* 1998; 18: 1402–12.
11. Grifo JA, Tang YX, Munne S, Alikani M, Cohen J, Rosenwaks Z. Healthy deliveries from biopsied human embryos. *Hum Reprod* 1994; 9: 912–6.
12. Findlay I, Ray P, Quirke P, Rutherford A, Lilford R. Allelic drop-out and preferential amplification in single cells and human blastomeres: Implications for preimplantation diagnosis of sex and cystic fibrosis. *Hum Reprod* 1995; 10: 1609–18.
13. Ray PF, Handyside AH. Increasing the denaturation temperature during the first cycles of amplification reduces allele dropout from single cells for preimplantation genetic diagnosis. *Mol Hum Reprod* 1996; 2:213–8.
14. Ao A, Wells D, Handyside AH, Winston RM, Delhanty JD. Preimplantation genetic diagnosis of inherited cancer: Familial adenomatous polyposis coli. *J Assist Reprod Genet* 1998; 15: 140–4.
15. Rechitsky S, Strom C, Verlinsky O, Amet T, Ivakhnenko V, Kukharenko V, Kuliev A, Verlinsky Y. Allele dropout in polar bodies and blastomeres. *J Assist Reprod Genet* 1998; 15: 253–7.
16. Sherlock J, Cirigliano V, Petrou M, Tutschek B, Adinolfi M. Assessment of diagnostic quantitative fluorescent multiplex polymerase chain reaction assays performed on single cells. *Ann Hum Genet* 1998; 62: 9–23.
17. Dreesen JC, Bras M, de Die-Smulders C, Dumoulin JC, Cobben JM, Evers JL, Smeets HJ, Geraedts JP. Preimplantation genetic diagnosis of spinal muscular atrophy. *Mol Hum Reprod* 1998; 4: 881–5.
18. El-Hashemite N, Delhanty JD. A technique for eliminating allele specific amplification failure during DNA amplification of heterozygous cells for preimplantation diagnosis. *Mol Hum Reprod* 1997; 3: 975–8.
19. Harper JC, Coonen E, Handyside AH, Winston RM, Hopman AH, Delhanty JD. Mosaicism of autosomes and sex chromosomes in morphologically normal, monospermic preimplantation human embryos. *Prenat Diagn* 1995; 15: 41–9.
20. Sermon K, De Vos A, Van de Velde H, Seneca S, Lissens W, Joris H, Vandervorst M, Van Steirteghem A, Liebaers I. Fluorescent PCR and automated fragment analysis for the clinical application of

preimplantation genetic diagnosis of myotonic dystrophy (Steinert's disease). *Mol Hum Reprod* 1998; 4: 791–6.

21. Wells D, Sherlock JK. Strategies for preimplantation genetic diagnosis of single gene disorders by DNA amplification. *Prenat Diagn* 1998; 18: 1389–401.
22. Eggerding FA. A one-step coupled amplification and oligonucleotide ligation procedure for multiplex genetic typing. *PCR Methods Appl* 1995; 4: 337–45.
23. Blake D, Tan SL, Ao A. Assessment of multiplex fluorescent PCR for screening single cells for trisomy 21 and single gene defects. *Mol Hum Reprod* 1999; 5: 1166–75.
24. Kuliev A, Rechitsky S, Verlinsky O, Ivakhnenko V, Evsikov S, Wolf G, Angastiniotis M, Georghiou D, Kukharenko V, Strom C et al. Preimplantation diagnosis of thalassemias. *J Assist Reprod Genet* 1998; 15: 219–25.
25. Wells D. Advances in preimplantation genetic diagnosis. *Eur J Obstet Gynecol Reprod Biol* 2004; 115: S97–101.
26. Fragouli E. Preimplantation genetic diagnosis: present and future. *J Assist Reprod Genet* 2007; 24: 201–7.
27. Xu K, Shi ZM, Veeck LL, Hughes MR, Rosenwaks Z. First unaffected pregnancy using preimplantation genetic diagnosis for sickle cell anemia. *JAMA* 1999; 281: 1701–6.
28. Hattori M, Yoshioka K, Sakaki Y. High-sensitive fluorescent DNA sequencing and its application for detection and mass-screening of point mutations. *Electrophoresis* 1992; 13: 560–5.
29. Mansfield ES. Diagnosis of Down syndrome and other aneuploidies using quantitative polymerase chain reaction and small tandem repeat polymorphisms. *Hum Mol Genet* 1993; 2: 43–50.
30. Ferre F. Quantitative or semi-quantitative PCR: Reality versus myth. *PCR Methods Appl* 1992; 2: 1–9.
31. Verma L, Macdonald F, Leedham P, McConachie M, Dhanjal S, Hulten M. Rapid and simple prenatal DNA diagnosis of Down's syndrome. *Lancet* 1998; 352: 9–12.
32. Zhang L, Cui X, Schmitt K, Hubert R, Navidi W, Arnheim N. Whole genome amplification from a single cell: Implications for genetic analysis. *Proc Natl Acad Sci USA* 1992; 89: 5847–51.
33. Paunio T, Reima I, Syvanen AC. Preimplantation diagnosis by whole-genome amplification, PCR amplification, and solid-phase minisequencing of blastomere DNA. *Clin Chem* 1996; 42: 1382–90.
34. Sermon K, Lissens W, Joris H, Van Steirteghem A, Liebaers I. Adaptation of the primer extension preamplification (PEP) reaction for preimplantation diagnosis: single blastomere analysis using short PEP protocols. *Mol Hum Reprod* 1996; 2: 209–12.
35. Tsai YH. Cost-effective one-step PCR amplification of cystic fibrosis delta F508 fragment in a single cell for preimplantation genetic diagnosis. *Prenat Diagn* 1999; 19: 1048–51.
36. Snabes MC, Chong SS, Subramanian SB, Kristjansson K, DiSepio D, Hughes MR. Preimplantation single-cell analysis of multiple genetic loci by whole-genome amplification. *Proc Natl Acad Sci USA* 1994; 91: 6181–5.
37. Kristjansson K, Chong SS, Van den Veyver IB, Subramanian S, Snabes MC, Hughes MR. Preimplantation single cell analyses of dystrophin gene deletions using whole genome amplification. *Nat Genet* 1994; 6: 19–23.
38. Telenius H, Carter NP, Bebb CE, Nordenskjöld M, Ponder BA, Tunnacliffe A. Degenerate oligonucleotide-primed PCR: General amplification of target DNA by a single degenerate primer. *Genomics* 1992; 13: 718–25.
39. Voullaire L, Wilton L, Slater H, Williamson R. Detection of aneuploidy in single cells using comparative genomic hybridization. *Prenat Diagn* 1999; 19: 846–51.
40. Dean FB, Hosono S, Fang L, Wu X, Faruqi AF, Bray-Ward P, Sun Z, Zong Q, Du Y, Du J et al. Comprehensive human genome amplification using multiple displacement amplification. *Proc Natl Acad Sci USA* 2002; 99: 5261–6.
41. Spits C, Le Caignec C, De Rycke M, Van Haute L, Van Steirteghem A, Liebaers I, Sermon K. Whole-genome multiple displacement amplification from single cells. *Nat Protoc* 2006; 1: 1965–70.
42. Lage JM, Leamon JH, Pejovic T, Hamann S, Lacey M, Dillon D, Segraves R, Vossbrinck B, González A, Pinkel D et al. Whole Genome Analysis of Genetic Alterations in Small DNA Samples Using Hyperbranched Strand Displacement Amplification and Array-CGH. *Genome Res* 2003; 13: 294–307.
43. Hughes S, Lim G, Beheshti B, Bayani J, Marrano P, Huang A, Squire JA. Use of whole genome amplification and comparative genomic hybridisation to detect chromosomal copy number alterations in cell line material and tumour tissue. *Cytogenet Genome Res* 2004; 105: 18–24.
44. Cheung VG, Nelson SF. Whole genome amplification using a degenerate oligonucleotide primer allows hundreds of genotypes to be performed on less than one nanogram of genomic DNA. *Proc Natl Acad Sci USA* 1996; 93: 14676–9.
45. Telenius H, Pelmear AH, Tunnacliffe A, Carter NP, Behmel A, Ferguson-Smith MA, Nordenskjold M, Pfragner R, Ponder BA. Cytogenetic analysis by chromosome painting using DOP-PCR amplified flow-sorted chromosomes. *Genes Chromosomes Cancer* 1992; 4: 257–63.
46. Coskun S, Alsmadi O. Whole genome amplification from a single cell: A new era for preimplantation genetic diagnosis. *Prenat Diagn* 2007; 27: 297–302.

47. Blanco L, Bernad A, Lazaro JM, Martin G, Garmendia C, and Salas M. Highly efficient DNA synthesis by the phage phi 29 DNA polymerase. Symmetrical mode of DNA replication. *J Biol Chem* 1989; 264: 8935–8940.
48. Rodríguez I, Lázaro JM, Blanco L, Kamtekar S, Berman AJ, Wang J, Steitz TA, Salas M, de Vega M. A specific subdomain in phi29 DNA polymerase confers both processivity and strand-displacement capacity. *Proc Natl Acad Sci USA* 2005; 102: 6407–12.
49. Hellani, A., Coskun, S., Benkhalifa, M., Tbakhi, A., Sakati, N., Al-Odaib, A., Ozand, P. Multiple displacement amplification on single cell and possible PGD applications. *Mol Hum Reprod* 2004; 10: 847–52.
50. Handyside AH, Robinson MD, Simpson RJ, Omar MB, Shaw MA, Grudzinskas JG, Rutherford A. Isothermal whole genome amplification from single and small numbers of cells: A new era for preimplantation genetic diagnosis of inherited disease. *Mol Hum Reprod* 2004; 10: 767–72.
51. Renwick PJ, Trussler J, Ostad-Saffari E, Fassihi H, Black C, Braude P, Ogilvie CM, Abbs S. Proof of principle and first cases using preimplantation genetic haplotyping—A paradigm shift for embryo diagnosis. *Reprod Biomed Online* 2006; 13: 110–9.
52. Pickering SJ, McConnell JM, Johnson MH, Braude PR. Use of a polymorphic dinucleotide repeat sequence to detect non-blastomeric contamination of the polymerase chain reaction in biopsy samples for preimplantation diagnosis. *Hum Reprod* 1994; 9: 1539–45.
53. Harton GL, Tsipouras P, Sisson ME, Starr KM, Mahoney BS, Fugger EF, Schulman JD, Kilpatrick MW, Levinson G, Black SH. Preimplantation genetic testing for Marfan syndrome. *Mol Hum Reprod* 1996; 2: 713–5.
54. Lee SH, Kwak IP, Cha KE, Park SE, Kim NK, Cha KY. Preimplantation diagnosis of non-deletion Duchenne muscular dystrophy (DMD) by linkage polymerase chain reaction analysis. *Mol Hum Reprod* 1998; 4: 345–9.
55. Sermon K, Lissens W, Joris H, Seneca S, Desmyttere S, Devroey P, Van Steirteghem A, Liebaers I. Clinical application of preimplantation diagnosis for myotonic dystrophy. *Prenat Diagn* 1997; 17: 925–32.
56. Daniels R, Holding C, Kontogianni E, Monk M. Single-cell analysis of unstable genes. *J Assist Reprod Genet* 1996; 13: 163–9.
57. El-Hashemite N, Wells D, Delhanty JD. Single cell detection of beta-thalassemia mutations using silver stained SSCP analysis: An application for preimplantation diagnosis. *Mol Hum Reprod* 1997; 3: 693–8.
58. Vrettou C, Palmer G, Kanavakis E, Tzetis M, Antoniadi T, Mastrominas M, Traeger-Synodinos J. A widely applicable strategy for single cell genotyping of beta-thalassaemia mutations using DGGE analysis: Application to preimplantation genetic diagnosis. *Prenat Diagn* 1999; 19: 1209–16.
59. Kanavakis E, Vrettou C, Palmer G, Tzetis M, Mastrominas M, Traeger-Synodinos J. Preimplantation genetic diagnosis in 10 couples at risk for transmitting beta-thalassaemia major: Clinical experience including the initiation of six singleton pregnancies. *Prenat Diagn* 1999; 19: 1217–22.
60. Scobie G, Woodroffe B, Fishel S, Kalsheker N. Identification of the five most common cystic fibrosis mutations in single cells using a rapid and specific differential amplification system. *Mol Hum Reprod* 1996; 2: 203–7.
61. Bermudez, M.G., Piyamongkol W, Tomaz s, Dudman E, Sherlock JK, Wells D. Single-cell sequencing and mini-sequencing for preimplantation genetic diagnosis. *Prenat. Diagn* 2003; 23: 669–677.
62. Hassold T, Chen N, Funkhouser J, Jooss T, Manuel B, Matsuura J, Matsuyama A, Wilson C, Yamane JA, Jacobs PA. 1980 A cytogenetic study of 1000 spontaneous abortions. *Ann Hum Genet* 1980; 44: 151–78.
63. Chandley AC. Infertility and chromosome abnormality. *Oxf Rev Reprod Biol* 1984; 6: 1–46.
64. Jacobs PA. The chromosome complement of human gametes. *Oxf Rev Reprod Biol* 1992; 14: 47–72.
65. Kallioniemi A, Kallioniemi OP, Sudar D, Rutovitz D, Gray JW, Waldman F, Pinkel D. Comparative genomic hybridization for molecular cytogenetic analysis of solid tumors. *Science* 1992; 258: 818–21.
66. Wells D, Delhanty JD. Comprehensive chromosomal analysis of human preimplantation embryos using whole genome amplification and single cell comparative genomic hybridization. *Mol Hum Reprod* 2000; 6: 1055–62.
67. Voullaire L, Slater H, Williamson R and Wilton L. Chromosome analysis of blastomeres from human embryos by using comparative genomic hybridization. *Hum Genet* 2000; 106: 210–217.
68. Wilton L, Williamson R, McBain J, Edgar D, Voullaire L. Birth of a healthy infant after preimplantation confirmation of euploidy by comparative genomic hybridization. *N Engl J Med* 2001; 345: 1537–41.
69. Wells D, Escudero T, Levy B, Hirschhorn K, Delhanty JD, Munné S. First clinical application of comparative genomic hybridization and polar body testing for preimplantation genetic diagnosis of aneuploidy. *Fertil Steril* 2002; 78: 543–9.
70. Fragouli E, Wells D, Thornhill A, Serhal P, Faed MJ, Harper JC, Delhanty JD. Comparative genomic hybridization analysis of human oocytes and polar bodies. *Hum Reprod* 2006; 21: 2319–28.
71. Le Caignec C, Spits C, Sermon K, De Rycke M, Thienpont B, Debrock S, Staessen C, Moreau Y, Fryns JP, Van Steirteghem A et al. Single-cell chromosomal

imbalances detection by array CGH. *Nucleic Acids Res* 2006; 34: e68.

72. Wilton L. Preimplantation genetic diagnosis and chromosome analysis of blastomeres using comparative genomic hybridization. *Hum Reprod Update* 2005; 11: 33–41.
73. Bejjani BA, Shaffer LG. Application of array-based comparative genomic hybridization to clinical diagnostics. *J Mol Diagn* 2006; 8: 528–33.
74. Hu DG, Webb G, Hussey N. Aneuploidy detection in single cells using DNA array-based comparative genomic hybridization. *Mol Hum Reprod* 2004; 10: 283–9.
75. Fiorentino F, Bono S, Biricik A, Nuccitelli A, Cotroneo E, Cottone G, Kokocinski F, Michel CE, Minasi MG, Greco E. Application of next-generation sequencing technology for comprehensive aneuploidy screening of blastocysts in clinical preimplantation genetic screening cycles. *Hum Reprod* 2014; 29:2802–13.
76. Yang Z, Lin J, Zhang J, Fong WI, Li P, Zhao R, Liu X, Podevin W, Kuang Y, Liu J. Randomized comparison of next-generation sequencing and array comparative genomic hybridization for preimplantation genetic screening: A pilot study. *BMC Med Genomics* 2015 Jun 23; 8:30.
77. Konstantinidis M, Prates R, Goodall NN, Fischer J, Tecson V, Lemma T, Chu B, Jordan A, Armenti E, Wells D et al. Live births following Karyomapping of human blastocysts: Experience from clinical application of the method. *Reprod Biomed Online* 2015; 31: 394–403.
78. Wells D, Alfarawati S, Fragouli E. Use of comprehensive chromosomal screening for embryo assessment: microarrays and CGH. *Mol Hum Reprod* 2008; 4: 703–10.
79. Basille C, Frydman R, El Aly A, Hesters L, Fanchin R, Tachdjian G, Steffann J, LeLorc'h M, Achour-Frydman N. Preimplantation genetic diagnosis: state of the art. *Eur J Obstet Gynecol Reprod Biol* 2009; 45: 9–13.
80. Handyside AH, Harton GL, Mariani B, Thornhill AR, Affara N, Shaw MA, Griffin DK. Karyomapping: A universal method for genome wide analysis of genetic disease based on mapping crossovers between parental haplotypes. *J Med Genet* 2010; 47: 651–8.
81. Natesan SA, Bladon AJ, Coskun S, Qubbaj W, Prates R, Munne S, Coonen E, Dreesen JC, Stevens SJ, Paulussen AD et al. Genome-wide karyomapping accurately identifies the inheritance of single-gene defects in human preimplantation embryos in vitro. *Genet Med* 2014; 16: 838–45.
82. Thornhill AR, Handyside AH, Ottolini C, Natesan SA, Taylor J, Sage K, Harton G, Cliffe K, Affara N, Konstantinidis M et al. Karyomapping-a comprehensive means of simultaneous monogenic and cytogenetic PGD: Comparison with standard approaches in real time for Marfan syndrome. *J Assist Reprod Genet* 2015; 32: 347–56.
83. Giménez C, Sarasa J, Arjona C, Vilamajó E, Martínez-Pasarell O, Wheeler K. et al. Karyomapping allows preimplantation genetic diagnosis of a de-novo deletion undetectable using conventional PGD technology. *Reprod Biomed Online* 2015; 31: 770–5.
84. Findlay I, Quirke P, Hall J, Rutherford A. Fluorescent PCR: A new technique for PGD of sex and single-gene defects *J Assist Reprod Genetics* 1996; 13: 96–103.
85. Holding C, Bentley D, Roberts R, Bobrow M, Mathew C. Development and validation of laboratory procedures for preimplantation diagnosis of Duchenne muscular dystrophy. *J Med Genet* 1993; 30: 903–9.
86. Ioulianos A, Wells D, Harper JC, Delhanty JD. A successful strategy for preimplantation diagnosis of medium-chain acyl-CoA dehydrogenase (MCAD) deficiency. *Prenat Diagn* 2000; 20: 593–8.
87. Hussey ND, Donggui H, Froiland DA, Hussey DJ, Haan EA, Matthews CD, Craig JE. Analysis of five Duchenne muscular dystrophy exons and gender determination using conventional duplex polymerase chain reaction on single cells. *Mol Hum Reprod* 1999; 5: 1089–94.
88. Ventura M, Gibaud A, Le Pendu J, Hillaire D, Gérard G, Vitrac D, Oriol R. Use of a simple method for the Epstein-Barr virus transformation of lymphocytes from members of large families of Réunion Island. *Hum Hered* 1998; 38: 36–43.
89. Van de Velde H, Sermon K, De Vos A, Lissens W, Joris H, Vandervorst M, Van Steirteghem A, Liebaers I. Fluorescent PCR and automated fragment analysis in preimplantation genetic diagnosis for 21-hydroxylase deficiency in congenital adrenal hyperplasia. *Mol Hum Reprod* 1999: 5: 691–6.
90. Salido EC, Yen PH, Koprivinkar K, Yu LC, Shapiro LJ. The human enamel protein gene amelogenin is expressed from both X and Y chromosomes. *Am J Hum Genet* 1992; 50: 303–316.
91. Ao A, Handyside AH. Cleavage stage human embryo biopsy. *Hum Reprod Update* 1995; 1:3.
92. Ao A, Ray P, Harper J, Lesko J, Paraschos T, Atkinson G, Soussis I, Taylor D, Handyside A, Hughes M et al. Clinical experience with preimplantation genetic diagnosis of cystic fibrosis (delta F508). *Prenat Diagn* 1996; 16: 137–42.
93. Cui XF, Li HH, Goradia TM, Lange K, Kazazian HHJr, Galas D, Arnheim N. Single-sperm typing: Determination of genetic distance between the G gamma-globin and parathyroid hormone loci by using the polymerase chain reaction and allele-specific oligomers. *Proc Natl Acad Sci USA* 1989; 86: 9389–93.
94. Han S, Zhong XY, Troeger C, Burgemeister R, Gloning K, and Holzgreve W. Current application of single-cell PCR. *Cell Mul Life Sci* 2000; 57: 96–105.

95. Wells D, Sherlock JK, Handyside AH, Delhanty JD. Detailed chromosomal and molecular genetic analysis of single cells by whole genome amplification and comparative genomic hybridization. *Nucleic Acids Res* 1999; 27: 1214–8.

96. Findlay and Quirke Fluorescent polymerase chain reaction: Part I. A new method allowing genetic diagnosis and DNA fingerprinting of single cells. *Human Reprod Update* 1996; 2: 137–152.

Diagnosis of endometrial receptivity and the embryo–endometrial dialog

29

FRANCISCO DOMÍNGUEZ, MARIA RUIZ-ALONSO, FELIPE VILELLA, and CARLOS SIMÓN

INTRODUCTION

The human endometrium is a complex tissue, predominantly composed of epithelial and stromal cells, that is cyclically and primarily regulated by steroid hormones (estrogens and progesterone). Endometrial receptivity is a self-limited period during which the endometrium transiently transforms to acquire the ability to receive a blastocyst and support implantation, a process that is mediated by immune cells, cytokines, growth factors, chemokines, adhesion molecules, and many other compounds (1–3). This transient period, called the window of implantation (WOI), has been postulated to open five days after endogenous or exogenous progesterone action and to close two days later (4,5). A receptive endometrium and a functionally normal blastocyst, as well as an exquisitely coordinated cross-communication between them, are required for implantation, the process by which the embryo attaches and invades the underlying maternal endometrial tissue.

Despite increasing interest in the regulation of endometrial receptivity, the role of the endometrium in successful implantation remains incompletely understood. During the WOI, the endometrium acquires the receptive phenotype, which involves both morphological and molecular changes such as plasma membrane transformation (6). Pinopodes, or epithelial protrusions, are also formed during this period (7), but their functional role is questioned (8). Although hundreds of biochemical molecules have been proposed as markers of endometrial receptivity—such as cytokines and their receptors (9), adhesion molecules and their receptors, cyclins (10–12), and classical hormonal receptors (13–15)—none has been clinically consolidated into a diagnostic tool (15). Thus, we still rely on inmunohistochemistry of the endometrial tissue based on the work of Noyes and colleagues in the 1950s. However, the dawn of the new "omics" (genomics, proteomics, lipidomics, and secretomics) techniques and the interrogation of the vast amount of data obtained with complex bioinformatics could advance our understanding of the black box that is endometrial receptivity.

In this chapter, we will discuss how to molecularly characterize and diagnose endometrial receptivity using a transcriptomic approach, and we will place emphasis on its clinical translation by means of the endometrial receptivity array (ERA) test. Later, we will focus on the embryo–endometrial dialog, with special attention on the proteomics, secretomics, and lipidomics of the human endometrium and the novel development of noninvasive biomarkers of endometrial receptivity in endometrial fluid.

MOLECULAR DIAGNOSIS OF UTERINE RECEPTIVITY

The molecular approach leads to an objective evaluation of the endometrium. At this level, many different molecules have been proposed as endometrial receptivity markers. However, none of them has had clinical applicability, probably due to attempts aiming to simplify a complex process into a single molecule (16). On the other hand, transcriptomics enables identification of a specific gene expression profile of a tissue under concrete conditions or treatments, providing a holistic view to address endometrial diagnosis (17). Several studies have assessed endometrial transcriptomes using microarray technology (reviewed by Díaz-Gimeno et al. [17] and Altmae et al. [18]). Early studies sought to identify genes that are differentially expressed between endometrial stages, revealing the existence of specific expression profiles for each stage (19–22). Further, focusing on the mid-secretory phase when the WOI opens has revealed upregulation of genes involved in processes of cell communication and cell adhesion, among others.

The goal of applying transcriptomic analysis to endometrial evaluation has been to develop an objective test that enables classification of endometrial receptivity for the synchronization of embryo transfer (23,24). These studies have resulted in one clinical application, the ERA, a customized microarray covering 238 genes that are differentially expressed between receptive and non-receptive endometria (17,25). This molecular test has revealed the necessity of personalizing embryo transfer according to the endometrial evolution during the menstrual cycle. In particular, some patients with recurrent implantation failure (RIF) exhibit a displacement of their WOI, which is advanced or delayed compared to the timing in the cycle during which it has classically been thought to be open (26). Once the WOI has been located, a personalized embryo transfer (pET) can be performed by synchronizing the ready-to-implant embryo with an endometrium that sends the proper signals to allow implantation (Figure 29.1). Synchronization depends on the timing of progesterone exposition, since not all women respond in the same way to similar progesterone dosages. This finding promotes a significant improvement in the clinical process; molecular evaluation of the endometrium can resolve RIF by correcting the day on which the embryo must be transferred. For example, in the study by Ruiz-Alonso et al. (26),

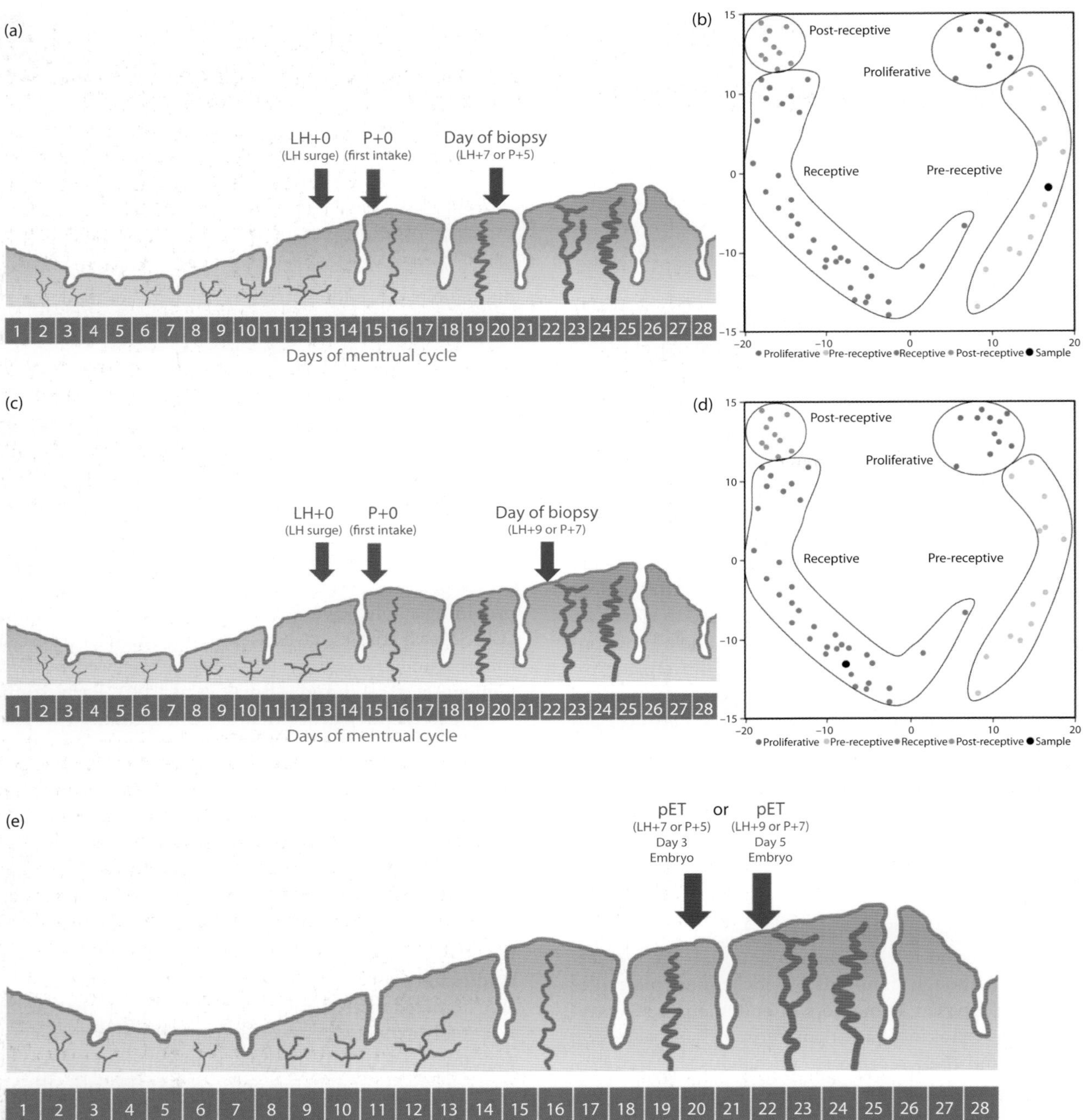

Figure 29.1 Endometrial receptivity array procedure. (a) First biopsy taken seven days after LH surge in a natural cycle or five days after the first intake of progesterone in a hormone replacement therapy cycle. (b) Principal component analysis (PCA) shows a pre-receptive profile. (c) Second biopsy taken in a new menstrual cycle, following the recommendation, two days after the first and under the same conditions (type of cycle). (d) PCA shows a receptive profile after the second biopsy. (e) pET must be done on the same day and under the same conditions as the biopsy with a "receptive" result. *Abbreviation*: LH, luteinizing hormone; P, progesterone; pET, personalized embryo transfer.

25.9% of RIF patients had a displaced WOI. In those cases, pET was performed on the day of the cycle in which a second ERA test obtained a receptive result, resulting in a 50% pregnancy rate (PR) and a 39% implantation rate (IR). A description of such patients is published in a recent case report (27), which presents the clinical history of a woman with seven failed embryo transfers in a pre-receptive endometrium (at P+5 [5 days after progesterone administration]). Once the WOI was discovered to begin two days later (P+7), pET resulted in healthy twins born alive (27).

The sensitivity and specificity of pET in the clinic have been calculated. Considering non-receptivity as the "positive" condition and receptivity as the "negative" one, the clinical outcomes were determined after routine embryo

Table 29.1 Clinical outcomes and efficiency of personalized embryo transfer according to endometrial receptivity array diagnosis

Clinical outcome	NR (52)	R (205)
IR first attempt	13% (12/90)	45% (161/355)
IR total attempts	10% (17/174)	41% (182/441)
PR first attempt	23% (12/52)	60% (123/205)
PR total attempts	17% (17/100)	55% (140/253)
OPR first attempt	0% (0/12)	74% (91/123)
OPR total attempts	0% (0/100)	74% (103/140)
Clinical efficiency	Positive (52)	Negative (205)
True	40	123
False	12	82
Sensitivity (TP / TP + FN)	0.33	
Specificity (TN / TN + FP)	0.91	
PPV (TP / TP + FP)	0.77	
NPV (TN / TN + FN)	0.60	

Abbreviations: FN, false negative; FP, false positive; IR, implantation rate; NPV, negative predictive value; NR, non-receptive; OPR, ongoing pregnancy rate; PPV, positive predictive value; PR, pregnancy rate; R, receptive; TN, true negative; TP, true positive.

transfer or pET, respectively (Table 29.1). A total of 257 patients was analyzed; 80% were receptive (n = 205) and 20% were non-receptive (n = 52). The specificity was 0.91, indicating that most of the patients that achieved pregnancy had embryo transfer to a receptive endometrium. On the other hand, sensitivity was 0.33, indicating that, even with a receptive endometrium, implantation was not always achieved. This likely resulted from the multifactorial nature of the implantation process. Finally, the positive predictive value was 0.77, while the negative predictive value was 0.60 (28). These data highlight the clinical relevance of the endometrial factor and how the molecular approach can help overcome infertility by correcting for a desynchronized embryo transfer, allowing higher PRs and IRs.

THE EMBRYO–ENDOMETRIAL DIALOG

The implantation process represents the first major physical embryo–maternal interaction, requiring synchronized, bidirectional communication, followed by adhesion and subsequent invasion of the decidualized uterine stroma (29). The WOI appears to play a critical role in establishing this bidirectional communication.

The knowledge of the signaling pathways that mediate human preimplantation embryo development and the embryo–maternal dialog has gradually improved (6,30–32); however, many parts of the process remain unknown. Human preimplantation embryos are programmed to produce soluble proteins, receptors, and other molecules that act as autocrine and paracrine factors. *In vitro* studies show that known levels of such factors can elicit changes in embryo developmental phenotypes. By inference, embryo development should respond to soluble factors of maternal origin by regulating proliferation, differentiation, adhesion, and invasiveness (33).

A range of ligands (mainly cytokines and growth factors) and their receptors are produced by the human endometrium during the receptive phase (34). At the same time, the receptive endometrium is "aware" of the embryo, modulating local immune responses to embryo-specific factors. A hypothetical embryo–maternal "cross-talk" or molecular dialog is therefore postulated to exist during the peri-implantation period. These signaling pathways are highly complex, often described as regulatory "circuits" (35).

Recently, evidence has emerged to support the existence of cross-talk between the mother and the embryo. Endometrial cells secrete exosome-associated microRNAs (miRNAs) into the endometrial fluid, where they can be internalized by the embryo and modify its transcriptome (36). miRNAs are short, 21–25-nucleotide RNA molecules that can regulate gene expression at a post-transcriptional level through degradation, repression, or silencing (37–39). A single miRNA can regulate up to hundreds of mRNA targets via the establishment of a perfect or imperfect complementation with the 3′-untranslated regions of their target transcripts (40). Four miRNAs have been identified as being regulated in receptive endometrium (miR-30b, miR-30d, miR-494, and miR-923) at the time of implantation. In particular, miR-30b and miR-30d are up-regulated, whereas miR-494 and miR-923 are down-regulated in receptive endometrium (41).

Our laboratory took a step forward in studying the role of miR-30d as a transcriptomic modifier of the preimplantation embryo. Specifically, we observed that, before its release into the endometrial fluid, miR-30d is incorporated into exosomes secreted by human endometrial epithelial cells. Exosomes are nanoscale-sized, phospholipid bilayer-enclosed particles (50–120 nm in diameter) actively released from cells into the extracellular space and body fluid under physiological and pathological conditions (42). Exosomes contain not only proteins and bioactive lipids, but also mRNAs, cytokines, growth factors, miRNAs, and double-stranded or genomic DNA (33,43–47). We found that exosomes secreted into the endometrial fluid contain miR-30d and can be taken up by trophectoderm cells of murine embryos, which triggers indirect over-expression of certain genes involved in embryo adhesion (i.e., *Itgb3*, *Itga7*, and *Cdh5*) (36). These results not only demonstrate the up-regulation of miR-30d in endometrial fluid during the WOI, but also describe a novel cell-to-cell communication mechanism involving the delivery of endometrial miRNAs from the maternal endometrium to the preimplantation embryo.

PROTEOMICS, SECRETOMICS, AND LIPIDOMICS OF ENDOMETRIAL RECEPTIVITY

To develop a complete view of endometrial receptivity, we must advance beyond transcriptomics; indeed, proteomics should be considered the next step in the study of biological systems (48). Proteomic analyses reflect what is really happening in the tissue at the cellular level, and a global study of the proteomics of the endometrium will reveal the molecular changes that occur in the endometrium. Several attempts have been made to determine the proteomic patterns of the human endometrium. DeSouza et al. (49) employed the first quantitative approximation to assess the proteome using isotope-coded affinity tags, affinity purification, and liquid chromatography coupled online with mass spectrometry. Later, Parmar et al. (50) published a prospective study identifying proteins with differential expression throughout the menstrual cycle. Our group also investigated the proteomics of endometrial receptivity by comparing the pre-receptive versus the receptive human endometrium proteome (51). In this study, endometrial biopsies were obtained from the same fertile woman in the same menstrual cycle. Protein extracts were analyzed using two-dimensional fluorescence difference gel electrophoresis and matrix-assisted laser desorption/ionization time-of-flight mass spectrometry. The results show 32 differentially expressed proteins in the receptive versus the pre-receptive endometrium, highlighting two proteins, Annexin A2 and Stathmin 1 (52). These cytoskeleton-related proteins display consistent opposite regulation in the receptive versus the pre-receptive endometrium and seem to play important roles in acquiring endometrial receptivity. This finding is not surprising since the receptive phenotype is associated with the remodeling of epithelial organization, primarily as a result of the disruption of the cytoskeleton in response to hormones (32).

Having established the ERA test for identifying the endometrial WOI, we applied a new proteomic approach to explore the protein content of endometria that have been diagnosed with the ERA test. We assessed whether any proteomic differences existed between receptive and non-receptive ERA-diagnosed endometria obtained on the same day of a hormone-replacement therapy treatment cycle (53). In this study, we detected 24 differentially expressed proteins in receptive versus non-receptive samples. *In silico* analysis identified several pathways and protein networks (Figure 29.2) that differ significantly between phenotypes, highlighting two proteins, PGRMC1 (a non-classical progesterone receptor) and ANXA6 (a transmembrane protein associated with cytoskeleton reorganization). Using this *in silico* approach, we were able to develop a complex proteomic signature of endometrial receptivity (53).

Proteomic and lipidomic techniques have also been used to analyze endometrial fluid to study endometrial receptivity. Endometrial fluid is a complex biological fluid secreted by the endometrial glands to provide nutrients for blastocyst survival and constitutes the microenvironment in which the embryo–endometrial dialog occurs before implantation (10,13,14). The advantage of working with endometrial fluid is that it can be collected easily and painlessly by aspiration using noninvasive methods (15). Furthermore, endometrial secretions are less complex compared to other biological fluids such as blood or urine in terms of their protein repertoire, and may serve as a pool of biomarkers for functional endometrium assessment.

Endometrial secretion has been shown to contain products of apoptotic epithelial cells, proteins originating from the transudation of serum, and proteins secreted from the glandular epithelium. This secretion undergoes significant changes in protein content during the transition from the proliferative phase to the secretory phase (54). Further, the endometrial secretion composition varies during the menstrual cycle as a result of changes in ovarian steroid serum concentration (55). In the past, protein variations in uterine secretions throughout the menstrual cycle were analyzed by electrophoresis. These studies revealed three different protein patterns that are typical of the phases of the menstrual cycle: intermediate phase, proliferative phase, and secretory phase. The results present characteristic “families” of protein bands corresponding to 63 proteins, some of which were identified by their molecular weight (56).

In another work (57), endometrial fluid obtained transcervically by aspiration immediately before embryo transfer was analyzed, and the protein profile in each sample was determined. These studies also demonstrated that endometrial secretion can be obtained for analysis immediately before embryo transfer in *in vitro* fertilization (IVF) cycles without lowering IRs. Although endometrial fluid aspiration is safe, sometimes the material obtained is insufficient for its analysis or it may be diluted as a result of uterine washing, thus making it difficult to interpret the results (58). More recently, an integral work (59) identified the catalog of proteins present in an endometrial fluid aspirate during the secretory phase of the menstrual cycle. A combination of different proteomic strategies led to the successful identification of 803 different proteins. This catalog of proteins provides a valuable reference for the study of embryo implantation and for the future discovery of the biomarkers involved in pathologic alterations of endometrial function.

The endometrium contains lipid compounds whose importance in reproduction has long since been known. Lipidomics can serve to unravel the specific lipid composition of endometrial fluid throughout the menstrual cycle and also to elucidate whether a particular lipid makeup is predictive of endometrial receptivity (60).

Some recent reports have applied lipidomics to studying reproductive function by assessing the lipid content of endometrial biopsies during pregnancy (61). However, these works neither refer to endometrial fluid in humans nor assess whether a particular lipid profile is distinctive of the WOI in relation to the rest of the cycle. Our lab reported that PGE_2 and $PGF_2\alpha$ concentrations increase significantly in the endometrial fluid during the WOI in normal-cycling women, during IVF, and in ovum donation. This profile is abrogated in the refractory endometrium with the insertion of an intra uterine device (IUD). Further, prostaglandins (PG) synthases, required for the production of PGE_2 and $PGF_2\alpha$, are localized in the endometrial epithelium and are hormonally regulated during the WOI, while PG receptors are localized at the trophectoderm of the human embryo. Using an *in vitro* model of embryo adhesion, we demonstrated that inhibition of PGE_2 and $PGF_2\alpha$ or blockade of PG receptors (EP2 and FP) prevents embryo adhesion, which can be overcome by adding back these molecules or using EP2 and FP agonists.

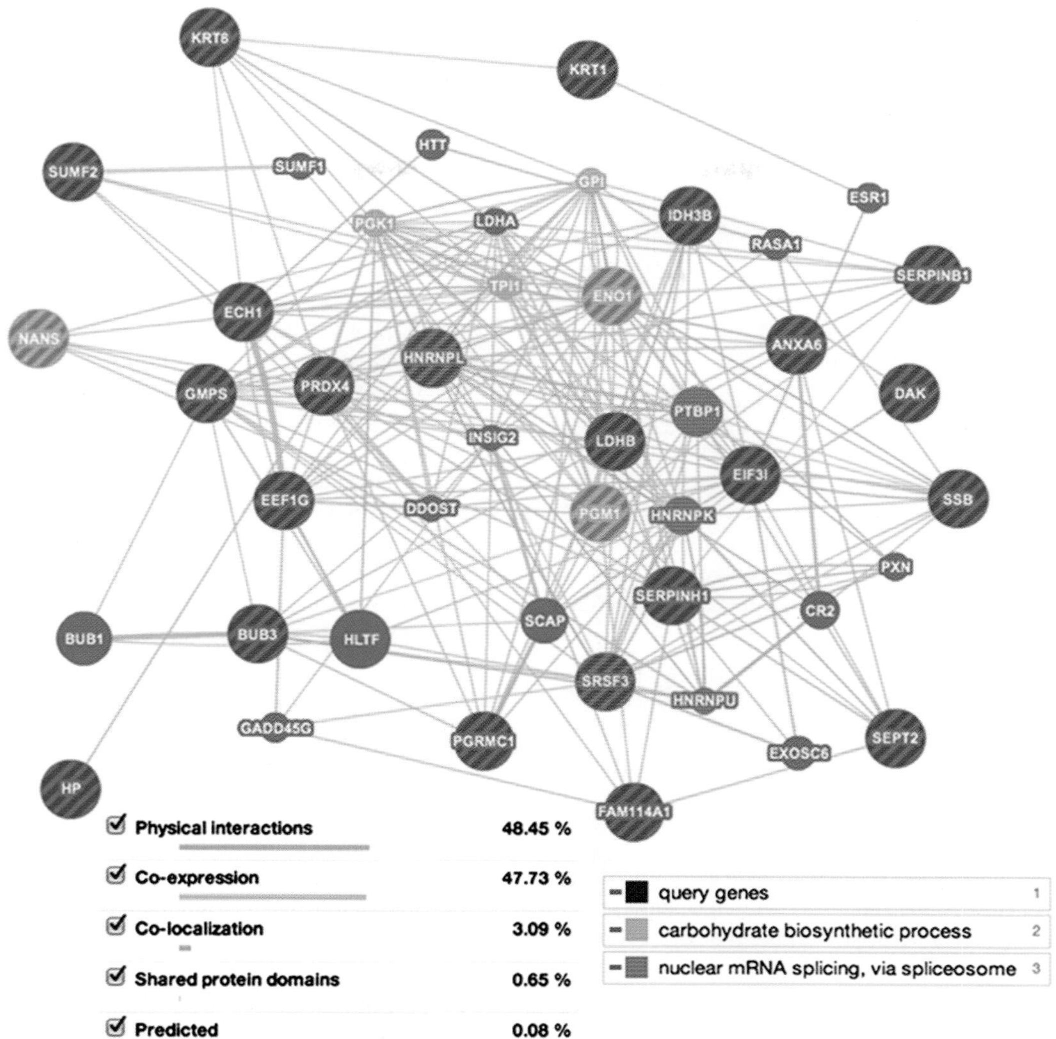

Figure 29.2 Proteomic network of deregulated proteins between receptive and non-receptive endometria diagnosed by endometrial receptivity array. All proteins are represented by their gene symbol name. Different-colored lines connecting proteins represent the relationships between them (physical interaction, co-expression, co-localization, shared protein domains, and predicted protein domains). Spheres represent proteins obtained in our proteomic study, while squares represent link nodes between them. Two statistically significant pathways were identified in the network: proteins integrated in the "carbohydrate biosynthetic processes" are represented in orange, while proteins related to "nuclear mRNA splicing via the spliceosome" are represented in red.

Finally, in a pilot study, we demonstrated that PGE_2 and $PGF_2\alpha$ concentrations in endometrial fluid (EF) aspirated 24 hours before embryo transfer predict pregnancy outcome. A receiver operating characteristic (ROC) curve was used in day-3 embryo transfer to analyze the sensitivity and specificity of this technique. We found 80% sensitivity and 86.7% specificity for PGE_2, and 100% sensitivity and 93.3% specificity for $PGF_2\alpha$ (Figure 29.3). Similar results were obtained for blastocyst transfer, in which the ROC curve showed 75% sensitivity and 77.8% specificity for PGE_2, and 37.5% sensitivity and 100% specificity for $PGF_2\alpha$ (62).

The results described above are meaningful for two reasons: first, they represent a proof of principle that endometrial fluids are suitable for lipidomic analyses, a possibility that has never been investigated before; and second, they illustrate how lipid changes actually occur in endometrial fluid throughout the cycle, increasing the likelihood of developing noninvasive methods to assess endometrial receptivity.

CONCLUSION

New molecular methods based on transcriptomics to identify endometrial receptivity have been introduced into the clinical routine in recent years. Thus, we now have molecular tools to date the WOI and thereby improve IVF success. Several other "omics" approaches are now being applied in order to unravel the complex process of acquiring endometrial receptivity. Although some technical limitations still exist, we believe that integrative sciences are the future of diagnosing the correct timing for embryo implantation. Furthermore, the application of these new technologies should be used to improve our knowledge of endometrial receptivity and the critical dialog between

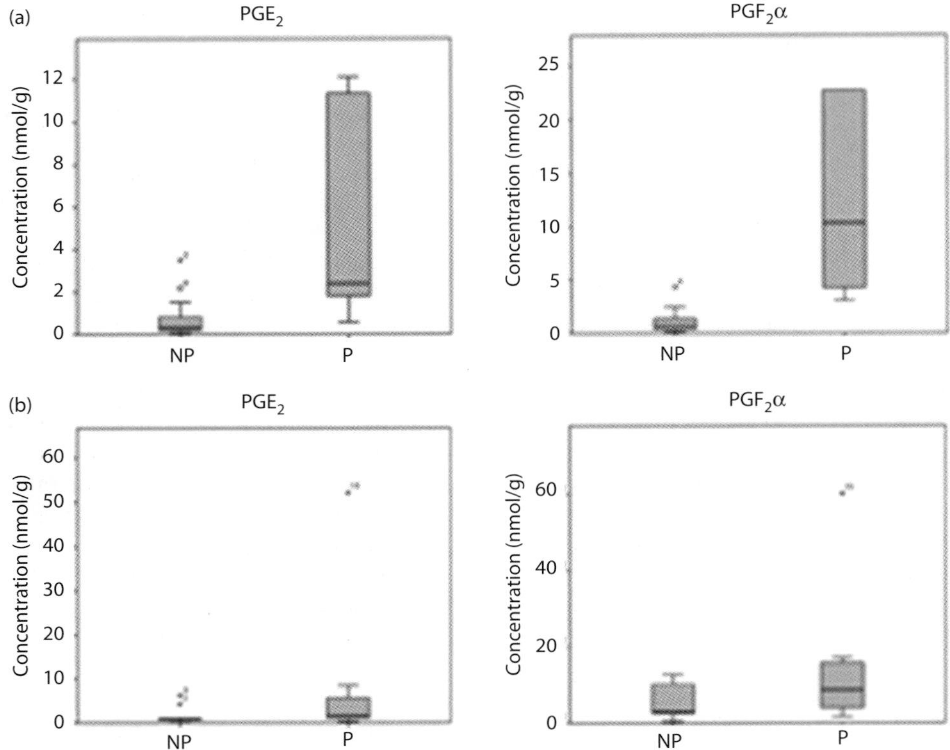

Figure 29.3 PGE_2 and $PGF_2\alpha$ concentrations in endometrial fluid (EF) predict successful pregnancy outcome. Pilot study to determine the detection sensitivity and specificity of PGE_2 and $PGF_2\alpha$ concentrations in endometrial fluid obtained 24 hours before embryo transfer in NP and P women. (a) In *in vitro* fertilization patients undergoing day-3 embryo transfer, measurement is taken 24 hours before embryo transfer. (b) In ovum recipients undergoing day-5 embryo transfer, measurement is taken 24 hours before embryo transfer. *Abbreviations*: NP, non-pregnant; P, pregnant.

embryo and endometrium, enabling the discovery of the main causes of implantation failure and opening up a new field for investigating interceptive molecules to aid and/or prevent embryo implantation.

REFERENCES

1. Kämmerer U, von Wolff M, Markert UR. Inmunology of human endometrium. *Inmunobiology* 2004; 209: 569–74.
2. Giudice LC. Implantation and endometrial function. In: *Molecular Biology in Reproductive Medicine*. Fauser BCJM (ed.). London, UK: Parthenon Publishing Group, 1999.
3. Dimitriadis E, White CA, Jones R et al. Cytokines, chemokines and growth factors in endometrium related to implantation. *Hum Reprod Update* 2005; 11: 613–30.
4. Finn CL, Martin L. The control of implantation. *J Reprod Fertil* 1974; 39: 195–206.
5. Martín J, Dominguez F, Avila S et al. Human endometrial receptivity: Gene regulation. *J Reprod Immunol* 2002; 55: 131–9.
6. Murphy CR. Uterine receptivity and the plasma membrane transformation. *Cell Res* 2004; 14: 259–67.
7. Nikas G. Cell-surface morphological events relevant to human implantation. *Hum Reprod* 1999; 14: 37–44.
8. Quinn CE, Casper RF. Pinopodes: A questionable role in endometrial receptivity. *Hum Reprod Update* 2009; 15: 229–36.
9. Giudice LC, Saleh W. Growth factors in reproduction. *Trends Endocrinol Metab* 1995; 6: 60–9.
10. Lessey BA. Endometrial integrins and the establishment of uterine receptivity. *Hum Reprod* 1998; 13: 247–58.
11. Dubowy RL, Feinberg RF, Keefe DL et al. Improved endometrial assessment using cyclin E and p27. *Fertil Steril* 2003; 80: 146–56.
12. Kliman HJ, Honig S, Walls D et al. Optimization of endometrial preparation results in a normal endometrial function test (EFT) and good reproductive outcome in donor ovum recipients. *J Assist Reprod Genet* 2006; 23: 299–303.
13. Lessey BA, Killam AP, Metzger DA et al. Immunohistochemical analysis of human uterine estrogen and progesterone receptors throughout the menstrual cycle. *J Clin Endocrinol Metab* 1988; 67: 334–40.
14. Develioglu OH, Hsiu JG, Nikas G et al. Endometrial estrogen and progesterone receptor and pinopode expression in stimulated cycles of oocyte donors. *Fertil Steril* 1999; 71: 1040–7.
15. Aghajanova L, Simon C, Horcajadas JA. Are favourite molecules of endometrial receptivity still in favour? *Expert Rev Obstet Gynecol* 2008; 3: 487–501.

16. Lessey BA. Assessment of endometrial receptivity. *Fertil Steril* 2011; 96: 522–9.
17. Díaz-Gimeno P, Ruiz-Alonso M, Blesa D, Simón C. Transcriptomics of the human endometrium. *Int J Dev Biol* 2013; 58: 127–37.
18. Altmae S, Esteban FJ, Stavreus-Evers A et al. Guidelines for the design, analysis and interpretation of "omics" data: Focus on human endometrium. *Hum Reprod Update* 2013; 20: 12–28.
19. Carson DD, Lagow E, Thathiah A, Al-Shami R, Farach-Carson MC, Vernon M, Yuan L, Fritz MA, Lessey B. Changes in gene expression during the early to mid-luteal (receptive phase) transition in human endometrium detected by high-density microarray screening. *Mol Hum Reprod* 2002; 8: 871–9.
20. Riesewijk A, Martin J, Van Os R, Horcajadas JA, Polman J, Pellicer A, Mosselman S, Simón C. Gene profiling of human endometrial receptivity on days LH+2 versus LH+7 by microarray technology. *Mol Hum Reprod* 2003; 9: 253–64.
21. Ponnampalam AP, Weston GC, Trajstman AC, Susil B, Rogers PA. Molecular classification of human endometrial cycle stages by transcriptional profi ling. *Mol Hum Reprod* 2004; 10: 879–93.
22. Talbi S, Hamilton AE, Vo KC et al. Molecular phenotyping of human endometrium distinguishes menstrual cycle phases and underlying biological processes in normo-ovulatory women. *Endocrinology* 2006; 147: 1097–121.
23. Tseng LH, Chen I, Chen MY, Yan H, Wang CN, Lee CL. Genome-based expression profiling as a single standardized microarray platform for the diagnosis of endometrial disorder: An array of 126-gene model. *Fertil Steril* 2010; 94: 114–9.
24. Díaz-Gimeno P, Horcajadas JA, Martínez-Conejero JA, Esteban FJ, Alamá P, Pellicer A, Simón C. A genomic diagnostic tool for human endometrial receptivity based on the transcriptomic signature. *Fertil Steril* 2011; 95: 50–60.
25. Díaz-Gimeno P, Ruiz-Alonso M, Blesa D et al. The accuracy and reproducibility of the endometrial receptivity array is superior to histology as a diagnostic method for endometrial receptivity. *Fertil Steril* 2013; 99: 508–17.
26. Ruiz-Alonso M, Blesa D, Díaz-Gimeno P, Gómez E, Fernández-Sánchez M, Carranza F, Carrera J, Vilella F, Pellicer A, Simón C. The endometrial receptivity array for diagnosis and personalized embryo transfer as a treatment for patients with repeated implantation failure. *Fertil Steril* 2013; 100: 818–24.
27. Ruiz-Alonso M, Galindo N, Pellicer A, Simón C. What a difference two days make: "Personalized" embryo transfer (pET) paradigm: A case report and pilot study. *Hum Reprod* 2014; 29: 1244–7.
28. Alonso MR, Díaz-Gimeno P, Gómez E, Rincón-Bertolín A, Vladimirov Y, Garrido N, Simón C. Clinical efficiency of embryo transfer performed in receptive vs non-receptive endometrium diagnosed by the endometrial receptivity array (era) test. *Fertil Steril* 2014; 3: e292.
29. Tabibzadeh S, Babaknia A. The signals and molecular pathways involved in implantation, a symbiotic interaction between blastocyst and endometrium involving adhesion and tissue invasion. *Hum Reprod* 1995; 10: 1579–602.
30. Hardy K, Spanos S. Growth factor expression and function in the human and mouse preimplantation embryo. *J Endocrinol* 2002; 172: 221–36.
31. Richter KS. The importance of growth factors for preimplantation embryo development and *in-vitro* culture. *Curr Opin Obstet Gynecol* 2008; 20: 292–304.
32. Martin JC, Jasper MJ, Valbuena D et al. Increased adhesiveness in cultured endometrial-derived cells is related to the absence of moesin expression. *Biol Reprod* 2000; 63: 1370–6.
33. Kahlert C, Melo SA, Protopopov A et al. Identification of doublestranded genomic DNA spanning all chromosomes with mutated KRAS and p53 DNA in the serum exosomes of patients with pancreatic cancer. *J Biol Chem* 2014; 289: 3869–75.
34. Thouas GA, Dominguez F, Green MP, Vilella F, Simon C, Gardner DK. Soluble ligands and their receptors in human embryo development and implantation. *Endocr Rev* 2015; 36: 92–130.
35. Kaye PL. Preimplantation growth factor physiology. *Rev Reprod* 1997; 2: 121–7.
36. Vilella F, Moreno-Moya JM, Balaguer N, Grasso A, Herrero M, Martínez S, Marcilla A, Simón C. Has-miR-30d, secreted by the human endometrium is taken up by the pre-implantation embryo and might modify its transcriptome. *Development* 2015; 142: 3210–21.
37. Ambros V. MicroRNA pathways in flies and worms: Growth, death, fat, stress, and timing. *Cell* 2003; 113: 673–6.
38. Bartel DP. MicroRNAs: Genomics, biogenesis, mechanism, and function. *Cell* 2004; 116: 281–97.
39. Lai EC. microRNAs: Runts of the genome assert themselves. *Curr Biol* 2003; 13: R925–36.
40. Lim LP, Lau NC, Garret-Engele P et al. Microarray analyses shows that some microRNAs downregulate large numbers of target mRNAs. *Nature* 2005; 433: 769–73.
41. Altmäe S, Martinez-Conejero JA, Esteban FJ, Ruiz-Alonso M, Stavreus-Evers A, Horcajadas JA, Salumets A. MicroRNAs miR-30b, miR-30d, and miR-494 regulate human endometrial receptivity. *Reprod Sci* 2013; 20: 308–17.
42. Barkalina N, Jones C, Wood MJ, Coward K. Extracellular vesicle-mediated delivery of molecular compounds into gametes and embryos: Learning from nature. *Hum Reprod Update* 2015; 21: 627–39.
43. Théry C. Exosomes: Secreted vesicles and intercellular communications. *F1000 Biol Rep* 2011; 3: 15.

44. Lee Y, El Andaloussi S, Wood MJ. Exosomes and microvesicles: Extracellular vesicles for genetic information transfer and gene therapy. *Hum Mol Genet* 2012; 21: R125–34.
45. Valadi H, Ekström K, Bossios A, Sjöstrand M, Lee JJ, Lötvall JO. Exosome-mediated transfer of mRNAs and microRNAs is a novel mechanism of genetic exchange between cells. *Nat Cell Biol* 2007; 9: 654–9.
46. Thakur BK, Zhang H, Becker A et al. Double-stranded DNA in exosomes: A novel biomarker in cancer detection. *Cell Res* 2014; 24: 766–9.
47. Cai J, Han Y, Ren H et al. Extracellular vesicle-mediated transfer of donor genomic DNA to recipient cells is a novel mechanism for genetic influence between cells. *J Mol Cell Biol* 2013; 5: 227–38.
48. Shankar R, Cullinane F, Brennecke SP et al. Applications of proteomics methodologies to human pregnancy research: A growing gestation approaching delivery? *Proteomics* 2004; 4: 1909–17.
49. DeSouza L, Diehl G, Yang EC et al. Proteomic analysis of the proliferative and secretory phases of the human endometrium: Proteinidentification and differential protein expression. *Proteomics* 2005; 5: 270–81.
50. Parmar T, Gadkar-Sable S, Savardekar L et al. Protein profiling of human endometrial tissues in the mid-secretory and proliferative phases of the menstrual cycle. *Fertil Steril* 2009; 92: 1091–103.
51. Domınguez F, Garrido-Gomez T, Lopez JA et al. Proteomic analysis of the human receptive versus non-receptive endometrium using differential in-gel electrophoresis and MALDI-MS unveils stathmin 1 and annexin A2 as differentially regulated. *Hum Reprod* 2009; 24: 2607–17.
52. Garrido-Gomez T, Dominguez F, Ruiz M, Vilella F, Simon C. In: *The Analysis of Endometrial Receptivity. Textbook of Assisted Reproductive Techniques: Laboratory Perspectives.* Gardner D, Weissman A, Howles CM, and Shoham Z (eds.). 4th edition. Vol. 1. Boca Raton, FL: Taylor & Francis Group, pp. 366–79.
53. Garrido-Gómez T, Quiñonero A, Antúnez O, Díaz-Gimeno P, Bellver J, Simón C, Domínguez F. Deciphering the proteomic signature of human endometrial receptivity. *Hum Reprod* 2014; 29: 1957–67.
54. Maathuis JB, Aitken RJ. Protein patterns of human uterine flushings collected at various stages of the menstrual cycle. *J Reprod Fertil* 1978; 53: 343–8.
55. Beier HM, Beier-Hellwig K. Molecular and cellular aspects of endometrial receptivity. *Hum Reprod* 1989; 4(8 Suppl): 115–20.
56. Beier-Hellwig K, Sterzik K, Bonn B, Beier HM. Contribution to the physiology and pathology of endometrial receptivity: The determination of protein patterns in human uterine secretions. *Reprod Biomed Online* 2003; 7: 105–9.
57. van der Gaast MH, Beier-Hellwig K, Fauser BC, Beier HM, Macklon NS. Endometrial secretion aspiration prior to embryo transfer does not reduce implantation rates. *Fertil Steril* 2003; 79: 900–4.
58. Olivennes F, Lédée-Bataille N, Samama M, Kadoch J, Taupin JL, Dubanchet S, Chaouat G, Frydman R. Assessment of leukemia inhibitory factor levels by uterine flushing at the time of egg retrieval does not adversely affect pregnancy rates with *in vitro* fertilization. *Fertil Steril* 2003; 79: 900–4.
59. Casado-Vela J, Rodriguez-Suarez E, Iloro I et al. Comprehensive proteomic analysis of human endometrial fluid aspirate. *J Proteome Res* 2009; 8: 4622–32.
60. Wenk MR. The emerging field of lipidomics. *Nat Rev Drug Discov* 2005; 4: 594–610.
61. Durn JH, Marshall KM, Farrar D et al. Lipidomic analysis reveals prostanoid profiles in human term pregnant myometrium. *Prostaglandins Leukot Essent Fatty Acids* 2010; 82: 21–6.
62. Vilella F, Ramirez L, Berlanga O et al. PGE2 and PGF2 concentrations in human endometrial fluid as biomarkers for embryonic implantation. *J Clin Endocrinol Metab* 2013; 98: 4123–32.

Artificial gametes
The oocyte

EVELYN E. TELFER and KELSEY M. GRIEVE

30

The ability to produce mature *in vitro*-derived gametes, either starting from immature gametes or obtaining them from alternative sources such as embryonic stem cells (ESCs), would allow insights into the basic science of oogenesis, folliculogenesis, and meiosis and may also offer the potential for new assisted reproduction technologies (ARTs). Gametes derived in this way have been described as "artificial gametes," and if they are shown to be safe, they would alleviate the need for donor eggs and sperm and would provide people who cannot produce mature gametes with the possibility of genetically related children. This chapter will cover the progress in producing so-called "artificial oocytes" from a range of cell types and will consider the technology of growing oocytes *in vitro* from the most immature stages to maturity.

SOURCE OF ARTIFICIAL OOCYTES

A major requirement of any cell type used to form artificial gametes would be that they can be collected from adult tissue, as this eliminates the use of primordial germ cells, which are only present during fetal life (1). Research has focused on obtaining artificial oocytes from three main cell types: ESCs, induced pluripotent stem cells (iPSCs) and oogonial stem cells (OSCs) or germline stem cells (GSCs). Stem cells are undifferentiated or differentiation-limited, self-renewing cells within a distinct niche responsible for renewal. Pluripotent stem cells have the ability to differentiate into all the cells of a mammalian embryo and therefore harbor the potential to generate germ cells. Mammalian oogenesis *in vivo* is a tightly coordinated process that requires the transient switching on and off of regulatory genes and molecular processes, of which we still have limited knowledge (Figure 30.1).

OOCYTES FROM ESCs

Artificial oocytes have been derived from mouse ESCs (2,3), but have not produced viable embryos. ESCs derived from the inner cell mass of a developing blastocyst (4) have been shown to differentiate into numerous cell types *in vitro*, including hematopoietic, endothelial, muscle, and neuronal cells (5), thus ESCs have been candidate progenitor cells for *in vitro* oogenesis despite ethical concerns surrounding their use. Mouse ESCs (mESCs) reported the first early differentiating germ cells within *in vitro* cultures (2); however, these experiments have been difficult to replicate. Isolation of these cells based on Oct4 and cKit expression identified different stages of germ cell development (migratory primordial germ cells and post-migratory germ cells) determined by the expression levels of the germ cell marker Vasa, which is expressed in post-migratory germ cells (Figure 30.1).

The identification of early germ cells within culture demonstrates recapitulation of the earliest stages of the complex pathway for germ cell development; however, prior to germ cell migration, germ cell fate is induced in the epiblast cells in mice by bone morphogenetic protein 4 (BMP4) signaling from the surrounding soma (6). Epiblast-like cells (EpiLCs) have been induced from mESCs with gene expression consistent with pre-gastrulating epiblasts. BMP4 induced expression of Blimp1 in EpiLCs and further gene expression analysis also showed up-regulation of Nanos3, Dppa3 and Prdm14 associated with primordial germ cell specification and down-regulation of somatic markers Hoxa1, Hoxb1, and Snail—these observations were seen in conjunction with epigenetic changes (7), replicating *in vivo* differentiation of epiblast cells into primordial germ cells. These results suggest successful differentiation of EpiLCs to primordial germ cell-like cells (PGCLCs) *in vitro* in a similar fashion to the *in vivo* situation. BMP4-dependent differentiation of PGCLCs could be inhibited by Noggin (a BMP4 antagonist), whereas Wnt3a—another mesoderm-promoting factor—also induced PGCLCs in culture (8), illustrating the importance of somatic factors in *in vitro* differentiation of germ cells. PGCLCs derived from embryoid bodies (EBs) differentiated into oocyte-like cells with expression of oocyte-specific genes (*Figα*, *GDF9*, *ZP1*, *ZP2*, and *ZP3*) and an early meiotic marker (*SCP3*) when co-cultured with granulosa cells (9); similar results were observed when PGCLCs were co-cultured with Chinese hamster ovary cells (10). However, these results could not be replicated with granulosa cell-conditioned medium (9), suggesting an important role for cell–cell interactions with ovarian somatic cells. Using a reconstituted ovary model, PGCLCs combined with embryonic ovarian somatic cells and xeno-transplanted to the ovarian bursa of immune-deficient recipient mice generated oocyte-like cells within developing follicles (Figure 30.2).

Oocyte-like cells were matured and fertilized *in vitro* and transferred to foster mothers for fetal development, which generated healthy offspring with normal imprinting patterns and full fertility (11). These results together demonstrate the potential of ESCs to undergo differentiation to all stages of oogenesis and subsequent embryonic development, and as with *in vivo* oogenesis, interactions with surrounding somatic cells are essential for successful *in vitro* oogenesis. Less success has been achieved with ESCs from other species. BMP4 exposure induced germ

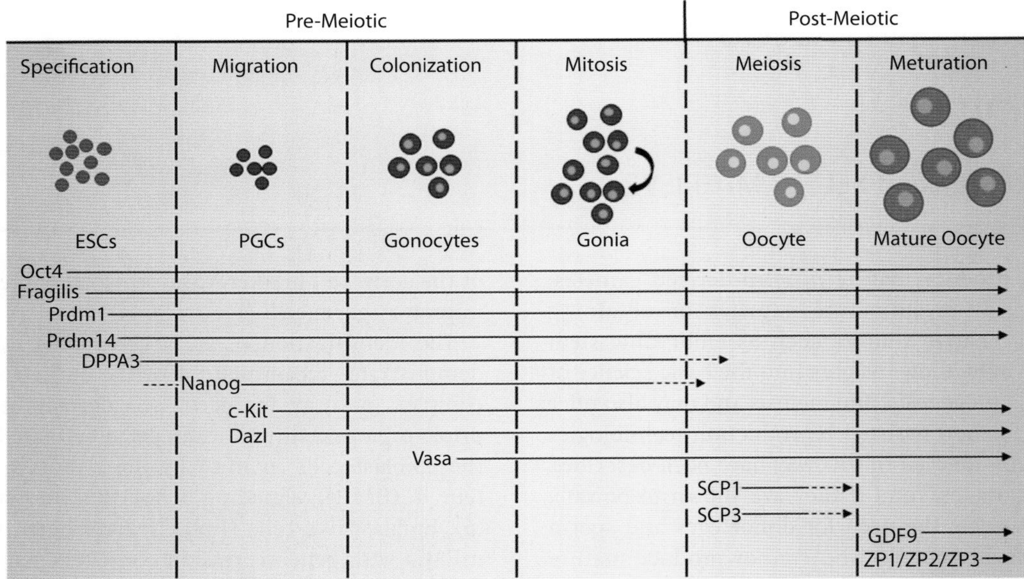

Figure 30.1 The different stages of germ cell development and expression levels of germ cell markers. *Abbreviations*: ESC, embryonic stem cell; PGC, primordial germ cell.

cell differentiation in buffalo ESCs in culture, which were morphologically similar to oocytes and expressed germ cell (cKit, Dazl, and Vasa), meiosis (SCP3), and oocyte (Gdf9, ZP2, ZP3, and ZP4) specific genes and proteins. Buffalo oocyte-like cells subsequently underwent parthenogenetic activation, extruding a polar body and developing to an eight-cell embryo within a ZP4 coat (12).

Germ cell differentiation of human ESCs has also been investigated and PGCLCs have been derived from human ESCs with gene expression patterns similar to PGCs. Activin A supplementation of blastocysts prior to derivation of hESC lines increased PGCLC differentiation from human embryonic stem gells (hESCs); furthermore, BMP4 also directed hESC differentiation to PGCLCs as seen in the mouse (13). Expression of germ cell and oocyte (ZP1 and GDF9) specific markers was observed in EBs derived from hESCs, and follicle-like structures were observed within EBs; however, a zona pellucida could not be detected (14).

Whilst this research gives us insight into cell lineage development, the clinical use of human ESCs is fraught with difficulties. A major concern is that derivation of oocytes from human ESCs for clinical application would be dependent on somatic cell nuclear transfer (15), and many ethical concerns surround this. Therefore, it is unlikely that derivation of gametes by this route would be used clinically, and a more likely route would be to utilize iPSCs.

OOCYTES FROM iPSCs

It is well accepted that cells can be de-differentiated and regain pluripotency. Mouse fibroblasts under the

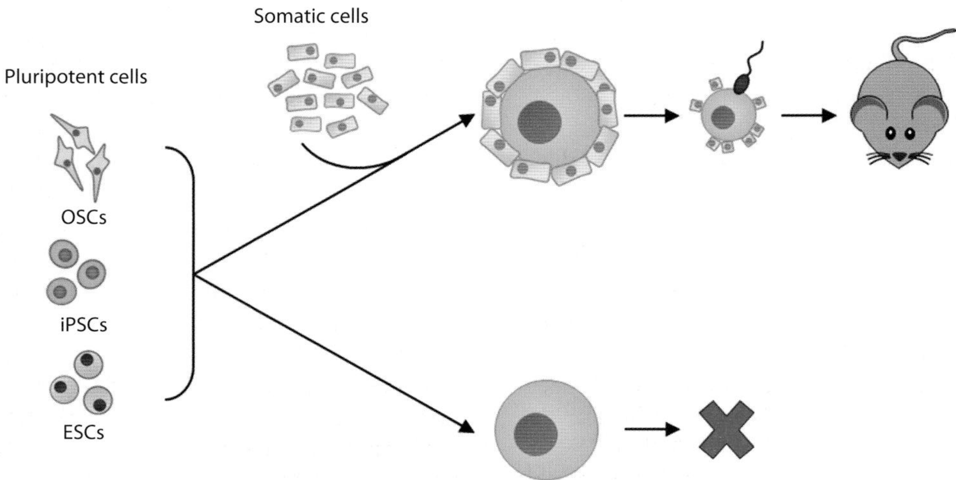

Figure 30.2 The different results of primordial germ cell-like cell trials. *Abbreviations*: ESC, embryonic stem cell; iPSC, induced pluripotent stem cell; OSC, oogonial stem cell.

expression of four crucial pluripotency genes—*Oct3/4*, *Klf4*, *Sox2*, and *c-Myc*—were induced to a pluripotent state and termed iPSCs (16), and have since been derived from numerous species, including humans (17). iPSCs do not raise the same ethical concerns as ESCs and they may offer a more likely clinical option for artificial gametogenesis.

Using a tetraploid complementation assay, mouse iPSCs have demonstrated their ability to generate all cell types, including germ cells (18,19), similarly to ESCs. Mouse iPSCs can be derived *in vitro* to EpiLCs and PGCLCs and utilized in the reconstituted ovary xeno-transplant model to generate oocytes. These oocytes have been shown to be meiotically and developmentally competent and offspring have been produced (11). Currently, no success has been achieved with human iPSCs in generating artificial oocytes.

OOCYTES FROM SOMATIC CELL TRANSFORMATION

The hierarchical stem cell differentiation model has recently been challenged by the cell plasticity model, which states that cells possess the ability to cross traditional lineage barriers (20). The ability to manipulate a somatic cell to transdifferentiate (conversion of a differentiated cell of one lineage to a differentiated cell of another lineage without reinstating pluripotency) by direct reprogramming could also allow the *in vitro* generation of new oocytes. Skin-derived stem cells (SDSCs) isolated from neonatal mice have also been shown to differentiate into PGCLCs *in vitro* (21,22). SDSC-derived PGCLCs also underwent epigenetic changes similar to PGCs *in vivo*, and activin A promoted PGCLC differentiation (22), similarly to human ESCs. SDSCs also generated aggregates, morphologically similar to follicles, containing large cells with expression of oocyte-specific markers, when cultured alone and with dissociated murine neonatal ovarian cells. The large oocyte-like cells also expressed meiotic markers, but SCP3 showed discontinuous staining patterns, which is consistent with the cells' inability to progress through meiosis. SDSCs that were aggregated with neonatal ovarian somatic cells and transplanted to the kidney capsules of recipient mice generated oocyte-like cells in developing follicles through to antral stages of development (21), suggesting SDSCs can differentiate and generate cells that have morphological similarities to oocytes, indicating the separation of oocyte development and meiotic/developmental potential.

Fetal porcine SDSCs have also demonstrated a potential for germ cell differentiation *in vitro*. PGCLCs derived from fetal porcine SDSCs express germ cell markers (Dppa3, Dazl, Vasa, and cKit) and also show imprint erasure (23). Further development of these PGCLCs to oocyte like cells (OLCs) in aggregates demonstrates the presence of a zona pellucida and expression of oocyte and meiotic markers. These aggregates also produced estrogen and progesterone from the surrounding cells and underwent parthogenetic activation, implicating a necessary role for somatic cells in germ cell differentiation. Rat pancreatic stem cells have also generated oocyte-like cells in culture with structures similar to a zona pellucida in aggregation with smaller cells, and they share gene expression patterns with oocytes, with oocyte and meiotic markers expressed (24). Human amniotic fluid stem cells have also been able to recapitulate this differentiation pathway *in vitro*, generating aggregates with large central cells (OLCs) surrounded by a zona pellucida structure and smaller cells that produced estrogen during culture. Analysis of the OLCs showed the expression of oocyte-specific and meiotic markers and underwent parthenogenetic activation during prolonged culture (25,26), consistent with previous reports from other cell types and species. Although these reprogrammed cells show many of the steps of germ cell differentiation *in vitro*, as identified by differentiation of true pluripotent ESCs and iPSCs, generated oocyte-like cells have not been fully tested and the meiotic and developmental competence of these cells has not been fully evaluated. It is clear that some cells under certain conditions can form morphological oocytes, but these do not enter meiosis. The process of oocyte differentiation can be dissociated from meiosis (27), so if functional artificial oocytes are to be obtained, then it will be essential to understand the connection between oocyte differentiation and entry into meiosis.

OOCYTES FROM OSCs

In recent years, there have been some exciting and controversial developments in female germ cell biology relating to an increasing body of evidence that shows oocytes may be formed by a rare population of putative GSCs that can be isolated from the adult ovary (reviewed in [28–30]). These are proposed to be germ lineage-specific rather than being pluripotent cells, but their contribution to the pool of oocytes is still unclear. This chapter will not deal with their potential physiological role and will only consider their potential *ex vivo*.

The isolation and identification of oocyte-producing GSCs—also referred to as OSCs—from adult mammalian ovaries remained elusive until 2009, when putative GSCs were isolated from adult mouse ovaries (31), then followed by isolation of similar cells from adult human ovaries (32). These cells have now been isolated from the ovaries of adult mice (31,32), rats (33), humans (32), and non-human primates (34). The isolation of these cells has been based on magnetic or fluorescent cell sorting utilizing an antibody to the germ cell marker DEAD box polypeptide 4 (DDX4) (28,31). The isolation process has led to controversy, as DDX4 is assumed to be internal rather than surface, and other groups have failed to isolate the cells using similar methodologies (35). Nonetheless, several groups have isolated a population of cells that have a molecular signature that includes germ cell (Mvh and fragilis/Ifitm3) and stem cell (e.g., Oct4/Pou5f1) markers. Injection of fluorescently labeled mouse OSCs into recipient fertile and infertile mouse ovaries has generated green fluorescent protein (GFP)-positive oocytes within host somatic cells, and these have been capable of ovulation, fertilization, and embryonic development (31,32), and in some cases live young have been produced (31,33). Human OSCs have also generated oocyte-like cells enclosed in host somatic cells, as assessed

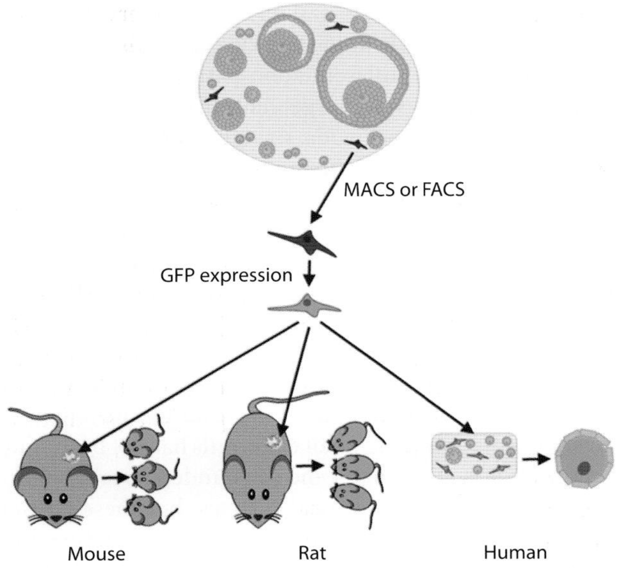

Figure 30.3 Results of identifying the oogenic potential of oogonial stem cells from adult mammalian ovaries as currently reported. Cells isolated either by magnetic activated cell sorting (MACS) (31) or fluorescent activated cell sorting (FACS) (32) and transfected with green fluorescent protein (GFP) for tracing.

by morphology and expression of oocyte-specific markers, after injection into adult human ovarian cortical tissue and xeno-transplantation into an immune-deficient mouse for seven days (30,32). For more details, see Figure 30.3.

Whilst identifying cells with apparent germline potential in the human ovary represents a major development, it has also led to a great deal of controversy. The methods used to isolate these cells still need to be clarified, but there is now too much evidence to dismiss them. These cells present an opportunity to learn more about germ cell development and the processes involved.

The "oocyte-like" cells derived from each of the cell types discussed require somatic cell support of paracrine and junctional communication to form follicles and to support development into functional oocytes. Combining these "oocyte-like" cells with ovarian culture models may facilitate follicle formation and growth (36).

SUPPORTING OOCYTE FORMATION AND GROWTH *IN VITRO*

The idea of obtaining viable oocytes by growing immature oocytes *in vitro* has been the subject of a great deal of research for almost 30 years. Whilst this is not the production of "artificial gametes," the techniques to support *in vitro* oocyte growth are essential to the development of a gamete being developed from any source. Complete growth *in vitro* from the most immature oocytes (primordial stages) with subsequent *in vitro* fertilization (IVF) and production of live young has only been achieved in mice (37,38). Early work on this two-step culture system resulted in only one live offspring being obtained, and this mouse had many abnormalities as an adult (37). Following improvements in the technique and after alterations to the culture medium, several mouse embryos and offspring have been obtained using oocytes that have been *in vitro* grown (IVG) combined with *in vitro* maturation (IVM) and IVF (38). This work has provided proof of concept that complete oocyte development can be achieved *in vitro* and has driven the development of culture systems that could be applied to other species, particularly humans. Advances in culturing follicles from humans, non-human primates, and domestic species have been made, bringing the prospect of achieving an *in vitro* system that supports complete human oocyte development closer (39–41).

IN VITRO GROWTH SYSTEMS

The generation of artificial gametes from any cell type requires the support of somatic cells in order to develop further into a mature gamete. Therefore, these cells need to be combined with somatic cells to form primordial follicles (Figure 30.2). Activation and growth of primordial follicles is marked by the transformation of the flattened epithelial cells surrounding the oocyte into cuboidal cells that proliferate, forming a multilaminar structure in which the germ cell will develop. Normal follicle/oocyte development is critically dependent upon intercellular communication between the growing oocyte and the developing granulosa cells; therefore, support and maintenance of these connections are essential (42). Whilst growing within the follicle, the oocyte is held in meiotic arrest, but as it grows it must acquire the ability to resume meiosis (meiotic competence) and the ability to support fertilization and embryonic development (developmental competence). The development of culture conditions to support germ cell development is an enormous challenge, and an understanding of the physiological requirements of each component of the developing follicle is needed.

Several culture systems have been developed that have been optimized for a range of different animal models (39,40,43). Whilst some are more advanced than others, there is not a single system that has been fully optimized to support the complete *in vitro* growth and maturation of human follicles and oocytes. All of the published systems have strengths and weaknesses that may be usefully exploited to meet the challenges of human follicle culture, but there is a consensus that in order to achieve complete *in vitro* growth, a dynamic culture system is required to support the three main transition steps (39,40,43). Developing each of these steps in human tissue has been slow because of the difficulty in obtaining experimental tissue, but progress has been made in three main steps in human tissue: (1) activation of primordial follicles (44–47); (2) isolation and culture of growing follicles to achieve oocyte growth and development (41,44–48); and (3) aspiration and maturation of oocyte cumulus complexes (49–53).

ACTIVATING PRIMORDIAL FOLLICLES

The regulation of follicle activation involves a combination of inhibitory, stimulatory, and maintenance factors (54). Recent work using knockout mouse models has highlighted the importance of the PI3K–AKT signaling pathway within the oocyte in regulating follicle activation (55). PTEN acts as a negative regulator of this pathway and suppresses initiation of follicle development (55). Follicle activation is also affected by other components of this pathway, namely mTORC1, a serine/threonine kinase that regulates cell growth and proliferation in response to growth factors and nutrients.

Disruption of the PI3K pathway using knockout models (55,56) and pharmacological stimulators and/or inhibitors (57) promotes activation of follicle growth in mice and xeno-transplanted human ovarian tissue and enhances ovulation in mice. These studies suggest that whilst PTEN within the oocyte suppresses activation of primordial follicles, mTORC1 promotes it. By using pharmacological inhibitors of PTEN *in vitro*, increased activation of human primordial follicles has been demonstrated (46,57), and treatment with rapamycin (an inhibitor of mTORC1) results in decreased activation of primordial follicles (58).

A human live birth has been reported following treatment of ovarian tissue for 48 hours *in vitro* with bpV(HOpic) and 740YP, an AKT stimulant, followed by replacement and IVF (59). This is an extremely encouraging development but needs to be treated with caution, as the use of similar inhibitors *in vitro* whilst increasing activation of primordial follicles results in poor-quality oocytes at later stages (46).

Primordial follicles can be activated to grow within mechanically loosened cortical pieces, developing to multilaminar preantral (secondary) stages within six days (Figure 30.4) (45). A key step in this process is tissue preparation, which involves removal of most of the underlying stromal tissue and any growing follicles so that the cultured tissue consists of predominantly ovarian cortex containing primordial and primary follicles. When these small fragments of human ovarian cortex are cultured, there is a significant shift of follicles from the quiescent to the growing pool over short culture periods of 6–10 days (45). This observation has been repeated in cattle, where

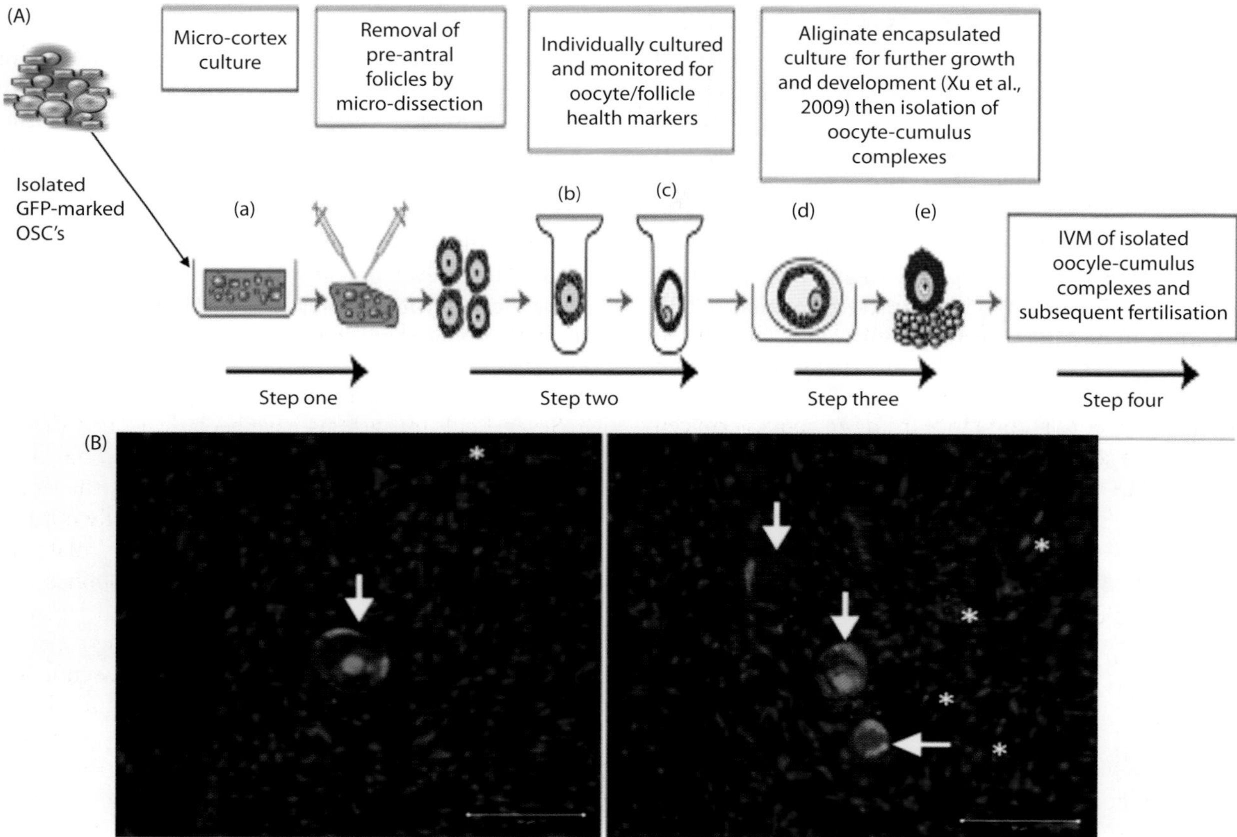

Figure 30.4 (A) Illustrates the potential use of an in vitro growth system to trace the development of human oogonial stem cells (OSCs) (32). Isolated OSCs can be transfected with green fluorescent protein (GFP) and injected into flattened strips of ovarian tissue (a) cultured in medium containing human serum albumin, ascorbic acid and basal levels of FSH [45–47]. Once follicles have reached multi-laminar stages they are isolated mechanically using needles and then cultured individually (b). Isolated follicle culture supports development from pre-antral to antral stages (c). The final stages of oocyte growth and development are achieved by removing the oocyte-cumulus complex from the antral follicle (d) and culturing the oocyte and its surrounding somatic cells (e). (B) Illustrates human OSCs containing GFP (asterix) injected into human ovarian cortical tissue and cultured for 7 days. Injected cells increase in size and develop into oocyte like structures (white arrows).

extensive primordial activation has been reported within two days *in vitro* (60–62), indicating that activation results from a release from intra-ovarian factors that act to inhibit the initiation of follicle growth. Tissue shape and stromal density are emerging as important factors that contribute to the regulation of follicle growth initiation *in vitro*, as solid cubes of cortical tissue show less growth initiation (44) than cortex cultured as flattened "sheets," where much of the underlying stroma is removed (45). The physical environment of the follicles within the cortical tissue affects their response to stimulatory and inhibitory factors and therefore influences their ability to grow.

Once follicle growth has been initiated within cortical tissue, follicles can develop to multilaminar stages. Large, multilaminar follicles do not survive well within the cortical environment and appear to be inhibitory to further growth, resulting in a loss of follicle integrity and oocyte survival (44,45). Therefore, in order to support further development, follicles need to be released from the cortical stromal environment and cultured individually to limit the effect of follicle interactions (45,60).

GROWING PRE-ANTRAL FOLLICLES *IN VITRO*

Once follicles have reached the multilaminar preantral stage of development, there are several culture systems that support further growth. The key to successful growth is maintaining oocyte–somatic cell interactions, and this is influenced by the physical environment. Placing preantral follicles in V-shaped microwell plates has allowed maintenance of the three-dimensional follicular architecture *in vitro* whilst promoting growth and differentiation in human follicles (45–47), with antral formation occurring within 10 days. Follicle differentiation has also been reported in bovine follicles embedded in collagen gels and cultured for 13 days (63), and by using a combination of media thickened with polyvinylpyrrolidone, a macromolecular supplement, and microporous membranes, two live calves have been produced from immature bovine follicles cultured for 14 days (64). In addition to V-shaped microwell culture plates, follicle encapsulation in alginate hydrogels has been used to support secondary human follicle growth *in vitro* (41,48), as well as rhesus monkey follicles (65). Alginate encapsulation is believed to mimic the extracellular matrix *in vivo* in terms of its ability to facilitate molecular exchange between the follicle and the culture medium; its flexibility can accommodate cell proliferation, but its rigidity prevents dissociation of the follicular unit.

The progression of human follicles following isolation from the cortex is remarkable. In the presence of follicle-stimulating hormone (FSH), enzymatically isolated secondary human follicles can differentiate, become steroidogenically active, and complete oocyte growth in 30 days (48), and these have been shown to be capable of meiotic maturation (41).

Quiescent follicles activated to grow within cultured fragments of cortex and mechanically isolated as secondary follicles become steroidogenic and undergo differentiation after a 10-day *in vitro* period with and without activin (Figure 30.5) (45). These observations confirm that local ovarian factors inhibit follicle development *in vivo*; however, the question remains as to whether the growth rate observed *in vitro* is accelerated or whether it represents growth without the brakes that are required *in vivo* to regulate follicle development within the context of the reproductive cycle. The next step is to demonstrate whether the oocytes produced in these systems are capable of *in vitro*

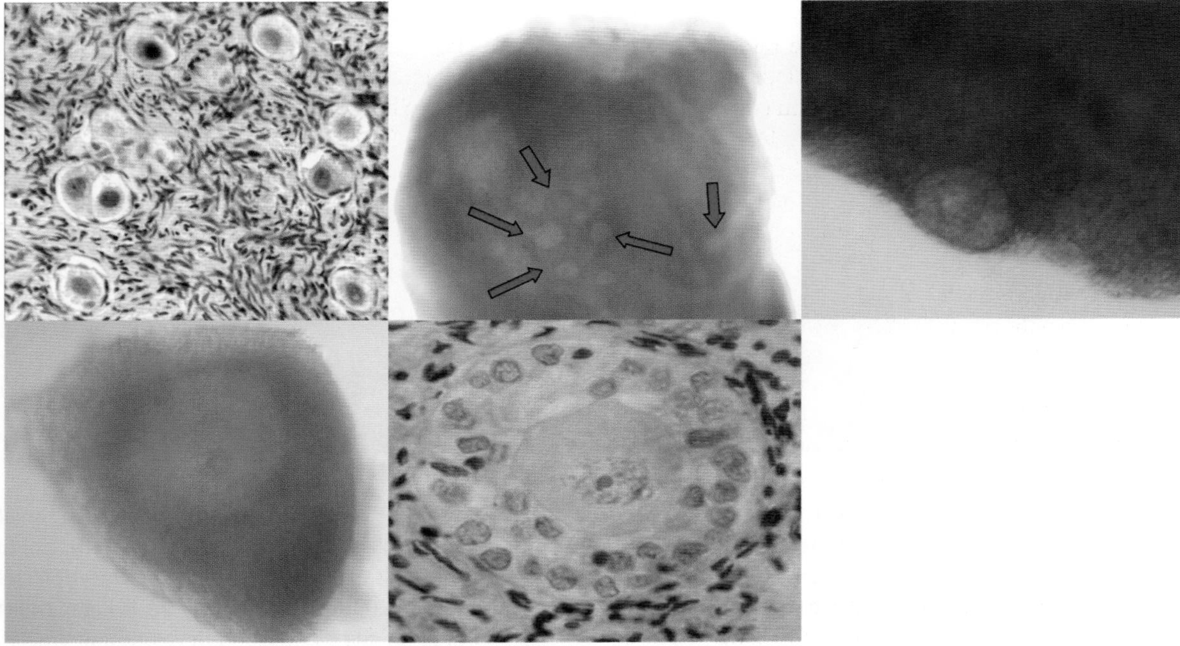

Figure 30.5 Development and differentiation of quiescent follicles. The arrows represent growing follicles in the cultured ovarian cortex.

maturation and to determine whether the growth pattern *in vitro* is deleterious to oocyte function, epigenetic changes, and health.

FINAL STAGES OF GROWTH AND MATURATION

The final goal of an *in vitro* system is to produce oocytes that can be fertilized and produce developmentally normal embryos. In order to achieve this, IVG human oocytes need to be matured *in vitro*. It is widely accepted that whilst 40%–80% of immature human oocytes can successfully complete *in vitro* maturation and fertilization and so give rise to live births, the rate of maturation of immature oocytes is still well below that of oocytes harvested from stimulated ovaries, indicating that the protocols are sub-optimal or that many of the harvested oocytes are intrinsically unable to undergo maturation (66).

Progress has been made in large mammalian species, with IVM achieved and live births reported using bovine oocytes of <100 μm that were aspirated from immature follicles and grown for 14 days until the oocyte was large enough to be matured *in vitro* (64). Oocyte growth within IVG preantral bovine follicles has shown that oocytes increase in size from <50 to >90 μm over a 15-day *in vitro* period whilst maintaining morphological normality (60). This suggests that an *in vitro* growth system is capable of supporting oocyte development initially within immature follicles and then as oocyte–somatic cell units outside the follicle until oocytes are large enough to undergo IVM. These results give encouragement that a similar system could be applied to human oocyte granulosa cell complexes aspirated from IVG follicles.

IVG oocytes may require a further period of growth within the cumulus complex before maturation (60). To achieve this final growth phase, the oocyte cannot be considered separately from its companion somatic cells, but this oocyte–somatic cell unit needs to be removed from the antral follicle. In order to achieve developmental competence, an oocyte must maintain close and constant contact with its companion innermost granulosa cells, the cumulus, as it is via the junctions established between the oocyte and the cumulus that the complex process is mediated (reviewed in [42]). Maintenance of oocyte–somatic cell interactions and cytoskeleton stability is important at this stage, and in bovine follicles, it has been demonstrated that the correct balance of activin and FSH *in vitro* affects these processes (67).

NEXT STEPS

The safety of developing gametes entirely *in vitro* needs to be a major consideration and appropriate testing for epigenetic and meiotic normality need to be applied (68,69). Recent studies in mice have demonstrated that complete oocyte formation and development can been achieved entirely *in vitro* from induced pluripotent stem cells and embryonic stem cells (70,71). These *in vitro* derived oocytes can be fertilised and result in apparently healthy offspring. A major factor in achieving this success is in combining the appropriate somatic cells to support germ cell development and with these systems (70,71). It is clear that if human oocytes are to be developed entirely *in vitro* from stem cells the somatic cell contribution will be a major determinant of success (72,73).

REFERENCES

1. Hendriks S, Dancet EAF, Van Pelt AMM, Hamer G, Repping S. Artificial gametes: A systematic review of biological progress towards clinical application. *Human Reproduction Update* 2015; 21: 285–96.
2. Hubner K, Fuhrmann G, Christenson LK, Kehler J, Reinbold R, De La Fuente R, Wood J, Strauss JF 3rd, Boiani, M., Scholer, HR. Derivation of oocytes from mouse embryonic stem cells. *Science* 2003; 300: 1251–6.
3. Salvador LM, Silva CP, Kostetskii I, Radice GL, Strauss JF, 3rd. The promoter of the oocyte-specific gene, Gdf9, is active in population of cultured mouse embryonic stem cells with an oocyte-like phenotype. *Methods* 2008; 45: 172–81.
4. Evans MJ, Kaufman MH. Establishment in culture of pluripotential cells from mouse embryos. *Nature* 1981; 292: 154–6.
5. Keller GM. *In-vitro* differentiation of embryonic stem-cells. *Curr Opin Cell Biol* 1995; 7: 862–9.
6. Lawson KA, Dunn NR, Roelen BA, Zeinstra LM, Davis AM, Wright CV, Korving JP, Hogan BL. Bmp4 is required for the generation of primordial germ cells in the mouse embryo. *Genes Dev* 1999; 13: 424–36.
7. Hayashi K, Ohta H, Kurimoto K, Aramaki S, Saitou M. Reconstitution of the mouse germ cell specification pathway in culture by pluripotent stem cells. *Cell* 2011; 146: 519–32.
8. Wei W, Qing T, Ye X, Liu H, Zhang D, Yang W, Deng H. Primordial germ cell specification from embryonic stem cells. *PLoS One* 2008; 3: e4013.
9. Qing T, Shi Y, Qin H, Ye X, Wei W, Liu H, Ding M, Deng H. Induction of oocyte-like cells from mouse embryonic stem cells by co-culture with ovarian granulosa cells. *Differentiation* 2007; 75: 902–11.
10. Eguizabal C, Shovlin TC, Durcova-Hills G, Surani A, McLaren A. Generation of primordial germ cells from pluripotent stem cells. *Differentiation* 2009; 78: 116–23.
11. Hayashi K, Ogushi S, Kurimoto K, Shimamoto S, Ohta H, Saitou M. Offspring from oocytes derived from *in vitro* primordial germ cell-like cells in mice. *Science* 2012; 338: 971–5.
12. Shah SM, Saini N, Ashraf S, Singh MK, Manik RS, Singla SK, Palta P, Chauhan MS. Bone morphogenetic protein 4 (BMP4) induces buffalo (*Bubalus bubalis*) embryonic stem cells differentiation into germ cells. *Biochimie* 2015; 119: 113–24.
13. Duggal G, Heindryckx B, Warrier S et al. Influence of activin A supplementation during human embryonic stem cell derivation on germ cell differentiation potential. *Stem Cells Dev* 2013; 22: 3141–55.

14. Aflatoonian B, Ruban L, Jones M, Aflatoonian R, Fazeli A, Moore HD. *In vitro* post-meiotic germ cell development from human embryonic stem cells. *Hum Reprod* 2009; 24: 3150–9.
15. Tachibana M, Amato P, Sparman M et al. Human embryonic stem cells derived by somatic cell nuclear transfer. *Cell* 2013; 153(6): 1228–38.
16. Takahashi K, Yamanaka S. Induction of pluripotent stem cells from mouse embryonic and adult fibroblast cultures by defined factors. *Cell* 2006; 126: 663–76.
17. Takahashi K, Tanabe K, Ohnuki M, Narita M, Ichisaka T, Tomoda K, Yamanaka S. Induction of pluripotent stem cells from adult human fibroblasts by defined factors. *Cell* 2007; 131: 861–72.
18. Boland MJ, Hazen JL, Nazor KL, Rodriguez AR, Gifford W, Martin G, Kupriyanov S, Baldwin KK. Adult mice generated from induced pluripotent stem cells. *Nature* 2009; 461: 91–4.
19. Zhao XY, Li W, Lv Z, Liu L, Tong M, Hai T, Hao J, Wang X, Wang L, Zeng F, Zhou Q. Viable fertile mice generated from fully pluripotent iPS cells derived from adult somatic cells. *Stem Cell Rev* 2010; 6: 390–7.
20. Estrov Z. Stem cells and somatic cells: Reprogramming and plasticity. *Clin Lymphoma Myeloma* 2009; 9(Suppl 3): S319–28.
21. Dyce PW, Liu J, Tayade C, Kidder GM, Betts DH, Li J. *In vitro* and *in vivo* germ line potential of stem cells derived from newborn mouse skin. *PLoS One* 2011; 6: e20339.
22. Sun R, Sun YC, Ge W et al. The crucial role of Activin A on the formation of primordial germ cell-like cells from skin-derived stem cells *in vitro*. *Cell Cycle* 2015; 14: 3016–29.
23. Linher K, Dyce P, Li J. Primordial germ cell-like cells differentiated *in vitro* from skin-derived stem cells. *PLoS One* 2009; 4: e8263.
24. Danner S, Kajahn J, Geismann C, Klink E, Kruse C. Derivation of oocyte-like cells from a clonal pancreatic stem cell line. *Mol Hum Reprod* 2007; 13: 11–20.
25. Cheng X, Chen S, Yu X, Zheng P, Wang H. *BMP15* gene is activated during human amniotic fluid stem cell differentiation into oocyte-like cells. *DNA Cell Biol* 2012; 31: 1198–204.
26. Yu X, Wang N, Qiang R, Wan Q, Qin M, Chen S, Wang H. Human amniotic fluid stem cells possess the potential to differentiate into primordial follicle oocytes *in vitro*. *Biol Reprod* 2014; 90: 73.
27. Dokshin GA, Baltus AE, Eppig JJ, Page DC. Oocyte differentiation is genetically dissociable from meiosis in mice. *Nat Genet* 2013; 45: 877–83.
28. Woods DC, Telfer EE, Tilly JL. Oocyte family trees: Old branches or new stems? *PLoS Genet* 2012; 8: e1002848.
29. Dunlop CE, Telfer EE, Anderson RA. Ovarian stem cells—Potential roles in infertility treatment and fertility preservation. *Maturitas* 2013; 76: 279–83.
30. Grieve KM, McLaughlin M, Dunlop CE, Telfer EE, Anderson RA. The controversial existence and functional potential of oogonial stem cells (OSCs). *Maturitas* 2015; 82: 278–81.
31. Zou K, Yuan Z, Yang Z et al. Production of offspring from a germline stem cell line derived from neonatal ovaries. *Nat Cell Biol* 2009; 11: 631–6.
32. White YA, Woods DC, Takai Y, Ishihara O, Seki H, Tilly JL. Oocyte formation by mitotically active germ cells purified from ovaries of reproductive-age women. *Nat Med* 2012; 18: 413–21.
33. Zhou L, Wang L, Kang JX et al. Production of fat-1 transgenic rats using a post-natal female germline stem cell line. *Mol Hum Reprod* 2014; 20: 271–81.
34. Hernandez SF, Vahidi NA, Park S, Weitzel RP, Tisdale J, Rueda BR, Wolff EF. Characterization of extracellular DDX4- or Ddx4-positive ovarian cells. *Nat Med* 2015; 21: 1114–6.
35. Zhang H, Panula S, Petropoulos S et al. Adult human and mouse ovaries lack DDX4-expressing functional oogonial stem cells. *Nat Med* 2015; 21: 1116–8.
36. Telfer EE, Albertini DF. The quest for human ovarian stem cells. *Nat Med* 2012; 18: 353–4.
37. Eppig JJ, O'Brien MJ. Development *in vitro* of mouse oocytes from primordial follicles. *Biol Reprod* 1996; 54: 197–207.
38. O'Brien MJ, Pendola JK, Eppig JJ. A revised protocol for *in vitro* development of mouse oocytes from primordial follicles dramatically improves their developmental competence. *Biol Reprod* 2003; 68: 1682–6.
39. Smitz J, Dolmans MM, Donnez J et al. Current achievements and future research directions in ovarian tissue culture, *in vitro* follicle development and transplantation: Implications for fertility preservation. *Hum Reprod Update* 2010; 16: 395–414.
40. Telfer EE, Zelinski MB. Ovarian follicle culture: Advances and challenges for human and nonhuman primates. *Fertil Steril* 2013; 99: 1523–33.
41. Xiao S, Zhang J, Romero MM, Smith KN, Shea LD, Woodruff TK. *In vitro* follicle growth supports human oocyte meiotic maturation. *Sci Rep* 2015; 5: 17323.
42. Li R, Albertini DF. The road to maturation: Somatic cell interaction and self-organization of the mammalian oocyte. *Nat Rev Mol Cell Biol* 2013; 14: 141–52.
43. Telfer EE, McLaughlin M. Strategies to support human oocyte development *in vitro*. *Int J Dev Biol* 2012; 56: 901–7.
44. Hovatta O, Wright C, Krausz T, Hardy K, Winston RM. Human primordial, primary and secondary ovarian follicles in long-term culture: Effect of partial isolation. *Hum Reprod* 1999; 14: 2519–24.
45. Telfer EE, McLaughlin M, Ding C, Thong KJ. A two-step serum-free culture system supports development of human oocytes from primordial follicles in the presence of activin. *Hum Reprod* 2008; 23: 1151–8.

46. McLaughlin M, Kinnell HL, Anderson RA, Telfer EE. Inhibition of phosphatase and tensin homologue (PTEN) in human ovary *in vitro* results in increased activation of primordial follicles but compromises development of growing follicles. *Mol Hum Reprod* 2014; 20: 736–44.
47. Anderson RA, McLaughlin M, Wallace WH, Albertini DF, Telfer EE. The immature human ovary shows loss of abnormal follicles and increasing follicle developmental competence through childhood and adolescence. *Hum Reprod* 2014; 29: 97–106.
48. Xu M, Barrett SL, West-Farrell E, Kondapalli LA, Kiesewetter SE, Shea LD, Woodruff TK. *In vitro* grown human ovarian follicles from cancer patients support oocyte growth. *Hum Reprod* 2009; 24: 2531–40.
49. Alak BM, Coskun S, Friedman CI, Kennard EA, Kim MH, Seifer DB. Activin A stimulates meiotic maturation of human oocytes and modulates granulosa cell steroidogenesis *in vitro*. *Fertil Steril* 1998; 70: 1126–30.
50. Cha KY, Chian RC. Maturation *in vitro* of immature human oocytes for clinical use. *Hum Reprod Update* 1998; 4: 103–20.
51. Mikkelsen AL, Smith SD, Lindenberg S. *In-vitro* maturation of human oocytes from regularly menstruating women may be successful without follicle stimulating hormone priming. *Hum Reprod* 1999; 14: 1847–51.
52. Cavilla JL, Kennedy CR, Byskov AG, Hartshorne GM. Human immature oocytes grow during culture for IVM. *Hum Reprod* 2008; 23: 37–45.
53. Chian RC, Uzelac PS, Nargund G. *In vitro* maturation of human immature oocytes for fertility preservation. *Fertil Steril* 2013; 99: 1173–81.
54. Hsueh AJ, Kawamura K, Cheng Y, Fauser BC. Intraovarian control of early folliculogenesis. *Endocr Rev* 2015; 36: 1–24.
55. Reddy P, Liu L, Adhikari D et al. Oocyte-specific deletion of Pten causes premature activation of the primordial follicle pool. *Science* 2008; 319: 611–3.
56. Fan H-Y, Liu Z, Cahill N, Richards JS. Targeted disruption of Pten in ovarian granulosa cells enhances ovulation and extends the life span of luteal cells. *Mol Endocrinol* 2008; 22: 2128–40.
57. Li J, Kawamura K, Cheng Y, Liu S, Klein C, Liu S, Duan EK, Hsueh AJ. Activation of dormant ovarian follicles to generate mature eggs. *Proc Natl Acad Sci USA* 2010; 107: 10280–4.
58. McLaughlin M, Patrizio P, Kayisli U, Luk J, Thomson TC, Anderson RA, Telfer EE, Johnson J. mTOR kinase inhibition results in oocyte loss characterized by empty follicles in human ovarian cortical strips cultured *in vitro*. *Fertil Steril* 2011; 96: 1154–9.
59. Kawamura K, Cheng Y, Suzuki N et al. Hippo signaling disruption and Akt stimulation of ovarian follicles for infertility treatment. *Proc Natl Acad Sci USA* 2013; 110: 17474–9.
60. McLaughlin M, Telfer EE. Oocyte development in bovine primordial follicles is promoted by activin and FSH within a two-step serum-free culture system. *Reproduction* 2010; 139: 971–8.
61. Wandji SA, Srsen V, Voss AK, Eppig JJ, Fortune JE. Initiation *in vitro* of growth of bovine primordial follicles. *Biol Reprod* 1996; 55: 942–8.
62. Wandji SA, Srsen V, Nathanielsz PW, Eppig JJ, Fortune JE. Initiation of growth of baboon primordial follicles *in vitro*. *Hum Reprod* 1997; 12: 1993–2001.
63. Itoh T, Kacchi M, Abe H, Sendai Y, Hoshi H. Growth, antrum formation, and estradiol production of bovine preantral follicles cultured in a serum-free medium. *Biol Reprod* 1999; 67: 1099–105.
64. Hirao Y, Itoh T, Shimizu M, Iga K, Aoyagi K, Kobayashi M, Kacchi M, Hoshi H, Takenouchi N. *In vitro* growth and development of bovine oocyte-granulosa cell complexes on the flat substratum: Effects of high polyvinylpyrrolidone concentration in culture medium. *Biol Reprod* 2004; 70: 83–91.
65. Ting AY, Yeoman RR, Lawson MS, Zelinski MB. *In vitro* development of secondary follicles from cryopreserved rhesus macaque ovarian tissue after slow-rate freeze or vitrification. *Hum Reprod* 2011; 26: 2461–72.
66. Nogueira D, Sadeu JC, Montagut J. *In vitro* oocyte maturation: Current status. *Semin Reprod Med* 2012; 30: 199–213.
67. McLaughlin M, Bromfield JJ, Albertini DF, Telfer EE. Activin promotes follicular integrity and oogenesis in cultured pre-antral bovine follicles. *Mol Hum Reprod* 2010; 16: 644–53.
68. Anckaert E, De Rycke M, Smitz J. Culture of oocytes and risk of imprinting defects. *Hum Reprod Update* 2013; 19: 52–66.
69. Handel MA, Eppig JJ, Schimenti JC. Applying "gold standards" to *in-vitro*-derived germ cells. *Cell* 2014; 157: 1257–61.
70. Morohaku K, Tanimoto R, Sasaki K, Kawahara-Miki R, Kono T, Hayashi K, Hirao Y, Obata Y. Complete in vitro generation of fertile oocytes from mouse primordial germ cells. *Proc Natl Acad Sci USA* 2016; 113(32): 9021–26.
71. Hikabe O, Hamazaki N, Nagamatsu G et al. Reconstitution in vitro of the entire cycle of the mouse female germ line. *Nature* 2016; 539(7628): 299–303. doi: 10.1038/nature20104.
72. Hummitzsch K, Anderson RA, Wilhelm D et al. Stem cells, progenitor cells, and lineage decisions in the ovary. *Endocr Rev* 2015; 36: 65–91.
73. Truman AM, Tilly JL, Woods DC. Ovarian regeneration: The potential for stem cell contribution in the postnatal ovary to sustained endocrine function. *Mol Cell Endocrinol* 2017; 445: 74–84.

Microfluidics in assisted reproduction technology

Towards automation of the in vitro fertilization laboratory

31

JASON E. SWAIN

Optimized production of preimplantation embryos for use in assisted reproduction technologies (ARTs) has been a central goal of reproductive scientists since the inception of the field, and, subsequently, methodologies have continually been refined to aid in this endeavor. For example, skilled technicians meticulously handle gametes and embryos in prescribed manners, extensive research has refined culture media formulations to cater to the changing metabolic needs of gametes and embryos, and commercial manufacturers have produced specialized equipment to meet the specific needs of cells in ART. Though approached from different perspectives, the commonality between these advancements is the pursuit of minimizing external stresses imposed upon gametes and embryos due to artificial manipulation within the *in vitro* fertilization (IVF) laboratory. Environmental and intracellular factors influenced by these manipulations, such as osmotic imbalances, shifts in temperature, mechanical stress, and pH fluctuations, can all have negative effects on embryo quality. However, even with these tremendous improvements, relatively little attention has been paid to the platform on which gametes and embryos are manipulated and cultured.

Modification of the platform on which gametes and embryos are handled may present an opportunity to further improve the culture conditions *in vitro*. Clinical embryology laboratories have historically selected between polystyrene test tubes, Petri dishes, organ culture wells, or four-well plates to accommodate varying numbers of cells and volumes of media used. However, this is a vast departure from the physical conditions presented by the female reproductive tract.

In the quest to optimize embryo development *in vitro*, a "back to nature" ideology has been adopted by some when formulating embryo culture media (1). To the best of its ability, this approach attempts to base culture media formations on the composition of fluids in the female reproductive tract in order to chemically manipulate embryo development *in vitro*. Similarly, this same biomimetic approach may also be applied to culture platforms, attempting to recapitulate the conditions experienced by the embryos *in vivo*. *In vivo*, gametes and embryos are exposed to the constricted "moist" environment of the female reproductive tract and are surrounded by variously oriented glycoproteins as they are gently moved via ciliated epithelium. This is in stark contrast to the expansive, largely static environment gametes and embryos are exposed to *in vitro*, resting on inert synthetic polymers, bathed in a relative ocean of media. Microfluidic technology and other novel culture platforms offer a means to further manipulate culture conditions *in vitro* in the hopes of creating an environment that is more suitable to gamete and embryo development and function. Furthermore, these platforms offer the potential to revolutionize the fundamental approaches currently utilized within IVF laboratories, allowing for the replacement of manual manipulations with automation of specific procedural steps.

BASIS AND APPEAL OF MICROFLUIDICS

Though a few dynamic culture platforms have emerged, many utilizing fluid movement on the macro-level, the focus of this review will be largely on those approaches or platforms employing microfluidics. While vibrational embryo culture and titling embryo culture have both yielded some promising preliminary results (2–8), these are large-scale devices that may not fully capitalize on approaches to pheno-mimic the female reproductive tract.

The term "microfluidic" refers to technology utilizing characteristics of fluid movement in a micro- or nano-environment. These characteristics, discussed in depth elsewhere (9,10), rely heavily on variables such as fluid density, viscosity, velocity, and size/geometry of the environment. At the macro-level, fluid flow results in chaotic particle movement within the fluid stream, leading to turbulence. In contrast, in the decreasing dimensions of microfluidic channels, fluid is imparted with streamlined and predictable flow patterns. These predictable flow patterns conferred by microfluidic devices impose laminar flow upon fluids, allowing parallel movement of multiple streams of media through the same microchannel with no mixing, except by diffusion across the fluid–fluid interface (Figure 31.1). It is at these extremely small scales that fluid viscosity and surface tension become increasingly important considerations for fluid flow. As a result, microfluidic approaches offer certain advantages, as well as disadvantages, over larger dynamic fluid movement approaches, and may also yield differing results in regard to gamete and embryo culture.

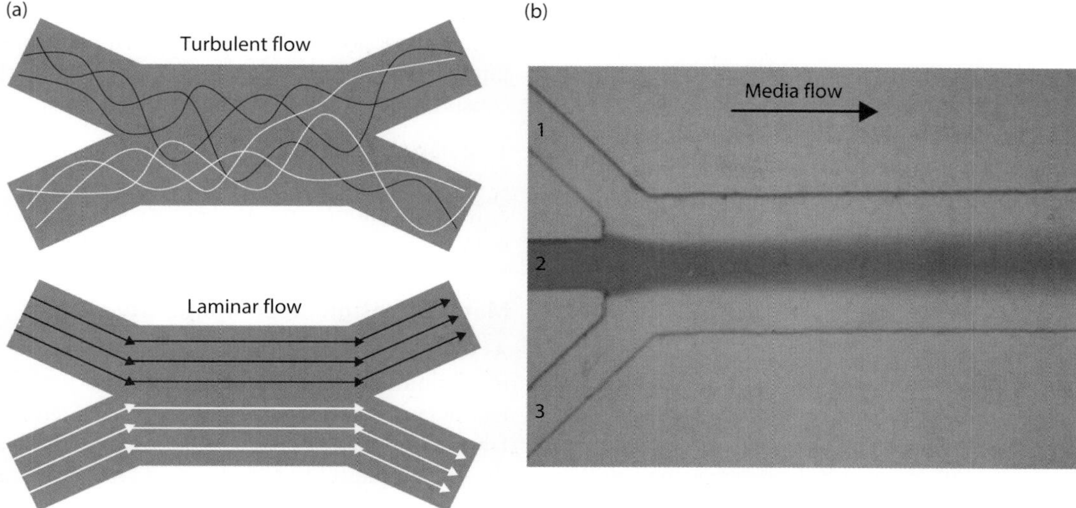

Figure 31.1 (a) Illustration of turbulent versus laminar flow. Laminar flow is one of the inherent properties of microfluidic platforms, which allows for unique applications in assisted reproduction technology. (b) Microfluidic device demonstrating laminar flow. Fluid from channels 1, 2, and 3 flows in parallel with no mixing, except by simple diffusion.

FABRICATION OF MICROFLUIDIC DEVICES FOR USE IN ART

Fabrication of microfluidic devices for use in ART has been covered elsewhere in reference to biocompatible materials and manufacturing approaches (11–13). A practical guide of considerations in regard to fabricating perfusion-based microfluidic platforms for adherent cell culture also exists (14), and key issues must be addressed for application in ART. To summarize, various materials have been found to be adequate for gamete and embryo culture, and currently tested devices are composed of polydimethylsiloxane (PDMS), silicone, borosilicate glass, Pyrex, quartz, or combinations of these materials (15–24). Materials selected for the construction of microfluidic channels may differ from materials selected for cell substrate or the actual surface on which cells lie. Though the cell substrate surface is a critical consideration for adherent cell culture to ensure cell attachment, it is not as crucial a factor for culture of non-adherent oocytes or embryos. Manufacturing techniques for microchannels involve molding, photolithography, and chemically or mechanically etching channels into suitable materials. The most commonly used material for microchannel fabrication is the polymer PDMS, which is selected due to its inherent use and fabrication advantages, such as flexibility, ease of soft-lithography patterning, and low autofluorescence for use with microscopy (14). Subsequently, compatible microchannel components are bonded to companion components/platforms with non-toxic adhesives or epoxies. Benefits of these materials and manufacturing processes include rapid, repeatable, precise, and inexpensive production, necessities for use in clinical ART, as devices should be disposable to ensure sterility.

MEDIA FLOW AND DYNAMIC APPROACHES IN ART MICROFLUIDIC DEVICES

As mentioned, one benefit of microfluidics for use in ART is the ability to achieve dynamic media flow on a culture platform. Although the approach of dynamic media flow in embryo culture is not new, prior attempts at perfusion systems, which remove or renew media on the macroscale, has proved inefficient and subsequently not been implemented on a large scale (25–27). Other simplified approaches using gentle media agitation on the macroscale are receiving more widespread attention, but lack the power for media removal or renewal and associated potential benefits. Fortunately, the unique nature of microfluidic platforms allows for alternative approaches to accomplishing media perfusion and movement that are more amenable to widespread use. These methods are often dictated by constraints of platform design, which is dependent upon whether perfusion systems are recirculating or non-recirculating. Furthermore, the ability of perfusion systems to operate over long periods of time with minimal manipulation is essential. In adherent cell systems, perfusion devices have been operated successfully for over one week (28,29).

Early devices for ART applications have employed gravity-driven passive flow, with hydrostatic pressure in media reservoirs as an important variable to drive media flow down microchannels (17,18,21,24,30,31). While the simplicity of the approach is advantageous, it is difficult to regulate flow speed or volume changes, especially over time, when the height of media columns diminishes. Others have utilized manually applied pressure via externally attached syringes to input/output ports to cause media flow through microfluidic devices (32). Again, the simplicity of this approach is attractive; however, it is difficult to regulate pressure precisely and manual methods to regulate flow are not feasible for use over the long periods of time required for embryo culture. A variation of the syringe-driven flow approach has been further adapted through use of Hamilton syringes attached to a programmable infusion pump (23). Although more precise and feasible for use over time, the required external tubing and machinery are problematic for use within a closed incubator environment. Additionally, at least one study has used a tilting culture system in conjunction with microfluidic channels, which, while still using gravity, offers more consistent control over flow gravity-driven hydrostatic pressure approaches. Titling devices may offer an improved means of providing gentle media and embryo movement, thereby possibly conveying any associated benefits, but have only been examined with use of larger-volume microdrops (3,33). Furthermore, tilting approaches and simple agitation do not necessarily remove or replenish the existing media. Regardless, this approach appears promising and warrants future study. Similar methods of combining simplified, constrictive microchannels with other dynamic methods of inducing fluid movement/flow, such as vibration (7,8,34), may be helpful, as gentle agitation appears to be beneficial for human embryos. Application of shaking or rotating platforms (35–39) with constrictive culture approaches remains to be explored and offers a seemingly simple way of introducing gentle physical stimulation to developing embryos. Importantly, use of these approaches needs to be validated, as sheer forces and other factors become relevant with embryo motion in small, confined areas. Finally, a Braille pumping system using tiny electric piezo-actuators has been used successfully to peristaltically move media along microchannels during embryo culture, while the embryos remain largely undisturbed (40–43). This approach not only allows for precise computerized regulation of speed and flow patterns, but also the devices are compact enough to fit multiple units within a single incubator. It should be noted, however, that the Braille system, like most other dynamic culture devices, is an electronic device, and special precautions must be taken to account for the humid incubator environment. Other possible approaches yet to be explored for ART to regulate fluid flow in microfluidic devices include pneumatics or magnetic gates/actuators. In addition, perhaps the most intriguing concept for regulating media flow within a microfluidic device entails use of the expansive characteristics of a three-dimensional matrix—a hydrogel—to regulate flow through channels (44). This technology offers the ability to control media flow through mechanical responses in the hydrogel due to external stimuli such as temperature, light, pH, and biological cues.

REQUIREMENTS OF MICROFLUIDICS FOR ART

Although the theoretical advantages of microfluidics platforms in ART should be apparent, it is important to recognize that several potential issues must be addressed in order to achieve widespread acceptance. Many of these issues exist regardless of the cell system cultured within microfluidic devices; however, reproductive applications of microfluidic platforms also require unique considerations. These considerations can be grouped into four major categories:

1. Material/design biocompatibility
2. Device operation/failure
3. Manipulation/removal of embryos
4. IVF laboratory/embryologist compatibility

Material/design biocompatibility

As with other embryo culture dishes, it must be shown that microfluidic devices are non-toxic and pass quality control assays. Though initial testing has identified suitable fabrication materials, in-house testing must also verify the biocompatibility of individual lots, ensuring contaminants were not introduced during production. Paramount in ensuring biocompatibility is the ability to sterilize devices following fabrication. Current studies have utilized devices treated with UV light, ethanol or ethylene oxide, or autoclaving (23,24). Although these approaches do not appear to affect the properties of PDMS (14,45), high heat or chemical sterilization can warp or change the biochemical properties of other polymers. Future exploration of more traditional sterilization methods, such as γ-irradiation, should be explored.

The fabrication materials used in current microfluidic devices display unique properties that must also be addressed before implementation into IVF labs. Although these properties may be conducive for fabrication purposes, materials such as PDMS are absorptive and can alter media characteristics, including media flow and osmolarity, thereby impeding subsequent embryo development (46). Fortunately, surface modification to fabrication materials, including parylene coating or bonding with poly(ethylene glycol) methyl ether methacrylate (PEG-MA), may alleviate some of these concerns (47,48).

Another important consideration is the small amount of medium present when using microfluidic platforms. Properties such as medium viscosity, pH, and density of cells become important factors in platform design.

Device operation/failure

Microfluidic devices employing dynamic culture must incorporate reliable mechanisms for imparting media flow. This requires a safe and effective interface between the microchannel platform and the perfusion regulatory device. Furthermore, a key consideration in regard to the operation of dynamic flow is the ability to avoid bubble formation within microchannels. Construction of a bubble trap along the microfluidic channel may help alleviate this concern (49). Alternatively, larger-scale dynamic platforms may be used, though these may ameliorate the benefits of the small scale. Fortunately, if devices fail and media flow halts, the result is the current default static system. However, it is essential that devices possess methods to easily determine if flow has been interrupted, and if so, easy correction or repair should be available.

Manipulation/removal of embryos

Perhaps the most difficult criterion to address in regard to the construction and implementation of microfluidic technology in the IVF lab is the ability to easily manipulate or remove gametes/embryos, a limitation not often considered in the devices currently used for adherent somatic cell culture or diagnostic assays. Furthermore, daily observation and manipulation of embryos cannot be a labor-intensive process, as increased time to view, add, or remove embryos will adversely stress blastomeres. Detriments with prolonged manipulation are exacerbated by the inherent problems that exist when dealing with extremely small volumes of liquid in microfluidics, such as rapid evaporation, resulting osmolarity shifts, and rapid shifts in pH and temperature. Thus, the design must incorporate a user-friendly interface through which the embryologist can access cells. A current approach that seems to work well is to culture cells within funnels (40), or to simply place a larger traditional static culture dish on a platform that moves or agitates the media. Furthermore, paramount in minimizing risks with prolonged handling is the ability to easily visualize cells within the device. Therefore, the materials used must possess optical properties for visualizing and tracking individual cells within the device for grading purposes. Optical properties should also be compatible with emerging technologies, such as polarized microscopy.

IVF laboratory/embryologist compatibility

Importantly, to gain widespread acceptance in clinical IVF, microfluidic devices need to be compatible with current IVF lab setups and practices. Thus, devices must fit into contemporary incubators without external or bulky tubing or apparatus. Though much of the prospective power of microfluidic technology resides in more advanced analytical and automated processes that can be resident on the platform, these advancements cannot be realized without strong initial acceptance by the practicing embryologist. Cost of implementation also becomes a consideration when attempting to bring new technology to the lab.

MICROFLUIDICS IN ANDROLOGY

Though future refinement is still required, addressing the key issues of microfluidics has progressed enough to begin to take advantage of the unique applications offered by microfluidic platforms in areas of reproduction, such as andrology (50).

Sperm movement and function

As early as 1993, microchannel devices made of silicone were used to evaluate sperm function via interactions with cervical mucus, hyaluronan, spermicide, and anti-sperm antibody beads (51). The same group later published a report demonstrating sperm count and motility assessment performed on etched glass microchannel devices (52). More recent devices composed of PDMS have proven useful for computerized analysis of pig sperm linear velocity and head displacement (53), and automated imaging software has been developed for use in assessing sperm motion with microfluidics (54).

Sperm separation

The first peer-reviewed publication on the use of microfluidic technology for separation of motile sperm from semen samples utilized a PDMS passive gravity-driven device where the hydrostatic pressure of two separate inlet reservoirs drove media flow down a converging microfluidic channel (Figure 31.2) (30). The principle of the device took

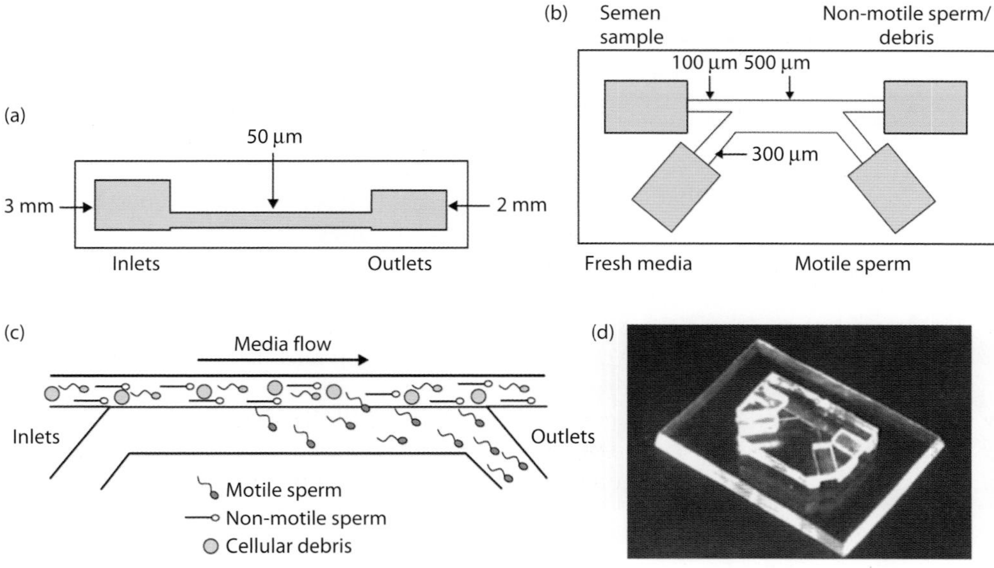

Figure 31.2 Illustration of a microfluidic sperm sorter. (a) Top view. (b) Side view. (c) Illustration demonstrating how laminar flow allows motile sperm to swim away from non-motile sperm and debris to collect in a separate reservoir. (d) Image of a sperm sorter device composed of polydimethylsiloxane.

advantage of the fact that only motile sperm can traverse the border that separates the parallel streams of diluted semen and fresh medium. Thus, the laminar flow properties exhibited by media in microchannels allowed motile sperm to swim away from non-motile sperm, debris, and seminal plasma and collect in a separate outlet reservoir. Follow-up experiments demonstrated that this microfluidic device design was not only biocompatible with human sperm, but that it could isolate motile, morphologically normal cells (17). Furthermore, surface modification of PDMS microfluidic sperm sorter devices to increase hydrophilicity with a coating such as PEG-MA may further improve this technology (47). Although limitations exist with the current device, including an inability to process large sample sizes, clogging, and sample viscosity issues, this novel approach provides a feasible alternative to isolating sperm from oligozoospermic patients for use in intracytoplasmic sperm injection (ICSI). Indeed, one microfluidic platform was shown to help isolate motile sperm and reduce the time needed for sperm processing to perform ICSI using porcine sperm by improving sperm recovery in oligospermic samples (Figure 31.3) (55).

Another approach employing microfluidics for sperm sorting utilized mouse sperm placed into a PDMS/glass device to isolate sperm based on motility, but also via chemotaxis towards cumulus cells (56). Sperm were placed into an inlet reservoir (2-mm radius) and allowed to swim down a straight channel, whose dimensions were optimized for motile sperm recovery at 1 × 7 mm

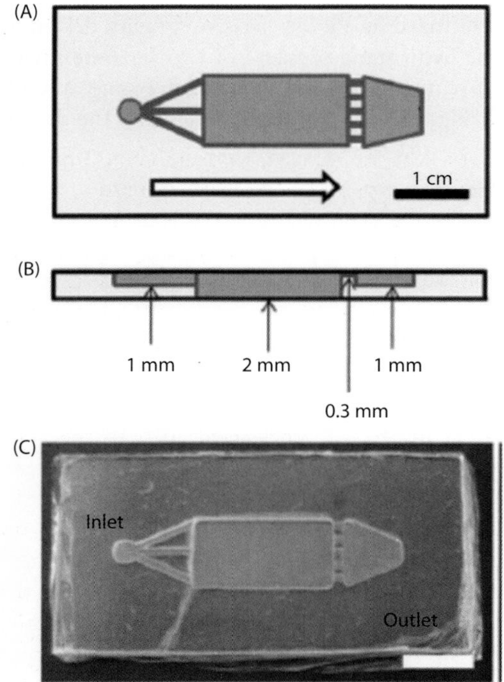

Figure 31.3 Images of a microfluidic sperm sorter that has been used to enrich sperm populations and reduce the time needed to perform intracytoplasmic sperm injection using poor-quality specimens. (A) Top view schematic. (B) Side view. (C) Image of the device composed of polydimethylsiloxane.

(width × length). Sperm then collected in a small central reservoir (1.25-mm radius), where video imaging could occur, before swimming onward into one of two branching channels (1 × 5 mm, width × length), each leading to separate collection reservoirs (2-mm radii). Other microfluidic devices to explore sperm chemotaxis exist and offer further methods to explore sperm function (57,58). Devices also exist to examine rheotaxis in sperm (59,60).

In another use of microfluidic technology for andrology, a PDMS/glass device has been constructed that directs sperm flow within oriented microchannels in order to separate, align, and orient sperm of mice, bulls, and humans (Figure 31.4) (61). Utilizing that facts that motile sperm orient themselves against media flow within these devices and that motile sperm can swim against media flow of a certain velocity, a series of three reservoirs and four microfluidic channels allow processing of sperm via hydrostatic media flow. Though this device requires precise regulation of media volumes in order to regulate hydrostatic pressure, the authors have designed devices with the future intent of exploring the implementation of a means of sorting X- and Y-bearing sperm, as well as the ability to add a "laser cutting" component in order to separate sperm heads from tails for ICSI.

Due to the limitations inherent in a microfluidic sperm sorting device, utilization of the technology must provide some added benefit over conventional processing methods. Conventional sperm preparation methods, such as serial centrifugation, density gradient separation, or swim up, are reported to induce sperm DNA damage, perhaps due to exposure to reaction oxygen species (ROS) (62–64). Preliminary data indicate that sperm isolated using a microfluidic sperm sorting device had significantly lower levels of DNA damage and higher motility compared to those isolated using more conventional approaches (31,65). Thus, microfluidic sperm sorting may allow for the selection of higher-quality sperm, potentially leading to improved embryo quality.

By utilizing these advantages of a microfluidic device for sperm isolation, implementation of a microfluidic sperm sorter manufactured out of quartz has begun in clinical IVF. A preliminary report indicates human semen can be processed rapidly and isolated motile sperm can be used to successfully fertilize human oocytes following ICSI (18). Continued research will determine if this technology results in improved embryo development and/or implantation rates.

MICROFLUIDICS IN EMBRYOLOGY

As mentioned, employing microfluidic technology for embryology applications requires considerations that are distinct from microfluidic devices utilizing adherent cells, including the ability to isolate or manipulate individual cells. In addition, the sensitivity of reproductive cells demands specialized precautions. Thus, progress implementing these devices has been slow. However, as with andrology applications, refinement of microfluidic designs has resolved several long-standing issues, and platforms

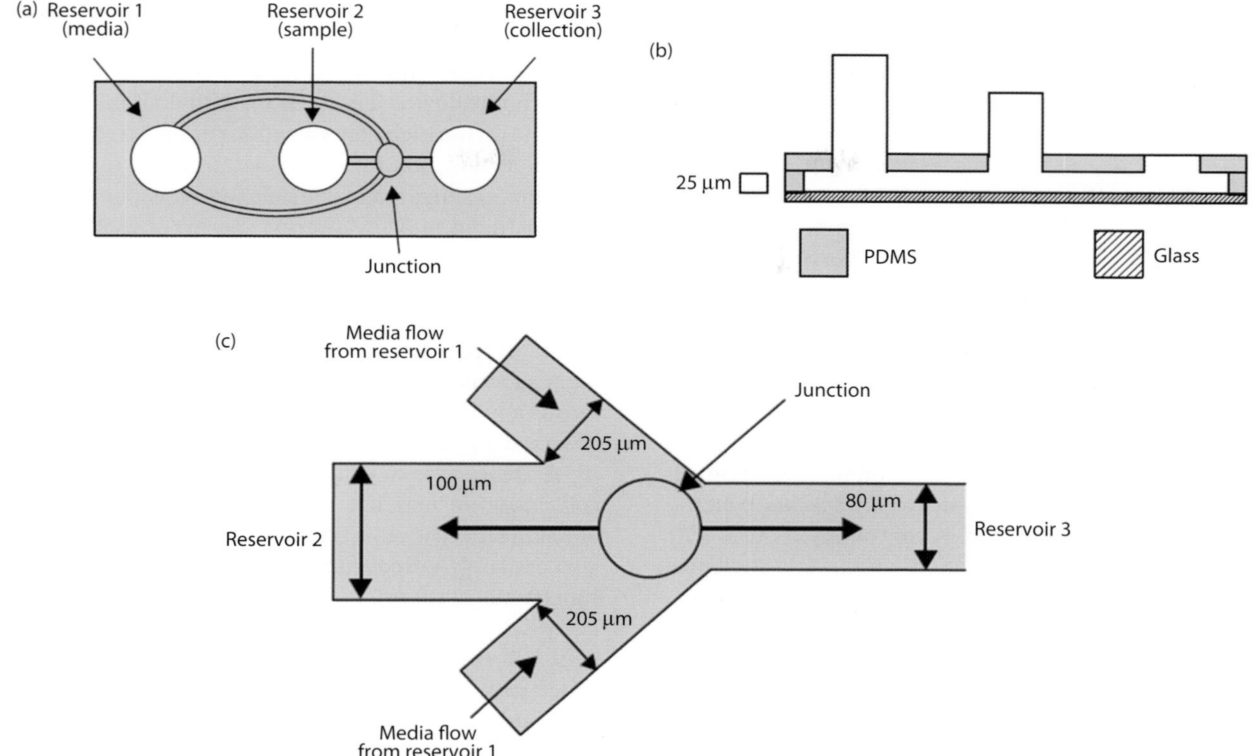

Figure 31.4 Diagram illustrating a microfluidic device for separation, orientation, and alignment of motile sperm from bulls, mice, and humans. Fresh medium is loaded into reservoir 1, while semen samples are loaded into reservoir 2. Hydrostatic pressure differences due to differences in height of the media columns in the three reservoirs cause media flow in various indicated directions. These media streams converge at a point known as the "junction." Motile spermatozoa orient themselves against the direction of media flow and are able to swim through the current to collect in reservoir 3. (a) Top view, (b) side view, and (c) dimensions of channel junction. *Abbreviation*: PDMS, polydimethylsiloxane.

have begun to receive initial testing in all aspects of embryology, including *in vitro* maturation (IVM), IVF, and embryo culture.

In vitro maturation

IVM is an especially appealing approach for human ART considering the tremendous advantages it offers, including reduced cost and reduced health risk regarding disorders such as ovarian hyperstimulation syndrome (66). However, IVM is still an inefficient practice. Fortunately, microfluidic approaches offer the potential to improve current IVM success rates. Preliminary data suggest that while porcine oocytes do not mature efficiently in silicone devices (2% development to metaphase II [MII]), they can indeed be matured successfully in PDMS microchannels (71% development to MII) (19). Oocytes matured in 200-μM wide PDMS microchannels containing approximately 8 μL of media displayed comparable development to MII as control oocytes matured in 8- or 500-μL drops. However, oocyte maturation consists of two components: nuclear and cytoplasmic maturation. Interestingly, cumulus cell expansion was noticeably diminished in oocytes matured in microchannels and 8-μL microdrops. This observation may be indicative of quality oocyte cytoplasmic maturation, as oocytes regulate cumulus cell development and function (67). Thus, the size and/or volume limitations of microchannels may have some limiting effect on porcine oocyte cytoplasmic properties or may physically restrict cumulus expansion. In contrast, subsequent follow-up experiments by Walters and co-workers from the same research group suggest that oocyte cytoplasmic maturation may actually be enhanced in static microchannels (22). Pig oocytes matured in 250-μM wide PDMS/borosilicate glass microchannels produced significantly higher numbers of two-cell embryos following IVF and embryo culture in microdrops compared to oocytes matured in 500-μL drops (67% vs. 49%) (22). Unfortunately, pronuclear formation, embryo development past the maternal–zygotic transition, or blastocyst cell numbers were not reported. Additionally, it should be noted that the chips utilized in these studies were not engineered with active media flow. Though some passive gravity-driven media flow may have been present, this parameter was not measured nor recorded in the experiments. Interestingly, preliminary studies indicate bovine oocytes matured in dynamic microfluidic devices with Braille pin-regulated media flow actually yield improved blastocyst development following IVF compared to static matured oocytes (personnel communication, Dr. Gary Smith). Despite these preliminary findings, the field awaits peer-reviewed publications examining the effects of fluid flow in microfluidic devices on more informative markers of oocyte cytoplasmic maturation, including genomic, proteomic, or metabolomic profiles.

In vitro fertilization

Another demonstration of microfluidic application in ART can be seen in IVF performed "on chip." The first attempt at this procedural step was performed using porcine oocytes placed into PDMS/borosilicate microchannels. Sperm was added in a manner in which pressure differences created from the volume of media added resulted in gravity-driven flow of sperm past oocytes (Figure 31.5). It was shown that the oocyte numbers used in experiments had no effect on sperm penetration. Further, fertilization in microchannels resulted in significantly lower rates of polyspermic penetration compared to fertilization in control microdrops (21). Reduced polyspermic penetration rates were attributed to the physical characteristics of the microfluidic device, mimicking the environment *in utero*. It is thought that microfluidic devices serve to limit the time of oocyte exposure to sperm, as sperm were not confined to the vicinity of the oocytes, as in microdrop culture, but allowed to flow past the eggs along the length of the microchannel. Further examination of sperm motility characteristics and interactions with oocytes during attempted fertilization in microfluidic channels demonstrated that flow rate is extremely important in regulating sperm motion, as a threshold exists where sperm are no longer capable of independent movement (68). Furthermore, sperm motion paths were influenced by the contours of the device. These qualities have immense implications for the success of fertilization in microfluidic device.

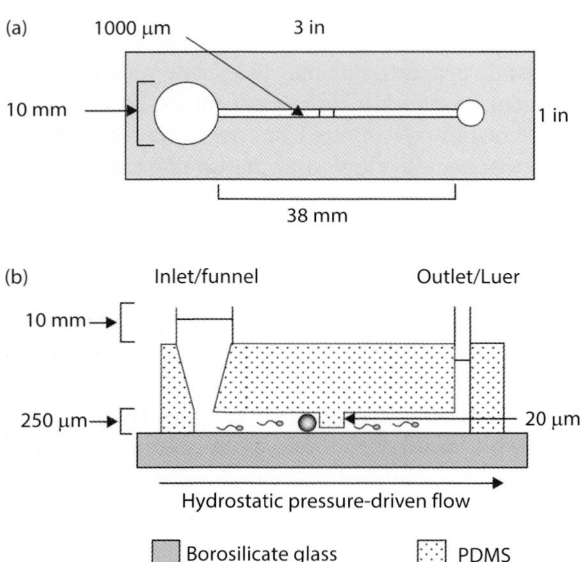

Figure 31.5 Illustration of a PDMS/borosilicate microfluidic device used to perform *in vitro* fertilization "on-chip." (a) Top view. (b) Side view. *Abbreviation*: PDSM, polydimethylsiloxane.

By utilizing cleavage of mouse embryos to two cells as an indicator of successful fertilization, Suh et al. (24) demonstrated that fertilization of mouse oocytes can occur in a microfluidic device (Figure 31.6). Although initial experiments utilizing high concentrations of sperm revealed that overall fertilization rates were decreased on the microfluidic device compared to controls, subsequent experiments demonstrated that, by lowering sperm concentration, fertilization rates in microfluidic devices were actually higher than fertilization rates in control drops. Fertilization rates obtained at these lower sperm concentrations in microfluidic devices were comparable to rates obtained with higher sperm concentrations in control microdrops. These results appear to be the result of chip design, as the authors observed increased concentration of sperm in the vicinity of the oocyte in microfluidic devices. This increased concentration may not only explain the increased rates of fertilization at reduced sperm concentrations, but may also explain the reduced fertilization rates at high concentrations of sperm. Increased sperm concentration may potentially result in decreased availability of local metabolic substrates, or result in detrimental shifts in culture conditions, such as pH or localized buildup of metabolic by-products.

Clark and co-workers presented preliminary data demonstrating both IVM and IVF of porcine oocytes could be performed in the same microfluidic device without removal of the cells between procedures (20). Media within devices were changed and sperm was added via manual pipetting without disturbing oocytes. Although there were no observable benefits in achieving cleavage to two cells compared to control treatments (49% vs. 51%), this was the first demonstration of multiple tasks of *in vitro* embryo production performed upon the same microfluidic platform. Such a realization has tremendous potential for performing multiple sequential steps "on chip" and minimization of stress to gametes/embryos.

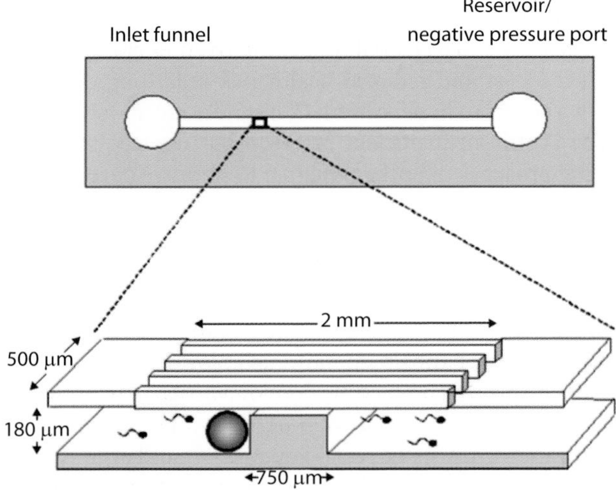

Figure 31.6 Microfluidic device composed of polydimethylsiloxane utilized to perform mouse *in vitro* fertilization "on chip."

More recently, fertilization has been performed on a microfluidic microwell device (69,70). Devices made of PDMS were constructed consisting of an inlet and outlet reservoir, which generated media flow using gravity. Microchannels (1 mm × 200 μm, width × height) leading from each reservoir connected to a larger microchamber (3 × 10 mm, width × length), which housed individual square microwells (200 × 200 × 200 μm, length × width × height), which contained individual oocytes (Figure 31.7). Microwell depth was optimized to permit retention of oocytes while allowing adequate debris removal and sperm interaction with oocytes. Media and sperm (1 ×10^6/mL) could then be flowed over the microwell housing the oocytes at ~2.5 mm/second. With oocytes settled in the bottom of microwells and out of the direct fluid stream, sheer forces are reduced, while permitting retention of any local autocrine/paracrine factors. Using this approach, similar rates of mouse oocyte fertilization were obtained compared to controls (69.0% vs. 71.4%) (71). An alternative device from the same research group with a differing design also yielded promising fertilization results and is discussed later (70).

IVF not only entails mixing of sperm and eggs, but also requires manipulation of presumptive zygotes to move cumulus cells in order to visualize pronuclei. Microfluidic devices do exist that can remove cumulus cells (72,73), and even zona pellucidae (74) by controlling media flow manually via attached syringes, exposing oocytes to chemical and physical manipulation. However, subsequent assessment of developmental competence, implantation, and live birth rates of microfluidic-derived IVF embryos is required to determine the efficacy of this approach. These efforts, though, are important, as this approach may offer substantial benefit to patients undergoing infertility treatment due to conditions such as oligozoospermia.

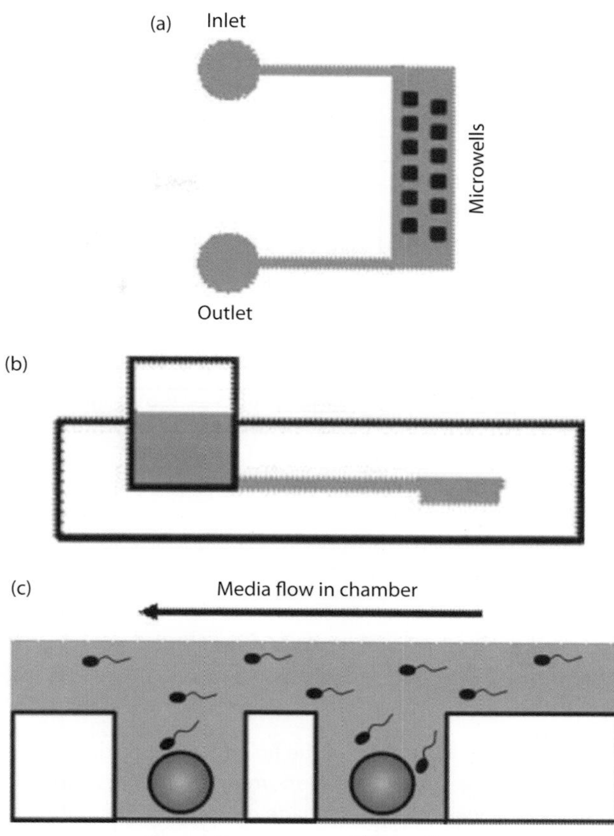

Figure 31.7 Microfluidic polydimethylsiloxane device utilizing gravity-driven media flow to pass sperm over mouse oocytes for *in vitro* fertilization. Oocytes are housed individually within microwells (200 × 200 × 200 μm, length × width × height) to prevent sheer stress, maintain autocrine/paracrine factors, and permit tracking of individual cells. (a) Top view. (b) Side view. (c) Close-up of microwells.

Embryo culture

Exhaustive studies have been conducted aimed at optimizing preimplantation embryo culture *in vitro*, and, similarly to IVM and IVF, a microfluidic platform may aid in this endeavor. The initial report on embryo culture using microfluidics by Raty and colleagues indicated that two-cell mouse embryos can be cultured to the blastocyst stage within static microchannels (Figure 31.8) (16,75). These experiments demonstrated that, compared to 30-μL control microdrops, culture within microchannels containing about 500 μL of media (10 μL within the actual channel itself) resulted in significantly greater 16-cell/morula formation at 24 hours, greater blastocyst formation at 48 and 72 hours, and a greater portion of hatched blastocysts at 72 and 96 hours. Subsequent experiments utilizing a similar device by Walters and co-workers from the same research group showed that *in vivo*-derived four-cell porcine embryos could be cultured to blastocyst and transferred, resulting in live birth (76). However, in these experiments, no observable beneficial effects on embryo development were seen when compared to culture in control organ-well dishes.

Building upon the initial chip-based static embryo culture studies, Hickman et al. examined mouse embryo development in microchannels with media flow controlled via a syringe infusion pump (Figure 31.9) (23). Flow rates examined in this study (0.1 and 0.5 μL/hour) did not enhance development compared to static culture. In fact, a flow rate of 0.5 μL/hour resulted in significantly lower development of two-cell mouse embryos to morula and blastocyst stages, while producing higher numbers of abnormal embryos compared to controls. Thus, flow rate and manner of flow delivery may be important variables for embryo culture in microfluidic devices. Indeed, embryos sense sheer stress, which can induce apoptosis and be detrimental to embryo development (77). However, it is questionable whether the flow rates necessary for dynamic fluid flow in microfluidic channels would approach velocities high enough to cause concern. Additionally, it should be noted that these data on the impact of media flow and flow rate on embryo development should be reassessed, as culture conditions may have been suboptimal. In this particular study, control mouse embryos cultured

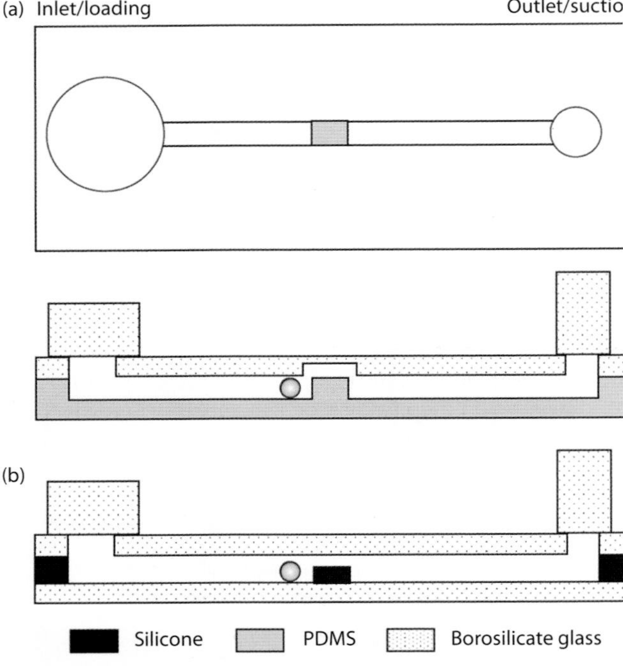

Figure 31.8 Illustration of the first microfluidic device created to culture preimplantation mouse embryos. (a) Top view. (b) Side view of devices made out of differing materials. *Abbreviation*: PDSM, polydimethylsiloxane.

in control static microchannels did not improve embryo development as previously reported by Raty et al. from the same research group (16). One possible source of variation requiring future study was the increased number of embryos cultured in each device.

Interestingly, by utilizing an alternative chip design, Cabrera and co-workers presented preliminary data

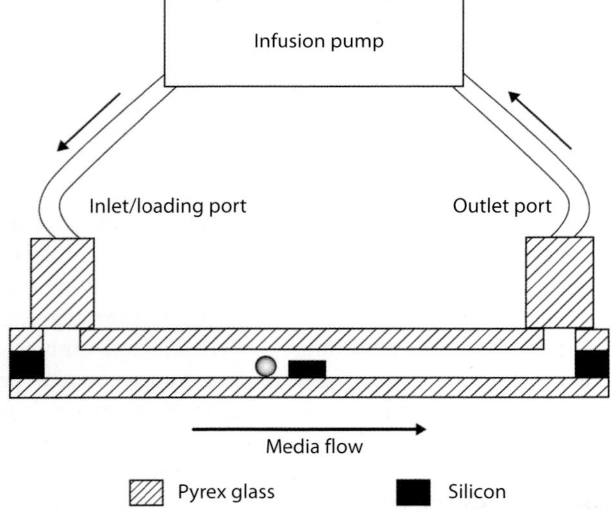

Figure 31.9 Diagram depicting a microfluidic perfusion system utilizing a syringe infusion pump to regulate media flow to culture preimplantation embryos.

showing that one-cell mouse embryos could be cultured efficiently within microfluidic devices offering media flow (42). Embryos were loaded into a funnel reservoir, while medium was added and removed via a microfluidic channel connected to the bottom of the funnel via the actions of a Braille actuator (Figure 31.10). It was demonstrated that regardless of media flow pattern (back and forth vs. flow-through) or speed (fast vs. slow), one-cell mouse embryos cultured in dynamic devices showed greater hatching of blastocysts and significantly higher cell numbers than static controls, yielding numbers similar to those obtained from *in vivo*-derived blastocysts.

Bormann and colleagues subsequently presented preliminary data validating the beneficial effects of Braille-driven media flow in a microfluidic device on murine and bovine embryo development (41). Greater numbers of mouse embryos reached morula stage at 48 hours, blastocyst stage at 72 hours, and hatched blastocyst stage at 96 hours compared to control static chips, while significantly more bovine embryos reached the blastocyst stage at 144 hours in microfluidic devices compared to control static devices. Follow-up experiments by Bormann and colleagues indicated that the beneficial effects of embryo culture in the dynamic culture device are additive and require a minimum of 48 hours of culture at the beginning or end of 96-hour culture periods (40). Importantly, more recent studies indicate not only that there is a benefit on preimplantation embryo development, but also that the quality of embryos cultured in a microfluidic device with media flow is superior to that of those grown in static systems, as evidenced by increased implantation rates, lower rates of absorption, and higher ongoing pregnancy rates in mice (Figure 31.11) (43).

Using a similar actuator platform based on the Braille system, but modified for clinical use, it was shown that human embryos grown in a pulsatile microfluidic device yielded lower amounts of fragmentation in cleavage-stage embryos compared to control sibling counterparts grown in static conditions (78). No advantages in terms of blastocyst development or clinical outcomes have been reported.

Yet another approach to culturing embryos within microfluidic devices has employed not only dynamic media flow, but also co-culture. Mizuno and co-workers have adopted a "womb-on-a-chip" design, in which endometrial cells are grown in a lower chamber while embryos are cultured in an upper chamber, separated from the lower chamber by a thin membrane (15,79), thus allowing embryos to interact with secreted factors from the endometrial cells (Figure 31.12). In this preliminary report, the authors demonstrated that mouse ova fertilized on and resulting embryos cultured in these devices showed similar cleavage to two cells and similar blastocyst formation rates compared to 50-μL control microdrops (79). Furthermore, cell number was significantly higher in blastocysts fertilized/cultured in microfluidic devices. Subsequently, blastocysts obtained from microfluidic devices were transferred to recipient female mice and resulted in live offspring at rates similar to embryos

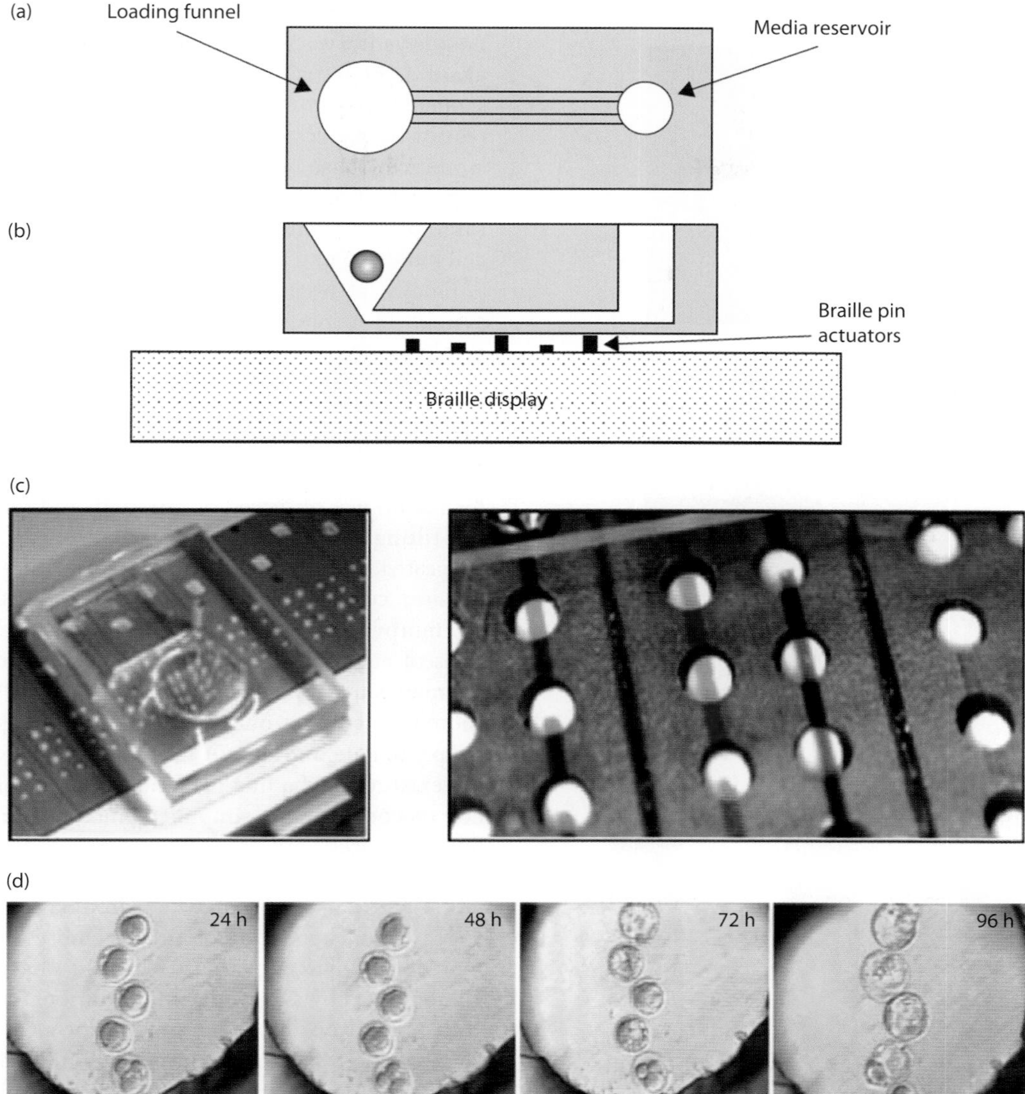

Figure 31.10 Microfluidic device composed of polydimethylsiloxane (PDMS) utilizing Braille actuators to drive media flow through two microchannels. Media flow is accomplished via Braille pin deflection of the thin bottom of the PDMS platform. Coordinated pin rise/fall allows peristaltic movement of a media bolus along the length of the microfluidic channels. (a) Top view. (b) Side view. (c) Image of a Braille pin PDMS device and demonstration of Braille pin rise/fall used to control fluid flow through microfluidic channels. (d) Images of mouse embryos cultured in the device over 96 h.

cultured in static microdrops. Though these experiments are still preliminary, they add to the advancement of microfluidic technology in ART, showing that both IVF and embryo culture can be performed in the same device, and that resulting embryos yield live offspring. A similar co-culture approach was undertaken by the same group, culturing two-cell mouse embryos to the blastocyst stage on the refined Opticell™ microfluidic device. Opticell microfluidic co-culture yielded chromosomally normal embryos capable of yielding live offspring (80).

Mizuno and colleagues published an abstract reporting the first instance of human embryo culture within microfluidic devices. Donated two- to four-cell-stage frozen human embryos were cultured to the blastocyst stage, resulting in significantly higher rates of blastocyst development from microfluidic devices compared to control microdrops (15). Additionally, visual scoring of microfluidic-derived blastocyst development revealed higher-quality blastocysts with significantly higher cell numbers compared to static controls. Unfortunately, co-culture confounds interpretation of the results obtained, as it is impossible to discern if the effects are attributed to co-culture or microfluidic design. As the goal of embryo culture has been the development of defined culture media, it will be interesting to see if similar studies can be performed without the use of co-culture.

Recently, mouse embryos have been cultured successfully in microwells housed in the same microfluidic

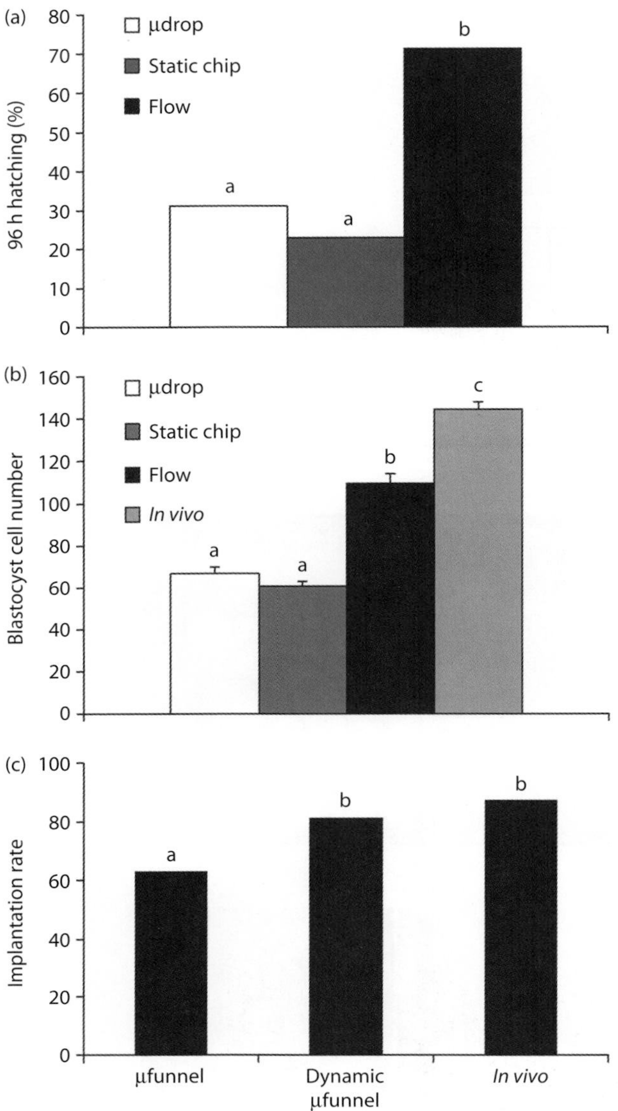

Figure 31.11 Microfluidic culture in a microfunnel improves mouse embryo development compared to static culture techniques resulting in (a) increased rates of blastocyst hatching at 96 hours, (b) increased blastocyst cell numbers, and (c) increased implantation rates following embryo transfer. Different superscripts (a,b,c) between columns within the same graph represent statistically significant differences, $P < 0.05$. (Adapted from Heo YS et al. *Hum Reprod* 2010; 25(3): 613–22.)

device where fertilization occurred. Han et al. (71) demonstrated that oocytes could be fertilized in microwells using media and sperm movement via gravity-driven hydrostatic pressure (Figure 31.7). Fertilization media were then replaced with embryo culture media by flowing media though the channels on the same device and embryos were cultured. Though there was no active media flow during the 96 hours of embryo development, similarly high rates of blastocyst formation were obtained following culture in microwells compared to controls (87.5% vs. 87.8%). Similarly, using a revised device design employing the "octacolumn" to house oocytes/embryos rather than microwells, the same group again demonstrated mouse oocyte fertilization and subsequent embryo development on the same microfluidic platform, yielding high rates of blastocyst formation similar to those of controls (86.9% vs. 85.3%) (70). This approach of combining multiple steps successfully on the same platform offers tremendous potential to minimize cell handling and associated stress.

Finally, at least one study has used a tilting culture system in conjunction with microfluidic channels to gently agitate embryos during culture. Bovine embryos were tilted by 10° over 1 minute and cultured inside straight microchannels (200 µm × 50 mm × 200 µm, width × length × height) or microchannels with a 150–160-µm constriction. Though no difference in blastocyst formation was observed or reported, and the influence of the tilting system alone was not examined, the authors suggested that combining an embryo tilting system with 169-µm constricted microchannels may offer a means of improving bovine embryo cleavage, yielding higher rates of eight-cell development after 44 hours of culture compared to straight channels (56.7% vs. 23.9%) (81). It should be pointed out, however, that tilting approaches simply agitate and do not necessary remove or replenish the existing media like perfusion systems. Similar methods of combining a simplified microchannel or microfluidic devices with other dynamic methods of inducing fluid movement generally used at the macro-level, such as vibration or agitation, may be helpful, as gentle agitation appears to be beneficial for human embryos (7,8). Though more recent dynamic culture platforms that agitate media and embryos by simply placing traditional culture dishes with microdrops or larger volumes of media on moving or vibrating platforms have been examined and appear promising (26–31), in the context of this review, these are not considered to be microfluidic culture platforms and may not utilized the full potential of the constrictive environment offered by other microfluidic approaches.

WHY DO OOCYTES/EMBRYOS BENEFIT FROM MICROFLUIDICS?

How do microfluidic approaches work to improve embryo development? It has been hypothesized that unknown autocrine/paracrine factors secreted by gametes or embryos are localized due to the confining nature of microfluidic devices, and that this localization of factors may carry certain benefits. Indeed, oocytes and embryos do secrete various factors, and research is ongoing to identify components of this secretome as noninvasive markers of embryo developmental competence (82,83). If secretion of beneficial factors from cultured cells is responsible for improved development, then quantity of embryos, volume of media, and surface area occupied would be extremely important factors to consider. Discussion of these issues in traditional culture platforms has been eloquently reviewed (84). Indeed, several studies have examined the beneficial effects of group embryo culture and media volume on traditional static culture platforms of

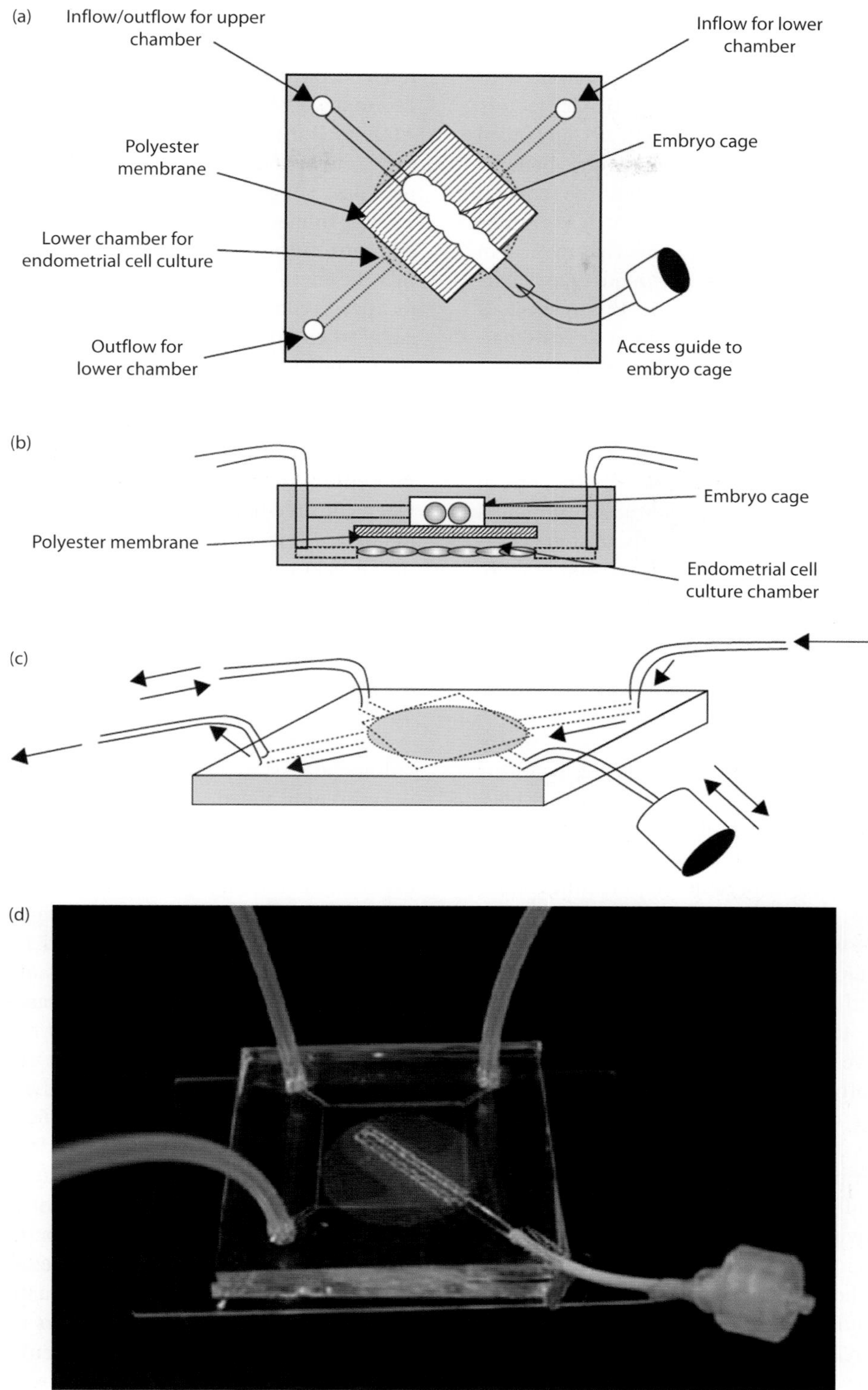

Figure 31.12 Illustrations of the "womb-on-a-chip" microfluidic perfusion system. Embryos are grown in a co-culture system separated from endometrial cells by a thin polyester membrane. (a) Top view. (b) Side view. (c) Indication of media flow. (d) Image of a polydimethylsiloxane "womb-on-a-chip" microfluidic device. (Photograph courtesy of Dr. Teruo Fujii.)

several species, including humans (85–88). Though direct comparisons are difficult due to differences in experimental parameters, it appears that in certain instances group culture does provide beneficial effects. Furthermore, in dealing with group culture, another important variable to consider is quality of companion embryos (89,90). However, experiments exploring the effects of embryo density within microfluidic devices are lacking.

Although the autocrine/paracrine debate offers an attractive means by which embryo development may benefit from microfluidic culture, secretion of trophic factors from embryos does not necessarily explain improved embryo development within microfluidic devices with dynamic conditions. With media flow, tropic factors would presumably be diluted or removed, yet advanced development is still observed. Alternatively, benefits within dynamic devices could be the result of the removal of harmful embryo metabolic by-products, such as ammonia (91), or the disruption of any gradients that may form (92,93). Shape of culture area can impact media flow characteristics (43) and may be important in this respect. If this is indeed the case, then undoubtedly a delicate balance exists regarding the correct number of embryos to culture in static devices in order not to negate any potential benefits of group autocrine/paracrine factors. However, it should be noted that studies removing spent culture media and replacement with fresh media from microdrops at various intervals show no benefit to embryo development (94,95). Thus, removal of by-products or disruption of gradients may not be the only reasons for improved embryo development within microfluidic devices.

A common denominator of static and flow devices is the constrictive nature of the microdevices, confining embryos to a very small area. Thus, benefits may somehow be related to cell proximity and spacing. Indeed, spacing of embryos during group culture affects development. Two innovative studies attached either pig or cattle embryos to culture dishes at measurable distances and assessed whether blastocyst development was not achieved if embryo spacing was too great (96,97). This spacing theory is supported by studies showing advanced embryo development in confining ultra-microdrops (95), culture within glass capillary tubes (87,98), culture within small concave wells (GPS dish) (1), small static microfluidic devices with no media flow (99), and culture within extremely small volumes/areas in the "well of a well" technique (100). If spacing is important and can improve embryo development when cultured in groups, then another variable to consider in designing microfluidic devices for ART is the shape of the culture area (84), which can dictate whether embryos are in direct contact or maintain physical separation. It remains to be seen whether microfluidic embryo culture improves the development of individually cultured embryos.

In terms of gradients formed in culture, it has been suggested by some that the benefits of culturing embryos within extremely small volumes, including microfluidic culture, may result from a reduction in localized oxygen tension due to culture in these confined spaces. In traditional culture approaches, reduced oxygen levels from atmospheric levels of around 20% to around 5%–7% are beneficial for embryo development and quality (101–103). Interestingly, the majority of reported microfluidic culture experiments were performed in 5% CO_2 in air, and thus reduction in localized oxygen would appear to be a plausible theory. However, bovine embryos cultured in dynamic microfluidic devices in 5% O_2 still showed improved development over static culture in the same device (41). Also, it should also be noted that hypoxic conditions are detrimental to oocytes and embryos (102,104). Thus, if localized oxygen depletion is occurring in microdevices, culturing in reduced oxygen tension could in fact result in hypoxia, decreasing embryo development. Fortunately, as the bovine study by Bormann and colleagues indicated, this does not appear to be the case (40). In support of this, mathematical modeling suggests oxygen depletion does not appear to be a factor in microdrops, regardless of the number of mouse embryos cultured, as diffusion and convection currents mix the environment to prevent anoxic regions (105). Thus, localized reduction in oxygen levels is questionable, especially when one considers the microfluidic devices used in ART studies are composed of PDMS, which is extremely gas permeable. However, at least one mathematical modeling study by Byatt-Smith et al. suggested that, due to their slightly larger size, culture of human embryos within static microdrops may become marginally hypoxic, especially when cultured in 5% O_2 (106). As a preventative measure to hypoxia, these same authors hypothesized that "embryos may develop more successfully in stirred, as opposed to still medium." Therefore, in studies utilizing dynamic microfluidic devices, media renewal due to flow should prevent any localized buildup or depletion of factors, including oxygen, thereby alleviating the possibility that advanced development is due to oxygen depletion.

Yet another possibility for the benefits of microfluidic culture, at least in dynamic flow devices, is gentle agitation of embryos or the media surrounding embryos. When considering the growing amount of data from both micro- and macro-dynamic culture devices, this seems like a plausible explanation. It is known that embryos can sense sheer stress and activate various intracellular signaling pathways in response, which leads to apoptosis (77,107). However, there may be a range of gentle agitations that permit intermediate activation of trophic signaling cascades that promote embryo development. Physiologically, this "active embryo hypothesis" makes sense, as gentle stimulation may be mimicking the vibrating actions of the ciliated epithelium within the female reproductive tract (8,34).

Unfortunately, each microfluidic device utilized to date is different in its construction (culturing in channels, culturing in funnels, culturing with/without flow, using co-culture, and utilizing different numbers of embryos/volume), thereby making it difficult to ascertain where the benefit to embryo development actually lies. Regardless, it is obvious that a number of factors is dictating embryo development and quality within any culture device, including microfluidic platforms. Further research examining the divergence of gene expression patterns, molecular signaling pathways, or other biochemical endpoints is required in order to begin to elucidate possible explanations for the observed effects in microfluidic culture and to optimize this promising technology for use in ART (Table 31.1).

MICROFLUIDICS AND VIABILITY ASSESSMENT

Perhaps the most important benefit of implementing a microfluidic platform for ART is the ability to integrate diagnostic tools in order to monitor gamete and embryo

Table 31.1 Practical considerations that must be addressed in order for microfluidic devices to gain widespread acceptance into *in vitro* fertilization laboratories

Biocompatibility	Operation	Manipulation of cells	Laboratory compatibility
Non-toxic fabrication materials Packaging to pass "in-house" quality control Disposable Design issues (volume, embryo number)	Perfusion system (recirculating vs. non-recirculating) Ability to be used over 5–6 days Detection of failure (air bubbles) Easy rectification of failure	Easy visualization Rapid loading/unloading Ability to isolate/monitor individual cells	Fit in conventional incubators User-friendly external apparatus Short set-up time

environmental conditions and physiologic processes. Though environmental monitoring has not yet received attention in ART, as an example, by using a nano-sized optical sensor, it is possible to monitor the pH of interstitial fluid flowing through a microfluidic device (108). Using nano- or micro-sensors, one can monitor temperature fluctuations (109,110), media flow rate (111), and volume of the cell to indicate shifts in media osmolarity (112). Additionally, electrical sensors have been developed to measure real-time changes in levels of ROS as indicators of oxidative stress in microfluidic devices (113,114). Conceivably, any one or a combination of these approaches could be adapted for use with ART microfluidic devices, as measurement of any of these environmental parameters may provide insight into the improvement of culture conditions and current IVF lab practices.

Furthermore, it has long been the goal of reproductive investigators to discover a means by which to interrogate gametes and embryos in order to identify markers of physiologic processes as a noninvasive means of predicting developmental competence and implantation potential. Current research is examining secreted proteins from embryos in the hopes of relating this information to cell quality (82,83). Implementation of enzyme-linked immunosorbent assays "on-chip" have met with some success in adherent cell systems (115,116), and may prove useful in analyzing embryo secretomic profiles. Additionally, examination of oocyte or embryo metabolomic activity and profiles has also showed promise for offering a noninvasive predictor of embryo quality (117–119). A silicone microfluidic device has been designed to measure oxygen consumption rates as indicators of mouse preimplantation embryo metabolic activity (120), and preliminary data measuring glucose, lactate, and pyruvate levels of spent embryo culture media in a pneumatic-controlled microfluidic device exist (121). Although embryos were not grown in microfluidic devices in these studies, ideally these types of analysis system will be constructed in the same device as cultured cells, allowing rapid, real-time analysis without additionally stressing embryos by further manipulation or removing them from the incubator environment. To this end, at least one device has assessed mouse embryo glucose metabolism on the same microfluidic platform on which they were cultured (Figure 31.13) (122).

Unique IVF-specific incubator and imaging systems now exist and have received widespread clinical implementation. These imaging systems each utilize customized culture platforms. While not utilizing microfluidics per se, these devices often use microwells and could conceivably be adapted to incorporate microfluidic aspects. Importantly, automation of the image analysis of developing embryos and morphokinetic patterns is now a reality in at least two of these clinical imaging systems (123–125), helping to move ART another step closer to automation within the clinical laboratory.

Finally, with increasing use of chromosome analysis and application of comprehensive chromosome screening as a means of selecting euploid embryos for transfer, the ability to perform rapid chromosome analysis within the IVF lab is attractive for turnaround times and cycle logistics. Furthermore, implementation of biopsied cell loading and subsequent analysis on the same platform on which embryos are cultured/biopsied offers the ability to reduce cell handling and potential introduction of lab errors. "On-chip" chromosome analysis has been performed in other cell types using polymerase chain reaction-based analysis (126) and could perhaps be applied to biopsied trophectoderm cells as well.

TOWARD LABORATORY AUTOMATION?

Many of the aforementioned studies implement a single procedural step on a microfluidic device. However, microfluidic technology offers the ability to implement multiple procedural steps on a single platform, which may be advantageous as it would reduce manual cell handling and the associated environmental stressors. Keeping the delicate cells in place while gradually changing media or gently rolling the cell to a new location may produce a less stressful environment and help optimize growth conditions.

One of the first examples of the integration of multiple procedural steps on a single microfluidic platform was presented by Clark and co-workers. Their preliminary data demonstrated that both IVM and IVF of porcine oocytes could be performed in the same microfluidic device without removal of the cells between procedures (20). Another example of multiple IVF procedures on a single platform entails separation of porcine sperm and then fertilizing

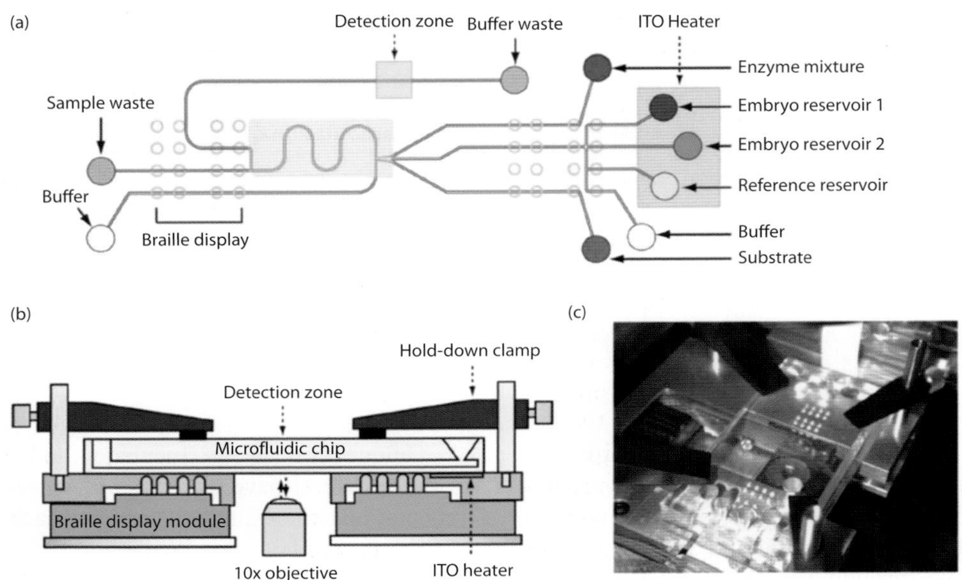

Figure 31.13 Schematic of a microfluidic device used to culture mouse embryos and noninvasively assess glucose metabolism as a potential indicator of embryo quality. (a) Detailed schematic of the microfluidic device showing the culture area and various channels and reservoirs for performing reagent mixing in order to assess glucose metabolism. (b) Schematic demonstrating how the microfluidic device mounts onto a microscope and Braille pin device to facilitate fluid flow and assessment of colorimetric changes for measuring metabolism. (c) Image of the microfluidic device. *Abbreviation:* ITO, Indium tin oxide transparent heater.

oocytes (127). More recently, mouse embryos have been cultured successfully on the same platform where fertilization occurred without removing cells between the procedural steps (69,70,79).

More ambitious and complex devices are emerging. Recently, a miniaturized array has been developed that can hold multiple zebrafish embryos, holding them in individual locations while utilizing microfluidic perfusion to supply fresh media or pharmacologic compounds in order to examine effects over time (128). Integrated with a perfusion pump, stage heater, and valves to help regulate flow and remove waste, this platform is also combined

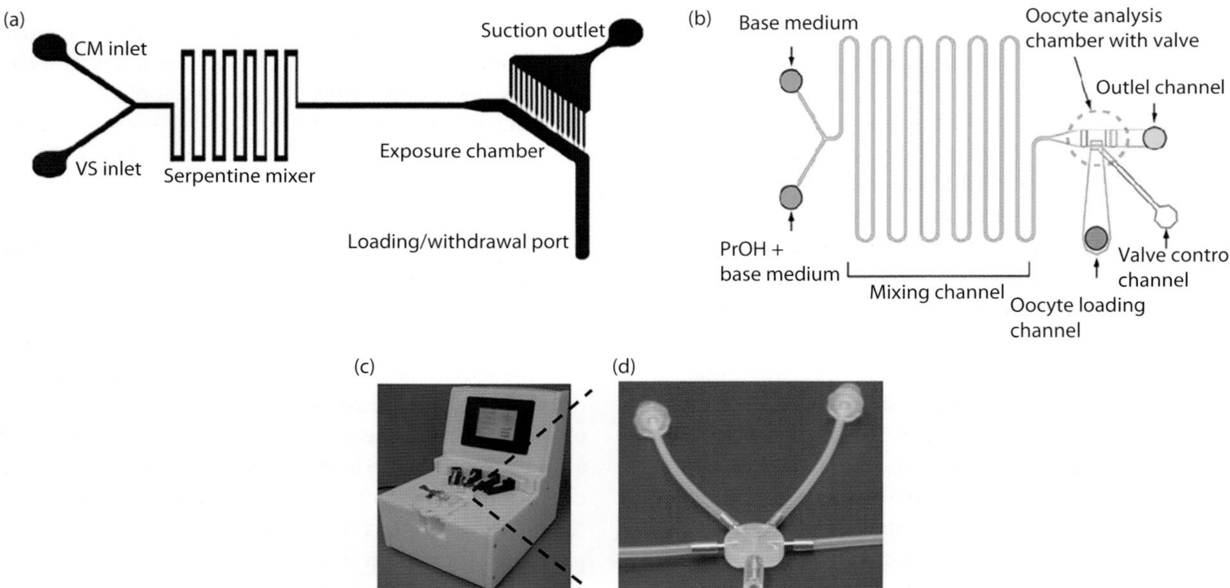

Figure 31.14 Microfluidic devices exist to gradually expose cells to gradients of cryoprotectant in order to reduce osmotic shock and improve outcomes. (a) Schematic of a microfluidic, gradual-mixing device used with cow and mouse oocytes and zygotes. (b) Schematic of a microfluidic device used to automate cryoprotectant exposure to oocytes. (c and d) Images of the suction device and microfluidic device.

with real-time video analysis. A similar approach could be envisioned for use in mammalian embryo culture.

Already, the field of IVF has seen many labs adopt the use of an uninterrupted culture system, leaving embryos in a single culture medium on a single dish in attempts to reduce handling and stress. Coupled with the rapid adaption of time-lapse imaging in IVF-specific incubators with novel culture platforms, this represents a potential platform that is conducive to automation of laboratory procedural steps. Indeed, automation of image analysis on at least two clinical time-lapse systems is already a reality (123–125,129).

Several examples of microfluidic platforms aimed at automating more complex procedures, such as sperm immobilization and microinjection, have been explored (130–135). Additionally, automated devices have been designed to flow cryoprotectant over cells in a gradual manner, reducing osmotic shock and offering a potential improvement to manual step-wise approaches (Figure 31.14) (136–138). Utilizing this approach with existing semi-automated vitrification systems (139) may offer the opportunity to further improve success rates.

CONCLUSION

To date, most of the procedural steps involved in IVF have already been accomplished on microfluidic platforms, though integration of multiple procedural steps on a single easy-to-use device still remains a work in progress. Coupled with automation of key procedures, it is clear that microfluidics offers many opportunities to revolutionize the ART laboratory through streamlining methods, reducing variability, and optimizing environmental conditions for gametes and embryos.

REFERENCES

1. Leese HJ. Human embryo culture: Back to nature. *J Assist Reprod Genet* 1998; 15(8): 466–8.
2. Hara T et al. A tilting embryo culture system increases the number of high-grade human blastocysts with high implantation competence. *Reprod Biomed Online* 2013; 26(3): 260–8.
3. Koike T et al. *In-vitro* culture with a tilting device in chemically defined media during meiotic maturation and early development improves the quality of blastocysts derived from *in-vitro* matured and fertilized porcine oocytes. *J Reprod Dev* 56(5): 552–7.
4. Matsuura K et al. Improved development of mouse and human embryos using a tilting embryo culture system. *Reprod Biomed Online* 20(3): 358–64.
5. Smith GD, Takayama S, Swain JE. Rethinking *in vitro* embryo culture: New developments in culture platforms and potential to improve assisted reproductive technologies. *Biol Reprod* 2012; 86(3): 62.
6. Swain JE, Smith GD. Advances in embryo culture platforms: Novel approaches to improve preimplantation embryo development through modifications of the microenvironment. *Hum Reprod Update* 2011; 17(4): 541–57.
7. Isachenko E et al. Mechanical agitation during the *in vitro* culture of human pre-implantation embryos drastically increases the pregnancy rate. *Clin Lab* 2010; 56(11–12): 569–76.
8. Isachenko V et al. *In-vitro* culture of human embryos with mechanical micro-vibration increases implantation rates. *Reprod Biomed Online* 2011; 22(6): 536–44.
9. Beebe D et al. Microfluidic technology for assisted reproduction. *Theriogenology* 2002; 57(1): 125–35.
10. Swain JE et al. Thinking big by thinking small: Application of microfluidic technology to improve ART. *Lab Chip* 2013; 13(7): 1213–24.
11. Bormann C et al. Microfluidics for assisted reproductive technologies. In: *Micro- and Nanoengineering of the Cell Microenvironment: Technologies and Applications*, Borenstein J, Khademhosseini A, Takayama S, Toner M (eds.), 2007.
12. Wheeler MB, Walters EM, Beebe DJ. Toward culture of single gametes: The development of microfluidic platforms for assisted reproduction. *Theriogenology* 2007; 68(Suppl 1): S178–89.
13. Glasgow IK et al. Handling individual mammalian embryos using microfluidics. *IEEE Trans Biomed Eng* 2001; 48(5): 570–8.
14. Kim L et al. A practical guide to microfluidic perfusion culture of adherent mammalian cells. *Lab Chip* 2007; 7(6): 681–94.
15. Mizuno J et al. Human ART on chip: Improved human blastocyst development and quality with IVF-chip. *Fertil Steril* 2007; 88(1): S101.
16. Raty S et al. Embryonic development in the mouse is enhanced via microchannel culture. *Lab Chip* 2004; 4(3): 186–90.
17. Schuster TG et al. Isolation of motile spermatozoa from semen samples using microfluidics. *Reprod Biomed Online* 2003; 7(1): 75–81.
18. Shibata D et al. Analysis of sperm motility and fertilization rates after the separation by microfluidic sperm sorter made of quartz. *Fertil Steril* 2007; 88(1): S110.
19. Walters E, Beebe D, Wheeler M. *In vitro* maturation of pig oocytes in polydimethylsiloxane (PDMS) and silicon microfluidic devices. *Theriogenology* 2001; 55: 497.
20. Clark S et al. A novel integrated *in vitro* maturation and *in vitro* fertilization system for swine. *Theriogenology* 2003; 59: 441.
21. Clark SG et al. Reduction of polyspermic penetration using biomimetic microfluidic technology during *in vitro* fertilization. *Lab Chip* 2005; 5(11): 1229–32.
22. Hester P et al. Enhanced cleavage rates following *in vitro* maturation of pig oocytes within polydimehtylsiloxane-borosilcate microchannels. *Theriogenology* 2002; 57: 723.
23. Hickman D et al. Comparison of static and dynamic medium environments for culturing of pre-implantation mouse embryos. *Comp Med* 2002; 52(2): 122–6.

24. Suh RS et al. IVF within microfluidic channels requires lower total numbers and lower concentrations of sperm. *Hum Reprod* 2006; 21(2): 477–83.
25. Lim JM et al. Perifusion culture system for bovine embryos: Improvement of embryo development by use of bovine oviduct epithelial cells, an antioxidant and polyvinyl alcohol. *Reprod Fertil Dev* 1997; 9(4): 411–8.
26. Lim JM et al. Development of *in-vitro*-derived bovine embryos cultured in 5% CO2 in air or in 5% O_2, 5% CO_2 and 90% N_2. *Hum Reprod* 1999; 14(2): 458–64.
27. Goverde HJ, Peeters RH, Willems PH. The development of a superfusion system for studying intracellular and secretory processes in embryos. *In Vitro Cell Dev Biol Anim* 1994; 30A(12): 819–21.
28. Chung BG et al. Human neural stem cell growth and differentiation in a gradient-generating microfluidic device. *Lab Chip* 2005; 5(4): 401–6.
29. Hung PJ et al. A novel high aspect ratio microfluidic design to provide a stable and uniform microenvironment for cell growth in a high throughput mammalian cell culture array. *Lab Chip* 2005; 5(1): 44–8.
30. Cho BS et al. Passively driven integrated microfluidic system for separation of motile sperm. *Anal Chem* 2003; 75(7): 1671–5.
31. Schulte R et al. Microfluidic sperm sorting device provides a novel method for selecting motile with higher DNA integrity. *Fertil Steril* 2007; 88(1): S76.
32. Davis J et al. Development of microfluidic systems for the culture of mammalian embryos. *First International IEEE EMBS Special Topic Conference on Microtechnology in Medicine and Biology*, 2000.
33. Matsuura K et al. Improved development of mouse and human embryos using a tilting embryo culture system. *Reprod Biomed Online* 2010; 20(3): 358–64.
34. Mizobe Y, Yoshida M, Miyoshi K. Enhancement of cytoplasmic maturation of *in vitro*-matured pig oocytes by mechanical vibration. *J Reprod Dev* 2010; 56(2): 285–90.
35. Hoppe PC, Pitts S. Fertilization *in vitro* and development of mouse ova. *Biol Reprod* 1973; 8(4): 420–6.
36. Isachenko V et al. Effective method for *in-vitro* culture of cryopreserved human ovarian tissue. *Reprod Biomed Online* 2006; 13(2): 228–34.
37. Oakes M et al. Effects of 3-dimensional topography, dynamic fluid movement and an insoluble glycoprotein matrix on murine embryo development. *Proceedings from the SGI Annual Meeting*, Glasgow, U.K., 2009.
38. Zeilmaker GH. Fusion of rat and mouse morulae and formation of chimaeric blastocysts. *Nature* 1973; 242(5393): 115–6.
39. Cohen J, Ooms MP, Vreeburg JT. Reduction of fertilizing capacity of epididymal spermatozoa by 5 alpha-steroid reductase inhibitors. *Experientia* 1981; 37(9): 1031–2.
40. Bormann C et al. Dynamic microfluidic embryo dynamic microfluidic embryo culture enhances blastocyst development of murine and bovine embryos. *Proceedings from the 14th World Congress on In vitro Fertilization*, 2007.
41. Bormann C et al. Dynamic microfluidic embryo culture enhances blastocyst development of murine and bovine embryos. *Biol Reprod* 2007; 77(Suppl_1): 89–90.
42. Cabrera L et al. Improved blastocyst development with microfluidics and braille pin actuator enabled dynamic culture. *Fertil Steril* 2006; 87(1): S43.
43. Heo YS et al. Dynamic microfunnel culture enhances mouse embryo development and pregnancy rates. *Hum Reprod* 2010; 25(3): 613–22.
44. Eddington DT, Beebe DJ. Flow control with hydrogels. *Adv Drug Deliv Rev* 2004; 56(2): 199–210.
45. Simmons A, Hyvarinen J, Poole-Warren L. The effect of sterilisation on a poly(dimethylsiloxane)/poly(hexamethylene oxide) mixed macrodiol-based polyurethane elastomer. *Biomaterials* 2006; 27(25): 4484–97.
46. Toepke MW, Beebe DJ. PDMS absorption of small molecules and consequences in microfluidic applications. *Lab Chip* 2006; 6(12): 1484–6.
47. Wu JM et al. A surface-modified sperm sorting device with long-term stability. *Biomed Microdevices* 2006; 8(2): 99–107.
48. Heo YS et al. Characterization and resolution of evaporation-mediated osmolality shifts that constrain microfluidic cell culture in poly(dimethylsiloxane) devices. *Anal Chem* 2007; 79(3): 1126–34.
49. Kim L et al. Microfluidic arrays for logarithmically perfused embryonic stem cell culture. *Lab Chip* 2006; 6(3): 394–406.
50. Suh R, Takayama S, Smith GD. Microfluidic applications for andrology. *J Androl* 2005; 26(6): 664–70.
51. Kricka LJ et al. Micromachined analytical devices: Microchips for semen testing. *J Pharm Biomed Anal* 1997; 15(9–10): 1443–7.
52. Kricka LJ et al. Applications of a microfabricated device for evaluating sperm function. *Clin Chem* 1993; 39(9): 1944–7.
53. Matsuura K et al. Hydrophobic silicone elastomer chamber for recording trajectories of motile porcine sperms without adsorption. *J Reprod Dev* 57(1): 163–7.
54. Elsayed M, El-Sherry TM, Abdelgawad M. Development of computer-assisted sperm analysis plugin for analyzing sperm motion in microfluidic environments using Image-J. *Theriogenology* 2015; 84(8): 1367–77.
55. Matsuura K et al. A microfluidic device to reduce treatment time of intracytoplasmic sperm injection. *Fertil Steril* 2013; 99(2): 400–7.
56. Xie L et al. Integration of sperm motility and chemotaxis screening with a microchannel-based device. *Clin Chem* 56(8): 1270–8.

57. Koyama S et al. Chemotaxis assays of mouse sperm on microfluidic devices. *Anal Chem* 2006; 78(10): 3354–9.
58. Zhang Y et al. Generation of gradients on a microfluidic device: Toward a high-throughput investigation of spermatozoa chemotaxis. *PLoS One* 2015; 10(11): e0142555.
59. El-Sherry TM et al. Characterization of rheotaxis of bull sperm using microfluidics. *Integr Biol (Camb)* 2014; 6(12): 1111–21.
60. Kantsler V et al. Rheotaxis facilitates upstream navigation of mammalian sperm cells. *Elife* 2014; 3: e02403.
61. Seo D et al. Development of sorting, aligning, and orienting motile sperm using microfluidic device operated by hydrostatic pressure. *Microfluidics and Nanofluidics* 2007; 3(5): 561–70.
62. Agarwal A, Ikemoto I, Loughlin KR. Effect of sperm washing on levels of reactive oxygen species in semen. *Arch Androl* 1994; 33(3): 157–62.
63. Shekarriz M et al. A method of human semen centrifugation to minimize the iatrogenic sperm injuries caused by reactive oxygen species. *Eur Urol* 1995; 28(1): 31–5.
64. Fraczek M, Sanocka D, Kurpisz M. Interaction between leucocytes and human spermatozoa influencing reactive oxygen intermediates release. *Int J Androl* 2004; 27(2): 69–75.
65. Shirota K et al. Separation efficiency of a microfluidic sperm sorter to minimize sperm DNA damage. *Fertil Steril* 2015; 105(2): 315–21.e1.
66. Chian RC, Lim JH, Tan SL. State of the art in *in-vitro* oocyte maturation. *Curr Opin Obstet Gynecol* 2004; 16(3): 211–9.
67. Gilchrist RB et al. Molecular basis of oocyte-paracrine signalling that promotes granulosa cell proliferation. *J Cell Sci* 2006; 119(Pt 18): 3811–21.
68. Lopez-Garcia MD et al. Sperm motion in a microfluidic fertilization device. *Biomed Microdevices* 2008; 10(5): 709–18.
69. Han C et al. Integration of single oocyte trapping, *in vitro* fertilization and embryo culture in a microwell-structured microfluidic device. *Lab Chip* 2010; 10(21): 2848–54.
70. Ma R et al. *In vitro* fertilization on a single-oocyte positioning system integrated with motile sperm selection and early embryo development. *Anal Chem* 2011; 83(8): 2964–70.
71. Han C et al. Integration of single oocyte trapping, *in vitro* fertilization and embryo culture in a microwell-structured microfluidic device. *Lab Chip* 2010; 10(21): 2848–54.
72. Zeringue HC, Beebe DJ. Microfluidic removal of cumulus cells from Mammalian zygotes. *Methods Mol Biol* 2004; 254: 365–74.
73. Zeringue HC, Rutledge JJ, Beebe DJ. Early mammalian embryo development depends on cumulus removal technique. *Lab Chip* 2005; 5(1): 86–90.
74. Zeringue HC, Wheeler MB, Beebe DJ. A microfluidic method for removal of the zona pellucida from mammalian embryos. *Lab Chip* 2005; 5(1): 108–10.
75. Raty S et al. Culture in microchannels enhances *in vitro* embryonic development of preimplantation mouse embryos. *Theriogenology* 2001; 55(1): 241.
76. Walters E et al. Production of live piglets following *in vitro* embryo culture in a microfluidic environment. *Theriogenology* 2003; 59: 441.
77. Xie Y et al. Shear stress induces preimplantation embryo death that is delayed by the zona pellucida and associated with stress-activated protein kinase-mediated apoptosis. *Biol Reprod* 2006; 75(1): 45–55.
78. Alegretti JR et al. Microfluidic dynamic embryo culture increases the production of top quality human embryos through reductin in embryo fragmentation. *Fertil Steril* 2011; 96(3): s58.
79. Mizuno J et al. Human ART on chip: Development of microfluidic device for IVF and IVC. *Proceeding from ESHRE*, 2007.
80. Nakamura H et al. New embryo co-culture system for human assisted reproductive technology (ART) by OptiCell. *Hum Reprod* 2007; 22(1): i170.
81. Kim MS et al. A microfluidic *in vitro* cultivation system for mechanical stimulation of bovine embryos. *Electrophoresis* 2009; 30(18): 3276–82.
82. Bormann C et al. Preimplantation embryo secretome identification. *Fertil Steril* 2006; 86(Suppl 2): s116.
83. Katz-Jaffe MG, Schoolcraft WB, Gardner DK. Analysis of protein expression (secretome) by human and mouse preimplantation embryos. *Fertil Steril* 2006; 86(3): 678–85.
84. Reed M. Communication skills of embryos maintained in group culture—The autocrine paracrine debate. *The Clinical Embryologist (Online)* 2006; 9(2): 5–19.
85. Moessner J, Dodson WC. The quality of human embryo growth is improved when embryos are cultured in groups rather than separately. *Fertil Steril* 1995; 64(5): 1034–5.
86. Almagor M et al. Pregnancy rates after communal growth of preimplantation human embryos *in vitro*. *Fertil Steril* 1996; 66(3): 394–7.
87. Lane M, Gardner DK. Effect of incubation volume and embryo density on the development and viability of mouse embryos *in vitro*. *Hum Reprod* 1992; 7(4): 558–62.
88. Canseco RS et al. Embryo density and medium volume effects on early murine embryo development. *J Assist Reprod Genet* 1992; 9(5): 454–7.
89. Spindler RE et al. Improved felid embryo development by group culture is maintained with heterospecific companions. *Theriogenology* 2006; 66(1): 82–92.
90. Spindler RE, Wildt DE. Quality and age of companion felid embryos modulate enhanced development by group culture. *Biol Reprod* 2002; 66(1): 167–73.

91. Lane M, Gardner DK. Ammonium induces aberrant blastocyst differentiation, metabolism, pH regulation, gene expression and subsequently alters fetal development in the mouse. *Biol Reprod* 2003; 69(4): 1109–17.
92. Trimarchi JR et al. Noninvasive measurement of potassium efflux as an early indicator of cell death in mouse embryos. *Biol Reprod* 2000; 63(3): 851–7.
93. Trimarchi JR et al. Oxidative phosphorylation-dependent and -independent oxygen consumption by individual preimplantation mouse embryos. *Biol Reprod* 2000; 62(6): 1866–74.
94. Fukui Y, Lee ES, Araki N. Effect of medium renewal during culture in two different culture systems on development to blastocysts from *in vitro* produced early bovine embryos. *J Anim Sci* 1996; 74(11): 2752–8.
95. Ali J. Continuous ultra microdrop culture yields higher pregnancy and implantation rates than either large-drop culture or fresh-medium replacement. *The Clinical Embryologist (Online)* 2004; 7(2): 1–23.
96. Stokes PJ, Abeydeera LR, Leese HJ. Development of porcine embryos *in vivo* and *in vitro*; evidence for embryo 'cross talk' *in vitro*. *Dev Biol* 2005; 284(1): 62–71.
97. Gopichandran N, Leese HJ. The effect of paracrine/autocrine interactions on the *in vitro* culture of bovine preimplantation embryos. *Reproduction* 2006; 131(2): 269–77.
98. Thouas GA, Jones GM, Trounson AO. The 'GO' system—A novel method of microculture for *in vitro* development of mouse zygotes to the blastocyst stage. *Reproduction* 2003; 126(2): 161–9.
99. Kieslinger DC et al. *In vitro* development of donated frozen–thawed human embryos in a prototype static microfluidic device: A randomized controlled trial. *Fertil Steril* 2015; 103(3): 680–6.e2.
100. Vajta G et al. New method for culture of zona-included or zona-free embryos: The Well of the Well (WOW) system. *Mol Reprod Dev* 2000; 55(3): 256–64.
101. Gardner DK, Lane M. Alleviation of the '2-cell block' and development to the blastocyst of CF1 mouse embryos: Role of amino acids, EDTA and physical parameters. *Hum Reprod* 1996; 11(12): 2703–12.
102. Feil D et al. Effect of culturing mouse embryos under different oxygen concentrations on subsequent fetal and placental development. *J Physiol* 2006; 572(Pt 1): 87–96.
103. Rinaudo PF et al. Effects of oxygen tension on gene expression in preimplantation mouse embryos. *Fertil Steril* 2006; 86(Suppl 4): 1252–65, 1265.e1–36.
104. Banwell KM et al. Oxygen concentration during mouse oocyte *in vitro* maturation affects embryo and fetal development. *Hum Reprod* 2007; 22(10): 2768–75.
105. Baltz JM, Biggers JD. Oxygen transport to embryos in microdrop cultures. *Mol Reprod Dev* 1991; 28(4): 351–5.
106. Byatt-Smith JG, Leese HJ, Gosden RG. An investigation by mathematical modelling of whether mouse and human preimplantation embryos in static culture can satisfy their demands for oxygen by diffusion. *Hum Reprod* 1991; 6(1): 52–7.
107. Xie Y et al. Pipetting causes shear stress and elevation of phosphorylated stress-activated protein kinase/jun kinase in preimplantation embryos. *Mol Reprod Dev* 2007; 74(10): 1287–94.
108. Baldini F, Giannetti A, Mencaglia AA. Optical sensor for interstitial pH measurements. *J Biomed Opt* 2007; 12(2): 024024.
109. Chang YH et al. Integrated polymerase chain reaction chips utilizing digital microfluidics. *Biomed Microdevices* 2006; 8(3): 215–25.
110. Lucchetta EM, Munson MS, Ismagilov RF. Characterization of the local temperature in space and time around a developing *Drosophila* embryo in a microfluidic device. *Lab Chip* 2006; 6(2): 185–90.
111. Lien V, Vollmer F. Microfluidic flow rate detection based on integrated optical fiber cantilever. *Lab Chip* 2007; 7(10): 1352–6.
112. Ateya DA et al. Volume cytometry: Microfluidic sensor for high-throughput screening in real time. *Anal Chem* 2005; 77(5): 1290–4.
113. Amatore C et al. Monitoring in real time with a microelectrode the release of reactive oxygen and nitrogen species by a single macrophage stimulated by its membrane mechanical depolarization. *Chembiochem* 2006; 7(4): 653–61.
114. Amatore C et al. Electrochemical detection in a microfluidic device of oxidative stress generated by macrophage cells. *Lab Chip* 2007; 7(2): 233–8.
115. Eteshola E, Balberg M. Microfluidic ELISA: On-chip fluorescence imaging. *Biomed Microdevices* 2004; 6(1): 7–9.
116. Herrmann M et al. Microfluidic ELISA on non-passivated PDMS chip using magnetic bead transfer inside dual networks of channels. *Lab Chip* 2007; 7(11): 1546–52.
117. Gardner DK et al. Noninvasive assessment of human embryo nutrient consumption as a measure of developmental potential. *Fertil Steril* 2001; 76(6): 1175–80.
118. Lane M, Gardner DK. Selection of viable mouse blastocysts prior to transfer using a metabolic criterion. *Hum Reprod* 1996; 11(9): 1975–8.
119. Seli E et al. Noninvasive metabolomic profiling of embryo culture media using Raman and near-infrared spectroscopy correlates with reproductive potential of embryos in women undergoing *in vitro* fertilization. *Fertil Steril* 2007; 88(5): 1350–7.
120. O'Donovan C et al. Development of a respirometric biochip for embryo assessment. *Lab Chip* 2006; 6(11): 1438–44.
121. Urbanski J et al. Development of a microfluidic platform to measure metabolic activity of preimplantation embryos. *Fertil Steril* 2007; 88(1): S36.

122. Heo YS et al. Real time culture and analysis of embryo metabolism using a microfluidic device with deformation based actuation. *Lab Chip* 2012; 12(12): 2240–6.
123. Paternot G et al. Semi-automated morphometric analysis of human embryos can reveal correlations between total embryo volume and clinical pregnancy. *Hum Reprod* 2013; 28(3): 627–33.
124. Wong C et al. Time-lapse microscopy and image analysis in basic and clinical embryo development research. *Reprod Biomed Online* 2013; 26(2): 120–9.
125. Wong CC et al. Non-invasive imaging of human embryos before embryonic genome activation predicts development to the blastocyst stage. *Nat Biotechnol* 2010; 28(10): 1115–21.
126. Fan HC et al. Microfluidic digital PCR enables rapid prenatal diagnosis of fetal aneuploidy. *Am J Obstet Gynecol* 2009; 200(5): 543.e1–7.
127. Sano H et al. Application of a microfluidic sperm sorter to the *in-vitro* fertilization of porcine oocytes reduced the incidence of polyspermic penetration. *Theriogenology* 2010; 74(5): 863–70.
128. Akagi J et al. Miniaturized embryo array for automated trapping, immobilization and microperfusion of zebrafish embryos. *PLoS One* 2012; 7(5): e36630.
129. Chavez SL et al. Dynamic blastomere behavior reflects human embryo ploidy by the four-cell stage. *Nat Commun* 2012; 3: 1251.
130. Lu Z et al. Robotic ICSI (intracytoplasmic sperm injection). *IEEE Trans Biomed Eng* 2011; 58(7): 2102–8.
131. Mattos LS et al. Blastocyst microinjection automation. *IEEE Trans Inf Technol Biomed* 2009; 13(5): 822–31.
132. Liu X et al. Automated microinjection of recombinant BCL-X into mouse zygotes enhances embryo development. *PLoS One* 2011; 6(7): e21687.
133. Leung C et al. Automated sperm immobilization for intracytoplasmic sperm injection. *IEEE Trans Biomed Eng* 2011; 58(4): 935–42.
134. Graf SF et al. Fully automated microinjection system for *Xenopus laevis* oocytes with integrated sorting and collection. *J Lab Autom* 2011; 16(3): 186–96.
135. Park J et al. Design and fabrication of an integrated cell processor for single embryo cell manipulation. *Lab Chip* 2005; 5(1): 91–6.
136. Lai D et al. Slow and steady cell shrinkage reduces osmotic stress in bovine and murine oocyte and zygote vitrification. *Hum Reprod* 2015; 30(1): 37–45.
137. Heo YS et al. Controlled loading of cryoprotectants (CPAs) to oocyte with linear and complex CPA profiles on a microfluidic platform. *Lab Chip* 2011; 11(20): 3530–7.
138. Meng L et al. Development of a microfluidic device for automated vitrification of human embryos. *Fertil Steril* 2011; 96(3): s207.
139. Roy TK et al. Embryo vitrification using a novel semi-automated closed system yields *in vitro* outcomes equivalent to the manual Cryotop method. *Hum Reprod* 2014; 29(11): 2431–8.

Epigenetic considerations in preimplantation mammalian embryos

32

HEIDE SCHATTEN and QING-YUAN SUN

INTRODUCTION

The development of a mammalian embryo includes a number of critical stages in which epigenetic programming and reprogramming are important aspects for development into a healthy offspring. Implications resulting from abnormal epigenetic reprogramming have been reviewed (1) and are not addressed here. This review is focused on the basic epigenetic mechanisms that take place during preimplantation mammalian development, which is briefly described in the following.

Mammalian oocytes are arrested at the germinal vesicle (GV) stage in the ovary at birth and remain at this stage until puberty. Follicle-stimulating hormone induces development of small antral follicles, resulting in one oocyte and its follicle becoming ovulatory. Meiotic resumption occurs after GV breakdown induced by luteinizing hormone and starting the process of oocyte maturation. Growth of the oocyte is associated with significant remodeling on cellular and molecular levels, resulting in the oocyte becoming fertilization-competent (reviewed in [2–12]). The first meiotic spindle forms, followed by second meiosis, during which the oocyte becomes arrested at metaphase II (MII) to await fertilization in order for development to continue. The meiotic stages encompass two successive, highly asymmetric cell divisions that result in small polar bodies and a large polarized oocyte. Fertilization after sperm incorporation triggers egg activation and formation of one male and one female pronucleus (zygote stage, day 1 in humans) that become appositioned and undergo chromosomal reorganizations before the mitotic spindle forms and separates chromosomes equally to the dividing daughter cells. Cell divisions continue, and at the eight-cell stage (day 3), embryos start to undergo compaction, a process during which the blastomeres become flattened and polarized. Blastocyst development continues with cellular differentiation when inner cells are formed (day 5; 32-cell stage) resulting in the inner cell mass (ICM) cells and the outer cells that form the trophectoderm (TE).

Epigenetic modifications are generally referred to as biochemical mechanisms that affect gene expression and regulation without changing the sequence of DNA itself. Genome-wide epigenetic reprogramming takes place during mammalian development when cells undergo cascades of irreversible cell fate decisions. These epigenetic alterations include DNA methylation and several histone modifications that influence the higher order of chromatin structure and allow selective activation or silencing of subsets of genes.

The history and milestones achieved in the field of epigenetics have been well reviewed by Rivera (13), and progress is being made consistently and rapidly to more fully uncover the mechanisms of specific epigenetic modifications in specific cells. New genome-wide technologies, such as chromatin immunoprecipitation followed by next-generation sequencing (as well as highly specific antibody detection for epigenetic modifications and bisulfite sequencing), have provided detailed information on epigenetics, but new methods are still in demand in order to fully understand the epigenetic landscape in single cells as diverse as sperm cells, oocytes, and specific cells comprising the preimplantation embryo so as to fully understand its developmental complexities.

DNA methylation

The primary classes of epigenetic modifications are DNA modification by cytosine methylation at CpG dinucleotides, with the best-studied form being 5-methylcytosine (5-mC) and also 5-hydroxymethylcytosine. 5-mC typically marks genes for transcriptional inactivity. *De novo* methyltransferases such as DNMT3a are required for the 5-mC marks, while maintenance of the marks through cell division requires the methyltransferase DNMT1.

Histone modifications

Histone modifications include highly dynamic post-translational modifications of histones. Four histones (H2A, H2B, H3, and H4) are typically assembled into a nucleosome, while the linker histone H1 associates with non-nucleosomal DNA that is localized between nucleosomes and plays a role in chromatin compaction.

Each histone contains N-terminal tails that protrude from the nucleosome core particle; they are enriched in lysine and arginine residues. The amino acid residues are modified by methylation (using histone methyltransferases as enzymes) and acetylation (using histone acetyltransferases as enzymes). These modifications influence the transcriptional activity of the gene they are associated with.

The nomenclature generally used to describe the specific histone modification activities first specifies the histone, then the specific amino acid, then the specific modification. For example, H3K27me3 indicates that histone H3 is trimethylated at lysine 27. These histone modifications exert either positive or negative effects on transcription. For example, H3K4me3 functions as a transcriptionally activating mark, while H3K27me3 marks repress transcription. There are, however, complexities that are still under current investigation involving molecular competition between methylation and acetylation.

SECTION 1: EARLY PREIMPLANTATION DEVELOPMENT FROM GV BREAKDOWN TO FERTILIZATION TO EARLY EMBRYONIC CELL DIVISIONS

As will be detailed below, early development is dominated by erasure of DNA methylation in the paternal zygotic pronucleus shortly after fertilization. A gradual loss of DNA methylation takes place during the cleavage stages and reactivation of the inactive X chromosome takes place in the female.

In germ cells, heterochromatin undergoes significant changes in terms of epigenetic modifications, with major changes in down-regulation of H3K9me2 and up-regulation of H3K27me3 and an increase in histone acetylation and H3K4me3, which are histone marks associated with euchromatin (14). Changes in germ cells have been reviewed previously (15,16) and are not specifically addressed here. These changes are likely to prepare the germ cells to successfully undergo subsequent epigenetic reprogramming after moving into the genital ridges. In the gonads (embryonic day 11.5 = E11.5 in the mouse), germ cells undergo a series of epigenetic reprogramming steps including DNA methylation, changes in chromatin structure, and genome-wide histone replacement, resulting in loss of a variety of histone modification marks (14,17). Genome-wide DNA demethylation is an active process and is independent of replication (14), as evidenced by it occurring during the G2 cell cycle stage. It occurs prior to the onset of global chromatin changes and includes transient loss of H3K9me3, H3K27me3, and H2A/H4 R3me2s, as well as other histone modification marks.

Sperm and eggs have very different configurations of CpG methylation and they differ significantly in their overall 5-mCpG content. As will be detailed below, sperm DNA is more methylated than egg DNA, but rapid active demethylation of sperm DNA follows after fertilization. The TET family of proteins has been identified as consisting of relevant 5-mCpG demethylases (18–20).

In the sperm head, paternal DNA is highly compacted using protamines, while these protamines are replaced by acetylated histones (21) when sperm DNA starts to decondense shortly after fertilization. For example, the histone variants H2L1/L2, which are present at the pericentric heterochromatin regions in sperm DNA (22), are removed from sperm chromatin shortly after fertilization (23). A small number of histones are retained in the sperm (~4% of the haploid sperm genome), which are transmitted to the embryo (24). Specifically transmitted are the sperm-specific histone variants H2AL1, H2HL2, and tH2B and the widely expressed H3.3, H2A.X, and H2A.Z (25), although the functions of these histones are not yet clear.

In oocytes, maternal DNA is wrapped around histones carrying several post-translational modifications. Differently from somatic cells, in which somatic H1 linker histones are present, the oocyte contains the H1oo subtype. The female haploid genome organized in the MII meiotic spindle is already associated with histones, but significant remodeling of the histone landscape occurs. Histone variants derived from the oocytes, including the linker histone H1FOO, are removed from the female genome and replaced with canonical linker H1 histones (26,27).

While both sperm and egg cells are transcriptionally silent prior to fertilization, fertilization triggers a significant reorganization of chromatin in both. During fertilization, mature gametes display distinct epigenetic information when paternal and maternal DNA start to decondense. Some of the RNA and proteins stored in the oocyte are used following fertilization. The protamines that had compacted the paternal genome are removed and replaced by histones produced and stored in the oocyte, which occurs before DNA replication (28). Specifically, the replication-independent H3.3 histone variant becomes deposited in the male pronucleus, thereby contributing to the epigenetic differences and epigenetic asymmetry between the male and female pronuclei (29,30). The variants heterochromatin histone marks H3K9me2, H3K9me3, and H3K27me3 are not present in the decondensing male pronucleus (31,32), while they are present in the female pronucleus. The female chromatin at the zygote stage is modified by the transient loss of the histone variant H3.3, while H3.2 is incorporated into the female chromatin (33).

The dynamics and regulatory mechanisms of pronuclear H3k9me2 asymmetry have recently been shown for mouse oocytes (34,35), and the molecules and mechanisms controlling the active DNA demethylation of the mammalian genome have recently been reviewed by Ma et al. (36,37).

Differences in histone modifications are found in male and female pronuclei from fertilization to the four- to eight-cell stages in the mouse embryo. DNA methylation is also asymmetric in male and female pronuclei. It is initially present at high levels in both paternal and maternal pronuclei, but it begins to disappear from the paternal pronucleus shortly after fertilization (38–40). 5-mC in the paternal genome but not the maternal genome is lost within 4 hours of fertilization in the mouse in a DNA replication-independent process (39). The DNA demethylation process is guided by the maternally inherited Stella protein (41), as evidenced by oocytes lacking Stella showing DNA demethylation in maternal and paternal pronuclei.

The differences in global levels of DNA methylation can be detected only to the two-cell stage of mouse embryo development (38). After this stage they become diluted as a result of passive loss of DNA methylation, which takes place until the late morula stages.

SECTION 2: PREIMPLANTATION DEVELOPMENT TOWARD THE FORMATION OF ICM AND TE CELLS AT THE BLASTOCYST STAGES

In mammals, about 200 cell types comprising multiple tissues are established from the zygote to the adult stages. All these cells carry identical genetic information, but become functionally divergent through selective activation and inactivation of subsets of genes.

While the genome itself remains constant, the transcriptome changes considerably in divergent cell types. The diversity of cell types is achieved through key transcription factors and unique epigenetic landscapes. In early preimplantation embryo development, changes in the epigenome include alterations in the methylation of CpG dinucleotides and post-translational modifications in the chromatin.

Epigenetic modifications are important for the establishment of cell lineages. As indicated above, developmentally asymmetric cells emerge at the morula stages and during formation of the blastocyst embryo when ICM and TE cells form. The ICM gives rise to the embryo, while the TE gives rise to the extraembryonic tissue of the placenta.

A series of epigenetic modifications takes place at the blastocyst stages when ICM and TE cells form. At this stage, the X chromosome (Xi) becomes reactivated in the ICM cells of female embryos, which is associated with the loss of Xi-linked polycomb silencing and elimination of *Xist* transcription driven by Xi (42–44). The passive DNA demethylation process is completed when histone polycomb marks are removed during the late blastocyst stages.

Both maternal and paternal imprinted genes typically maintain their methylation states through the fertilization process, but significant changes in CpG methylation take place following fertilization and during subsequent cleavage stages. Extensive epigenetic remodeling takes place throughout early embryogenesis.

During the cleavage stages of embryogenesis, levels of 5-mCpG decrease and *de novo* methylation takes place using DNMT3a and DNMT3b. Methylation is maintained by the CpG methyltransferase DNMT1.

The enhancer of zeste 2 (EZH2) is a polycomb group 2 (PcG2) histone methyltransferase that is stored in mature oocytes and produces H3K27me3. It is critical for development, as depletion of EZH2 from the maternal store results in delayed development. EZH2 is thought to play a role in epigenetic histone methylation affecting H3K27 patterning in the early preimplantation embryo (45,46). The H3K27me demethylase JmJD3 is strongly expressed in the four-cell embryo stage as shown in porcine embryos, but it is decreased in blastocysts (47).

Polycomb group 1 (PcG1) is required for embryo formation. It is present in maturing oocytes while histone modification plays a role in zygotic totipotency (48). In two-cell embryos, each one of the blastomere cells is totipotent, which has also been shown for human embryos (49). Each cell can produce an embryo, as well as extraembryonic placenta cells and TE cells. Specification into cell lineages with epigenetic reprogramming continues throughout development (reviewed in [1]).

Taken together, the field of epigenetics has contributed significant insights to mammalian embryo development and to diseases associated with developmental abnormalities. As the field is still relatively young, it can be expected that new methods and new technologies will allow us to further our understanding of the role of epigenetics in single cells including sperm, eggs, and early embryo cells.

Important new insights into the role of epigenetics in oocyte aging have been gained and addressed in detail in recent papers (50–53), and the effects of metabolic diseases such as diabetes on epigenetics have been reported (54–57). Furthermore, it has been shown that epigenetic effects can be inherited by gametes and can affect human reproduction for generations (58–61). These studies are of critical importance for reproduction and are worth pursuing given the high percentage of our population affected by diabetes and obesity worldwide.

REFERENCES

1. Rivera RM, Ross J. Epigenetics in fertilization and preimplantation embryo development. Special issue on Systems Biology and Reproductive Biology. *Prog Biophys Mol Biol* 2013; 113(3): 423–32.
2. Fan HY, Huo LJ, Meng XQ, Zhong ZS, Hou Y, Chen DY, Sun QY. Involvement of calcium/calmodulin-dependent protein kinase II (CaMKII) in meiotic maturation and activation of pig oocytes. *Biol Reprod* 2003; 69: 1552–64.
3. Fan H-Y, Liu Z, Shimada M, Sterneck E, Johnson PF, Hedrick S, Richards JS. MAPK3/1 (ERK1/2) in ovarian granulosa cells are essential for female fertility. *Science* 2009; 324: 938–41.
4. Voronina E, Wessel GM. The regulation of oocyte maturation. *Curr Top Dev Biol* 2003; 58: 53–110.
5. Brunet S, Maro B. Cytoskeleton and cell cycle control during meiotic maturation of the mouse oocyte: Integrating time and space. *Reproduction* 2005; 130: 801–11.
6. Sirard MA, Richard F, Blondin P, Robert C. Contribution of the oocyte to embryo quality. *Theriogenology* 2006; 65: 126–36.
7. Liang C-G, Su Y-Q, Fan H-Y, Schatten H, Sun Q-Y. Mechanisms regulating oocyte meiotic resumption: Roles of mitogen-activated protein kinase. *Mol Endocrinol* 2007; 21: 2037–55.
8. Ai J-S, Wang Q, Li M, Shi LH, Ola SI, Xiong B, Yin S, Chen DY, Sun QY. Roles of microtubules and microfilaments in spindle movements during rat oocyte meiosis. *J Reprod Dev* 2008; 54: 391–6.
9. Ai J-S, Wang Q, Yin S, Shi L-H, Xiong B, Ouyang Y-C, Hou Y, Chen D-Y, Schatten H, Sun Q-Y. Regulation of peripheral spindle movement and spindle rotation during mouse oocyte meiosis: New perspectives. *Microsc Microanal* 2008; 14: 349–56.
10. Ai J-S, Li M, Schatten H, Sun Q-Y. Regulatory mechanism of spindle movements during oocyte meiotic division. *Asian Aust J Anim Sci* 2009; 22: 1447–86.
11. Schatten H, Sun QY. Centrosome and microtubule functions and dysfunctions in meiosis: Implications for age-related infertility and developmental disorders. *Reprod Fertil Dev* 2015; 27(6): 934–43.

12. Schatten H, Sun Q-Y. Centrosome–microtubule interactions in health, disease, and disorders. In: *The Cytoskeleton in Health and Disease*. Schatten H (ed.). New York, NY: Springer Science and Business Media, 2015; pp. 119–146.
13. Rivera RM. The epigenetic story. *Mol Reprod Dev* 2014; 81(2). doi: 10.1002/mrd.22304.
14. Hajkova P, Ancelin K, Waldmann T, Lacoste N, Lange UC, Cesari F, Lee C, Almouzni G, Schneider R, Surani MA. Chromatin dynamics during epigenetic reprogramming in the mouse germ line. *Nature* 2008; 452: 877–81.
15. Hajkova P. Epigenetic reprogramming—Taking a lesson from the embryo. *Curr Opin Cell Biol* 2010; 22: 342–50.
16. Rasmussen TP. The epigenetics of early development: Inferences from stem cells. *Mol Reprod Dev* 2014; 81: 194–201.
17. Hajkova P, Erhardt S, Lane N, Haaf T, El-Maarri O, Reik W, Walter J, Surani MA. Epigenetic reprogramming in mouse primordial germ cells. *Mech Dev* 2002; 117: 15–23.
18. Cimmino L, Abdel-Wahab O, Levine RL, Aifantis I. TET family proteins and their role in stem cell differentiation and transformation. *Cell Stem Cell* 2011; 9: 193–204.
19. Guo JU, Su Y, Zhong C, Ming GL, Song H. Emerging roles of TET proteins and 5-hydroxymethylcytosines in active DNA demethylation and beyond. *Cell Cycle* 2011; 10: 2662–8.
20. Tan L, Shi YG. Tet family proteins and 5-hydroxymethylcytosine in development and disease. *Development* 2012; 139: 1895–902.
21. Rousseaux S, Reynoird N, Escoffier E, Thevenon J, Caron C, Khochbin S. Epigenetic reprogramming of the male genome during gametogenesis and in the zygote. *Reprod Biomed Online* 2008; 16: 492–503.
22. Govin J, Escoffier E, Rousseaux S et al. Pericentric heterochromatin reprogramming by new histone variants during mouse spermiogenesis. *J Cell Biol* 2007; 176: 283–94.
23. Wu F, Caron C, De Robertis C, Khochbin S, Rousseaux S. Testis-specific histone variants H2AL1/2 rapidly disappear from paternal heterochromatin after fertilization. *J Reprod Dev* 2008; 54: 413–7.
24. Hammoud SS, Nix DA, Zhang H, Purwar J, Carrell DT, Cairns BR. Distinctive chromatin in human sperm packages genes for embryo development. *Nature* 2009; 460: 473–8.
25. Kimmins S, Sassone-Corsi P. Chromatin remodeling and epigenetic features of germ cells. *Nature* 2005; 434: 583–9.
26. Gao S, Chung YG, Parseghian MH, King GJ, Adashi EY, Latham KE. Rapid H1 linker histone transitions following fertilization or somatic cell nuclear transfer: Evidence for a uniform developmental program in mice. *Dev Biol* 2004; 266: 62–75.
27. Teranishi T, Tanaka M, Kimoto S, Ono Y, Miyakoshi K, Kono T, Yoshimura Y. Rapid replacement of somatic linker histones with the oocyte-specific linker histone H1foo in nuclear transfer. *Dev Biol* 2004; 266: 76–86.
28. Rodman TC, Pruslin FH, Hoffmann HP, Allfrey VG. Turnover of basic chromosomal proteins in fertilized eggs: A cyto-immunochemical study of events *in vivo*. *J Cell Biol* 1981; 90: 351–61.
29. Torres-Padilla ME, Bannister AJ, Hurd PJ, Kouzarides T, Zernicka-Goetz M. Dynamic distribution of the replacement histone variant H3.3 in the mouse oocyte and preimplantation embryos. *Int J Dev Biol* 2006; 50: 455–61.
30. van der Heijden GW, Dieker JW, Derijck AA, Muller S, Berden JH, Braat DD, van der Vlag J, de Boer P. Asymmetry in histone H3 variants and lysine methylation between paternal and maternal chromatin of the early mouse zygote. *Mech Dev* 2005; 122: 1008–22.
31. Arney KL, Bao S, Bannister AJ, Kouzarides T, Surani MA. Histone methylation defines epigenetic asymmetry in the mouse zygote. *Int J Dev Biol* 2002; 46: 317–20.
32. Santos F, Peters AH, Otte AP, Reik W, Dean W. Dynamic chromatin modifications characterise the first cell cycle in mouse embryos. *Dev Biol* 2005; 280: 225–36.
33. Akiyama T, Suzuki O, Matsuda J, Aoki F. Dynamic replacement of histone H3 variants reprograms epigenetic marks in early mouse embryos. *PLoS Genet* 2011; 7: e1002279.
34. Ma JY, Zhao K, OuYang YC, Wang ZB, Luo YB, Hou Y, Schatten H, Shen W, Sun QY. Exogenous thymine DNA glycosylase regulates epigenetic modifications and meiotic cell cycle progression of mouse oocytes. *Mol Hum Reprod* 2015; 21(2): 186–94.
35. Ma XS, Chao SB, Huang XJ et al. The dynamics and regulatory mechanism of pronuclear H3k9me2 asymmetry in mouse zygotes. *Sci Rep* 2015; 5: 17924.
36. Ma JY, Liang XW, Schatten H, Sun QY. Active DNA demethylation in mammalian preimplantation embryos: New insights and new perspectives. *Mol Hum Reprod* 2012; 18(7): 333–40.
37. Ma JY, Zhang T, Shen W, Schatten H, Sun QY. Molecules and mechanisms controlling the active DNA demethylation of the mammalian zygotic genome. *Protein Cell* 2014; 5(11): 827–36.
38. Mayer W, Niveleau A, Walter J, Fundele R, Haaf T. Demethylation of the zygotic paternal genome. *Nature* 2000; 403: 501–2.
39. Oswald J, Engemann S, Lane N, Mayer W, Olek A, Fundele R, Dean W, Reik W, Walter J. Active demethylation of the paternal genome in the mouse zygote. *Curr Biol* 2000; 10: 475–8.
40. Santos F, Hendrich B, Reik W, Dean W. Dynamic reprogramming of DNA methylation in the early mouse embryo. *Dev Biol* 2002; 241: 172–82.

41. Nakamura T, Arai Y, Umehara H et al. PGC7/Stella protects against DNA demethylation in early embryogenesis. *Nat Cell Biol* 2007; 9: 64e71.
42. Okamoto I, Otte AP, Allis CD, Reinberg D, Heard E. Epigenetic dynamics of imprinted X inactivation during early mouse development. *Science* 2004; 303: 644–9.
43. Mak W, Nesterova TB, de Napoles M, Appanah R, Yamanaka S, Otte AP, Brockdorff N. Reactivation of the paternal X chromosome in early mouse embryos. *Science* 2004; 303: 666–9.
44. Silva J, Nichols J, Theunissen TW, Guo G, van Oosten AL, Barrandon O, Wray J, Yamanaka S, Chambers I, Smith A. Nanog is the gateway to the pluripotent ground state. *Cell* 2009; 138: 722–37.
45. O'Carroll D, Erhardt S, Pagani M, Barton SC, Surani MA, Jenuwein T. The polycomb-group gene *Ezh2* is required for early mouse development. *Mol Cell Biol* 2001; 21: 4330–6.
46. Erhardt S, Su IH, Schneider R, Barton S, Bannister AJ, Perez-Burgos L, Jenuwein T, Kouzarides T, Tarakhovsky A, Surani MA. Consequences of the depletion of zygotic and embryonic enhancer of zeste 2 during preimplantation mouse development. *Development* 2003; 130: 4235–48.
47. Gao Y, Hyttel P, Hall VJ. Regulation of H3K27me3 and H3K4me3 during early porcine embryonic development. *Mol Reprod Dev* 2010; 77: 540–9.
48. Posfai E, Kunzmann R, Brochard V et al. Polycomb function during oogenesis is required for mouse embryonic development. *Genes Dev* 2012; 26: 920–32.
49. Vassena R, Boue S, Gonzalez-Roca E, Aran B, Auer H, Veiga A, Izpisua Belmonte JC. Waves of early transcriptional activation and pluripotency program initiation during human preimplantation development. *Development* 2011; 138: 3699–709.
50. Ge ZJ, Schatten H, Zhang CL, Sun QY. Oocyte ageing and epigenetics. *Reproduction* 2015; 149(3): R103–14.
51. Liang XW, Ge ZJ, Guo L, Luo SM, Han ZM, Schatten H, Sun QY. Effect of postovulatory oocyte aging on DNA methylation imprinting acquisition in offspring oocytes. *Fertil Steril* 2011; 96(6): 1479–84.
52. Liang XW, Ge ZJ, Wei L, Guo L, Han ZM, Schatten H, Sun QY. The effects of postovulatory aging of mouse oocytes on methylation and expression of imprinted genes at mid-term gestation. *Mol Hum Reprod* 2011; 17(9): 562–7.
53. Liang X, Ma J, Schatten H, Sun Q. Epigenetic changes associated with oocyte aging. *Sci China Life Sci* 2012; 55(8): 670–6.
54. Ge ZJ, Liang QX, Luo SM, Wei YC, Han ZM, Schatten H, Sun QY, Zhang CL. Diabetic uterus environment may play a key role in alterations of DNA methylation of several imprinted genes at mid-gestation in mice. *Reprod Biol Endocrinol* 2013; 11: 119.
55. Ge ZJ, Liang XW, Guo L, Liang QX, Luo SM, Wang YP, Wei YC, Han ZM, Schatten H, Sun QY. Maternal diabetes causes alterations of DNA methylation statuses of some imprinted genes in murine oocytes. *Biol Reprod* 2013; 88(5): 117.
56. Ge ZJ, Liang QX, Hou Y, Han ZM, Schatten H, Sun QY, Zhang CL. Maternal obesity and diabetes may cause DNA methylation alteration in the spermatozoa of offspring in mice. *Reprod Biol Endocrinol* 2014; 12: 29.
57. Ge ZJ, Luo SM, Lin F, Liang QX, Huang L, Wei YC, Hou Y, Han ZM, Schatten H, Sun QY. DNA methylation in oocytes and liver of female mice and their offspring: Effects of high-fat-diet-induced obesity. *Environ Health Perspect* 2014; 122(2): 159–64.
58. Wei Y, Schatten H, Sun QY. Environmental epigenetic inheritance through gametes and implications for human reproduction. *Hum Reprod Update* 2015; 21(2): 194–208.
59. Chao SB, Guo L, Ou XH, Luo SM, Wang ZB, Schatten H, Gao GL, Sun QY. Heated spermatozoa: Effects on embryonic development and epigenetics. *Hum Reprod* 2012; 27(4): 1016–24.
60. Luo YB, Ma JY, Zhang QH, Lin F, Wang ZW, Huang L, Schatten H, Sun QY. MBTD1 is associated with Pr-Set7 to stabilize H4K20me1 in mouse oocyte meiotic maturation. *Cell Cycle* 2013; 12(7): 1142–50.
61. Zhu JQ, Zhu L, Liang XW, Xing FQ, Schatten H, Sun QY. Demethylation of LHR in dehydroepiandrosterone-induced mouse model of polycystic ovary syndrome. *Mol Hum Reprod* 2010; 16(4): 260–6.

Index